Seventh Edition

D1457971

Obstetric Nursing

Erna E. Ziegel, R.N., B.S., M.A.

*Emeritus Associate Professor, School of
Nursing of the University of Wisconsin–
Madison, Madison, Wisconsin*

Mecca S. Cranley, R.N., B.S., M.S.

*Lecturer, Perinatal Nursing, School of
Nursing of the University of Wisconsin–
Madison, Madison, Wisconsin
Formerly Clinical Nurse Specialist,
Maternal Intensive Care Team, University
of Wisconsin–Madison*

Macmillan Publishing Co., Inc.
NEW YORK
Collier Macmillan Publishers
LONDON

Earlier editions copyright 1922, 1928, 1933,
© 1957, and copyright © 1964 and 1972 by
Macmillan Publishing Co., Inc. Copyright
renewed 1950 and 1956 by Carolyn Conant Van Blarcom,
renewed 1961 by First Western Bank and Trust Company.

Macmillan Publishing Co., Inc.
866 Third Avenue, New York, New York 10022

Collier Macmillan Canada, Ltd.

Library of Congress Cataloging in Publication Data

Ziegel, Erna.
    Obstetric nursing.

    First–4th ed., by C. C. Van Blarcom, have title:
Obstetrical nursing.
    Includes bibliographies and index.
    1. Obstetrical nursing.   I. Cranley, Mecca,
joint author.   II. Van Blarcom, Carolyn Conant.
Obstetrical nursing.   III. Title. [DNLM:
1. Obstetrical nursing.   2. Pregnancy—Nursing
texts. WY157 Z66o]
RG951.V3   1978   618.2'0024'613   77-14082
ISBN 0-02-431560-5

Printing: 2   3   4   5   6   7   8   Year: 9   0   1   2   3   4

The seventh edition of *Obstetric Nursing* reflects an emphasis on the role of nurses as integral members of professional teams that deliver health care of increasing excellence. The nurse, with greater responsibility for health care, is in a key position to influence the kind of maternity care that will enable individuals and families to achieve their goals for health and for family unity. The nurse will serve the best interests of childbearing families when she continually pursues excellence through knowledge of the scientific basis for childbirth care—biologic, medical, and behavioral. He or she can then provide families with the sensitive care and homelike atmosphere they desire before, during, and after birth.

In their practices, nurses have the opportunity to be colleagues of both client and physician. Patient advocacy can involve defending patient rights. It can also involve patient education, providing women with information about all of their options and helping them make the best choices for themselves.

Believing the above, we have made an effort to include in this edition a balance of physiologic, technical, and psychosocial information—both the *science* and the *art* of perinatal nursing are essential to good care.

There has been some reorganization in this edition, mainly in placing all the high-risk conditions—maternal, fetal, and newborn—into one section following discussion of the normal events of pregnancy, labor, and the postpartum family. All chapters have been updated, many have been entirely rewritten, and there are several entirely new chapters.

Throughout this edition the fetus and the newborn are referred to as "he." The reader should not infer that this represents any preference on the part of the authors for boys rather than girls. It simply seemed less awkward to use this conventional grammatical form.

It is our hope that the nurses who read this book will be stimulated to synthesize the information into nursing care plans that meet the best interests of their patients, to make pertinent and insightful adaptations of care, and to seek new knowledge to enhance their professional practice. Although the contents of this book are as up-to-date as we could make them, perinatal nursing is a rapidly developing field. The excellent nurse will continually read and study the current journal literature.

Erna E. Ziegel
Mecca S. Cranley

Acknowledgments

The authors wish to acknowledge with sincere gratitude the assistance given to us by many individuals. We are grateful for the assistance and patience of Mr. T. P. McConahay, editor, Miss Lola Peters, and other members of the staff of Macmillan Publishing Co., Inc., during the preparation and production of this edition. We are particularly indebted to our colleagues in nursing, Dorothy M. Patteson and Sue A. Frazier, for their valuable suggestions regarding content of the manuscript. In addition, we wish to thank Mrs. Donna L. Weihofen, nutritionist, Luis B. Curet, M.D., Ronald W. Olson, M.D., and Phillip R. Hamilton, M.D., for the critical reading of certain portions of the manuscript, and Richard O. Friday, M.D., for providing us with the ultrasound photographs and helpful comments on the text on ultrasound. We thank Mr. Edwin Hord for assistance with illustrations, and Mr. Roger Pribbenow and Mr. Duane Hopps for taking some of the photographs.

Finally, we wish to take this opportunity to express our appreciation to Edward Cranley for xeroxing all of our material. Mrs. Cranley also appreciates his moral support and understanding that authors, not unlike pregnant women, are often preoccupied and irritable. In addition, she wishes to acknowledge the valuable experience with pregnancy and mothering provided by Martha, Patrick, Elizabeth, Paul, Anne, and Philip Cranley.

Erna E. Ziegel
Mecca S. Cranley

Contents

Part Four

The Postpartum Family **417**

Part Five

The High-Risk Mother and Baby **603**

Obstetric Nursing

Part One

Scientific Foundations for Perinatal Care

1

Anatomy of the Reproductive Organs

Although this book deals more specifically with the function of the female reproductive system, the anatomy and physiology of the male reproductive organs will be briefly discussed to add to an understanding of the total reproductive process. The physiologic processes of the female organs will be considered in more detail.

FEMALE REPRODUCTIVE ORGANS

The female reproductive organs are divided into two groups, the internal organs and the external genitalia. These organs, as well as other related structures, the bladder, urethra, rectum, pelvic diaphragm, and perineum, because of their close proximity, and the breasts, because of their functional relationship, will be discussed. The bony pelvis, in and below which the reproductive organs are situated, is described in Chapter 10, where the pelvis is considered as the birth canal or passage through which the baby moves during the birth process.

External Female Reproductive Organs

The external genitalia of the female, collectively, are commonly called the *vulva;* occasionally the term *pudendum* is used for this group of organs. The vulva includes all the externally visible organs, situated between the thighs, extending from the area over the symphysis pubis to the base of the perineal body,

which lies in front of the anus. The following structures are included in the vulva: mons veneris, labia majora, labia minora, clitoris, vestibule, urinary meatus, vaginal opening, and glandular structures.

Mons Veneris (Mons Pubis)

The mons veneris, which constitutes the upper aspect of the vulva, is the firm cushion of adipose and connective tissue that lies over the symphysis pubis and the adjoining pubic bones (Fig. 1-1). The overlying skin contains many sebaceous glands and after puberty is abundantly covered with hair.

Labia Majora (Singular: Labium Majus)

The labia majora are the two longitudinal, heavy ridges of adipose and connective tissue, covered with skin, that form the lateral boundaries of the vulva (Fig. 1-1). They are continuous with and extend downward on each side from the mons veneris, gradually become narrower, and disappear into the base of the perineal body posteriorly. The labia majora usually lie in close apposition, covering the structures between them, but they may gape in women who have had children.

Each labium has an inner and an outer surface. After puberty the outer aspect is covered with hair, which becomes more sparse toward the perineum. The inner surface of the labium is moist and has the appearance of a mucous membrane; it has numerous sebaceous glands, but is

3

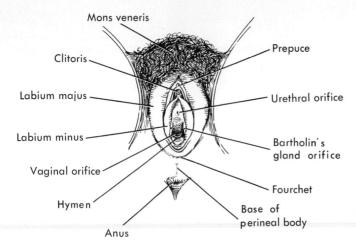

Figure 1-1. The external genitalia of a woman who has had children. All that remains of the hymen are a few fleshy projections at the orifice of the vagina. [*Modified from L. Brady, E. Kurtz, and E. McLaughlin,* Essentials of Gynecology, *2nd ed. Macmillan Publishing Co., Inc., New York, 1949.*]

not covered with hair. The labia contain an abundance of blood vessels. Varicose veins sometimes develop and may become markedly enlarged during pregnancy.

Labia Minora (Singular: Labium Minus)

The labia minora are two thin cutaneous folds lying between, and parallel to, the labia majora; they may be completely covered by the labia majora or may project from between them (Fig. 1-1). Resembling the inner surface of the labia majora, they are reddish in color, have the appearance of a mucous membrane, are moist, contain numerous sebaceous glands, and do not have a hair covering. The labia minora contain a number of blood vessels. An abundance of nerves makes them very sensitive.

Anteriorly each labium minus divides into two parts for a short distance and then joins at an angle with the other labium to form a double ridge of tissue around the clitoris, one ridge above and one below the clitoris. The labia minora thus form a hoodlike covering for the clitoris, termed the *prepuce* (Fig. 1-1), and a band of tissue below it, termed the *frenulum* of the clitoris. Like the labia majora, the labia minora taper as they extend posteriorly, where they join below the vaginal opening into a thin, flat, transverse fold of tissue called the *fourchet* (Fig. 1-1).

Clitoris

The clitoris is a small, cylindrical body located at the upper aspect of the vulva in the area where the labia minora join anteriorly (Fig. 1-1). The clitoris is the homologue of the penis of the male and, similar to it, is composed of erectile tissue, contains many blood vessels and nerves, and is extremely sensitive. The clitoris is 2 to 3 cm in length, but is almost entirely covered by the labia. Only the anterior end, the glans, is visible under the prepuce and above its frenulum. These tissues sometimes draw together over the end of the clitoris, cover it, and give this area the appearance of the opening to an orifice. This resemblance to an opening may cause confusion with the urethral orifice unless both are carefully identified and an attempt to insert a catheter here for bladder catheterization causes considerable discomfort.

Vestibule

The vestibule is the triangular area that becomes visible when the labia minora are spread apart; the clitoris is at the apex of this triangle and the fourchet at its base. The orifices of the urinary meatus, Skene's (paraurethral) ducts, vagina, and Bartholin's (vulvovaginal) glands are located in the vestibule. A depressed space in the tissue between the vaginal opening and the fourchet, termed the *fossa navicularis*, may be seen at the posterior end of the vestibule, but it is usually obliterated after the birth of a baby.

Urinary Meatus

The external urinary meatus, although not a part of the female genital organs, is described with the vulva because of its anatomic location. It is situated in the midline of the vestibule below the clitoris and above the vaginal orifice (Fig. 1-1). The urinary meatus varies considerably in appearance, ranging from an easily identifiable opening to a puckered elevation of tissue that appears to have no orifice. Separation of the labia minora, followed by slight upward traction on the labia, will usually reveal a triangular opening in the puckered membrane that surrounds the meatus.

The *paraurethral (Skene's) ducts*, which have a very small caliber, open just on each side of the urethral meatus. These ducts may become infected by the gonococcus.

Vaginal Opening and Hymen

The vaginal orifice is in the lower portion of the vestibule (Fig. 1-1). It is partly covered by the *hymen*, a membranous tissue which varies considerably in thickness and size in different women. The opening in the hymen is somewhat circular in outline; it may be so large that the vaginal orifice is almost completely open, or it may be very small and nearly close the orifice. The hymen may be quite elastic and stretch considerably with distention, or it may tear easily. After childbirth the remnants of the hymen are seen as small tags of mucous membrane around the vaginal orifice; these are termed *carunculae myrtiformes*.

Bartholin's Glands

Bartholin's glands, the largest of several vulvovaginal glands, are compound, racemose, mucus-secreting glands. They are situated at the base of the labia majora and their ducts open into the vestibule just outside the lateral margins of the vaginal orifice (Fig. 1-1). Their mucus secretion keeps the inner surfaces of the labia moist and provides lubrication to the vaginal orifice and canal, especially during coitus. Secretion is considerably increased during sexual excitement. These glands are normally small and are not palpable, but a gland may become so large as to distend a considerable part of the labium if it becomes infected or cystic.

The Pelvic Diaphragm and the Perineum

Pelvic Diaphragm

The pelvic diaphragm, made up of muscles and their fascial covering, stretches across the lowermost part of the pelvic cavity like a hammock. It almost completely closes the abdominal and pelvic cavities and serves as a slinglike support for the abdominal and pelvic organs. The urethra, vagina, and anal canal pass through this diaphragm to their external openings. In addition to the major supportive function of the pelvic diaphragm, its muscle fibers are important in assisting with constriction of the vagina, the rectum, and the anus.

The pelvic diaphragm is composed of two pairs of muscles, the levator ani and the coccygeus muscles (Fig. 1-2). The *levator ani*, the largest and most important component of the pelvic diaphragm, is in actuality a paired muscle, but the two sides join so closely that it functions as a single sheet of muscle. This broad, thin muscle stretches from the pubic bones to the spines of the ischial bones, with some fibers passing to the coccyx and the sacrum. The levator ani are often described as consisting of three parts, the pubococcygeus, iliococcygeus, and puborectalis muscles, all of which are closely joined. The other muscles of the pelvic diaphragm, the *coccygeus* muscles, are also paired and closely joined. They arise at the spines of the ischia and insert into the coccyx and lower part of the sacrum. The coccygeus muscles assist the levator ani in giving support to the abdominal and pelvic viscera.

Perineum

The perineum is the area between the thighs that extends from the pubic area to the coccyx

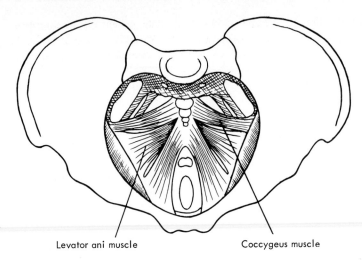

Levator ani muscle   Coccygeus muscle

Figure 1-2. Levatores ani and coccygei as seen from above.

and lies below and superficial to the pelvic diaphragm. The perineum is made up of several pairs of muscles and their fascia, among which are the bulbocavernosus (sphincter vaginae), the transverse perineal muscles, and those forming the anal sphincters (Fig. 1-3). The pelvic diaphragm and the muscles and fascia of the perineum are closely associated in structure and in function; the structures in the perineum reinforce the diaphragm by providing support and assisting in constricting the orifices passing through it.

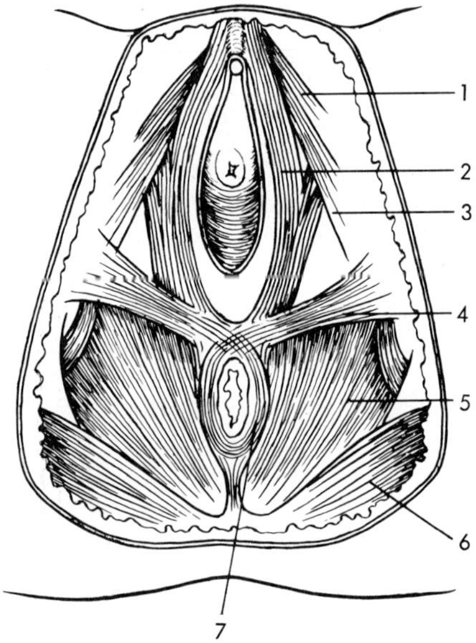

Perineal Body

The perineal body is a wedge-shaped mass of fibromuscular tissue that extends upward from the perineum and occupies the area between the vagina and the rectum. The lower and outer surface of this body, representing the base of the wedge, lies between the vaginal and anal openings and is covered with skin. This external surface, or base, is often called the perineum of the female and is the area referred to when the woman is said to have sustained a perineal laceration or incision.

The perineal body is about 4 cm in width and depth and is continuous, deep into the pelvis, with the rectovaginal septum. The levator ani and a number of muscles of the perineum, including the sphincter ani, meet and fuse in the center of this body.

The perineal body is stretched and flattened when the vagina is distended as the baby passes through the birth canal during delivery. Although this mass of tissue, largely made up of muscle, stretches to a considerable degree dur-

Figure 1-3. Dissection showing the muscles of the vulvar area and the pelvic floor. *1, 3.* Ischiocavernosus. *2.* Sphincter vaginae. *4.* Transversus perinei. *5.* Levator ani. *6.* Gluteus maximus. *7.* External anal sphincter.

ing the birth of a baby, it nonetheless is often lacerated, or it is incised to prevent tearing and to facilitate delivery. An incision or a laceration of more than minor extent must be repaired to reestablish the support that this structure gives to the pelvic organs. (See pages 351–52 for further discussion of perineal lacerations and episiotomy, and page 377 for perineal repair.)

Internal Female Reproductive Organs

The internal female reproductive organs are contained in the true pelvic cavity and comprise the *uterus* and *vagina* in the center, an *ovary* and a *fallopian tube* on each side, together with their various ligaments, blood vessels, lymph supply, and nerves and a certain amount of fat and connective tissue (Fig. 1-4).

Uterus

The uterus (womb) is the organ in which the fetus develops and from which menstruation occurs. It is a muscular structure that contains a cavity lined with mucous membrane. The uterus is situated in the pelvic cavity between the bladder and the rectum; it joins with a fallopian tube on each side near its upper part, and its lower end (the cervix) projects into the vagina (Figs. 1-4 and 1-5).

The uterus has the shape and approximate size of a somewhat flattened, inverted pear. Its size varies in different women, but measurements approximate 7.5 cm (3 in.) in length, 5 cm (2 in.) in width at the upper part, and 2.5 cm (1 in.) in anteroposterior diameter. It weighs approximately 60 gm (2 oz). The uterus enlarges tremendously during pregnancy, attaining a length of 30 to 35 cm (12 to 14 in.), a width of 20 to 25 cm (8 to 10 in.), and a weight of approximately 1000 gm (2 lb). After pregnancy the uterus returns almost, but not entirely, to its former size and shape.

The uterus is comprised of two parts: an upper triangular part termed the *corpus*, or *body*, and a lower cylindrical, and smaller, part designated the *cervix*, or *neck* (Fig. 1-4).

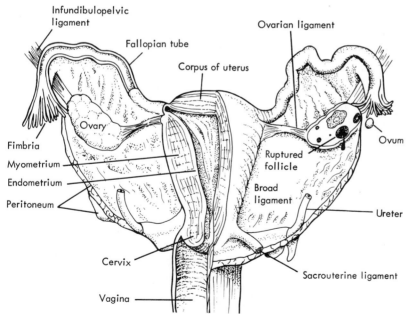

Figure 1-4. Uterus and associated organs. [*Reprinted with permission from Macmillan Publishing Co., Inc., from Sigmund Grollman,* The Human Body: Its Structure and Physiology, *4th ed. Copyright Sigmund Grollman 1978.*]

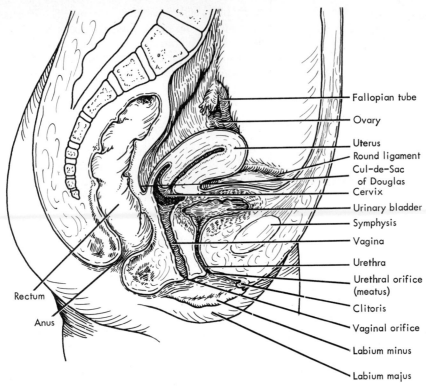

Figure 1-5.   The female reproductive system. Sagittal section. [*Adapted from W. B. Youmans,* Human Physiology, *rev. ed. Macmillan Publishing Co., Inc., New York, 1962.*]

CORPUS   The corpus narrows from above downward. Its upper, rounded portion, above the points of entrance of the fallopian tubes, is termed the *fundus uteri,* and the lower, narrowed portion where the corpus meets the cervix is called the *isthmus* (Fig. 1-6). The isthmus is significant during pregnancy when it forms the lower uterine segment; the remainder of the corpus makes up the upper uterine segment.

The cavity of the corpus of a nonpregnant uterus is small, since the major part of the corpus consists of thick muscular tissue and its anterior and posterior walls lie close together. The uterine cavity is somewhat triangular in shape with an opening at each of the three angles. The openings at the *cornua,* or two upper angles, join with the fallopian tubes, and the lower opening leads into the cavity of the cervix, which in turn opens into the vagina (Fig. 1-6).

The corpus of the uterus is a firm, hard mass, consisting of irregularly disposed, involuntary (nonstriated) muscle fibers, connective tissue, elastic fibers, nerves, and blood vessels and an inner lining of mucous membrane. It consists of three layers: the serous, the muscular, and the mucous.

1. The serous layer, also termed the *perimetrium,* is the external layer. It is derived from the peritoneum, which covers the uterus front and back, except along the lower part of the anterior wall, where it is reflexed up over the bladder (Fig. 1-6).
2. The muscular layer, designated as the *myometrium,* is the middle layer (Fig. 1-4). It makes up the largest part of the uterus.

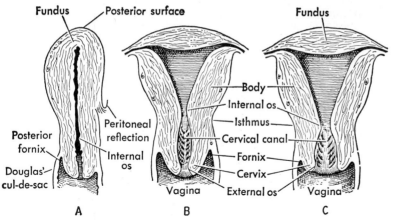

Figure 1-6. Diagrams of sections of virgin and multiparous uteri. *A.* Anteroposterior section. *B.* Lateral section of a virgin uterus. *C.* Lateral section of a multiparous uterus. Since Douglas' cul-de-sac lies beyond the upper portion of the posterior wall of the vagina, it is through the posterior fornix that pathology in the cul-de-sac often can be determined by palpation, by cul-de-sac puncture, or by insertion of a culdoscope for visualization.

This layer consists of muscular tissue through which are interspersed blood vessels, lymphatics, and nerves. The arrangement of the muscle fibers in the uterus is unique. They run longitudinally, circularly, spirally, and crisscross in every direction, forming a veritable network. Strong intermittent contractions of this muscular layer during labor dilate the cervical canal to permit the baby to pass through it and also serve as a major force in advancing the baby through the birth canal during delivery. Contraction of these unusually arranged muscle fibers around open blood vessels is the chief factor in prevention of hemorrhage after delivery of the placenta.

3. The mucous, internal layer, which lines the uterine cavity, is called the *endometrium* (Fig. 1-4). It is a pinkish, velvety, highly vascular mucous membrane which contains numerous uterine glands and is covered with ciliated columnar epithelium. This layer undergoes constant cyclic changes during the reproductive period and varies in thickness from 1 to 5 mm, depending on the period in the cycle. These changes are described under "The Endometrial (Menstrual) Cycle" on pages 31–33. This internal layer is continuous with the lining of the fallopian tubes and with the lining of the cervix.

CERVIX The cervix, which constitutes the smaller part of the uterus, measures from 2.5 to 3 cm long, about one third the length of the corpus. It is approximately an inch in diameter. About one half of the cervix protrudes into the vagina (Figs. 1-5 and 1-6). The attachment of the vagina at about the midpoint divides the cervix into two parts, a supravaginal and an infravaginal portion.

The cavity of the cervix, known as the *cervical canal,* is spindle-shaped, being expanded between its two somewhat constricted openings, the internal orifice or *internal os* above, by which it opens into the cavity of the uterine body, and the external orifice or *external os* below, opening into the vagina (Fig. 1-6). The external os, only a few millimeters in diameter, is a small round opening in the woman who has not borne children, but after childbirth is converted into a small transverse opening, bounded in front by the *anterior lip* and posteriorly by the *posterior lip* of the cervix. It is through the cervical canal that the baby passes during birth. Under the influence of strong uterine muscle contractions the cervix dilates sufficiently to permit a full-term baby to pass through it and thereafter returns to its original size and shape, with the exception of the change in the external os noted above.

The cervix consists largely of connective tissue, but contains some muscle fibers and elastic tissue. It has many blood vessels. The cervical canal is lined with a single layer of ciliated columnar epithelium, which contains numerous glands extending into the stroma of the cervix. These glands secrete a mucus with complex properties that vary considerably during the different phases of each ovarian cycle (see page 30). Near the external os the cervical lining changes to squamous epithelium, similar to the lining of the vagina.

BLOOD SUPPLY   The uterus has an excellent blood, lymph, and nerve supply. The abundant blood supply reaches the uterus principally through the uterine arteries from the internal iliac (hypogastric) arteries, but also to some extent through the ovarian arteries from the aorta. The arteries follow a tortuous course, and many of the branches anastomose. Arteries from both sides of the uterus are united by a branch vessel in the area where the cervix and corpus of the uterus meet, thus forming an encircling artery at this site. A deep cervical tear during delivery of a baby may break this vessel and result in profuse bleeding. Veins in the uterus are also large and tortuous. The uterine and ovarian veins empty into the internal iliac (hypogastric) veins and then into the common iliac veins.

POSITION   The uterus normally occupies an oblique or almost horizontal position in the body, with the corpus pointed forward. It is also slightly anteflexed, being somewhat bent forward on itself. In this position the fundus lies above the bladder, and the cervix points downward and backward toward the sacrum (Fig. 1-5). However, the position of the uterus is not firmly fixed, and it is easily subject to variations. A distended bladder may push the uterine body backward; a full rectum, forward. Changes of body posture may alter the position of the uterus, and during pregnancy it rises upward.

SUPPORT   The major support to the uterus comes from the muscles and fascia of the pelvic diaphragm, to which it is attached at the junction of the cervix and corpus. Several pairs of ligaments, described below, give additional support and help to maintain the uterus in its forward inclination.

The *broad ligaments,* one on each side, are in reality one continuous structure that is formed by a fold of the peritoneum, which drops down over the uterus, investing the corpus, part of the cervix, and part of the posterior wall of the vagina (Fig. 1-4). It unites on each side of the uterus to form a broad, flat membrane extending laterally to the pelvic wall, dividing the pelvic cavity into an anterior and posterior compartment, containing, respectively, the bladder and rectum. Between the folds of the broad ligament are situated the ovaries and ovarian ligaments, the fallopian tubes, the round ligaments, the cardinal ligaments, blood vessels, lymphatics, nerves, and a certain amount of muscle and connective tissue.

The *cardinal ligaments,* one on each side, are a part of the broad ligaments, making up their lower borders. They are bands of dense connective tissue attached to the supravaginal part of the cervix and extending to the lateral wall of the pelvis. These ligaments, along with the pelvic diaphragm and the perineum, keep the uterus from prolapsing by providing support from below.

The *round ligaments,* one on each side, are fibromuscular cords composed of muscle prolonged from the uterus and a small amount of connective tissue. They contain blood and lymph vessels and nerves. They extend upward and forward from their uterine origin just below and in front of the tubal entrance, pass through the inguinal canal, and merge into the mons veneris.

The *uterosacral ligaments*, again one on each side, extend backward from the cervix, pass on each side of the rectum, and insert at the posterior wall of the pelvis (Fig. 1-4). They connect the cervix with the fascia covering the sacrum and aid in keeping the uterus in its normal position by exerting traction on the cervix.

The *anterior ligament* is a portion of the peritoneum that forms a fold between the bladder and the uterus. The *posterior ligament* is formed in the same manner by a deep fold of peritoneum between the uterus and the rectum.

Vagina

The vagina is a musculomembranous canal which extends from the lower part of the vulva to the cervix and thus connects the external and internal reproductive organs (Fig. 1-5). It serves as the organ of copulation and as the passageway for menstrual blood and for the fetus during birth.

The axis of the vagina is pointed toward the first sacral vertebra and thus in the erect position of the body it is directed upward and backward from the vulva to the cervix, to which it joins at an angle (Fig. 1-5). Attachment to the cervix is near its midpoint. The cervix thus protrudes into the vagina for 1.0 to 1.5 cm (about ½ in.) at almost a right angle, with the external os pointing backward. The posterior wall of the vagina is about 8 to 9 cm (3.2 to 3.6 in.) long. The anterior wall is shorter, because of the angle of its attachment, measuring 6 to 7 cm (2.4 to 2.8 in.) in length (Fig. 1-5).

The vagina consists of a muscular layer, a loose connective tissue layer, and a mucous layer. It is abundantly supplied with blood vessels and lymphatics. The mucous layer is a thick, heavy, mucous membrane which normally lies in small transverse folds or corrugations called *rugae*. These folds are obliterated and the lining is stretched into a smooth surface as the canal distends during delivery; the folds may disappear after childbirth. The epithelial cells of the mucosa undergo changes in response to hormonal stimulation, showing different characteristics during the various phases of ovarian function. The mucosal cells contain a considerable amount of glycogen.

There are no glands in the vagina. The small amount of whitish secretion present in the vagina is derived from the epithelial cells, the mucus-secreting glands in the cervix, and from the bacteria that normally inhabit the vagina and their by-products. Nonpathogenic organisms are normally present in the vagina; among these the Döderlein bacilli are prevalent and important to maintenance of normal secretion and acidity. During the childbearing years of life the vaginal secretion is normally acid, with a pH ranging from 4.0 to 5.0. This acidic reaction is believed to be due to lactic acid resulting from breakdown of glycogen by the Döderlein bacilli. The pH varies with ovarian activity; the acidity is somewhat reduced by alkaline cervical secretions before the onset of menstruation and by menstrual flow during menstruation.

The vagina is somewhat flattened, since the anterior and posterior walls lie in apposition toward the middle; on cross section it resembles the letter H. The bore of the vaginal canal ordinarily permits introduction of a vaginal speculum for visualization of the cervix or introduction of one or two fingers for palpation of the pelvic organs. The vagina is capable of a great deal of distention, as is evident from the tremendous stretching it undergoes during the birth of a baby. Tissue changes occurring during pregnancy permit such distention. The levator ani muscle, through which the vagina passes, serves to constrict the vaginal opening to some extent, and the sphincter vaginae provides slight sphincter action, but the vagina is not tightly closed by a sphincter as are the urethral and anal openings.

The upper end of the vagina, which forms a circular cuff around the cervix, ends in a blind vault. This vault, or space between the cervix and vaginal wall, is termed the *fornix* (Fig. 1-6). It is in actuality a potential space, since the tissues lie in apposition; however, they are easily spread apart. For convenience of description, the fornix is divided into four sections or fornices: the anterior, the posterior, and the two lateral fornices. The posterior fornix is considerably deeper than the anterior, because the vagina is about 2 cm (¾ in.) longer posteriorly than anteriorly and it is attached higher up on the posterior wall of the cervix than on its anterior wall (Fig. 1-6). The fornices are important in pelvic examination, since the internal pelvic organs can usually be quite readily palpated through their relatively thin walls.

Other pelvic organs lie in close proximity to the vagina. The bladder and the urethra are situated immediately above it anteriorly. Posteriorly, the middle portion of the vaginal wall lies close to the rectum; at its lower end the perineal body and the rectovaginal septum separate the vagina and the rectum; and at its upper end a blind pouch in the peritoneal cavity, known as *Douglas' cul-de-sac*, lies between the vagina and the rectum (Figs. 1-5 and 1-6). In this cul-de-sac area the peritoneum is separated from the vagina by only a thin muscular wall.

Fallopian (Uterine) Tubes

The fallopian tubes, also known as oviducts, are two slender muscular tubes that extend laterally from the cornua of the uterine cavity, one from each side, to the ovaries (Fig. 1-4). They provide the passageway through which ova reach the uterus. After passing through the uterine muscle wall, the tubes extend between the folds of the upper margin of the broad ligaments, taking a somewhat tortuous course in an upward and outward direction. Their length varies from 7 to 14 cm (2.8 to 5.6 in.). Thickness also varies; at the juncture with the uterus the lumen of the tubes is so small as to admit the introduction of only a fine bristle, but there is a slight gradual increase in width distally.

The uterine tubes consist of a serous layer, made up of peritoneal covering, a muscular layer, and an inner mucous membrane, which lies in longitudinal folds (Fig. 1-4). The inner surface is lined by a single layer of epithelium composed in part of ciliated cells and in part of nonciliated, secretory cells. Rhythmic contractions of the musculature of the tube and probably also movement of the cilia effect transport of

ova and sperm in the tubes. Activity of tubal mucosa and muscle undergoes cyclic changes in response to the hormonal changes of the ovarian cycle.

Each fallopian tube is described in several parts: the portion that passes through the muscular wall of the uterus is termed the *interstitial;* the *isthmus* is immediately adjacent to the uterus; the *ampulla* is the expanded lateral portion; and the wide distal opening is called the *fimbriated end* or *infundibulum.* The distal, or fimbriated, end of the tube is a funnel-shaped opening surrounded by fringelike projections called *fimbriae* (Fig. 1-4). One of the fimbria, the *fimbria ovarica,* which has the form of a shallow gutter, or groove, extends to, or almost to, the ovary. The fimbriated ends of the fallopian tubes open into the peritoneal cavity. There is thus a small, but continuous opening from the vulva to the peritoneal cavity through the irregularly constructed muscular canal which passes through the vagina, the uterus, and the fallopian tubes. This canal is lined throughout its entire length with continuous mucous membrane.

Ovaries

The ovaries, the sex glands (gonads) of the female, are two small, flattened, oval-shaped organs, located one on each side of the uterus. They are attached to the back of the broad ligaments below the fimbriated end of the fallopian tubes (Fig. 1-4). The longest of the fimbria from each tube, the fimbria ovarica, reaches to, or nearly to, the ovary. Each ovary is attached to the lateral wall of the uterus by the *ovarian ligament* and to the pelvic wall by the portion of the broad ligament that continues beyond the fallopian tube; this portion is termed the *infundibulopelvic* or *suspensory ligament* (Fig. 1-4). The position of the ovaries is not fixed and will vary with positional changes of the uterus.

An ovary is usually described as having the size and shape of an almond; each is about 4 to 5 cm long, 2 cm wide, and 1 cm thick, and has a weight of 2 to 5 gm. It presents a glistening, more or less irregular, roughened surface externally, and is a dull white color. Size and external appearance of the ovaries vary according to the maturity of the woman, since the ovaries undergo constant change until after the menopause.

The ovary consists of two parts: a central portion or *medulla*, and an outer layer or *cortex*. The medulla is composed of connective tissue, blood and lymph vessels, and nerves. Embedded in the cortex, between connective tissue, are numerous minute follicles, each of which contains an oocyte, the germ cell of the female. These have been produced during the first five to six months of fetal life, at which time further development of germ cells ceases, and the individual's full quota of occytes is established. It is estimated that there are 200,000 or more primary oocytes present in each ovary at birth; many of these undergo degenerative changes early in life, leaving an estimated number of 50,000 or more in each ovary at the beginning of adolescence. During reproductive years, the follicles containing the oocytes are present in varying stages of development between a primary state, when the follicle is designated a *primary follicle,* and the mature stage, when it is termed *a graafian follicle* (Figs. 2-1 and 2-2, pages 22 and 24). Growth and development of the follicles are described under "The Ovarian Cycle" on pages 21–26.

The ovaries perform two vital functions: (1) they produce, mature, and extrude ova, and (2) they elaborate internal secretions or hormones. Because of this latter function, they are included in the group of glands classified as the endocrine, or ductless, glands of the body. Ovarian function is described in detail in Chapter 2.

Related Pelvic Organs

The bladder and the rectum are contained in the pelvic cavity and lie in close proximity to the reproductive organs. Thus pressure from one organ may exert an effect on another. A full bladder or full rectum may interfere with a satisfactory examination of the reproductive organs.

Pressure exerted during pregnancy by the enlarged uterus is felt in both the rectum and bladder at certain stages of pregnancy and may at these times cause a feeling of urgency to evacuate their contents frequently.

Bladder

The urinary bladder is a musculomembranous sac that serves as a reservoir for urine. It is situated behind the symphysis pubis and in front of the uterus and the vagina (Fig. 1-5). Urine is conducted into the bladder by the *ureters,* two slender tubes, one on each side, that pass downward from the kidney pelvis. The ureters pass across the brim of the bony pelvis, to the posterior part of the bladder, which they enter somewhat obliquely, at about the level of the cervix (Fig. 1-4). Pressure of an enlarged pregnant uterus on the ureters may be a contributing factor to pyelitis, sometimes a complication of pregnancy. The bladder empties through the *urethra,* a short tube about 3.8 cm (1½ in.) long that terminates in the *urinary meatus.* The meatus is a small opening situated in the middle of the vestibule between the clitoris and the vaginal orifice (Fig. 1-1).

Rectum

The rectum, the lowest segment of the intestinal tract, is situated behind and to the left of the uterus and vagina (Fig. 1-5). It extends downward from the sigmoid flexure of the colon to its termination in the anal opening. The *anus* is a deeply pigmented, puckered opening situated 4 to 5 cm (1½ to 2 in.) below the vaginal orifice. It is provided with bands of circular muscles, the *internal* and *external sphincter ani.* Normal contraction and relaxation of these muscles make possible retention and expulsion of rectal contents. The skin covering the surface of the body extends upward into the anus, where it becomes highly vascular, and merges into the mucous membrane lining of the rectum. Veins of the lower rectum and anal canal sometimes become engorged and inflamed during pregnancy, as a result of pressure exerted by the greatly enlarged uterus. The distended veins, called *hemorrhoids,* not infrequently protrude from the anus and may become very painful.

The Breasts

The breasts are large, specially modified skin glands of the compound racemose or grape-cluster type, embedded in fat and connective tissue, and abundantly supplied with nerves and blood vessels (Fig. 1-7). They are situated quite remote from the pelvic organs, but because of the intimate functional relation with these organs, the breasts of the female may be regarded as accessory glands of the reproductive system. Their function is to secrete, in the parturient woman, suitable nourishment for the human infant during the first months of life.

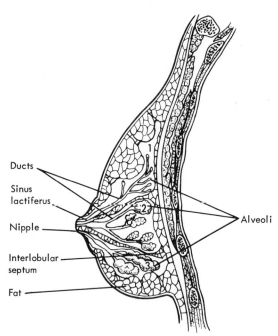

Ducts

Sinus
lactiferus

Nipple

Alveoli

Interlobular
septum

Fat

Figure 1-7. Cross section of mammary gland, showing the development of the alveolar system under different conditions. *1.* Nonpregnant woman. *2.* Middle pregnancy. *3.* During lactation. [*Reprinted with permission from Macmillan Publishing Co., Inc. from Sigmund Grollman,* The Human Body: Its Structure and Function, *4th ed. Copyright Sigmund Grollman 1978.*]

The breasts are symmetrically placed, one on each side of the chest, and occupy the space between the second and sixth ribs, extending from the margin of the sternum almost to the midaxillary line. A bed of connective tissue separates them from the underlying muscles and ribs. The breasts are usually hemispheric or conical in shape, but vary in size and shape at different ages and with different individuals, particularly in women who have borne and nursed children, when they tend to become pendulous.

A nipple protrudes from the apex of each breast for a distance of 0.6 to 1.3 cm (¼ to ½ in.). The nipples are composed largely of sensitive, erectile tissue and become more rigid and prominent during pregnancy and at menstrual periods. The nipple surfaces are pierced by the orifices of the milk ducts, which are 15 to 20 in number (Fig. 19-1, page 514).

The breasts are covered with delicate, smooth skin, except for the *areolae,* the circular, pigmented areas 2.5 to 10 cm (1 to 4 in.) in diameter that surround the nipples. The areolae are darker in brunettes than in blonds, and in all women become darker during pregnancy, gradually becoming paler again after delivery. The surface of the nipples and of the areolae is roughened by small, shotlike lumps or papillae known as the *tubercles of Montgomery* (Fig. 19-1). This roughness becomes more marked during pregnancy, since the papillae then become larger. The tubercles are sebaceous glands that secrete a lipoid material which lubricates the nipples and thus helps to protect them during the baby's sucking.

The small breasts of the child begin to develop markedly at puberty, due to hormonal stimulation. During pregnancy, hormones influence additional growth, as well as stimulate the secretion of milk after delivery of a baby.

The mammary glands first appear in the human embryo at 6 weeks as thickened bands of raised ectoderm. As the fetus grows the mammary glands continue to develop until at full-term birth they have become rudimentary mammary buds and nipples. Each breast consists of 15 to 20 epithelial tubules surrounded by connective tissue. Sometimes the glandular tissue of the newborn is developed sufficiently to secrete a small amount of fluid for a few days after birth. This is the result of stimulation from a high level of estrogens in the mother's blood, which crosses the placenta to the fetus. During infancy and childhood there is little development of the breasts other than normal growth along with the rest of the body.

In early puberty the breasts undergo extensive changes and rapid growth, characterized by a complex branching and lengthening of the mammary ducts. The nipples enlarge and the areolae become pigmented. Each breast is made up of 15 to 20 lobes of ductal systems and each lobe has an excretory duct that opens into the nipple. A large amount of connective tissue and adipose tissue surrounds each ductal system. True alveolar (secretory) cells are not formed in this first period of rapid growth and development.

Mammary growth is controlled by hormones. The combined influence of the ovarian hormones, estrogen and progesterone, and the anterior pituitary hormones, somatotropin (growth hormone) and prolactin, bring about normal growth of the breasts, providing that normal metabolism of the mammary cells is maintained by insulin. It is believed that estrogens are responsible for development of the mammary ducts, and progesterone stimulates lobuloalveolar development.

At the end of puberty the breasts reach a size that is characteristic for the individual woman. There is little change until pregnancy, when major changes take place, especially in development of secretory tissue (described on pages 114–16). Still other changes occur during lactation, when the glandular tissue secretes milk (Chapter 19).

Under hormonal influence the breasts continue internal changes during the first years after puberty until they reach maximum development. These changes alternate between proliferation and involution according to the alternating blood levels of hormones during the menstrual cycles. In the two-week period after ovulation, while progesterone predominates, the epithelial glandular tissue proliferates. Under the influence of adrenocorticoids, insulin, somatotropin, prolactin, estrogen, and progesterone the ducts lengthen and branch, some lobuloalveolar development takes place, and increased vascularization and blood flow occurs. The breasts may feel somewhat tender and heavy during this time.

With the onset of menstruation, and for the two weeks following, the ovarian hormonal influence is different. Estrogen levels are relatively higher than progesterone. During this period there is a regression in some of the cellular changes that took place in the previous two-week period. Involution of glandular tissue does not regress to the state of the previous proliferation, however, and there is always some advancement until the breasts have reached their maximum postpuberty development. An understanding of the cycling of the ovarian hormones, described in Chapter 2, will be helpful in understanding their influence on breast development.

MALE REPRODUCTIVE ORGANS

The male reproductive system consists of the testes (sex glands) in which the male germ cells and the sex hormones are formed; a series of ducts, continuous with one another, through which spermatozoa are transported from the testes to the exterior; accessory glands that produce secretions important to sperm nutrition, survival, and transport; and the penis which serves as the organ of copulation.

Testes

The testes, the sex organs, or gonads, of the male are two slightly flattened, ovoid, glandular bodies suspended by bilateral spermatic cords (Fig. 1-8). The spermatic cords originate just above the inguinal canal, pass through the canal, and down into the scrotum. The testes, epididymides, and parts of the spermatic cords are en-

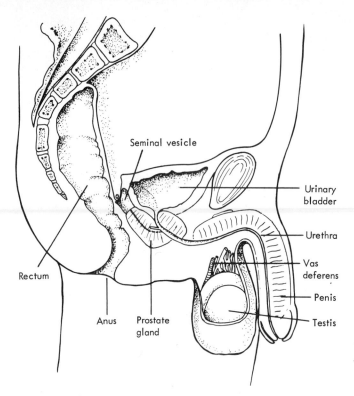

Figure 1-8. Male reproductive system. Sagittal section. [*Reprinted with permission from Macmillan Publishing Co., Inc. from William B. Youmans,* Human Physiology, *rev. ed. Copyright 1954 by Macmillan Publishing Co., Inc.*]

closed, supported, and protected in the *scrotum,* a pouchlike, double-chambered structure made up of skin, fascia, and muscle (Fig. 1-8).

Similar to the ovaries of the female, the glandular reproductive organs of the male have a twofold function. They produce germ cells, called *spermatozoa,* and they serve as an endocrine gland, producing a typically male hormone, called *testosterone.*

The testes are formed in the peritoneal cavity during fetal development and then normally migrate through the inguinal canal and into the scrotum during the eighth or ninth month of fetal life, or occasionally soon after birth. Descent into the scrotum by the age of puberty is essential for normal spermatogenesis, which is adversely affected by the relatively higher temperature within the body. Each testis is a mass of narrow, coiled tubules, called *seminiferous tubules* (Fig. 1-9). Partial septi, extending from a fibrous capsule covering the testis, divide its

substance into a large number of wedge-shaped lobules. Each lobule contains three or four seminiferous tubules. These tubules are from 1 to 3 ft long; the combined length of the many tubules in one testis equals almost 1 mile.

As the seminiferous tubules leave the lobules near their apexes, they join together with adjacent tubules to form ducts. These ducts come together to form a network of ducts, the *rete testis,* from which they lead out and converge into a single coiled tube, the epididymis.

Epididymides

The epididymides (sing., epididymis) are bilateral narrow bodies, situated along the upper posterior part of each testis. Each contains a narrow, tortuous tubule approximately 20 ft in length (Fig. 1-9). This tubule serves as the area to which the spermatozoa that have been released into the seminiferous tubules are con-

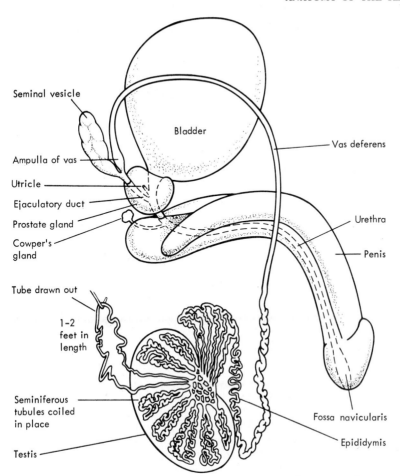

Figure 1-9. Diagrammatic representation of the testis, showing its duct system and the relation of the ducts to the accessory sex glands and penis. [*Reprinted with permission from Macmillan Publishing Co., Inc., from Sigmund Grollman,* The Human Body: Its Structure and Physiology, *4th ed. Copyright Sigmund Grollman 1978.*]

veyed, and where they may remain for about three weeks. Here they are retained until physiologic maturation is complete and until they become motile. As the tubule of the epididymis leaves this body it becomes known as the vas deferens.

Vasa Deferentia (Ductus Deferentia, Seminal Ducts)

The vasa deferentia (sing., vas deferens) are bilateral ducts, approximately 18 in. long, which

continue from each epididymis, and, after a devious course, terminate in the bilateral ejaculatory ducts, which open into the urethra (Figs. 1-8 and 1-9). A vas deferens ascends from each testis through a spermatic cord, passes through the inguinal canal, enters the pelvic cavity, and after coursing upward and medially, passes downward to the base of the bladder where it widens into an ampulla. This terminal end joins with a duct from the seminal vesicle and they become the ejaculatory duct. In addition to functioning as a part of the long excretory duct from the testis, the vas deferens serves as a storage site for sperm.

Seminal Vesicles

The seminal vesicles are two membranous pouches, situated between the lower part of the bladder and the rectum (Figs. 1-8 and 1-9). Through a short duct each vesicle joins the terminal end of a vas deferens and with it becomes an ejaculatory duct.

Ejaculatory Ducts

The ejaculatory ducts are paired, narrow, short tubes formed by the joining of the terminal ends of the vasa deferentia and the ducts from the seminal vesicles. These two ducts descend between the lobes of the prostate gland and open into the urethra into which they discharge sperm and secretions from the seminal vesicles and the epididymides (Fig. 1-9).

Prostate Gland

The prostate gland is located just below the bladder and surrounds the upper portion of the urethra (Figs. 1-8 and 1-9). It is generally described as being the size and shape of a chestnut. It secrets a thin, complex fluid that is discharged into the urethra through many small tubules that open into it.

Bulbourethral Glands (Cowper's Glands)

The bulbourethral glands are two small pea-sized bodies located below the prostate gland, within the pelvic floor. They secrete an alkaline, viscous fluid that is emptied into the urethra through a small duct from each gland.

Penis

The penis is the male organ of copulation. Semen is ejaculated through it into the vagina of the female during intercourse, and active sper-matozoa in the semen can enter the cervix and travel to the fallopian tubes where fertilization of an ovum may take place.

The penis is a cylindrical organ composed of three elongated masses of cavernous erectile tissue; two of these columns lie paired and anteriorly, and one lies medially and ventrally to the other two. The urethra passes through the medial column of tissue and opens at the tip of the penis. This organ is enclosed in fascia and is covered with skin (Figs. 1-8 and 1-9). Relatively large spaces in the cavernous tissue usually become distended with blood during sexual stimulation, causing this organ, which is otherwise flaccid, to become firm and erect.

A slight enlargement at the end of the penis, called the *glans penis,* contains the urethral opening and many very sensitive nerve endings. The skin of the penis extends over its end, covers the glans, and becomes folded upon itself. This is called the *prepuce* or *foreskin* (Fig. 1-8) and is the portion that is surgically removed when a circumcision is performed.

The male urethra, which extends from the neck of the bladder to the orifice in the glans of the penis, serves two purposes. It conveys urine from the bladder, and, at separate times, transmits semen containing spermatozoa to the outside of the body.

SUMMARY

The anatomic structure of the reproductive organs of the female and the male have been described and some reference has been made to their function. Chapter 2 gives a more detailed discussion of the physiology of the reproductive organs, especially function of the gonads in production of germ cells and hormones.

BIBLIOGRAPHY

Danforth, David N. (ed.), *Obstetrics and Gynecology,* 3rd ed. Harper and Row, New York, 1977, Chapters 3 and 4.

Goss, Charles Mayo (ed.), *Gray's Anatomy of the*

Human Body, 29th American ed. Lea & Febiger, Philadelphia, Pa., 1973.

Grollman, Sigmund, *The Human Body: Its Structure and Physiology*, 4th ed. Macmillan, New York, 1978.

Lapides, Jack (ed.), *Fundamentals of Urology*. Saunders, Philadelphia, Pa., 1976.

Miller, Marjorie, and Leavell, Lutie C., *Kimber-Gray-Stackpole's Anatomy and Physiology*, 16th ed. Macmillan, New York, 1972.

Reid, Duncan E., Ryan, Kenneth J., and Benirschke, Kurt, *Principles and Management of Human Reproduction*. Saunders, Philadelphia, Pa., 1972.

2

Physiology of the Reproductive Organs

During childhood the reproductive system undergoes gradual growth, along with other parts of the body, but it does not become physiologically mature until sometime during adolescence. About the age of 11 to 12 years the reproductive organs begin to undergo rapid development and in another two to three years they are physiologically capable of carrying out their reproductive function. This development is completed earlier today than in past generations and is accompanied by rapid physical growth of the entire body.

After the ability to reproduce has been attained, the reproductive organs of the female go through a series of cyclic changes each month throughout the childbearing years, with the exception of alterations during pregnancy and lactation. The many changes in each cycle include development of a graafian follicle, ovulation, formation of a corpus luteum, production of ovarian hormones, changes in the epithelial lining and secretions of the reproductive tract, and menstruation. Normal function of the reproductive organs is dependent on a complex interrelationship between the gonad-stimulating hormones from the anterior pituitary gland and the ovarian hormones.

ADOLESCENCE AND PUBERTY

Adolescence is the period of physiologic and psychologic growth and development during which an individual gradually progresses from the physical and emotional characteristics of a child to full maturation of the body and the traits and capabilities of an adult. The adolescent period covers a span of several years. The age at which adolescence begins and the rate of progression toward adulthood vary, depending upon constitutional traits, genetic influences, and other factors. Physical signs of adolescence often become noticeable by 10 to 11 years of age in girls and by 12 to 13 years of age in boys. Indications of approaching adolescence are present earlier but are not as distinctly identifiable as physical and behavioral signs.

The changes of adolescence are apparently dependent upon a number of interrelated factors, but especially rely upon changes in the function of the endocrine glands. It is at this time that the anterior pituitary gland begins secretion of appreciable amounts of gonadotropic hormones, which thereafter gradually rise to adult levels. These hormones, in turn, gradually stimulate the gonads to produce hormones and to mature germ cells. The typical sex hormones secreted by the gonads, estrogen in the female and testosterone in the male, stimulate growth and development of adult sexual characteristics. Adrenal androgen secretion also increases during adolescence and brings about further body development.

Adrenal androgen secretion stimulates the growth of pubic and axillary hair as well as the characteristic spurt in body growth, with a distinct increase in height and a still more marked increase in weight. Estrogen stimulation causes other changes that take place in girls during adolescence. The sexual changes in the female in their approximate order of appearance are (1) growth and reshaping of the bony pelvis, resulting in a widening and broadening of the hips, (2) characteristic feminine fat distribution, (3) development of the breasts, (4) growth and change to adult cell structure and glandular function of the internal and external reproductive organs, (5) appearance of pubic and axillary hair, (6) onset of menstruation, and (7) initiation of ovulation. With these many and rapid physical and physiologic changes, the importance of provision for good physical health through ample exercise, well-balanced diet, and adequate sleep is apparent.

Puberty usually refers to the time at which reproduction becomes possible; it is one stage in the maturation process of adolescence. In girls, the appearance of the first menstrual period, termed the *menarche*, is commonly accepted as evidence of puberty. However, reproduction may not be possible this early, since ovulation often does not occur during the first several menstrual cycles. In boys, puberty is defined as the time when spermatozoa make their appearance; this manifestation is not as clearly evident as the distinguishing characteristic of approaching sexual maturity in girls. Sexual maturation in boys usually occurs between the ages of 12 and 16 years. Hormonal function in the male and spermatogenesis are discussed on pages 37–40.

The age at which girls reach puberty (begin menstruation) is usually between 11 and 15 years, with 13 years considered the average age. Very occasionally menstruation appears as early as 10 years of age and as late as 17 years. Menstrual periods are often not well established at the beginning, and they may occur at irregular intervals during the first one to two years. Ovulation may or may not occur prior to these first menstrual periods. When menstruation occurs without prior ovulation, the bleeding is called anovulatory; it results from changes in estrogen level, with a temporary decrease or withdrawal

of estrogen causing partial desquamation of the endometrium and bleeding. Menstruation that follows ovulation is described later in this chapter.

Adolescence is a period of emotional growth of considerable magnitude as well as a time of many physiologic changes. An adolescent changes from a dependent child to a more independent individual, with an expanding social awareness requiring many social adjustments. An adolescent's ties with other persons change; these ties become strong with other adolescents of both sexes and are of a less dependent nature with parents. A striving for independence is strong in the adolescent, but this is interspersed with intervals of dependency. Periods of modesty, self-consciousness, uncertainty, and awkwardness are common during the adjustments the adolescent must necessarily make to rapid increase in body size and in sexual development. Confused feelings and attitudes regarding sex role arise. Understanding, support, and guidance by adults throughout the variety of changes that take place in adolescents can contribute much to their emotional growth.

The physiologic and emotional changes of adolescence require clear, frank, and dignified social and sex education. This education, variously known as sex education or in a broader context as family life education, is most effectively done over a period of years. It is best begun early, long before adolescence, and should always be done with recognition of the child's developmental stages. It is then continued in home, school, and church during the years of maturation toward adulthood. Effective education includes discussions of attitudes as well as factual information. The aims of this education are to increase knowledge of the reproductive system and the process of reproduction, to develop self-understanding and understanding of the opposite sex, and to prepare for family life.

THE OVARIAN CYCLE

The ovarian cycle consists of the series of changes in an ovary which are repeated at monthly intervals. These changes are under the influence of anterior pituitary gonadotropic hormones. Main phases of the cycle include the development of a graafian follicle, ovulation, and formation of a corpus luteum. The results of ovarian changes are the maturation and extrusion of an ovum, making one available for fertilization at monthly intervals, and the production of ovarian hormones.

Primary Follicle

The formation of each woman's full quota of ova is complete before birth. These *immature* or *primary oocytes,* as they are called, are single cells scattered throughout the connective tissue of the ovarian cortex. An oocyte is sometimes referred to as an ovum, although it is technically not an ovum until it has reached full maturation, as described on pages 55–58 and in Figure 3-8. Each oocyte is surrounded by a single layer of flattened cells. This structure of an oocyte and its surrounding single layer of epithelial cells is termed a *primary follicle* (Fig. 2-1). It is estimated that at birth each ovary contains 200,000, or even a larger number, of immature follicles closely packed together and separated by thin bands of connective tissue. Many of these disappear in early life by an atretic process, so that perhaps 50,000 or a somewhat larger number of oocytes are present in each ovary when puberty is reached.

Some of the immature follicles are always in a process of development toward a more mature state. Up to the age of puberty they develop mainly in the deeper portion of the cortex and do not reach the surface of the ovary and rupture, as does the mature follicle during reproductive years. After a certain stage of development has been reached, these partly matured follicles go through retrogressive changes. At birth the ovary is largely cortex, but the cortex gradually becomes thinner as the follicles go through development and then disappear.

Graafian Follicle

From puberty until menopause, some of the primary follicles, under the influence of follicle-stimulating hormone from the anterior pituitary gland, develop to full maturation. When a follicle matures, remarkable changes take place (1) in the oocyte, (2) in the cells of the follicle, and (3) in the connective tissue adjacent to the follicle.

As soon as a primary follicle begins maturation, two layers of cells derived from the adjacent ovarian stroma develop around it. The outer layer of cells is known as the *theca externa* and the inner layer the *theca interna.* The theca interna seems to be important in the formation of the hormone estrogen, which is derived from the follicle. The theca interna cells develop a

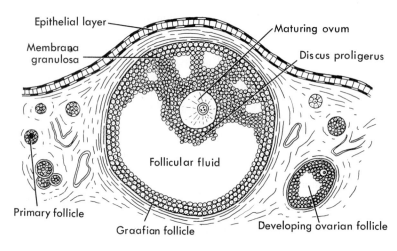

Epithelial layer

Membrana granulosa

Maturing ovum

Discus proligerus

Follicular fluid

Primary follicle

Graafian follicle

Developing ovarian follicle

Figure 2-1. Diagram of an ovary, highly magnified. [*Modified from C. Stackpole and L. Leavell,* Textbook of Physiology. *Macmillan Publishing Co., Inc., New York, 1958.*]

granular appearance due to fat and a yellow pigment. They are known as *theca lutein cells,* and have a role in the formation of the corpus luteum and in degeneration of follicles that do not develop to full maturity.

The single layer of cells of the primordial follicle, the layer surrounding the oocyte, proliferates during maturation of the follicle, with the result that the oocyte is surrounded by several layers of epithelial cells instead of only one layer. Fluid develops between the follicular cells, and, as this fluid accumulates in the center of the follicle, it forms a vesicle (Fig. 2-1). This fluid, known as *follicular fluid* or *liquor folliculi,* contains the ovarian follicular hormone *estrogen.* The epithelial lining of the follicle, which encloses the oocyte and the follicular fluid, having now developed to several layers of thickness, is termed the *membrana granulosa* (Fig. 2-1). This lining is much thicker at one point than in any other area; at this thickened point it forms a mass of cells in which the oocyte is included. This mass is called the *discus proligerus* or *cumulus oophorus* (Fig. 2-1).

The structure described above constitutes a *graafian follicle,* named for Dr. Reijnier de Graaf, who first described it (Fig. 2-1). In the course of its maturation the graafian follicle expands toward the surface of the ovary, where it resembles a clear blister. When fully developed and about to rupture, this blisterlike protrusion on the surface of the ovary measures 10 to 15 mm (roughly ½ in.) in diameter.

While the changes described above are taking place in the follicle, the oocyte grows and increases considerably in size; its diameter may reach a length of 0.2 mm. During this growth period yolk granules, known as *deutoplasm,* are being deposited in the cytoplasm (Fig. 4-3, page 63) to be available for nutriment during the early days of embryonic development, should fertilization occur. Just before rupture of the graafian follicle, the oocyte undergoes the first of the two maturational cell divisions that must take place in all germ cells before they are ready for fertilization. Maturation of germ cells is described on pages 50–58).

Maturation of a follicle, and finally rupture and extrusion of the ovum, occur regularly each month during the years from puberty to the menopause, except during pregnancy, and probably also during lactation, when this process is suspended. Several follicles begin to develop, but usually only one reaches maturity each month (Fig. 2-2). The others, after reaching partial development, undergo an atretic process. Occasionally, however, more than one follicle matures and ruptures at the same time, and if each extruded ovum is fertilized, this results in double-ovum twins or treble-ovum triplets.

Ovulation

When a graafian follicle, with its enclosed maturing oocyte, reaches the surface of the ovary, its wall becomes thinner and it finally ruptures. The follicle contents, the follicular fluid and the oocyte which has become separated from the discus proligerus, are extruded. This process of extrusion of a maturing oocyte from the ovary through rupture of a graafian follicle is called ovulation (Fig. 2-2). The ovum, with some adherent epithelial cells, is discharged near the fimbriated end of the fallopian tube, which it usually enters (Fig. 4-6, page 69).

Ovulation is the dividing period between two phases of an ovarian and a menstrual cycle. The preovulatory period, during which a graafian follicle and its hormone estrogen develop, is commonly termed the *follicular phase.* The postovulatory period, during which the corpus luteum and its hormones develop, is designated as the *luteal phase.*

The time of ovulation is approximately 14 days before the end of a cycle, which means about 14 days before the first day of the next menstrual period. In a 28-day cycle ovulation will therefore occur at approximately the middle of the cycle or usually between the twelfth and sixteenth days. In cycles that are shorter or longer than the average of 28 days, ovulation will occur before or after the middle of the cycle since the postovulatory period remains fairly constant at approximately 14 days.

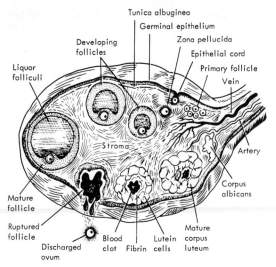

Figure 2-2. Cross section of ovary, showing the stroma and associated structures. [*Reprinted with permission from Macmillan Publishing Co., Inc. from Sigmund Grollman*, The Human Body: Its Structure and Physiology, *4th ed. Copyright Sigmund Grollman 1978.*]

Several signs and symptoms may give evidence that ovulation will or has probably taken place. Some are recognizable only after ovulation has occurred and thus do not predict when the follicle will rupture.

The cervical mucus alters considerably under estrogen stimulation as the graafian follicle proceeds in its development. This mucus reaches its maximum changes at ovulation and after ovulation returns to the characteristics prior to the stimulation by estrogen. The characteristics of cervical mucus and examinations for evidence of ovulation time are described on pages 30 and 586.

Midcycle abdominal pain, known as *mittel-schmerz*, may be felt by some women near the time of ovulation. This discomfort may vary in intensity or in its regularity of appearance, and many women rarely or never experience it.

Midcycle vaginal bleeding, amounting to no more than spotting, is also noted by some women at the time of ovulation.

A shift in basal body temperature occurs at approximately the time of ovulation or shortly thereafter. The body temperature is relatively higher during the postovulatory than the preovulatory phase of the cycle. A rise of a fraction of a degree takes place rather abruptly at this shift. Often there is a sharp drop just before the rise. Once risen, the higher temperature level is maintained until at or near the next menstrual period, when it again drops. The basal body temperature shift is a useful clinical method of determining the approximate time of ovulation. The woman is instructed to take her temperature daily, immediately after waking in the morning and before arising. She records these daily readings on a graph in order to visualize the pattern they are taking (Fig. 2-3).

Corpus Luteum

After ovulation the cavity of the ruptured graafian follicle is replaced by a compact mass of tissue termed the *corpus luteum* (yellow body), so named because of its yellow color (Figs. 2-2 and 2-5). The corpus luteum functions as an endocrine organ. It produces a typical or main hormone, *progesterone*, and also secretes the follicular hormone *estrogen*.

Rapid changes take place in development of the corpus luteum; these are under the influence of the luteinizing hormone of the anterior pituitary gland. After extrusion of the oocyte and the follicular fluid with ovulation, the walls of the follicle collapse; its cavity becomes smaller; and the space that remains is filled with a small blood clot, which is soon absorbed. Granulosa cells that remained adherent to the follicle wall and cells from the theca interna begin invasion of the clot-filled follicle (Fig. 2-2). The granulosa cells increase in size and number and assume a yellowish tint due to a yellowish pigment; these cells are then termed *granulosa lutein cells*. Connective tissue and blood vessels arising from the theca interna grow into the structure between the lutein cells.

The corpus luteum continues activity and growth for about eight days and reaches a diameter of 10 to 20 mm at the end of that time. Its

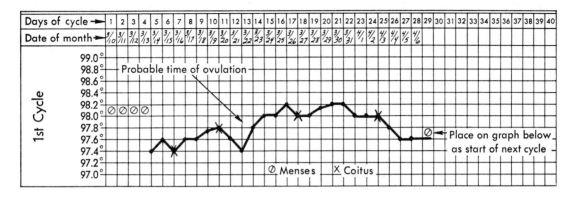

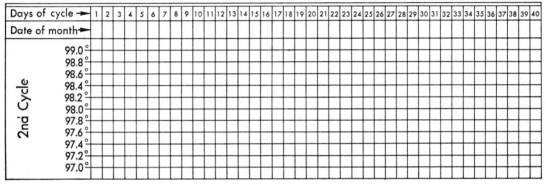

Figure 2-3. Basal body temperature record which may be used to determine the approximate time of ovulation.

course thereafter is determined by whether or not the ovum has been fertilized. If fertilization has not taken place, which is the common event, retrogressive changes begin after about the eighth day. This structure is then termed the *corpus luteum of menstruation.* Degenerative changes are rapid; secretory activity decreases; menstruation begins in about six days; and regression of the corpus luteum is soon complete. The degenerated cells are absorbed, and the corpus luteum is replaced by connective tissue. Late in its regressive phase, when the corpus luteum takes on a dull white appearance, it is termed a *corpus albicans* (Fig. 2-2).

If the ovum has been fertilized, existence and activity of the corpus luteum, which is now termed the *corpus luteum of pregnancy,* continue for approximately three months. It becomes larger than the corpus luteum of men-

struation and may occupy as much as one third of the ovary. The corpus luteum apparently functions at its highest level during the first two months of pregnancy, continues good function for another few weeks, and then, at about the third month of pregnancy, begins to undergo retrogressive changes and decrease in secretory activity. The placenta begins production of the corpus luteum hormones at a very early stage of development, secretes substantial amounts of hormones by the third month of pregnancy, and assumes the corpus luteum function as that structure regresses.

Follicular Atresia

The majority of primordial follicles that begin development do not reach maturity; they degenerate without rupture and disappear by a process termed *atresia*. When partly grown, the follicles undergo retrogressive changes, during which the oocyte undergoes cytolysis; the follicular fluid absorbs; and the follicle cells change until the structure takes on the characteristics of a degenerated corpus luteum. This atretic process begins during fetal life and continues until after the menopause. It is particularly active before puberty and during pregnancy.

The reason for the lavish provision of at least 200,000 or more oocytes for each woman, who uses only a few hundred in the course of her life, is not known. Whatever the purpose of this enormous supply, it makes possible the removal of a considerable amount of ovarian tissue, in case of disease, without loss of reproductive ability, provided the remaining tissue is normal.

INTERRELATIONSHIP OF ORGANS AND HORMONES INFLUENCING THE FEMALE REPRODUCTIVE CYCLE

The central nervous system, hypothalamus, anterior pituitary gland, and ovaries are all closely interrelated in the reproductive process. Interaction between hormones released into the bloodstream from these organs follows a monthly cyclic pattern in which the proportion of each hormone present in the blood varies at different periods in each cycle. Levels of one hormone influence production of the others. The level of these hormones at different periods of the cycle in turn produce the cyclic changes that occur in all of the female reproductive organs each month, such as ovulation, changes in cervical secretion, changes in the endometrial lining, and menstruation.

CNS and Hypothalamus Control

Certain stimuli activate specialized neurons in the brain to release neurotransmitter molecules that reach neurosecretory cells in the hypothalamus, which is located at the base of the brain. These stimuli may be sensory from the external environment and/or humoral from the internal

environment, such as a change in hormone levels.

When the hypothalamus receives the neurotransmitter message it responds by releasing the appropriate releasing factor (Fig. 2-4). The hypothalamus synthesizes and releases several different neurohormones that stimulate pituitary secretion; among these are a thyrotropin-releasing factor and a corticotropin-releasing factor. In responding to a message concerning the reproductive cycle the hypothalamus discharges a gonadotropin-releasing factor (GnRF), which is a small polypeptide hormone composed of 10 amino acids. These hormones from the hypothalamus reach the anterior pituitary gland in high concentration through a short local circulatory system of small blood vessels, the portal vessels of the hypothalamopituitary stalk.

Pituitary Gonadotropic Hormones

The GnRF causes the anterior lobe of the pituitary gland to discharge two gonadotropic hormones. These are large glycoproteins called follicle-stimulating hormone (FSH) and luteinizing hormone (LH), which enter the bloodstream and are carried to the gonads where they exert their influence (Fig. 2-4).

In the female the two gonadotropic hormones act together in stimulating the ovaries, but each also has a specific effect. Although both hormones are present in fairly large amounts in the early part of a cycle, FSH is the hormone that causes growth and maturation of an ovarian follicle, changing it into a graafian follicle as described on page 22. As the follicle grows, its hormone-secreting cells increase the level of the estrogens, principally estradiol (Fig. 2-5).

The gonadotropin LH reaches a midcycle peak level about the time the graafian follicle and its enclosed oocyte are mature. The declining FSH level resurges at this time (Fig. 2-5). The surge of hormones, mainly LH, is responsible for triggering ovulation within 24 hours of this peak production.

After ovulation the empty follicle is changed to a corpus luteum. LH stimulates these new lu-

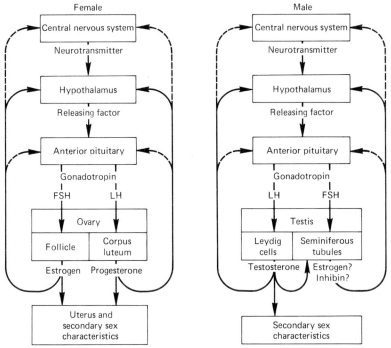

Figure 2-4. Interrelations of organs involved in the reproductive process are shown in this flow diagram. The central nervous system, prompted by external or internal stimuli, causes the hypothalamus to secrete a releasing factor that stimulates the anterior pituitary gland. The pituitary thereupon releases the gonadotropic hormones FSH and LH, which stimulate specific structures in the gonads to secrete the steroid hormones: either estrogen and progesterone or testosterone. The gonadal steroids affect reproductive organs and feed back to the hypothalamus and perhaps to other structures to stimulate and/or inhibit their activity. [*Reproduced with permission from Sheldon J. Segal, "The Physiology of Reproduction." Copyright September 1974 by* Scientific American, Inc. *All rights reserved.*]

teal cells to produce the ovarian hormone progesterone in increasing amounts. At this time ovarian hormonal production is reversed from a predominance of estrogens to a predominance of progesterone (Fig. 2-5).

Ovarian Hormones

The ovaries produce two steroid hormones, estrogen and progesterone, which exert a major influence on preparation of the endometrium for implantation of a fertilized ovum. In addition, these hormones have an effect on many other systems, including bone, muscle, blood, and metabolic processes. These two hormones are also produced in abundance by the placenta; their production and actions in pregnancy is described on pages 120–24.

Estrogen

Estrogen, which may be considered the characteristic female sex hormone, is important to growth and development of the reproductive organs and the mammary glands and to their maintenance in a normally mature state. It is also obligatory for the maturation of secondary

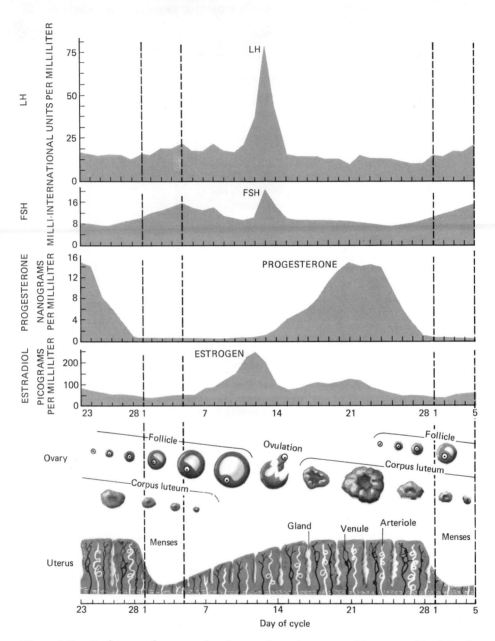

Figure 2-5. Ovulatory and menstrual cycles are charted in terms of fluctuating blood levels of gonadotropins and gonadal steroids, development of a follicle and corpus luteum in the ovary, and changes in the thickness and in the blood vessels and glands of the endometrial lining of the uterus. A rising FSH level stimulates follicular development, causing the ovaries to secrete estrogen (primarily estradiol), which, once menstruation is over, promotes anew the thickening and vascularization of the endometrium. Estradiol also signals a peak in LH release that brings on ovulation: an egg is released from the developed follicle, which is converted into a corpus luteum. The corpus luteum now secretes the steroid progestrone,

female sex characteristics. Estrogen stimulates many of the cyclic changes in the reproductive organs; changes in cervical secretions and growth of the endometrium during the follicular phase of each menstrual cycle are described on pages 30 and 32. In addition to influence on the reproductive organs, estrogen is involved in a number of systemic processes, such as fluid and electrolyte balance and body temperature, described on page 24.

Estrogen is responsible for (1) changing the cervical mucus to favor migration of sperm, (2) stimulating mobility of the fallopian tubes to propel matured ova through the tube, and (3) bringing about proliferation of the endometrium as one phase in its preparation for implantation of a fertilized ovum.

Estrogen plays a major role in growth of the uterus during pregnancy, and it influences a number of metabolic processes during that time. Along with progesterone, it is important to ensure proper function of the uterus and development of the breasts in pregnancy. Production and function of estrogen in pregnancy is further described on pages 121–24.

Estrogen is produced in increasing amounts in the first half of a cycle with a surge of hormone production at midcycle. Thereafter the level diminishes. The surge of estrogens at midcycle signals the hypothalamus, which in turn induces the surge of LH that will trigger ovulation and initiate development of a corpus luteum.

Progesterone

The corpus luteum secretes its typical hormone progesterone in large amounts (Fig. 2-5) and also some estrogen.

Progesterone is a progestational hormone, which induces changes in the endometrium to prepare the uterus for implantation of a fertilized ovum and maintenance of a pregnancy.

This hormone, along with estrogen, is responsible for many of the cyclic changes in the reproductive tract, and is necessary for complete development of the mammary glands. Progesterone also has some effect on metabolic processes, such as its influence on basal body temperature, described on page 24, and has considerable influence on a number of body processes during pregnancy. Its production and function in pregnancy are described on pages 120–21.

After proliferation of endometrium under the influence of estrogen, progesterone causes the secretory changes necessary for pregnancy. The endometrium becomes spongy and highly vascular with an increased glandular secretion by the twentieth day of a cycle, ready for implantation and nourishment of a fertilized ovum (Fig. 2-5).

When a fertilized ovum imbeds in the endometrium, progesterone maintains the pregnancy through support of the endometrium in its secretory state. It also reduces the contractions that normally recur in the uterine muscle, thereby allowing the fertilized ovum to implant and develop, protected against expulsion.

If the ovum is not fertilized, the luteal cells decrease their production of progesterone. In 4 to 5 days the endometrium, no longer receiving adequate support from the diminishing amount of progesterone, sloughs off, and menstruation occurs (Fig. 2-5). Buildup of endometrium and its regression leading to menstruation is described below.

CYCLIC CHANGES IN THE FEMALE REPRODUCTIVE ORGANS

The cyclic changes in the ovaries have been described on pages 21–26. Simultaneous with, and in response to, changes in the ovarian cycle, all the other reproductive organs undergo cyclic

which further prepares the endometrium for pregnancy. In the absence of fertilization, however, progesterone production falls and the endometrium is sloughed off with menstruation.

variations. Alterations in the endometrium are most apparent; those of the cervix can readily be observed; others are more obscure. These cyclic changes take place in response to the level of ovarian hormones in the body. The changes that are easily detected clinically can be studied for assessment of hormone secretion, for evidence of normal ovarian function, and for indication of ovulation. Of the many changes that take place in the reproductive system, only a few will be described below.

The ovarian cycle may be divided by the event of ovulation into a follicular phase, characterized by graafian follicle development, and a luteal phase, characterized by development of the corpus luteum.

Vaginal Mucosa

The mucosal cells and the secretions of the vagina undergo regular cyclic changes during each ovarian cycle, with the type of epithelial cells and the content of the secretions dependent upon the level of estrogen and progesterone. The vaginal epithelium thickens under the influence of estrogen, and the glucose excretion is maximal at the time that the estrogen level is highest, about the time of ovulation. Vaginal smears may be used to estimate estrogen activity.

Cervical Mucus

The cervical mucus is a complex secretion at all times, but, in addition, varies considerably in its characteristics during the course of each ovarian cycle. Estrogen stimulation during the preovulatory or follicular phase of a cycle causes increased activity of the cervical glands and changes in their secretion. These changes are progressive, reach their maximum at the time of ovulation, and then regress, returning to the characteristics of the beginning of the cycle (Fig. 2-6).

During much of the ovarian cycle cervical mucus is relatively scant in amount, opaque in appearance, and viscous in consistency. In mid-cycle, corresponding to the ovulatory period, cervical mucus is considerably increased in amount, is clear in appearance, and of low viscosity. A thin clear mucus secretion from the vagina may be noted at this time. The pH of cervical mucus, which may be slightly below 7.0 before and after ovulation, rises to near 7.5 at the time of ovulation. Changes in the cervical mucus during the ovulatory period make it most receptive to sperm at this time, enhancing sperm penetration of the mucus and migration through it.

Cervical mucus can be examined and evaluated for its qualities to determine the approximate time of ovulation and to assess ovarian function. Two properties which can easily be investigated clinically are termed spinnbarkheit and ferning or arborization. These properties develop under estrogen stimulation, are maximal at ovulation, and decrease after progesterone appears.

Spinnbarkheit relates to the elasticity of cervical mucus, a property that permits it to be drawn into a long, thin strand. Spinnbarkheit can be measured by placing a drop of mucus on a glass slide and then drawing it out into a thread with another slide, a cover glass, or a small wooden spatula. Elasticity of cervical mucus increases progressively during the follicular phase and reaches a maximum at the time of ovulation. Threads of mucus from 15 to 20 cm in length can be drawn from cervical mucus examined at ovulation as compared to threads from 1 to 2 cm long when estrogen stimulation of the cervical glands is minimal (Fig. 2-6).

Fern pattern or *arborization* refers to the pattern into which cervical mucus dries when it is under estrogen stimulation. Examination for this characteristic aids in assessment of ovulation time. To observe cervical mucus for ferning, a drop of mucus is spread on a glass slide, allowed to dry, and examined microscopically for pattern. The pattern of dried cervical mucus results from crystallization of the sodium chloride in the mucus and is determined by the environment (the other components of the mucus) from which

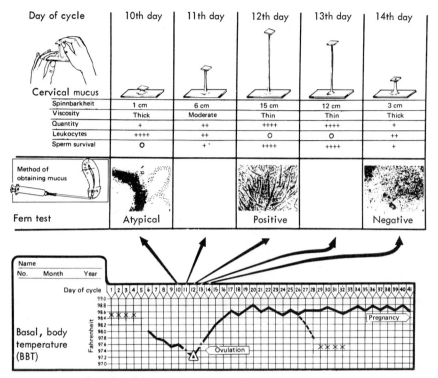

Day of cycle	10th day	11th day	12th day	13th day	14th day
Cervical mucus					
Spinnbarkheit	1 cm	6 cm	15 cm	12 cm	3 cm
Viscosity	Thick	Moderate	Thin	Thin	Thick
Quantity	+	++	++++	++++	+
Leukocytes	++++	++	O	O	++
Sperm survival	O	+	++++	++++	+
Fern test	Atypical		Positive		Negative

Method of obtaining mucus

Name / No. / Month / Year

Basal body temperature (BBT) — Ovulation — Pregnancy

Figure 2-6. Clinical and laboratory criteria of ovulation. [*Reproduced with permission from Melvin R. Cohen, "Methods of Determination of Ovulation,"* Lying-In: The Journal of Reproductive Medicine, *1 (No. 2):181–86 (Mar.–Apr.) 1968, p. 182.*]

the sodium chloride crystallizes. When the concentration of sodium chloride in the mucus is relatively high, ferning takes place. Ferning is dependent upon estrogen stimulation, which increases the content of sodium chloride in the mucus, provided the mucus is not simultaneously under progesterone influence. Progesterone lowers the sodium chloride content of the mucus and when progesterone is present ferning does not occur. The presence of a ferning pattern of cervical mucus is thus determined by the hormones present.

The fernlike pattern of cervical mucus progressively increases during the preovulatory phase, becoming more full and complete, and it is most pronounced about the time of ovulation. The fernlike pattern is replaced by a cellular pattern when progesterone appears, beginning one to two days after ovulation. This cellular pattern persists during the postovulatory period (Fig. 2-6).

The Endometrial (Menstrual) Cycle

As the ovary undergoes cyclic changes, so the endometrial lining of the uterus also undergoes a series of changes, repeated at monthly intervals. These endometrial changes are under the influence of ovarian hormones and thus progress concurrently with changes in the ovarian cycle. As the amount and kind of ovarian hormones change during the cycle, the endometrial characteristics typical of each ovarian hormonal action appear. Since the ovarian cycle is under the influence of anterior pituitary gonadotropic hormones, there is a close correlation between the pituitary gonadotropic hormones, the ovarian cycle and its hormones, and the endometrial cycle.

The endometrial cycle may be described in three main phases:

1. The follicular or preovulatory phase, during which the endometrium grows under the influence of estrogen
2. The luteal or postovulatory phase, during which there is a progressive increase in secretory activity of the endometrium, as it is influenced by progesterone as well as estrogen
3. The menstrual phase, during which regression and partial desquamation of the endometrium occurs as a result of regression of the corpus luteum and withdrawal of its hormones

The Follicular Phase

The follicular phase immediately follows a menstrual period. It coincides with the preovulatory period of the ovarian cycle, at which time the graafian follicle develops and produces increasing amounts of estrogen (Fig. 2-5). Under the influence of estrogen the endometrium, which was partly desquamated during the preceding menstrual period, regenerates and grows. This follicular phase, during which proliferation of endometrium takes place, may be termed the *proliferative phase* of the cycle.

At the beginning of the follicular phase the endometrium is from 1 to 2 mm thick and its glands are short, straight, and narrow. During this phase cells proliferate; the uterine glands increase in size; and the mucosa reaches a thickness of about 3 mm by the end of the period of proliferation.

The Luteal Phase

The luteal phase begins after ovulation and coincides with the period of corpus luteum development and progesterone secretion (Fig. 2-5). In response to progesterone the glands of the endometrium begin to secrete; this phase may therefore be termed the *secretory phase* of the cycle.

The luteal phase is characterized by increasing endometrial secretory activity, as well as continuing increase in thickness. The glands become longer, wider, and tortuous, and they secrete large quantities of glycogen. Vascularity increases and the arterioles become coiled and tortuous. The stroma increases and becomes edematous.

At the end of the luteal phase the endometrium is soft, velvety, and edematous and measures 4 to 6 mm in thickness. This vascular, spongy, glycogen-rich endometrium is ready for implantation and nourishment of a fertilized ovum. Because of this preparation for pregnancy, the luteal phase may also be termed the *progestational phase*. If pregnancy occurs, endometrial development continues under the influence of progesterone to an even thicker tissue which is termed the *decidua* of pregnancy. When pregnancy does not occur, the endometrium regresses along with the corpus luteum.

The Menstrual Phase

The menstrual phase is a period of regression during which the previously well-developed endometrium becomes ischemic, degenerates, and desquamates with moderate bleeding. This phase coincides with regression of the corpus luteum and withdrawal of its hormones, progesterone and estrogen (Fig. 2-5).

The menstrual phase begins several days before the actual onset of menstrual bleeding and may be divided into a premenstrual and menstrual period. During the few days preceding menstruation, concurrent with corpus luteum regression, circulation in the endometrium decreases and shrinkage due to loss of tissue fluids and secretions takes place. There is a period of vasoconstriction, then relaxation of, and bleeding from, the vessels, and thereafter desquamation of the upper layers of tissue begins. Bleeding and tissue loss continue during the next several days, which are termed the menstrual period. Regeneration begins in the lower layer of the endometrium even before the menstrual phase is completed.

Menstruation normally recurs throughout the

childbearing period, from puberty to menopause, except during pregnancy and lactation. Although menstruation is usually preceded by ovulation and corpus luteum formation, periodic bleeding without prior ovulation sometimes occurs. Such anovulatory periods are physiologically different from true menstrual periods, but do not necessarily vary much clinically.

The interval from the onset of one menstrual period to the onset of the next period is termed the *menstrual cycle*. A cycle is usually considered to be 28 days in length, but there are many variations from this, not only in different women, but also in the same individual. Such variations in interval usually range between 21 and 32 days. Regularity of menstrual periods may be temporarily disturbed, or the periods may be completely absent for a few months, as a result of a marked change in a woman's daily regime of living due to either physical or emotional factors. After adjustment to the disturbing cause, gradual resumption of normal menstrual periods follows.

The duration of a menstrual period is usually from four to six days, but lengths from two to eight days are considered within normal range.

The amount of menstrual flow varies from 60 to 180 ml (2 to 6 oz), but actual blood loss is less, usually from 30 to 60 ml (1 to 2 oz). In addition to blood, the menstrual discharge consists of fragments of endometrium, secretions from uterine glands, and mucus. The menstrual flow is scant at the beginning, gradually increases, is usually greatest on the second day, and then gradually diminishes. Menstrual discharge is ordinarily dark red in color. It normally does not clot. The rather offensive odor from menstrual discharge is caused by decomposition of blood and increased secretions from the sebaceous glands of the vulva.

Clinical Aspects

A menstrual period may be preceded and/or attended by a certain amount of emotional and physical disturbance. A few days before bleeding begins, certain premonitory signs are frequently noticed. Common signs are abdominal distention, headache, backache, breast fullness, and premenstrual tension, characterized by depression or anxiety.

While many women may observe little or no physical change during menstruation, others are somewhat uncomfortable at this time. They may be tired and may have less endurance and resistance than usual. Headaches, with a sense of fullness, dizziness, and heaviness, are sometimes accompaniments. Backache is a frequent source of distress. Abdominal discomfort may vary from an uncomfortable sense of dragging heaviness to pain. There may be pain in the hips and thighs. Occasionally there is a loss of appetite or sometimes nausea. Slight bladder irritability and a tendency to constipation may be noted. If breast changes occur, they are much the same as, though slighter than, those occurring during pregnancy. The breasts may become firmer and somewhat increased in size; a burning, tingling sensation and soreness may accompany these changes. The nipples may be turgid and prominent, and the pigmented areas may temporarily become darker. The skin over other parts of the body sometimes changes in appearance, possibly accompanied by circles under the eyes and pimples. Some women are pale and others are flushed during their menstrual period.

In addition to the physical discomfort that may be coincident with menstruation, there is sometimes evidence of emotional and nervous instability. This may be characterized by irritability, lack of poise and control, and a state of depression or of tension. Drowsiness and mental sluggishness are not uncommon.

The disturbances accompanying menstruation, described above, vary widely in different women, and in the same woman at different times and under different conditions. Several symptoms may persist with more or less severity throughout the menstrual life of one woman, while perhaps only one or two will occasionally disturb another. Discomfort usually begins from one to several days before the menstrual flow appears, is at its height during the following day, and then subsides steadily and progresses to a feeling of well-being. Many women feel better at the end of their menstrual period and during the days immediately following than at any other time during the cycle.

It is believed that an attitude that regards menstruation as a normal physiologic process often reduces its discomforts. When discomfort appears to be greater than that which may normally be expected to accompany menstruation, a medical examination is indicated.

Under normal circumstances it is seldom necessary for a woman to depart markedly from her usual mode of living during a menstrual period. Exercise in moderation and all other normal activities may be performed as usual.

Personal hygiene during menstruation is not necessarily different from daily hygiene at any other time. Frequent bathing and frequent changes of perineal pads are important. Many women use a vaginal tampon to absorb the menstrual flow. The tampon is comfortable when worn properly, has certain advantages over the perineal pad, and in most instances there is no objection to its use. The tampon eliminates the bulk and irritation of the external pad. It overcomes the problem of the unpleasant odor that accompanies the menstrual flow, since menstrual discharge is almost entirely odorless unless exposed to air.

Heat to the abdomen and lumbar region, warm baths, rest and quiet, and good posture will usually give relief from menstrual discomfort. Cold baths are not advisable during painful menstruations since they may increase distress. If the woman understands that premenstrual tension and general irritability may appear, she may more readily accept this discomfort and plan according to her ability to cope with it.

Menstrual Irregularities

The most common menstrual irregularities are as follows. *Dysmenorrhea* is painful menstruation. *Menorrhagia* is an abnormally copious menstrual flow. *Metorrhagia* is bleeding between the menstrual periods. *Amenorrhea* is absence of menstruation. Common causes are pregnancy, lactation, and endocrine disturbances.

Menstrual irregularities require medical attention. Endocrine disturbances can often be corrected. Pathologic conditions require early diagnosis and treatment, this being especially important for diagnosis and treatment of malignancy.

THE CYCLIC INTERRELATIONSHIPS OF EVENTS IN THE FEMALE REPRODUCTIVE PROCESS

The hypothalamus, the gonadotropic hormones of the anterior pituitary, the ovarian hormones, maturation of an ovum, ovulation, and preparation of the endometrium for a fertilized ovum are all very finely integrated.

At the beginning of a cycle, follicles in the ovary develop in response to an increase in FSH and LH from the pituitary gland. As these follicles grow toward maturation they produce increasing amounts of estrogens, which cause the endometrium to proliferate. The ovum develops simultaneously (Fig. 2-5).

When follicular development nears its maximum and estrogen production is high, FSH secretion decreases somewhat, but LH secretion gradually increases. At the maximal estrogen level there is a moderate surge of FSH and an enormous surge of LH, which stimulates ovulation (Fig. 2-5). Usually only one of the follicles reaches complete maturity and ruptures. This rupture, termed ovulation, marks the dividing period between the preovulatory or follicular phase and the postovulatory or luteal phase.

The luteinizing hormone influences development of the corpus luteum and, concomitantly, the production of progesterone as well as estrogen. These hormones stimulate the endometrial glands to secrete abundantly; this is called the secretory phase.

After ovulation, just past midcycle, estrogen and progesterone feed back to the hypothalamus and the anterior pituitary to suppress secretion of FSH and LH (Fig. 2-4), thereby preventing further follicle development and ovulation.

After 8 to 10 days the corpus luteum degenerates, unless pregnancy has occurred; its hormones are gradually withdrawn; the endometrium regresses; and menstruation takes place. When the corpus luteum hormones decrease in the late luteal phase, a stimulus to the hypothalamus and the anterior pituitary brings about a rise in FSH and LH. These hormones then stimulate development of another cycle even before menstruation from the last cycle has taken place (Fig. 2-5). Apparently, if an ovum has not been fertilized, a signal to the brain initiates the series of events that will lead to another series of hormonal production (Fig. 2-4). Feedback between the ovarian hormones and the hypothalamus, with its gonadotropic releasing factor, appears to regulate synthesis and release of FSH and LH. The anterior pituitary and its hormones appear to regulate the sequence of events surrounding ovulation.

The above-described cycle changes continue from puberty to menopause, with the exception of interruptions during pregnancy and lactation. Both the ovary and the endometrium are in a constant state of change, and each day is different from the preceding one. This is also true, to a less apparent degree, of the other reproductive organs. Although the changes described above have been presented in phases, they are not so distinctly divided, but rather are on a continuum, and one phase may begin before another ends.

If the mature ovum that was expelled from the graafian follicle at midcycle is fertilized, a new series of events must take place to prevent menstruation and expulsion of the embryo. An uninterrupted supply of progesterone is necessary to maintain endometrial attachment (Fig. 2-7).

A blastocyst soon develops from the fertilized ovum. Even before implantation into the endometrium, the outer cells of this blastocyst, the

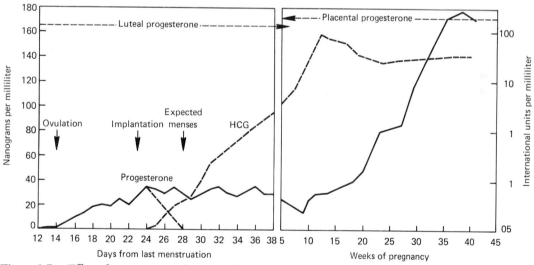

Figure 2-7. Effect of pregnancy on the cycles illustrated on page 28 is essentially to maintain progesterone production, which would otherwise fall off (*broken line*), leaving the implanted blastocyst to be sloughed off with the menstrual flow. Instead the trophoblast (the outer cells of the fertilized egg) secretes the hormone HCG, which is similar to LH and causes the corpus luteum to keep secreting progesterone. Beginning at about the fifth week of pregnancy the placenta takes over the task of progesterone production. [*Reproduced with permission from Sheldon J. Segal, "The Physiology of Reproduction." Copyright September 1974 by* Scientific American, Inc. *All rights reserved.*]

trophoblastic cells, produce a hormone called human chorionic gonadotropin (HCG). This hormone, which is very similar to LH in function and structure, signals the corpus luteum to continue producing progesterone (Fig. 2-7). With continuing production of progesterone the events of menstruation and the beginning of a new cycle are suspended.

The corpus luteum is limited in its ability to survive and produce, but by about the fifth week the placenta begins to take over production of progesterone (Fig. 2-7). Soon thereafter the corpus luteum does not appear to be essential to maintenance of pregnancy. Placental production of HCG is described on page 118 and its production of the hormone progesterone on page 120.

The Climacteric or Menopause

The *climacteric*, frequently termed the *menopause* and sometimes called "the change of life," is the period of life at which ovarian function gradually decreases and eventually stops. Menopause, which means the permanent cessation of menstruation, is one of the easily distinguishable signs of the climacteric. Menopause is only one of the physiologic changes of the climacteric, but it is the term that is commonly used for all or any part of this transitional period.

The climacteric occurs ordinarily between the ages of 45 and 50, but there is a considerable variation of time. In some women menstruation normally ceases before the age of 45, while in others it continues after age 50. The climacteric is not abrupt; it involves a change covering a period of several years.

Just as adolescence is a normal developmental process during which ovarian activity begins and becomes well established, so the climacteric is a normal retrogressive change in which there is a gradual physiologic decline in ovarian activity. A period of anovulatory function, with follicular development and estrogen secretion, but without ovulation, may precede cessation of activity. During the climacteric, ovulation stops and the childbearing period ends; menstruation ceases; the reproductive organs undergo atrophic changes; and the body makes adjustments to hormonal alterations. The climacteric is a physiologic process, and the entire organism is gradually prepared for cessation of ovarian function, both physically and psychologically. Since the transition of the climacteric is made slowly, it should not be greatly disturbing, but women often experience a certain amount of nervous instability, and some discomfort from "hot flashes," until a physiologic adjustment has been made.

As menopause approaches, menstruation often occurs irregularly; the flow sometimes temporarily increases slightly, but usually begins to diminish in amount. Menstrual periods may stop abruptly, but the process is more likely to be gradual, with periods of fairly regular menstrual cycles alternating with periods of amenorrhea. Eventually menstruation does not reappear.

Vasomotor changes—hot flushes of the face and neck, sweats, and flashes of heat which may involve the entire body—are the most characteristic symptoms of the climacteric. Severity of these symptoms varies, being almost absent in some women, moderate in others, and severe in a few. Other effects of menopause are vulvovaginal changes. Atrophy of the epithelium, which may become traumatized easily, vaginal dryness, and pruritis may cause discomfort.

During the reproductive years there is a close interrelation between pituitary gonadotropic and ovarian hormone production. The decrease in ovarian function during the climacteric disturbs this relationship and may, for a variable period of time, result in an imbalance in the relationship. The vasomotor phenomena that often accompany the climacteric may be produced by an excess of gonadotropic hormones, or the symptoms may be caused primarily by the decrease in estrogens. The reason is not quite clear. There is an upset in the feedback mechanism. The close interrelationship of these hormones with the CNS may also have an influence on some of the symptoms attributed to the menopause.

Many women have little or no discomfort during the climacteric, but if or when symptoms become severe enough to merit the risks, estrogen replacement therapy may be used to treat the estrogen deficiency. Estrogen may be administered only during the period of transition, until adjustment to the changes in endocrine function have been made, or it may be continued longer. It is used in the lowest therapeutic dose possible. An increased incidence in osteoporosis in postmenopausal women is one reason for prophylactic estrogen therapy. Reports linking the use of estrogen to endometrial carcinoma make prophylactic use risky, especially in anything more than minimal dose.

Unfortunately, many unrelated symptoms are often ascribed to the menopause, with the result that symptoms of serious organic diseases may erroneously be attributed to it. Excessive menstrual flow, for example, may be accepted as normal prior to menopause and accordingly neglected. A change in menstruation, with increased or prolonged bleeding, cannot be accepted as a normal forerunner of menopause, and any bleeding, however slight, occurring after the menopause demands medical attention.

REPRODUCTIVE FUNCTION IN THE MALE

Spermatogenesis

The lining of the seminiferous tubules contains two types of cells important for sperm production. (The terms sperm and spermatozoa will be used interchangeably; sperm may be considered as a shortened term for spermatozoa.) Many of the lining cells are germinal epithelium or *spermatogenic cells*, which produce immature germ cells, spermatogonia, continuously after sexual maturity. Thus, the male produces billions of spermatozoa in a lifetime. This process differs from formation of oogonia in the ovaries,

in that the latter activity ceases during fetal life, and the full quota of immature germ cells is established before birth. A significant depletion of germ cells, characteristic of the ovaries, never occurs in the testes.

Other cells in the lining of the seminiferous tubules, called *Sertoli cells,* are supportive in function. These cells are tall and extend from the basement membrane of the tubules to the lumen. They provide a place for the germ cells that have reached the spermatid stage to attach and receive nutritive material during their further development into spermatozoa (Fig. 2-8). Spermatozoa that have matured become detached from the Sertoli cells, are released into the lumen of the seminiferous tubules, and are conveyed through this duct system to the epididymis. These sperm are not motile at this stage of development and are believed to be transported by mechanical pressure from more sperm released into the tubules and possibly by movement of cilia in the tubular lining.

The testes begin their function of producing mature germ cells and sex hormones at the age of puberty, between 12 and 16 years. (Maturation of germ cells begins at puberty in both sexes. This process is described on pages 50–58). The testes continue to function into advanced years, or throughout life in many individuals. Whereas cessation of ovarian function occurs between the fourth and fifth decade of life, testicular function ordinarily does not show a sharp decline or cessation at a definite age. A very gradual decline in function with advancing age may result in decreased or incomplete spermatogenesis and also a lowering of hormone production, but often without evidence of distinct change.

Maturation of germ cells in the male is not cyclic, as in the female, but rather is a continuous process. Many germ cells, in various stages of development, are always present in the lining of the seminiferous tubules and are released into the lumen when they have reached the spermatozoan stage of development (Fig. 2-8). A great number are constantly matured and released, in

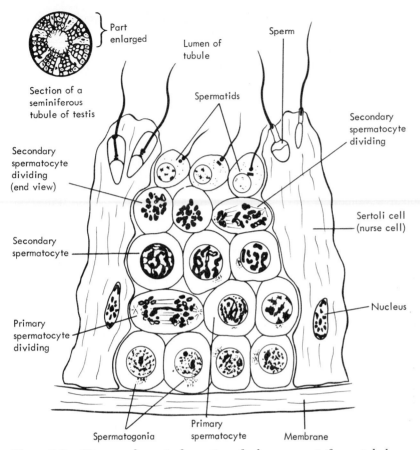

Figure 2-8. Diagram of a part of a section of a human seminiferous tubule arranged to show the different stages of spermatogenesis. [*Reprinted with permission from Macmillan Publishing Co., Inc., from James Watts Mavor and Harold W. Manner*, General Biology, 6th ed. *Copyright Macmillan Publishing Co., Inc., 1966.*]

contrast to maturation and release of one germ cell from the ovaries during each monthly cycle.

Interrelationship of Organs and Hormones Influencing the Male Reproductive Cycle

In the male, as has been described above for the female, the CNS, the hypothalamus, and the anterior pituitary gland are closely integrated with function of the reproductive organs. The CNS sends out a neurotransmitter to the hypothalamus to discharge a releasing factor. This gonadotropin-releasing factor (GnRF) causes the anterior pituitary to discharge the two gonadotropic hormones which then stimulate the testes to produce testosterone and mature sperm.

In the testes a framework of connective tissue between the seminiferous tubules contains specialized cells, called *interstitial cells* or *Leydig cells*. These cells produce the male sex hormone, *testosterone*, under the influence of the pituitary gonadotropic hormones. Testosterone is necessary for normal development and activity of the male genital organs, development and maintenance of masculine secondary sex characteristics, and normal spermatogenesis.

The testes, similar to the ovaries, are under the influence of the pituitary gland for normal function, both for spermatogenesis and for hormone production. The pituitary gonadotropic (gonad-stimulating) hormones, which are the same in both sexes, are named according to their influence on the ovaries, but they also influence testicular function.

The follicle-stimulating hormone (FSH), the hormone that stimulates growth of ovarian follicles, stimulates spermatogenesis from the germinal cells in the lining of the seminiferous tubules. The hormone known as the luteinizing hormone (LH), named for its influence in the female on the corpus luteum, stimulates the interstitial cells (Leydig cells) in the testes to produce testosterone. The luteinizing hormone, because of its influence on the interstitial cells, is sometimes called the interstitial cell-stimulating hormone (ICSH), especially when referred to in the male.[1] In the female, both of the pituitary gonadotropic hormones are involved in ovarian hormone secretion; only one, ICSH, is believed to influence testicular hormone secretion. However, both gonadotropic hormones are necessary for sperm development. Although FSH is primarily the spermatogenic hormone, ICSH is necessary for spermatogenesis, since adequate development of sperm cannot take place without a normal level of testosterone.

In the male as in the female, there is a reciprocal relationship between the gonadotropic hormones of the anterior pituitary gland and the hormones of the gonads, with the activity of either gland responding to an increase or a decrease in the activity of the other. The feedback

mechanism functions in the manner illustrated in Figure 2-4.

Semen

Semen is a viscous, slightly yellowish or grayish fluid consisting of spermatozoa, produced and released from the testes, suspended in secretions derived from the male accessory glands. The seminal fluid, or plasma, is a complex mixture of secretions produced primarily by the seminal vesicles, the prostate gland, and the bulbourethral glands, and to a smaller extent by the epididymides. The combined secretion of the several glands provides a fluid that serves as a medium for sperm transport and as a substance favorable to sperm fertility.

The seminal vesicles secrete a slightly yellowish, complex fluid that contains, among a number of substances, a rich supply of fructose. This fluid is discharged during ejaculation and becomes available to the sperm at that time, when both are simultaneously being discharged from the vas deferens. This secretion increases the bulk of the seminal plasma (the fluid in which the sperm are suspended), thus adding to the fluid medium in which sperm are transported. The high fructose content in the secretion is an important source of nutritive material, which enables the sperm to develop good motility and fertilizing ability.

The secretion from the prostate gland is also added to the semen during ejaculation, being discharged at the same time that sperm are discharged from the vasa deferentia. This secretion is an addition to the bulk of the semen, and it adds substances important to sperm for good motility and fertility. Finally, the bulbourethral glands contribute an alkaline viscous fluid to the semen that is believed to aid in neutralization of the acidic vaginal secretions.

Among the many components of seminal fluid are water, fructose, sodium, potassium, chloride, bicarbonate, acid-soluble phosphate, proteins, citric acid, acid phosphatase, and proteolytic enzymes. The pH of semen varies from 7.35 to 7.50. Its phosphate and bicarbonate

[1] Traditionally ICSH has referred to action in the testes and LH to action in the ovaries. Recent investigations have established that these substances are the same chemically, and therefore the term LH is more commonly used today.

components provide a buffer action that protects sperm from the acidity of vaginal secretions. The function of the glands that secrete the seminal fluid, and the concentration of some of its substances, is dependent upon and closely related to androgenic activity.

Semen is ejaculated from the male genital tract in an average volume of 3 ml. Each milliliter of semen normally contains from 50 to 150 million spermatozoa, with a range from below 40 to over 160 million. A count of 20 million or less sperm per milliliter is considered to be unfavorable for fertility. Semen analysis for fertility assessment includes, in addition to sperm count per milliliter, examination of sperm morphology, degree of motility, percentage of motile sperm, and volume of ejaculate.

Route of Sperm Through the Male Reproductive System

Spermatozoa develop from the spermatogenic cells in the lining of the seminiferous tubules of the testes. When mature, they separate from the Sertoli cells to which they have been attached, fill the tubules, and are pushed into the epididymides where they accumulate until they reach physiologic maturity and become motile. They may remain there for several weeks. From the epididymides they enter the vasa deferentia, which also serve as a storage site.

Sperm transport through the epididymides and the vasa deferentia is accomplished by their own motility, cilia on the tubular lining, and muscular contraction of the tubules, with the relative significance of each not certain. Passage of sperm from the lower ends of the vasa deferentia through the ejaculatory ducts, into the urethra, and to the exterior of the body occurs during ejaculation. During this reflex act, at the climax of coitus, involuntary muscle contractions, chiefly those of the perineum, forcibly eject the sperm and the secretions of the accessory glands (the semen) through the urethra. As the sperm are discharged from the vasa deferentia into the urethra the secretions of the bulbourethral glands, the prostate, and the seminal

vesicles are added in rapid succession and provide the sperm with the vehicle and the nutritive and protective substances that these glands supply. The route of the sperm and the points at which glandular secretions are added to the semen can be traced in Figure 1-9, page 17.

Spermatozoa can live in the ducts of the male reproductive tract for several weeks, but once they are discharged to the exterior, their life is short. They may survive in the female reproductive tract for two to three days, but their ability to fertilize is lost even sooner. When sperm are not ejaculated, they disintegrate and are reabsorbed from the reproductive tract.

SUMMARY

A number of the physiologic events in the reproductive process have been described. The complex interrelationship of the organs involved in reproduction are similar in many respects in both male and female.

In both sexes, the series of events that lead to maturation of germ cells and production of hormones begins at puberty. The initiating factor remains obscure. The changes that start the process appear to be in the brain. Current evidence suggests that an increase in gonadotropin-releasing factor is responsible for the onset of puberty, but this is not certain. An increase in GnRF is in turn dependent upon maturation of the brain.

The series of interrelationships of the hormones begins with specialized nerve cells in the brain. In response to stimuli they send a neurotransmitter to the hypothalamus, which then discharges a stored supply of two gonadotropic hormones, FSH and LH. These two hormones, similar in both sexes, are carried to the gonads by the bloodstream.

The gonadotropic hormones stimulate the ovaries to produce two hormones, estrogen and progesterone, and maturation and release of an ovum each month. In the male, they stimulate production of one hormone, testosterone, and maturation and release of millions of sperm.

The sex hormones influence a number of target cells. Under hormone influence in the female, release of a mature ovum is coordinated with changes in the cervix, which permit passage of sperm, changes in the fallopian tubes to assist ovum transport, and development of the endometrium for implantation. In the male the sex hormone influences maturation and transport of spermatozoa and the components of the secretions that make up the semen as a medium for transport.

The process described above is cyclic in the female and noncyclic in the male. Also, this process ends between ages 45 and 50 years in the female, but continues throughout life in the male.

BIBLIOGRAPHY

Abraham, Guy E., Marshall, John R., and Daane, Thomas A., Disorders of ovulation, in *Pathophysiology of Gestation*, Vol. I. *Maternal Disorders*, edited by Nicholas S. Assali. Academic Press, New York, 1972, pp. 1–61.

Banner, Edward A., The menopause and thereafter, *Postgrad. Med.* 59:174–178 (June) 1976.

Barnes, H. Verdain, Physical growth and development during puberty, *Med. Clin. North Am.* 59:1305–1317 (Nov.) 1975.

Brobeck, John R. (ed.), *Best and Taylor's Physiological Basis of Medical Practice*, 9th ed. Williams and Wilkins, Baltimore, Md., 1973.

Chiazze, Leonard, Jr., Brayer, Franklin T., Macisco, John J. Jr., Parker, Margaret P., and Duffy, Benedict J., The length and variability of the human menstrual cycle, *JAMA* 203:377–380 (Feb. 5) 1968.

Cohen, Melvin R., Methods of determination of ovulation, *J. Reprod. Med.* 1:181–186 (Mar.–Apr.) 1968.

Danforth, David N. (ed.), *Obstetrics and Gynecology*, 3rd ed. Harper and Row, New York, 1977.

Griffiths, Mary, *Introduction to Human Physiology*. Macmillan, New York, 1974.

Grollman, Sigmund, *The Human Body: Its Strucutre and Physiology*, 4th ed. Macmillan, New York, 1978.

Guillemin, Roger, Hypothalamic hormones: Releasing and inhibiting factors, *Hosp. Pract.* 8:111–118 (Nov.) 1973.

Judd, Howard L., Hormonal dynamics associated with the menopause, *Clin. Obstet. Gynecol.* 19:775–788 (Dec.) 1976.

Kistner, Robert W., The menopause, *Clin. Obstet. Gynecol.* 16:106–129 (Dec.) 1973.

Marshall, W. A., Variations in pattern of pubertal changes in girls, *Arch. Dis. Child.* 44:291–303 (June) 1969.

———, and Tanner, J. M., Variations in the patterns of pubertal changes in boys, *Arch. Dis. Child.* 45:13–23 (Feb.) 1970.

Miller, Marjorie, and Leavell, Lutie C., *Kimber–Gray–Stackpole's Anatomy and Physiology*, 16th ed. Macmillan, New York, 1972.

Newton, Niles, *Maternal Emotions*. Hoeber, New York, 1955.

Novak, Edmund R., Jones, Georgeanna Seeger, and Jones, Howard W., *Gynecology, Condensed From Novak's Textbook of Gynecology*, 9th ed. Williams and Wilkins, Baltimore, Md., 1975.

Page, Ernest W., Villee, Claude A., and Villee, Dorothy B., *Human Reproduction*, 2nd ed. Saunders, Philadelphia, Pa., 1976.

Reid, Duncan E., Ryan, Kenneth J., and Benirschke, Kurt, *Principles and Management of Human Reproduction*. Saunders, Philadelphia, Pa., 1972.

Reiter, Edward O., and Root, Allen W., Hormonal changes of adolescence, *Med. Clin. North Am.* 59:1289–1304 (Nov.) 1975.

Root, Allen W., Endocrinology of puberty. II. Observations of sexual maturation, *J. Pediatr.* 83:187–200 (Aug.) 1973.

———, Endocrinology of puberty. I. Normal sexual maturation, *J. Pediatr.* 83:1–19 (July) 1973.

Segal, Sheldon J., The physiology of human reproduction, *Sci. Am.* 231:52–62 (Sept.) 1974.

Strickler, Ronald C., The climateric woman: To replace or not to replace estrogens, *Contemp. Ob/Gyn* 8:100–103 (Aug.) 1976.

Tichy, Anna M., and Malasanos, Louis J., The physiological role of hormones in puberty, *MCN. Am. J. Maternal Child Nurs.* 1:384–88 (Nov.–Dec.) 1976.

Youmans, William B., *Human Physiology*, rev. ed. Macmillan, New York, 1962.

3

Genetic Factors in
Perinatal Care

Basic knowledge of genetic mechanisms and of cell reproduction is important to an understanding of embryology and development of the fetus. This chapter will describe the chromosomes, the genes, and the genetic information they carry; the manner in which this genetic material is replicated and divided during cell divisions; and the way in which the hereditary material carried by parents is transmitted to another generation.

CHROMOSOMES AND GENES

Chromosomes

The nuclei of all cells contain certain characteristic and very important bodies of variable size and shape, called *chromosomes*, so named because of their ability to take up certain dyes. The chromosomes are composed of nucleic acids and special proteins, complexes that are referred to as nucleoproteins. All body cells in an organism have an identical number of chromosomes which is characteristic for the organism in which they exist. Human cells contain 46 chromosomes.

Chromosomes normally occur in pairs. With the exception of the sex chromosomes in the male, each member of the pair is similar to the other member in size and shape and is said to be homologous with the other member. One chromosome of each pair is of maternal origin, having been contributed by the ovum, and the

other one of paternal origin, contributed by the sperm at the time of fertilization. The 46 chromosomes in human cells appear as 23 pairs consisting of 22 pairs of homologous *autosomes* and 1 pair of *sex chromosomes*. The sex chromosomes differ in the sexes; they are designated XX in female cells and XY in male cells.

Chromosomes are sometimes spoken of as appearing in sets, with one member of each pair making up one set. Each set in a human cell consists of 23 chromosomes. Cells with two sets (double set) of chromosomes, which is characteristic of body cells, are referred to as *diploid* cells. Mature germ cells (ova and sperm) are an exception to all other cells in that they contain only a single set of chromosomes; such cells are referred to as *haploid cells*. The fusion of the nuclei of an ovum and a sperm at fertilization brings together two sets of chromosomes, one of maternal and one of paternal origin, and produces the diploid cell from which the individual will develop.

Chromosomes change in characteristics during different stages of activity of a cell. During the periods between one cell division and the next, each chromosome is represented by a long, thin, threadlike structure. The threads are difficult to recognize, but prior to division of the cell nucleus, they condense and change into compact bodies of different sizes and shapes. With special techniques the individual chromosomes can be visualized during the phase of cell division in which they are compact (Fig. 3-1).

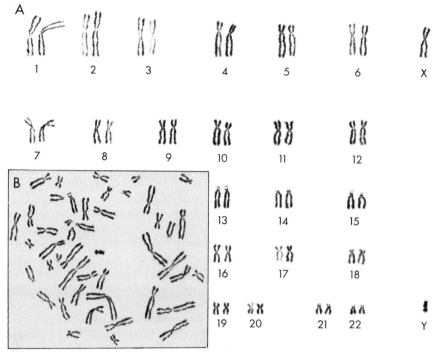

Figure 3-1. Normal human male chromosomes as they appear during metaphase. Cell division has been arrested by treatment with colchicine; hypotonic salt solution then is added to swell and disperse the chromosomes and make them more visible. *B.* Inset: chromosomes as they appear under the microscope following this treatment. *A.* Karyotype: chromosomes are paired and arranged according to a standard classification based on the size, position of the centromere, and other characteristics. The normal human has 22 somatic pairs plus two sex chromosomes (an *X* and *Y* in males, two *X*'s in females). [*Courtesy of Dr. James L. German III, Cornell University Medical College, New York City.*]

Each individual chromosome has a characteristic size and shape. They are rodlike structures either straight or bent and of varying size. Each has, somewhere along its length, an area of constricture. This constricture is called the *centromere* or *kinetochore* (Fig. 3-1), and the portions above or below this point are called *arms*. The centromere is situated in a different position in different chromosomes, but it is in a constant position in any one chromosome. In some chromosomes the centromere is placed near the center, and in others it is located near one of the ends.

Chromosomes have been identified, grouped, and numbered on the basis of decreasing size, position of the centromere, and length of arms above and below the centromere. Specially prepared and enlarged pairs of chromosomes of a single cell may be photographed or drawn, placed in order of decreasing size, and numbered from 1 to 23. Such a picture is called a *karyogram* or *karyotype* of the cell from which the preparation was made (Fig. 3-1). Those chromosomes with similarities can be classified into a group according to their size and the position of the centromere. These groups and the chromosomes that make up the groups are as follows:

Group A   (I) Chromosomes 1, 2, 3
Group B   (II) Chromosomes 4, 5
Group C   (III) Chromosomes 6, 7, 8, 9, 10, 11,
                 12, and X
Group D   (IV) Chromosomes 13, 14, 15
Group E   (V) Chromosomes 16, 17, 18
Group F   (VI) Chromosomes 19, 20
Group G (VII) Chromosomes 21, 22, and Y

A more precise identification of individual chromosomes is possible with the use of banding techniques. It has been found that certain stains or dyes bind differentially, giving the stained chromosome a striped appearance. Although the exact mechanism for the banding is conjectural, the pattern of the bands is consistent for any one chromosome. These patterns, unique for each chromosome, make it possible to distinguish all 23 pairs of human chromosomes, and are significant in identifying abnormal chromosome complements, especially structural variations.

Genes

Within each chromosome there is a string of a large number of molecules called *genes*. Genes, as well as chromosomes, appear in pairs, with one member of each pair of maternal origin and one of paternal origin. Genes are arranged in a linear order in the chromosomes, with each gene of a pair occurring at a given and constant position on a chromosomal pair. Genes are too small to be exactly identified microscopically but are estimated to occur in tens of thousands, making a tremendously large number of pairs.

Genes are the basic units of heredity. The genes that an individual inherits regulate the traits that will develop in that individual, with each gene performing its specific function. Genes which occur at the same position or locus on homologous chromosomes are concerned with the same trait. These genes are said to be *alleles*. The alleles may be *alike*, producing the same effect on a particular body characteristic, or they may be *different*, with each controlling a contrasting variation of the same characteristic.

When a pair of genes or alleles is alike in an individual, he is said to be *homozygous* for that trait. When the alleles differ, the individual is *heterozygous* for the trait influenced by those genes. When the individual is heterozygous, one of the two genes of the pair may be *dominant* to the other and exert its influence strongly enough to mask the other. The gene of a pair that is unexpressed is *recessive*. A recessive gene can be carried for many generations and may ultimately find expression when a mating occurs which matches it with another gene recessive for the same trait.

Genotype is a description of the genetic makeup (kinds of genes) of an individual with respect to a given characteristic. Genes are assigned letters for symbols (see Fig. 3-6). A capital letter is traditionally used to designate a gene that is dominant and a lowercase letter for one that is recessive. If the letters D (dominant) and d (recessive) are used for genes governing a particular characteristic, then individuals with a DD pair would be of homozygous genotype for the dominant genes, those with dd would be homozygous for the recessive genes, and those with Dd would be heterozygous.

An observable physical or chemical characteristic, one that develops under the control of an individual's genotype, is termed his *phenotype* for that characteristic. Observation of a characteristic often does not reveal the genotype, but may provide a clue. When the observable characteristic is known to be produced by a dominant gene, at least one of the genes of the pair is dominant. From the example given above it could be a DD or Dd genotype. If the phenotypic characteristic is known to be governed by a recessive gene, then both of the individual's genes are recessive, from the example above, a dd genotype.

Each gene has its own particular chemical structure, and, according to that structure, directs a biochemical process of development. The chemical components of genes and the way in which they give their directions for development of body characteristics are described below under "Genes and the Genetic Code."

CELL DIVISION

The usual form of cell division, termed mitosis, is the means by which cells reproduce themselves. *Mitosis* is a process of cell division that results in the formation of two daughter cells from one parent cell, with each of the daughter cells receiving a complete set of chromosomes that are identical in both of the new cells and identical to those of the original cell before its division. In the process of mitosis the chromosomes are exactly duplicated in the parent cell and then separated into two new nuclei. Immediately after the nucleus has divided, the cytoplasm divides. This results in the formation of two separate cells which can each undergo a period of growth and another similar division. Mitosis is a continuous process, but is divided into stages for descriptive purposes (Fig. 3-2). A different form of cell division, termed meiosis, one that occurs only in maturation of germ cells, will be described on pages 51–53.

GENES AND THE GENETIC CODE

Genes consist of segments of a long-chain chemical compound, a nucleic acid known as deoxyribonucleic acid (DNA). Each chromosome is made up of many of these segments forming a single long chain of DNA. (It is estimated that the length of DNA in each human chromosome is approximately 4 cm.) In addition, the chromosome contains a protein, usually histone, which has a high concentration of basic amino acids. Histone attaches to the acidic phosphate groups of the DNA strand forming a DNA-histone thread. There are also a variety of nonbasic proteins whose function is unknown.

Although it is known that there are a large number of genes in each chromosome, the detailed arrangement of these genes within the chromosome is still largely unknown. Geneticists are now able to map some genes according to their relative closeness on the chromosome by studying some of their behavior in meiosis. This is, however, a slow and tedious process.

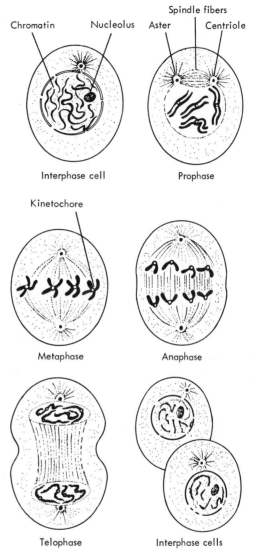

Figure 3-2. Schematic summary of mitosis in animal cells, showing chromosomes, spindle, and asters. [*Reprinted with permission from Macmillan Publishing Co., Inc., from Karl F. Guthe,* The Physiology of Cells. *Copyright Karl F. Guthe 1968.*]

It was formerly thought that DNA occurred only in chromosomes, but recent studies have shown that a certain amount of DNA is also present in some of the bodies of the cytoplasm, as in the mitochondria.

The DNA Molecule

A DNA molecule is composed of a series of units called *nucleotides*. A nucleotide is made up of three components: a sugar (deoxyribose, from which deoxyribonucleic acid derives its name), a phosphate, and a nitrogenous base. The base may be one of four kinds; an adenine or a guanine (purine bases) or a cytosine or a thymine (pyrimidine bases). These bases may be represented by the letters A, G, C, and T.

The DNA molecule consists of two long strands of nucleotides which lie adjacent to one another and are linked together by hydrogen bonds between the bases of each strand. The two long strands are made up of a series of successive nucleotides. The nitrogenous bases of the nucleotides of one strand pair with complementary bases of the other strand and hydrogen bonds form between the members of the pair. Thus each nucleotide is joined to a successive nucleotide in its own strand and hydrogen-bonded by its base to the base of a nucleotide of the adjacent strand (Fig. 3-3).

The construction of the DNA molecule gives it a ladderlike appearance. The two sides of the ladder are composed of sugar and phosphate units which are repeated over and over. These sides are connected by a series of steps. Each step is made up of a pair of complementary bases with a hydrogen bond between them. This ladder is not straight, as could be assumed from the above description. The molecule is arranged spirally, with the two long strands of nucleotides twisted around each other. This form or shape is referred to as a double helix and may be compared to the appearance of a twisted rope ladder (Fig. 3-3).

Binding between the nitrogenous bases of the nucleotides of one strand to those of the adjacent strand, referred to above as pairing of complementary bases, is restricted to specific combinations. An adenine base (purine) is always bound to a thymine (pyrimidine), and a guanine (purine) to a cytosine (pyrimidine). Thus, if the base in the nucleotide on one chain is an adenine, the nucleotide paired with it from the adjacent chain can only contain thymine or it may be a vice versa arrangement. The sequence of bases in one strand determines the sequence of bases in the adjacent strand. The four possible combinations of bases are A-T, T-A, C-G, and G-C (Fig. 3-3).

The four different bases named above, one of which appears in each nucleotide, makes four varieties of nucleotides that can appear along one strand of a DNA molecule (and also four varieties of nucleotide pairs along the two adjacent strands). Although there are only four varieties of nucleotides, the order in which these varieties may be arranged in any one strand is not limited. The total number of sequential arrangements of successive nucleotides, and therefore of successive bases, is very great. Strands of different DNA molecules may be made up of a variable, but very large, number of nucleotides, which in turn can be placed in an endless variety of different arrangements along the strand. Thus each gene represented on a DNA molecule can have its individual sequential arrangement of nucleotides (which may number several hundred), and therefore of bases, an arrangement that is different from that of all other genes.

The DNA molecules carry the genetic code, or the instructions for the production of the particular body characteristics of an individual. The arrangement of the nucleotides in a DNA molecule gives a particular sequence to the bases. This sequence provides the genetic code, or set of instructions, from the gene.

Each gene has a different arrangement of nucleotides from the other genes and each sends out its particular chemical instructions according to its own special code. Thus, genes for brown eyes carry the instructions that bring about the production of the pigment that gives a brown color to the eyes. Variations in the nucleotide arrangement in the DNA molecule of the genes of different individuals for color of eyes or any other characteristic make possible the genetic differences of individuals. A very slight variation

A. Hydrogen bonding between complementary base pairs

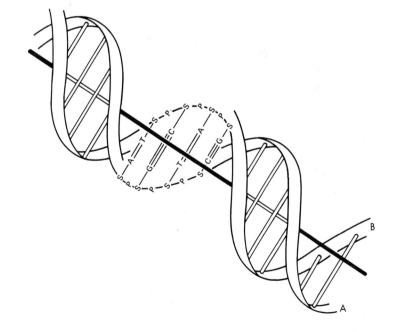

B. Complementary sequences of bases in the 2 strands of DNA

C. The arrangement of the 2 strands in the DNA double helix.

Figure 3-3. The structure of DNA from complementary base pair to double-stranded helix. [*Reprinted with permission from Macmillan Publishing Co., Inc., from Richard A. Goldsby, Cells and Energy. Copyright Richard A. Goldsby 1967.*]

in the pattern of a gene can make a tremendous difference in the chemical code.

DNA molecules must duplicate themselves to provide for an exact replica in each daughter cell that results from cell division. A hypothesis suggested by James Watson and Francis Crick, known as the Watson–Crick hypothesis, proposes how duplication of DNA takes place. According to this hypothesis, the bonds between the complementary bases separate at one point

of the "ladder" and the separation continues all along the line until the double helix has separated into two single strands of DNA with open, exposed bases (bases unattached to another) (Fig. 3-4). The exposed bases of the single strands then form hydrogen bonds with free nucleotides that are present in the surrounding matter of the cell. They specifically attach to nucleotides with bases that are exactly like the ones from which they separated; an A attracts a

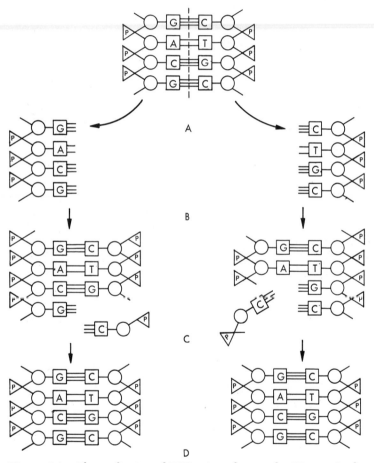

Figure 3-4. The replication of DNA. According to the Watson–Crick theory, the parental double strand separates and, by addition of complementary nucleotides to each strand, forms two identical daughter DNA molecules. [*Reprinted with permission from Macmillan Publishing Co., Inc., from Richard A. Goldsby, Cells and Energy. Copyright Richard A. Goldsby 1967.*]

T and a C attracts a G. With attachment of free nucleotides to the exposed bases of the two single strands of DNA two double strands are formed and the DNA is exactly duplicated (Fig. 3-4). There are now two double helixes where there formerly was one, each identical to the other and identical to the original one.

As each DNA molecule exactly duplicates, all of the chromosomes are exactly duplicated and doubled. After doubling, mitosis proceeds and two daughter cells are formed, each with a complement of chromosomes exactly like that of the parent cell.

Cell divisions of the new daughter cells can continue by repetition of the process described above; first replication of the DNA molecules and then separation of the doubled DNA molecules, and thus of the doubled genes and chromosomes, to form two new daughter cells from each dividing cell. Through replication of DNA and separation of the doubled molecules, the information in the DNA of the chromosomes of each parent cell is given to the daughter cells resulting from mitosis. Every cell does not continue to divide indefinitely. Those cells that have become differentiated in specialized organs and will not proceed through another division do not go through a process of replication of DNA.

RNA

For the code messages, or instructions, of DNA to be utilized, they must be transferred to the cytoplasm of the cells. Another type of nucleic acid, ribonucleic acid (RNA), acts as the intermediate substance in the transfer of messages. RNA can move out of the nucleus and into the cytoplasm, whereas the DNA cannot.

RNA molecules are made up of nucleotides that are structurally very similar to those of DNA molecules. The messenger RNA (mRNA), within the nucleus of a cell, is formed as a single strand alongside the DNA molecule. Its formation is very similar to replication of a strand of DNA. As the RNA strand is synthesized along a strand of the DNA molecule, the DNA bases at-

tract the nucleotides that will compose the RNA strand. Only one of the two DNA strands is used in producing mRNA. It is not known how the system knows which strand it will be. Complementary bases are attracted by the DNA bases just as if exact replication was taking place, with the exception that each adenine base attracts a uracil instead of a thymine. This process makes the mRNA strand complementary in base sequence to the DNA strand; the DNA has specified the sequence of the mRNA bases. In this synthesis, the DNA codes the mRNA so that it has the instructions of the DNA molecule. This process may be referred to as transcription of the code.

After the mRNA is formed, it leaves the nucleus and passes into the cytoplasm to the site of protein synthesis, the ribosomes. From its genetic information it directs synthesis of the protein appropriate to the message code. Similar to DNA, mRNA has only four different bases but these also appear in a large variety of sequences, with the sequence in each RNA molecule having been directed by the DNA molecule that synthesized it.

Since protein is the basic structural unit of all cells, and also of enzymes, which direct metabolic reactions, the structure and physiology of the body are determined by production of proteins according to the messages carried on the DNA molecules. In addition to the genes that specify sequences of amino acids, there are some genes that direct the amount of protein assembled, or that function in other controlling roles, and there are some genes that govern or regulate the action of other genes.

As cells of the body multiply to many millions in number, they become specialized, form the many different tissues and organs, and carry on the specialized functions of the various parts of the body. At all times, these many different cells have an exact replica of the genes in the original one cell from which the body began. They all contain the same genetic material, but the information in the DNA of each of these cells is not all expressed at any one time. That information which is needed is selected as and when necessary for specific purposes. Each gene has its own specific time for action; that of some is essential at the beginning of embryonic development and that of others may not appear until late in adult life. Some genes may direct development of several characteristics, or the influence of several genes may be essential for development of one characteristic. Environmental conditions may change or modify the manner in which a gene is expressed.

Specialization of cells is determined by selection of the genetic information that will be transcribed and translated into the development of the kind of special cells needed for a certain part of the body or a certain function. Such critical selection of thousands of different crucial processes requires coordination between the genes and a great interdependence between the many regulatory mechanisms and reactions in the total body metabolism.

Mutations

A mutation is a heritable change in the structure of the genetic material in a gene. This variation changes the genetic code and results in an alteration in the kind of protein that is synthesized or in the amount that is produced. Mutations may involve (1) a loss of part of a DNA molecule (deletion); (2) an addition of a new base (insertion); or (3) a variation in the sequential intramolecular arrangement of the bases (substitution).

It is important to note that a mutation is a *heritable* change. Unless it is passed on to an offspring it cannot be accepted as a mutation, since its genetic implication cannot be established.

As a chemical substance, DNA is subject to chemical reactions with other substances which change its structure and, often, the genetic code. This is most likely to occur during replication of the DNA molecule as the long strands of nucleotides separate to form two new molecules. At this time mutagens (substances which cause mutations) may bring about alterations in the base-pair sequences by substituting, adding,

or deleting bases to the DNA molecule. Other mutagens, such as ionizing radiation, cause changes by altering the covalent structure of the DNA, thereby leading to chromosomal breakage.

Mutations may appear to arise spontaneously or they may be attributable to certain factors in the environment, such as radiation or pharmacologic agents. In either event the exact duplication of the DNA is altered and the genes carry a set of instructions that differ from those of the original cell. A mutation may cause only a very slight variation in a body characteristic, or it may produce a major alteration. A significant number of mutations are thought to be lethal and therefore are never detected in offspring, since they result in early embryologic death. Most mutations which involve a change from function to nonfunction are recessive and therefore will not be detected unless there is a chance mating with another individual carrying an identical mutant gene. Needless to say, this may not occur for many generations, if ever. Some mutations have barely detectable effects; a few may be useful; others are undesirable and harmful.

On rare occasions, somatic cell mutations can be detected. When mutation occurs in such a cell it gives rise to a clone of cells which differ from the nonmutant surrounding cells. Usually this difference can be detected only if there is a visible change such as in pigmentation. Because somatic cell mutations are not transmissible to offspring, it is difficult to determine their genetic implications, if any.

MATURATION OF GERM CELLS

Before the germ cells, the ovum and the sperm, are fully developed and ready for fertilization, they must undergo developmental changes termed *maturation*. In the maturation process the number of chromosomes in the germ cell is reduced to one half the original number, decreased to one member of each pair, 22 autosomes and 1 sex chromosome. This reduction process is necessary to keep the number of chromosomes in the cells of each new human being constant, since the nuclei of two germ cells unite during fertilization. If the number of chromosomes in each germ cell were not reduced to one half, the new cell resulting from the union of these two cells would have double the number of chromosomes typical for man.

Meiosis

It will be recalled that in mitosis, the characteristic form of cell division of somatic cells, the chromosomes are first duplicated and then divided, with the result that the two daughter cells each receive a full and equal complement of chromosomes. Germ cells, as they mature, divide by a different and special process termed meiosis.

Meiosis is the reduction cell division, a process which results in daughter cells that have only a single set of chromosomes, or only one member of each pair of chromosomes present in the parent cell. This may be either the maternal or the paternal member of the pair. It is a process which reduces the chromosomes in the cells from a diploid (double) set to a haploid (single) set. Immature (primary) germ cells are diploid cells with 23 pairs of homologous chromosomes and are thus identical to somatic cells in their genetic makeup. These primary cells undergo meiosis. The daughter cells of the division, with only a single set of chromosomes, are the mature germ cells.

Meiosis, or maturation division, takes place in two successive stages, termed the first and the second meiotic division or the first and the second maturation division. The second division rapidly follows completion of the first division.

First Meiotic Division

In the first meiotic division the chromosomes duplicate to form two chromatids joined at a centromere. Each duplicated chromosome then moves toward its homologue until the two homologous chromosomes of each pair come to lie very closely side by side, a process that is called *pairing* (Fig. 3-5). Since the chromosomes are

doubled, each represented by two chromatids, each pair of homologous chromosomes now consists of four chromatids. This step of pairing occurs only in meiosis and is different from any process in mitosis, during which homologous chromosomes do not pair. There are also progressive shortening and thickening of chromatids, separation of centrioles, formation of the spindle, and disappearance of the nuclear membrane, as in mitosis.

Each doubled chromosome then comes to lie on the equator of the spindle and becomes attached to it by its centromere, as in mitosis, but different from mitosis in that the pairs arrange coupled. The previously paired homologous chromosomes remain side by side and occupy the same position on the equatorial plane, with one chromosome of the pair on one side of the plane and the other chromosome of the pair on the other side. In mitosis, where the chromosomes do not pair, each chromosome lines up on the equator of the spindle independent of the others, and the homologous chromosomes may occupy different positions of the equatorial plane.

Nuclear membranes then form around each of the two groups of chromosomes and the cytoplasm divides. Two haploid cells have been produced. Thus the first meiotic division reduces the chromosome number in each daughter cell to one half and separates homologous chromosomes in such a manner that each of the new cells contains one member of each pair of the chromosomes present in the parent cell (Fig. 3-5). The chromosomes in these new cells are composed of two chromatids. Since the chromatids remained together during this cell division, the chromosomes moved to opposite ends of the cell in a doubled state, with the identical chromatids remaining together. The cells produced by the first meiotic division are ready to undergo the next stage of meiosis, the second meiotic division.

Second Meiotic Division

The second meiotic division of each of the two cells produced by the first division begins im-

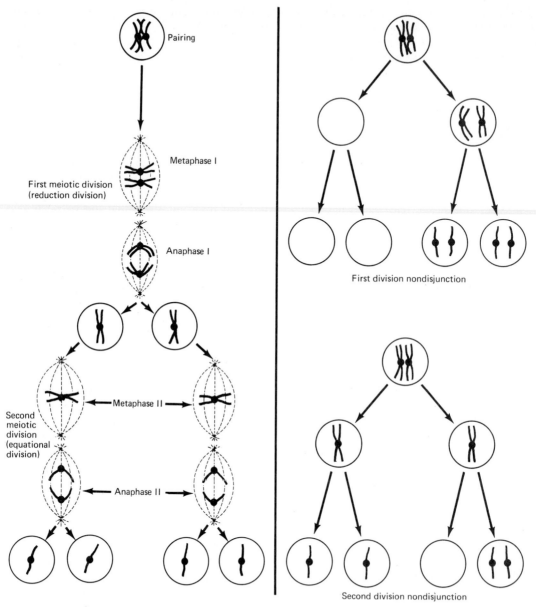

Figure 3-5. Schematic diagram of meiosis showing one chromosome is illustrated on the left. The original cell gives rise to four haploid cells or gametes. Not all of the steps recognized by cytologists are shown. On the right, first and second division nondisjunction are diagrammed. Such accidents of meiosis result in offspring having too many or too few chromosomes. The most commonly recognized example is Down's syndrome where nondisjunction of chromosome 21 results in the individual having three no. 21 chromosomes and 47 rather than 46 total chromosomes.

Labels within figure: Pairing; Metaphase I; First meiotic division (reduction division); Anaphase I; Metaphase II; Second meiotic division (equational division); Anaphase II; First division nondisjunction; Second division nondisjunction mediately after completion of the first division. The second division is shorter and less complicated than the first. The chromosomes are already present in a duplicated state and they are less threadlike than after a mitotic division.

Many of the events of the second meiotic division are similar to mitosis, but there are two major differences. Similar to mitosis, a spindle forms; the chromosomes consisting of two identical chromatids joined at a centromere attach on the equatorial plane of the spindle; the centromeres and chromatids separate and go to opposite poles of the cell; and the cytoplasm divides. One difference from mitosis is that the chromosomes enter the second meiotic division in a duplicated state as two identical chromatids, this duplication having taken place early in the first meiotic process. A second difference is the number of chromosomes involved in the division. As in mitosis, duplicates of the original chromosomes separate in the second meiotic division, but there are only one half as many chromosomes present in the cells. After separation of the chromatids, each new cell of the second meiotic division has one half the number of chromosomes typical for the species, 23 chromosomes in the human cell.

The two successive divisions of meiosis produce four cells from each parent cell. The first division divides the paired homologous chromosomes between two cells, each cell receiving one member of each pair of chromosomes. In human cells, each receives 23 chromosomes. The second division divides the identical chromatids of the 23 chromosomes in each of the two cells of the first division. The result of the maturation divisions is the formation of four haploid cells from one diploid cell (Fig. 3-5).

Distribution of Genetic Material During Meiosis

The genetic material (genes) that any one sperm or ovum carries does not include all that was present in the parent from which the germ cell was derived. Immature germ cells, from which sperm and ova develop, contain all the genetic information present in the parent, but meiosis of these cells changes the number and the distribution of the genes that are present in the cells produced by the maturation divisions.

Distribution of Chromosomes and Genes

Each pair of homologous chromosomes in immature germ cells, as in all somatic cells, is composed of one chromosome derived from the father and one derived from the mother of the individual in whom the cell exists. In the first meiotic division the chromosomes of an immature germ cell are divided between two cells which will each undergo the second meiotic division to become gametes. Due to this first division, each gamete carries only one half of the chromosomal material present in the individual from whom the gamete is derived.

Reduction division is precise in that pairing is always between homologous chromosomes, and division of the pair assures that one chromosome of each pair occurs in each of the gametes. Each cell will have 23 chromosomes, one of each pair, but how many of these 23 will be the maternal member of a pair and how many of the paternal member is chance. As the paired chromosomes arrange on the equatorial plane of the spindle and then divide, the maternal members of all pairs could be on one side of the plane and go to one cell. All the paternal members would then be on the other side of the plane and go to the other cell. However, it is *very unlikely* that all maternal members of a pair would go to one cell and all paternal members to the other cell. The chromosomal pairs can arrange so that any combination of maternal and paternal members can go to each cell as long as there is one of every original pair in the two cells resulting from the first meiotic division. If the homologous pairs of chromosomes arrange so that the maternal members of 10 pairs are on one side of the equatorial plane and the paternal members of the other 13 pairs are on the same side, then one cell of the division will receive 10 maternal and 13 paternal chromosomes and the other cell will receive 13 maternal and 10 paternal chromosomes. The different kinds of gametes that can be formed, with respect to chromosomal combinations of maternal and paternal origin, is very great; over 8 million kinds are possible.

When the homologous chromosomes are divided into two cells at the first meiotic division, the homologous genes are of necessity also divided. If the genes in any one homologous pair are alike, controlling reactions that produce similar characteristics of a trait, the four cells resulting from meiotic division of a cell will carry the same characteristics. If these genes are contrasting, two of the cells resulting from meiosis will carry a different variation of the characteristic from those of the genes in the other two cells. This may mean that two of the gametes resulting from meiosis will carry a dominant gene and the other two a recessive gene.

Crossing-over of Chromosome Parts

Crossing-over refers to an exchange of segments between two homologous chromosomes as they are paired during the first meiotic division. In the process of pairing, the chromatids of homologous chromosomes tend to twist around each other. As the chromosomes move apart, the point or points where chromatids have crossed over each other may not separate as readily as the centromeres or as easily as the parts that are not closely entwined. The chromatids may break apart at the crossover points and the broken off segments may interchange and combine with the homologous chromatid involved in the crossover (Fig. 3-6).

An interchange of chromosome parts at cross-

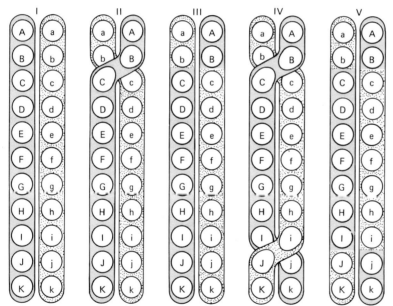

Figure 3-6. Diagram illustrating the crossing-over of pieces of chromosomes with their genes. The bars represent the chromosomes and letters the genes. A single crossover is shown in I–III, a double crossover in IV and V. This diagram shows only the two chromatids that have participated in a crossover of chromosomes and omits the other two that have not made an exchange. [*Reprinted with permission from Macmillan Publishing Co., Inc. from Alfred F. Huettner,* Comparative Embryology of the Vertebrates, *rev. ed. Copyright 1941 by Macmillan Publishing Co., Inc., renewed 1969 by Mary A. Huettner.*]

over does not change the number of, or the position of, genes in the chromosomes. Genes each have their own particular position on a chromosome; homologous genes occur at corresponding positions on homologous chromosomes. When the chromosomes pair, they do so very precisely, with homologous chromosomes coming together so that all corresponding parts of the chromosomes lie exactly side by side. Crossing-over, therefore, will involve exchange of exactly the same parts of homologous chromosomes and exchange of the genes involved in those particular segments of the chromosomes. The mechanism of crossing-over is quite mysterious at present. It is not known if crossing-over takes place only between genes, or happens regularly within genes.

Crossing-over changes the distribution of maternal and paternal chromatin material within the germ cell before it divides. The reshuffling or interchange of genes between any two homologous chromosomes produces two chromosomes that are different from the original two in the pair but which are still homologous. Together the two chromosomes of a pair have the same amount and kind of genetic material that they had before crossover, but as they separate, they will carry to each gamete a different genetic material than they would have carried if crossover had not taken place.

Crossing-over is an important feature of meiosis. It provides an additional opportunity for redistribution of maternal and paternal genes in the mature germ cells and thus another possibility for variation in the characteristics a germ cell may carry.

Spermatogenesis

Maturation of spermatozoa, termed *spermatogenesis*, takes place before the sperm are separated from the seminiferous tubules. Germ cells in the lining of the seminiferous tubules divide by mitotic division to form many *spermatogonia*. Spermatogonia grow to become *primary spermatocytes* and then undergo meiosis. Each primary spermatocyte divides into two smaller cells, *sec-*

ondary spermatocytes, by reduction meiosis, which results in cells with only 23 chromosomes. The two secondary spermatocytes quickly undergo the second maturational division, each resulting in two *spermatids* containing 23 chromosomes. Thus four spermatids are produced from one primary spermatocyte (Fig. 3-7). Hundreds of primary spermatocytes may be undergoing meiosis at the same time in order to produce the large number of mature sperm that are present in the adult male reproductive tract at any one time.

Spermatids become attached to, or are engulfed into, the Sertoli cells present in the lining of the seminiferous tubules; from these cells, they appear to receive nutriment. The spermatids gradually develop into very specialized cells, the *spermatozoa*. At this time it will be useful to review Figure 2-8, page 38, which diagrammatically shows the different stages in spermatogenesis in a section of a seminiferous tubule.

When the maturing germ cells have reached the spermatozoan stage of development, approximately 64 days after spermatogenesis begins, they are detached or freed from the Sertoli cells and are released into the lumen of the seminiferous tubules. Spermatozoa are functional when released into the tubular lumen, but appear to undergo additional maturation as they progress through the reproductive tract.

Oogenesis

Similar to maturation of spermatozoa, maturation of ova, termed *oogenesis,* also takes place by meiosis. However, the division of the cytoplasm of the female germ cells is very uneven in each of the two maturational divisions, and only one of the four cells resulting from the divisions is functional.

Unlike production of spermatogonia, development of oogonia (female immature germ cells) does not take place during sexual maturity. Oogonia multiply by mitosis during early fetal life, but this process ceases by the fifth to sixth month of fetal life, at which time the full quota

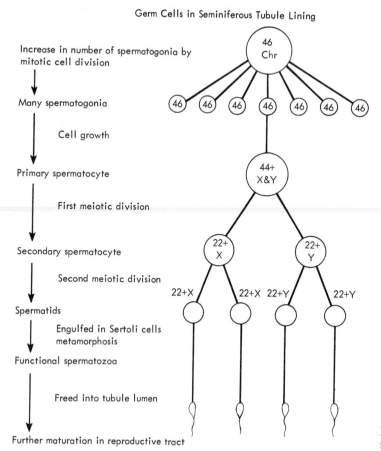

Germ Cells in Seminiferous Tubule Lining

Increase in number of spermatogonia by mitotic cell division

Many spermatogonia

Cell growth

Primary spermatocyte

First meiotic division

Secondary spermatocyte

Second meiotic division

Spermatids

Engulfed in Sertoli cells metamorphosis

Functional spermatozoa

Freed into tubule lumen

Further maturation in reproductive tract

Figure 3-7.   Diagram illustrating maturation of spermatozoa.

of oogonia has been reached. Many of the oogonia undergo degenerative changes during the early years of life, but there is still an ample supply for the childbearing years.

Oogonia become differentiated into oocytes during fetal life. These primary oocytes enter the first meiotic division before birth of the infant, but after proceeding through the early stages, the process ceases for a number of years and meiosis does not go on to completion until sometime during the years of sexual maturity. With sexual maturity further development of oocytes will proceed, and, in most circumstances, one oocyte progresses through the complete process of maturation during each ovarian cycle. (The ovarian cycle is described on pages 21–26.) Some oocytes will not resume the meio-

tic division that was begun in fetal life until late in the childbearing years of life, and some will never mature.

When a *primary oocyte* proceeds in its development toward complete maturation during the years of sexual maturity, it grows considerably in size and accumulates yolk in its cytoplasm. Meiosis, which was begun prior to birth, is resumed and the first maturational division is completed about the time of ovulation. The primary oocyte divides into two *secondary oocytes*, each receiving 23 chromosomes but a very unequal amount of cytoplasm. One of the secondary oocytes of this division is much larger than the other, having received practically all of the yolk material of the primary oocyte. The secondary oocyte, termed the first polar body, receives very little of the cytoplasm and is a very small cell (Fig. 3-8). The polar body becomes functionless. It may undergo a second maturation division or it may degenerate before division takes place.

At the same time that the primary oocyte is developing and increasing in size, the graafian follicle is also developing (page 22), and the membranes that surround the mature ovum are being formed. Polar bodies are enclosed in

these membranes and thus, although functionless, are not completely cast off (Fig. 3-8).

The large secondary oocyte begins a second maturational division, probably after ovulation, but this division may not be completed until after a sperm enters the ovum at fertilization. As in the first division, the cytoplasm is very unevenly divided in the second division. One cell of the second division, the ovum, receives most of the cytoplasm and is relatively large. It is a

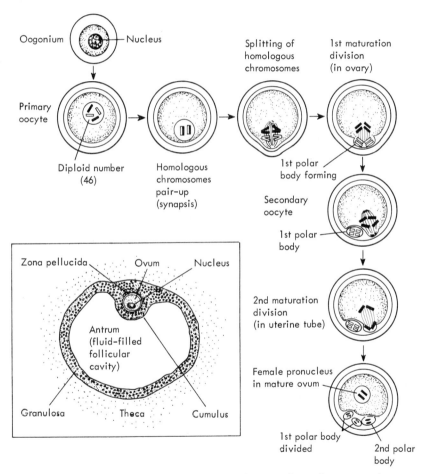

Figure 3-8. Diagram illustrating oogenesis, showing the reduction in chromosomes to form a mature female ovum. For simplification only two pairs of homologues are included. Insert illustrates the mature ovum located within the graafian follicle. [*Reprinted with permission from Macmillan Publishing Co., Inc. from Sigmund Grollman,* The Human Body: Its Structure and Physiology, *4th ed. Copyright Sigmund Grollman 1978.*]

cell with one half the characteristic number of chromosomes (23) and a relatively large amount of yolk material. This cell is ready for fertilization. The other cell of the division, *the second polar body,* is very small, has virtually no cytoplasm, and soon degenerates (Fig. 3-8).

Maturation of each oogonium results in one ovum and two polar bodies, or three polar bodies, if the first polar body undergoes cell division. These four cells correspond to the four spermatids that result from maturation of a spermatogonium. Unlike the spermatids, which all become functional, only one of the four cells of oogenesis, the ovum, which received all of the yolk material of the primary oocyte, is capable of fertilization. An advantage of only one functional ovum among four cells is that the amount of nutritive material available to the zygote if fertilization takes place is considerably greater than if the yolk had been equally distributed to four cells.

After the germ cells have undergone maturation, both ovum and spermatozoon now termed gametes, are ready for fertilization. Each gamete carries one chromosome of each pair and thus one gene of each pair. Entry of a sperm into an ovum and union of their nuclei, termed fertilization, results in a new cell called a zygote. Fertilization is described on pages 64–66.

SEX DETERMINATION

Two of the 46 chromosomes in human cells are termed sex chromosomes. These two appear alike in female cells, and therefore in the ovum, and are designated as XX. In male cells the two chromosomes in the sex pair differ in size and shape and are known as the X and Y chromosomes. The gamete resulting from meiotic division of an oogonium always has an X chromosome since division of the pair of sex chromosomes results in X and X, one X going to the functional cell and the other X to the polar body. Meiotic division of male germ cells gives rise to two varieties of spermatozoa, one half with 22 autosomes and one X chromosome and the other half with 22 autosomes and a Y chromosome (Figs. 3-7 and 3-9A).

Sex is determined by the type of spermatozoon fertilizing the ovum. If it is fertilized by a spermatozoon with an X chromosome, the zygote will have 22 pairs of autosomes and one pair of X chromosomes and will produce a female. If the ovum is fertilized by a Y chromosome, the sex chromosomes will be an X and Y pair and will produce a male. Although the number of males and females should be equal, because there are an equal number of sperm with an X and a Y chromosome, more male than female babies are born, the usual proportion being about 105 boys to 100 girls.

Sex Chromatin or Barr Body

Somatic cells of a normal female differ from those of a normal male by the presence of a chromatin mass, a small dark body, in the nuclei of many of the cells. This chromatin mass is called the *sex chromatin,* or *chromatin-positive body,* or the *Barr body.* It is derived from one of the X chromosomes. The number of chromatin-positive bodies in the nuclei of cells is one less than the number of X chromosomes in the cells. Normal females, with XX sex chromosomes, have one Barr body in many of the cell nuclei, and normal males, with XY chromosomes, have none. Somatic cells of individuals with sex chromosome abnormalities (as shown in Fig 3-9B) will show Barr bodies according to their sex chromosomal composition. Cells of females with XO sex chromosomes do not have a Barr body and those with XXX have two chromatin-positive bodies. Cells of males with XYY composition have no Barr body and those with XXY chromosomes will show one sex chromatin mass.

The number of Barr bodies is one less than the number of X chromosomes. This implies that regardless of the number of X chromosomes in the cell, there is only one *active* X, and this "explains" why males with one X chromosome and females with two are alike for traits (except sex) carried by genes on the X chromosome.

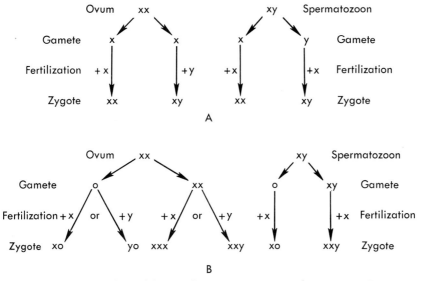

Figure 3-9. *A.* Separation of the sex chromosomes in normal meiosis. *B.* One possible mechanism of unequal distribution of the chromosomes in an ovum and a sperm. Nondisjunction may occur in any pair of autosomes in a manner similar to that shown above for the sex chromosome pair.

The sex chromosome composition of an individual can be determined indirectly by examination of somatic cells for sex-chromatin bodies as well as directly through analysis of the chromosomes. The X chromosome may be difficult to distinguish from other chromosomes similar in size and shape, and examination for Barr bodies is useful in interpretation of abnormal karyotypes.

Epithelial cells taken from the lining of the cheek are an easily available source of somatic cells for examination for chromatin-positive bodies. Study of sex chromosomal composition becomes important when there are body characteristics that suggest a sex anomaly.

ALTERATIONS IN CHROMOSOMAL DISTRIBUTION

Chromosomes sometimes accidentally become unequally distributed at some point during cell divisions, with the result that the daughter cells have an imbalance of genetic material.

Such abnormal chromosome distribution may occur during meiosis or during mitosis.

In normal meiosis homologous chromosomes first pair and then separate and distribute equally to two cells (Figs. 3-9A and 3-10A). Normal separation of a pair of chromosomes during the first meiotic division is designated *disjunction,* meaning separation or disjoining. Sometimes a coupled pair of chromosomes does not separate; this lack of separation or nondisjoining is termed *nondisjunction.* With nondisjunction one daughter cell receives an extra chromosome and the other lacks one, and the gametes resulting from such an abnormal cell division will have an atypical number of chromosomes (Figs. 3-9B and 3-10B). In nondisjunction during maturation of an oogonium the extra chromosome may go to either the ovum or the polar body. Nondisjunction during spermatogenesis results in some sperm with an extra chromosome and some lacking one.

Another mechanism resulting in an unequal distribution of chromosomes is a lack of pairing of two homologous chromosomes during meio-

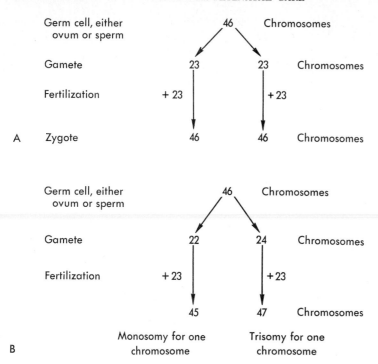

Figure 3-10. *A*. The number of chromosomes in gametes and zygotes when meiosis has taken place normally. *B*. The number of chromosomes in gametes and zygotes when a pair of chromosomes does not separate during maturation of a germ cell. In addition to the unequal distribution of chromosomes shown in this illustration, a chromosome may get lost and not get into either cell, resulting in gametes with 22 and 23 chromosomes. For this reason monosomy is more frequent than trisomy; although this is not ordinarily detected because most monosomics lead to embryonic death.

sis, with the possibility of both of the unpaired chromosomes going to the same cell (Fig. 3-5). Also, a part of a chromosome may break off and relocate elsewhere, with the chance that a daughter cell may have a part of a chromosome added to its normal quota.

Fertilization of a gamete that has an extra chromosome or that lacks one by a gamete that has the normal number of 23 results in a zygote with an abnormal number of chromosomes, either 45 or 47 instead of the typical number of 46. Lack of a chromosome in a zygote is termed *monosomy*, for whichever chromosome is lacking. An extra chromosome, making three of one kind, is termed *trisomy*, as, for example, trisomy for no. 18 (Fig. 3-10B). If a zygote receiving an abnormal number of chromosomes continues cell division, all cells of the developing embryo contain the abnormal number of chromosomes, since cell division proceeds by mitosis, with duplication of the original cell.

The genetic balance of a zygote with an abnormal number of chromosomes is upset, and development is not normal. The effect of the genetic imbalance depends largely on the particular chromosome that is lacking or that is extra. However, any genetic imbalance of itself may bring about certain nonspecific manifestations of abnormality. The effect of an abnormal number of chromosomes may be so severe that survival of the zygote is impossible, either from the beginning or after a certain stage of development, possibly accounting for some spontaneous abortions. If the chromosomal abnormality is not incompatible with life, it alters development of the embryo. This produces body anomalies, sometimes multiple and gross, and frequently results in mental retardation. It appears that the brain especially needs a normal balance of genes for normal development.

In addition to abnormalities caused by incomplete duplication of a chromosome, abnormalities may arise from breakage of a segment of a chromosome. Such a segment may be lost, may reattach in an inverted position, or may attach to another chromosome. Most changes, perhaps all, are reciprocal; a broken end most likely attaches to another broken end. Such a change is known as a *translocation*. If no chromosomal material is lost, merely rearranged, it is said to be a *balanced translocation*. Changes in placement of chromosomal parts also frequently give rise to abnormalities in body development or function.

A chromosomal abnormality may also occasionally arise during cell division of a normal zygote or developing embryo, either at the first division or later. In these cases the abnormality occurs in mitosis, in the separation of two chromatids of a doubled chromosome, rather than in the separation of a pair. Such an abnormality results in two, or sometimes more, types of body cells, since each cell resulting from an abnormal division of a chromosome reproduces like cells. The effect of this mosaic pattern of mixed cell types will depend on the parts of the body that develop from the involved cells.

Chromosomal aberrations are very complex. The above description provides only a very brief introduction to a few of these aspects. Knowledge about chromosomal and gene action is advancing rapidly, and much new information is continuously forthcoming. The student is urged to read new publications for advances in this field.

BIBLIOGRAPHY

Crow, James F., *Genetic Notes*, 7th ed. Burgess, Minneapolis, Minn., 1976.

McKusick, Victor A., *Human Genetics*, 2nd ed. Prentice-Hall, Englewood Cliffs, N.J., 1969.

Scheinfeld, Amram, *Your Heredity and Environment.* Lippincott, Philadelphia, Pa., 1965.

Sutton, H. Eldon, *An Introduction to Human Genetics,* 2nd ed. Holt, Rinehart, and Winston, New York, 1975.

4

Development of the Embryo and Accessory Structures

Development of the fetus and the accessory structures vital to its intrauterine existence proceeds from a single cell resulting from fusion of an ovum and a sperm. The new cell, termed a zygote, carries all the traits and characteristics of the parent cells. Through cell divisions of the zygote, and differentiation and specialization of these cells, the entire complex human body develops. In addition, the fetal portion of the placenta, the umbilical cord, and the fetal membranes arise from the zygote. These accessory structures become functionless at birth and are cast off when they serve no further purpose.

THE GERM CELLS

Ovum

The ovum is a large round cell measuring approximately 0.2 mm in diameter. It is the largest cell in the body, being just barely visible to the naked eye. The nucleus of the ovum contains the 23 chromosomes that were distributed to it during the first maturational division. The second maturational division has probably begun but is not completed until a sperm enters the ovum.

The ovum contains a relatively large amount of cytoplasm, which accounts for its size. The cytoplasm contains small yolk granules. A thin membrane, termed the *vitelline membrane*, forms the outside boundary of the cytoplasm (Fig. 4-1).

The ovum is surrounded by a thick, tough, semitransparent membrane termed the *zona pellucida* (Fig. 4-1). This membrane also contains the polar bodies (Fig. 4-4). Encircling the zona pellucida are the follicle cells that adhered when the ovum was discharged from the graafian follicle. These adherent follicle cells, termed the *corona radiata* (Fig. 4-1), disintegrate and separate from the ovum soon after it has entered the fallopian tube. The zona pellucida persists through several days of development of a fertilized ovum.

Most ova discharged from the graafian follicles enter the fimbriated end of the fallopian tube nearby. Various factors may assist the ovum to enter this small opening, but the relative importance of each is not clear. Muscular action at the time of ovulation appears to move both the tube and the ovary to a position that facilitates the ovum's entry into the tube. Also, the rhythmic contractions of the tubal musculature are frequent at the time of ovulation, and cilia on the fimbriated end of the tube may produce a current that carries the ovum toward the tube. In the fallopian tube the ovum either disintegrates, as most do, or meets and fuses with a spermatozoon, resulting in a cell that will proceed to further development.

Spermatozoon

A spermatozoon does not resemble a typical cell in appearance. It is a slender, elongated

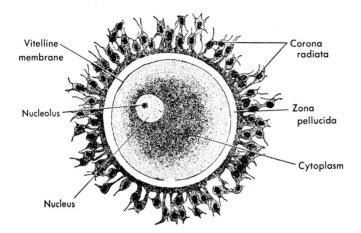

Figure 4-1. Diagram of human ovum.

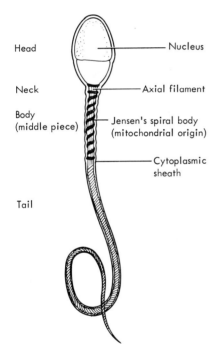

Figure 4-2. Mature sperm cell (spermatozoon). [*Reprinted with permission from Macmillan Publishing Co., Inc. from Sigmund Grollman, The Human Body: Its Structure and Physiology, 4th ed. Copyright Sigmund Grollman 1978.*]

structure having the shape of a microscopic tadpole, with a flat, oval head, a neck, a tapering body or middle piece, and a long tail (Fig. 4-2). A spermatozoon is very small as compared with an ovum, owing to its relatively small amount of cytoplasm. It is one of the smallest cells of the body, while the ovum is among the largest (Fig. 4-3). A spermatozoon measures about 0.06 mm in length, but its slenderness makes its total volume very small. The head of the spermatozoon comprises about one twelfth of its total length.

The nucleus of the sperm, containing 23 chromosomes, is located in the head of the sperm and makes up almost its entire bulk. The anterior half of the head is covered with a head cap, which includes a structure known as the acrosome. The long tail of the sperm makes

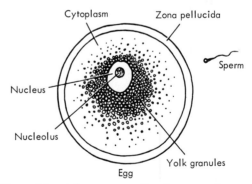

Figure 4-3. A human egg cell and a sperm drawn to the same scale. The actual diameter of the human egg is approximately 0.2 mm. [*Reprinted with permission from Macmillan Publishing Co., Inc. from James Watts Mavor and Harold W. Manner, General Biology, 6th ed. Copyright Macmillan Publishing Co., Inc. 1966.*]

lashing motions which propel the cell, resulting in the very rapid movements that are a striking characteristic of spermatozoa.

The motility of sperm, which gives them the ability to move rapidly, appears to be relatively unimportant to their passage through the female reproductive tract. Muscular contractions of the uterus and the fallopian tubes are apparently the major influence in moving sperm upward from the vagina. Motility does appear to be important to the sperm's approach to the ovum. Through what appear to be aimless movements, a number of sperm move toward the ovum. Then the tail aids the sperm that fertilizes the ovum in its penetration of the membranes surrounding the ovum.

FERTILIZATION

Passage of a spermatozoon into an ovum and fusion of their nuclei into a single cell is termed *fertilization* or, in lay parlance, *conception*. Fertilization usually takes place in the outer one third of the fallopian tube, where a number of sperm surround a recently discharged ovum (Fig. 4-6A).

It is estimated that as semen is ejected at the time of coitus, from 120 to 500 million sperm, suspended in the seminal fluid, are deposited in the upper part of the vagina. This lavish supply of sperm provides for the possibility of fertilization, since many are lost before they reach the site of fertilization. Of the millions of sperm deposited in the vagina, only a few hundred reach the fallopian tubes and of these only one enters the ovum.

When conditions are favorable for sperm movement through the female reproductive tract, especially around the time of ovulation, sperm may reach the fallopian tubes within a very few hours. Muscular contractions of the uterus and the fallopian tubes, ciliary action of the mucosa of the reproductive tract, and fluid currents within the fallopian tubes apparently transport the sperm quite rapidly. Motility of the sperm may assist to some degree in their

upward progress. In the fallopian tube, usually in the outer third, the spermatozoa may meet a discharged and matured ovum, and fertilization may take place.

The integrated hormonal actions, described in Chapter 2, synchronize ovulation, prepare the reproductive tract for final maturation and movement of sperm, and create appropriate conditions for fertilization of an ovum.

Fertilization must occur soon after the ovum and spermatozoa reach the fallopian tube, since the period of viability of ova and sperm is estimated to be relatively short. It is believed that an ovum is fertilizable for not more than 24 hours after extrusion from the ovary, and that the fertilizing capability of spermatozoa is not longer than 48 hours after they enter the female genital tract.

Random movements of sperm bring them to the nonmotile ovum. A number of sperm surround the ovum and several may become attached, but only one sperm penetrates it (Fig. 4-4). Changes in the ovum after entry of a sperm make it impervious to other spermatozoa. Entry of a sperm into an ovum through its relatively tough surrounding membranes is aided by action of an enzymatic substance, hyaluronidase, produced by the sperm. This substance dissolves a portion of the membranes and permits penetration of the corona radiata and the zona pellucida.

As soon as a sperm enters an ovum, marked changes take place in both structures. In the sperm, the head detaches from the body, increases in size, moves toward the center of the ovum, and takes on the appearance of a typical nucleus. At this stage it is termed the *male pronucleus* (Fig. 4-4). The body and tail of the sperm soon disappear, apparently through absorption by the cytoplasm of the ovum. After entry of a sperm, the ovum completes its maturation by separation of the second polar body. The chromosomes that remain in the ovum organize into a nucleus, which is now termed the *female pronucleus*. The two pronuclei move toward each other gradually and soon meet and unite (Fig. 4-4). The fertilization process that

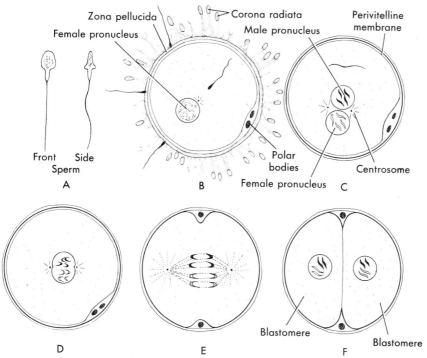

Figure 4-4. Diagram showing fertilization of an ovum, the joining of the male and female pronuclei, the chromosomes organized on the spindle, and the two-cell stage of blastomeres. [*Reprinted with permission from Macmillan Publishing Co., Inc. from M. Miller and L. Leavell,* Kimber-Gray-Stackpole's Anatomy and Physiology, *16th ed. Copyright Macmillan Publishing Co., Inc. 1972.*]

started when the sperm began to enter the ovum is complete with the joining of the male and female pronuclei.

Union of the nuclei of an ovum and a spermatozoon results in a cell, previously nonexistent, termed a *zygote*. It is the beginning of the embryo as a single cell and is ready for the first cell division of the many that will follow in the development of a new being.

With union of the nuclei of the ovum and the sperm, the unpaired chromosomes of both gametes are brought together, providing the zygote with the 23 pairs of homologous chromosomes characteristic of human cells. Both ovum and sperm carry maternal and paternal chromosomes of the parent from which they originated; when these chromosomes are brought to the zygote, those contributed by the ovum are all

designated as maternal and those provided by the sperm as paternal. When the male and female pronuclei have met, a spindle appears in the cell, the chromosomes of both pronuclei arrange on the spindle, and mitosis proceeds, resulting in the two-cell stage of development in about 36 hours (Fig. 4-4).

Fertilization has (1) provided the new cell with the characteristic number of chromosomes; (2) established the sex of the new being through the sex chromosome carried by the sperm; (3) determined the inherited traits and characteristics through the chromosomes brought to the zygote by both gametes; and (4) initiated the repetitive mitotic divisions that proceed soon after the male and female pronuclei join.

All inherited traits and characteristics are established at the time of union of the nuclei of the gametes. At this decisive moment the entire contribution of inheritance is made since the chromosomes in each nucleus are directly descended from the nuclear substance of the parents and their ancestors. They carry the intricate and elaborate material that the child inherits from his parents, grandparents, and yet more distant progenitors. After this the only contribution made to the fetus is in the form of suitable environment contributed by the mother's body. This is an important contribution, however, since the manner in which characteristics are developed may be tremendously influenced by environmental conditions.

The characteristics that an individual inherits from parents and ancestors are determined by the chromosomes and genes carried by the particular gametes that were fertilized. As the maturational process reduced the chromosomal number in the gamete to one half, certain characteristics of the parent were lost to it. In addition, the cell divisions of meiosis permitted a great many different combinations of chromosomes and an interchange of genes between homologous chromosomes. The result of the maturational process is that each mature germ cell produced by an individual may carry a different combination of the paternal and maternal genes of that person.

All the body characteristics of the individual that will develop from the zygote are influenced by the combination of the genes that were carried by the ovum and the sperm. Some genes will carry recessive traits and some traits that are completely or partly dominant. The recessive trait may not appear in an individual who also inherits a gene that is dominant for the same characteristic. This recessive gene may, however, be carried to another generation, and the trait may appear in an individual who lacks a dominant gene for that particular characteristic. For example, the gene for brown eyes is dominant to the gene for blue eyes. If one of the genes present is for brown eyes and one for blue eyes, the eyes will be brown. The gene for blue eyes is present in the individual's cells, however, and when it is passed on to an individual

in another generation who inherits two genes for blue eyes, that individual's eyes will be blue. The inheritance of all characteristics is much more complex, but this example shows that there may be great variation in characteristics inherited by different children of the same parents. It is through certain combinations of factors that it is apparently possible to skip the inheritance of certain characteristics from parents, but to inherit traits from grandparents or even more remote ancestors.

EARLY DEVELOPMENT OF THE EMBRYO

The single extraordinary cell resulting from the union of a male and female germ cell immediately begins a development leading toward the formation of the fetus, the fetal part of the placenta, the umbilical cord, and the fetal membranes. Growth occurs through cell proliferation, and groups of cells differentiate and specialize to develop into tissues and structures widely different from each other, but also capable of working together as a well-organized functioning body.

Cleavage, Morula, and Blastocyst

The zygote begins its development by undergoing a series of rapid mitotic cell divisions termed *cleavage*. The cells of these early divisions are called *blastomeres*. The zygote divides into two smaller cells, these two divide into four; the four into eight. Thus the process of division continues until a solid mass of blastomeres is formed, shaped something like a mulberry, and called the *morula* (Fig. 4-5). Since the zona pellucida still surrounds the zygote, this development takes place within its confines. There is actually no increase in mass during this very early development; the cells of these divisions become smaller, approximating more closely the size of the cells normally found in the body.

As cellular activity continues within the mor-

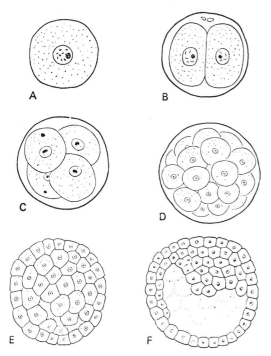

Figure 4-5. Diagram to show very early stages of mammalian development. *A.* One-celled embryo. *B.* Two-celled embryo. *C.* Four-celled embryo. *D.* Berrylike ball of cells or *morula.* *E.* Beginning formation of the blastocyst. *F.* Well-developed blastocyst, consisting of a hollow ball of *trophoblast* cells and an inner mass of cells known as the *embryoblast.* [*Reprinted with permission from Macmillan Publishing Co., Inc. from M. Miller and L. Leavell, Kimber-Gray-Stackpole's Anatomy and Physiology, 16th ed. Copyright Macmillan Publishing Co., Inc. 1972.*]

ula, fluid appears in the center, with the result that the cells are rearranged toward the periphery, thus forming a sac. At this stage the embryo is called a *blastocyst.* At one point within the blastocyst, some of the cells remain grouped into a cluster of cells, termed the *inner cell mass* or the *embryoblast.* The cells of this mass will develop into the body of the embryo. A single layer of cells, known as *trophoblasts,* comprises the vesicular wall (Fig. 4-5). The trophoblastic cells in this outer layer are nourishing cells. They have the ability to cause cytolysis of

the endometrial cells and thus invade the endometrium for implantation of the blastocyst. These outer cells will contribute to the formation of the placenta.

Sometime during the blastocyst stage, the cells and the membrane that originally surrounded the ovum and then remained around the zygote will disappear. The corona radiata is lost by the time the developing zygote reaches the uterine cavity and the zona pellucida becomes thinner and disintegrates shortly before implantation.

Development from the one-celled zygote to the blastocyst stage probably takes place during the course of several days; the exact time of each stage is not certain. During this early period the developing zygote is advancing through the fallopian tube toward the uterus, where it will implant (Fig. 4-6). Muscular contractions of the fallopian tube, increased ciliary action, and an increased flow of glandular fluids move the developing zygote along. Movement through the tube covers a period of three to four days. The developing zygote is then free in the uterus for another two or three days, continuing its existence as a floating blastocyst, and thereafter attaches to the endometrium.

Implantation

On about the seventh day after fertilization, while in the blastocyst stage, the embryo begins to implant into the endometrium, which has been prepared for its reception by the premenstrual swelling described on page 32. Even before implantation, the trophoblastic cells begin producing the hormone HCG to protect the developing embryo from being lost. The HCG stimulates the corpus luteum to continue producing progesterone, which will support the endometrial attachment and make possible maintainance of the pregnancy until the placenta produces an adequate amount of progesterone (Fig. 2-7, page 35). Just before implantation the endometrium undergoes vascular changes similar to those occurring immediately prior to menstruation. Implantation depends on these vascular changes and the power of the tropho-blastic cells surrounding the blastocyst to invade and destroy tissue.

The point at which the embryo attaches is somewhat a matter of chance, but is usually somewhere in the upper part of the uterine cavity on either the anterior or posterior wall. There it destroys the minute underlying area of tissue—capillaries, venous sinuses, glands, and stroma—by digestive action and burrows into the endometrium. Although this seems to imply extensive tissue destruction, it actually involves only the width of a few cells. The endometrium fuses above the blastocyst, and the embryo is soon completely encapsulated in a cavity of its own that has no connection with the uterine cavity (Fig. 4-6).

Differentiation of Cells

At the time of implantation the blastocyst is about 0.25 mm ($^1/_{100}$ in.) in diameter. The product of conception has increased very little in size up to this time. After implantation, the tropho-blastic cells multiply and enlarge, and the inner cell mass begins a rapid increase in size, with its cells increasing both in number and in specialization. Differentiation of cells, which already began in the morula, now progresses rapidly. Very early the specialized cells begin organ formation.

A detailed description, tracing the intricate development of the embryo through its various stages, will not be given. However, in addition to the brief description that follows, certain aspects of fetal development are presented in the following chapter.

The cells of the inner cell mass are arranged very early into three primary germ layers, a stage of development termed *gastrulation*. The outer layer is termed the *ectoderm* and the inner layer the *entoderm*. These two layers are well defined several days after implantation. A third layer, which appears a little later between the other two, is called the *mesoderm* (Fig. 4-6). Although these three primary germ layers origi-nate from the single-celled zygote, they are dif-ferent in character. The difference steadily in-creases until finally all of the complex fetal organs and tissues evolve from their further specialization and development.

From the ectoderm arise the skin with its appendages, the salivary and mammary glands, the nasal passages and upper part of the pharynx, the anus, the crystalline lens, the external ear, and the entire nervous system.

From the mesoderm are derived the urinary and reproductive organs, the muscles, bones, and connective tissues, and the circulatory system.

From the entoderm are developed the alimentary canal, the thymus, thyroid, liver, lungs, pancreas, bladder, and the various small glands and tubules.

It is apparent that embryonic development comprises both growth and evolution. The early stages of development consist of (1) proliferation of, and alterations in, the kinds of cells, (2) their arrangement into groups, and (3) a differentiation of the functional activity of these groups of cells before the mass assumes human form and develops organs. The developing organism is called the embryo during this stage of grouping and differentiation, which takes place in the first eight weeks of pregnancy. Thereafter it is termed the fetus until the time of birth.

Differentiation of cells of the growing zygote, in addition to development of the embryo, leads to formation of those structures that are not a part of the embryo itself, but essential to its development and survival. The amnion, chorion, umbilical cord, and placenta are formed very early in embryonic life and continue to develop in complexity and function as this is necessary to meet the needs of the fetus.

THE DECIDUA

The decidua is the altered mucous membrane (endometrium) of the pregnant uterus. Although not a product of the fertilized ovum, this membrane is described here because of its function

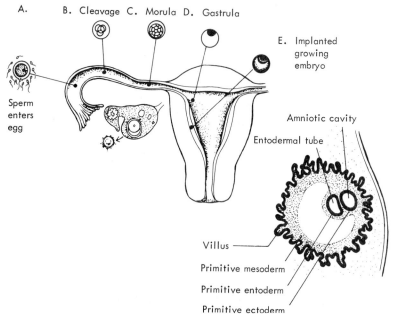

A.
B. Cleavage C. Morula D. Gastrula

E. Implanted
growing
embryo

Sperm
enters
egg

Amniotic cavity

Entodermal tube

Villus

Primitive mesoderm

Primitive entoderm

Primitive ectoderm

Figure 4-6. Implantation of the fertilized ovum (nidation). Approximate location of fertilized egg at various stages of development (*A, B, C, D, E*). Lower right-hand illustration shows cross section of gastrula implanted within the uterine endometrium. [*Reprinted with permission from Macmillan Publishing Co., Inc. from Sigmund Grollman, The Human Body: Its Structure and Physiology, 4th ed. Copyright Sigmund Grollman 1978.*]

in protection and nourishment of the developing embryo.

Several days after implantation of the embryo, changes begin to take place in the endometrium, already hypertrophied as a result of the premenstrual swelling. Increased thickening takes place, producing deep furrows in the uterine mucosa. The stroma cells increase in size, and the glands become markedly distended, hyperplastic, and secretory. These changes convert the uterine lining into decidua, which reaches its height, a thickness of about 10 mm, at the third or fourth month of pregnancy. It then begins to thin with increasing distention of the uterus until it is only 1 to 2 mm thick at the end of pregnancy. The decidua separates and is expelled after delivery of the fetus, with the exception of a basal layer from which the endometrium is regenerated after pregnancy.

After the embryo has implanted, the decidua consists of three portions: (1) The hypertrophied membrane that lines the uterus as a whole is called the *decidua vera (parietalis)*. (2) The *decidua basalis (serotina)* is that portion lying directly beneath the embryo which later enters into the formation of the placenta. (3) The *decidua capsularis (reflexa)*, which surrounds and covers the buried embryo, consists of the fused margins of mucosa that have grown over the embryo (Figs. 4-7 and 4-10).

THE AMNION

The amnion is the inner of two fetal membranes; the outer membrane is termed the chorion (Figs. 4-7 and 4-10). The amnion begins to develop very early in embryonic life, appearing in the second week (Fig. 4-9). It invests the embryo completely in a membranous sac, even

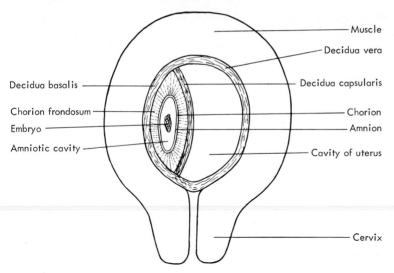

Figure 4-7. Diagram of a longitudinal section of a pregnant uterus showing the implanted embryo and the relationship between the fetal membranes and the uterine mucosa soon after implantation. This diagram may be compared with Figure 4-10, a later stage of development.

before the body has form. This sac is reflected up around the umbilical cord, thus forming its outer covering. At first there is an appreciable space with some fluid between the two fetal membranes, but with the advance of pregnancy, the amnion comes in contact with and is loosely adherent to the chorion.

THE AMNIOTIC FLUID

Very early in its development, during the second week, the double-layered membranous sac formed by the amnion and chorion contains a slightly opaque fluid, known as *amniotic fluid* (Fig. 4-8). This fluid surrounds the embryo, and as the embryo grows, the amniotic cavity and the fluid increase (Figs. 4-7 and 4-10). The amount of fluid at the end of pregnancy averages 850 ml (29 oz).

The source of amniotic fluid is not definitely known. It is ultimately derived from the mother, but its exact site of origin is in question. It has been postulated that the fluid, which is present in early pregnancy, is a transudate of maternal plasma across the placenta and the fetal membranes. Also, the fetal skin may make a contribution, and the umbilical cord may be considered a possible source in fluid production. The amniotic fluid in early pregnancy is very similar to maternal plasma. From about the fourth month of life to term, the fetus modifies the composition and volume of amniotic fluid. The fetus swallows the fluid and voids hypotonic urine into it in increasing amounts. Movement of fluid in and out of the respiratory tract also adds secretions. The quantity of fetal urine and of secretions from the respiratory tract and the skin is unknown.

Amniotic fluid is continuously replaced at a very rapid rate, but its routes of disappearance, like its origin, are uncertain. This is not a static collection of fluid around the fetus; there is apparently a constant exchange of the fluid and of at least some of the constituents of the fluid between the maternal and the fetal circulation and the amniotic fluid itself. Bidirectional turnover of water between mother and fetus and amniotic fluid is very rapid. It has been determined that water is exchanged at a rate of 500 ml/hr at full-term pregnancy, and the amniotic fluid is completely replaced about once every 3 hours.

The continual circulation of amniotic fluid may involve several possible sites for its removal. The amnion may actively remove the fluid, the fetal skin may absorb it, and absorption from the gastrointestinal tract may play a major role. The relative importance of any of these sites is not known.

Amniotic fluid consists of over 98 percent water and between 1 and 2 percent organic and inorganic solids. The composition of the fluid changes as pregnancy advances. In the first half of pregnancy the fluid is essentially the same composition as maternal plasma, but with a lower protein concentration. Later in the pregnancy the fluid becomes progressively hypotonic, presumably from the addition of very hypotonic fetal urine.

The amniotic fluid contains electrolytes, glucose, lipids, proteins, enzymes, hormones, and an increasing concentration of urea, uric acid, and creatinine as term approaches. It also con-

tains fetal urine and secretions from the respiratory tract. Variable amounts of particulate matter also accumulate in the amniotic fluid. There are desquamated fetal cells, sebaceous material, epithelial cells, lanugo and scalp hair, and vernix caseosa. The fluid is fairly clear except for the flecks of solid material cast off from the fetal skin.

The volume of amniotic fluid increases as pregnancy advances. The volume increases at a rate of about 25 ml per week from 11 to 15 weeks and at a rate of 50 ml per week from 15 to 28 weeks. There is an average volume of 50 ml at 12 weeks, 400 ml at midpregnancy, and a variable volume with a mean of 850 ml in the last trimester. Volume reaches a peak of about 1000 ml at 38 weeks and then begins to de-

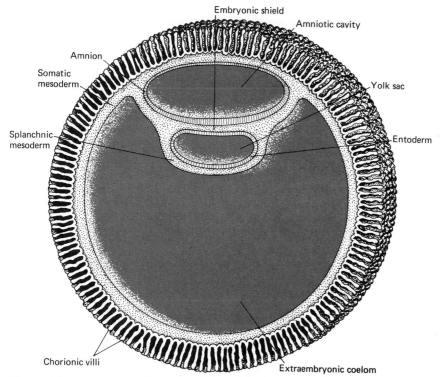

Figure 4-8. Stereogram of a human blastocyst containing an embryo of approximately 14 to 15 days. [*Reprinted with permission from Macmillan Publishing Co., Inc. from Alfred F. Huettner,* Comparative Embryology of the Vertebrates, *rev. ed. Copyright 1941 by Macmillan Publishing Co., Inc., renewed 1969 by Mary A. Huettner.*]

crease somewhat. In the woman who progresses to a postterm pregnancy, the fluid may be well below the mean of 850 ml by 42 or 43 weeks gestation.

An excessive amount of amniotic fluid, called polyhydramnios, or an unusually small amount of fluid, termed oligohydramnios, are sometimes present. These conditions may be associated with congenital anomalies in which the fetus cannot swallow fluid, or cannot produce urine, or in which the membranes produce excessive amounts of fluid, or various other conditions. Sometimes there is no apparent defect with polyhydramnios or oligohydramnios.

Amniotic fluid serves a variety of purposes, all of which appear to be mainly directed toward providing an optimal environment for the fetus during intrauterine development. The fetus begins to swallow amniotic fluid by the fourth month of development, and it has been calculated that by the time he reaches full term, he swallows as much as 500 ml per day. This may indicate that the fluid is important to fetal metabolism. The fluid helps to dispose of secretions from the kidneys and the respiratory tract. The fluid permits the fetus to move with ease in the uterus. It protects him against possible injury, by equalizing the pressure of any sudden force, and it keeps him at a uniform temperature. By acting as a water wedge, forced down by uterine contractions at the time of labor, the fluid may be important in dilating the cervix.

Since the amniotic fluid contains cells and secretions that originate with the fetus, analysis of the fluid gives valuable information concerning fetal health and maturity. When necessary for diagnosis, a sample of fluid can easily be withdrawn. Removal of fluid and the examinations which may be performed on it are described on pages 610–14.

THE CHORION AND THE CHORIONIC VILLI

The chorion is the outer of the two fetal membranes (Figs. 4-7 and 4-10). It is formed as implantation of the embryo is completed, arising from a modification of the trophoblasts. After

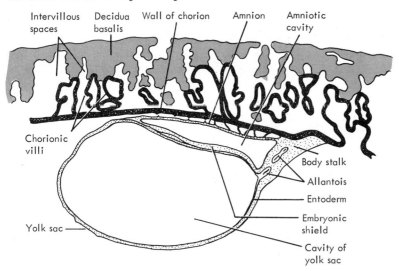

Figure 4-9. Human embryo (Mateer) described by Streeter, estimated to be 17 days old and 0.92 mm long. Formation of the body stalk. The amnion is detaching itself from the chorion. [*Reprinted with permission from Macmillan Publishing Co., Inc. from Alfred F. Huettner,* Comparative Embryology of the Vertebrates, *rev. ed. Copyright 1941 by Macmillan Publishing Co., Inc., renewed 1969 by Mary A. Huettner.*]

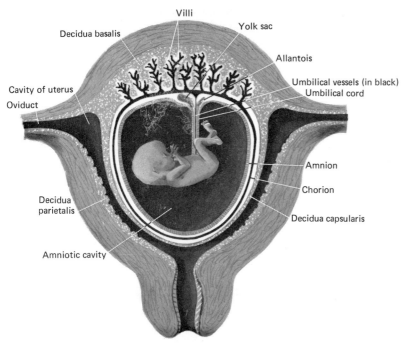

Figure 4-10. Sectional diagram of human uterus with fetal membranes and their relationship to the uterus and the embryo. (Adapted from Longet.) [*Reprinted with permission from Macmillan Publishing Co., Inc. from Alfred F. Huettner,* Comparative Embryology of the Vertebrates, *rev. ed. Copyright 1941 by Macmillan Publishing Co., Inc., renewed 1969 by Mary A. Huettner.*]

the chorion is formed, the implanted blastocyst is called the *chorionic vesicle.* This vesicle is surrounded by a "lake" of maternal blood created by erosion of maternal tissues and vessels during implantation.

The chorionic vesicle enlarges, and toward the end of the second week tiny, threadlike projections, termed *chorionic villi,* begin to form. These villi, which soon cover the entire surface of the chorion vesicle, give it the shaggy appearance of a chestnut bur. The villi enlarge the surface area of the chorionic vesicle and thus increase the absorption of nutrients from the maternal lake of blood (Fig. 4-8).

The chorionic villi grow and extend to the maternal tissues, and their trophoblastic cells erode additional areas of endometrium. Blood vessels soon appear in the chorionic villi, and at about the beginning of the fourth week after fer-

tilization fetal blood circulates through the villi. Some of the villi, known as *fastening villi,* extend far enough into the decidua to attach the vesicle to it, while the rest dip freely in the pools of maternal blood.

The chorionic villi are equally distributed over the chorion at first (Fig. 4-8). As the chorionic vesicle increases in size and the decidua capsularis is pushed outward and farther away from the uterine vessels, the villi in contact with the capsularis gradually atrophy and disappear. Over the relatively small area beneath the vesicle, where the chorion is in contact with the decidua basalis, the villi become much more abundant. The placenta develops at this site (Figs. 4-9 and 4-10). After the greater part of the surface of the chorion, which is in contact with the decidua capsularis, has become denuded of villi, it is known as the *chorion laeve,* or bald chorion. The chorion lying against the decidua basalis where the villi are well developed is termed the *chorion frondosum,* or tufted chorion.

As pregnancy advances and the fetal sac enlarges, the chorion laeve, covered by the decidua capsularis, is pushed farther out into the uterine cavity. Finally it reaches the opposite wall, meets the decidua vera, and obliterates the entire space that had existed between the two membranes (Fig. 4-10). This means that, instead of a uterine cavity lined with decidua and a tiny capsule somewhere off to the side lined with chorion, the latter has distended until it completely fills and becomes the cavity within the uterine walls. The decidua capsularis and decidua vera fuse early in the fourth month, and eventually the decidua capsularis degenerates and almost entirely disappears.

THE PLACENTA

The placenta (afterbirth), vital to fetal life, is formed as a special organ to serve the fetus. It serves as lungs, intestinal tract, and kidneys for the fetus throughout intrauterine life, functioning as an organ for exchange of nutrients and waste products between mother and fetus. It also functions as an endocrine organ, producing hormones that will serve the fetus and that are necessary to maintenance of the pregnancy. The health, and sometimes survival, of the fetus is dependent on how efficiently the placenta functions throughout pregnancy.

The placenta's unique functional characteristics include such diverse activities as transport of oxygen and metabolites from mother to fetus, elimination of waste products from the fetus to the maternal circulation, and production of protein and steroid hormones for the needs of the fetus and the pregnancy.

Placental Growth

The amount of yolk accompanying the human ovum is very small, and the fetus is soon dependent on the mother for nutrition. The embryo receives nutritive material from the mother as soon as it reaches the uterine cavity. Even before implantation, the trophoblasts serve as a membrane through which nutritive material in the uterine cavity reaches the embryonic cells. This early supply comes from the secretion of the uterine glands, which are rich in glycogen. After implantation of the embryo, the products of the cells that were broken down by the erosive trophoblasts during entry of the blastocyst into the endometrium—blood, glandular secretion, and tissue fluids—surround the vesicle. These nutritive substances reach the embryonic cells by diffusion.

After the above two stages of nourishment, the placenta and its circulation begin to develop. Villi begin to form over the chorion during the second week of embryonic development, and they involve more and more of the endometrium (Figs. 4-8 and 4-9). These villi arise from the trophoblasts. As the trophoblasts proliferate they differentiate into two layers: an inner cellular layer of trophoblasts called the *cytotrophoblast* or *Langhans' layer* and an outer layer called the *syncytiotrophoblast,* which is a layer of protoplasm without cell margins (Fig. 4-13). Isolated spaces, called lacunae, appear in the syncytiotrophoblast. These lacunae soon become filled with (1) blood from opened-up maternal capillaries, and (2) secretions from eroded maternal glands. This fluid in the lacunae provides nourishment to the embryo.

Development of villi continues rapidly and intervillous spaces filled with maternal blood from small vessels opened by trophoblastic cells are soon formed (Fig. 4-9). The overall intervillous space is thus derived from the lacunae that developed in the second week. These spaces enlarge through further erosion by the trophoblasts. Together they form a large blood-filled sinus, known as the *intervillous space,* located between the chorionic plate and the decidua basalis. This space, which does not have clearly defined boundaries, connects the maternal arterial input with the venous outflow (Fig. 4-13). The space becomes more and more occupied with chorionic villi as pregnancy progresses until the space becomes more virtual than real.

Growth continues and maternal blood begins to flow through the intervillous space, entering from the arterial capillaries of the endometrium that have been opened by trophoblastic cells and returning through opened venous capillaries (Fig. 4-13). A maternal circulation, a rather primitive uteroplacental circulation, is thus established around the chorionic vesicle in a period of slightly over two weeks, and there is continual replacement of blood in the intervillous space.

Blood vessels appear in the villi very soon after they are formed. Blood vessels simultaneously begin to form in the yolk sac and the connecting stalk (Fig. 4-9), and very soon blood vessels, heart tubes, and primitive plasma and blood cells develop in the embryo. Isolated vessels then fuse and form a network to establish a circulation between the embryo and the chorionic vesicle and the embryo and the yolk sac. By the end of the third week after fertilization blood is flowing through vessels connecting the villi and the embryo. Thus, within less than one month, both a fetal and a maternal circulation have been established. Exchange of nutritive material and waste takes place between the maternal blood circulating in the intervillous space and the fetal blood circulating in the villi that dip into this space.

At the end of the first month of development the chorionic villi lying over the decidua basalis have developed into an early placenta. The placenta, developing at the site of implantation, is partly fetal and, to a smaller extent, maternal in origin. It arises jointly from the chorion frondosum and the underlying decidua basalis. The free villi of the chorion frondosum grow and branch, increasing the absorptive surface; the anchoring villi that serve to attach the chorionic vesicle to the decidua grow and multiply, and the decidua basalis increases in thickness (Fig. 4-10).

As pregnancy advances the placenta continues to enlarge. It covers nearly one third of the internal surface of the uterus at any stage of its de-velopment. Although the placenta is growing throughout pregnancy, its growth is not as rapid as that of the fetus. Before the fourth month of gestation, the placenta is heavier than the fetus; at the fourth month the weights of the placenta and the fetus are approximately equal; and at full term, the weight of the placenta is about one sixth to one seventh that of the fetus.

To meet the demands of the increasingly greater size of the fetus as compared to that of the placenta, the villi increase in size and complexity by branching in a treelike fashion. With the villi internally supplied with a circulatory system that carries fetal blood and externally surrounded by maternal blood, the ever increasing branches of villi enlarge the surface area through which exchange can take place (Fig. 4-10). Most of the bulk of the placenta is made up of the chorionic villi and the blood in the intervillous space. In addition to the expanding surface area of the villi, exchange is also increased as pregnancy advances by progressive thinning and permeability of the membranes making up the villi.

Separated from the uterine wall, at term the placenta is a flattened, fairly round, spongy mass 15–20 cm (6–8 in.) in diameter, and about 2–3 cm (1 in.) thick near the center, with thinning out toward the margin. Continued from the margin are the filmy fetal membranes. A rupture in these membranes during labor provides the opening through which the amniotic fluid escapes and the fetus passes during birth (Fig. 4-11). The placenta weighs about 500 gm (about 1 lb), or one sixth to one seventh as much as the baby, and accordingly varies in size and weight with the baby.

After detachment from the uterine wall, the maternal surface of the placenta is rough, bloody, and dark red and is irregularly divided into lobes, termed *cotyledons* (Fig. 4-12A). These maternal cotyledons or placental lobes are filled with the highly developed villi of the placenta. Septa that appear in the placenta during its development separate it into 15 to 30 units or large cotyledons, which are further subdivided into smaller units. This separation is incomplete,

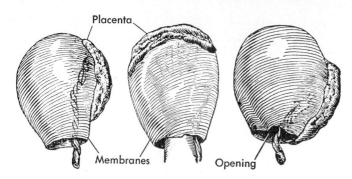

Figure 4-11. Diagram showing general structure and relation of fetal membranes, placenta, and umbilical cord. Three different areas of placental development, representing three different sites of implantation of the blastocyst, are shown.

and the cotyledons are therefore only partly divided from one another.

The inner, or fetal, surface of the placenta is smooth and glistening, of a bluish color, and covered with the amnion (Fig. 4-12B). The fetal surface is traversed by a number of large blood vessels which arise from the umbilical cord blood vessels and spread out from the point of insertion of the umbilical cord (Fig. 4-12B). These vessels branch and divide until their termination in the innumerable chorionic villi dipping into the intervillous space.

Placental Circulation

As implied above, the placenta contains both a fetal and a maternal circulation. Fetal blood flows to the placenta through two umbilical arteries, which branch and divide until they terminate in the innumerable chorionic villi dipping into the intervillous space. This blood returns to the fetus through a single umbilical vein (Fig. 4-13).

On the maternal side of the circulation, blood spurts into the intervillous space of the placenta from the spiral arteries and drains back into endometrial veins (Fig. 4-13). Maternal arterial blood from the spiral arteries enters the intervillous space in "spurts" that are produced by the maternal arterial blood pressure. The entering blood is propelled into the intervillous space, which has a low pressure, in funnel-shaped streams, which are driven high up toward the chorionic plate (Fig. 4-14). As the head

of pressure is reduced the blood disperses laterally. When this happens blood flows around the chorionic villi, enhancing metabolic exchange through the capillaries of the villi. Continuing influx of arterial blood exerts pressure on that which is already in the intervillous space, pushing it out. The blood drains out through peripherally located endometrial veins, and from there into the uterine and pelvic veins (Fig. 4-14).

Each cotyledon is supplied by a spiral artery, which carries the maternal blood through the myometrium and the basal plate and then enters the intervillous space in a centrally located, relatively empty space in the cotyledon. This permits the jets of maternal blood to enter the middle of the cotyledon where there is a space that is relatively empty of villi. Among factors that influence flow of blood in the intervillous space are intermittent uterine contractions of the Braxton-Hicks quality (page 162). These contractions temporarily compress veins, preventing drainage of blood. Then, when the uterine muscle relaxes, drainage of blood from the intervillous space takes place rapidly. Other factors are shown in Figure 4-15.

It is estimated that the intervillous space can hold about 150 ml of blood at any one time and that from 500 to 700 ml of maternal blood circulates through the placenta every minute, permitting a replacement of the blood in the intervillous space every two to three minutes. The fetal circulation through the placenta is estimated to be from 300 to 400 ml per minute.

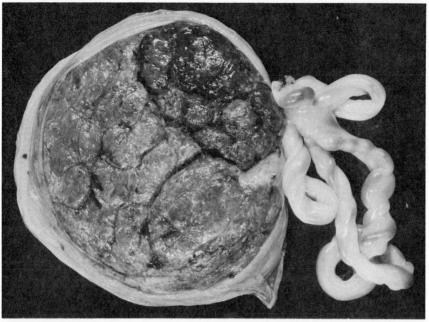

A

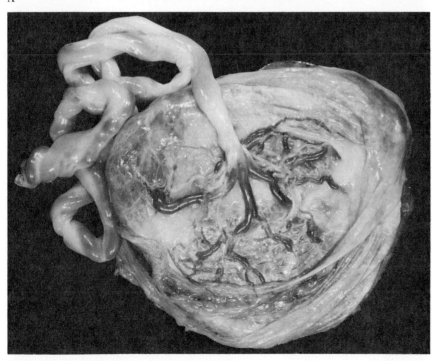

B

Figure 4-12. **A.** Maternal surface of the placenta, surrounded by the membranes. The umbilical cord arises from the fetal surface. **B.** Fetal surface of the placenta, showing some of the membranes and the origin of the umbilical cord.

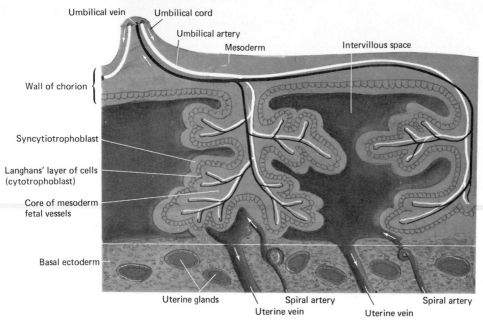

Figure 4-13. Schematic drawing of the structure of the villi at an early stage of development. The capillaries of the fetal circulation are separated from maternal blood in the intervillous space by surrounding layers of mesoderm, cytotrophoblast, and syncytiotrophoblast. After the fifth month only a single layer, that of the syncytiotrophoblast, lies between the fetal capillary wall and the maternal blood. Note the umbilical cord containing one umbilical vein and two arteries. Two uterine spiral arteries emptying into the intervillous space and two veins returning maternal blood are shown. [*Reprinted with permission from Macmillan Publishing Co., Inc. from M. Miller and L. Leavell,* Kimber-Gray-Stackpole's Anatomy and Physiology, *16th ed. Copyright Macmillan Publishing Co., Inc. 1972.*]

The total absorbing surface of the villi of a full-term placenta is very large, with estimates of this surface as high as 10 square yards. Owing to a copious maternal circulation through the placenta, an extensive absorbing area, and a large volume of fetal blood flowing through the villi, the exchange of substances between the two bloodstreams is usually very efficient.

It is apparent that the maternal and fetal bloodstreams are in close relation, being separated by only the thin tissues that form the walls of the villi and the walls of the blood vessels within the villi. This arrangement makes it possible for the villi to discharge their function of receiving nourishment for the embryo from the maternal blood and releasing to the mother waste products from the fetal blood.

Transfer of Substances Across the Placenta

Transfer of substances from mother to fetus and from fetus to mother takes place through the chorionic villi. These villi, dipping into the intervillous space which is continuously filled with blood, can take from and give substances to the maternal blood according to the needs of the fetus (Fig. 4-13). From the time the first fetal blood vessels appear in the early floating villi, until the baby is born, when many complex villi make up the placenta, there is a constant exchange of nutriment and waste material between the maternal and fetal blood. The maternal blood in the intervillous space gives to the fetal blood in the villi the oxygen and other substances necessary to nourish and build the grow-

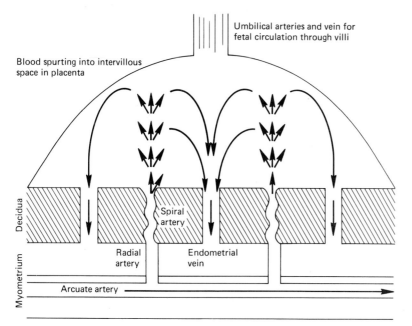

Figure 4-14. Diagrammatic representation of the maternal circulation in the placenta. Blood spurts into the intervillous space of the placenta from the spiral arteries and drains back into endometrial veins. Reference should be made to Figure 4-13 to visualize how the fetal circulation relates to the maternal circulation in the placenta.

ing body. It receives the broken-down products of fetal metabolism. The waste is carried by the maternal bloodstream to the mother's lungs and kidneys for excretion. Adequate exchange across the placenta between maternal and fetal circulation is essential to normal growth and development of the fetus. The placenta is a very active organ. Its growth is ongoing, at least until near the end of pregnancy, and its function changes when necessary as pregnancy advances in order that it may adequately serve the fetus.

Three microscopic tissue layers separate the fetal and maternal circulation, and it is across this placental "membrane" that exchange takes place. The tissue layers of this membrane consist of (1) a first layer, the trophoblast which covers the villi and consists of a layer of cytotrophoblast and a layer of syncytiotrophoblast; (2) a second layer of connective tissue; and (3) a third layer composed of the endothelium of the fetal capillaries (Fig. 4-13). As maturation of the villi continues, the placental membrane becomes progressively thinner until finally only a very thin layer of tissue separates the maternal and fetal blood.

Transfer of substances across the biologic membrane in the placenta may take place by six different mechanisms: simple diffusion, facilitated diffusion, active transport, pinocytosis, bulk flow, and breaks in the placental villi. Different from other organs of the body, placental transfer of substances takes place by several different mechanisms simultaneously. Respiratory gases transfer by simple diffusion; carbohydrate exchange is by facilitated diffusion; amino acids are actively transported; large molecules, such as immunoglobulins, are probably transported by pinocytosis; and osmotic pressure changes probably facilitate water exchange. Exchange rates and transfer mechanism vary for different substances and they may be affected by physiologic limitations and pathologic changes in the placenta.

Simple Diffusion

Simple diffusion of a substance takes place when that substance moves across a membrane from an area of high concentration to one of lower concentration (Fig. 4-16). It depends upon a concentration difference. It is a passive

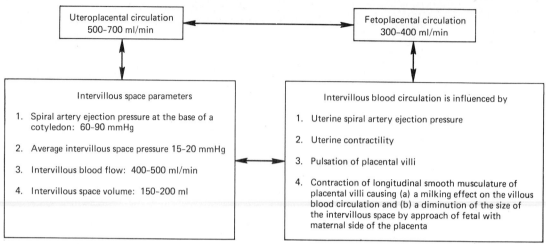

Figure 4-15.   Parameters and interrelationships of uteroplacental circulation near term. The figures listed in this chart represent average values as derived from various reports in the literature; they serve only to give an idea of the uteroplacental and fetoplacental circulatory interrelationships near term. [*Reproduced with permission from Nicholas S. Assali (ed.),* Pathophysiology of Gestation, *vol. I.* Maternal Disorders, *Academic Press, New York, 1972, p. 159.*]

process that requires no energy and it continues only until an equilibrium is reached. The amount of exchange per unit of time is influenced by the concentration or electrochemical difference of the substance on each side of the membrane and by characteristics of the membrane, such as its permeability and thickness and the area of exchange.

Oxygen and carbon dioxide, small ions such as sodium and chloride, and fatty acids cross the placenta by simple diffusion. In general, substances of small molecular size, such as oxygen, diffuse more rapidly than those of a larger size. High molecular weight substances such as protein cross the placental membrane slowly or not at all.

Facilitated Diffusion

Facilitated diffusion differs from simple diffusion in that the rate of transfer is faster than would be predicted on the basis of concentration difference of the substance on each side of the membrane, on the thickness and permeability of membrane, and on area of exchange. The exact mechanism of transfer is not clear, but it is as-

sumed that the substance to be transferred combines with a carrier in the membrane and then the carrier–substance complex crosses the membrane at a faster rate than the substance would be able to cross alone (Fig. 4-16). Carrier-mediated facilitated diffusion takes place only until an equilibrium of the substance on both sides of the membrane is reached. Glucose crosses the placenta by facilitated diffusion.

Active Transport

Active transport is the transfer of molecules from a low concentration on one side of the membrane to a higher concentration on the other side. This is a transfer in a direction opposite of the concentration gradient. It is an uphill process and requires metabolic energy.

Active transport is believed to occur when a carrier in the membrane combines chemically with the substance to be carried. It goes through some kind of a process that changes the carrier's relative high affinity for the substance on one side of the membrane to a lower affinity on the other side of the membrane, where it then releases the substance (Fig. 4-16). Amino

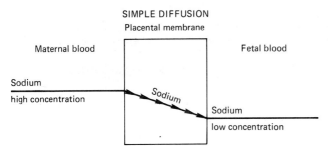

SIMPLE DIFFUSION

Simple diffusion is a passive process that continues until an equilibrium on both sides of the membrane is reached.

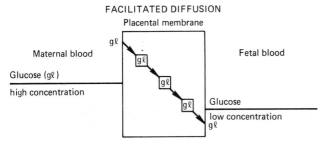

FACILITATED DIFFUSION

Carrier-mediated facilitated diffusion assists a substance to cross the placental membrane faster than by simple diffusion. It does not require expenditure of energy. It continues only until an equilibrium on both sides of the membrane is reached.

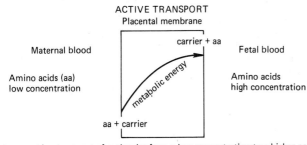

ACTIVE TRANSPORT

Active transport is a transport of molecules from a low concentration to a higher concentration. It is an uphill process and requires metabolic energy.

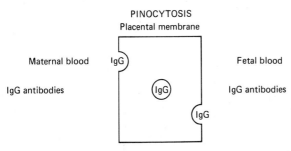

PINOCYTOSIS

In pinocytosis the substance is engulfed by the membrane and then slowly moved across the placental membrane and released on the other side.

Figure 4-16. Diagrammatic representation of placental transfer mechanisms.

acids, water-soluble vitamins, and some of the large ions (calcium, iron, iodine) are thought to cross the placenta by active transport.

Pinocytosis

In pinocytosis, invaginations of cell membrane engulf minute droplets of substance and water, forming small vesicles, cross the membrane with the vesicles, and release the droplets on the other side (Fig. 4-16). This is a relatively slow process, but it takes care of transfer of large particles such as immunoglobulins, large proteins, and certain drugs.

Bulk Flow

Differences in hydrostatic or in osmotic pressure on each side of the membrane will cause water molecules to transfer. This process is referred to as bulk flow. Water movement also carries dissolved particles with it, a process called *solvent drag.* An increased hydrostatic pressure on one side of the membrane results in more solvent crossing the membrane than could be expected by diffusion. An osmotic pressure difference brought about by a higher concentration of solute on one side than on the other will have the same result.

Breaks in Placental Villi or Leakage

Breaks in placental villi will result in transfer of substances in small amounts. Such transfer is not one of the normal physiologic processes, but rather an unusual event that may lead to a pathologic problem. An important example of this is passage of fetal red cells into the maternal circulatory system. Under certain conditions such breaks initiate a series of events that induce an Rh-negative mother to develop antibodies to Rh-positive blood cells (see page 645).

It is also considered possible for blood cells to be transferred from the fetal to the maternal circulation through an intact placenta, by leakage of cells through the chorionic villi when intracapillary pressure in a villus is transiently elevated.

The mechanisms described above explain how substances transfer across the placental membrane. Several mechanisms may function for different substances simultaneously, and a certain substance may be transferred by more than one mechanism at the same time. For example, amino acids may be transferred mainly by active transport, but at the same time may also cross to some extent by simple diffusion and by pinocytosis.

Transfer of Specific Substances (Figure 4-17)

OXYGEN AND CARBON DIOXIDE   Oxygen and carbon dioxide are presumed to cross the placenta by simple diffusion. An uninterrupted oxygen flow is vital to the fetus because he cannot store oxygen. The oxygen diffuses from a high partial pressure in maternal blood to a lower partial pressure in fetal blood. Other factors, however, also influence placental diffusing capacity. The oxygen must dissociate from maternal hemoglobin and combine with fetal hemoglobin. Fetal blood has a higher affinity for oxygen.

Thickness of membrane, permeability, and surface area are also important in rate of diffusion. Placental diffusing capacity may be reduced by pregnancy complications that thicken placental membranes or reduce the area of exchange through infarcts.

Decreased uterine blood flow, either through a decrease in uterine perfusion pressure or an increase in resistance to blood flow, may seriously interfere with oxygen transfer. Hypotension from any cause results in decreased uterine blood flow. Certain complications of pregnancy, such as hypertensive disorders, are likely to decrease uterine blood flow. Hemoglobin concentrations of maternal and fetal blood also exert an influence; anemia may decrease the capacity of the blood to carry oxygen. Any adverse factor will result in a lessened amount of oxygen transferred, unless compensation can be made in some of the other factors.

Exchange of carbon dioxide from fetal to maternal blood also takes place by passive diffusion and is affected by the same factors that affect ox-

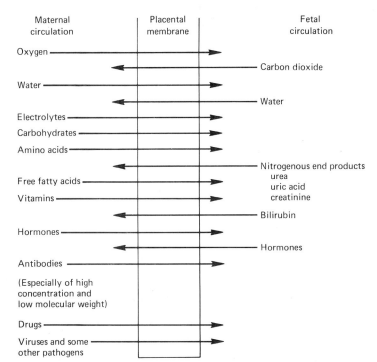

Figure 4-17. Interchange of substances between mother and fetus.

ygen exchange. However, the carbon dioxide exchange is not as critical as that of oxygen.

WATER Water is absolutely essential to cells and is continuously exchanged between mother and fetus. Although many studies have been done, the mechanism of water transfer is not clear. Simple diffusion and osmosis and hydrostatic pressure differences between maternal and fetal blood are thought to be means of water transfer. Pressure differences between the two circulations cannot be great and may only be intermittent, but they apparently move a large amount of water to and from the fetus.

ELECTROLYTES Electrolytes apparently cross the placenta freely. Sodium, potassium, and other univalent ions are assumed to cross by simple diffusion and some may cross by "solvent drag" along with water movement. Iron is apparently actively transported and calcium may also cross in that way. Fetal blood levels of iron and calcium are higher than maternal levels,

and it may be assumed that transfer is against a gradient.

CARBOHYDRATES The transfer rate of glucose is necessarily high, since it is the fetus' principal metabolic fuel, and he is in need of a continuous supply. Fetal blood glucose concentration is normally approximately 70 to 75 mg/100 ml of blood as compared to a normal mean maternal blood glucose concentration of 90 to 100 mg/100 ml of blood. Since the blood glucose level in the fetus is 20 to 30 mg/100 ml of blood lower than maternal blood glucose, it would appear that transfer could take place by simple diffusion. It is believed, however, that transfer is at a faster rate than simple diffusion would permit and takes place mainly by carrier-mediated facilitated diffusion.

In addition to utilization of glucose for energy, the fetus needs glucose for glycogen storage in the liver in the last few weeks of gestation. The placenta contains large amounts of glycogen, most of which is synthesized from maternal glucose. The role of the placental glucose is not clear.

AMINO ACIDS   Amino acids are transferred very freely from mother to fetus. They are moved across the placenta by active transport and are found in higher concentration in fetal than in maternal blood. The plasma amino acid concentration is also found to be lower in pregnant than in nonpregnant women. It appears that the fetus synthesizes most of its own proteins from the amino acids transferred from the mother.

FREE FATTY ACIDS   Free fatty acids cross the placenta by simple diffusion. Large amounts of free fatty acids are potentially available to the fetus, but the amount actually transferred is rather low. Transfer is less than required for fat deposition in the fetus in the last trimester; fetal synthesis of fat apparently accounts for much of the fetal adipose tissue.

VITAMINS   Transfer of vitamins across the placenta occurs by several different mechanisms—simple diffusion, facilitated diffusion, active transport, and pinocytosis. The B and C vitamins have been found to be present in a higher concentration in fetal blood than in maternal blood. This implies that these vitamins are actively transported. The concentration of the lipid-soluble vitamins (A, D, and K) in the fetal blood is generally the same as maternal blood levels, but occasionally it is lower. Vitamin E is present in a lower concentration in fetal than in maternal blood.

HORMONES   Estrogens, progesterone, and other steroids appear to cross the placenta easily and are found in relatively high amounts in fetal blood. Hormones administered to the mother have been found to cross the placenta readily and sometimes adversely affect the fetus (page 201).

A number of steroids appear to undergo enzymatic alteration as they move across the placenta, and this may have a major influence in their transport. The placenta also changes steroids produced by the fetus, which move to the maternal circulation. An example is conversion of steroids produced by the fetal adrenal glands to the hormone estriol, which is then transferred from the placenta to the maternal circulation (page 122).

Placental transfer of anterior pituitary and thyroid hormones from the mother is too limited to influence the fetus. The fetal endocrine system appears to mature early and function autonomously. Fetal insufficiency of anterior pituitary or thyroid is not compensated by maternal transfer of hormones. A small amount of insulin is probably transferred across the placenta from the mother, but the fetus apparently responds to insulin need with its own production.

The placenta is thus relatively impermeable to the protein hormones. The protein hormones synthesized in the placenta itself, e.g., HCG, are secreted into maternal blood in considerably higher concentration than into fetal blood.

ANTIBODIES   Antibodies to some diseases, such as diphtheria, tetanus, measles, mumps, scarlet fever, polio, and smallpox, if present in the maternal blood, will pass through the placenta and give the baby a certain amount of passive immunity for a short time. A baby born prematurely receives fewer antibodies than a full-term baby. Immunoglobulins are present in the fetal blood in very small amounts in the first half of gestation. In the latter half, fetal and maternal concentration of gamma-G (IgG) are about the same. This may be evidence of increasing pinocytosis in late gestation.

Delivery of maternal IgG to the fetus is of major importance to survival, since the fetus ordinarily lacks exposure to antigens and must get antibodies from the mother. Only insignificant amounts of immunoglobulins other than IgG reach the fetus.

There is great variability in the amount of antibody transferred from mother to fetus. Much depends on the amount of antibody in the maternal circulation and on its molecular size. Those of high concentration and of low molecular weight, such as antibody to rubella, are readily transferred. One of higher molecular weight, such as antibody to pertussis, is transferred poorly.

DRUGS The placenta is permeable to most and probably all drugs, especially when present in high concentration. It should be assumed that any drug or chemical that enters the maternal circulatory system will reach the fetus. Most drugs transfer by simple diffusion, but occasionally by another mechanism.

The molecular size of the substance is important in its transfer. In general, the smaller the molecular weight the easier the transfer. Drugs with a molecular weight of less than 600 cross easily, and those with a molecular weight of over 1000 cross less effectively. As the molecular weight increases, other factors, such as lipid solubility, degree of ionization, and protein-binding, become very important, but all of these factors have a different influence on drug transfer through the placenta than they do on transfer through other biologic membranes.

VIRUSES AND BACTERIA Viruses associated with influenza, rubella, rubeola, variola, varicella, mumps, cytomegalovirus, encephalitis, Coxsackie B, and other infections may pass through the placenta and cause infection in the fetus. Bacteria and protozoa such as *Toxoplasma* may infect the placenta and thereafter the fetus. Syphilis is transmitted after the fifth month of gestation. The exact mechanism by which pathologic organisms pass the placenta is not known, and it appears that the placenta is a barrier against some infecting agents.

Transfer of Substances from Fetus to Mother

The end products of fetal metabolism—carbon dioxide, water, and nitrogenous products (urea, uric acid, creatinine)—and bilirubin pass across the placenta from the fetal to the maternal circulation. Urea, the major end product of protein catabolism, and creatinine probably transfer by simple diffusion and at term are present in the same concentration in both circulations. Fetal bilirubin, a metabolite of

hemoglobin, is transferred from fetal serum through the placenta to maternal serum to be conjugated and excreted. Transfer of carbon dioxide was described above.

Production of Hormones

The physiologic function of the placenta is very complex. In addition to its manifold transfer and transport functions, the placenta has a very important endocrine function, producing both protein and steroid hormones, which are apparently essential to the pregnancy. The placental endocrine role was suspected as far back as 1905, but was first ascertained in 1927, when Dr. Ashheim and Dr. Zondek discovered human chorionic gonadotropin.

The placenta produces its hormones in abundance; their functions are primarily concerned with pregnancy. The protein hormones, chorionic gonadotropin, chorionic somatomammotropin, and chorionic thyrotropin, are unique substances that are basically present only in pregnancy. These may be considered analogues of pituitary hormones.

The steroid hormones, estrogen and progesterone, are not peculiar to pregnancy, since they are ordinarily produced by the ovaries, but they are present in much larger amounts in pregnant than in nonpregnant women. Production of these steroid hormones is dependent upon precursors from both the mother and the fetus.

The placental hormones, their production and their function, are described in further detail on pages 118–24.

The Placenta at Term

Having served its purpose, the placenta is cast off from the uterine wall, along with the fetal membranes, almost immediately after birth of the baby. At this time it has the appearance of the term placenta described on page 75 (Fig. 4-12A, B). The maternal side is rough, bloody, and dark red, and the fetal side is smooth and shiny with the umbilical cord centrally attached.

The fetal membranes extend from all around the margin of the placenta. These consist of the amnion and chorion, with a small amount of decidua attached. They are broken at the area where the fetus passed through them during birth (Figs. 4-11 and 12A, B). The two membranes are somewhat adherent but can usually be separated from one another. The amnion is paper thin, transparent, and glistening. The chorion, which is the chorion laeve, is somewhat thicker, but usually not over 1 mm in thickness, and is slightly opaque. A small amount of decidua is attached to the chorion. The remainder of the decidua, except the basal layer adjacent to the uterine wall, will be cast off during the following several days.

THE UMBILICAL CORD

Circulation between the embryo and the chorionic villi is established very early through the yolk sac, the allantois, and the body stalk, which is the forerunner of the umbilical cord (Fig. 4-9). As the embryo grows, the amnion envelops the body stalk and the umbilical cord develops. It extends from the umbilical area of the fetus to the center of the fetal surface of the placenta (Fig. 4-12B). The umbilical cord grows with the fetus. At term it measures about 55 cm (22 in.) in length, but may vary from 30 to 100 cm (12 to 39 in.). Diameter of the cord at term varies from 1 to 2.5 cm (⅓ to 1 in.). The umbilical cord appears moist, is dull white in color, and often has a twisted or spiral appearance all along its length (Fig. 4-12A, B). The blood vessels of the cord, which also spiral, can often be seen bulging the surface of the cord.

The umbilical cord contains three blood vessels, two arteries and one vein. A gelatinous substance, termed *Wharton's jelly,* consisting of a mucoid connective tissue, surrounds the blood vessels and makes up the remainder of the interior of the cord. Contrary to the usual pattern, the arteries carry venous blood and the vein oxygenated blood. Blood from the fetus flows through the two umbilical arteries to the placenta, where it gives up its waste products, and the vein carries oxygenated, nourishment-bearing blood from the placenta to the fetus (Fig. 4-13). It is apparent that the life of the fetus is contingent on an uninterrupted, two-way flow of blood through the umbilical cord.

Occasionally an umbilical cord has only two blood vessels, one artery and one vein. This abnormality is sometimes associated with congenital anomalies. The number of umbilical vessels can be seen when the umbilical cord is severed after the birth of the baby. The cut end is examined in order to be alert to possible anomalies.

MULTIPLE PREGNANCY

A multiple pregnancy is one in which the pregnant uterus contains two or more embryos. They are termed twins when there are two embryos and triplets when there are three and quadruplets, or quintuplets, when there are four, or five, embryos, respectively. Occasionally there are even a larger number of fetuses in a multiple pregnancy.

Twin pregnancies may result from the fertilization of two separate ova or of a single ovum. Fertilization of two ova gives rise to double-ovum, dizygotic, or fraternal twins. Fertilization of one ovum results in single ovum, monozygotic, or identical twins. With dizygotic or fraternal twins, both ova may come from the same ovary or one may come from each ovary. The babies may or may not be of the same sex and do not resemble each other more than they resemble any other brother or sister. There are two placentas, although they may be fused, two amnions, and two chorions. Biologically, dizygotic twins are not really twins, but rather the result of the maturation and fertilization of two ova at a single ovulation period.

Monozygotic or identical twins are truly twins. They arise from the union of a single ovum and a single sperm. Separation of the cells of the developing zygote results in formation of two embryos. This separation may take place in an early blastomere stage, or the inner cell mass may separate into two, or occasionally the embryonic disc may be duplicated. Beginning but incomplete separation of the embryonic disc results in conjoined (Siamese) twins. Approximately one out of three sets of twins are identical twins.

Monozygotic twins have an identical genetic pattern. They are of the same sex and resemble each other closely in structure and appearance. These twins usually have one placenta, one chorion, and two amnions, but when division of the developing zygote takes place very early, two placentas and two chorions are formed.

Triplets may derive from one ovum, as in the case of twins, or from two or three ova. Accordingly there may be single-, double-, or triple-ovum triplets. The same is true of quadruplets, the number being carried to four ova.

It is estimated that twins occur about once in every 90 pregnancies and triplets once in about every 9000 births. Twins are born more frequently in the black than in the white race and are least common in the oriental race.

Hereditary influence in the tendency toward multiple pregnancies is not certain. The occurrence of a single pair of twins in a family where single pregnancies have been the rule does not suggest hereditary influence, but if several sets of twins occur in the same family, the tendency is believed to be inherited, through either maternal or paternal transmission.

Twins are likely to be smaller than a baby of the same age resulting from a single pregnancy, but their combined weight is usually greater than that of a single infant. Sometimes twins differ considerably in size, one being much larger than the other. Single ovum twins do not always have a completely separate circulatory system through the placenta and this permits their blood to intermingle. This can result in an imbalance in circulation and a decreased blood supply to one fetus, a condition that may be hazardous to the fetus. Multiple pregnancies are likely to give rise to more complications during the antepartum period and during labor and delivery than single pregnancies, and the greater distention of the uterus tends toward premature delivery.

The likelihood of twins or triplets living is affected by the same general factors as those influencing survival of a single baby, that is, the length and quality of intrauterine life and development at birth. The chances of all the babies of a quadruplet or quintuplet pregnancy surviving are rather small.

BIBLIOGRAPHY

Allen, Robert D., The moment of fertilization, *Sci. Am.* 201:124–134 (July) 1959.

Arey, Leslie B., *Developmental Anatomy*, 7th ed. Saunders, Philadelphia, Pa., 1965.

Benirschke, Kurt, and Kim, Chung K., Multiple pregnancy, *N. Engl. J. Med.* 288:1276–1284 (June 14) and 1329–1336 (June 21) 1973.

Brosens, I. A., Robertson, W. B., and Dixon, G. (eds.), *Human Placentation*. Proceedings of an International Symposium 29–30 July 1974, Leuvens, Belgium. Excerpta Medica, Amsterdam, 1975.

Corliss, Clark Edward, *Patten's Human Embryology*. McGraw-Hill, New York, 1976.

Corner, George W., *Ourselves Unborn*. Yale University Press, New Haven, Conn., 1945.

Dancis, Joseph, Feto-maternal interaction, in *Neonatology*, edited by Gordon B. Avery. Lippincott, Philadelphia, Pa., 1975.

Ebert, James D., The first heartbeats, *Sci. Am.* 200:87–96 (Mar.) 1959.

Flanagan, Geraldine L., *The First Nine Months of Life*. Simon and Schuster, New York, 1962.

Gilbert, Margaret S., *Biography of the Unborn*, rev. ed. Hafner, New York, 1963.

Greenhill, J. P., and Friedman, Emanuel A., *Biological Principles and Modern Practice of Obstetrics*. Saunders, Philadelphia, Pa., 1974.

Hamilton, William J., Boyd, J. D., and Mossman, H. W., *Hamilton, Boyd and Mossman's Human Embryology*, 4th ed. Williams and Wilkins, Baltimore, Md., 1972.

Huettner, Alfred F., *Fundamentals of Comparative*

Embryology of the Vertebrates, rev. ed. Macmillan, New York, 1949.

Longo, Lawrence D., Placental transfer mechanisms—An overview, *Obstet. Gynecol. Annu.* 1:103–138, 1972.

Miller, Marjorie, and Leavell, Lutie C., *Kimber–Gray–Stackpole's Anatomy and Physiology,* 16th ed. Macmillan, New York, 1972.

Moore, Keith L., *The Developing Human: Clinically Oriented Embryology,* 2nd ed. Saunders, Philadelphia, Pa., 1977.

Ostergard, Donald R., The physiology and clinical importance of amniotic fluid. A review, *Obstet. Gynecol. Surv.* 25:297–319 (Apr.) 1970.

Parer, J. T., Normal and impaired placental exchange, *Contemp. Ob/Gyn* 7:117–127 (Feb.) 1976.

Potter, Edith L., *Fundamentals of Human Reproduction.* McGraw-Hill, New York, 1948.

Pritchard, Jack A., and MacDonald, Paul C., *Williams Obstetrics,* 15th ed. Appleton-Century-Crofts, New York, 1975.

Rock, John, and Hertig, Arthur, The human conceptus during the first two weeks of gestation, *Am. J. Obstet. Gynecol.* 55:6–17 (Jan.) 1948.

Shettles, Landrum B., Human fertilization, *Obstet. Gynecol.* 20:750–754 (Dec.) 1962.

———, The living human ovum, *Obstet. Gynecol.* 10:359–365 (Oct.) 1957.

Tredway, Donald R., Rapidity of sperm transport in the female reproductive tract, *Contemp. Ob/Gyn* 7:89–90 (Feb.) 1976.

Trichmann-Duplessis, H., David, G., and Haegel, P., *Illustrated Human Embryology,* Vol. I. *Embryogenesis.* Springer-Verlag, New York, 1972.

Woodling, B. A. *et al.,* Gross examination of the placenta, *Clin. Obstet. Gynecol.* 19:21–44 (Mar.) 1976.

5

Growth and Development of the Fetus

When the developing embryo reaches an age of eight weeks, it is commonly termed a *fetus*. The distinction between embryo and fetus is largely based on a difference in the developmental process of these two periods. The embryonic stage is primarily a period of organogenesis. The fetal period is characterized by growth and further development of the organs and systems established during the embryonic stage. A division between these two periods, made on the basis of development, cannot be distinct, since all body structures do not develop at the same time or at the same rate. Some parts of the developing body may be in an embryonic period at the time that others have reached the fetal period. Some structures continue development into infancy.

Intrauterine development, considered in broad terms, may be divided into three phases, which are not sharply divided. In the first, or embryonic, period differentiation of cells proceeds rapidly, and organs and systems are established. Development is so rapid that there are distinct differences in an embryo from one day to the next. At the end of this period, the beginning of the fetal period, the developing organism has the external features of a human body, and all of the internal body organs are established and functioning in a limited way (Figs. 5-1 and 5-2).

The main features of the second phase of development, the first half of the fetal period, are continuing growth and further tissue differentiation of body structures. Although still limited, there is a gradual increase in functional ability of all body structures and systems. Growth in length is rapid during this time, but the body mass remains relatively small. At the end of the sixth lunar month the fetus has attained approximately 60 percent of his length, but only about 20 percent of his anticipated weight at full term. In the third phase, or latter part of the fetal period, organs and systems develop to the stage where they can function outside of the uterus. Body weight increases more rapidly than body length in the latter part of the fetal period.

The fetal period changes into the newborn period at the time of birth, which usually occurs at approximately the end of the tenth lunar month, considered full-term gestation. Normally a fetus is best ready to begin extrauterine life when full term is reached, but the transition from intrauterine to extrauterine existence can often be satisfactorily made at an earlier time. The end of the seventh lunar month is considered to be the earliest that the fetus has a fair chance of survival outside of the uterus. Unless conditions are unfavorable to intrauterine development, every week within the uterus from the seventh lunar month to full term increases the fetus' likelihood of survival.

Development begins with fertilization and the age of the embryo or fetus begins with this date. Since the time of fertilization cannot be precisely known, the age of the embryo can be calculated with fair reliability from the fourteenth day after the onset of the last menstrual

TIMETABLE OF HUMAN PRENATAL DEVELOPMENT
1 to 6 weeks

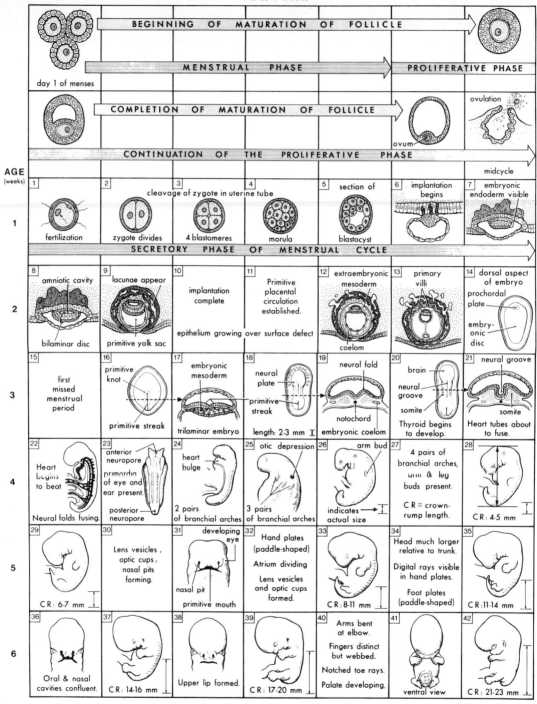

TIMETABLE OF HUMAN PRENATAL DEVELOPMENT
7 to 38 weeks

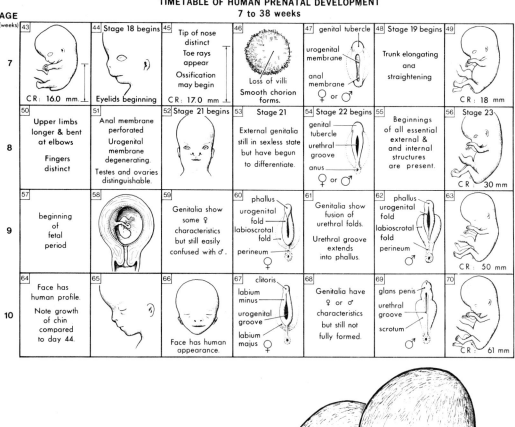

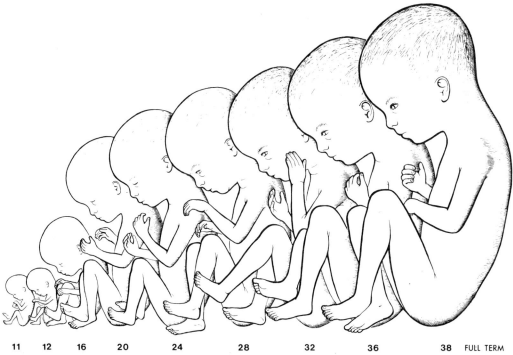

Figure 5-2. A table which illustrates the progressive development of the human fetus. [*Reproduced with permission from Keith L. Moore,* The Developing Human. Clinically Oriented Embryology, *2nd ed. W. B. Saunders Co., Philadelphia, Pa., 1977.*]

period, assuming that day to be the approximate date of ovulation. Duration of pregnancy is usually computed from the date of onset of the last menstrual period (see page 165). Age of an embryo computed from approximate time of ovulation would be two weeks less than age calculated from the last menstrual period. This difference ordinarily presents no major concern. Since development of the embryo proceeds rapidly and many changes take place in a two-week period, it is of interest to know the developmental age in describing the embryo's development at an early stage of pregnancy. As growth of the fetus advances and developmental changes are less rapid, the difference between "ovulation age" and "menstrual age" lessens.

DEVELOPMENT OF THE FETUS

Some of the developmental features of the embryo and fetus are described below in both text and illustrations.

The First Four Weeks

Development of the zygote from a one-cell stage through the morula and the blastocyst stage and its implantation has been described on pages 66–68. Development of the blastocyst continues rapidly. During the early days following implantation, the chorion and early villi develop, the amnion and yolk sac become differentiated, the body of the embryo appears as a flat embryonic disc, and a body stalk connects the embryo to the chorion (Fig. 4-9).

The flat embryonic disc, composed of two layers, embryonic ectoderm and embryonic endoderm, soon becomes a trilaminar (three-layered) embryo. Early in the third week of development a primitive streak appears as a midline thickening of the ectoderm. It gives rise to cells that migrate between the ectoderm and endoderm and form the mesoderm, the third germ layer. These three primary germ layers will give rise to all of the tissues and organs of the body.

A cellular rod, the notochord, develops from the primitive streak. The notochord forms the midline axis of the embryo and its primitive skeleton support. Later the skull and vertebral column develop around it, and it then disappears.

A longitudinal neural groove develops along the line of the notochord. Neural folds from the sides of the neural groove meet and fuse to form the neural tube, which will later give rise to the brain and spinal cord.

The mesoderm on each side of the notochord and the neural tube thicken to form two longitudinal columns. By the end of the third week these columns of mesoderm begin to divide and become segmented to form 42 to 44 pairs of cuboidal bodies of mesoderm, known as *somites*. The somites appear first in the occipital area, and then gradually continue to develop caudally.

Between 20 and 30 days of development, called the somite period, the stage of development of an embryo is often described by the number of somites present. Development proceeding from the somites includes the vertebrae and ribs, muscles associated with the axial skeleton, and the dermis of the skin. Spinal nerves enter the portions of the somites that will form the muscles.

The primitive streak, the notochord, and the somites all develop in a cephalocaudal progression pattern. This pattern can also be noted in development of other structures. Development of the lower limbs occurs later than the upper limbs.

As the embryonic disc, which has no characteristics of a human body, rapidly continues its development, it begins to take a form that shows a head and a body and then more and more develops into a shape that resembles a human embryo (Fig. 5-3). During this very early development of the embryo, all future parts of the body are laid down, at least in rudimentary form.

At the end of the fourth week of development, the embryo, although still very small, has increased in size tremendously from its beginning of one cell. It has taken form from the em-

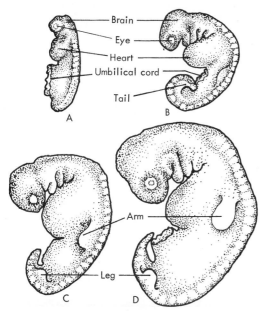

Figure 5-3. Development of the human embryo during the fourth week of life. Each embryo is drawn ten times its actual size, and is shown from its left side. The umbilical cord has been cut off near the belly of the embryo. The drawings are based on photographs of embryos described by Streeter. *A.* Twenty-four days. *B.* Twenty-six days. The flat embryonic disc has been converted into a C-shaped cylindrical embryo. *C.* Twenty-eight days. Somites are visible as surface elevations. *D.* Thirty days. Note the rapid growth and also the change in shape that results from folding in of both the longitudinal and transverse planes. [*By permission from Margaret S. Gilbert,* Biography of the Unborn, *rev. ed. Hafner Publishing Company, New York, 1962.*]

bryonic disc, but does not yet have clearly defined structures. It becomes somewhat elongated and curved upon itself with its two extremities almost in contact. Most of the body systems have begun to appear in rudimentary form at the end of the first month. The cardiovascular system, which develops more rapidly than the others, is functioning. The alimentary canal exists as a straight tube, and the thymus, thyroid, lungs, kidneys, and liver begin to develop. The brain, spinal cord, eyes, nose, and ears appear in rudimentary form. The ex-

tremities begin to be evident as tiny, budlike projections on the surface of the embryo (Figs 5-3 and 5-4).

The heart, bloodstream, and blood cells develop in the third week. The heart, a very simple but relatively large structure (Fig. 5-4) begins beating by the end of the third week, and blood flows through the simple vessels established by this time. The circulatory system must begin to function very early in order to transport the food that is absorbed from the maternal blood, by the chronic villi, to the tissues of the embryo.

The yolk sac (Fig. 4-9), which forms very early in gestation, serves several important functions in the first two to four weeks of embryonic development. It is a yolk sac in appearance only, without yolk or nutrients, but it seems to have an essential function in transfer of nutrients to the embryo during the second and third weeks while the uteroplacental circulation is being established. It develops a large circulation, and its blood vessels are a part of the early circulatory system of the embryo.

The yolk sac is also essential for blood development in the early weeks. Blood forms on its walls, beginning in the third week, and blood cell formation continues there until the liver takes on this function in the sixth week of fetal development.

Primordial germ cells appear in the wall of the yolk sac early in the third week. These cells migrate to the developing sex glands and they become the primitive germ cells, which will later become the sperm or ova in the sex glands.

During the fourth week the posterior part of the yolk sac is incorporated into the embryo and becomes the primitive gut. That part of the yolk sac that is not included in the embryo decreases in size as pregnancy advances and soon becomes a small remnant, which is attached to the gut by a narrow yolk stalk. This stalk later detaches from the gut.

By the end of the fourth week the chorionic sac is 20 mm or slightly larger in diameter, and it is large enough to begin bulging the uterine mucosa out into the uterine cavity (Fig. 5-5).

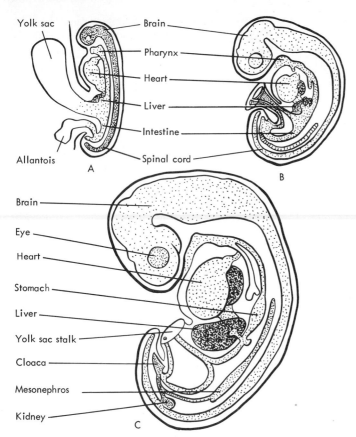

Yolk sac — Brain — Pharynx — Heart — Liver — Intestine — Spinal cord — Allantois

A

B

Brain — Eye — Heart — Stomach — Liver — Yolk sac stalk — Cloaca — Mesonephros — Kidney

C

Figure 5-4. Development of the internal organs of the human embryo during the fourth week. Each embryo is outlined in profile from the left side and the internal organs are shown in their proper places within the embryonic body. The three embryos are drawn to the same magnification (ten times actual size), so comparison of the three diagrams shows the great growth that occurs in the brain and heart. (Based on Streeter.) *A.* Twenty-four days; same embryo pictured in Figure 5-3*A*. *B.* Twenty-six days; same embryo pictured in Figure 5-3*B*. *C.* Thirty days; same embryo pictured in Figure 5-3*D*. [*By permission from Margaret S. Gilbert*, Biography of the Unborn, *rev. ed. Hafner Publishing Company, New York, 1962.*]

The sac has two walls, an outer wall, or chorion, covered with villi, and a smooth inner wall, the amnion, and it contains amniotic fluid which surrounds the embryo. The placenta has begun development and the umbilical cord is taking form from the body stalk (Fig. 5-5). The embryo measures 4–5 mm (0.2 in.) from crown to rump.

The Second Lunar Month of Development

During the second lunar month embryonic development is very rapid, and, beginning with week four, this period is especially critical to the development of all major structures. Any disturbance from drugs, viruses, or other environmental factors may give rise to congenital anomalies.

During the second month the embryonic body cavity is divided into three—the pericardial, the pleural, and the peritoneal cavities. The rapid growth of the brain causes an increase in head size. The extremities show considerable development, more so in the arms than in the legs.

By the end of the eighth week, the head end of the embryo has greatly increased in size and is about as large as the rest of the body (Fig. 5-6). The central nervous system is growing rapidly. Neuromuscular development is sufficient to permit some fetal movements. The body is covered with a thin skin. The facial features are more distinct. Bone centers appear in the rudimentary clavicles, the limbs are more developed, and the hands and feet are forming (Fig.

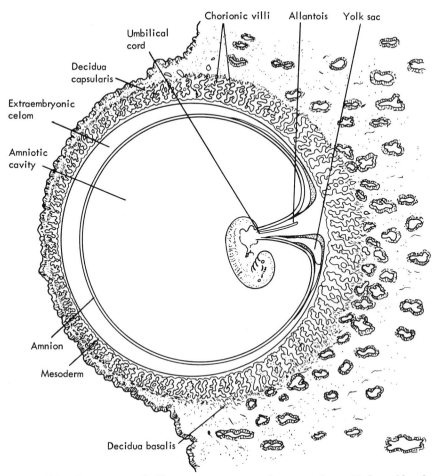

Figure 5-5.   Stereogram of a blastocyst containing a human embryo, 33 days old and 5 mm long. The blastocyst has formed an elevation on the surface of the uterine mucosa. The extraembryonic celom has been almost entirely replaced by the amniotic cavity. The body stalk has been converted into the umbilical cord by being covered with the amnion. The rudimentary umbilical cord contains the allantois, yolk sac, and the umbilical vessels. The latter are not shown. The chorionic villi in the decidua capsularis begin to atrophy, and those in the decidua basalis are growing larger and show a greater branching. [*Reprinted with permission from Macmillan Publishing Co., Inc. from Alfred F. Huettner,* Comparative Embryology of the Vertebrates, *rev. ed. Copyright 1941 by Macmillan Publishing Co., Inc., renewed 1969 by Mary A. Huettner.*]

5-6). The external genitalia appear but do not yet show definite sex characteristics. The umbilical cord has definite form. The approximate weight of the embryo is 5 gm, and its crown–rump length is about 30 mm.

The Third Lunar Month of Development

By the end of the twelfth week, the neck is longer; teeth are forming under the gums, and centers of ossification have appeared in most of the bones. The fingers and toes are well differentiated and bear nails in the form of fine membranes. The eyes have lids, which now fuse and do not reopen until during the sixth month. Growth in body length is rapid, but development of the head advances relatively more slowly than the rest of the body.

The lungs take definite shape, although their development continues throughout intrauterine life. The fetus may begin to make respiratory-like movements. The kidneys are able to secrete early in this third month, although kidney tubule formation is continued until term. The digestive system develops more completely. The fetus can now swallow, and he begins to take in the amniotic fluid, which he will con-

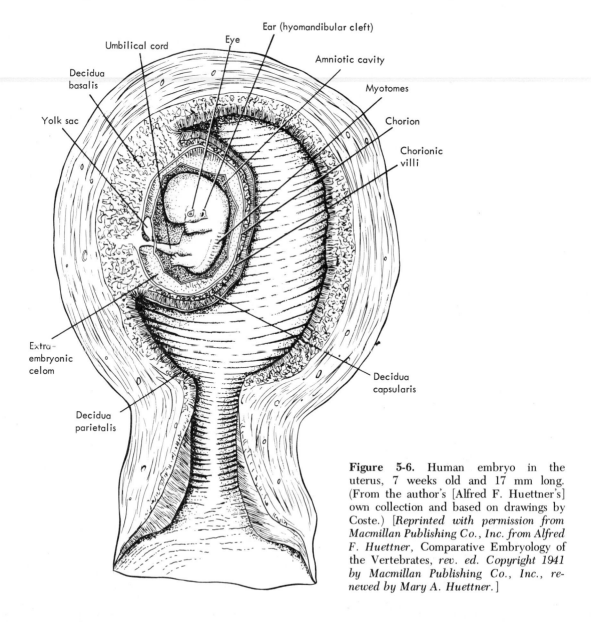

Figure 5-6. Human embryo in the uterus, 7 weeks old and 17 mm long. (From the author's [Alfred F. Huettner's] own collection and based on drawings by Coste.) [*Reprinted with permission from Macmillan Publishing Co., Inc. from Alfred F. Huettner,* Comparative Embryology of the Vertebrates, *rev. ed. Copyright 1941 by Macmillan Publishing Co., Inc., renewed by Mary A. Huettner.*]

tinue to swallow in large amounts for the remainder of his intrauterine life. Nasal septum and palate fusion is completed. Nucleated red blood cells predominate in the blood, and the liver begins blood formation. Sex is now distinguishable.

Neuromuscular development increases rapidly during the third month. The fetus moves easily and becomes active, although his mother does not feel these movements because he is still very small and his movements are weak. The fetus responds to stimulation, and some of his reflexes, such as the grasp reflex, are developing.

The amnion and chorion are now in contact. The villi are disappearing except at the point where there is a small, but complete and well-delineated placenta. The fetus is about 8 to 9 cm (3 to 3.5 in.) long from crown to rump and weighs about 45 gm (1½ oz) (Fig. 5-7).

The Fourth Lunar Month of Development

By the end of the sixteenth week, the fetus has increased considerably in size, since this, as well as the third month, is one of rapid growth (Fig. 5-8 and Table 5-1). The fetus is now about 15 cm (6 in.) long and weighs about 200 gm (7 oz). A downy hair, termed *lanugo*, appears over the body. There is tarry fecal material, called *meconium*, in the intestines.

The size of a fetus' head in relation to his body decreases with growth. By the sixteenth week the fetus' head and body have become a more proportionate size. Also, the face has developed a more human appearance.

The Fifth Lunar Month of Development

By the end of the twentieth week, the fetus has made additional marked advances in growth and development (Fig. 6-5, p. 117, and Table 5-1).

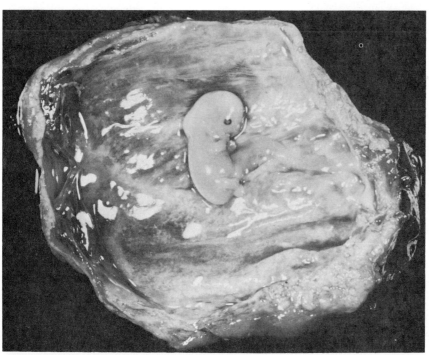

Figure 5-7. Embryo in amniotic sac. This photograph is of a spontaneous complete abortion at 12 weeks of gestation. [*Courtesy of Dr. Madeline J. Thornton.*]

Table 5-1. Characteristics of Developmental Progress in the Fetal Period
(Note the cepalocaudal progression in structural development.)

Gestational Age	Selected Developmental Characteristics	Mean Weight*	Mean Length
8 weeks	All major internal and external structures have begun development. Heart has been beating since three weeks. Facial features becoming distinct. Hands and feet are forming. Eyes open but will soon close. Head almost as large as rest of body.	5 gm	30 mm crown–rump
12 weeks	Head and body more proportioned. Arms almost final relative length. Legs still relatively short. Sex distinguishable externally. Fingernails developing. Teeth are forming under gums. Sucking and swallowing reflexes appear, but not strong and not synchronized. Kidneys begin producing urine. New nerve cells are forming rapidly in the brain.	45 gm	8–9 cm crown–rump
16 weeks	Head erect and now relatively small. Legs well developed. Skeleton will show on x-ray films. Meconium appearing in intestines.	200 gm	14 cm crown–rump
20 weeks	Skin completely covered with lanugo and vernix caseosa. Eyebrows and hair on head visible. Toenails developing. Mother recognizes fetal movements. Beginning of rapid brain growth. Grasp reflex good but not strong.	450 gm	19 cm crown–rump
24 weeks	Skin pink and wrinkled. Beginning a deposit of fat beneath skin. Respiratory movements quite well developed. Surfactant production in lungs begins. Swallows large amounts of amniotic fluid. Capable of crying.	800 gm	34 cm crown–heel
28 weeks	Eyes have reopened. Eyelashes present. Skin wrinkled. Hair on head well developed. Beginning descent of testicles into scrotum. Reacts to auditory stimuli. Lungs developed sufficiently to permit exchange of gas. Is capable of surviving if born prematurely.	1100 gm	37 cm crown–heel
30 weeks	Subcutaneous fat deposition accelerated from now until term.	1300 gm	39.75 cm crown–heel
32 weeks	Skin pink and smooth. Lanugo hair begins to disappear. Fingernails reach fingertips. Suck and swallow may be coordinated by this time. Nipple buds visible.	1600 gm	42.5 cm crown–heel
34 weeks	Rooting reflex good. Sucking reflex strong. Beginning surge of stable surfactant in lungs. Plantar creases fine and indistinct. Ear returns slowly from folding.	2050 gm	45 cm crown–heel

Table 5-1. (*Continued*)

Gestational Age	Selected Developmental Characteristics	Mean Weight *	Mean Length
36 weeks	Lanugo hair almost gone. Toenails reach tips of toes. Grasp reflex strong—may lift baby off bed. Plantar creases show indentation on anterior one third of sole only. Flat breast areola of 1–2 mm. Labia majora widely separated. Scrotum small; few rugae.	2600 gm	47 cm crown–heel
38–40 weeks	Body is plump. Skin whiter, less red. Fingernails extend beyond fingertips. Plantar creases deep over most of foot. Ears firm and erect. Chest is prominent. Mammary glands protrude and have a raised areola of 4 mm or greater. Labia majora completely cover labia minora. Scrotum full; many rugae. Testes in scrotum or in inguinal canal.	2950–3200 gm	48–49 cm crown–heel

*Mean measurements for 24 to 40 weeks are the 50th percentile on the intrauterine growth chart from Lula O. Lubchenco, Charlotte Hansman, and Edith Boyd, "Intrauterine Growth in Length and Head Circumference as Estimated from Live Births at Gestational Ages from 26 to 42 weeks," *Pediatrics* 37:403–408 (Mar.) 1966. See Figure 18-2 on page 475. There is a wide range in measurements of individual fetuses depending upon genetic factors, nutritional adequacy, and general environmental influences.

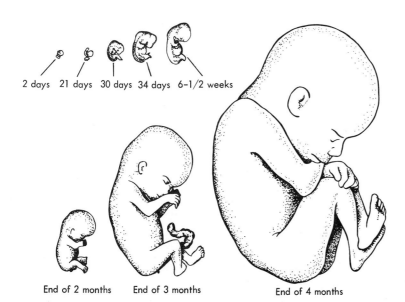

2 days   21 days   30 days   34 days   6-1/2 weeks

End of 2 months   End of 3 months   End of 4 months

Figure 5-8. Diagram showing appearance of fetus at different stages in its development.

The body is about 25 cm (10 in.) long and weighs about 450 gm (16 oz). The skeleton hardens. The buds for the permanent teeth begin to develop. The commissures of the brain are complete, and myelinization of the spinal cord begins. The skin is less transparent. *Vernix caseosa*, a greasy, cheesy substance consisting of secretion of the sebaceous glands of the skin, makes its appearance. It covers the skin from now until birth. Hair appears on the head.

Fetal movements are stronger, and it is usually sometime during the fifth lunar month, though occasionally earlier, that they are first felt by the mother. This early detection of fetal movement by the mother is commonly referred to as *quickening*, or perception of life. It is also during this month that the fetal heartbeat can be heard through a stethoscope placed against the mother's abdomen.

The Sixth Lunar Month of Development

By the end of the twenty-fourth week, the skin is markedly wrinkled, but there is a beginning deposit of fat beneath it, which produces a substantial weight gain. The body is better proportioned, but it is thin, and the head is still large compared with the rest of the body. Growth in the fetus proceeds more rapidly at the head end than the caudal end. Thus the fetal head constitutes a large part of the body throughout embryonic and fetal development. The eyebrows and eyelashes are appearing by the end of the sixth month. The skin is varying shades of pink to red because blood is visible in the capillaries. The fetus is about 34 cm (13 in.) long and weighs about 800 gm (1 lb 12 oz). If born at this time it will attempt to survive, but often dies shortly after birth.

The Seventh Lunar Month of Development

By the end of the twenty-eighth week, the fetus still appears thin and scrawny, the skin is reddish and is well covered with vernix caseosa, and the intestines contain an increased amount of meconium. He is about 37 cm (14.5 in.) long and weighs about 1100 gm (2 lb 7 oz). Hair on the head is well developed. The fetus' eyes reopen during this month. The CNS has developed sufficiently to maintain rhythmic breathing and a relatively stable body temperature if supplied with some additional warmth.

If born at the end of seven lunar months the baby may move and cry quite vigorously. An infant this size is very immature, but his organs are sufficiently developed to make his chances for survival not entirely unfavorable if he is given expert care, and if he has not been handicapped during his intrauterine life.

The Eighth Lunar Month of Development

By the end of the thirty-second week, the fetus has grown to about 42 cm (16.5 in.) in length and 1600 gm (3 lb 9 oz) in weight. He still appears thin and old and wrinkled. The nails extend to the ends of the fingers, and are firmer in texture. The lanugo begins to disappear from the face. The hair on the head is more abundant. If born at this age, the baby has a good chance to live. This is true in spite of the ancient superstition, still current, that a seventh-month baby is more likely to live than one born at eight months (meaning calendar months). The fact is that after the eighth lunar month, a little more than seven calendar months, the probability of the baby's living increases with each day spent within the uterus, unless that environment is unfavorable to good development.

The Ninth Lunar Month of Development

By the end of the thirty-sixth week, an increased deposit of fat under the skin has given a plumper, rounder contour to the entire body and the aged look has passed. The baby now weighs about 2600 gm (5¾ lb) and is about 47 cm (18.5 in.) long. If he is born at this time, his chances of living are good.

The Tenth Lunar Month of Development

During the tenth month, the fetus reaches full-term development (Fig. 6-6, page 117). Accumulation of fat continues, the body becomes plumper, and weight increases. The skin is now smooth, with little or no lanugo hair, and is whiter, less red. The fingers and toes have well-developed nails which extend beyond their tips. The bones of the skull are firmer and come close together at the suture lines. The chest is prominent and the mammary glands protrude. The average normally developed, full-term baby has attained a length of about 50 cm (20 in.) and a weight of approximately 3300 gm (about 7¼ lb), boys usually being several ounces heavier than girls.

All figures on weight and length represent averages, and there is considerable individual variation in antenatal growth. The weight of normal healthy babies varies from 2500 gm (5½ lb) to 4080 gm (9 lb), or more. Although there is marked normal variation, a full-term baby weighing under 2500 gm (5½ lb) is considered a low-birth-weight infant (page 744), and one weighing over 4080 gm (9 lb) is considered excessive in size.

FETAL BODY SYSTEMS

Development and function of body systems have been referred to in the above description of development of the embryo and fetus during the 10 lunar months of intrauterine growth. Additional information about some of the fetal systems will clarify their function before birth.

Cardiovascular System

The cardiovascular system is the first organ system to become functional in the fetus. Blood begins to circulate at the end of the third week of life. Such early development of the circulatory system is necessary for growth and development of all other systems, since they are dependent on adequate circulation for acquiring nutrients and eliminating waste products.

Heart development is first indicated at 18 or 19 days of life. Initially there are a pair of heart tubes. Blood vessels begin to form early in the third week in the yolk sac, the connecting stalk,

the chorion, and then the embryo. Primitive plasma and blood cells are derived mainly from endothelial cells of the blood vessels in the yolk sac and the allantois. The heart tubes join the blood vessels to form a primitive cardiovascular system, and circulation of blood starts by the end of the third week.

In further development of the heart, the paired heart tubes fuse into a fairly straight tube. This tube then bends upon itself forming a U-shaped tube which takes on more of the external appearance of a heart. Partitioning for development of atria and ventricles takes place during the fourth and fifth week of gestation, becoming relatively complete by the end of the fifth week. Certain morphologic alterations continue to take place, and important adjustments in the circulatory system occur at birth.

The locus of blood cell formation in the embryo and fetus changes as development progresses. Primitive blood cells are first formed from blood islands in the yolk sac and from endothelial cells of primitive blood vessels. In the second lunar month, blood formation takes place in the liver, and this remains the chief organ of blood formation until the sixth month. The spleen, lymph glands, and thymus pass through a peak of blood formation and gradually lose this ability. Hematopoiesis in bone marrow begins during the fourth to fifth fetal month, and then becomes the dominant site of blood cell formation during the last months of gestation.

Fetal blood circulation and the changes in circulation at birth will be described at the end of this chapter.

Respiratory System

The respiratory system is in a continuous stage of maturation throughout fetal life and on into childhood. The first indication of development of the respiratory system appears in the fourth week, when the earliest stages of the larynx and trachea appear and lung buds begin to develop. Lung development then proceeds through several stages. From 5 to 17 weeks the lung is in a very early developmental phase during which the bronchi and bronchioles form, and the lung resembles a gland microscopically. From 13 to 25 weeks alveolar ducts develop, lumina of bronchi and bronchioles enlarge, and the lung tissue becomes highly vascular.

Beginning at about 24 weeks and continuing to birth the alveolar ducts develop into primitive alveoli, or saccules, and the capillary network grows closer to the air sacs. By 26 weeks of fetal life the primitive alveoli and the pulmonary vasculature may be sufficiently developed to permit adequate exchange of gas in the lungs and survival of a prematurely born infant. Also beginning with 23 to 24 weeks of fetal life the alveolar cells produce surfactant, a surface-active material, in increasing amounts. This material is necessary to maintenance of good lung expansion. Birth prior to adequate production of surfactant leads to respiratory distress.

The last period of development, the alveolar period, begins in late fetal life and continues until eight years of age. During this time the lining of the air sacs becomes very thin and indents further, developing into characteristic pulmonary alveoli with larger and better surface area for gas exchange. The number of alveoli that are characteristic of adult life is only one eighth to one sixth complete at birth.

Present-day fetal monitoring by ultrasound has shown that the fetus makes respiratory movements *in utero*. Fetal breathing is episodic, and is present as much as 70 percent of the time, with a frequency of 30 to 70 times per minute. Fetal breathing has been detected as early as 13 weeks gestation. The fetal lungs are partially inflated with fluid derived from the lungs themselves. At birth, when gas exchange must take place through the lungs, ongoing respiration quickly becomes established, and the lung fluid is rapidly replaced by air.

Gastrointestinal System

The primitive gut or digestive system forms during the fourth week of fetal life as the dorsal part of the yolk sac is incorporated into the embryo. The intestines project into the umbilical cord during the fifth week because of inadequate room in the abdomen. They return to the abdomen during the tenth week when the liver and kidneys occupy less space than they did previously and when the abdominal cavity enlarges. A membrane that separates the rectum from the exterior ruptures at the end of the seventh week, opening the anal canal. Characteristic coiling of the bowel begins with its return to the abdominal cavity, and it takes on normal configuration and relative size by the twentieth week.

Most of the digestive enzymes are present quite early, beginning their appearance at 3 to 4 months, and mobility of the intestinal tract develops early. Peristalsis of the small intestine appears by the eleventh week.

Swallowing and sucking are apparently first elicited in the fetus at 12 to 13 weeks. The sucking reflex is quite well developed, albeit weak, at 24 weeks, and at 30 weeks or earlier the fetus can suck food. Sucking and swallowing, however, may not be well integrated before 32 to 36 weeks, and sometimes not until several days after full-term birth.

By 24 weeks of life the fetus can swallow amniotic fluid at the rate of 5 ml/kg-hour. This means that at full term the fetus swallows almost 500 ml of amniotic fluid per day. This fluid is reabsorbed from the fetal gastrointestinal tract.

After swallowing begins, the intestines start to fill with a tarry fecal material. This intestinal content, called *meconium,* consists of desquamated cells, digestive secretions, mucus, bile pigments, and lanugo and vernix caseosa swallowed in the amniotic fluid. The bowels are normally inactive and do not empty until after birth. If there is interference with fetal oxygenation, the sphincter ani muscles may relax and allow meconium to escape. The amniotic fluid may then become deeply stained by the black, sticky meconium.

The liver, gallbladder, and pancreas develop from buds off the foregut. The liver grows rapidly and fills a good deal of the abdominal cavity.

Hematopoiesis in the liver begins during the

sixth week. The liver is the chief organ of blood formation from the third to the sixth month of fetal life. A decline in blood formation in the liver then takes place, so that at birth most of the blood is formed in the bone marrow.

Many hepatic enzymes are delayed in maturing. A bilirubin load is not easily handled by newborns, especially prematures, because of immature or inadequate development of the enzyme glucuronyl transferase. This enzyme is necessary to convert bilirubin into an excretable variety. The level of the enzyme increases rapidly in the first few days after birth, and the ability of the liver to handle bilirubin does not reach full capacity until after birth.

Insulin is present in the fetal pancreas at the eleventh week. The amount increases with fetal age and is believed to become excessive if stimulated by hyperglycemia in the mother.

Urinary System

The excretory system and the reproductive system are closely associated developmentally, but they will be described separately.

The permanent kidneys appear in the fifth week of fetal life and assume functional form in the eighth week. There have been two sets of rudimentary, transitory kidneys prior to the permanent ones, but it is not known if they are functional in the human.

Although the fetal kidneys are not essential to intrauterine life, they develop early and soon function to a limited degree. A certain amount of glomerular filtration and tubular activity has begun by the end of the first trimester of gestation. Development of the kidneys, however, is quite prolonged. It continues throughout fetal life and into the postnatal period. Function is fairly adequate at the time of birth, but the kidneys must continue to develop greater efficiency postnatally. Thus at birth there is still an appreciable immaturity of the kidneys in both structure and function, and development will continue into infancy.

The fetal kidneys apparently produce a large amount of urine beginning in the early months

of life. In fetuses of only a few centimeters in length the bladder is filled with a clear fluid which is voided into the amniotic sac. It is believed that human amniotic fluid is largely derived from fetal urine, at least in the latter months of pregnancy.

During development the kidneys undergo a relative ascent from a pelvic position to the lumbar region. Some of this apparent ascent occurs because of further growth of the caudal part of the fetus.

Reproductive System

Genetic sex is determined at fertilization by the kind of sperm that fertilizes the ovum, but gonadal sex is not at first apparent. Gonadal development first becomes evident in the fifth week, appearing identical in both sexes. In this stage an embryo has the potential to develop into either sex. Indication of sex is not evident before the seventh week, at which time the indifferent gonads begin to become recognizable as testes in the male. Ovaries develop more slowly and are not identifiable until about the tenth week.

Gonadal sex is controlled by the Y chromosome, which exerts a strong influence on the indifferent gonads to develop them into testes. In embryos that do not have a Y chromosome the indifferent gonads develop into ovaries, but at a much slower rate than testicular development.

The genital ducts and the external genitalia also pass through an indifferent stage of development. The fetal testes soon produce masculinizing hormones that stimulate development of the primordial ducts into the male reproductive tract and the indifferent genitalia into penis and scrotum. In the absence of androgens, the primordial ducts develop into uterus, fallopian tubes, and vagina, and the indifferent genitalia into those of a female.

The external genitalia are not distinguishable as male or female at first. They begin to take on some sexual characteristics in the early fetal period but appear somewhat similar until the end of the ninth week. Final form of distinctly male or female is not established until the twelfth week.

Descent of the testes through the inguinal canal usually begins during the twenty-eighth week. Entry into the scrotum ordinarily occurs several weeks later.

Skeletal and Muscular Systems

The skeletal and muscular systems develop from mesoderm, with the vertebral column, the ribs, and much of the skeletal muscle developing from cells that are derived from the somites. Much of the skeleton, bone, cartilage, and connective tissue develop from multiple areas of condensed mesenchyme (embryonic mesodermal tissue).

The trunk is quite well formed by the end of the third week. Cartilagenous models of bone begin to develop toward the end of the first month. The limb buds appear about the thirtieth day, with the arm buds growing a few days ahead of the leg buds. Ossification centers appear in the long bones by the eighth week.

From the eighth week onward into postnatal life the amount of calcium in the bone increases as the bones grow and calcify when cartilage is transformed into bone. The skeleton continues to grow in postnatal development and bony tissues continue to mature until adulthood.

Functionally, immature muscle contractions take place early in embryogenesis, but it is felt that effective neuromuscular activity does not occur until motor end plates are formed. Thus, consistent reflex movements do not occur before 12 weeks. Sometime during the fifth lunar month the mother begins to feel fetal movement, which becomes stronger with age of the fetus.

Skeletal muscles grow by increase in number of muscle fibers and in size of individual fibers. Increase in number of fibers is greatest in fetal life.

The skeletal muscles are not mature at birth. Growth of muscle fibers in the fetus, and postnatally, appears to be related to functional need. Muscle fibers in the diaphragm of the newborn are larger than in the limb muscles, presumably because respiration is the main form of muscular activity in the neonatal period. In older children fibers in limb muscles and the diaphragm are the same size.

Nervous System

The nervous system is one of the first of the body systems to appear in the embryo and is the one that grows most rapidly but, with the exception of the reproductive system, is the last to mature. The area from which the brain and spinal cord will develop appears very early in embryonic development. A neural plate appears during the third week. A neural tube and a neural crest soon develop from the neural plate. The neural tube is temporarily open at both ends. These openings, called neuropores, close during the fourth week. The neural tube differentiates into the central nervous system, with the cranial end developing into the brain and the remainder into the spinal cord. Defects in closure of the neural tube account for many of the congenital malformations of the CNS. The neural crest gives rise to the peripheral nervous system.

The CNS goes through rapid development of structure and function and is very easily subject to insult. Teratogenic agents may interfere with many sensitive processes in the early weeks of development and may lead to gross malformations. Later, during the third trimester, and in the perinatal period, hazards such as hypoxia, malnutrition, and hypoglycemia can cause irreversible changes. Also, interference of any kind as the brain goes through a rapid growth spurt may leave harmful effects.

Study of the brain is obviously difficult in the human, but inferentially from animal studies and from observations of children, a certain amount of information on developmental progress can be obtained.

The cerebral cortex is still in a relatively primitive state at the beginning of the fetal period, but thereafter brain development proceeds rapidly. Development from that time can be arbitrarily divided into two phases: an early period of neuronal development, and a later period of rapid brain growth.

The formation of new nerve cells occurs primarily between 10 and 18 weeks of gestation. This is the major period of multiplication of neuroblasts, and an adult number of neurons is established quite early. Any interference with brain growth during this time may lead to a reduced number of brain cells. Viral infections, chromosomal anomalies, and maternal medication could have an adverse influence on neuron multiplication.

The next phase of brain development begins with the second half of pregnancy and continues into the second postnatal year. This is the period of the brain growth spurt, which is arbitrarily defined as the transient period when the brain is growing most rapidly. The human brain growth spurt appears to run from midpregnancy to about 18 months of postnatal age. Thereafter there is some further gradual growth until maturity.

At midpregnancy active multiplication of new nerve cells declines, being almost complete, and glial division takes over. The glial cells actively multiply and lay down a delicate fibrous network of supporting substance for the nerves and cells of the brain. Myelination also takes place during this growth spurt, and nerve cells branch and grow, and synapses rapidly form between nerve cells.

It is during this critical period of rapid growth that fetal malnutrition is most likely to affect brain development. Maternal undernutrition, or placental insufficiency that reduces supplies to the fetus, may interfere with such important processes as myelination, growth of the neurons, and establishment of synaptic connections.

The time at which function of the various regions of the nervous system is established is not well known, but some movements and reflex activities can be observed by the end of the second month of development. The first reflex observed, which consists of bending the head to the side opposite the area stimulated, has been noted at 7.5 weeks menstrual age. Local reflexes may begin to appear by 9.5 weeks of menstrual age, first in the face by squinting, swallowing, tongue retraction, mouth opening and then in the upper and lower extremities and body. Motor responses distal to the point of stimulation are not observed until 9.5 weeks, and these responses are not refined. They are mass movements with flexion of contralateral neck and trunk muscles.

Sensory end organs are not complete when some of the early reflexes appear. A reflex is thus at first limited because only the earliest matured part of the neuromuscular system can respond. With further development and maturity, more parts of the body respond and the reflex becomes more complete.

At 12 weeks the fetus turns toward a stimulus with lip and head movements. A little later sucking movements appear. The swallowing reflex appears between 12 and 13 weeks and first sucking movements are also noted about this time. The sucking reflex is quite well developed at 24 weeks but is not strong. However, the ability to coordinate suck and swallow does not develop until 6 to 8 weeks later. The grasp reflex first appears at 12 to 13 weeks; true grasp is present at 18 weeks.

Respiratory movements occur *in utero*. They have been detected as early as 13 weeks, and are apparently quite well developed by 22 to 24 weeks. The fetus is capable of crying by 24 weeks and perhaps earlier. Fetal reaction to auditory stimuli has been noted at 29 to 30 weeks.

Maturation of the fetal nervous system and its functional development proceeds in an orderly fashion and at a fairly constant rate. Numerous reflexes appear during fetal maturation and they are well-developed by full-term gestation, many of them much earlier. Since various reflexes begin to appear at a fairly set time in development, a number of them are used in examination of the newborn to assess gestational age.

Motor behavior of the newborn seems to be mainly under control of the spinal cord and the medulla. Cortical activity does, however, appear to have some influence on an infant's motor behavior at the time of birth. Although myelination and branching of nerve cells and synaptic connections occur mainly postnatally, these processes have started before birth, and it could be expected that cortical activity could influence behavior. Maturation of the brain continues postnatally and more and more regulation is taken over by the cerebral cortex and becomes voluntary.

Newborns are capable of turning toward sounds and can follow objects with their eyes to some extent. They have a strong grasp, they can bring their hands to their mouth, they can suck and swallow, and they can cry when hungry or in pain. A crying baby will become quiet when picked up and held even before a conditioned response has had time to develop. It is possible that conditioning can already be developing during the first week after birth.

FETAL CIRCULATION

After the first month of development, the placenta serves the fetus as an organ for exchange of gases, for obtaining nutrients, and for elimination of waste products. It is in the placenta that the oxygen and nutrients requisite for life and growth pass from the mother's blood into the fetal circulation, and carbon dioxide and fetal waste products pass from the fetal blood to the mother's circulation. The fetus must therefore possess a circulatory mechanism by which its blood flows through the placenta. The fetal circulatory system is peculiar to it, differing from that of the independently existing human body, in which lungs and other body systems are fully functioning.

Fetal circulation is made possible through certain structures existing in the fetal circulatory system that become obliterated after birth. These structures, necessary to fetal circulation, but useless after birth, are as follows:

1. Placenta, one umbilical vein, and two umbilical arteries
2. Foramen ovale, a direct opening between the right and left atrium of the heart

3. Ductus arteriosus, a fetal vessel connecting the pulmonary artery and the aorta
4. Ductus venosus, a fetal blood vessel connecting the umbilical vein and the inferior vena cava

Course of the Fetal Blood

There are three blood vessels in the umbilical cord: one umbilical vein, which in spite of its name, conveys aerated blood to the fetus, and two umbilical arteries, which carry deoxygenated blood from the fetus. Blood flows from the fetus to the placenta by way of the umbilical arteries. After this fetal blood has given up its carbon dioxide and other waste products to the maternal blood and taken up oxygen and nutritive material, it returns to the fetus through the umbilical vein (Fig. 5-9).

The umbilical vein passes to the liver of the fetus where it joins the ductus venosus, the fetal blood vessel connecting the umbilical vein and the inferior vena cava, and also gives off branches to the liver. Blood traversing the umbilical vein flows to the inferior vena cava, in part directly through the ductus venosus and in part indirectly through the liver, entering the inferior vena cava by the hepatic veins.

The blood flowing into the inferior vena cava from the ductus venosus and the hepatic veins becomes mixed with a small amount of blood that is returning along the inferior vena cava from the lower part of the body. Although this mixing of deoxygenated blood from the portal veins and from the lower part of the body and oxygenated blood directly from the placenta takes place, the blood in the inferior vena cava is still relatively well oxygenated because of the large amount of blood that comes directly from the placenta.

As the blood that is flowing up the inferior vena cava reaches the heart, it divides into two streams, one large and one small. The large stream, the major portion of this relatively well-oxygenated blood, is emptied from the inferior vena cava into the right atrium from where it passes directly through the foramen ovale into the left atrium. The smaller stream joins the flow from the superior vena cava, through which deoxygenated blood is returning from the head and upper extremities. This oxygen-poor blood from the superior vena cava is also emptied into the right atrium, but it then passes into the right ventricle. The two streams of blood, one entering from the inferior vena cava and the other entering from the superior vena cava, cross in the right atrium, but they do not mix

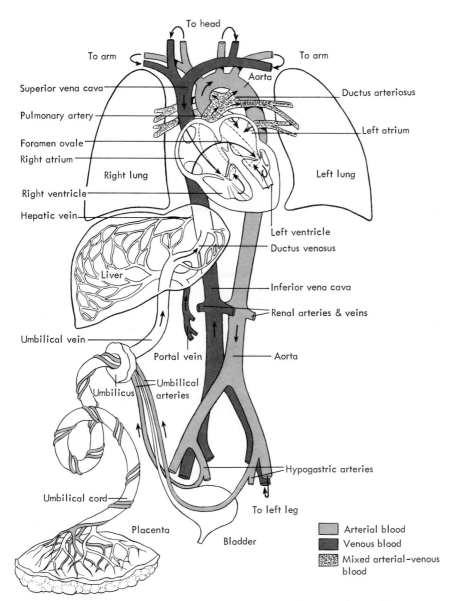

Figure 5-9. Fetal circulation. [*Adapted by permission from* Fetal Circulation, *Ros. Clinical Education Aid No. 1, 1963. Ross Laboratories, Columbus, Ohio.*]

(Fig. 5-9). The continuing path of each of the streams of blood that enters the right atrium is described below.

The blood that enters the right atrium from the superior vena cava and goes to the right ventricle is ejected into the pulmonary artery. Some of this blood goes to the nonfunctioning lungs, but the greatest part of it (85 to 90 percent) flows directly from the pulmonary artery into the aorta, passing through the ductus arteriosus, the fetal vessel that connects the pulmonary artery and the aorta (Fig. 5-9). The pulmonary blood vessels are constricted in the nonaerated lungs. They do not permit the large volume of circulation essential after birth but not necessary in the fetus. Circulation through the lungs before birth is for the nourishment of the lungs only.

The relatively well-oxygenated blood that enters the right atrium from the inferior vena cava moves across the right atrium, through the foramen ovale, into the left atrium, and from there into the left ventricle. This blood is then pumped into the ascending aorta. From there it is distributed principally to the coronary arteries, the head, and the arms, although some also flows into the descending aorta. The route taken by the blood from the inferior vena cava, which comes quite directly from the placenta, assures that the heart and the brain receive the blood when it is still well oxygenated.

The blood in the descending aorta, a mixture coming from both the right and left ventricle, is distributed to the abdominal viscera, the pelvis, and the lower extremities. From the lower part of the body the blood is conveyed to the placenta for reoxygenation. The largest amount of this blood flows from the hypogastric arteries into the umbilical arteries and on into the placenta. A small amount passes into the inferior vena cava, where it mixes with the blood that has just returned from the placenta by way of the umbilical vein.

From this description it is apparent that the blood circulating in the fetus is never entirely oxygenated. The blood in the inferior vena cava and that distributed to the heart, head, and upper extremities is more directly from the placenta than that distributed to the lower part of the body.

Changes in the Circulatory System at Birth

As soon as the baby is born, he loses the placental circulation and must obtain oxygen through his lungs. The pulmonary circulation of necessity becomes immediately more important and greatly increases in volume. In fact, the entire fetal circulation is readjusted to meet the needs of the new and independent functions that the body now assumes. The changes that take place in the circulatory system at, and shortly after, birth are described in detail on pages 424–26.

SUMMARY

In the course of 10 lunar months the single cell resulting from fertilization of an ovum has developed into the complex structures of a full-term fetus ready to begin life as a separate entity. The periods of embryonic and fetal development are characterized by rapid growth which involves active protein synthesis, differentiation of various tissues and organs, and development of organ function.

Development during the embryonic period is multiple and very rapid. The beginning of all major internal and external structures takes place during this time. This is a critical period of development, and exposure to adverse environmental influences, such as drugs or viruses, may cause major congenital malformations.

The fetal period begins about eight weeks after fertilization and ends with birth. By the time this period begins the fetus has features that are recognizably human. This period is characterized by growth and maturation of the tissues and organs that began their development in the embryonic period. Body growth is rapid and body fat is deposited during the last 6 to 8 weeks.

During the latter part of the fetal period the fetus increases its capacity to perform many of the biochemical and physiologic functions typical for the systems and organs of the body. Some of this maturation occurs around the time of birth, and some continues into the postnatal period.

Although the fetal organs and systems have functioned only to a limited degree in the protective intrauterine environment, they have developed to the capacity for independent function by the time of full-term birth at the end of the tenth lunar month, and often much earlier. Babies born prematurely are often able to function quite well with good supportive care. The longer the intrauterine period, however, the better the chances for survival, providing the intrauterine environment is good. Until at least 26 weeks gestational age a fetus is unable to survive extrauterine because of immaturity of the respiratory system.

Major adjustments must be made immediately after birth. With loss of placental circulation, the baby must begin breathing immediately to obtain oxygen, and sudden alterations in the circulatory system are essential when oxygen is obtained through the lungs. All other body systems must also adjust to extrauterine life, but may do so at a slower rate. The physiologic changes made by the newborn are described in Chapter 17.

BIBLIOGRAPHY

Allan, Frank D., *Essentials of Human Embryology*, 2nd ed. Oxford University Press, New York, 1969.

Arey, Leslie B., *Developmental Anatomy*, 7th ed. Saunders, Philadelphia, Pa., 1965.

Boddy, K., and Mantell, C., Observation of fetal breathing movements transmitted through maternal abdominal wall, *Lancet* ii:1219–1220 (Dec. 2) 1972.

Corliss, Clark Edward, *Patten's Human Embryology*. McGraw-Hill, New York, 1976.

Corner, George W., *Ourselves Unborn*. Yale University Press, New Haven, Conn., 1945.

Davis, John A., and Dobbing, John (eds.), *Scientific Foundations of Paediatrics*. Heinemann, London, 1974.

Dawes, G. S., Fetal circulation and breathing, *Clin. Obstet. Gynaecol.* 1:139–149 (Apr.) 1974.

Flanagan, Geraldine L., *The First Nine Months of Life*. Simon and Schuster, New York, 1962.

Gilbert, Margaret S., *Biography of the Unborn*, rev. ed. Hafner, New York, 1962.

Hamilton, William J., Boyd, J. D., and Mossman, H. W., *Hamilton, Boyd, and Mossman's Human Embryology*, 4th ed. Williams and Wilkins, Baltimore, Md., 1972.

Huettner, Alfred F., *Fundamentals of Comparative Embryology of the Vertebrates*, rev. ed. Macmillan, New York, 1949.

Moore, Keith L., *The Developing Human: Clinically Oriented Embryology*, 2nd ed. Saunders, Philadelphia, Pa., 1977.

———, *Before We Are Born*, rev. reprint. Saunders, Philadelphia, Pa., 1977.

Potter, Edith L., *Fundamentals of Human Reproduction*. McGraw-Hill, New York, 1948.

Smart, Mollie S., and Smart, Russell C., *Children, Development and Relationships*, 2nd ed. Macmillan, New York, 1972.

Stave, Uwe (ed.), *Physiology of the Perinatal Period*, Vols. I and II. Appleton-Century-Crofts, New York, 1970.

Walsh, S. Zoe, Meyer, W. W., and Lind, John, *The Human Fetal and Neonatal Circulation*. Charles C Thomas, Springfield, Ill., 1974.

6

Maternal Physiologic Changes During Pregnancy

Profound physiologic changes take place in the maternal body during pregnancy, involving all systems. These functional adjustments, in response to the increased physiologic load, begin in the first weeks of pregnancy and continue throughout. Upon delivery of the baby and placenta, the mother's body begins to return to its nonpregnant state. Some changes reverse rapidly. Those that occur more slowly are completed in approximately six weeks, with the exception of the breasts, which continue milk secretion for some months if the mother nurses her baby.

CHANGES IN THE REPRODUCTIVE ORGANS

Uterine Body

The most remarkable gestational changes occur in the uterus, which is transformed from a small, almost solid organ to one that will hold a full-term fetus, a placenta, and 500 to 1000 ml of amniotic fluid.

The weight of the uterus increases about 20-fold during pregnancy, 60 gm (2 oz) before pregnancy to about 1000 gm (2 lb) at the end of full-term gestation, and it increases five to six times in size. At the end of pregnancy the uterus is 30 to 35 cm (12 to 14 in.) long, from 20 to 25 cm (8 to 10 in.) wide, and about 22 cm (8.8 in.) deep. Its capacity has increased from 700 to 1000 times, from approximately 4 ml to 4000–5000 ml.

The uterine muscle wall is greatly enlarged due to a marked hypertrophy of the muscle cells already present and the development of new muscle cells during the early part of pregnancy. There is also a marked development of connective and elastic tissue, an increase in the size and number of blood vessels, and hypertrophy of the lymphatic tissue. Later in pregnancy uterine size increases through stretching of the myometrial fibers by the growth of the products of conception.

During the first half of pregnancy the walls of the uterus thicken to approximately 2 cm. This phase of myometrial growth is one of hypertrophy and hyperplasia stimulated by estrogens, progesterone, and chorionic somatomammotropin. Evidence of this is seen in tubal pregnancies in which there is definite enlargement of the uterus during the early weeks, although the fetus is not contained within it.

From midpregnancy into the last trimester the uterus enlarges as a result of both hormonal and mechanical stimulation. Hypertrophy is predominant in these myometrial changes; the muscle fibers increase in both length and thickness. The fetus causes some mechanical distention during this time.

In the third trimester the increase in uterine size is brought about by mechanical distention. As the fetus grows rapidly during this time it exerts pressure on the uterine walls, which begin to stretch and thin out. Toward the latter part of pregnancy the uterine walls are only about 5 mm ($^{1}/_{5}$ in.) thick. This allows for easy palpation of the fetus through the stretched uterine and abdominal tissues.

During pregnancy the uterine blood supply increases from 20 to 40 times. The uterine arteries, which are the major source of the uterine blood supply, branch off the internal iliacs, pass into and along the broad ligaments, and enter the uterus at about the level of the internal os of the cervix. They then ascend on each side of the uterus and form a network of spiral arterioles, which provide an ample blood supply to the uterus.

The uterine blood vessels increase considerably in both size and number in pregnancy. The uterine arteries enlarge several times and coiling of their arterioles permits them to adapt easily to growth of the myometrium. There is also increasing vascularization of the uterine corpus and cervix. Changes in the uterine vessels are probably brought about, in part at least, by the increase in estrogens and progesterone. Changes also develop in response to the tremendous increase in uterine blood flow and decrease in uterine vascular resistance that accompanies development of the uteroplacental circulation.

The uterine venous system is also greatly enlarged in pregnancy. The uterine veins increase in size and dilate to a diameter that may be up to 60 times larger than their nonpregnant diameter. Such enlargement is necessary to provide adequate venous drainage for the large uteroplacental blood flow. The ovarian veins also enlarge a great amount in pregnancy. Connection between the uterine and ovarian veins and other venous systems in the body is good and this assures good blood return to the heart.

Changes in the blood vessels are quickly reversed after delivery. Within one week post partum the uterine vessels have returned to their prepregnant size.

The musculature of the uterus is a heavy network of interlacing muscle fibers. The many blood vessels of the uterus extend throughout this network. Each muscle fiber has a double curve, and as any two fibers interlace, they form an arrangement similar to a figure 8. Contraction of the fibers in such an arrangement following delivery of the baby and placenta constricts the blood vessels that pass between them. These fibers act as ligatures around the blood vessels, a most important factor in control of bleeding from the placental site and control of hemorrhage (Fig. 6-1).

The pregnant uterus increases in its contractility. Contractions of the uterine muscle occur throughout pregnancy. These are very mild at first, but increase in strength, so that later in pregnancy the uterus can be felt to contract when a hand is placed on the abdomen. These irregular painless uterine contractions, termed *Braxton-Hicks* contractions, become more regular toward the end of pregnancy and sometimes become painful (see page 259).

As the uterus increases in size, its shape and position change. From a firm, thick-walled, somewhat flattened body in its nonpregnant state, the gravid uterus assumes a globular outline. After the first few weeks and later, owing to a more rapid increase in length than width, it becomes oval in shape. Enlargement is greatest in the fundus. The uterus begins to rise out of the pelvis to above the symphysis pubis during

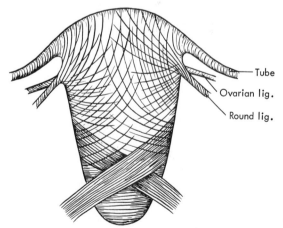

Figure 6-1. Diagram showing interwoven pattern of uterine muscle fibers. [*Reproduced with permission from J. Robert Willson, Clayton T. Beecham, and Elsie Reid Carrington,* Obstetrics and Gynecology, *5th ed. The C. V. Mosby Co., St. Louis, Mo., 1975, p. 224.*]

the third month of pregnancy and continues a steady upward rise into the abdominal cavity as the pregnancy continues. Early in pregnancy, as the body of the uterus becomes larger, the anteflexion normally present in the nonpregnant state increases. As the uterus rises out of the pelvis, slight rotation to the right is common.

As the uterus grows and rises out of the pelvis, it lies against the abdominal wall, displacing the intestines to the sides of the abdomen, especially when the woman is in the upright position. With the upper part of the pregnant uterus lying freely in the abdomen, and the lower portion anchored quite firmly by the cervical connections, it is quite mobile. This permits it to move forward against the abdominal wall when the woman stands up and fall back against the vertebral column when she is in the supine position.

Ligaments

As the uterus rises into the abdominal cavity considerable tension is placed on the broad ligaments and changes take place in the round ligaments. These become hypertrophied and elongated during pregnancy. They help to stabilize the uterus, and, since they lie somewhat anterior to the fundus, tend to keep it close to the abdominal wall. Since the round ligaments are composed principally of smooth muscle extending from the uterus, they contract whenever the uterine muscle contracts. The woman may feel some discomfort during pregnancy from tension on, and contraction of, the round ligaments. Such discomfort is commonly called round ligament pain. During labor, the contraction of these ligaments simultaneously with the uterine muscle may help to pull the uterus forward during each contraction and align its long axis with the birth canal.

Cervix

The cervix also undergoes radical changes during pregnancy. The cervix is composed mainly of connective tissue; only 5 to 10 percent of the cervical tissue in pregnancy is made up of myometrial fibers. The cervical connective tissue is composed of collagenous microfibrils that are mainly responsible for elasticity and resistance to tearing and of ground substance that permits and supports tissue distensibility and stretching. The ground substance acts as the adhesive between fibers of collagenous tissue.

In pregnancy the connective tissue ground substance in the cervix is considerably increased. There is an increase in connective tissue cells in both size and number. The ratio of ground substance to collagenous microfibrils is doubled in pregnancy and the connective tissue becomes looser. This increases the ease with which the cervix can be stretched in pregnancy and aids in cervical dilation during labor. With a normal balance between the ground substance and the microfibrils, the collagen fibers of the cervix, along with the small number of myometrial fibers, will provide adequate cervical support to the products of conception. Occasionally there may be an imbalance, in favor of an excessive amount of ground substance, which leads to cervical insufficiency. This usually becomes apparent between the fourth and sixth month of gestation as described on page 641.

The connective tissue of the cervix becomes edematous in pregnancy. This occurs because estrogens and progesterone, which are greatly increased in pregnancy, increase the water and electrolyte uptake and retention in this tissue. The blood supply to the cervix also increases considerably.

Another cervical change is a marked thickening of the mucous lining and a proliferation of the glands of the endocervix. The cervical glands proliferate so much in pregnancy that they make up almost one half of the cervix by the end of pregnancy. The spaces between the glands become progressively thinner and finally have the appearance of a honeycomb structure, which becomes filled with mucus. This tenacious mucus acts to close the cervical canal during pregnancy. It is called a mucous plug and is expelled when the cervix begins to shorten and dilate during labor.

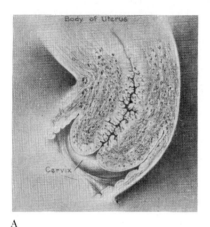 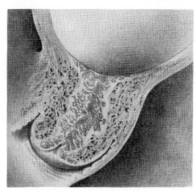

A   B

Figure 6-2. **A.** Cervix in the nonpregnant woman. **B.** Cervix in pregnancy. Note the elaboration of the mucosa into a honeycomblike structure, the meshes of which are filled with a tenacious mucus—the so-called mucous plug. [*Reproduced with permission from Jack A. Pritchard and Paul C. MacDonald,* Williams Obstetrics, *15th ed. Appleton-Century-Crofts, New York, 1975, p. 174.*]

As a result of changes in pregnancy the cervix becomes softer, relatively shorter, more elastic, and larger in its diameter, and its glandular secretion is greatly increased (Fig. 6-2A, B). The softening of the cervix and a bluish color from the increased vascularity are often noticeable very early in pregnancy and are used as presumptive signs of pregnancy.

Ovaries and Tubes

The fallopian tubes and ovaries show changes in their position during pregnancy. They are carried up by the enlarging uterus from the pelvis into the abdominal cavity, and, owing to the traction, their long axis becomes nearly vertical instead of at right angles to the uterus. Because the enlargement of the uterus is more marked in the fundus, the tubes and the ovarian ligaments appear to be attached more nearly to the middle of the uterus during pregnancy than in its nonpregnant state. There is a great increase in vascularity in these organs. Ovulation does not occur during pregnancy; the follicles which begin to develop undergo atretic changes. Usually there is only one large corpus luteum of pregnancy present in one of the ovaries.

Vagina

The changes in the vagina are chiefly due to increased vascularity. The blood vessels actually become larger. This change causes the normal pinkish tint of the mucous lining of the vagina to deepen to red or even purple, the deepest color being termed *Chadwick's sign*. To prepare the vaginal wall for the distention it must undergo during delivery, certain other changes take place. The mucosa increases in thickness, hypertrophy of the muscles takes place, and the connective tissue becomes looser.

Vaginal discharge, arising from the cervical glands, is more profuse. It is thick, white, and of a crumbly consistency. It has a strong acid reaction due to lactic acid which, it is believed, helps to keep the vagina relatively free of pathogenic bacteria.

Perineum

The perineal tissues show changes similar to those of the vagina—increased vascularity, hypertrophy of the skin and muscles, and loosening of the connective tissues.

CHANGES IN THE BREASTS

Marked changes take place in the breasts during pregnancy due to development of quiescent glandular tissue. The breasts increase in size and firmness and become nodular. Striations of the skin often appear. Enlargement is noticeable within weeks after conception and continues throughout gestation. There is also a considerable increase in vascularity of the breasts early in pregnancy and the superficial veins grow more prominent. These changes are often accompanied by a feeling of tenderness, tingling, and heaviness of the breasts early in pregnancy and are considered presumptive signs of pregnancy.

The nipples and the surrounding areolae be-

come larger and more prominent and their color becomes darker in pregnancy. The nipples become more mobile and will be easier for the baby to grasp for nursing. The glands of Montgomery enlarge.

There is a wide range of individual difference in the increase in breast size, but the average increase will be about 700 gm (1½ lb) for each breast.

Considerable alteration takes place within the breast tissue itself: (1) there is proliferation of the glandular tissue, and (2) the alveolar cells become differentiated so that they become secretory (see Fig. 6-3). As the proliferative changes take place the ducts within the breasts lengthen and branch to many times their prepregnancy size. Alveoli and lobules develop at

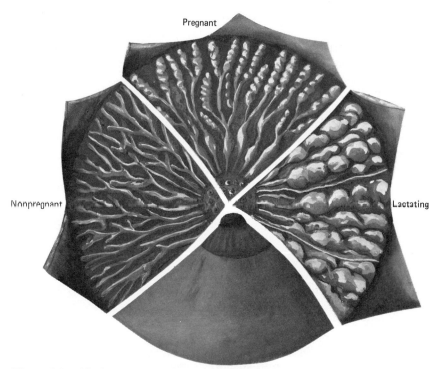

Figure 6-3. The breast in pregnancy and lactation. There is progressive proliferation of glandular tissue during pregnancy. Ducts lengthen and branch extensively, and alveoli and lobules develop at the tips of many of the branches. With increasing secretory activity toward the end of pregnancy the alveoli and ducts become distended with colostrum. In the lactating breast the alveoli and ducts are distended with milk.

the tips of many of the branches until finally there is a large compound gland in each breast with many lobules and alveoli (Fig. 19-3A, page 518).

After a certain stage of proliferation of glandular tissue during the first trimester, the alveolar cells begin to differentiate in the second trimester. Many of these cells will become secretory and able to secrete milk. By the end of the second trimester a small amount of thin yellowish fluid, called *colostrum*, is secreted into the ducts.

Enlargement of the breasts continues for the remainder of pregnancy due to a combination of ongoing proliferation of cells and an increasing amount of secretion from the alveolar cells as they advance in their development. By the time of delivery a considerable amount of colostrum fills the alveoli, ducts, and ampullae.

Near to the time of term delivery, growth and development of the breasts is close to maximum. The alveoli and ducts are distended with

colostrum and the alveoli are ready to secrete milk. The circulatory bed is enlarged and the blood flow is increasing, ready to bring a good supply of hormones and milk precursors to the glandular tissue. The glands are functionally ready, but secretion is inhibited, presumably by the high level of progesterone in pregnancy and by the lack of stimulation. Hormonal changes take place as soon as the baby is born and milk secretion will begin in a few days. In the event of a premature birth, the breasts will be sufficiently developed to take on the function of lactation a few weeks early.

Breast development in pregnancy is under the control of hormones, which include ovarian and placental hormones: estrogen and progesterone; anterior pituitary hormones; somatotropin, prolactin, and adrenocorticotropin; and insulin. As the placenta develops it provides the estrogens and progesterone which were secreted by the ovaries earlier in pregnancy. In addition, a placental hormone, called human

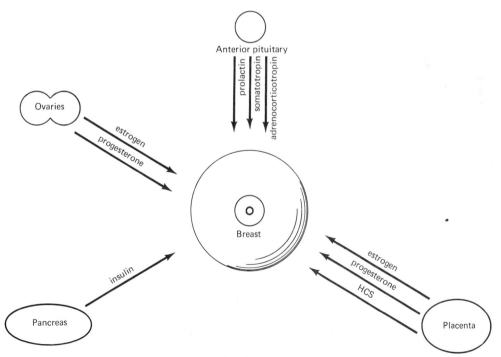

Figure 6-4.   Hormonal influence on breast development in pregnancy.

chorionic somatomammotropin (HCS), assists in preparation for milk secretion (Fig. 6-4). The placental hormones are discussed in more detail below.

Growth of the breasts is greater in a first pregnancy than in subsequent ones, because they start with less development. Regression of breast development after delivery or after a period of lactation is not entirely back to the original prepregnancy state, and therefore growth is not as great in subsequent pregnancies. Some additional mammary development does take place, however, in a second and probably also in the third pregnancy.

CHANGES IN THE ABDOMEN

The abdomen changes in contour as the enlarging uterus extends into the abdominal cavity, filling it more and more, until the baby within the uterus lies completely within the abdominal cavity (Figs. 6-5 and 6-6). The abdominal muscles support much of the weight of the baby.

Toward the end of pregnancy the fundus of the uterus has risen so that it puts pressure against the diaphragm. The upper abdominal organs are crowded into the upper part of the abdominal cavity, and the intestines lie above, behind, and to the sides of the uterus (Fig. 6-6).

During the latter part of pregnancy, irregular, wavy, slightly depressed streaks or striations frequently develop in the skin of the abdomen and sometimes also in the skin of the breasts, hips, and upper part of the thighs. These striations are termed *striae gravidarum*. Fresh striae are pale pink or bluish in color. After delivery they take on the silvery, glistening appearance of scar tissue. In a woman who has borne children there may be both new and old striae, those resulting from former pregnancies are silvery and shining and are termed *striae albicantes*, while the fresh striae are pink or blue.

Two factors are involved in the formation of striae and it appears that both factors need to be present. The skin is primed for separation of its collagen fibers by hormones of pregnancy, and

the primed skin then gets tension (stretch) placed on it by the enlarging uterus.

Estrogens, corticosteroids, and relaxin, hormones that are formed in increasing amounts in pregnancy, produce changes in the connective tissue of the skin. Under this hormonal influence the cohesive force between the collagen fibers of the skin relaxes, allowing the fibers to separate easily. When the primed skin is subjected to stretching some of the collagen fibers pull apart, resulting in a thinning of the skin (striae), which appear pinkish or bluish depending on the vascular bed.

Striae develop in areas of maximum stretch: the abdomen, breasts, and thighs. Subcutaneous fat increases in pregnancy and stretches the skin above it. Considerable weight gain in pregnancy, obesity from the beginning of pregnancy, unusual stretching of the abdominal skin, and fluid retention and generalized edema are all likely to increase stretching of the skin. Some women are much more susceptible than others to separation of the connective tissue of the skin; thus some women have many striae and others with a similar amount of stretching have few or none.

Abdominal striae in nonpregnant women may occasionally be associated with abdominal distention, a marked increase in fat, or an abdominal tumor. Those on the hips and thighs may be due to normal postpubertal changes.

The abdominal distention with pregnancy sometimes causes a separation of the recti muscles. This separation, known as *diastasis*, is sometimes slight but occasionally very marked. The space between the muscles is easily felt through the thinned abdominal wall.

The umbilicus is deeply indented during about the first three months of pregnancy, then grows steadily shallower, and becomes level with the surface, or it may protrude.

CHANGES IN THE ENDOCRINE GLANDS

A large number of the physiologic changes that take place in pregnancy are attributed to

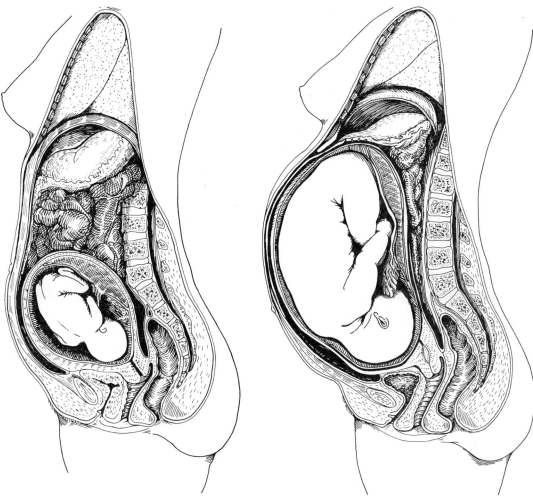

Figure 6-5. A semidiagrammatic drawing of the abdominal cavity of a woman as seen from the left at the end of the fifth lunar month of pregnancy. [*Adapted with permission from* Charts of Relation of Growing Uterus to Other Organs. *Maternity Center Association, New York, 1963, Plate 2.*]

Figure 6-6. A semidiagrammatic drawing of the abdominal cavity of a woman as seen from the left at the end of the ninth lunar month of pregnancy. [*Adapted with permission from* Charts of Relation of Growing Uterus to Other Organs. *Maternity Center Association, New York, 1963, Plate 3.*]

the endocrine glands. Secretions from most of these glands—the pituitary, thyroid, adrenal, and others—is altered in pregnancy, and often there is an increasing amount of hormone production. In addition, the placenta serves as an endocrine organ. It produces several hormones, some of which are present only in pregnancy. The physiologic purpose of this large increase in most of the hormones in maintenance of the pregnancy, in metabolic homeostasis, and perhaps in many other important functions is as yet not clear in many respects.

The Placental Hormones

Some of the most important endocrine changes of pregnancy are those brought about by the development of the placenta. The placental hormones are produced by the trophoblasts, beginning early in pregnancy and generally continuing in ever increasing amounts as the placenta grows. Two categories of hormones, protein hormones and steroid hormones, are manufactured. The protein hormones, chorionic gonadotropin, chorionic somatomammotropin, and chorionic thyrotropin are substances present only in pregnancy, playing a specific role during gestation and then disappearing with separation of the placenta. These hormones may be considered analogues of pituitary hormones. The steriod hormones, estrogen and progesterone, are ordinarily present in mature nonpregnant women, being produced by the ovaries, but they are also synthesized by the placenta in much larger amounts during the course of pregnancy. Production of these steroids by the placenta relies on precursors derived from the fetal and maternal circulations.

Placental hormones are released into both the maternal and the fetal circulation by way of the intervillous space and the umbilical vein. Hormonal levels of each of the hormones in the fetal circulation may be very small or may be unknown. The hormones are also released into the amniotic fluid in small amounts.

Human Chorionic Gonadotropin

Human chorionic gonadotropin (HCG) is a hormone of pregnancy produced by the trophoblastic cells. It has many similarities to luteinizing hormone. It appears very early in pregnancy and continues to be secreted into the maternal circulation; some of it is excreted in the urine. The urinary excretion level reflects the serum concentration.

By sensitive radioimmunoassay methods of examination HCG has been detected in the serum as early as 8 days after ovulation and only 1 day after implantation. With conventional, less sensitive, testing HCG is first detectable in the urine at about 26 days after conception, which corresponds to approximately six weeks after the onset of the last menstrual period. There is then a rapid increase with a peak concentration at 60 to 70 days of pregnancy. Thereafter the concentration falls, reaching a lower level of about one third of the peak, between 100 and 130 days of gestation. It then rises slowly again until the end of pregnancy but does not reach the earlier peak level (Fig. 6-7). The hormone disappears rapidly, within three to four days, after delivery.

A major physiologic role of chorionic gonadotropin appears to be maintenance of the corpus luteum during early pregnancy when the corpus luteum is thought to be essential to the pregnancy. By maintaining the corpus luteum and keeping it from degenerating at the end of its usual active span, production of progesterone and maintenance of the endometrium for implantation and early development of the zygote is assured. It serves until placental production of progesterone is sufficient to maintain the pregnancy and prevent separation of the decidua (see Figure 2-7, page 35).

Chorionic gonadotropin is the pregnancy hormone that is the basis for any of the biologic or immunochemical pregnancy tests, described on pages 162–64.

Human Chorionic Somatomammotropin

Human chorionic somatomammotropin (HCS), discovered in the early 1960s, is a protein hormone synthesized by placental trophoblasts. Since it has both strong lactogenic properties and a resemblance to pituitary growth hormone it was first called human placental lactogen (HPL) or chorionic growth hormone-prolactin (CGP). More recently the term human chorionic somatomammotropin (HCS) has been used, since that term emphasizes its two major influences, as derived from animal studies— stimulation of growth and lactation.

HCS is detectable in minimal amounts in the serum of pregnant women by one to two weeks after implantation. Serum levels of the hormone rise steadily, keeping pace with placental growth, and reach a high concentration in late pregnancy (Fig. 6-7). Fetal serum levels are very small compared to maternal. The half-life of HCS is very short, so production must be great and blood levels should closely reflect the rate of production. Serial determinations of blood levels of HCS are sometimes used as one means of monitoring placental function and fetal well-being. HCS disappears very rapidly after separation of the placenta.

HCS appears to be an important metabolic hormone of pregnancy, affecting carbohydrate and fat metabolism so as to assure a good supply of nutrients for the fetus. It has two opposing effects on carbohydrate metabolism, promoting secretion of insulin and also antagonizing the insulin, diminishing its peripheral effectiveness. This tends to raise the blood sugar and contribute to a diabetogenic state in pregnancy. HCS induces mobilization of free fatty acids. This action appears to favor growth of the fetus by providing the mother with a source of energy that decreases her utilization of carbohydrates and

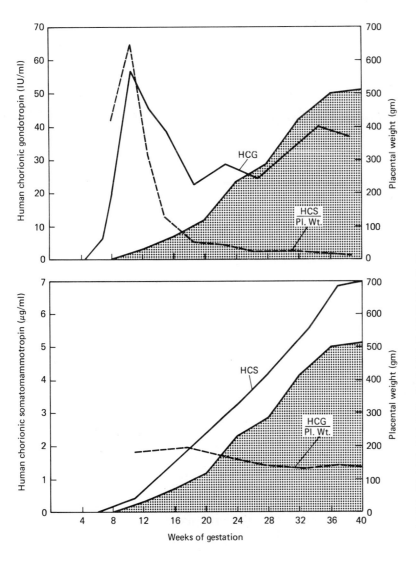

Figure 6-7. Changes in serum levels of HCG and HCS, two placental protein hormones, show marked differences during pregnancy. Drop in production of HCG after early-pregnancy peak, emphasized by ratio of hormone levels to placental weight, is masked and compensated by placental growth. In contrast, rise in HCS levels almost keeps pace with placental growth, with ratio remaining relatively constant until delivery. [*Reproduced with permission from Robert B. Jaffe, "Endocrine Interactions and the Placenta,"* Hosp. Pract. *6(12):71–82 (Dec.) 1971.*]

increases glucose availability to the fetus. HCS also has some effect on protein metabolism, reducing the mother's use of breakdown products and enhancing amino acid availability to the fetus.

HCS influences breast growth and development in pregnancy, thus assisting in preparation for milk secretion, but actual latogenic properties have not been demonstrated in humans. The hormone has disappeared from the circulation by the time lactation begins. HCS may also stimulate the acromegaloid changes, or coarsening in features, that some women develop in pregnancy.

Human Chorionic Thyrotropin

The most recently described protein placental hormone is human chorionic thyrotropin (HCT). The exact structure and the determination of maternal serum levels of the hormone remain to be defined, but it appears to have thyrotropic properties, with some similarity to pituitary thyroid-stimulating hormone.

The physiologic role of HCT is not known. It may play a role in the thryoid function changes observed in pregnancy, such as enlargement of the thryoid gland and increase in maternal thryoid activity.

The same protein hormones, HCG, HCS, and HCT, that are secreted in normal pregnancy appear to be elaborated by all varieties of trophoblastic tissue. They are not restricted to trophoblasts and have been found in certain malignancies.

Progesterone

The placenta produces a very large amount of progesterone during normal pregnancy. The level of progesterone in the plasma and in urinary excretion as pregnanediol, the main metabolite of progesterone, increases steadily during gestation (Fig. 6-8). Only a very small amount of the total production of progesterone comes from the ovary after the first few weeks of pregnancy. In the first several weeks of gestation progesterone from the corpus luteum may be vital to maintenance of the pregnancy. Between six and nine weeks of gestation placental production takes over and becomes the main source of this hormone. Thereafter the corpus luteum appears to have little further influence on the successful course of pregnancy.

Production of progesterone is apparently brought about by placental utilization of precursors from both the mother and the fetus, but synthesis of progesterone does not seem to be as intimately associated with the well-being of the fetus as is the production of estrogens, described below.

Progesterone, generally regarded as the hormone that preserves pregnancy, is responsible for some of the characteristic changes of pregnancy.

Under the influence of progesterone, in the second half of the menstrual cycle, the endometrium is changed from proliferative to secretory, the stroma becomes edematous, and the glycogen content of the endometrial cells increases. With these changes the endometrium is ready for implantation and nourishment of the blastocyst.

A major function of progesterone during pregnancy is believed to be its quieting effect on uterine myometrial contractions. By reducing muscle tone in the uterus and decreasing the inherent contractility of the muscle, the blastocyst is allowed to implant and develop, and it is protected against expulsion by uterine myometrial activity. Administration of progesterone to women with uterine contractions in early pregnancy with a threatened abortion or at any other stage of pregnancy is not advised, however, unless a deficiency in progesterone production can be demonstrated. Although the progesterone theoretically decreases uterine contractions, there is no good evidence that it has been useful in treating threatened abortion, and there is concern that it may harmfully decrease uterine blood flow. Administration of progesterone may also adversely affect fetal development.

Progesterone is believed to have a relaxing effect on smooth muscles in several other parts of the body in pregnancy. Poor muscle tone might

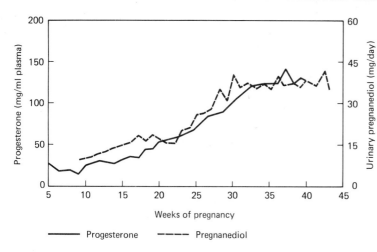

Figure 6-8. Progesterone production during pregnancy can be monitored directly by measuring serum levels of the hormone. However, it can be followed more easily through measurements of its excreted end-product, pregnanediol; the similar shape of the two curves suggests that they are measuring the same basic phenomenon. The data for the pregnanediol curve are from multigravidas. [*Reproduced with permission from Robert B. Jaffe, "Endocrine Interactions and the Placenta,"* Hosp. Pract. *6(12):71–82 (Dec.) 1971.*]

explain slow emptying of the stomach, regurgitation and heartburn, and constipation, all common occurrences in pregnancy. Similarly, the relaxation and dilatation of the ureters in pregnancy may be an effect of progesterone.

Progesterone is believed to have an influence on the central nervous system that results in a listless, sleepy feeling which makes concentration on work difficult. This is a common complaint of women in early pregnancy. There is evidence that progesterone induces hyperventilation in pregnancy, which reduces alveolar and arterial P_{CO_2} This effect may be brought about by a progesterone influence on the respiratory center.

The large amount of progesterone in pregnancy appears to have a number of metabolic effects. The reason for many of these influences are obscure and most of them have not been fully explored. There is a suggestion that the considerably large amount of fat the mother stores in pregnancy may be governed by progesterone. This hormone may also influence the rate of protein catabolism and the lowering of amino acids in the plasma. Progesterone influences fluid and electrolyte homeostasis in pregnancy. It enhances sodium and chloride excretion in pregnancy, which then results in a compensatory rise in aldosterone to overcome the effects of progesterone and prevent a dangerous sodium loss. Another general metabolic

effect is the rise in basal body temperature after ovulation in each normal menstrual cycle. If conception occurs, the elevated temperature of 0.4 to 0.6°C is maintained until midpregnancy when it returns to normal.

Progesterone, along with estrogen and other hormones, is responsible for growth of the breasts; progesterone is thought to be necessary for alveolar development.

Progesterone action often appears to be combined with the estrogens or it may be modified by the estrogens, which have an opposing influence and probably balance its action. An example of combined action is the influence of both hormones on breast development. The quieting effect of progesterone on the myometrium as opposed to the enhancement of uterine muscular activity by estrogen is an example of opposing hormonal influence with a balancing of action. The large amount of progesterone production in pregnancy also influences other hormone production, sometimes being matched by large amounts of other hormones, as, for example, by secretion of aldosterone in large amounts.

Estrogens

In the mature, nonpregnant woman estrogens are produced cyclically by the ovary. In pregnancy the principal source of an ever increasing level of estrogens in the body is the placenta.

The ovary does not appear to be an important source of estrogens after the first few weeks of pregnancy. In nonpregnant women the ratio of urinary estriol to estrone plus estradiol is about equal. In pregnancy there is a very large increase in the ratio of estriol to the other estrogens. This disproportionate rise in estriol excretion in pregnancy is from a second independent pathway for estriol biosynthesis— the placenta.

Production of estrogens in the placenta is different than in the ovary in that its biosynthesis depends primarily on an increasing supply of a steroid precursor that is produced mainly by the fetal adrenals. Enzyme systems necessary for the production of estrogens are present in the fetal liver and the fetal adrenal glands and in the placenta.

The estrogen precursor from the fetal adrenal goes to the fetal liver where it is hydroxylated. From there it passes to the placenta where it is changed by an enzyme and converted to estriol. Some of the precursor from the fetal adrenal also goes directly to the placenta and is converted to estrone and estradiol. The placenta also receives a precursor from the maternal adrenal, which accounts for about 10 percent of the estrogens excreted in late pregnancy. All the other precursors needed arise in the fetal adre-nal. Estrogens formed in the placenta are secreted into the maternal circulation, and before excretion in the urine they are conjugated in the maternal liver (Fig. 6-9).

It is apparent that there is considerable interdependence between the fetus and the placenta in the production of estrogens. The production and excretion of the hormone is dependent on the integrity of the fetal adrenal, the fetal pituitary gland which appears responsible for development of the fetal adrenal, the fetal liver, and the placenta, and excretion in the mother's urine involves prior conjugation in the maternal liver.

Placental production of estrogens, largely estriol, is high. This is reflected in maternal urinary estriol excretion, which rises progressively in pregnancy. The tremendous rise in estrogen production in pregnancy reflects increasing production of precursors by the fetal adrenals. The fetal adrenal glands grow rapidly and by four months of fetal life have reached a size that is larger than the fetal kidneys. The glands are very active in steroid metabolism, providing the hormonal precursors to the placenta for estrogen and progesterone production. The fetal adrenals rapidly decrease in size as full-term growth is approached and continue a rapid involution after birth.

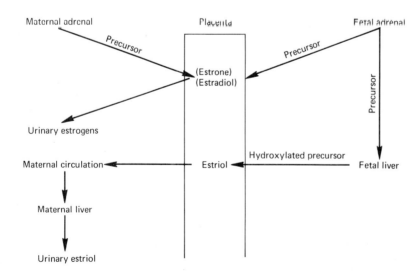

Figure 6-9. Simplified scheme of biosynthesis of placental estrogens in pregnancy.

Urinary excretion of estriol rises slowly until about the twelfth week of gestation and then increases more rapidly in a steady upward curve (Fig. 21-2, page 615). Since estriol originates predominantly in the fetal–placenta unit and adequate function of both fetus and placenta are necessary for its production, measurement of maternal urinary estriol level may be used as one clinical index of the condition of the fetus and the placenta. A single measurement of urinary estriol excretion does not accurately reflect the status of the fetal–placental unit because variations in estriol production occur normally from day to day, but daily or several times weekly readings are valuable. Serial measurements are necessary with the expectation that there will be fluctuations in values, but the trend will constantly be upward. Falling values of 50 percent or more would indicate fetal–placental impairment. Use of estriol studies as one measure of assessment of fetal status in high-risk pregnancies is described on pages 614–15.

Many phenomena of pregnancy have been attributed to estrogens, but clear evidence of their action on many processes, at least in the human, is lacking. Many of the functions attributed to estrogens seem to be combined with progesterone action. It seems that the two hormones may exert an influence on a number of processes, such as development of the uterus and the breasts, at different stages in the development of these organs, and that both hormones are necessary for their adequate function. Also estrogens often appear to oppose the influence of progesterone and thus balance the end result.

It is generally believed that a major role of estrogens is control of growth and function of the uterus. After implantation of the blastocyst, estrogen brings about the hyperplasia and hypertrophy of the uterine muscle that permits the growth of the uterus that is necessary to accommodate the growing fetus. Estrogens also have the effect of enhancing the activity of the myometrium, the opposite effect of progesterone. Estrogens bring about vasodilation of the myometrium, important to good uterine blood flow.

Paradoxically, progesterone appears to constrict arterioles. A proper ratio, of some unknown quantity, of estrogen to progesterone appears to be important to uterine muscle tone and to uterine blood flow.

Estrogens may have a softening effect on the substance between the fibers of collagen tissues of the cervix and thus permits easy stretching of the cervix in late pregnancy. Changes in connective tissue may also bring about the increased mobility of the nipples of the breasts that occurs in pregnancy, and also permit striae (stretch marks) in the skin to develop over several parts of the body.

Estrogen, along with progesterone, is important to development of the breasts, with estrogen believed to be responsible for development of the alveolar ducts.

Estrogen has an influence on the respiratory center. It seems that, while progesterone lowers the threshold of the respiratory center to carbon dioxide, estrogen increases the sensitivity of the center.

A number of generalized metabolic effects are attributed to the influence of estrogens, at least in part. Estrogens appear to be responsible for some of the changes in the blood picture in pregnancy. The fall in total plasma proteins, mostly in serum albumin; the increase in a variety of serum-binding proteins, which bind with increased hormones of other glands such as the thyroid; the rise in fibrinogen concentration; and the characteristic leukocytosis of pregnancy are attributed to estrogen influence.

Changes in a number of other endocrine glands in pregnancy occur as a result of estrogens.

In closing this discussion on placental hormones it can be said that much has been learned in recent years about the biochemistry of many of the hormones and also of some of their biologic actions, some of this from animal studies. Conclusions from animal evidence, cannot, however, be easily transferred to the human. Thus many important questions remain concerning placental hormones. The physiologic function of the large amount of hormones is as yet not clearly understood in such important aspects of pregnancy as control of uterine muscle contractions and uterine blood flow, action in onset and control of labor, influence on general metabolic function, and maintenance of electrolyte balance.

Although the fetus is intimately involved in production of the placental hormones, very little is known about their role in fetal development.

The existence of more placental hormones, in addition to those described above, has been suggested, and others may yet be discovered.

The Thyroid Gland

The thyroid gland shows increased vascularity, hyperplasia, and a tendency to moderate enlargement in pregnancy, and the serum concentration of thyroid hormones, thyroxine (T_4) and triiodothyronine (T_3), is increased during gestation. Changes in thyroid function in pregnancy suggest hyperthyroidism, but in actuality thyroid hormone activity remains normal, and the normal pregnant woman remains euthyroid.

In pregnancy the general picture of thyroid activity is modified by the hormones of pregnancy. Estrogens increase the thyroid-binding globulin in the blood by a considerable amount and progesterone is associated with a low level of arterial Po_2, which in turn is associated with a low level of free hormone. As thyroid hormone is released from the thyroid gland into the plasma, most of it is bound to a thyroid-binding globulin and becomes inactive. It then acts as a storage source for ready availability. The free or unbound circulating hormone, the metabolically active hormone, is not increased above nonpregnant normal values. Thus in pregnancy the total amount of hormone is increased, but the free amount is normal, remaining relatively constant, and the peripheral thyroid activity remains normal.

The usual clinical criteria of hyperthyroidism can be misleading in pregnancy and interpretation of thyroid function tests is difficult. There is a rise in BMR of 15 to 20 percent in pregnancy, but most of this increase in oxygen consumption is due to metabolic activity of the fetus and the increased maternal tissues. A rapid pulse and warm skin are normal pregnancy changes. The bound thyroid hormone, measured as protein-bound iodine (PBI), or in other tests that measure bound hormone, show increased levels in pregnancy, similar to levels in hyperthyroidism, but these values do not reflect the free hormone level in the same way as they do in the nonpregnant state. The only useful test of thyroid function in pregnancy is one that ascertains the amount of free hormone by determining the free thyroxine concentration (FT_4) in the serum or by calculation of the free thyroxine index (FTI) of the serum.

Available evidence suggests that thyroxine (T_4) crosses the placenta but does so with some difficulty. Crossing-over may change with duration of pregnancy and with aging of the placenta, but exact changes are not clear.

Radioactive iodine is not used in pregnancy for studying thyroid function through measurement of uptake in the thyroid gland, or for treatment of hyperthyroidism, because of its radiation effects, particularly to the fetus. Iodine quickly crosses the placenta. The fetal thyroid gland has a very special affinity for iodine. It readily takes up the iodine and concentrates it in the gland in large amounts beginning as early as the twelfth week of gestation.

When antithyroid drugs must be used for treatment of hyperthyroidism, the mother is closely monitored by frequent thyroid function studies to keep the drug used at an optimal level, one that keeps her at an upper range of normal values. Antithyroid drugs cross the placenta and they have the potential of adversely affecting fetal thyroid function, inducing fetal hypothyroidism and causing goiter in the fetus. When drugs have been used to treat the mother, the infant is closely monitored for both early and delayed signs of drug influence.

The Parathyroid Glands

Parathyroid hyperplasia occurs during pregnancy, suggesting increased hormone production. The reason for such increased function is not clear. Parathyroid hormone has an important function in calcium metabolism, and it has been hypothesized that the hyperparathyroidism occurs as a physiologic response to the demands of the growing fetus on maternal calcium stores.

The Adrenal Glands

The blood levels of cortisol (free and bound) and of aldosterone are considerably increased in pregnancy, and there are major changes in their metabolism. Plasma levels of cortisol rise progressively. An increase in the plasma level of cortisol-binding globulin results in a considerable increase in the circulating level of bound cortisol, but there is also a rise in free cortisol (the metabolically active hormone), approaching two to three times normal. There appears to be evidence that the increase in cortisol in pregnancy may be the result of a slowed rate of metabolism and prolonged half-life of the hormone as well as, or instead of, increased production.

The clinical effects of increased plasma cortisol are uncertain but appear to show some evidence of mild adrenocortisol hyperfunction. Maternal carbohydrate metabolism may be affected by the increased level of cortisol, which induces mobilization of protein and fat when food carbohydrate is not available. It increases the synthesis of glucose by the liver from the amino acids that become available and thus contributes to the tendency of hyperglycemia in pregnancy.

In addition to the effect on glucose metabolism, the adrenocortical hyperactivity is thought to be one of the predisposing factors in the development of striae in the skin, the stretch marks of pregnancy. It is also thought that increased cortisol may suppress inflammatory reactions in pregnancy.

Another hormone of the adrenal glands, aldosterone, is greatly increased in pregnancy. It is secreted in response to the threat of sodium loss, which is promoted by progesterone and increased glomerular filtration. Aldosterone secretion increases as necessary to maintain sodium balance as described on page 142.

Prostaglandins (PGs)

Prostaglandin is a generic term for a number of closely related fatty acid derivatives of prostanoic acid. The different members of the groups of prostaglandins are designated by letters, numbers, and Greek letters as, for example, PGE_2 and $PGF_{2\alpha}$. PGs are widely distributed in the body, and they have a great variety of actions. Some of these actions are of special interest to reproductive physiology, and some of their biologic activity is related to many nonreproductive physiologic mechanisms.

Prostaglandins were originally isolated from seminal fluid, which has a high concentration of these substances, but they are now known to be widely distributed in all tissues of the body including lungs, kidneys, brain, and reproductive organs. They occur in amniotic fluid, decidua, and in umbilical and placental vessels. The uterine endometrium and myometrium produces PGs and the placenta probably does also.

PGs have a potent stimulating effect on the contractility of the myometrium at any stage of pregnancy. A finding of a greater amount of PGs in amniotic fluid in women in labor than otherwise suggests a relationship of these agents to spontaneous abortion and spontaneous labor. They have been used for induction of labor, but whether they are safe or superior to oxytocin has not been determined. Uterine contractions sometimes have episodes of incoordination and hypertonic action with the use of prostaglandins.

Administration of PGs is associated with a number of side effects of which frequent episodes of vomiting and diarrhea are very distressing. Currently, use of PGs for termination of pregnancy in the second trimester seems to be a reasonable alternative to other methods. There is an ongoing search for a compound that will have fewer disadvantages than those named above when it is used clinically.

Pituitary Prolactin

Prolactin has only recently been identified as a separate pituitary hormone—separate from human growth hormone, which has some pro-lactin-like activity.

Prolactin has many known functions in birds and mammals, but at present the only certain action in humans is its role in initiation of lactation and possibly maintenance of breast milk secretion. Its action also apparently influences the considerable breast growth and development of the alveolar system that takes place in pregnancy, possibly in conjunction with chorionic somatomammotropin.

An increased level of prolactin is first observed in pregnancy at about eight weeks gestation. There is then a steady rise of prolactin to a maximum by the end of pregnancy, reaching a mean level of 200 ng/100 ml. The normal serum prolactin level is below 20 ng/ml.

If the level of prolactin alone was the stimulating factor for lactation it could be expected that the rise in prolactin in pregnancy would result in lactation. There is reason to believe that the high level of steroid hormones in pregnancy, especially progesterone, block prolactin action until these hormones decrease post delivery. By the time breast engorgement occurs in the postpartum period the level of prolactin has already decreased to one half the concentration it was at the time of delivery.

In women who do not nurse their babies, serum levels of prolactin are back to about pre-pregnancy levels in three weeks. In women who do nurse, prolactin levels also decrease and reach about 20 ng/ml in four weeks, but each sucking stimulus produces large transient increases within 15 to 30 minutes, which again fall back to baseline in about the same length of time. After three to four months nursing the baby no longer produces the transient increases. The level of prolactin apparently does not need to be elevated for lactation to continue after it is well established.

Amniotic fluid contains a very high concentration of prolactin and high levels are also found in the newborn. The possible role of prolactin in the life of the fetus and the newborn is not known.

CHANGES IN THE CARDIOVASCULAR SYSTEM

Some of the most significant and extensive adaptations in maternal physiology during pregnancy occur in the cardiovascular system. Circulatory system adjustments are important to both mother and fetus. They protect the mother's normal functions by adapting her body to the demands of pregnancy, performing a major function in meeting her metabolic needs. They provide for adequate fetal growth and development by assuring efficient delivery of nutrients and removal of wastes. The cause of the altered circulation in pregnancy is obscure and may be multifactorial. At present, it seems reasonable to suppose that the dramatic changes in hormonal production in early pregnancy play an important part in bringing about circulatory adaptations.

Blood Volume—Plasma and Erythrocytes

The maternal blood volume increases considerably in pregnancy. It begins to expand by the tenth to twelfth week of gestation, reaches a maximum volume over nonpregnant levels by 32 to 34 weeks of pregnancy, and then plateaus and remains constant until delivery. Blood volume returns to the nonpregnant level within two to three weeks after delivery (Fig. 6-10).

The increase in total blood volume during pregnancy averages 30 to 40 percent, but the range is wide and varies from only a moderate amount to nearly a double volume in different individuals. The increase in amount of blood in the body is between 1 and 1½ liters. This hypervolemia of pregnancy serves to fill the greatly enlarged vascular system of the uterus and the expanded venous capacity of the legs. It meets the demands of the pregnant uterus and helps to protect the mother and the fetus against the poor venous return from the lower extremities that is common in pregnancy.

The increase in blood volume during pregnancy results from an increase in both plasma and erythrocyte volumes, but the increase in plasma volume is greater than that of the red cell mass (Fig. 6-10). Although there is considerable increase in erythrocyte production during pregnancy (an average increase of 250 to 450 ml of red blood cells, depending upon the amount of iron available), the disproportionate increase in plasma volume leads to a decrease in hemoglobin and erythrocyte concentrations and thus a fall in hematocrit value during pregnancy.

The above changes in the blood picture in pregnancy have often been called "physiologic anemia of pregnancy." This is an erroneous statement, since the physiologic blood changes do not result in a true anemia. Anemia may, however, be present during pregnancy from another cause, usually iron deficiency. There does seem to be some increased liability to iron-deficiency anemia during pregnancy and it must be considered when hematocrit value, hemoglobin level, and erythrocyte count fall below the minimum levels of normal.

An anemia, rather than a change due to increased blood volume, is suggested when the hematocrit value is less than 34 percent, or the hemoglobin level drops below 11 gm/100 ml of blood, or the red blood cell count is less than 3,750,000/ml blood. Medicinal iron is administered prophylactically to meet the demand for iron that is created by the increased erythropoiesis or it is started at the appearance of ane-mia. Iron administration will increase the likelihood of the pregnant woman having a normal level of hemoglobin and erythrocytes at the end of pregnancy. Iron requirements in pregnancy are discussed on page 183.

Cardiac Output

Cardiac output, the volume of blood distributed by the heart to the body per minute, increases tremendously during pregnancy. This rise in cardiac output is important not only in meeting the demands of the enlarging uterus and growing placenta, but also that of other organs with increased functions, as, for example, the kidneys. It has generally been understood that a peak in the resting cardiac output of 30 to 35 percent over nonpregnant levels is reached at 30 to 32 weeks gestation, after which the cardiac output remains at a plateau for the remainder of pregnancy and then returns to nonpregnant levels within the first six weeks after delivery. Increase in cardiac output during pregnancy would then progress at approximately the same rate as increase in blood volume (Fig. 6-10).

Information has been accumulating that strongly suggests that the increase in cardiac output in pregnancy is much faster than stated above and that it reaches a maximum early in pregnancy. Frank E. Hytten and Isabella Leitch

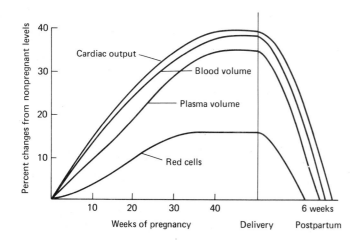

Figure 6-10. Changes in blood volume, plasma volume, red cell volume, and cardiac output during pregnancy and in the puerperium. The curves were constructed from various reports in the literature. They serve to illustrate the trend of changes rather than absolute values. [*Reproduced with permission from Nicholas S. Assali (ed.)*, Pathophysiology of Gestation, *Vol. I.* Maternal Disorders. *Academic Press, New York, 1972, p. 280.*]

state: "A wholly satisfactory study has yet to be made. . . . Yet the circumstantial evidence is strong that for the normal pregnant woman at rest, but not lying on her back, cardiac output rises within the first ten weeks of pregnancy by about 1.5 litre per minute and that rise is maintained for the remainder of the pregnancy." [1]

The increase in cardiac output during pregnancy is brought about by both an increase in the heart rate and in stroke volume, that volume of blood that is expelled from the left ventricle with each beat.

Increased cardiac output during pregnancy imposes an increased work load on the mother's heart. Since this work load is proportional to the cardiac output and the mean arterial blood pressure, which is altered very little during pregnancy, the basal work of the heart will have increased 30 to 35 percent by the beginning of the second trimester of pregnancy.

Added to the increase in basal work load is the additional work of physical activity, since the pregnant woman's activity demands more work of the heart than does the identical activity performed by the nonpregnant woman, especially as pregnancy advances and maternal weight increases. The normal heart of a healthy mother is not affected by this additional work load, but if the pregnant woman has heart disease, the added work may cause cardiac complications, especially between the twenty-eighth and thirty-fifth weeks of gestation, when blood volume reaches its peak and cardiac load reaches a high level.

During labor and delivery and the immediate puerperium, there are sudden changes in hemodynamics. Cardiac output is difficult to study during labor but is known to increase. Up to 300 ml of blood is expelled from the uterus with each uterine contraction, temporarily increasing systemic blood volume and raising cardiac output. There is a definite but lesser increase in

cardiac output during labor in the intervals between contractions.

Immediately after delivery there is also a rise, at least transient, in cardiac output, as the contracted uterus expels blood from the uterine vessels into the systemic circulation. In addition, pressure of the heavy uterus on the abdominal and pelvic veins is relieved as the uterus is emptied, blood flow from the lower extremities is improved, and venous return to the heart is increased. At the same time that the amount of circulating blood is increased by the above changes, it is modified to a variable degree by blood loss at the time of delivery. A loss of 200 to 300 ml, the amount associated with a normal delivery, reduces the volume of blood that would otherwise be available to the circulation. Larger blood loss can markedly reduce total blood volume. Cardiac output quickly decreases in the postpartum period, returning to the nonpregnant level within a few weeks.

Heart Rate

Heart rate is difficult to study during pregnancy because of the influence of many stimuli, but there is fairly general agreement that there is a distinct increase in pulse rate early in pregnancy, in the first trimester. Thereafter, the pulse rate may gradually rise even more to an overall increase in rate of at least 15 beats per minute over nonpregnant levels by late pregnancy. This means a rise from a nonpregnant mean of 70 beats per minute to a rate of approximately 85 beats per minute by late pregnancy. Many minor stimuli may temporarily increase the heart rate.

Position and Size of the Heart

Alterations in the heart during pregnancy involve a change in position of the heart, altered cardiac sounds, a slight increase in cardiac filling volume, and possibly slight hypertrophy or dilation of the heart, or both, resulting from the increased volume. As the diaphragm is progres-

[1] Frank E. Hytten and Isabella Leitch, *The Physiology of Human Pregnancy*, 2nd ed. Blackwell Scientific Publications, Oxford, London, and Edinburgh, 1971, p. 75.

sively elevated during pregnancy, the heart is gradually pushed upward and to the left and rotated forward (Fig. 6-13). With this shift, changes in cardiac outline can be expected, and the apical impulse moves upward and laterally. The amount of change depends upon the size and position of the uterus and the extent to which it pushes on the diaphragm.

Auscultatory changes are common during pregnancy. Systolic murmurs over the base of the heart are common, some cardiac sounds are accentuated, and split sounds may develop. Changes in heart sounds and development of murmurs become evident in the first half of pregnancy, and most disappear one week after delivery. The physiologic changes in heart sounds and in size and position of the heart during pregnancy are sometimes difficult to interpret, since they may be sufficiently altered to be considered pathologic when they are present at any other time.

Blood Pressure

The exact influence of pregnancy on blood pressure has been difficult to assess, but there is fairly general agreement that arterial blood pressure readings during pregnancy are somewhat below nonpregnant levels. Evidence from studies on arterial blood pressures suggests that the blood pressure falls early in pregnancy (first trimester), generally reaches its lowest readings in the second trimester (between 16 and 20 weeks according to Figure 6-11), and then rises slightly and progressively for the remainder of pregnancy toward the nonpregnant level (Fig. 6-11). According to Figure 6-11 the blood pressure was highest in the postnatal period, taken at 6 weeks after delivery. Prepregnancy readings had not been obtained in this study, but the postnatal readings can probably be assumed to be representative of the prepregnancy levels.

Changes in blood pressure during pregnancy are more marked in the diastolic than in the systolic readings. Whereas the fall in the systolic reading in early pregnancy may be only a few

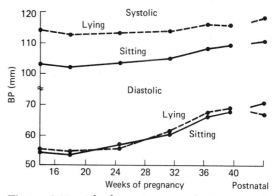

Figure 6-11. Blood pressure trends (sitting and lying) during pregnancy. [*Reproduced with permission from I. MacGillivray, G. A. Rose, and B. Rowe, "Blood Pressure Survey in Pregnancy,"* Clin. Sci. *37(2):395–407 (Oct.) 1969, p. 399.*]

millimeters of mercury, the diastolic reading may be from 10 to 15 millimeters lower. Subsequent rise of blood pressure in later pregnancy toward nonpregnancy levels is also more obvious and distinct in the diastolic readings (Fig. 6-11).

According to Figure 6-11, systolic pressure was 6 to 12 mmHg higher at all stages of pregnancy when the woman was recumbent than when she was sitting. Diastolic readings were similar in both positions.

The lowering of blood pressure during pregnancy results from a lowered vascular tone (a lower generalized systemic vascular resistance) and from the presence of the placental circulation, which is considered a low-resistance system. It is possible that, during the second trimester, the lowered vascular tone and a relative hypovolemia, due to a rapidly increasing uteroplacental vascular space, combine to reduce the blood pressure to its lowest level.

Knowing that there is a normal lowering of blood pressure during pregnancy has important clinical implications for observation and diagnosis. A woman with chronic hypertension may be normotensive during part of her pregnancy because of the physiologic fall, and it may be at a low level when she presents for antepartum care. Then when her pressure rises significantly, diagnosis is difficult if there is no prepregnancy record. Also a blood pressure of 140/90, which has often been considered the upper limit of normal, is likely to be too high for some women. Judgment of the significance of a rise in blood pressure in pregnancy should be related to the individual's previous readings rather than to an absolute figure.

Systemic Vascular Resistance

Systemic vascular resistance, the resistance offered by the vascular bed to the flow of blood, is decreased during pregnancy. Studies have shown that there is a considerable decrease in the midpregnancy period. This fall in systemic vascular resistance is responsible for the decrease in arterial blood pressure during pregnancy, and it probably also facilitates the increase in cardiac output. Although a number of factors may act to reduce peripheral vascular resistance in pregnancy, the two changes that exert the major effects are peripheral blood vessel dilation and the addition of the placental vascular system to the maternal circulation.

The placental vascular bed acts as a low-resistance network and takes on a relatively large portion of the maternal cardiac output. Uterine veins increase enormously in size and number during pregnancy. Uterine vascular resistance is greatly decreased during pregnancy, being at least ten times less than in the nonpregnant state. This marked decrease in uterine vascular resistance facilitates the tremendous increase in uterine blood flow during pregnancy, and it is also responsible for a considerable fall in systemic vascular resistance.

Pregnancy-associated changes in blood vessels lead to a generalized, progressive, peripheral blood vessel dilatation during gestation. There is relaxation of most or all smooth muscles during pregnancy, and this includes the muscular coat of all blood vessels. The vascular tone, maintained by the smooth muscle fibers, is thus decreased; the vessels have looser walls, an increased ability to dilate, and increased capacity.

This capacity for vasodilatation is probably a major factor in a greatly increased peripheral blood flow in pregnancy.

Since the total peripheral vascular resistance is dependent upon all factors that affect peripheral blood flow, the vasodilatation in pregnancy, which leads to an increased caliber of the terminal arteries, arterioles, and capillaries, is an important factor in the decrease in total peripheral vascular resistance.

Within a week after delivery the uterine blood flow, the uterine vascular resistance, the cardiac output, and the systemic vascular resistance all return to their nonpregnant levels.

Venous Pooling and Venous Pressure

Venous pooling, the capacity of the venous system of the lower part of the body, is expanded by several times above normal during pregnancy, especially when the woman is in an upright position. Pregnancy-associated changes in blood vessels lead to a progressive increase in venous distensibility as well as to the progressive peripheral blood vessel dilatation that was described above. The change takes place early in pregnancy. The looser walls of the veins permit a progressive increase in the capacity of the veins of the lower extremities to store blood. The velocity of venous blood flow may then be considerably reduced.

Under ordinary circumstances, in nonpregnant persons, the walls of veins, which are thin and flaccid, will yield to small pressure changes and easily increase their storage capacity. During pregnancy, this capacity for distensibility is greatly increased. Small increments of internal pressure will augment the capacity of the veins enormously. This means that the tendency to venous pooling on standing, which is present in all individuals, is aggravated in pregnancy. Venous capacity and venous pressure in the legs increase progressively throughout gestation, often becoming marked toward the end of pregnancy, as the enlarging uterus exerts more and more pressure on major abdominal and pelvic veins.

Both changes in the blood vessels themselves and mechanical factors appear to influence the distensibility of the veins. Although the hypervolemia of pregnancy tends to keep circulation normal by filling the enlarged vascular area in the legs, venous pooling does contribute to circulatory problems, such as postural hypotension, by reducing the amount of blood returned to the heart.

Venous pressure in the legs shows a marked increase during pregnancy. Pressures in the femoral and other leg veins are high. In the nonpregnant individual, venous pressure tends to be nearly equal in all parts of the body when the individual is in the horizontal position. During pregnancy, however, venous pressure in the legs is several times higher than in the upper extremities, even when the woman lies horizontally. This increase in femoral venous pressure is the result of venous obstruction brought about by mechanical pressure of the heavy uterus on the iliac veins and the inferior vena cava and by pressure of the fetal head on the iliac veins (Fig. 9-7, page 209.

High venous pressure in the legs and stagnation of blood contribute to the edema of the feet and legs common to pregnancy, and to increased incidence of varicosities. After delivery, the high pressure in the femoral veins drops abruptly.

Venous problems with *thrombosis* and *varicosities* may result, at least in part, from the venous dilatation, increased capacity of the veins, sluggish blood flow, and increased venous pressure. Venous thrombosis, which sometimes develops after birth of the baby and occasionally during pregnancy, is described on page 701.

Easy distention of the walls of the veins, along with the pressure and stagnation of blood that accompanies venous pooling in the legs, contributes to an increased incidence of problems with varicose veins and hemorrhoids in pregnancy. These problems arise from both preexisting varicose veins and from veins that develop incompetent valves during pregnancy. Vulvar varicosities, a problem unique to pregnancy, may also develop.

The veins return to normal during the first month after delivery, although some residual effects from venous problems may remain.

Edema of the Legs

When any individual stands or sits for long periods of time, the normally higher venous pressure in the legs, as opposed to the upper part of the body, increases capillary pressure in the legs. This results in a shift of fluid from the blood to the extravascular space and subsequently to edema of the feet and legs.

In the pregnant individual, the much higher than normal venous pressure in the legs, brought about by pressure of the heavy uterus on major abdominal and pelvic veins, increases capillary pressure. Also, a fall in plasma colloid oncotic pressure permits fluid to escape from the capillaries. Shift of fluid from the blood to the extravascular space in the legs is therefore much greater than normal in pregnancy. Dependent edema of the legs is very common and may be considered normal in pregnancy. Edema may be confined to the feet and ankles, or it may extend up the legs to the thighs and it may include the vulva.

To minimize lower extremity edema, the pregnant woman who must stand or sit a considerable amount of time should walk around frequently to improve circulation, through the massaging action of the muscles close to the veins. The edema also lessens when the effect of gravity is reduced. Sitting down with the feet resting on a chair or elevation of the feet for a short time several times daily may provide considerable relief of discomfort from swelling. Edema fluid from the lower extremities is redistributed when the woman lies down and frequently is mobilized and excreted to some extent while she is recumbent, especially in the lateral position.

Postural Hypotension and Fainting

As described above, when a recumbent person stands up, there is a normal tendency for blood to pool in the dependent distensible veins in the legs. This tends to decrease return of venous blood to the heart, diminish cardiac output, and lower the systemic arterial pressure. Under normal circumstances, compensatory factors will quickly counteract the effects of gravity and restore the circulation to normal.

With a greater than normal tendency to venous pooling in a pregnant woman upon assuming the upright position, compensatory mechanisms may not be able to restore adequate circulation quickly, especially when a large uterus has already exerted pressure on major veins and caused considerable pooling of blood while the woman was recumbent. With decreased blood return to the heart and decreased cardiac output as a result of the pooling, marked hypotension and fainting may occur when the pregnant woman stands up. Severe oliguria may also occur.

Supine Hypotension

A supine hypotensive syndrome, accompanied by dizziness, faintness, pallor, tachycardia, sweating and nausea, will occur in some pregnant women when they lie on their backs. In the supine position, the inferior vena cava and the major pelvic veins are compressed to varying degrees by pressure of the heavy pregnant uterus (Fig. 9-7, page 209). This results in the same pathophysiologic circulatory abnormalities as those that occur in assuming the upright position. There is pooling of blood in the lower extremities, a decrease in venous return to the heart, fall in cardiac output, and hypotension. It is possible for a very large amount of the circulating blood to be collected in the legs. The blood pressure may drop precipitously and hypotension, accompanied by shocklike signs and symptoms, may become severe.

Whenever signs of supine hypotension occur, it is very important for maternal and fetal well-being, as well as for maternal comfort, to have the mother turn to her side immediately. Such a change of position will remove pressure from the inferior vena cava and quickly restore the

pooled blood to the circulation. A mother is likely to recognize that turning to her side will relieve her faintness. If she becomes distressed while on her back during an examination or a treatment, she must be permitted to change her position immediately.

Since compression of major veins by the enlarged uterus will vary, all pregnant women do not develop signs of hypotension when they lie on their backs. Severe venous pooling may not occur when pressure on major abdominal veins is not great. The degree of pressure may depend upon the amount of pressure exerted by the abdominal wall or by a greatly enlarged uterus, or it may be determined by variations in position. A tight abdominal wall places more pressure on the uterus and the veins than a relaxed one. A uterus considerably distended with a large baby or a large amount of amniotic fluid is likely to exert more pressure than one of moderate enlargement. There is less likelihood of pressure on the vena cava when the woman lies on a soft flexible mattress than when she lies on a hard table.

Effects of Autonomic Block

Increased activity of the autonomic nervous system in pregnancy provides good control over the vasomotor tone of the circulatory system. This good tone possibly tends to counteract to some degree the increased vein distensibility and venous pooling. Blockage of the autonomic nervous system with spinal anesthesia or with drugs also blocks the increased venomotor tone present in pregnancy and leaves pregnant women especially susceptible to hypotension and circulatory shock.

Blockage of the autonomic nervous system leaves the veins with very little or no tone and greatly increases their capacity. Pooling of blood in the legs can become severe. Under such circumstances, even a small amount of compression of abdominal and pelvic veins by the uterus can lead to a great amount of venous pooling and severe hypotension. In administration of spinal anesthesia to a pregnant woman, it is essential to take measures that will prevent or minimize hypotensive problems. One such step is to position the woman on her side to prevent or reduce pooling of blood in the legs.

Advantages of the Lateral Position in Pregnancy

Regardless of whether or not a pregnant woman has signs of hypotension when she lies supine, it can be assumed that an enlarged uterus will compress the major abdominal and pelvic vessels (inferior vena cava, abdominal aorta, and iliac vessels) to some degree when she lies on her back. Such interference with circulation may reduce cardiac output significantly and be deleterious to both mother and fetus.

In the supine position an enlarged uterus may compress the aorta as well as the inferior vena cava. As a result, pressure in the uterine arteries and other vessels distal to the compression is reduced. Uterine arterial pressure may be considerably lower than that of the brachial artery when a pregnant woman lies supine. This decreased pressure results in decreased tissue perfusion, including poor placental perfusion. If, for some reason, the mother also has systemic hypotension, the arterial pressure distal to compression of the aorta may be markedly lowered. Perfusion of tissue may then be greatly reduced and be very harmful to both mother and fetus.

When a pregnant woman turns to her side (preferably left side) from a supine position, obstruction of the major abdominal veins is relieved, the pooled blood in the lower extremities quickly returns to the systemic circulation, and cardiac output and general circulation are improved. Blood flow to the placenta and the uterine tissues is significantly improved and maternal kidney function is greatly enhanced. It has been observed that there may be a 30 to 50 percent increase in cardiac output and in uterine and renal blood flow when a woman changes from the supine to the lateral position.

To assure that neither the inferior vena cava nor the abdominal aorta will be compressed,

that maternal circulation will be good, and that blood flow to the placenta will be adequate for fetal well-being, it is highly desirable for a pregnant woman to lie on her side rather than on her back at all times that she is recumbent. If, in addition, she has complications that may result in hypotension, such as bleeding or conduction anesthesia, the lateral position is especially important.

Regional Increases in Blood Flow

Uterus

The uterus with its tremendous growth, its greatly enlarged blood vessels, and its development of the placental circulation to serve the fetus, is a major target of an increased blood flow in pregnancy. Uterine blood flow increases tremendously, progressively becoming greater until it reaches a peak of 20 to 40 times nonpregnant values by the end of pregnancy. Measurements of uterine blood flow are very difficult, but estimates from observations that have been made indicate that there appears to be a steady increase during gestation. It is estimated that the uterine blood flow is around 200 ml/min by 28 weeks gestation, and at term the average from a wide range of figures is 500 ml/min (Fig. 6-12). This increased blood flow to the uterus is of prime importance in providing adequate oxygen and nourishment for the fetus and for the uterine tissues.

The increment in blood flow to the uterus during pregnancy is derived from the increment in cardiac output. It is facilitated by the low-resistance network of the uteroplacental circulation, which results in at least a tenfold decrease in uterine vascular resistance during pregnancy.

Skin

There is considerable evidence that blood flow in the skin is greatly increased in pregnancy, especially in the hands and feet. Clinically, pregnant women feel warm, frequently complain of heat, and feel quite comfortable in cold weather and cold rooms. Their skin feels warm to touch and their hands are often clammy.

Increased blood flow in the skin has been estimated to be around 500 ml/min (Fig. 6-12). Blood flow in the hands is probably six to seven times greater than in the nonpregnant state; flow in the feet is smaller but definitely increased. Increased blood flow to the skin begins early in pregnancy. Its purpose is elimination of heat from the body, dissipating heat generated by the fetus and by increased metabolism. The increased flow is brought about by peripheral vasodilation and also some increase in the number of capillaries. As a result of the increased blood flow, there is a considerable increase in skin temperature during pregnancy. Finger temperature reaches nearly physiologic maximum levels in late pregnancy.

As a result of the dilatation and increased number of capillaries, pregnant women may develop vascular spiders and palmar erythema. Hemangiomas that are present may increase in size and new ones may form, especially on the face and hands. Increased growth of fingernails of pregnant women has been reported, probably the result of increased blood flow. Hair growth has not been reported as increased in rate, but its character of growth has been found to be changed. It appears that in pregnancy the percentage of actively growing hair is greater and

that fewer hairs are ready to fall out. There are then more overaged hairs by the end of pregnancy, and these fall out in large numbers in the puerperium.

The nasal mucous membranes also appear to have an increased blood flow in pregnancy, causing congestion of the mucosa. The vasodilatation brings about a tendency to nose bleeds and it may cause blockage of narrow nasal passages.

Kidneys

The kidneys are an important target of increased blood flow during pregnancy. This increase begins early in pregnancy and the flow is up to 400 ml/min above nonpregnancy levels by the beginning of the second trimester (Fig. 6-12). The purpose of the increased blood flow to the kidneys is to enhance elimination, beginning early in pregnancy.

Breasts

The changes in the breasts in early pregnancy that include sudden enlargement, engorgement, sensation of tingling and heat, and dilated veins suggest that blood supply is considerably increased. Growth of the breasts during pregnancy would surely indicate that there would be a need for an increase in blood flow.

The Alimentary Canal

Measurements of blood flow to the alimentary canal during pregnancy have not been carried out, but the apparent increased efficiency of digestion and absorption of foods may mean an increased blood supply.

General Remarks

The increased cardiac output in pregnancy is distributed to a number of regions in the body. The mechanisms that control regional blood flow changes are not clear and are probably complex. A major change appears to be vasodilatation, with a lowering in peripheral vascular tone. Increased blood flow to the uterus is necessary for local growth needs and for needs of the fetus. Increased flow to the breasts is probably, at

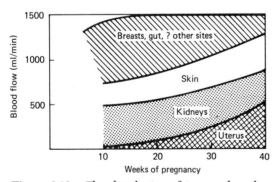

Figure 6-12. The distribution of increased cardiac output in pregnancy. [*Reproduced with permission from Frank E. Hytten and Isabella Leitch,* The Physiology of Human Pregnancy, *2nd ed. Blackwell Scientific Publications Ltd., Oxford, 1971, p. 106.*]

least in part, due to growth of tissue. Two other major regional increases, that of the kidneys and of the skin, serve to enhance elimination from the body. There may be other important areas of increased flow that are unknown at this time. The regional blood flow increases described above all begin early in pregnancy and reach their maximum early, with the exception of the uterus, which continues a gradual, progressive increase up to the end of pregnancy (Fig. 6-12).

CHANGES IN THE RESPIRATORY SYSTEM

Respiratory adjustments are made in pregnancy to provide for both maternal and fetal needs. The fetus must obtain oxygen and eliminate carbon dioxide through the mother, and the maternal oxygen requirements rise in response to the increase in tissues in the uterus and the breasts and to the greater metabolic activity of the maternal body in pregnancy.

Anatomic Changes

Capillary engorgement of the respiratory tract is common in pregnancy. The nose, nasopharynx, larynx, trachea, and bronchi become swollen. Nose breathing is difficult, nose bleed occurs easily, and voice changes frequently become apparent. Congestion of the larynx in pregnancy may adversely effect the voice of singers. Mild upper respiratory infections easily produce inflammatory manifestations in pregnancy.

Even before there is much upward pressure of the enlarging uterus the level of the diaphragm rises by as much as 4 cm in pregnancy, and there is an equal decrease in the length of the lungs. At the same time, the effect of this shortening is satisfactorily offset by a broadening of the chest as the anteroposterior and transverse diameters increase by 2 cm. The lower ribs flare out progressively in pregnancy, and the substernal angle widens about 50 percent, from approximately 68 degrees in the first tri-

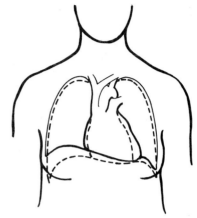

Figure 6-13. Changes in the position of the heart, lungs, and thoracic cage in pregnancy. *Broken line:* Nonpregnant. *Solid line:* Change that occurs in pregnancy.

mester to 103 degrees by the end of pregnancy. There is a 5- to 7-cm increase in thoracic cage circumference during pregnancy (Fig. 6-13).

Expansion of the thoracic cage is made possible, at least in part, by relaxation of the ligamentous attachment of the ribs, a change similar to that which takes place in other joints in the body. The ribs do not always return to their prepregnancy position after delivery. Changes in the chest begin early in pregnancy, before there is any significant enlargement in uterine size, and they are therefore not entirely produced by mechanical pressure.

Diaphragmatic movement is not decreased by encroachment of the full-term uterus. Breathing has been found to be more diaphragmatic and less costal at any stage of pregnancy than it is in nonpregnant women.

Lung Function

Vital capacity, the maximum volume of gas which can be expired after a maximum inspiration, and *maximum breathing capacity,* the maximum voluntary ventilation, are not significantly altered in normal pregnancy. There is, however, a rearrangement in pregnancy of the various components of lung function. Beginning at the first trimester there is a progressive increase in *tidal volume,* the volume of gas inspired or expired with each breath (the amount of gas that is exchanged with each breath), and there is a slight rise in respiratory rate, from 14 to 16 per minute. The pregnant woman increases her ventilation mainly by breathing more deeply and only slightly by increased respiratory rate. The increase in tidal volume and slight rise in respiratory rate means that the volume of gas expired per minute, the *minute ventilation,* increases to a peak level of close to 50 percent above normal by the end of pregnancy (Fig. 6-14). Clinically, this rise means hyperventilation.

Another progressive change during the second half of pregnancy is a considerably smaller *functional residual capacity,* the volume of gas that remains in the lungs at the end of a normal expiration. This means that the lungs of a preg-

nant woman are more collapsed and contain less residual gas at the end of a normal expiration than the lungs of a nonpregnant woman. Since the functional residual capacity is the volume of gas with which the tidal air must mix, the changes in pregnancy mean that an increased tidal volume of air is taken into a smaller volume of gas in the lungs. This means much more efficient gas mixing. The *alveolar ventilation* thus increases 65 to 70 percent (Fig. 6-14).

More rapid changes of gas in the lungs means that very rapid, deep breathing, as might occur during the stress of a labor contraction, could lower arterial P_{CO_2} and raise pH values to harmful levels. It also means that induction of and recovery from inhalation anesthesia are more rapid than in the nonpregnant woman.

Oxygen Consumption

Oxygen consumption in pregnancy, usually studied as basal metabolic rate, is difficult to determine, and studies have often been unsatisfactory. However, it has been estimated that a rise of 15 percent, or approximately 30 ml of oxygen per minute above nonpregnant oxygen consumption, seems to be reasonable and in accord with the increase in oxygen-carrying capacity of the blood.

A large part of the increment in oxygen consumption, at least as pregnancy advances, is related to the products of conception, the fetus and placenta. The increased metabolic activities of some parts of the mother's body, increased cardiac and respiratory work, and increased tissues of the uterus and the breasts account for the rest of the rise in oxygen consumption (Fig. 6-15).

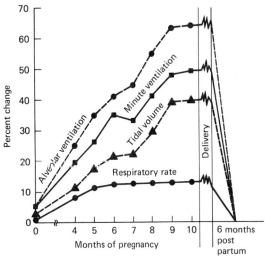

Figure 6-14. Changes in respiratory parameters during pregnancy. The curves for rate, tidal volume, and minute ventilation were developed from data of Cugell *et al.* Since the respiratory rate increases to a much lesser degree than tidal volume, percent increase in alveolar ventilation is greater than the percent increase in minute ventilation. [*Reproduced with permission from John J. Bonica,* Principles and Practice of Obstetric Analgesia and Anesthesia, *Vol. I. Fundamental Considerations. F. A. Davis, Philadelphia, Pa., 1967, p. 32.*]

Hyperventilation (Overbreathing)

A state of hyperventilation exists during pregnancy, beginning as early as the first trimester. Nonpregnant persons ordinarily do not hyperventilate until their P_{CO_2} reaches approximately 60 mmHg. Pregnant women hyperventilate at a normal P_{CO_2} level (38–40 mmHg).

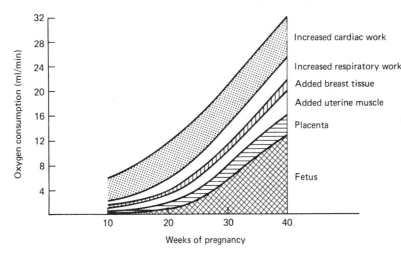

Figure 6-15. The components of increased oxygen consumption in pregnancy. [*Reproduced with permission from Frank E. Hytten and Isabella Leitch,* The Physiology of Human Pregnancy, *2nd ed. Blackwell Scientific Publications Ltd., Oxford, 1971, p. 125.*]

Overbreathing is not related to changed mechanics of breathing and is not necessary for adequate ventilation. Although oxygen consumption increases during pregnancy (approximately 15 percent), minute ventilation increases much more, up to 50 percent above normal by the end of pregnancy. In addition, ventilation is more effective. With alveolar ventilation increasing up to 65 to 70 percent it is approximately four times greater than the increase in oxygen consumption. Thus there is considerable hyperventilation in pregnancy. The increased ventilation is evidence of overbreathing, or a response of the body to a stimulus other than need.

Hyperventilation appears to be stimulated by a lowered threshold of the respiratory center to carbon dioxide, a response which is very likely brought about by the action of progesterone on the respiratory center. The respiratory center is also more sensitive, a reaction which may be influenced by estrogen. To some extent the hyperventilation and the changes that accompany it (such as a lowering of alveolar PCO_2) are a continuation of changes found in the luteal (progestational) phase of each menstrual cycle.

Carbon Dioxide Output

Overbreathing causes carbon dioxide to be washed out of the lungs, and because of this the alveolar concentration of carbon dioxide is significantly lower in the pregnant than in the nonpregnant woman. Accompanying this is a lowering of the arterial carbon dioxide tension from approximately 38 to 30 to 32 mmHg.

As the arterial PCO_2 level changes there is a transient respiratory alkalosis. Then renal excretion of bicarbonate appears to compensate for the lowered arterial carbon dioxide tension. Thus the decrease in arterial PCO_2 is accompanied by a parallel decrease in plasma bicarbonate, causing the pH to readjust to a normal nonpregnant level.

Dyspnea

Approximately 60 to 70 percent of normal pregnant women develop dyspnea, a conscious need to breathe. Dyspnea should be differentiated from hyperventilation, which is effortless breathing. Shortness of breath is a common complaint of pregnant women. This sensation of dyspnea is often present at rest and not when moving about. It may be episodic and it is likely to begin to occur in the first trimester.

The cause of dyspnea is obscure. It appears to be unrelated to the mechanics of breathing, but may be caused by changes in respiratory center sensitivity. It is believed that the lowered alveolar PCO_2 may contribute to dyspnea. Dyspneic women may have a tendency to hyperventilate more excessively than those who are nondyspneic, and they may either be more sensitive to progesterone or have a higher level of this hormone.

Although dyspnea is usually physiologic, it may at times be important to look for a pathologic reason. Common causes of dyspnea in pregnancy, other than excessive hyperventilation, include severe anemia, pulmonary edema, severe acidosis, and excessive pressure on the diaphragm as with hydramnios.

CHANGES IN THE URINARY SYSTEM

The kidneys, vital as excretory organs, have the very important function of maintaining the internal environment of the body in a relatively constant homeostatic state and in an optimal condition for the efficient functioning of body cells. They maintain electrolyte balance, control acid–base balance, regulate the extracellular fluid volume, excrete waste products, and conserve essential nutrients. To accomplish these very important functions approximately 1000 to 1200 ml of blood (about 500 to 600 ml of plasma) normally flow through both kidneys per minute. This is 20 to 25 percent of the total cardiac output. About 125 ml of plasma is filtered through the 2,000,000 glomeruli in one minute (170 to 180 liters per 24 hours). The glomerular filtrate, which is essentially protein-free plasma removed from the blood, is greatly modified, and, through a very complex process of tubular reabsorption and tubular secretion, most of the filtrate is selectively reabsorbed and other substances are secreted (excreted from the blood).

Tubular function includes all of the processes that change glomerular filtrate into urine. This includes the reabsorption of almost all of the filtered water, electrolytes, amino acids, inorganic salts, and other solutes. Unneeded substances are not absorbed and others that are unwanted or are waste products are actively excreted by the renal tubule cells. Thus the constancy of the internal environment of the body is maintained, and the volume of the filtrate is reduced from

the 180,000 ml, which pass through the glomeruli in 24 hours, to about 1500 ml of fluid, which is excreted as urine during the 24-hour period.

Renal function is greatly altered in normal pregnancy. During pregnancy the mother's kidneys must handle the increased metabolic and circulatory demands of the maternal body and also excretion of fetal waste products. In addition, there is a tremendous increase in stimuli that may affect renal function. Mechanisms which maintain homeostasis are changed and renal function and water and electrolyte distribution are considerably altered. Values from clinical tests of renal function and any seemingly pathologic changes in function must therefore be considered in light of the physiologic changes that are normally peculiar to pregnancy.

Anatomic Changes

During pregnancy the kidney pelves and the ureters, down as far as the pelvic brim, become dilated, starting as early as the tenth week of gestation. The ureters have been found to be of normal caliber below the pelvic brim. Dilatation of the ureters is accompanied by hypertrophy and hyperplasia of the ureteral smooth muscle. Later in pregnancy, dilatation of the renal pelvis and the ureter becomes more pronounced on the right side than on the left. Kinking of the ureters, often acute, has been found to occur on both sides.

The volume of urine contained in the renal pelves and ureters is greatly increased in pregnancy because of their dilatation. This means that there is considerable lag between the time urine is formed and the time it enters the bladder. This easily distorts clearance tests, particularly if the urine flow rate is low at the time of the test. If the urine flow is slow, the urine that is retained in the dilated kidneys and ureters and in the bladder may contain substances that were filtered through the glomeruli many hours previously.

For accurate testing, as much of the urine as possible that is produced in a unit of time should be obtained for analysis. Unless this is done errors may be significant even when 24-hour urine specimens are collected. Inaccuracies due to retained urine can be reduced in two ways: by producing a fairly adequate urinary flow with an increase in fluid intake (a water load) an hour before the beginning and the end of a test, and by requesting the woman to lie in the lateral recumbent position as much as possible during the collection period.

Stagnation of urine due to dilatation of the urinary tract may also be a factor in frequent urinary tract infections. There is an increased incidence in both asymptomatic bacteriuria and acute pyelonephritis in pregnancy. In addition to stagnation, the excretion of a large number of nutrients in the urine in pregnancy, especially glucose, provides a very favorable environment for bacterial growth.

The cause of dilatation of the renal collecting system is not clear. For many years it was believed that there was atony of tissues, largely a hormonal effect, possibly typical of smooth muscle relaxation in general, attributed to a progesterone effect. This concept has not been entirely

discarded, although there is some evidence to the contrary. Some believe that the dilatation is a purely mechanical effect and may be so even when it occurs early. There has been evidence that the ureters may be compressed by dilated blood vessels. Later the enlarging uterus compresses the ureters as they pass over the pelvic brim, placing more pressure on the right side than the left, possibly owing to uterodextrorotation. Also, the left side is believed to be somewhat protected by the sigmoid colon.

Renal Plasma Flow and Glomerular Filtration

Renal plasma flow (RPF) and glomerular filtration rate (GFR) are markedly increased in pregnancy. A rapid rise is evident very early in pregnancy, by the end of the first trimester, and is sustained to term (Fig. 6-16). According to data currently available it seems that the rise in blood flow through the kidneys is from a nonpregnant level of a mean of 1000 ml/min to a level that is between 25 to 50 percent higher. The renal plasma flow, which is the volume of

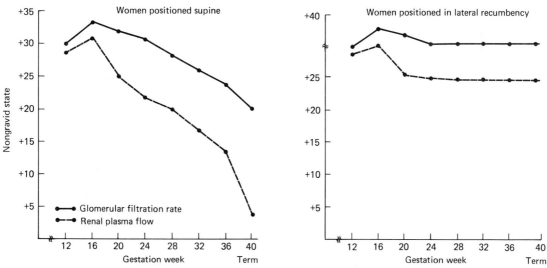

Figure 6-16. Renal hemodynamics in pregnancy. Increases in parameters of renal hemodynamics occur early in pregnancy and are sustained to term if subjects are tested in lateral recumbency. [*Reproduced with permission from Marshall D. Lindheimer and Adrian I. Katz, "Managing the Patient with Renal Disease," Contemp. Ob/Gyn 3(1):49–55 (Jan.) 1974, p. 51.*]

plasma flowing through the kidneys every minute, seems to rise by about 225 ml/min, from a level of 500 to 600 ml/min to between 700 and 900 ml/min. The glomerular filtration rate (GFR) rises from a nonpregnant level of 100 to 125 ml/min to as high as 140 to 170 ml/min, a rise of about 50 percent.

As the renal plasma flow increases approximately 35 percent the GFR rises to as much as 50 percent. The greater rise in glomerular filtration over that of plasma flow means that the filtration fraction, the proportion of the renal plasma flow that is filtered by the glomeruli, is greater than the nonpregnant level. The serum protein concentration in plasma is lower in pregnancy by about 1 gm per 100 ml. Such a change decreases the plasma oncotic pressure by about 20 percent, and it is likely that this decreased colloid oncotic pressure permits increased filtration of plasma in the kidneys.

The cause of the increases in renal blood flow and glomerular filtration in pregnancy is not known. It has been suggested that, with the rise in cardiac output early in pregnancy and the decrease in total peripheral vascular resistance, the resistance to blood flow through the kidneys may be specifically lowered and the flow easily increased. Progesterone and possibly estrogen may have an effect. Human growth hormone is known to increase renal plasma flow and glomerular filtration. This hormone remains at normal levels during pregnancy, but human chorionic somatomammotropin (HCS), a hormone present early in pregnancy and having similarities to growth hormone, has been considered a possible cause of increasing renal blood flow and glomerular filtration. Another consideration is that the increase in extracellular fluid volume in pregnancy may bring about an increase in renal hemodynamics.

Effect of Posture on Renal Function

Renal function of women in late pregnancy is considerably altered by position. The supine and the upright positions both bring about a reduction in renal blood flow and glomerular filtration and in excretion of water and sodium and chloride (Fig. 6-16). The rate of excretion may be less than half in either the supine or standing position. As described on page 130, women in late pregnancy are very likely to pool a large amount of blood in their legs. When they lie supine the heavy uterus compresses the inferior vena cava and the aorta, and when they sit or stand quietly the uterus compresses the common iliac veins. In either case venous return from the legs is impaired, the effective blood volume is decreased, cardiac output falls, and blood pressure falls.

A compensatory change in response to decreasing circulating blood volume and decreasing cardiac output is renal vasoconstriction. This response provides a better blood flow to areas more vital than the kidneys, but it also means a considerable reduction in renal blood flow and in glomerular filtration. Whenever renal function must be improved during gestation, it is essential that the pregnant woman lie in bed on her side, preferably her left side, as much as possible.

Diurnal Pattern of Renal Function

The normal nonpregnant individual has a lower excretion of water and electrolytes during the night than in the daytime. This pattern of urinary output is an established periodic alteration that is not merely a reflection of difference in fluid intake. In ambulatory pregnant women this usual pattern of urinary output is reversed. During the day pregnant women tend to collect fluid as dependent edema. At night, when they lie down, they mobilize this extracellular fluid and excrete it. Excretion of sodium and water is thus increased at night. This change in pattern of urinary output also leads to the common problem of nocturia in pregnant women.

Clearance of Waste Products

Creatinine, urea, and uric acid are excreted more effectively in pregnancy than in the nonpregnant state, owing to enhanced renal clearance. Since there is essentially no change in the production of these products in pregnancy, the result of this increased clearance is a lower level of nitrogenous breakdown products in the blood than in nonpregnant women. Concentrations of plasma urea nitrogen, creatinine, and uric acid are reduced to about two thirds of nonpregnant levels. Thus, values that are considered normal in nonpregnant women may signify decreased renal function in pregnancy. Concentrations of serum urea nitrogen over 13.0 mg percent or of serum creatinine over 0.8 mg percent require further evaluation of renal function.

Renal Sodium Excretion

The content of sodium in the body is kept within narrow limits by the regulatory functions of the kidneys. Under normal circumstances, threats to sodium balance are countered by quick physiologic adjustments, which keep the extracellular fluid (plasma and interstitial fluid) constant in volume and osmolarity. This is necessary, since any distortion in the composition of these extracellular fluids would soon have disastrous results.

Since sodium is freely filtered at the glomeruli and actively absorbed by the tubules, the amount of sodium excreted in the urine is the difference between the amount filtered and the amount reabsorbed. It could be assumed then that sodium excretion may be increased by an increase in GFR or by a decrease in reabsorption, or by a combination of both. Ordinarily, however, tubular reabsorption is quickly adjusted to the rate of glomerular filtration to maintain sodium in careful balance. More than 99 percent of the sodium filtered by the glomeruli is reabsorbed.

A number of factors control GFR and tubular reabsorption, but regulation of reabsorption seems to be of major importance. Reabsorption must be, and is, quickly adjusted to changes in the filtered load of sodium so that it keeps pace with that which is filtered out. Increases in sodium intake, or losses of sodium from the body, are accompanied by changes in tubular reab-

sorption. Thus, sodium and water balances, the balance between their intake and output, depend critically on tubular reabsorption.

In normal persons regulatory mechanisms are very precise and sodium balance varies very little despite marked changes in dietary intake or in losses due to sweating, vomiting, or diarrhea. Sodium balance may, however, become upset in disease or under certain circumstances in which sodium-retaining factors or sodium-losing factors are disrupted so that they operate out of proportion to normal.

Regulation of sodium excretion and sodium retention, a very complicated process under normal circumstances, appears to be even more so in pregnancy. Sodium-retaining factors and sodium-losing factors are sufficiently changed in pregnancy to bring about a tendency to sodium depletion. This can become a major problem if an inadequate amount of dietary sodium is ingested in pregnancy or if diuretics are used.

There is actually a very gradual cumulative retention of sodium during pregnancy, a total of 500 to 900 mEq, but this amount is only enough to meet the special needs of pregnancy and does not change the maternal electrolyte balance. This retained sodium is necessary to meet the requirements of the developing fetus and to provide for the mother's increased interstitial and intravascular fluid volumes. Considering the usual increase in extracellular fluids in pregnancy, it is apparent that additional sodium must be retained to permit expansion of fluid volume and to maintain an isotonic state.

Tendency to Promote Renal Excretion of Sodium

Of the several factors that tend to promote renal excretion of sodium in pregnancy the increased GFR and an increase in progesterone levels have the greatest influence. These tend to produce considerable sodium loss.

Increase in Glomerular Filtration

The tremendous rise in GFR in pregnancy, up to levels of 50 percent above nonpregnant values, results in a similar increase of filtered load of sodium. If this were not accompanied by an equal increase in tubular reabsorption of sodium, severe sodium depletion would quickly occur. The ability of the kidney to adjust to a large increase in reabsorption of sodium so that it can match the enhanced filtration of sodium is a major adaptation of pregnancy.

Progesterone

Progesterone may significantly promote sodium excretion. It antagonizes the effect of aldosterone, which enhances sodium reabsorption, and thus interferes with reabsorption. Since progesterone is greatly increased in pregnancy, anywhere from 10- to 100-fold, it can exert considerable influence.

Physical Factors

A decrease in both plasma albumin and vascular resistance in pregnancy may tend to enhance excretion of sodium. The low serum colloid oncotic pressure in pregnancy may tend to reduce reabsorption.

Factors Tending to Enhance Sodium Reabsorption

A compensatory mechanism, the renin–angiotensin–aldosterone system, that works toward overcoming sodium loss by enhancing its reabsorption, functions very well in pregnancy. Thus the influence of the increased GFR and the increased progesterone level in producing considerable sodium loss is offset by increased activity of the renin–angiotensin–aldosterone system. With such activity there is a marked increase in aldosterone secretion in normal pregnancies, an increase of severalfold. The aldosterone enhances sodium reabsorption and thus prevents excessive sodium wasting while the increased GFR is filtering it out in large amounts.

The Renin–Angiotensin–Aldosterone System

Renin is a proteolytic enzyme secreted into the blood by the kidneys, specifically by the cells of a specialized area of each nephron known as the juxtaglomerular apparatus, which is located in the walls of the renal afferent arterioles. It acts on a circulating renin substrate causing the formation of angiotensin. Angiotensin, the major regulator of aldosterone secretion, stimulates secretion of aldosterone by the adrenal cortex. Aldosterone enhances the tubular reabsorption of sodium, returning it to the circulation.

The marked increase in plasma renin activity and in aldosterone secretion in normal pregnancy apparently is not excessive but is an adaptation that is ready to prevent sodium depletion. It appears to be a compensatory response to the threat of sodium loss and to the need to retain additional sodium to meet the needs of the fetus and of the additional maternal extracellular fluids. Thus aldosterone secretion is regulated by normal mechanisms in pregnancy and increases only as necessary for maintenance of sodium balance.

As in normal nonpregnant persons, aldosterone secretion is easily influenced by changes in dietary sodium intake; its secretion increases with sodium deprivation and decreases with high salt intake. The difference is in the much greater levels of the hormone in pregnancy at all levels of dietary sodium intake. The renin–angiotensin–aldosterone system thus apparently adjusts to sodium restriction or to increased needs of pregnancy, but could possibly be severely stressed if necessary adjustments were prolonged or severe.

Other Hormones

Estrogen, which is considerably increased in pregnancy, tends to induce sodium retention. Other hormones tending to decrease sodium excretion are placental HCS, increased prolactin levels in pregnancy, and increased plasma cortisol concentration.

Effect of Posture on Sodium Excretion

The supine and upright positions tend to decrease renal excretion of sodium and water. The fall in GFR in these positions is accompanied by an equal fall in sodium excretion. In addition to this influence of posture, it appears that the supine and upright positions also cause an active reabsorption of sodium, independent of glomerular filtration. It has been suggested that the reduction in effective circulating plasma volume in these positions stimulates reabsorption of sodium.

SUMMARY

In summary, pregnancy results in a tendency to sodium depletion rather than excessive sodium retention. Restriction of dietary sodium or administration of diuretics in pregnancy may stress the renin–angiotensin–aldosterone mechanism and exaggerate the normal sodium-depletion tendency. If this became severe, it could cause excessive volume depletion and could even result in poor placental perfusion.

Excretion of Water

The capacity of the kidneys to deal with a water load changes as pregnancy progresses. The ability to excrete water is excellent in early pregnancy. This is also a time of thirst for many pregnant women. There is then a decline, and in later pregnancy excretion of a water load is considerably below the nonpregnant average. There is evidence to suggest that the ability to excrete a water load decreases in late pregnancy because the water then pools in the lower extremities and does not trigger a diuretic response. It is only mobilized when the woman lies down. It has also been suggested that there may be a new lower level of osmolarity in late pregnancy, or that increased oxytocin secretion in late pregnancy may cause some antidiuresis.

As with sodium excretion, the excretion of water is decreased in the upright and the supine positions. Also the nonpregnant diurnal variation is reversed and excretion of both sodium and water is greater at night during pregnancy.

Glucosuria

Under normal conditions almost all glucose filtered through the glomeruli is reabsorbed by the tubules and only minute amounts can be detected in the urine. Normally there is so little glucose in the urine that for clinical purposes it may be considered absent. Normal pregnancy, however, is frequently associated with glucosuria. Reabsorption of glucose in pregnancy is apparently not as efficient as reabsorption of sodium, and the glucose which is not absorbed is excreted in the urine. The amount of sugar lost can vary considerably from day to day, and individual urine specimens may be positive or negative to glucose at irregularly intermittent times.

Glucosuria in pregnancy seems to be due, in part, at least, to an increase in the filtration of glucose brought about by the increased GFR in pregnancy and an inability of the renal tubules to increase reabsorption as much as the glomerular filtration increases. More glucose is filtered out with the plasma filtrate and presented to the renal tubules than they can reabsorb.

There is also some evidence that maximum tubular glucose reabsorption may be lower in pregnant than in nonpregnant women. This would mean that pregnant women have a somewhat lower blood sugar value than nonpregnant at which reabsorption no longer takes place or at least is decreased. Sugar may then be excreted into the urine rather than be reabsorbed back into the bloodstream at blood values of considerably less than 160 to 180 mg/100 ml of blood. Such a loss of sugar appears to be a waste by the kidneys, but the same is true of amino acids and a number of other nutrients. The reason for such increased excretion by the kidneys and the apparent waste is not known.

The urine of pregnant women is tested for glucose at each antepartum visit. A dip stick, to which a reagent specific for reaction with glucose is affixed, is used for the testing. It is dipped into freshly voided urine, and the reagent is checked for a color change which will take place if glucose is present. The results are read by comparing the color change in the reagent with a color chart, which is read as negative, or light, medium, or dark, signifying varying degrees of positive reaction. The results are qualitative, indicating negative or the presence of glucose in relative amounts from small to large. Approximately 0.1 gm of glucose per 100 ml of urine is detectable.

Although glucosuria is common in normal pregnancy, it should not be ignored. The possibility of diabetes mellitus must be considered. All pregnant women, however, whether or not they have glucosuria should be screened for diabetes by blood testing according to the regimen described on page 172.

Proteinuria

Proteins (albumin, globulin) are abnormal constituents of the urine. Proteinuria is an important sign of renal disease, and it is commonly present in preeclampsia. Measurement of urinary protein excretion is therefore one of the most valuable tests of renal function. Although trace amounts of protein may normally be found in concentrated urine, it is difficult to detect in such small amounts. Protein excretion is abnormal in nonpregnant women when the total daily excretion exceeds 150 mg. Normal pregnant women may excrete slightly more because of their increased glomerular blood supply and their tendency to lordosis, but an amount over 250 mg per day is considered excessive.

Since proteinuria is an important sign of abnormal renal function and a characteristic sign in preeclampsia, measurement of urinary protein excretion is an essential test in pregnancy for both discovery of renal disease and detection of preeclampsia. The urine of pregnant women is therefore examined for protein at each antepartum visit.

A rapid, convenient, and sensitive method of detecting protein in urine is based on a color-producing reaction between albumin and a reagent dye at the end of a dip stick. The albumin reagent stick is a very satisfactory semiquantitative measure of small amounts of protein in the urine.

The reagent end of the dip stick is dipped into *freshly voided* urine, or the mother is asked to pass the reagent end of the stick through a stream of urine. A clean midstream voided specimen should be used to reduce the chance of contamination of the urine with vaginal discharge. The dip stick is read by comparison with a color chart. The protein reagent's color change may read negative, or trace (5 to 20 mg of albumin per 100 ml of urine), or present in 30, 100, 300, or 1000 or more mg of protein (albumin) per 100 ml of urine. When the dip stick reaction to protein is more than a trace, a 24-hour urine specimen may be necessary to assess accurately the total daily excretion.

Clinical Tests of Renal Function

Clinical tests of renal function and for evidence of renal disease include complete urinalysis, testing of urine for glucose and protein, and evaluation of glomerular filtration rate by creatinine clearance or urea clearance tests if this seems indicated.

Microscopic Examination

Microscopic examination of the urine is valuable in detecting renal disease. A morning, first-voided specimen is preferable, since it will be more concentrated than urine voided at other times of the day. Casts, red blood cells, white blood cells, and epithelial cells are abnormal constituents of the urine, are interpreted as evidence of renal lesions, and require further investigation. Testing for the presence of glucose and protein has been described above.

Glomerular Filtration Test

A commonly used clinical test for evaluation of glomerular filtration consists of measurement of blood creatinine and creatinine clearance in the urine. Measurement of plasma creatinine is made at the same time that urine is collected for the test because clearance is calculated from the amount excreted within a unit of time and its concentration in the plasma. Measurement of blood urea and urea clearance in the urine may be used in assessment of renal function, but these measurements are influenced by a number of factors that may adversely influence results and make interpretation difficult.

Creatinine is cleared primarily by glomerular

filtration, whereas urea clearance measures a composite of glomerular and tubular function. Creatinine clearance is a practical measure of GFR and therefore of renal function. It can be followed serially if necessary during pregnancy. With normal renal function, the results of urine clearance tests in pregnancy should be expected to average 30 to 50 percent above normal nonpregnant values. Normal creatinine clearance in the nonpregnant person is approximately 100 ml/min; normal pregnancy values will be 140 to 150 ml/min.

Other Clinical Function Tests

The phenolsulfonphthalein (PSP) test for renal plasma flow is invalid during pregnancy. Owing to the dilated ureters and the increased dead space of the urinary tract during pregnancy, there is often a lag in the appearance of the dye in the bladder. An apparent below-normal excretion of PSP is not meaningful because excretion of the dye may be normal but seem to be impaired, owing to the lag in appearance.

Urine concentration–dilution tests are occasionally used to measure kidney function. These tests are likely to give misleading results in pregnancy because of the diurnal pattern of urinary flow. Even when fluids have been properly withheld to test the ability of the kidneys to concentrate urine, mobilization of edema fluid at night causes the urine to be more dilute in the morning than in the nonpregnant state. If such tests are done during pregnancy, the woman should be in bed and lie in the lateral recumbent position in order to assure normal kidney function.

SUMMARY OF RENAL FUNCTION

Alterations in the renal system in pregnancy include both anatomic and functional changes. Dilatation of the kidney pelves and ureters brings about changes that result in stagnation of urine. Stasis of urine may interfere with accurate urine testing and it is a factor in the tendency to urinary tract infections in pregnancy.

Renal plasma flow and glomerular filtration rate increase markedly in pregnancy and bring about a great increase in filtration of a number of substances such as metabolic waste products, nutrients, and electrolytes.

Unless reabsorption of many of these substances is also increased, there will be a greater than normal output, and a deficit will quickly occur.

Enhanced renal clearance in pregnancy means more effective excretion of waste products, creatinine, urea, and uric acid. As a result blood level values of these products in pregnancy are normally two thirds of nonpregnant values and urine clearance tests of waste products in pregnancy should average 30 to 50 percent above normal nonpregnant values.

Enhanced renal clearance also means rapid clearance of sodium and water and of glucose and other nutrients. Tubular reabsorption must increase and keep pace with filtration of these substances to prevent their rapid depletion in the body.

Sodium is a substance that is freely filtered at the glomeruli, being promoted by increased GFR and an increase in progesterone, which antagonizes the effect of aldosterone. A quick adjustment in the reabsorption of sodium, equal to the amount filtered, is critical to maternal homeostasis. To overcome the increased excretion of sodium, a compensatory mechanism, the renin–angiotensin–aldosterone system, produces aldosterone in large amounts. The aldosterone enhances tubular reabsorption of sodium as necessary to prevent sodium depletion.

There is a tendency toward sodium depletion in pregnancy and yet also a need to accumulate a total of 500 to 900 mEq of sodium during pregnancy for fetal needs and for expansion of maternal fluid volume. Although aldosterone production adjusts to need, restriction of dietary sodium or use of diuretic drugs may unduly stress the system, interfere with sodium reabsorption, and exaggerate sodium depletion.

Water excretion is excellent in early pregnancy, but later declines. In late pregnancy water pools in the lower extremities and excretion is below nonpregnant averages.

The supine and upright positions (sitting and standing) reduce GFR and excretion of both water and sodium. In these positions, pooling of blood in the legs and decreasing circulating blood volume bring about renal vasoconstriction and a reduced renal blood flow. Pregnant women with edema may thus be advised to lie on their side, preferably left, to improve excretion of fluid and of sodium.

Glucosuria is common in pregnancy and may be present intermittently. It is due in part to increased GFR and an inability of the renal tubules to reabsorb all that is filtered. Maximum tubular reabsorption may also be lowered in pregnancy so that spillage of glucose begins at a lower blood sugar value than in nonpregnant persons. Glucosuria, although common, requires evaluation.

Proteinuria is abnormal in pregnancy, signifying the presence of preeclampsia, renal disease, or urinary tract infection. Measurement of urinary protein excretion is a very valuable test of renal function, and the urine should be examined for protein at each antepartum visit.

CHANGES IN THE GASTROINTESTINAL TRACT

Changes in the digestive tract during pregnancy are signified by nausea and possibly vomiting in early pregnancy; heartburn and eructations; flatulence; and constipation, which may be most troublesome during the latter part of pregnancy. The appetite may be very capricious during the early weeks of pregnancy or it may be increased. Cravings for, or aversions to, certain foods without apparent reason are common. *Pica*, a craving for unusual substances that are not considered food, such as chalk, laundry starch, or clay, is also sometimes present.

Nausea and *vomiting* are very common disturbances in early pregnancy, occurring to some degree in about 50 percent of expectant mothers. The symptoms vary from the slightest feeling of nausea when the woman first raises her head in the morning to persistent and frequent vomiting, which then assumes a serious condition. Nausea and/or vomiting may appear at any time of the day but is most common in the early morning upon arising. Nausea and vomiting will usually disappear at the end of the first trimester.

There may be changes in the mouth tissues in pregnancy. The gums often become swollen. Some women develop a pregnancy *gingivitis*, characterized by edematous spongy gums, which bleed easily and may show some detachment. The edema is believed to be a part of the general change in the connective tissue ground substance that is caused by the estrogens in the body. Pregnancy usually does not affect the teeth adversely, but an occasional woman has an increase in dental caries in pregnancy.

Heartburn, a painful retrosternal burning sensation, often described as a feeling of burning first in the stomach and then rising into the throat, and eructations are fairly common. Heartburn is caused by frequent regurgitations of gastric acid into the esophagus. This influx of secretions may be the result of general relaxation of the stomach in pregnancy and, along with it, relaxation of the cardiac sphincter, especially when intraabdominal pressure is raised.

Gastric secretion is reduced in pregnancy, a relative hypochlorhydria is present, and gastric tone and mobility are slowed. The enlarging uterus causes the stomach to be displaced upward and to rotate to the right. The large bowel and the cecum are also displaced upward, and the rest of the intestinal tract is pushed to the sides and behind the uterus (Figs. 6-5 and 6-6).

A *general relaxation of tone* of the entire gastrointestinal tract is characteristic of smooth muscle relaxation in pregnancy and appears concomitant with relaxation of smooth muscle of other parts of the body such as the uterus, the ureters, and the blood vessels. Large amounts of progesterone apparently contribute to this muscle relaxation. It is felt that the relaxation of the gastrointestinal tract may contribute to the common occurrences of nausea and constipation in pregnancy.

Constipation appears to be present in at least

one half of all pregnant women. It may become a considerable problem, especially for the woman who previously had a tendency to constipation. Bowel relaxation is considered a major cause of constipation in pregnancy, but impaired tone of the stretched abdominal muscles may also be a contributing factor. Decreased mobility of the gastrointestinal tract may also permit gas to accumulate in the bowel to an uncomfortable extent.

Digestion and absorption of foods seem to be very efficient in pregnancy and apparently are not adversely influenced by the poor tone of the intestinal tract.

CHANGES IN THE MUSCULOSKELETAL SYSTEM

Changes in the skeleton of pregnant women are characterized by softening of the pelvic cartilages and increased mobility of the joints of the sacroiliacs, the sacrococcygeal, and the symphysis pubis. These changes are presumably the result of hormonal influences.

The increased size and weight of the uterus during pregnancy shift the center of gravity forward, increasing the normal amount of lordosis as an effort is made to balance the body. If the abdominal muscles are relaxed and in poor tone before pregnancy, the abdomen may protrude markedly as the uterus enlarges. This is followed by a great increase in the forward tilt of the pelvis, an increased strain at the sacroiliac joints, and marked lordosis.

Change in posture during pregnancy, progressive lordosis, and increased mobility and instability of the pelvic joints tends to cause tripping and falling, results in a waddling gait, and commonly leads to backache. See page 209 for discussion of backache in pregnancy.

CHANGES IN THE SKIN

Skin changes in pregnancy consist of increased blood flow, appearance of vascular spiders, increased coloration of pigmented areas, appearance of striae, and possibly increased activity of the sebaceous and sweat glands and the hair follicles. The increase in blood flow, the possible appearance or increase in size of vascular spiders and hemangiomas, and increase in hair follicle activity has been described on page 133. Abdominal striae were discussed on page 116.

As a result of increased coloration, the nipples and areolar areas of the breasts grow darker. The umbilical area becomes more pigmented. The *linea alba*, a whitish line that divides the abdomen longitudinally from sternum to symphysis pubis, becomes darker and is then known as the *linea nigra*. This line grows progressively paler after delivery. Brownish, irregularly shaped blotches sometimes appear on the face and in a masklike distribution around the eyes and over the nose and cheekbones. These are termed *chloasma*, or mask of pregnancy. Dark circles under the eyes are common.

Changes in skin pigment are probably brought about by a pituitary hormone, the *melanocyte-stimulating hormone (MSH)*. The blood level of this hormone is greatly increased in pregnancy beginning with the second month of gestation. Estrogen and progesterone have also been reported to stimulate deposition of melanin.

The pigmented areas on the breasts and abdomen usually do not return completely to their original color. The mask of pregnancy usually disappears or at least becomes considerably lighter.

CHANGES IN CARBOHYDRATE METABOLISM

Pregnancy is associated with considerable change in carbohydrate metabolism. The following discussion of these changes begins with a brief account of some of the basic mechanisms in carbohydrate metabolism in the nonpregnant individual. This is followed by a description of how these mechanisms are altered by several factors in pregnancy.

Carbohydrate Metabolism in the Nonpregnant Individual

The intermittent ingestion of food and the steady requirement of the body for energy make some mechanism for metabolic homeostasis essential. Such homeostasis is achieved by a series of complex processes that function to keep the blood glucose level within a range of 70 to 110 mg per 100 ml of blood. The blood glucose is maintained at a relatively constant and appropriate level by metabolism and storage of the foods that are absorbed; by hormones, mainly insulin; and by liberation of glucose into the circulation by the liver to counterbalance the amount of glucose that is taken out of the blood by the tissues.

The level of blood glucose at any given time is the balance between sources of glucose to the blood and the demands made on it by the tissues. A change in one direction or the other toward hypoglycemia or hyperglycemia is normally counteracted by mechanisms that bring the blood sugar back to a normoglycemic range. As glucose is taken out of the circulation by the tissues, more glucose, although not necessarily a similar amount, is added through liberation by the liver. Many individuals, however, will experience hypoglycemia after a short fast that can be corrected by eating. The liver is the principal regulator of the blood sugar level. The blood sugar level has an important regulatory influence on protein and fat metabolism as well as carbohydrate metabolism.

Glucose is supplied to the blood from three general sources: (1) absorption of food carbohydrate from the small intestine, (2) breakdown of glycogen that is stored in the liver to glucose, and (3) formation of glucose by the liver from certain amino acids and a very small amount of glycerol. Glucose, obtained from breakdown of glycogen which has been stored in the liver, is liberated at times when food carbohydrate is not available. The glycogen reserve in the liver is a short-term source of blood glucose because it can be depleted within 24 hours if food is not taken. Manufacture of glucose by the liver from amino acid and glycerol precursors maintains the blood sugar when glycogen stores become exhausted and over a more sustained period of time.

Glucose is removed from the blood by (1) the cells that utilize it for energy, (2) the liver for storage as glycogen, and (3) conversion to fat for storage.

Immediately after a meal the blood sugar rises to 120 to 130 mg per 100 ml of blood. After several hours the blood glucose level is back to 70 to 100 mg percent and is maintained at that level between meals even though glucose is constantly used by the tissues. When a glucose load from food comes to the liver and into the circulation it is soon removed from the blood by utilization for cell energy and by conversion into stores of glycogen and fat. This assures that the blood sugar level does not stay elevated for very long and that stores are built up for later use.

In normal individuals the plasma insulin level rises and falls in response to increases and decreases in blood sugar. Increased blood glucose levels stimulate the beta cells of the islets of Langerhans in the pancreas to secrete insulin. In this way insulin regulates use and storage of food supplies. As the blood glucose level rises with a meal the plasma insulin level also rises. Absorption of a glucose load from the gastrointestinal tract is accompanied by a relatively large spurt of insulin, which is secreted in response to the hyperglycemia and to some undetermined intestinal factor.

Insulin stimulates the various processes that will lower the blood glucose level. It stimulates the tissues to utilize glucose as a major source of energy. An important and fundamental effect of insulin is to facilitate the entry of glucose into tissue cells and thus make possible the utilization of glucose by muscle and adipose tissue. Insulin also stimulates conversion of glucose to glycogen and to fat, each to be stored for later use. With these processes functioning adequately, production of glucose from protein and fat is not necessary at this time and protein is conserved, being made available for repair and growth of tissue. Insulin thus serves to promote storage of carbohydrate, protein, and fat during the hours of an abundant supply.

When the supply of glucose from food is diminished, there is a decrease in insulin secretion as well. Thus the plasma insulin level falls between meals. Low levels of insulin cause decreased use of glucose by muscle and adipose tissue cells; most tissues then begin to increase their utilization of fatty acids for their metabolic needs. Lipolysis of adipose tissue stores is very sensitive to drops in insulin; this then provides for an accelerated release of fatty acids for use for tissue energy. A decrease in insulin also shifts protein synthesis to a certain degree of protein breakdown. The amino acids thus released may then be used by the liver as precursors for synthesis of glucose.

The glucose synthesized by the liver is used mainly to meet the energy requirements of the brain. Other tissues are utilizing fatty acids for energy. They use only a minimal amount of carbohydrates during hypoinsulinemia. Central nervous system tissue depends on a continuous supply of glucose from the blood. These cells do not store glycogen, but glucose is indispensable to them for their fuel and to their function. Utilization of glucose by brain cells is not dependent upon insulin as it is for many other cells of the body and therefore the plasma insulin level is not important to them.

In certain circumstances, when there are insufficient carbohydrate supplies, metabolism of fatty acids may become excessive while meeting the body's energy needs and ketone bodies may accumulate in the tissues. As fatty acids are oxidized, formation of ketone bodies takes place. Ordinarily the rate of fat catabolism and ketone body formation is such that the ketone bodies are promptly and completely oxidized by the peripheral tissues. When fatty acid breakdown becomes excessive, formation of ketone bodies in the liver exceeds the rate by which the peripheral tissues can oxidize and dispose of them. Ketone bodies—beta-hydroxybutyric acid and acetoacetic acid—then accumulate in the blood and tissues and are also excreted in the urine. An accumulation of ketones in the blood above normal concentration is termed ketosis.

One condition in which ketone bodies increase to excess is fasting, a time during which the rate of catabolism of fatty acids is high in order to meet the body's energy needs. Such starvation ketosis can be corrected by an intake of carbohydrate. The carbohydrate will replenish the liver glycogen and restore normal carbohydrate metabolism, it will inhibit output of fatty acids, and the glucose will stimulate utilization of ketone bodies by the peripheral tissues.

Starvation ketosis differs from ketosis in a person with diabetes, who has an adequate supply of carbohydrates that cannot be properly utilized because of an inadequate supply of insulin. Excess fatty acid catabolism and ketone formation then takes place. Diabetic ketosis is corrected by administration of insulin, whereas starvation ketosis requires only carbohydrates. A diabetic could, however, also develop starvation ketosis if carbohydrate intake was not adequate. The results of both ketotic processes are the same on the developing fetus and should be avoided.

Carbohydrate Metabolism in Pregnancy

The fetus is totally dependent on the mother for his nutrition, and he receives a continuous supply of glucose from her for his energy needs. Also, in pregnancy a large amount of hormones that interfere with the action of insulin make their appearance. These two major factors, plus several others of lesser importance, alter carbohydrate metabolism and make adjustments a necessity.

Tendency to Hypoglycemia

FETAL GLUCOSE NEEDS   The fuel requirements of the fetus are met entirely by glucose obtained from the mother. The fetus uses glucose (1) for his maintenance energy needs, (2) to provide the energy necessary to synthesize proteins for his growth, (3) as a precursor in the synthesis of fat, and (4) for formation of his own glycogen stores. It has been estimated that the fetus utilizes glucose for his oxidation and synthesis needs at the rate of 6 mg per kg of body weight per minute, which is two to three times greater than that used by an adult per kilogram per minute.

Blood glucose level in the fetus is 20 to 30 mg per 100 ml of blood lower than maternal blood glucose. This would permit transfer of glucose by simple diffusion, but it is believed that glucose is transferred across the placenta from mother to fetus at a faster rate and that facilitated diffusion takes place at a fairly rapid rate. Insulin does not cross the placenta, but the fetus has his own insulin by 12 weeks of age. He can utilize maternal glucose independent of maternal insulin, and he can respond with his own insulin production, at least to some degree, to the amount of available glucose and amino acids.

Amino acids are actively transported across the placenta from the maternal to the fetal circulation. This results in a lowered level of blood amino acids in the mother. Since the mother uses amino acids, especially alanine, as precursors for glucose formation by the liver when she is in a fasting state, the fetus is drawing glucose precursors as well as glucose from the mother.

There is a distinct lowering of fasting blood glucose values in the mother beginning fairly early in pregnancy. As early as 15 weeks gestation the mother's blood sugar values after an overnight fast are 15 to 20 mg lower per 100 ml of blood than after a similar fast in a nonpregnant individual. Blood sugar level drops even a greater amount if the mother is without food for a longer period of time and hypoglycemia then becomes significant.

GLUCOSURIA   Loss of glucose in the urine is a possible factor in lowering blood sugar. An increased glomerular filtration rate in pregnancy means that an increased amount of glucose is filtered out. If the renal tubules cannot increase reabsorption of glucose at the same rate that it is filtered, some glucose will be lost in the urine. It is thought that maximum glucose tubular reabsorption may be lower in pregnancy than at other times. This would mean that glucose could be lost at a lower blood glucose level in pregnancy than in the nonpregnant state. Glucosuria is present intermittently in many pregnant women.

Tendency to Ketosis

Since insulin production is lowered as blood sugar is lowered, the mother whose blood sugar is falling will also have a fall in plasma insulin levels. Pregnancy exaggerates and accelerates the response to fasting. Both blood glucose and plasma insulin levels fall more rapidly than in the nonpregnant woman. This precipitates an acceleration of the processes that lead to ketosis during fasting.

The lowered insulin levels bring about utilization of fatty acids for energy and release of amino acids as described above. Metabolism of an excessive amount of fatty acids, especially in the absence of carbohydrates, results in release of a large number of ketone bodies. Blood levels of beta-hydroxybutyric acid and acetoacetic acid are two to four times higher in pregnancy after an overnight fast than in the nonpregnant individual.

Ketone bodies are transferred across the placenta, and they may help to meet fuel requirements in the fetus if the glucose supply is limited, but this may not be without danger. There is some evidence that use of ketones by the fetus, or possibly some of the metabolic changes that accompany ketosis, have an adverse effect on fetal brain development.

Tendency to Hyperglycemia

Maternal peripheral tissues become progressively resistant to the hypoglycemic effects of insulin in the course of pregnancy. This progressive insulin antagonism is the result of increased secretion of hormones, primarily by the placenta, that interfere with the action of insulin. Secretion of hormones increases as pregnancy advances and as the placenta grows, making their effect most noticeable in the latter half of pregnancy. Four hormones appear to exert a major influence on carbohydrate metabolism in pregnancy.

HUMAN CHORIONIC SOMATOMAMMOTROPIN HCS is known to exert a significant antiinsulin effect. It augments insulin secretion but diminishes its peripheral effectiveness. By diminishing the effect of insulin, HCS reduces utilization of glucose by the mother. It also causes a marked increase in mobilization of fatty acids from fat depots, and it appears to have some anabolic effect on protein metabolism.

HCS has been described as a hormone that enhances utilization of fatty acids by the mother and reduces her utilization of glucose and protein breakdown. In this way it enhances glucose and amino acid availability to the fetus, providing for a constant flow of these nutrients from mother to fetus. This promotion of lipid metabolism by HCS together with hypoinsulinemia also leads to increased production of ketone bodies.

HCS is secreted in increasing amounts in pregnancy, and its concentration in maternal plasma is especially high in the last trimester. Some studies have shown a rise in HCS during nutritional deprivation.

ESTROGEN AND PROGESTERONE The placental sex hormones, estrogen and progesterone, are secreted in increasing amounts in pregnancy. The exact influence of these hormones is not clear, but it appears that both augment insulin secretion and at the same time act as insulin antagonists.

CORTISOL Maternal carbohydrate metabolism may be influenced by increasing plasma levels of cortisol in pregnancy. This rise in cortisol has generally been attributed to a rise in the metabolically inactive bound hormone, but it is not known if the bound hormone is completely inactive. Also recent studies have indicated that the concentration of free cortisol promotes insulin secretion, but at the same time antagonizes peripheral insulin action. Cortisol induces mobili-

zation of protein during fasting thus increasing glucose production in the liver and contributing to hyperglycemia. Cortisol also contributes to mobilization of fat during fasting.

Maternal Insulin Secretion

A constant increase in hormones antagonistic to insulin as pregnancy progresses means that more and more insulin is needed to regulate the storage and utilization of the body's energy supplies and keep the blood sugar below a hyperglycemic level. There is a significant need for increased insulin by the middle of pregnancy and an even greater need in the last trimester when placental hormones reach peak concentrations.

As more insulin is needed in pregnancy to overcome the hormonal antiinsulin effects, the beta cells produce more and more insulin to attempt to maintain homeostasis of carbohydrate metabolism. The antiinsulin effects of the hormones are matched by insulin production.

Antiinsulin effects do not appear to be present in the first trimester of pregnancy. When exogenous insulin is used by diabetics its hypoglycemic effects appear to be slightly increased in the first trimester. Thereafter, however, the effect of insulin diminishes considerably and progressively.

Requirement for an increasing amount of insulin secretion in pregnancy places a stress on the beta cells, but they are usually able to meet the demand. For the woman who has a tendency toward a disordered carbohydrate metabolism the stress of providing more and more insulin may become too great during the latter half of pregnancy. She may develop hyperglycemia and have an abnormally high two-hour postprandial blood sugar. She is then identified as having gestational diabetes, described on page 683. The purpose of blood sugar screening in late second trimester of pregnancy as noted on page 172 is to identify the clients in whom the challenge to insulin production becomes too great.

For the pregnant diabetic, the increasing production of antiinsulin hormones and increasing need for insulin requires very frequent monitoring and insulin dosage adjustment throughout pregnancy to maintain homeostasis.

Although the increase in insulin production in pregnancy brings the postprandial plasma insulin level up, the fasting insulin level still tends to be quite low. This occurs because of the tendency toward fasting hypoglycemia, which is present at all times during pregnancy.

SUMMARY OF CARBOHYDRATE METABOLISM

Fuel metabolism in pregnancy is associated with marked alterations. There is an overall tendency to fasting hypoglycemia in pregnancy, which is characterized by low blood sugar, a lowered level of circulating amino acids, an increase in free fatty acids, a low level of plasma insulin, and an increase in ketone bodies. This metabolic condition has been described as one of "accelerated starvation," since it rapidly shows the characteristic responses to starvation.

Pregnancy is also said to have a diabetogenic influence on the mother. Her peripheral tissue response to insulin is decreased and two-hour postprandial blood glucose levels tend to be in the upper limits of normal.

The two seemingly opposite conditions of tendency to hypoglycemia and tendency to hyperglycemia are the result of the fetus continuously taking food supplies from the maternal circulation, producing a hypoglycemic state, and the placenta producing hormones that interfere with the action of insulin, especially in the last half of pregnancy. The beta cells produce an increasing amount of insulin to counterbalance the hormonal influence.

In the normal pregnant woman an equilibrium usually exists between the various factors that alter carbohydrate metabolism, and she remains nearly normoglycemic. If the client has a tendency to disordered carbohydrate metabolism she may show an abnormal glucose tolerance as pregnancy progress.

With the tendency to hypoglycemia in pregnancy, it is important to minimize the likelihood of starvation ketosis and its possible adverse effects on the fetus. Caloric restrictions or weight reduction programs should not be imposed on the mother at any time during pregnancy. It is advisable for her to eat food at fairly regular times; to avoid long periods of fasting, such as an overnight fast plus omitting breakfast; and to maintain a minimal intake of 150 gm of carbohydrate per day even when it may seem necessary for her to slow her rate of weight gain.

After delivery, placental antiinsulin hormones are rapidly metabolized and excreted from the body. Insulin requirements are quickly decreased. In the normal woman a physiologic adjustment in carbohydrate metabolism is apparently made without difficulty. For the diabetic, insulin sensitivity is considerably increased immediately after delivery. Her requirements for insulin probably fall well below prepregnancy levels in the first days of the puerperium. From there adjustments in insulin dosage are made according to blood and urine glucose determinations.

CHANGES IN BODY WEIGHT

An increase in body weight is one of the metabolic changes of pregnancy. The total weight gain of a well-nourished pregnant woman at 40 weeks gestation is usually between 10 and 12.5 kg (22 and 27.5 lb); the average is 11 kg (24 lb). Whether or not such a gain is optimal is not certain nor is it known if specific gains are likely to be optimal for all persons. Some healthy individuals with a normal pregnancy will gain considerably more than the above average.

The weight gain of pregnancy includes weight of the fetus of approximately 3400 gm (7½ lb), placenta of about 650 gm (1½ lb), and amniotic fluid of 800 to 1000 gm (1¾ to 2¼ lb). The increase in uterine muscle accounts for approximately 900 gm (2 lb), and an increase in the glandular tissue of the breasts adds from 400 to 500 gm (1 lb). The increase in maternal blood volume during pregnancy adds a weight of approximately 1300 to 1500 gm (3 to 3¼ lb), and an increase in extracellular fluid toward the end of pregnancy adds another 1500 gm (3¼ lb) or more to the total weight gain in pregnancy (Fig. 6-17).

Growth of the products of conception, growth of the maternal organs of reproduction, and increases in maternal blood volume and extracellular fluid account for approximately 9000 gm (20 lb). It is apparent from the components of weight gain listed above that a gain of 9 kg (20 lb) is the minimum that should be expected at term pregnancy. A gain of less than 9 kg (20 lb) means that the mother must be catabolizing her own tissues to some degree.

The weight gain not accounted for by the increases enumerated above appears to consist mainly of maternal stores of fatty tissue. In women with an average weight gain, the stores of fat may account for 2300 to 3300 gm (5 to 7¼ lb). Fat deposition begins early in pregnancy and slows late in pregnancy (Fig. 6-17). Most of the fat deposit apparently has been stored by 30 weeks gestation and little more is laid down thereafter. Weight gain after 30 weeks gestation is from growth of the products of conception and from fluid retention.

The reason for storage of fat in pregnancy is not exactly known, but it is believed that it serves as a potential energy supply which could be used in late pregnancy. Such use would probably become necessary only in a society where women work hard until the end of pregnancy and find food scarce. If the mother nurses her baby, this fat deposit may be used for some of the energy requirements of lactation. Although the exact reason for fat deposition in pregnancy is not clear it appears to be one of the normal physiologic processes of pregnancy. If fat storage and therefore weight gain becomes excessive and is not lost in the puerperium, it may become a significant component of excess weight later in life.

In enumerating the components of weight gain above, an increase of extracellular fluid was listed as accounting for an average of 1500 gm (3¼ lb) of the total weight. If the woman develops clinical edema, even when it is slight, she may have as much as 5 liters (11 lb) or even more of extra fluid in her tissues. Such retention of tissue fluid may add considerably to her weight in the last weeks of pregnancy. This weight, however, is quickly lost after delivery.

Weight gain during pregnancy follows a slightly sigmoid upward trend (Fig. 6-18). There is little gain during the first trimester, rapid increase during the second trimester, and a slightly slower increase during the third trimester. With an average weight gain of 11 kg (24 lb) the gain may be about 1 to 1½ kg (2¼ to 3¼ lb) during the first trimester, 5 to 6 kg (11 to 13 lb) during the second trimester, and 4 to 5 kg (9 to 11 lb) during the third trimester. At 20 weeks a

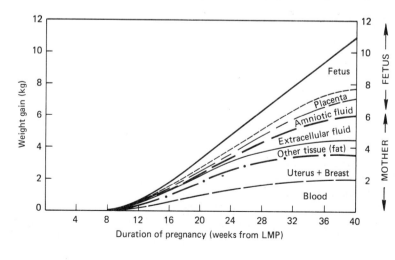

Figure 6-17. Patterns and components of average maternal weight gain during pregnancy. [*Reproduced with permission from Roy M. Pitkin, "Nutritional Support in Obstetrics and Gynecology," Clin. Obstet. Gynecol. 19(3):489–513 (Sept.) 1976, p. 491.*]

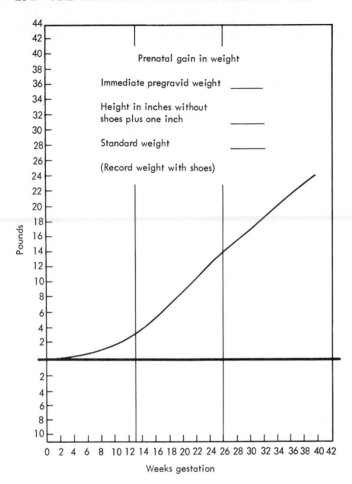

Prenatal gain in weight

Immediate pregravid weight _____

Height in inches without
shoes plus one inch _____

Standard weight _____

(Record weight with shoes)

Figure 6-18. Pattern of normal prenatal gain in weight. [*Reproduced with permission of the National Academy of Sciences from* Maternal Nutrition and the Course of Pregnancy, *National Academy of Sciences, Committee on Maternal Nutrition, Washington, D.C., 1970, p. 175.*]

gain of about 3¾ kg (8 lb) can be expected, and at 30 weeks approximately 8 kg (18 lb) will normally have been gained. During the second half of pregnancy a gain of 350 to 450 gm (¾ to 1 lb) per week will keep the weight gain within a favorable range. A weight gain of only 1000 gm (2¼ lb) per month is not adequate and one of 3000 gm (6½ lb) per month may be excessive for many women.

About 5 kg (11 lb) of the weight gain of pregnancy are lost at the time of delivery of the fetus, placenta, and amniotic fluid. Another 2 to 2½ kg (4½ to 5½ lb) are lost in the immediate puerperium, largely due to release and elimination of the extracellular fluid in the tissues. A still further reduction occurs during the suc-

ceeding weeks when the mother's body returns to approximately its prepregnant state. Most women, especially if they breast-feed their babies, continue to lose weight for at least three months after delivery, and all but a small number eventually lose all of the weight they gained during pregnancy. If there has been an excessive amount of fat storage and it is not lost between pregnancies, it may contribute to later obesity.

Edema

One of the metabolic alterations of pregnancy is an increased tendency of the body to retain water in all of its tissues. Total body water increases continuously throughout pregnancy. This includes water accumulated in the products of conception, the added maternal tissues and the blood, and water in the maternal extracellular tissue spaces. The extravascular, extracellular fluid may or may not be clinically apparent as edema. When edema does develop it is usually not evident until after 30 weeks gestation, and it is likely to be most obvious in the last few weeks of pregnancy.

A certain amount of edema seems to be a normal physiologic accompaniment of pregnancy. It is often confined to the lower extremities (see page 131) but may also be perceptible elsewhere, as in the face and hands, probably noticed mainly by tightness of the rings. An *abnormal* amount of generalized fluid retention is often associated with preeclampsia as described on page 654.

It has been estimated that women with no evidence of clinical edema, or with leg edema only, have an increase of 2½ to 3 liters of body water that cannot be accounted for in the fetal tissues and the added maternal tissues and blood. When generalized, although only slight, edema develops there appears to be an excess of body water that averages about 5 liters at term. This excess or surplus body water is assumed to be mainly fluid in the extracellular spaces. Retention of surplus water and edema will be reflected in the weight gain of the pregnant woman. Retention of even several liters of extracellular fluid may mean 2000 to 4000 gm (4 to 8 lb) of additional weight.

Although edema of the legs is common in late pregnancy, there is some evidence to suggest that the fluid in the legs represents only a small part of the total extracellular fluid increase in pregnancy. There is some reason to believe that much of the extracellular fluid is held in the skin. It is considered probable that estrogens bring about an increased mobility and distensibility of connective tissue in the body, and that the skin, which has large amounts of connective tissue, can hold much of the excess fluid. This may or may not appear as clinical edema.

In late pregnancy, especially when edema of the lower extremities is common, there may be fairly large diurnal variations in body fluid. Edema of the legs often decreases considerably after a period of rest in bed. Some of this change may be the result of redistribution of fluid, but often there is also a diuresis, especially when the woman assumes the lateral recumbent position.

Reversal of water retention, with release of accumulated extracellular fluid, occurs during the first few days after delivery. Diuresis is apparent during the first day or two post partum, and weight loss is greater during the first week of the puerperium than in the succeeding weeks.

SUMMARY

Pregnancy brings about dramatic alterations in maternal physiology which involve every system of the body. A number of these changes have been described in this chapter; many others have not been discussed.

Many physiologic adaptations of pregnancy begin very early, earlier than often appears necessary, and a number of them appear to be greater than essential to meet any immediate need. An example of a change that goes beyond the demands of pregnancy is the nearly 50 percent increase in respiratory minute volume, which is more than adequate to meet the 15 percent increase in oxygen consumption. Another example is the storage of fat early in pregnancy as a potential energy source in case of later need. Often the alterations of pregnancy appear to be exaggerated, perhaps to serve as safeguards.

The mechanisms that cause the dramatic changes in maternal physiology can sometimes be explained, at least partially. At other times the cause of the adaptations is not at all clearly understood. There is reason to believe that many of the alterations in pregnancy are triggered by hormones from the fetoplacental unit and are controlled by the fetus. Many of the adaptations of pregnancy represent changes important to adequate fetal development. In general, it can probably be said that the responses in the mother appear to work toward both facilitating growth and development of the fetus and safeguarding her own welfare.

BIBLIOGRAPHY

Assali, Nicholas S. (ed.), *Pathophysiology of Gestation*, Vol. I. *Maternal Disorders*. Academic Press, New York, 1972.

Bonica, John J., Maternal respiratory changes during pregnancy and parturition, *Clin. Anesth.* 10:1–19, 1973.

Burrow, Gerard N., and Ferris, Thomas F., *Medical Complications During Pregnancy*. Saunders, Philadelphia, Pa., 1975.

Danforth, David N. (ed.), *Obstetrics and Gynecology*, 3rd ed. Harper and Row, New York, 1977.

Ehrlich, Edward N., Sodium metabolism in pregnancy: Current views, *Contemp. Ob/Gyn* 4:17–20 (Dec.) 1974.

Felig, Philip; Maternal and fetal fuel homeostasis in human pregnancy, *Am. J. Clin. Nutr.* 26:998–1005 (Sept.) 1973.

Fournier, P. J. R., Desjardins, P. D., and Friesen, H. G., Current understanding of human prolactin physiology and its diagnostic and therapeutic applications: A review, *Am. J. Obstet. Gynecol.* 118:337–343 (Feb. 1) 1974.

Friesen, Henry G., Placental protein hormones and tissue receptors of hormones, in *Modern Perinatal Medicine*, edited by Louis Gluck. Year Book Medical Publishers, Chicago, Ill., 1974.

———, Fournier, P., and Desjardins, P. Pituitary prolactin in pregnancy and normal and abnormal lactation, *Clin. Obstet. Gynecol.* 16:25–45 (Sept.) 1973.

Goldberg, Vivian J., and Ramwell, Peter W., Role of prostaglandins in reproduction, *Physiol. Rev.* 55:325–351 (July) 1975.

Greenhill, J. P., and Friedman, Emanuel A., *Biological Principles and Modern Practice of Obstetrics*. Saunders, Philadelphia, Pa., 1974.

Hytten, Frank E., and Leitch, Isabella, *The Physiology of Human Reproduction*, 2nd ed. Blackwell Scientific Publications, Oxford, 1971.

Jaffe, Robert B., Endocrine interactions and the placenta, *Hosp. Pract.* 6:71–82 (Dec.) 1971.

Levine, Rachmiel, and Haft, David E., Carbohydrate homeostatis, *N. Engl. J. Med.* 283:175–182 (July 23) 1970 and 283:237–246 (July 30) 1970.

Lindheimer, Marshall D., and Katz, Adrian I., Managing the patient with renal disease, *Contemp. Ob/Gyn* 3:49–55 (Jan.) 1974.

———, Renal function in pregnancy, *Obstet. Gynecol. Annu.* 1:139–176, 1972.

Liu, David T. Y., Striae gravidarum, *Lancet* I:625 (Apr. 6) 1974.

MacGillivray, I., Rose, G. A., and Rowe, B., Blood pressure survey in pregnancy, *Clin. Sci.* 37:395–407 (Oct.) 1969.

Page, Ernest W., Villee, Claude A., and Villee, Dorothy B., *Human Reproduction*, 2nd ed. Saunders, Philadelphia, Pa., 1976.

Pritchard, Jack A., and MacDonald, Paul C., *Williams Obstetrics*, 15th ed. Appleton-Century-Crofts, New York, 1975.

Reid, Duncan E., Ryan, Kenneth J., and Benirschke, Kurt, *Principles and Management of Human Reproduction*. Saunders, Philadelphia, Pa., 1972.

Ross Conference, Report of the Third Ross Conference on Obstetric Research, *The Endocrine Milieu of Pregnancy, Puerperium and Childhood*. Ross Laboratories, Columbus, Ohio, 1974.

Shearman, Rodney P. (ed.), *Human Reproductive Physiology*. Blackwell Scientific Publications, Oxford, 1972.

Siiteri, Pentti, Steroid hormones in pregnancy, in *Modern Perinatal Medicine*, edited by Louis Gluck. Year Book Medical Publishers, Chicago, Ill., 1974.

Yen, S. S. C., Endocrine regulation of metabolic homeostasis during pregnancy, *Clin. Obstet. Gynecol.* 16:130–147 (Sept.) 1973.

Part Two

The Antepartum Period

7

Antepartum Care—
Data Collection and
Assessment

The antepartum period extends from conception until the onset of labor. The terms *prenatal* and *antepartum* are often used interchangeably. Strictly speaking, the meaning is not identical, but for practical purposes precise definition is not necessary. Antepartum means before labor. Prenatal means before birth and therefore includes the period of labor until the time of the baby's birth.

Antepartum care has traditionally been defined as the care given an expectant mother during her pregnancy. With increasing knowledge and sophistication in the science of fetology the developing fetus has become as much the focus of care as the woman herself. In addition, the birth of an infant has an impact not only on the mother but also on the father, other siblings, and grandparents, requiring adjustments in all of their roles and relationships. For this reason the nurse should most properly consider childbearing in the setting of the family to which the woman belongs and into which the infant will be introduced.

Although pregnancy is a biologically normal event, it is an unusual one in the life of a woman and as such requires some special adaptations for the promotion of her health and that of her fetus. Health professionals should view this time as an optimal opportunity for preventive health maintenance and client education. Often the woman has not had a complete physical examination or health history since childhood. In addition there is usually a need for instruction and

counseling in many health-related areas, such as pregnancy, nutrition, sexuality, and family relationships.

The following three chapters will explore in some detail the various aspects of antepartum care. Underlying the discussion is belief in the family-centered nature of pregnancy and childbearing, the importance of careful screening and continual vigilance in the areas of preventive medicine, and the necessity for a well-informed client who can be a knowledgeable participant in the decision making relative to her care. Emphasis will be on the role of the nurse as a provider of health care in colleagueship with professionals from other disciplines.

Confirmation of the fact of pregnancy is the first task of antepartum care for the health professional as well as for the woman and her family. Some women "just know" that they have conceived; rare others have reportedly remained ignorant of the pregnancy until delivery. For most women, however, diagnosis of pregnancy is made because of the manifestations of certain signs and symptoms.

So many signs of pregnancy are known to women that the majority recognize pregnancy quite early, particularly if they have borne children before. They will usually, however, seek confirmation of their opinion from other women or health professionals, probably as one way of working out the ambivalence so characteristic of early pregnancy.

Occasionally women approaching menopause,

or others who intensely desire to be pregnant, may experience an imaginary or spurious pregnancy. This condition, known as *pseudocyesis,* is characterized by many of the signs and symptoms of true pregnancy but usually can be readily ascertained by bimanual examination, revealing an unenlarged uterus. Psychiatric assistance may be necessary to support the woman in accepting this diagnosis.

SIGNS OF PREGNANCY

Traditionally the signs of pregnancy are classified under three self-explanatory headings: *presumptive* signs and symptoms, *probable* signs, and *positive* signs. The absolutely positive signs cannot be detected until the sixteenth to twentieth week of gestation; the probable signs are usually available earlier, and the presumptive signs may be present at varying times.

Presumptive Signs and Symptoms

The presumptive symptoms, which consist largely of subjective symptoms observed by the woman herself and which may be experienced at varying periods, are as follows.

Cessation of Menstruation

A menstrual period may be missed for any one of several causes, but in a healthy woman of the childbearing age, whose menses have previously been regular, missing two successive periods after intercourse is a strong indication of pregnancy. This is usually the first symptom noticed.

Changes in the Breasts

Early in pregnancy the breasts increase in size and firmness, and many women have a throbbing, tingling, or pricking sensation and a feeling of tension and fullness. The breasts may be so tender that even slight pressure is painful. The nipples are larger and more prominent, and along with the surrounding areolae, become darker. The veins under the skin are more apparent and the glands of Montgomery larger. If, in addition to these symptoms, it is possible to express a pale yellowish fluid from the nipples of a woman who has not had children, pregnancy may be strongly suspected. Practically all of these signs in the breasts can be due to causes other than pregnancy. A woman who has borne children may have milk present in her breasts for months after the birth of a baby even if she is not breast-feeding.

Nausea and Vomiting

"Morning sickness," as the name suggests, is nausea, sometimes accompanied by vomiting, which many pregnant women have immediately upon arising in the morning. It varies in severity from a mild attack when the woman first lifts her head to repeated and severe recurrences during the day, and even into the night. The morning nausea, lasting but a few hours, usually occurs daily for about six weeks, when it gradually disappears. When the vomiting is very severe and not relieved by simple remedies, it is termed "pernicious vomiting." Morning sickness may begin immediately after conception, but as a rule it starts about the sixth week of gestation and continues until the third or fourth month. It occurs in about half of all pregnancies and is particularly common among women pregnant for the first time. Many women go throughout the entire period of gestation without nausea and vomiting, while others are entirely comfortable in the morning and nauseated only during the latter part of the day.

Frequent Micturition

There is usually a desire to void urine frequently during the first three or four months of pregnancy, after which the tendency disappears, but recurs during the later months. Frequency of urination is largely caused by reduction in the capacity of the bladder, due to crowding by pressure exerted on it by the enlarging uterus while both organs remain within the unyielding bony pelvis. Pressure on the outside of the bladder gives much the same sensation as is experienced when the bladder is distended with urine. After the uterus and bladder rise from the pelvic cavity into the abdomen, the uterus no longer crowds the bladder. During the last month or six weeks of pregnancy the fetal head presses on the bladder, and again there is a desire to void frequently.

Other Signs and Symptoms

Increased discoloration of the pigmented areas of the skin and the appearance of abdominal striae are other presumptive signs.

Chadwick's sign, the dark bluish or purplish appearance of the vulval and vaginal lining, which is the result of the great increase in vascularity, is another early sign of pregnancy.

Quickening is the widely used term which designates the mother's first perception of fetal movements. This occurs about the sixteenth to eighteenth week of pregnancy. The sensation is comparable to a very slight quivering or tapping, or to the fluttering of a bird's wings imprisoned in the hand. Beginning very gently, these movements increase in intensity as pregnancy progresses. They may become very troublesome toward the latter part of pregnancy, amounting then to sharp kicks and blows.

Women who have had children can usually be relied upon to distinguish between quickening and the somewhat similar sensation caused by the movement of gas in the intestines, but a woman pregnant for the first time may be deceived. Women often use the term "feeling life" when they feel the fetus move, and physicians and nurses frequently use this term when questioning the expectant mother about the perception of fetal movements.

Fatigue may be one of the most prominent complaints of the woman during the first trimester.

There are other possible symptoms of pregnancy, but their value is uncertain. Even the ones described above are not entirely dependable, but if two or more of them occur coincidentally, they probably indicate pregnancy.

Probable Signs

The probable signs of pregnancy are chiefly discoverable by the physician or nurse after careful examination. They also are numerous and uncertain, but some are quite dependable. All of the probable signs of pregnancy, like the presumptive symptoms, may be simulated in nonpregnant conditions; hence the appearance of any one of them alone may not be deeply significant. Two or more occurring coincidentally constitute strong evidence of pregnancy.

Enlargement of the Abdomen

Enlargement of the abdomen begins to be apparent about the third month of gestation. At this stage, the growing uterus may be felt through the abdominal wall as a tumor that steadily increases in size as pregnancy advances. Rapid enlargement of the abdomen in a woman of childbearing age, therefore, may be taken as fair, but not positive, evidence of pregnancy. Too much reliance cannot be placed on this sign, as the abdomen may be enlarged by a tumor, fluid, or a rapid weight gain.

Changes in the Uterus

Changes in the size, shape, and consistency of the uterus which take place during the first three months of pregnancy are very important indications of pregnancy. These are discoverable upon vaginal examination. The uterus is found to be considerably enlarged, somewhat globular in shape, and of a soft, doughy consistency.

About the sixth week, the so-called *Hegar's sign* is perceptible through bimanual examination. This is discovered when the fingers of one hand are pressed deeply into the abdomen, just above the symphysis pubis, and two fingers of the other hand are passed through the vagina until they rest in the posterior fornix, behind the cervix. The isthmus of the uterus, which may be felt between the fingertips of the two hands, is extremely soft and compressible. Occasionally the change in consistency is so marked that there appears to be no connection between the cervix, which is felt below the fingertips, and the body of the uterus, which lies above them. This sign, named for the man who first described it, is one of the most valuable signs of early pregnancy.

Softening of the cervix occurs, as a rule, about the beginning of the second month of pregnancy. In some cases, such as certain inflammatory conditions and in carcinoma, this sign may not appear. This softening of the cervix is often called *Goodell's sign.*

Painless uterine contractions, called *Braxton-Hicks* contractions, from their first observer, begin during the early weeks of pregnancy and recur at intervals of 5 to 10 to 20 minutes throughout the entire period of gestation. These contractions may be observed during the early months by bimanual examination and subsequently by placing the hand on the abdomen. One feels the uterus growing alternately hard and soft as it contracts and relaxes. At first the mother is not conscious of these contractions, but as pregnancy progresses she may become aware of a periodic tightening of her abdomen. As term approaches, Braxton-Hicks contractions are sometimes mistaken by the mother for beginning labor.

Ballottement

During the fourth and fifth months of gestation the fetus can move freely in the amniotic fluid. If it is made to passively move in this fluid, it rebounds against the fingers. Ballottement is accomplished by giving a sharp or sudden push to the fetus and feeling it rebound in a few seconds to its original position. Such passive movements are among the most certain of the probable signs.

Ability to Palpate the Outline of the Fetus

When the outline of the fetus can be distinguished by feeling and pressing the abdomen, it is a fairly reliable sign of pregnancy. Since a tumor may occasionally simulate the fetal head or other parts of the body, this sign alone is not considered reliable for positive diagnosis.

Pregnancy Tests

Although pregnancy tests are quite reliable, they are not considered a positive sign of pregnancy, since both false-positive and false-negative results are possible, as well as laboratory errors.

The theory that something in the urine of pregnant women would cause plants to grow or seeds to germinate has been held since ancient time, but it was not until the twentieth century that any real scientific research was carried out. Several investigators discovered that the urine of pregnant women contained large amounts of a hormone that would stimulate the ovaries of animals to ovulate. This hormone, now known as *chorionic gonadotropin,* is one of the placental hormones elaborated by the chorionic villi. It is present in the blood and urine of pregnant women in fairly large concentration by the fifteenth day of pregnancy. The concentration increases, reaching a peak between 8 and 10 weeks of gestation. Then it slowly falls, reaching a low level between 14 and 18 weeks, after which it remains at a low level until separation of the placenta, when it disappears.

As a result of the early research, the first scientific test for pregnancy, known as the Aschheim-Zondek test, was demonstrated in 1928. In that test immature female mice were injected with urine from the woman in whom pregnancy was suspected. Further developments in pregnancy testing utilized rabbits, and in a later discovery the common North American male frog proved to be a very reliable test animal.

More recently *immunologic pregnancy tests,* dependent upon antigen–antiserum reaction, have replaced the biologic tests. These tests are based on the reaction of human urinary chorionic gonodatropin (HCG) to antiserum. The tests are easy to use clinically and are highly reliable, and the test material is readily available commercially.

For the immunologic pregnancy test, particles of latex coated with human chorionic gonadotropic hormone are used as the antigen. A drop of the urine to be tested is thoroughly mixed on a glass slide with a drop of antiserum against HCG. Next, two drops of a suspension of latex particles coated with HCG are added to the urine and antiserum mixture. After a few minutes of agitation, to ensure complete exposure of the latex particles, the slide is examined for agglutination. If the urine does not contain HCG, the antiserum is available to react with the HCG-coated latex particles and agglutination takes place. Visible agglutination is a negative test. If HCG is present in the urine, the hormone will neutralize the antiserum and prevent agglutination of the latex particles. Absence of agglutination means a positive pregnancy test (Fig. 7-1). Depending upon the commercial preparation used, the test results may be available in two minutes.

A hemagglutination inhibition test may also be used as a pregnancy test. For this test urine and antiserum are mixed, and a suspension of sheep erythrocytes coated with HCG is added. Results are not available for two hours.

Urine for a pregnancy test should be collected in a laboratory urine specimen bottle. Any container considered suitable for collection of a specimen at home is *not* satisfactory. Residue of former contents, which may remain in such a container even after careful washing, and traces of detergent may interfere with agglutination results and give erroneous values.

Soon after fertilization of an ovum the trophoblastic cells begin to secrete chorionic gonadotropin. Since conception would have taken place approximately two weeks after the last menstrual period, there may be sufficient chorionic gonadotropin in the urine to detect pregnancy by the time the woman realizes that she has missed her first menstrual period. The assurance of accuracy of a pregnancy test is high after six weeks have elapsed since the first day of the last menstrual period. The test is thus a fairly reliable means of diagnosis of early pregnancy.

False-negative pregnancy tests are more common than false-positive tests. False-negative results may be obtained when the test is done so early that there is insufficient hormone or when the urine is greatly diluted. A positive pregnancy test only indicates that chorionic gonadotropic hormone is present. This may or may not be produced by a normal pregnancy.

A pregnancy test may be a valuable aid in diagnosis of complications in which it is essential to know whether or not conception has oc-

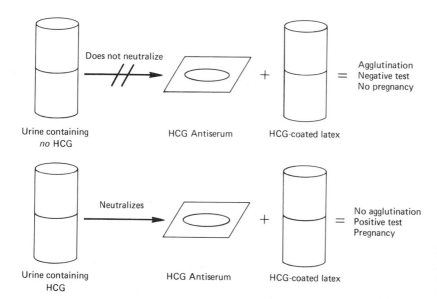

Figure 7-1. Diagram illustrating the mechanism of immunologic pregnancy tests.

curred. Tumors and cysts can simulate or mask pregnancy, and this test may help in making a final diagnosis. The test is one of several findings that may confirm or rule out the suspicion of an ectopic pregnancy when a tubal mass is discovered, although a negative test does not exclude the possibility of an ectopic pregnancy. When an abortion has threatened, the test may be valuable in determining whether or not the placenta has separated and may thus be important when a decision must be made on further treatment.

The pregnancy test is very strongly positive in such abnormal conditions as hydatidiform mole and choriocarcinoma. On this basis it may be an aid in making the diagnosis and also in determining whether or not all abnormal tissue has been expelled or removed.

A radioreceptorassay of HCG, the Saxena test, is available for the diagnosis of pregnancy as early as two weeks after conception. Although it is not ordinarily necessary to have such an immediate diagnosis it does have benefits for determining the presence of an ectopic pregnancy, in situations following infertility treatment or artificial insemination, or when the pregnancy would be high risk (to initiate early care of the diabetic, for example).

Until recently a *hormone-induced withdrawal bleeding test* was sometimes used to differentiate early pregnancy from amenorrhea of a functional nature in a woman who previously had regular menses. This test is based on the physiologic effect on the development of the endometrium when the ovarian hormones, estrogen and progesterone, are administered. If the woman is not pregnant the discontinuance of the medication after a few days results in endometrial desquamation and withdrawal bleeding or menstruation. If the woman is pregnant, the corpus luteum of pregnancy or, later, the placenta are producing sufficient hormones to maintain the decidua and no bleeding will occur. Both animal and clinical studies now suggest that there is a teratologic risk to the developing embryo when these hormones are administered during pregnancy, especially during the first trimester. Therefore, their use as an aid in the diagnosis of pregnancy is not warranted.

Positive Signs

The three positive signs of pregnancy are not apparent until the eighteenth to twentieth week of pregnancy. All emanate from the fetus.

Hearing and Counting the Fetal Heartbeat

The fetal heartbeat is unmistakable evidence of pregnancy. The sound of the fetal heartbeat is usually likened to the ticking of a watch under a pillow. It should be counted and recorded. The rate varies from 120 to 160 beats per minute in different babies, but tends to remain at nearly the same rate in an individual baby. To ensure that the fetal heart and not the maternal pulse is being counted, the mother's radial pulse may be palpated while counting.

With a stethoscope the fetal heartbeat is usually heard between 18 and 20 weeks gestation. Ultrasonic equipment permits detection of heart movement by 10 weeks of gestation. Ultrasonic equipment is generally not necessary in normal pregnancy but may be used when auscultation of the fetal heart is questionable at a time when it could be expected to be audible.

Perception of Active Movement of the Fetus

Active movement of the fetus is accepted as a second incontrovertible sign of pregnancy if the fetal movements are perceived by an objective observer other than the mother. Active fetal movements may be felt at intervals after the fifth month of pregnancy by placing a hand over the abdomen. They are very faint at first, but become strong later and are easily felt and sometimes seen.

Ability to Visualize the Fetal Skeletal Outline by X-ray or by Ultrasound

Because x-ray exposure of the fetus is not without risk, particularly early in pregnancy, it is advisable to avoid x-ray studies unless absolutely essential for diagnosis. This may be necessary, however, in order to differentiate between a normal pregnancy and a tumor, or for diagnosis in a very obese woman. Since the fetal skeleton can only be seen after some calcification has taken place, it is not visible before the fourteenth week and usually 18 weeks is the earliest it can be seen with reasonable certainty.

With the use of *ultrasound* pregnancy can be diagnosed as early as the sixth week of gestation when the gestational sac appears as a white ring in the fundus of the uterus (Fig. 7-2). Since there are no known ill effects of ultrasonography on the products of conception this method not only permits earlier diagnosis but also appears to be safer.

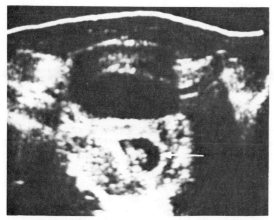

Figure 7-2. The arrow is pointing to the gestational sac and the embryo is seen as the white area in the dark sac. The large black area above the developing embryo is an ovarian cyst.

ESTIMATING THE PROBABLE DATE OF DELIVERY

The exact duration of pregnancy cannot be ascertained, since the time when the ovum was fertilized is not known. It is impossible, therefore, to know the exact length of pregnancy, but labor usually begins about 10 lunar months, 40 weeks, or from 273 to 280 days after the onset of the last menstrual period.

The approximate date of delivery may be estimated by counting forward 280 days or backward 85 days from the first day of the last menstrual period. What is perhaps simpler, and gives approximately the same date, is to add seven days to the onset of the last period and count back three months. For example, if the last period began on June 3, the addition of seven days gives June 10, while counting back three months indicates March 10 as the approximate date on which the delivery may be expected. Designating the months by numbers the foregoing example would be as follows: 6/3 plus 7 days = 6/10 minus 3 months = 3/10. This method of computation, known as *Naegele's rule*, is probably as satisfactory as any, being accurate within 10 days before or after the estimated date in about two thirds of all deliveries.

Another method sometimes employed to determine the duration of pregnancy is to estimate the gestational age to which pregnancy has advanced by measuring the height of the uterine fundus. This may be done by palpating the abdomen and noting the height of the fundus in relation to other abdominal landmarks or by measuring the distance from the superior edge of the symphysis pubis to the top of the fundus, using either calipers or an ordinary tape measure (Fig. 7-3).

The growth of the uterus should be fairly uniform throughout pregnancy. When palpating the abdomen it is observed that the fundus is palpable as a firm, rounded organ just above the symphysis pubis at approximately 12 to 14 weeks gestation. By 16 weeks it is halfway between the symphysis and the umbilicus, and by 20 weeks it is at the level of the umbilicus. At 28 weeks gestation the fundus is halfway between the umbilicus and the xiphoid process, and it is at the level of the xiphoid by about the 36th week. At the 40th week, or term, the fundus in primigravidas frequently sinks downward to about the position it occupied at the 32nd to 34th week (Fig. 7-4). This descent is more common among primigravidas, since the head enters the pelvis earlier than in the multigravida. In primigravidas this descent usually occurs in the last weeks of pregnancy, but in women who have had children the head may not enter the pelvis until the onset of labor.

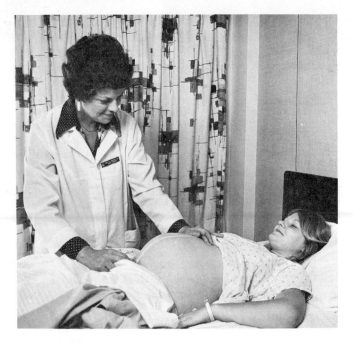

Figure 7-3.   The nurse is measuring the height of the uterine fundus to determine the duration of pregnancy.

Various formulas or rules have been devised to estimate the gestational age from measurements of fundal height. The most convenient rule of thumb to bear in mind, however, is that the distance in centimeters from the symphysis pubis to the top of the fundus, when measured with an ordinary tape measure, is approximately the same as the weeks of gestation. In other words, if the height of the fundus is 28 cm by tape measure, the weeks gestation will also be approximately 28 (Fig. 7-5).

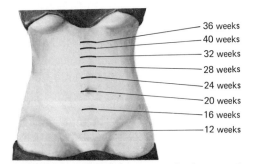

36 weeks
40 weeks
32 weeks
28 weeks
24 weeks
20 weeks
16 weeks
12 weeks

Figure 7-4.   Height of the uterine fundus at each of the 10 lunar months of pregnancy.

Still another method of estimating the duration of pregnancy is to count forward 22 to 24 weeks from the day on which the expectant mother first feels fetal movement. This experience, termed "quickening," usually occurs about the eighteenth to twentieth week, but is so irregular that it is unreliable as a basis for computation.

Dates when pregnancy tests are positive in relation to the last menstrual period and the time when fetal heart tones are first heard with an ordinary fetoscope may also be valuable information in estimating the gestational age and therefore the probable date of delivery.

All of these estimations may be further complicated by variations in the size of fetuses and amounts of amniotic fluid at the same periods of gestation in different pregnancies, an unknown date of onset of the last menses, or conception occurring during a period of amenorrhea, as in the nursing mother. For this reason, no one piece of information is relied upon as a sufficient estimator; rather a combination of all available data is analyzed in order to arrive at the most

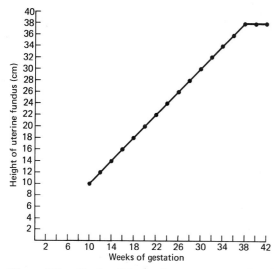

Figure 7-5. Height of the fundus at various weeks of gestation, showing that the growth of the uterus is fairly uniform throughout pregnancy.

reasonable assessment of gestational age. Occasionally it is necessary to utilize laboratory studies of fetal lung maturity and/or fetal biparietal diameter measurements to substantiate the expected date of confinement. This is particularly true in the case of high-risk pregnancies.

INITIATING ANTEPARTUM CARE

As soon as a woman suspects herself to be pregnant she should make an appointment with a clinic or physician's office to initiate antepartum care for herself and her fetus. Although pregnancy is a normal physiologic process, the many changes taking place in the woman's body result in a narrower borderline between health and illness than is present when she is not pregnant. Prevention—or at least early detection—of abnormal signs, followed by prompt and efficient treatment, will avert many complications associated with childbearing, not only throughout the antepartum period but also during labor and delivery and afterward. Thus antepartum care is essentially preventive care for mother and fetus.

The first antepartum visit should be primarily one of assessment for both the woman and the health professionals. This is the woman's opportunity to evaluate for herself the health care system she has entered. She should become aware of the basic philosophy of the health care providers, the number and qualifications of the personnel, general policies and procedures, and costs of care. The nurse has a responsibility to facilitate this introduction to the system. This can often be accomplished in informal conversation and by supporting the client in asking questions of others. The woman may wish to know if she will be examined by the same physician at each visit, if nurses will do some or all of the antepartum care including physical assessments, if the physician "approves" of natural childbirth, how frequently she will have to visit, and which hospital or maternity center she will use for delivery. The most satisfying childbearing experiences are generally provided in settings where the health professionals encourage the development of knowledge which enables clients to participate actively in making decisions about their own care.

COLLECTION OF DATA

In addition to becoming acquainted with the office or clinic, the main purpose of the first antepartum visit is a thorough health assessment of the newly pregnant woman. Three methods of data collection are utilized: the health history, the physical examination, and laboratory screening procedures.

The Health History

The health history is perhaps the most important of the three data collection methods. A carefully elicited history will provide not only objective facts but also valuable information concerning the client's beliefs and feelings and ways in which she prefers to be helped.

The interview for a health history should take place in a comfortable, homelike environment

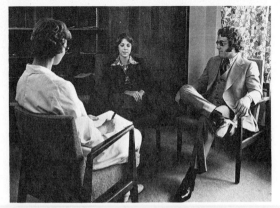

Figure 7-6. Nurse taking a health history from a couple at the woman's first antepartum visit.

removed from the disquieting sight of examination tables and gleaming instruments. The presence of her husband or other supportive person may help the woman to feel more at ease and will make the family feel included and important (Fig. 7-6).

For a thorough review of history-taking procedures the reader is referred to one of the basic texts on this subject. Outlined below are selected portions of the history which are of particular importance to the perinatal practitioner.

1. Menstrual History
   A. Age at time of onset of menses (menarcho)
   B. Regularity, interval, and duration of flow
   C. Dysmenorrhea or other complications
   D. Date of first day of last menstrual period

These data provide valuable gynecologic information. In addition, the nurse who is sensitive to affect and terminology can often pick up significant clues about the client's feelings about her own femininity and self-worth. This will be an important foundation for how she feels about herself as a pregnant woman and, ultimately, as a mother. For example, women who regard menstruation as a "curse" or who are repulsed by this bodily function may need special help to

cope with the physical changes and increased body awareness that are characteristic of pregnancy.

The first day of the last menstrual period (LMP) is important in order to make use of Naegele's rule in estimating the expected date of confinement (EDC). Of equal importance in interpreting the estimated date of confinement is the information concerning the interval between menses. Naegele's rule is based on the presumption of a 28-day cycle with ovulation and fertilization occurring on approximately day 14 of the cycle. If an individual woman's cycle is not 28 days this method of estimation will be less accurate. Although this is seldom of significance in the normal pregnancy, it could assume major importance in a pregnancy at risk where the determination of gestational age of the fetus is an essential diagnostic requirement. Such should be the case if, for example, the fetus were suspected of intrauterine growth retardation or malnutrition.

2. Obstetric History
   A. Past pregnancies
      1. Date
      2. Course of pregnancy, labor, and post partum
      3. Sex, name, birthweight, and gestational age of infant
      4. Neonatal course and present health of child
   B. Present pregnancy
      1. Planned vs. unplanned
      2. Subjective signs and symptoms

Certain terms commonly used to designate a woman's previous childbearing experience are defined here for use in the obstetric history.

Gravid refers to a pregnancy regardless of its duration.

Para refers to past pregnancies that continued to the period of viability.

A *primigravida* is a woman who is pregnant for the first time.

A *multigravida* is a woman who is in her second or any subsequent pregnancy.

A *nullipara* (para O) is a woman who has not had children.

A *primipara* (para I) is a woman who has given birth to one child of viable age. However, this term is often used interchangeably with primigravida.

A *multipara* (para II, para III, para IV) is a woman who has given birth to two or more children. This term is also often used loosely and applied to the woman who is pregnant for the second time or is in her second labor, at which time she is still a para I.

A *parturient* is a woman in labor.

The past obstetric history of a woman is probably more completely described by the use of the terms gravida and para than by the terms primipara and multipara. A woman pregnant for the first time is a primigravida or a gravida I, para O, during her pregnancy and labor. Once delivered she is a gravida I, para I. A woman whose first pregnancy ended in abortion and who is now pregnant a second time is a gravida II, para O. Para refers to pregnancies terminated beyond 20 weeks, not to babies. The woman who delivers twins from her first pregnancy remains a para I in spite of having two babies. She is also a para I if the baby was stillborn or died soon after birth, since para refers to a pregnancy that has progressed to the period of viability regardless of the condition of the baby.

Discussing past pregnancies with the woman and her family may help to anticipate needs as well as expectations during the present pregnancy. Certainly medical complications should be noted. Among these are excessive nausea and vomiting, preeclampsia/eclampsia, bleeding during pregnancy, labor, or post partum, and premature labor. Although the woman may not recall (or, unfortunately, may never have known) medical diagnoses, she may describe symptoms and/or treatments which will be suggestive of certain situations. These can later be reviewed with her previous medical record if one is available. In addition, information should be elicited about those things during the pregnancy which

were pleasant as well as those which were irritating and how the family adapted their living patterns to accommodate.

Information about the weight, gestational age, and neonatal course of other children may have important predictive value. For example, weights of other infants in the family may suggest a normal, genetic explanation for smallness, thus allaying concerns about pathologic growth retardation. Women who have had previous unexplained premature deliveries are at increased risk for future premature deliveries. Neonatal illness or anomalies may suggest a need for parent education, anticipatory guidance, or genetic counseling. Additionally it is useful to have data about the present age, developmental status, and general health of the other children. This can form the basis for helping parents prepare the children for a new baby as well as indicate possible family stressors and needs for referral and/or consultation with other members of the health team.

In talking about whether the present pregnancy was planned or not the nurse can also obtain information about contraceptive practices. This will be helpful in assisting the couple with decision making in this area during the postpartum period. If oral contraceptives have been used it is well to note if the last menstrual period was a "bleed-off" from the last cycle of pills. If it was, Naegele's rule for estimating the date of confinement may be less accurate. It should also be determined if any oral contraceptives were taken following conception, since recent research indicates a possible teratologic effect of such drugs.

3. Medical History
   A. Family
   B. Personal

The medical history should not be limited to a litany of past diseases but should be systematically elicited to meet three major objectives. The first of these objectives is to obtain data concerning medical or surgical conditions of the woman or of her family which are likely to have a direct bearing on this pregnancy. Among such conditions would be those of a hereditary nature, such as diabetes mellitus, cystic fibrosis, or mental retardation. Also important are past illnesses of a chronic or recurring nature, such as frequent urinary tract infections or monilial vaginitis.

Second, information about drugs taken is important. If a woman does not know what a particular prescription drug is she should bring it with her for identification. It is preferable for all drugs to be labeled by name so that the consumer is aware of what is being taken. Nonprescription drugs are often not mentioned unless the interviewer specifically questions about such things as vitamins, aspirin, alcohol, marijuana, laxatives, and so on.

The third objective is to gain insight into the woman's previous experience with pain and hospitalization and what coping strategies she has used to deal with these. Finally, it is useful to be aware of any current family illness—either chronic or acute—which may be an added stressor during the pregnancy.

4. Personal/Social History
   A. Education and occupation of the couple
   B. Available support persons from kinship or friendship groups
   C. Marital and sexual history
   D. General health habits regarding rest and sleep, nutrition, elimination, recreation

The educational achievement and occupation of the couple give clues to their level of understanding and their financial resources. If the woman is employed outside the home assistance may be required to integrate her present career with her new one as parent. If she plans to stop working there may be financial difficulties as a result of losing her salary. In addition, the occupation and work environment may provide information about possible health risks to either parent or to the fetus. Lead is probably the most publicized toxic chemical that causes birth defects, but there is a growing list of industrial and agricultural materials that can produce genetic damage to both men and women as well as to a developing fetus.

A diet history, which is a part of this data collection, will be discussed more fully in the chapter on nutrition during pregnancy (Chapter 8).

It will be apparent to the reader that all of the information which comprises the health history will not be gathered at the initial antepartum visit. There is a time limitation as well as the fact that the client may not recall all of the facts at once. For this reason, some agencies are finding it helpful to use a printed checklist which can be completed by the client prior to the interview and can save time by focusing the interview on the more significant aspects of the individual history. Even so, it should be realized that some of the data of a more personal nature will not be divulged unless and until a relationship of trust is established between client and nurse. Nevertheless, a history should be initiated at this visit, recorded in orderly fashion on the agency records and updated as additional data become available during subsequent months. Only in this way can it form a useful basis for individualized planning and care for each pregnant woman.

The Physical Examination

A complete general examination should be performed by a qualified practitioner. It is most usual for at least the first physical examination of the pregnancy to be done by a physician, although nurses or midwives may follow the physical progress throughout most or all of the remainder of a normal gestation.

As with any procedure the woman who is advised about what is to be done and what sensations she is likely to experience will be more comfortable and at ease.

In addition to the general physical examination, an obstetric evaluation of the abdomen and pelvis should be accomplished. The abdomen is palpated to determine the height of the uterine fundus and, if gestation has progressed far enough, the outline of the fetus. In addition to the usual gynecologic examination of the reproductive organs, a study of the size and shape of the pelvis is included to help determine adequacy for delivery. (See Chapter 10 for a more complete discussion of pelvic measurements.)

Laboratory Screening Procedures

The reader is referred to Figure 7-7 for an outline of laboratory screening tests during pregnancy and the usual time at which they are obtained. A brief description of the rationale for their use follows.

Hematocrit or *Hemoglobin:* This test is performed to detect anemia at the intial visit, at the

```
         LABORATORY SCREENING TESTS

I.   First Antepartal Visit

     Blood Studies

          Hematocrit
          WBC and differential
          Blood typing (ABO and Rh)
          Atypical antibody screen
          Serology
          Rubella screen
          2-hour postprandial blood sugar (if client history warrants)

     Urine Studies

          Routine urinalysis
          Urine culture

     Cervical Studies

          "Pap" smear
          Gonococcus culture

II.  28 Weeks Gestation

     Blood Studies

          Hematocrit
          Atypical antibody screen
          2-hour postprandial blood sugar

     Urine Studies

          Urine culture

III. 36 Weeks Gestation

     Blood Studies

          Hematocrit
```

Figure 7-7. Laboratory screening tests required during pregnancy. Some tests are performed only once, at the first antepartum visit. Others are repeated at 28 and 36 weeks gestation, when altered physiology may exert its influence on particular organ systems.

end of the second trimester, and again at 36 to 37 weeks gestation. Women who are taking iron supplementation and eating an adequate diet will rarely become anemic if their hematocrit is greater than 34 percent at 28 weeks gestation (hemoglobin greater than 11 gm/100 ml of blood). The hematocrit may also provide a clue to hidden bleeding, malabsorption, or failure to take iron.

White Blood Cell Count and Differential: As in any client, these tests detect rare abnormalities which are not necessarily pregnancy related. It should be remembered that there is an increased WBC count during pregnancy up to approximately 12,000/mm³ with levels as high as 20,000 to 25,000 during labor and immediately post partum.

Blood Typing: Both ABO and Rh typing is done in order to detect rare groups and, for the Rh determination, to advise the client whether or not she is a potential candidate for Rhogam (Rh immunoglobulin) after delivery.

Antibody Screen: This test will determine whether antibodies are present to any clinically significant antigens involved in erythroblastosis fetalis. (See Chapter 22 for a more complete discussion of isoimmune disease as a complication of pregnancy.)

Urinalysis and Urine Culture: Evidence of acute or chronic kidney or bladder disease is revealed by these tests. It is particularly important to note the results of the urine culture, since asymptomatic bacteriuria is not an unusual finding in pregnancy and can lead to more serious urinary tract disease as well as complications of pregnancy itself.

Serology: Many states in the United States require a serologic examination for syphilis. It is best done prior to 16 to 18 weeks gestation in order that syphilis, if present, can be treated before the fetus is affected. Tests are almost always positive within 4 to 6 weeks after infection.

Cervical Smear for Neisseria gonorrhoeae: Gonorrhea appears to be an increasingly prevalent community health problem in the United States. This may be due, in part, to changing patterns of sexual activity as well as the development of penicillin-resistant strains of the bacteria. For this reason many health officials are recommending that all antepartum clients be screened.

Papanicolaou Smear of Cervix: This test for atypical cells, often called the cancer test, should be an annual part of every woman's health supervision whether she is pregnant or not. Squamous cell cancer of the cervix has an incidence of 1 in 500 in women of childbearing age.

Rubella Screen: A positive blood antibody titer for rubella will reassure the woman that she is protected against this disease. If no antibody titer is present, plans should be made for immunization in the early postpartum period. Rubella immunization should NOT be undertaken during pregnancy since it utilizes a live virus vaccine which is very teratologic.

Blood Sugar Screen: All clients should be screened for blood glucose composition in the late second trimester. This is the time when the pregnancy begins to present the greatest challenge to maternal insulin production. In addition, some women are at increased risk to develop diabetes mellitus during pregnancy and consequently should be screened at the first antepartum visit as well as in the second trimester. These women include those having a positive family history of diabetes, obesity (greater than 20 percent over recommended weight for age and height), recurrent infections, previous large-for-gestational-age infant (greater than 4300 gm at term). A convenient and commonly used laboratory test is the two-hour postprandial blood sugar. Blood is drawn two hours after eating a meal of known carbohydrate content, usually 100 gm. Blood sugar values less than 140 mg/100 ml of blood are considered normal.

MAKING AN ASSESSMENT

After the data have been collected and analyzed, an assessment or diagnosis can be made. The nurse may do this independently or in conjunction with other professionals involved in the care of the client. Ideally the key health professionals in the care delivery system, usually the nurse and the physician, will sit down with the pregnant woman and her family to discuss the assessment and its implications and to plan together for her care.

A particularly important aspect of the assessment process is the determination of whether or not there are data to suggest that the pregnancy is at risk for the mother, fetus, or newborn.

Figure 7-8 lists factors which may predispose the mother and/or her fetus to complications of the gestational and neonatal periods. Women whose histories, physical examinations, and/or

```
                FACTORS IN HIGH-RISK PREGNANCY

 I.  Personal/Social/Economic

       Age — under 15 or over 35
       Parity — primigravida or greater than gravida V
       Single parent
       Nutrition — obesity, underweight, inadequate caloric and/or protein intake
       Drug usage — nicotine, alcohol, and other habituating or addictive drugs
       Unusual stress or anxiety
       Environment and occupation

 II. Medical

       Diabetes mellitus
       Hypertension
       Cardiac disease
       Renal disease
       Endocrine dysfunction
       Malignancy
       Anemia
       Positive serology for syphilis
       Acute viral infections
       Urinary tract infections
       Psychiatric disorders

 III. Obstetric

       History of previous high risk pregnancy
           Premature labor
           SGA or LGA infants
           Cesarean section or other operative delivery
           Abortion or stillbirth
           Neonatal morbidity
           Maternal complications during pregnancy, labor, or post partum
       Present pregnancy
           Exposure to teratogens (radiation, chemicals)
           Hyperemesis gravidarum
           Vaginal bleeding
           Isoimmune disease
           Preeclampsia/eclampsia
           Polyhydramnios or oligohydramnios
           Multiple gestation
           Abnormal presentation
           Inappropriate fetal growth for gestational age
           Premature labor

 IV. Genetic

       Family history of inheritable disorder
       Previous infant with congenital anomalies
       Maternal age greater than 40
       Parents known carriers of recessive disorder
       Consanguinity
```

Figure 7-8. Factors which may predispose to complications in pregnancy.

WISCONSIN PERINATAL CENTER SOUTH CENTRAL REGION
WISCONSIN FETAL RISK PROJECT
OFFICE – CLINICAL FORM

PATIENT'S NAME *J. R. L.* L.M.P. *4 Apr 77* E.D.C. *11 Jan 78*
DOCTOR *R. F.* HOSPITAL *M G H*
MOTHER'S BIRTH DATE *12-7-41* MARITAL STATUS: S (M) D W
DATE OF TERMINATION OF LAST PREGNANCY _____ PARA *1/0*
PREPREGNANCY WEIGHT *125* lb INFERTILITY WORKUP: YES ☐ NO ☒
YEARS OF SCHOOL COMPLETED *14* HEIGHT *5* FT. *6* IN.
PREVIOUS PRENATAL CARE FOR THIS PREGNANCY: YES ☐ NO ☒

A BASELINE DATA: | e.g. Age 35+ . . . 1 ☑ | **PREVIOUS OBSTETRICAL HISTORY:**

Age 35+ . . . . 1 ☑
  40+ . . . . 2 ☐
Para 0 . . . . 1 ☑
  6+ . . . . 2 ☐
Interval Less Than 2 Yrs . . . . 1 ☐
Obesity 200 Lb+ . . . . 1 ☐
Diabetes Mild-Moderate . . . . 2 ☐
  Severe . . . . 3 ☐
Chronic Renal Disease . . . . 1 ☐
with Diminished Renal Function . . . . 3 ☐
Preexisting Hypertension
  140+/90+ . . . . 1 ☐
  160+/110+ . . . . 2 ☐

Abortion . . . . ☐
Stillbirth . . . . ☐
Neonatal Death . . . . ☐
Surviving Premature Infant . . . . ☐
Antepartum Hemorrhage . . . . ☐
Toxemia . . . . ☐
Mid-Forceps Delivery . . . . ☐
Cesarean Section . . . . ☐
Major Congenital Anomaly . . . . ☐
Baby 10 Lb + ... ☐
  One Instance of Above . . . . 1 ☐
  Two or More Instances of Above . . . . 2 ☐

  RH Isoimmunized Mother . . . . 2 ☐
  + History of Erythroblastosis . . . . 3 ☐

B PRESENT PREGNANCY: | e.g. Hydramnios . . . 3 ☑ |

       MO/DAY/YEAR   MO/DAY/YEAR

Bleeding, Before 20 Weeks
  Alone . . . . 1 ☑ *7-19-77* Toxemia Mild-Moderate . . . . 1 ☐ _____
  With Pain . . . . 2 ☐ _____   Severe . . . . 3 ☐ _____

Bleeding, After 20 Weeks   Hydramnios (Single Fetus) . . . . 3 ☐ _____
  Ceased . . . . 1 ☐ _____
  Continues . . . . 2 ☐ _____ Multiple Pregnancy . . . . 2 ☐ _____
  With Pain . . . . 3 ☐ _____ Abnormal Glucose Tolerance . . . . . . 1 ☐ _____
  With Hypotension . . . . 3 ☐ _____
                Decreasing Insulin Requirement . . . . 3 ☐ _____
Spontaneous Premature
  Rupture of Membranes . . . . 1 ☐ _____ Maternal Diabetic Acidosis . . . . 3 ☐ _____
  Latent Period 24 Hr + ... 2 ☐ _____
                Maternal Pyrexia . . . . 1 ☐ _____
Anemia 8 to 10 Gm . . . . 1 ☐ _____ Pyrexia + FHR Greater than 160 . . . . 2 ☐ _____
  Less than 8 Gm . . . . 2 ☐ _____
                RH Negative
42 Wks . . . . 1 ☐ _____ Pos. Antibody Titer . . . . 2 ☐ _____
43 Wks OR More . . . . 2 ☐ _____ Amniotic Fluid Liley Zone 111 . . . . . 3 ☐ _____

A prenatal score of 3 or more in parts A and B mark a high-risk pregnancy.

LATE PREGNANCY DATA
Antibody Screen at 28 weeks ± 1 week Pos. _____ Neg. _____
Hemoglobin/Hct at 28 weeks ± 1 week _____ gm%
2 Hr P.P. Sugar at 28 weeks ± 1 week _____ mg%
Weight at 37 weeks ± 1 week _____ lb
Presentation at 37 weeks ± 1 week _____

PRENATAL VISITS   **(GOODWIN, DUNNE AND THOMAS FETAL RISK SCORING SYSTEM)**

e.g. Jan. 2/75	DATE 1 *June 14/77*	2 *July 11/77*	3 *July 25/77*	4	5	6
Gestation / Fetal in Weeks / Risk Score **29/40** **4/6**	*10* /40 *2* /6	*14* /40 *2* /6	*16* /40 *3* /6	/40 /6	/40 /6	/40 /6

DATE 7	8	9	10	11	12	13
/40 /6	/40 /6	/40 /6	/40 /6	/40 /6	/40 /6	/40 /6

Figure 7-9. Example of a risk scoring form for use during the antepartum period. A hypothetical client is used to illustrate how the form is utilized. At the initial antepartum visit on 6/14/77 Mrs. L. is found to be 10 weeks gestation and to have a fetal risk score of 2 out of 6. On her third visit the fetal risk score is increased to 3 out of 6 because of painless vaginal bleeding which occurred on 7/19/77. Because of age, parity, and first trimester bleeding, this pregnancy is at increased risk for toxemia, intrauterine growth retardation, and placenta previa, as well as intrapartum complications.

laboratory findings reveal the presence of one or more of these factors should receive appropriate consultation from specialists in high-risk obstetrics and neonatology. Although statistically there is a significant increase in both maternal and infant mortality and morbidity in each of these conditions, there is much that can be done to prevent or treat problems and therefore appreciably improve the prognosis.

It seems apparent that all the factors listed in the table in Figure 7-8 do not threaten to the same degree. For this reason various investigators have attempted to devise a means of scoring a woman according to the severity of her risks. Such a scoring system would serve a dual function. First, it would identify those women in need of special surveillance and possible referral to a tertiary care center. Second, a systematic method of record keeping would provide a mechanism for peer review and other studies of quality of care, morbidity, and mortality.

Figure 7-9 illustrates one such scoring system which is being used to detect pregnancies at risk. The form, designed to be part of the woman's medical record, is filled out by the nurse or physician during pregnancy. This record is then forwarded to the inpatient setting where the woman will deliver, thus providing baseline data with which the intrapartum staff can begin their care plan. Similar forms have been developed to be completed at the time of admission to the labor suite and are intended to be predictive of the probability of complications during this critical period.

SUMMARY

Women are usually able to diagnose their own pregnancy but typically seek confirmation of the fact from others. Signs and symptoms of pregnancy are classified according to whether they are presumptive, probable, or positive.

When conception has occurred, antepartum care should be initiated to provide health maintenance, education, counseling, and appropriate intervention for complications. The first visit is one of assessment. The woman and her family assess the health care system, and a health history, a physical examination, and laboratory studies are completed.

The collected data are analyzed; then the professionals responsible for care discuss their findings with the client, and a plan for care is agreed upon.

An essential part of the assessment is the identification of the woman whose pregnancy may be at risk because of her history, chronic or acute illness, and/or genetic conditions. Scoring systems have been devised to help in the systematic evaluation of risk factors.

BIBLIOGRAPHY

Aubry, Richard H., and Pennington, John C., Identification and evaluation of high-risk pregnancy: The perinatal concept, *Clin. Obstet. Gynecol.* 16:3–27 (Mar.) 1973.

Auger, Jeanine Roose, Behavioral assessment and nursing, in *Behavioral Systems and Nursing*, edited by J. R. Roose. Prentice-Hall, Englewood Cliffs, N. J., 1976, pp. 144–170.

Contemporary Ob/Gyn, Discriminating against mother? Guarding fetus?, 8:129 (Aug.) 1976.

GPO Perinatal News, Prevention of congenital rubella syndrome, 4(2):7–8, 1974. (Great Plains Organization for Perinatal Health Care, Wisconsin Perinatal Center, Madison, Wis.)

Habel, Calvin *et al.*, Prenatal and intrapartum high-risk screening, *Am. J. Obstet. Gynecol.* 117:1–9 (Sept.) 1973.

Hricko, Andrea, and Brunt, Melanie, *Working for Your Life: A Woman's Guide to Job Health Hazards.* University of California Labor Occupational Health Program, Berkeley, Calif., 1976.

Kitay, David Z., Assessing anemia in the pregnant patient, *Contemp. Ob/Gyn* 2:17–24 (Oct.) 1973.

Schneider, Jan, The high-risk pregnancy, *Hosp. Pract.* 6:133–136; 141–143 (Oct.) 1971.

Skinner, Rebecca, Stat answer to "Am I pregnant?" *Patient Care* 11:110–112 (Jan.) 1977.

WPC News, Rationale for prenatal screening tests 3(7):5–6 and 3(8):5, 1973. (Wisconsin Perinatal Center, Madison, Wis.).

8

Nutrition During the Childbearing Period

Food, and the nutrients it contains, are necessary for life and growth. The human embryo and fetus can obtain food only from the mother through placental transfer. If the mother is malnourished, adequate nutrients will not be available and intrauterine growth retardation will occur.

Growth failure may occur in two ways: there may be a failure of cells to multiply, resulting in a smaller number of cells, or there may be multiplication of cells without individual cell growth. A combination of these two may also occur. The consequences of fetal malnutrition may be reversible if growth in cell size (hypertrophic growth) is primarily affected but may be permanent if hyperplastic (cell number) growth is affected. The severity of the consequences is proportional to the timing, duration, and severity of the malnutrition and depends upon the particular nutrient involved.

DIETARY MODIFICATIONS DURING PREGNANCY

Both science and folklore have recognized the important relationship between food and pregnancy for as long as history has been recorded. Indeed many of the ancient rituals and taboos about eating during pregnancy were more beneficial for the developing fetus than some of the restrictive dietary regimens that were prevalent through much of the twentieth century.

It seems reasonable that the dramatic growth and development of the fetus places demands on the mother's body and her nutrition. A variety of research findings supports the idea that a woman who is in a good nutritional state prior to pregnancy, and who maintains adequate nutrition throughout gestation, significantly improves her chances for a healthy baby. Thus an important dimension of antepartum care is the special consideration given the woman's diet.

The Diet History

Just as it is necessary to obtain a health history prior to initiating the antepartum plan of care, so it is useful to obtain a diet history before beginning dietary instruction or counseling. Many forms or outlines, such as the one illustrated in Figure 8-1, are available. Although they vary in detail, they usually have in common a list of food likes and dislikes, a 24-hour recall of food eaten, and an average number of times per week that a client eats certain basic foods such as bread, milk, meat, and so on. In addition, it is helpful to obtain data relative to the client's cultural, religious, and family food customs. Food is important not only for its nutrient value; it also plays a significant role in society as a symbol of warmth, love, and good fellowship. In the Judeo-Christian tradition, family or community meals are very much interwoven with religious ceremonies. Some religious practices and some cultures forbid the

DIET HISTORY

Date _____

Name _____Age_____Height _____ Wt. before Preg. _____

Physician's name _____ Due Date _____ Present Wt. _____

How much weight do you expect to gain during your pregnancy? _____

Have you ever had problems with your weight? _____ If yes, describe. _____

_____

_____

Please list all the food and beverages you had yesterday. Include the time you ate the food, the place, and an estimate of the quantity of food.

For example: 2:30 p.m.   home   apple   1 small
                                        cheddar cheese   1 ounce
                                        tea   1 cup

TIME	PLACE	FOOD EATEN	AMOUNT

Figure 8-1. Example of a form used to record a diet history.

DIET HISTORY (Page 2)

What beverages do you drink frequently (3 times a week or more)? Coffee _____   Tea _____   Milk _____

      Soft drinks such as Coke _____   Fruit juice _____   Wine _____   Beer _____

      Other alcoholic drinks _____

List any foods you do *not* like:

      Meat _____

      Vegetables _____

      Fruits _____

      Milk and dairy foods _____

      Others _____

Are you presently taking any vitamins or iron or other minerals? _____

Are you allergic to any foods? No _____   Yes _____   List _____

_____

Have you had cravings for any particular foods since you have been pregnant? _____   If so, which foods? _____

_____

Do you have cravings for starch, clay, or other substances? _____

Are you bothered by nausea? _____   indigestion? _____   "gas"? _____   constipation? _____

      loss of appetite? _____   excessive thirst? _____   excessive appetite? _____

Number of people in your household: Adults over 18 _____

                               Children 12-18 _____

                               Children under 12 _____

Who does most of the cooking at your house? _____

Who does the grocery shopping? _____

How often is grocery shopping done? _____

Are you receiving either of the following: Food stamps? _____   WIC vouchers? _____

What questions do you have about your diet during pregnancy or about the diets of any of your family members? _____

_____

_____

_____

Figure 8-1. *Continued*

177

eating of certain foods either absolutely or at certain seasons or in certain circumstances. It would be useless to instruct a client in a diet which violated any of these beliefs, regardless of how nutritionally sound it might be.

It is also necessary to be aware of the financial resources available for the purchase of food so that the recommendations can be practical. If the pregnant woman is not the person responsible for the purchase and preparation of food, it is advisable to include the one who is responsible in the diet instruction and counseling.

Identification of Nutritional Risk

Using the diet history as a screening tool, certain women can be identified as being nutritionally at risk, and particular attention can be directed toward helping them meet the dietary needs of pregnancy. Several groups of women at increased risk are discussed here.

1. Those who are underweight prior to conception (that is, their prepregnant weight was 10 percent or more below ideal weight for height and age). These individuals are more likely to have insufficient nutrient stores and to maintain these deficits throughout childbearing. They have an increased incidence of small-for-gestational-age infants.

2. Obese women (that is, their prepregnant weight was more than 20 percent above ideal weight for their height and age). It is not uncommon for the obese to be poorly nourished because of the kinds of foods they eat. These women will need special help in eating quality foods rather than a quantity of calories, and in resisting the temptation to try to lose weight during pregnancy. There is a tendency among physicians and nurses to advocate caloric restriction for these women so that there will be a net loss of weight at the end of pregnancy. This is probably not advisable for several reasons: first, severe caloric restriction often results in insufficient intake of other essential nutrients; second, calo-

ries (energy) are needed for amino acid utilization; and third, in the absence of caloric intake fat deposits are metabolized to provide energy needs. This latter phenomenon results in ketonuria, which has been associated with lower IQ scores in offspring when measured at four years of age.[1] For these reasons, the obese woman, like her thinner sister, should gain approximately 24 pounds during pregnancy.

3. Those who fail to gain weight during pregnancy or who gain 1 kg or less per month during the second or third trimester. The less the weight gain the greater the risks of prematurity and small-for-gestational-age infants. These women should be helped to increase food intake and bring their weight gain up to normal.

4. Those who have excessive weight gains of 3 kg or more per month. Several obstetric complications, notably preeclampsia, have traditionally been attributed to excessive weight gain during pregnancy. It is now evident that increased caloric intake (as reflected in weight gain) does not cause preeclampsia. However, when calories are eaten in excess of energy needs the excess is stored as fat. If this is not lost after pregnancy it could contribute to obesity, which has implications for the woman's health far beyond childbearing. For this reason, it is probably desirable to keep weight gain within the normal range.

5. Those with hematocrits of less than 35 percent. These women will probably need iron and/or folic acid supplements as well as help in selecting foods which are good iron sources.

6. Those who limit their intake to certain kinds of foods because of personal preference or religious conviction (for example, vegetarian diets). These women, like those

[1] J. A. Church and H. W. Berendes, Intelligence of children whose mothers had acetonuria during pregnancy, in *Perinatal Factors Affecting Human Development*, Pan American Health Organization, Scientific Publication No. 185. Washington, D.C., 1969, pp. 30–35.

on therapeutic diets for various illnesses, must be helped to meet the nutritional demand of pregnancy as well as possible within the confines of their dietary restrictions. The protein needs are usually the most difficult to meet with restricted diets.

8. Adolescents. Teenage girls who have not reached their full development need nutrients for their own growth as well as the growth of their fetuses. They may not be the ones responsible for purchase and preparation of food, or, if they are, their inexperience may result in uneconomical shopping and use of many prepackaged foods. Occasionally a young girl may attempt to hide her pregnancy from school officials, family, or friends by weight reduction.

9. Multigravidas with closely spaced pregnancies. The interconceptional period may not have been sufficient for the replenishing of maternal stores. In addition, a woman with several small children may need help in planning not only what foods she will eat but also the time for relatively quiet, organized meals.

10. Those on low incomes. Concrete, practical examples of low-cost foods with high nutritional value are helpful, especially if accompanied by serving suggestions and meal planning, which includes combinations of foods which augment each other in nutrients.

11. Healthy women who have some misinformation or old wives' tales about what to eat and not to eat in pregnancy, how much weight to gain, and so on.

Dietary Instructions

The recommended diet for pregnancy is, in general, an increase in all nutrients over prepregnant levels. In addition, since pregnant women may be at risk for hypoglycemia and ketonuria following periods of fasting, they should avoid skipping meals and develop a habit of late evening snacks to carry them through the night.

Calories should be increased to permit the progressive gain during pregnancy of approximately 11 kilograms (24 pounds).

Protein intake should be increased to provide the extensive amino acids needed for fetal growth and development, as well as for building and maintenance of maternal tissues during gestation and lactation.

The recommended daily allowance (RDA) for virtually every vitamin and mineral is also increased for this period. These substances are best provided by dietary sources. Blanket prescriptions for vitamin supplements should be avoided, since there is at least a theoretical possibility of hypervitaminosis. An important exception is the need for supplemental iron and possibly folacin. These substances are very difficult to ingest in sufficient quantities from food sources alone.

Dietary instruction should, of course, be modified to suit the individual circumstances of each woman as indicated in her diet history. Many nurses and nutritionists, however, find it convenient to use the Basic Four Food Groups as identified by the U.S. Department of Agriculture as the framework for their teaching (Fig. 8-2). Women should be encouraged to adapt a menu pattern to their families' schedule rather than to adhere to any stereotyped meal plan. Opportunities for group discussion of nutrition are often very profitable as women are able to share ideas for "quick" meals, sack lunches, high-protein snacks, new recipes to add variety, and so on.

The nutrients required to maintain the pregnant and lactating woman in a state of good nutrition and to supply the needs of the fetus are listed in Table 8-1. The reasons for an increase in most nutrients and the foods that will best supply those nutrients are discussed below.

Energy Requirements (Calories)

In all people energy sources are necessary for body maintenance and physical activity. During pregnancy there are additional energy expenditures for growth of the fetal–placental unit and

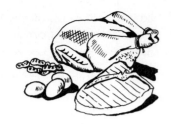

Meat Group: beef, veal, pork, lamb, poultry, fish, or eggs

3 or more servings per day
1 serving equals: 2–3 oz. lean meat
                       1/2 cup canned tuna
                       2 frankfurters
                       2 eggs
                       1 cup cooked diced peas, beans, or lentils
                       4 tablespoons peanut butter

Fruit and Vegetable Group

4 or more servings including one good source vitamin C and one
                good source vitamin A
1 serving equals: 1/2 cup vegetable
                       1 apple, banana, orange, potato
                       1/2 grapefruit

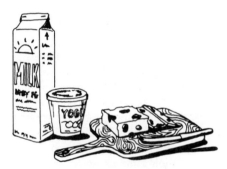

Milk Group

Adults — 4 or more cups
Under 17 — 6 or more cups
1 cup of milk equals: 1 cup buttermilk, yogurt, baked custard
                        2 inch cube of cheese
                        1-1/2 cups cottage cheese
                        1/3 cup dried milk powder

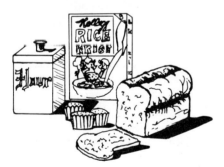

Cereal–Bread Group

4 or more servings (include one serving of iron-enriched food
                daily)
1 serving equals: 1 slice bread
                       1 roll, muffin, pancake, waffle
                       1 ounce ready-to-eat cereal
                       1/2–3/4 cup cooked cereal, rice, macaroni,
                                grits, cornmeal, spaghetti
If made with enriched flour count
                       1 taco shell, 1 wedge pizza crust, 1 doughnut,
                       1 serving of cake

Other Foods

Add variety and calories by using foods such as butter, margarine,
salad dressing, jellies, candies, syrups, carbonated beverages,
gravies, and sauces

Figure 8-2. Basic Four Food Groups as a guide to meal planning in pregnancy and lactation.

Table 8-1.   Recommended Dietary Allowances
Food and Nutrition Board, National Academy of Sciences–
National Research Council, Eighth Edition, 1974

| | Nonpregnant Females | | | | | |
	11–14 yr [a]	15–18 yr [b]	19–22 yr [c]	23–50 yr [c]	Pregnancy	Lactation
Energy (kcal)	2,400	2,100	2,100	2,000	+300	+500
Protein (gm)	44	48	46	46	+30	+20
Vitamin A (IU)	4,000	4,000	4,000	4,000	5,000	6,000
Vitamin D (IU)	400	400	400		400	400
Vitamin E (IU)	12	12	12	12	15	15
Ascorbic acid (mg)	45	45	45	45	60	80
Folacin (μg)	400	400	400	400	800	600
Niacin (mg)	16	14	14	13	+2	+4
Riboflavin (mg)	1.3	1.4	1.4	1.2	+0.3	+0.5
Thiamin (mg)	1.2	1.1	1.1	1.0	+0.3	+0.3
Vitamin B_6 (mg)	1.6	2.0	2.0	2.0	2.5	2.5
Vitamin B_{12} (μg)	3	3	3	3	4	4
Calcium (mg)	1,200	1,200	800	800	1,200	1,200
Phosphorus (mg)	1,200	1,200	800	800	1,200	1,200
Iodine (μg)	115	115	100	100	125	150
Iron (mg)	18	18	18	18	*	18
Magnesium (mg)	300	300	300	300	450	450
Zinc (mg)	15	15	15	15	20	25

[a] Weight 44 kg (97 lb), height 155 cm (62 in.).
[b] Weight 54 kg (119 lb), height 162 cm (65 in.).
[c] Weight 58 kg (128 lb), height 162 cm (65 in.).
*The increased requirements of pregnancy cannot usually be met by ordinary diets; therefore, the use of supplemental iron is recommended.

added maternal tissues (such as in the breasts and uterus) as well as to support an increased maternal metabolic rate. It is apparent from a consideration of the overall physiology of pregnancy that energy requirements are not constant throughout gestation. Rather, there is a minimal increase in the first trimester, with a sharp rise in the second trimester, which then continues fairly constant to term. While maternal factors are chiefly responsible for the energy requirements of the second trimester, the growth of the fetus and placenta account for most of those of the third trimester.

To meet these energy needs of pregnancy the Food and Nutrition Board, National Academy of Sciences–National Research Council, recommends the intake of an additional 300 calories per day over and above the prepregnant diet throughout pregnancy. The Food and Agriculture Organization of the World Health Organization, taking into account the differential energy needs of the three trimesters, recommends an increase of 150 calories per day for the first trimester and 350 calories per day for the last two trimesters. These increases are necessary for the energy expenditures of pregnancy alone. Additional dietary modifications may be needed to accommodate growth requirements of an adolescent pregnant woman, or in the presence of physical exercise, climatic differences, and so on.

Obviously, caloric intake will have to be individualized according to the needs of each pregnant woman. Probably the easiest method of evaluating the adequacy of caloric intake is to observe weight gain systematically during pregnancy. If this follows a pattern of accumulation of 1–2 kg (2–4½ lb) in the first trimester and then a fairly linear progression of 0.35–0.4 kg (0.77–0.88 lb) per week until term, the caloric intake is appropriate. For a more complete discussion of weight gain during pregnancy see pages 152–54.

Proteins

Additional protein is required during pregnancy for growth and maintenance of the fetus and for formation of new maternal tissues. It has been estimated that about 950 gm of new protein is formed during pregnancy. Nearly one half of this amount is accumulated in the fetus; the remainder is needed for development of the placenta, growth of the uterus and the breasts, and increase in the maternal blood. From this estimate it is determined that about 950 gm of additional protein is needed during pregnancy to meet its demands.

The amount of protein deposited daily during pregnancy is relatively small during the first trimester, and then gradually increases as the pregnancy advances. The average daily amount of protein added to the fetal and maternal tissues is computed to be 0.8, 4.4, and 7.2 gm for the first, second, and third trimesters, respectively, with some individual variation.

To meet the protein needs of pregnancy the Food and Nutrition Board of the National Research Council recommends an additional 30 gm of protein per day during pregnancy. This additional allowance takes into account individual variability of mothers and variability in the quality of protein ingested. If the expectant mother is an adolescent whose growth is not complete, the total recommended protein allowance for pregnancy may be too low for her. She will need protein to meet her own growth needs as well as the demands of pregnancy. This may raise her requirements for protein above the recommended allowance of 76 gm daily during pregnancy.

If the woman's protein intake is normally high she may need to make little or no adjustment in her diet to meet the protein needs of pregnancy. For example, a diet that includes 1 quart of milk, ¼ pound of lean meat, 2 slices of bread, and a 1-ounce slice of cheddar cheese furnishes approximately 76 grams of protein and thus meets most or all of the daily requirements of pregnancy. Animal proteins (meat, fish, eggs, milk) are said to have high biologic value, since they contain all of the eight essential amino acids and therefore furnish the best building materials available.

Most vegetables and cereal proteins are low in some of the essential amino acids, and some are also low in digestibility. These proteins are said to have low biologic value when eaten alone. However, if they are supplemented with animal protein they make valuable additions to the diet, since they add variety and are usually less costly than animal protein. It can be seen that a vegetarian diet presents a real challenge to a woman to meet protein requirements. It is important that she have counseling about the specific amino acid content of various foods so that these can be combined to form a total diet of protein of high biologic value.

Carbohydrates and Fats

Carbohydrates and fats serve as important sources of food energy for the body. When it is necessary to increase or decrease caloric intake during pregnancy this can best be done by altering carbohydrate and fat intake. When a decrease in caloric intake is desirable, the daily intake of fat, the most concentrated form of food energy, must be carefully considered. However, a moderate amount of fat is important in the pregnant woman's diet to provide her with essential fatty acids, and its intake should not be severely curtailed. Fat in the form of dairy products, meat, poultry, and fish will supply some important nutrients as well as energy. Carbohydrate in the form of milk, fruits, vegetables, and whole-grain cereals and breads will provide protective substances and bulk as well as energy.

Calcium and Phosphorus

Calcium and phosphorus are essential in the diet as tissue-building material. The requirement for these minerals is increased during pregnancy to meet the needs of the fetus. There is evidence that about 30 gm of calcium is required for pregnancy; all except about 2 gm is utilized by the fetus, mainly during the latter half of gestation at the time of calcification of the fetal skeleton. A good calcium intake will provide for the needs of the fetus, and, in addition, permit the mother to store some calcium in preparation for lactation. Despite evidence of increased intestinal uptake and conservation of calcium during pregnancy, additional dietary calcium is important to meet the increased requirements.

The recommended increase of calcium during pregnancy is 400 mg per day, which raises the total daily recommended intake to 1200 mg. Increase in the phosphorus requirement is probably even greater than increase in calcium need, but when calcium requirements are met, the phosphorus will be adequately supplied. Foods that are high in calcium are also high in phosphorus.

Milk is the best food source of calcium and phosphorus; 1 quart of milk supplies 120 mg of calcium. Since it is virtually impossible to ingest sufficient calcium without adequate milk, and since milk is an inexpensive source of many other dietary essentials (protein, carbohydrates, fats, vitamins, and fluid), many authorities consider milk to be an indispensable part of the diet for pregnancy. Milk may be used in any form, but, as it is difficult to use a whole quart in cooking, some should be taken as a beverage, as whole milk, low-fat milk, skimmed milk, buttermilk, or cocoa. Using skimmed milk instead of milk with fat is a means of reducing caloric intake should this be necessary because of a tendency toward excessive weight gain. Unless fortified with vitamin A, skimmed milk cannot be considered a source of vitamin A, but this vitamin can be supplied by other foods as necessary.

Ingestion of large amounts of milk has been implicated in the tendency toward leg cramps experienced by some pregnant women. The rationale is that the high phosphorus content of milk results in high phosphorus concentration in blood and a relative hypocalcemia. According to this theory, treatment of leg cramps consists of curtailing milk consumption, supplementing the diet with nonphosphate calcium salts, and taking an aluminum antacid, which tends to remove some of the dietary phosphorus from the alimentary tract. This relationship remains controversial, however, since not all studies confirm these findings. For the woman bothered by leg cramps this approach may be tried for relief.

The calcium needs of the pregnant teenager may not be met as easily as stated above. During the rapid growth period of puberty a high level of calcium retention (approximately 400 mg/day) appears to be necessary for adequate mineralization of the skeleton.[2] With the added burden of the developing fetal skeleton the adolescent's calcium needs range between 1200 and 1600 mg/day with individual requirements being determined by her own rate of growth at the time of pregnancy. Foods other than dairy products contribute only from 200 to 300 mg of calcium daily. To assure that the pregnant teenager has an adequate calcium intake from food, she needs an extra glass of milk, or some other dairy products, in addition to the 1 quart of milk recommended for the adult woman during pregnancy. Emotional distress is likely to disturb calcium metabolism. In this event, it may be difficult for the teenager to meet the calcium requirements of her own body and those of her pregnancy.

Iron

The demands for iron are considerably increased during pregnancy. In the entire course of a pregnancy an additional 600–800 mg of elemental iron is required to meet fetal and in-

[2] Bonnie S. Worthington, Joyce Vermeersch, and Sue Rodwell Williams, *Nutrition in Pregnancy and Lactation.* Mosby, St. Louis, Mo., 1977, p. 125.

creased maternal needs. About 300 mg, or more, of iron is transferred to the fetus and the placenta. The fetus needs iron to form hemoglobin and to build a store of iron for the first three months after birth, when a baby's iron intake from food is low. Up to 500 mg of iron is incorporated into maternal hemoglobin as the red blood cell volume expands. This large requirement of iron is to some extent offset by cessation of menstruation which reduces the woman's ordinary loss. There is an estimated saving of about 120–140 mg of iron due to the amenorrhea of pregnancy. Thus the iron requirements increase from the average of 1.5 mg per day for the nonpregnant female of childbearing age to about 3.5 mg per day during pregnancy, with a range of need up to 6.0 mg per day. The additional requirements are greatest during the latter part of pregnancy and may be as high as 6.0 to 7.0 mg per day during the last four to five months of pregnancy.

Absorption of food iron varies both according to the type of food eaten and the individual eating it. On the average, healthy persons absorb approximately 10 percent of the iron ingested in food. For this reason the RDA of food iron must be 10 times greater than the daily requirement to insure sufficient absorption. The recommended allowance of food iron during pregnancy is 18 mg per day, the same as for the nonpregnant woman of childbearing age. This should be sufficient to permit the accumulation of iron stores which would then be available to meet *some* of the needs of pregnancy, assuming the woman's iron stores were adequate at the time of conception.

It is difficult to obtain an adequate amount of iron from food. Usual diets contain about 6 mg of iron per 1000 calories and dietary surveys indicate that the ordinary American diet contains 10–15 mg of food iron daily.[3] Careful selection of food and use of foods enriched with iron can enhance this amount. Liver is an excellent source of iron; other organ meats, eggs, green leafy vegetables, and certain fruits, such as prunes, peaches, apricots, grapes, and raisins are good sources if eaten often. Iron-enriched cereals, breads, and flour can also significantly improve the iron intake. Even with all this, the iron intake will most likely be inadequate for pregnancy.

In addition to food a potential source of iron for pregnancy is that stored in the reticuloendothelial cells of the bone marrow. However, most women of childbearing age have inadequate iron stores, so this backup system is not likely to be sufficient to meet the needs of pregnancy.

For the reasons suggested above, supplemental iron is usually required to meet the needs of gestation, especially during the latter half. Medicinal iron in the form of ferrous fumarate, ferrous sulfate, or ferrous gluconate may be prescribed as a prophylaxis against iron deficiency. Supplemental iron is not recommended, however, during the first trimester because of suspected teratogenicity, as well as aggravation of gastrointestinal symptoms common during this period of gestation. In 1970 the Committee on Maternal Nutrition, National Academy of Sciences, National Research Council recommended that all women receive 30 to 60 mg of ferrous iron as a daily oral supplement during the second and third trimesters, in order to build and protect their iron stores. It has been found that with the ingestion of supplemental iron the hemoglobin concentration at the end of pregnancy averages 12.0 gm or more per 100 ml of blood.

In women who do not receive iron supplements, the iron stores decrease as pregnancy advances because of the effective parasitism of the fetus. Without adequate stores or adequate intake, sufficient iron will not be available to increase the hemoglobin mass, and the maternal hemoglobin and hematocrit values will fall. Depletion of maternal iron stores may result in an iron deficiency of a nonanemic nature or in an iron-deficiency anemia. The baby of a mother with severe iron-deficiency anemia will have adequate neonatal hemoglobin, but he may have a low store of iron, thus placing him at risk for

[3] Roy M. Pitkin, Nutritional support in obstetrics and gynecology, *Clin. Obstet. Gynecol.* 19:489–513 (Sept.) 1976.

anemia later in infancy. Unless the mother loses an excessive amount of blood at or following delivery, some of the iron that was added to her own blood cells may later be available for her own stores.

Folacin

Folacin, a water-soluble vitamin normally stored in the body, is required in increased amount during pregnancy. Unless intake of folacin is ample, a moderate folacin deficiency may appear during the last trimester of pregnancy, caused by increasing demands of the growing fetus and depletion of maternal stores.

Folacin deficiency results in megaloblastic anemia. Such anemia may be induced by pregnancy when dietary intake is inadequate. A significant number of cases of megaloblastic anemia of pregnancy occur. Overt evidence is apparently less common in the United States than in other parts of the world.

An allowance of 800 μg (micrograms) of folacin per day, from dietary sources, is recommended during pregnancy. This is 400 μg above the normal needs of the nonpregnant woman. Pure forms of folacin are effective in much smaller doses. With dietary sources, the absorption of the total amount of ingested food folacin averages only 10 percent, with wide variations, in which absorption may be much higher.

Folacin occurs in a wide variety of animal and vegetable foods, particularly in glandular meats and green leafy vegetables. However, a considerable amount, and sometimes practically all, of the folacin in food may be lost in cooking. Dietary intake is likely to be inadequate in women who do not eat raw, green, leafy vegetables, or foods high in animal protein. Vitamin B_{12} appears to be important to folate metabolism. Vitamin B_{12} is quite stable during cooking and is adequately provided by a diet that includes animal protein.

Prophylactic administration of an oral folic acid preparation to all pregnant women may be desirable, but the optimal dose is controversial. However, if a multivitamin supplement is pre-

scribed during pregnancy, it is considered advisable to use a preparation that includes folacin. When oral folic acid is administered prophylactically to pregnant women a dose varying from 200 to 400 mg may be used daily throughout pregnancy. Vitamin supplementation should not be a substitute for helping the woman improve her general nutrition.

Iodine

In certain geographic regions, where soil and water are low in iodine content, the diet is likely to be deficient in this mineral. Pregnancy may require an increased amount of iodine. Lactation increases the need for iodine, since it is excreted in the milk. Iodized salt usually supplies this need adequately. Seafoods are another rich source of iodine.

Vitamin A

Need for vitamin A is increased to 5000 IU daily during pregnancy. This vitamin is essential to the nutritional well-being of the rapidly growing fetus, and furnishes the mother with good resistance to infection. It is fat-soluble and readily stored in the body. Whole milk, green leafy vegetables, yellow vegetables, fruits, and liver are the best sources of vitamin A. Vegetable sources should be used freely, especially if the woman drinks only skimmed milk, as it contains little vitamin A. Eating raw carrots for snacks is a convenient way to meet the daily requirement.

Mineral oil in the gastrointestinal tract interferes with the absorption of fat-soluble vitamins and also of calcium and phosphorus. It should therefore not be used with foods (e.g., as an ingredient in salad dressing) and should never be taken as a laxative near a mealtime.

Vitamin D

Since vitamin D is necessary for proper utilization and retention of calcium and phosphorus, it is important during pregnancy. Vitamin D is present in significant amounts in only a few foods—fish, liver, whole milk, cream, butter, and eggs—and even then varies with the seasons. Some foods, especially milk, are enriched with vitamin D. Their use aids in meeting requirements. Vitamin D is also acquired by exposure to sunlight and for some persons this may be a good source.

Vitamin C

This water-soluble vitamin is poorly stored in the body and should be included in the diet daily for good nutrition. The recommended daily dietary allowance for pregnancy and lactation is increased above that of the woman's usual needs (see Table 8-1). Ascorbic acid is present in liberal quantity in fresh fruits (especially citrus), tomatoes, and raw green leafy vegetables. There is seldom a deficiency of ascorbic acid in the summer when fresh fruits and vegetables are readily available and used freely. With a daily intake of orange juice or tomato juice it is possible to maintain an adequate intake of vitamin C during the winter months.

Niacin

The recommended allowance for niacin is 6.6 mg per 1000 calories, but not less than 13 mg for caloric intakes of less than 2000 calories. The recommended allowance for pregnancy is increased by 2.0 mg, based on the increased energy need and caloric intake. Since the recommended caloric intake of the teenage expectant mother is higher than that for the adult, the niacin allowance is increased accordingly, being raised to 16–18 mg per day during pregnancy. Most diets in the United States supply an adequate amount of niacin.

Riboflavin

The increase in metabolic size during pregnancy, owing to growth of the fetus and accessory structures, increases riboflavin requirements. An additional intake of 0.3 mg per day is considered to meet this requirement. The recommended allowance during pregnancy is thus raised to 1.7 mg per day. A considerable amount of the requirement for riboflavin is met when 1 qt of milk, which contains 1.6 mg riboflavin, is consumed daily. Other foods, especially meat, will help to ensure an adequate intake of riboflavin.

Thiamin

Thiamin needs appear to be increased during pregnancy. The requirement has been established to be 1.4 mg per day. This is a 0.3 mg increase over the woman's ordinary allowance and is in accord with the slight increase in caloric requirements during pregnancy. On the basis of a higher caloric intake of the teenage expectant mother her total daily allowance may be considered to be 1.5 mg.

Whole-grain cereals and breads and enriched cereals and breads are the most important sources of food thiamin. Meat is a relatively good source of thiamin; lean pork is especially high. Milk is a fair source when it is consumed in quantity, such as 1 qt per day.

Vitamin B$_6$

Vitamin B$_6$ is actively transported by the placenta to the fetus, but it is not definitely known how much of the vitamin the mother needs to meet the fetal requirements. On the assumption that an additional 0.5 mg in the mother's diet would meet fetal requirements, a total of 2.5 mg of vitamin B$_6$ per day is considered a safe allowance for a pregnant woman.

Sodium

Additional sodium is needed during pregnancy to maintain the osmolarity of the expanding maternal interstitial and intravascular fluid volumes as well as to meet the requirements of the developing fetus. This additional sodium would appear to be supplied by the physiologic adjustments in tubular reabsorption (see pages

141–43). For this reason it is probably most appropriate neither to increase nor restrict sodium intake during pregnancy but simply to advise the woman to salt her food to taste.

Water

Under normal conditions thirst is a good guide to intake of water. It is suggested that coffee, tea, and alcohol be used with moderation.

Residue

The expectant mother should make certain that her food contains considerable residue such as is provided by fruit, especially raw; coarse vegetables, particularly uncooked; and whole-grain cereals and bread. This residue increases the bulk of the intestinal contents, stimulating peristaltic action and thus helping to overcome the tendency toward constipation.

SUMMARY

It has been seen that pregnancy is characterized by the need for increased amounts of all nutrients. For the woman who enters pregnancy in a state of good nutrition and is accustomed to eating a well-balanced diet, the change will not seem great. Indeed, her increased appetite will probably serve as an accurate gauge for increased intake. However, if her dietary habits have been poor every effort must be made to encourage her to eat the proper food. Poor food habits are frequently of long standing and difficult to change, but the pregnant woman is often highly motivated to improve her diet to provide the best opportunities for her baby's growth and development. For this reason the nurse should consider pregnancy a good opportunity to influence the formation of good eating habits, which will carry beyond childbearing. Moreover, since it is usually the mother who selects and prepares food for the family, it is an opportunity to contribute to the nutritional health of the next generation.

DIETARY MODIFICATIONS DURING LACTATION

The diet demands special consideration during lactation, just as it did during pregnancy, since the normal physiologic processes are now also altered and additional demands are placed on the body. Nutritional requirements are considerably increased above normal needs. Throughout the entire nursing period the mother's diet must be such that it will nourish her adequately and also aid in producing milk. The mother should be advised early in the postpartum period about the foods to include in an optimum diet. The physiologic costs of lactation in terms of many dietary needs are not completely clear and utilization of certain foods may be altered during pregnancy and lactation. It appears, however, that nutritional requirements are increased.

Lactating women should receive substantially more calories, proteins, and calcium as well as modest increases in most other nutrients (Table 8-1). Milk production will not be good if there is any marked deficiency of protein or caloric intake. If the woman is able to sustain good milk production in the presence of nutritional deficiencies she does so at a cost to herself.

Calories

Energy needs during lactation may be increased as much as 50 percent above the mother's normal requirements. Her diet must be sufficiently high in calories to meet the needs of her own body, to meet the caloric value of the milk secreted, which is 70 cal/100 ml, and to furnish the energy that is used in the actual production of milk. Thus a mother who is secreting 850 ml of breast milk per day, the average amount secreted during established lactation, would need nearly 800 cal. In addition, she needs energy to produce milk. The caloric cost of lactation is uncertain. It has been estimated to be somewhere between 150 and 400 cal for production of 850 ml of breast milk. The additional caloric requirement is thus proportional to the actual amount of breast milk produced. When caloric requirements are not met, the mother must use her body stores to subsidize her caloric needs. The 1974 recommended daily allowance of calories for the lactating woman is 500 cal above her usual nonpregnant intake (Table 8-1). During pregnancy 2–4 kg (5–10 lb) of fat was stored and is available to produce an additional 200–300 calories per day for about three months to assist in meeting the energy needs of lactation. For the mother who continues to breast-feed after three months, or for the woman who is underweight or feeding more than one infant, more than 500 calories may need to be added. Additionally, individual needs may require adjustment up or down depending on how the woman is able to maintain her weight.

Protein

The estimated additional requirement for protein during lactation is based on the amount of milk excreted and on the amount of protein in the milk. Human milk averages 1.2 gm of protein per 100 ml. Assuming that the mother secretes an average of 850 ml (30 oz) of breast milk per day, with an upper limit of 1200 ml (42 oz), her daily output of protein may be as high as 15 gm per day. This means that the mother who is producing a large amount of breast milk needs to add to her own body's protein requirements an additional 15 gm of ideal protein each day. This allowance, based on a high milk secretion, should be ample for all mothers. However, to allow for variability in the quality of protein eaten, an additional 20 gm of protein per day is recommended for the period of lactation.

Although overall protein content of breast milk does not appear to be altered by deficient maternal diet, there is evidence that protein-deficient diets result in lowered amounts of lysine and methionine, two essential amino acids.[4]

[4] B. S. Lindblad and R. J. Rahimtoola, A pilot study of the quality of human milk in lower socio-economic groups in Karachi, Pakistan, *Acta Paediatr. Scand.* 63:125, 1974.

Thus maternal protein deficiency may result in a qualitatively poorer milk.

Calcium and Phosphorous

As in pregnancy, some physiologic adjustment which increases calcium uptake and calcium conservation also takes place during lactation. However, since calcium will be excreted in breast milk, an intake of dietary calcium above the mother's ordinary daily needs is important during lactation. The recommended calcium intake of the nursing mother is increased by 400 mg per day, which makes a recommended total intake of 1200 mg per day during lactation. One quart of milk per day will provide 1200 mg of calcium. Other foods in the daily diet will provide some additional calcium if needed.

Dietary phosphorus intake ordinarily equals or exceeds calcium intake. Phosphorus, therefore, is recommended in an amount equal to that of calcium. This increases the recommended allowance of phosphorus by 400 mg during lactation.

Other Minerals

Maternal sodium intake will directly influence the amount of sodium secreted in breast milk. On the other hand, maternal intake does not appear to affect the concentration in breast milk of iron, copper, or fluoride. The amount of iron in breast milk is fairly constant at 0.5 to 1.0 mg per day. For this reason iron deficiency is not uncommon in breast-fed infants, particularly as the period of breast feeding is lengthened. Iron supplementation of breast-fed infants is thus commonly recommended. Iron supplementation of the lactating woman is also common as a means of building up stores depleted by pregnancy, even though such supplementation does not affect milk levels.

Fat-soluble Vitamins

Vitamins A and E are present in breast milk in appreciable amounts, thus suggesting a need for increased dietary intake (Table 8-1). The vitamin D requirement is uncertain and the breast milk content of vitamin D is low. Some authorities have recommended vitamin D supplementation for breast-fed infants, but it would seem that exposure to sunlight is almost universally practical and a preferred method.

Water-soluble Vitamins

The recommended daily allowance for each of these vitamins is somewhat increased over non-pregnant, nonlactating levels. In addition, the amount of maternal intake is directly related to the amount secreted in the milk. Deficient maternal intake can produce deficiency diseases in the infant.

Fluids

A fluid intake up to 2500 or 3000 ml is important for adequate milk production. To facilitate adequate intake it is a good plan to keep a pitcher or Thermos bottle of water on the bedside table and replenish it every 4 hours. Some mothers have experienced great thirst during nursing. Fluids during nursing relieve thirst, increase the amount of milk, and often stimulate the letdown of milk.

Restricted Foods

The mother may eat any food that agrees with her. The belief that certain substances from highly flavored vegetables such as onions, cabbage, turnips, and garlic are excreted through the milk to upset the baby's digestion is not given general credence. Some physicians believe that cabbage and members of the cabbage family have a tendency to give the baby colic. Others think that chocolate or certain berries may produce signs of allergy, such as rashes. Ordinarily the mother may eat any kind of food she wishes unless she finds that her baby is disturbed by a particular one. Any food, of course, that causes her to have indigestion should be avoided.

SUMMARY

Increase in the intake of all nutrients is necessary during lactation in order to maintain the maternal bodily needs and/or to supply appropriate levels of nutrients to the infant in breast milk. As during pregnancy, all of these increased needs may be met by increasing the quantity of a well-balanced diet. Should the quality of the diet be poor, nutritional counseling, not unlike that of pregnancy, is indicated. The lactating mother may have an additional difficulty in learning to schedule her time to allow herself opportunity for rest and adequate mealtimes.

NUTRITION DURING THE INTERCONCEPTIONAL PERIOD

The periods of pregnancy and lactation are short, albeit important, times compared to the lifetime of a woman. Attention to good nutrition should be an integral part of health care throughout the life cycle. The interval between pregnancies is especially important for the replenishing of stores depleted during pregnancy and lactation and for establishing optimum weight levels. It is appropriate that nutrition counseling be directed toward maintaining or improving the total family dietary habits.

Recently considerable attention has been directed at the nutritional needs unique to women receiving hormonal therapy, specifically those women taking oral contraceptives. Most information to date is of a biochemical nature and its clinical implications are somewhat speculative. Tests indicating vitamin B deficiency are consistently reported in oral contraceptive users. It has been suggested that this may be a mechanism in the development of depression, and, although this information remains controversial, it is probably reasonable to consider B_6 deficiency as one possible cause of depression if a woman is taking oral contraceptives.

Other biochemical studies have suggested the need for increased folic acid, vitamins C, B_6, B_{12}, and certain trace elements for women taking oral contraceptives. On the other hand, requirements for iron, niacin, vitamin K, copper, and calcium may be diminished. It should be emphasized that the significance of these chemical findings is unclear at present; therefore dietary alterations or supplementation should not be recommended until further investigations clarify the issues.

Because some women who use the intrauterine device for contraception have increased menstrual flow, it is advisable to follow hematocrit levels in this group of women. Dietary counseling should emphasize foods rich in iron, and iron supplementation may even be considered.

BIBLIOGRAPHY

Abel, Marjorie, Nutrition. Part I: Implications for maternal, fetal, and neonatal systems, in *Childbearing: A Nursing Perspective,* edited by Ann L. Clark and Dyanne D. Affonso. F. A. Davis, Philadelphia, Pa., 1976, pp. 165–188.

Bergner, L., and Susser, M. W., Low birth weight and prenatal nutrition: An interpretive review, *Pediatrics* 46:946–966 (Dec.) 1970.

Bernhardt, I. R., and Dorsey, D. J., Hypervitaminosis A and congenital renal anomalies in a human infant, *Obstet. Gynecol.* 43:750–755 (May) 1974.

Committee on Maternal Nutrition, *Maternal Nutrition and the Course of Pregnancy: Summary Report.* Food and Nutrition Board, National Academy of Sciences, Washington, D.C., 1970.

Committee on Nutrition of the Mother and Preschool Child, *Oral Contraceptives and Nutrition—A Statement.* Food and Nutrition Board, National Academy of Sciences, Washington, D.C., 1975.

Esterly, John R., and Oppenheimer, Ella H.; Intrauterine rubella infection, in *Perspectives in Pediatric Pathology*, Vol. 1, edited by Harry S. Rosenberg and Robert P. Bolande. Yearbook Medical Publishers, Chicago, Ill., 1973, pp. 313–338.

Filer, L. J., Maternal nutrition in lactation, *Clin. Perinatal.* 2:353–360 (Sept.) 1975.

Hytten, F. E., and Leitch, I., *The Physiology of Human Pregnancy*, 2nd ed. Blackwell Scientific Publications, Oxford, 1971.

Pitkin, R. M., Kaminetzky, H. A., Newton, M., and Pritchard, J. A., Maternal nutrition: A selective review of clinical topics, *Obstet. Gynecol.* 40:773–785 (Dec.) 1972.

9

Clinical Management of the Antepartum Client

Pregnant women have several needs which the nurse must be prepared to meet during the course of gestation. These include:

1. Health history and physical assessment
2. Ongoing assessment of the mother's physiologic status and that of her fetus
3. Adequate nutition to maintain the mother's health and assure optimum development of the infant
4. Emotional/psychological support
5. Education and information concerning what is happening to the mother's body as well as immediate preparation for labor and delivery and care of an infant

Since history and physical assessment and nutrition have been discussed in Chapters 7 and 8, this chapter will focus on the remaining three needs.

It should be kept in mind that the perinatal practitioner can never deal with a single client. At the minimum there are two clients: a mother and a fetus. In all but exceptional circumstances there is also a father, and frequently there are others such as grandparents, siblings, and close friends. Sometimes the nurse may serve all of these people directly, particularly if she practices in a small community or rural setting or has opportunities for home visits. More often she must try to meet their needs relative to the pregnancy indirectly through the pregnant woman. Whenever possible, particular effort should be made to give at least the father direct

contact with the health care professionals. This may require evening or weekend office hours to avoid conflict with his work schedule. Since the family needs tend to be primarily in the area of education, information, and emotional support, interventions specific to the family will be discussed in that context.

ONGOING ASSESSMENT OF MATERNAL–FETAL PHYSIOLOGIC STATUS

Monitoring of the physical–physiologic changes of pregnancy and the growth and development of the fetus is accomplished by a series of office (clinic) visits at intervals throughout gestation. A typical schedule for these visits is once a month for the first seven months, then every two weeks until the last month, and, finally, every week until the onset of labor. The visits are scheduled more frequently as term approaches because of the increasing chance of complications (especially toxemia) during the third trimester.

Care should be taken in scheduling appointments to avoid long waiting periods which are inconvenient and annoying. Sometimes particular days of the week are set aside to see only antepartum clients, thus permitting more accurate scheduling. Nurses have also found ways to utilize waiting room time very profitably for informal teaching and group discussion when only pregnant women are present.

The sequence of events during an antepartum visit will obviously vary, depending on the needs of the client, the style of the nurse, and the setting in which it occurs. For instance, a visit to a private obstetrician is usually different than one to a university teaching clinic or to a clinic where nurse practitioners or midwives give the majority of care. Ideally, each woman would have an opportunity to select the setting and the philosophy of care best suited to her needs. Since this is rarely possible in reality, a certain flexibility is essential in all types of health care delivery.

One way of organizing an antepartum visit is outlined in Figure 9-1 and discussed below.

1. *Determine the woman's (family's) agenda for this visit.*

It is common for clients having frequently scheduled appointments, as women do during pregnancy, to "save up" questions and concerns from one visit to the next. Very often it is helpful to encourage them literally to make a list as things occur to them. It is appropriate then that these items be the first order of business at the time of the visit. Some questions can be quickly and immediately answered, some may require referral to the physician, while still others may involve obtaining additional data from the client and scheduling a longer time for talking later in the appointment.

Suggested Outline for Return Antepartum Visits

1. Determine the woman's (family's) agenda for this visit.

2. Review the present plan of care with the client.

3. Collect subjective data.

4. Collect objective data.

5. Obtain necessary assessment and/or intervention by consultants.

6. Validate or modify plan of care together with the client.

7. Do appropriate teaching/counseling.

Figure 9-1. Suggested outline for a return antepartum visit. This will necessarily be modified depending on the individual needs of the client and the setting in which care is given. For a more complete discussion, see text.

2. *Review the present plan of care with the client.*

This gives the nurse the opportunity to refamiliarize herself with this particular client's situation and to determine if the client's understanding, the nurses' understanding, and the written client record are all in agreement. It will also reveal parts of the plan which are no longer appropriate or are not working and therefore need revision. For example, the care plan may call for the woman to take ferrous sulfate twice daily, but, because of nausea and constipation, she has not been taking it regularly. Clearly a new plan must be made. In another situation a woman may have been following certain precautions to relieve the nausea of early pregnancy and now finds they are no longer necessary as her nausea has subsided. Furthermore, new situations may arise which require additions to the plan of care. For example, instruction about labor and delivery is inappropriate for the first trimester, but becomes necessary during the second half of pregnancy. New dietary patterns may need to be worked out as the enlarging uterus makes it uncomfortable to eat three large meals a day.

3. *Collect subjective data.*

Although this part of the visit may overlap the discussion of the woman's questions and concerns in step 1 above, it is important to consider it separately. The nurse should systematically inquire about symptoms or events which give evidence of the normal progression of the pregnancy. For example, has the woman felt fetal movement? If so, when did she first note this event and, as gestation progresses, is there any change in the character of the movement? (See Chapter 21, page 610.)

The nurse should also note those symptoms or events which might indicate a developing complication. One useful guide to a systematic collection of data is to use the order of a review of systems, often employed in medical history-taking. That is, beginning at the head and progressing to the feet, determine if there are any symptoms associated with any body system.

It is usually worthwhile to anticipate the more

common discomforts of pregnancy so the woman can be prepared to care for herself. Also, some women may assume that nausea or constipation or other symptoms are necessary evils to be tolerated when pregnant. For this reason they may not spontaneously mention them and therefore will not get help to correct them unless the information is elicited by the nurse. On the other hand, some women may not mention these problems because they are managing them very capably on their own. In this instance the nurse can learn a good deal from her clients.

4. *Collect objective data.*

At each visit the woman is weighed, her blood pressure is checked, and her urine examined for protein and glucose. The abdomen is palpated to determine the position of the fetus, the fundal height is measured, and the fetal heart tones are auscultated. The feet, legs, hands, and face are observed for the presence of edema.

In the past the "weighing-in" ritual in the obstetrician's office was a highly stressful event as rigid weight restrictions were advocated and nurses and physicians were often punitive toward women who gained "too much." It was not uncommon for women to fast for two or three days before their appointment or even to take diuretics in an attempt to please the physician with their lack of weight gain. It is now known that weight restriction is inappropriate during pregnancy and that excessive weight gain is problematic only to the woman who tries to lose it post partum.

It is still important, however, to have a record of weights throughout pregnancy to be sure that weight gain is occurring and to be able to observe the pattern of that gain. It is helpful to the woman as well as to the health professionals to graph her weight on a weight chart as illustrated in Figure 6-18. Deviations from this pattern may indicate the need for special nutrition counseling. A sudden increase in weight of more than 500 gm or 1 lb per week without any other explanation may indicate edema and, possibly, preeclampsia. This is often the earliest sign of impending preeclampsia and, as such, is a very important observation.

Blood pressure should be accurately measured and recorded at each visit in order to establish the individual woman's baseline reading by which deviations can be judged. Errors in blood pressure measurement most often occur from using a cuff that is too narrow for the size of the arm or not wrapping the cuff snugly enough before inflating. This may result in falsely high readings and unnecessary concern about hypertension and toxemia. The American Heart Association recommends using a cuff 20 percent wider than the diameter of the arm. Figure 9-2 illustrates a convenient method of estimating the appropriate cuff width.

At a visit between 28 and 32 weeks gestation a "rollover test" may be done to identify more specifically those women who are likely to develop preeclampsia. (See Chapter 22, page 657.)

Urine tests for protein and glucose may be done very simply by using test papers or "dip sticks" impregnated with the appropriate re-

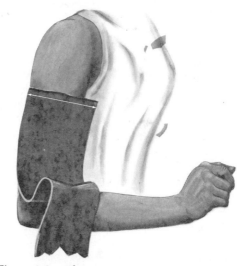

Figure 9-2. The appropriate width blood pressure cuff can be readily estimated by comparing the cuff width with the arm to be used. The cuff should be approximately 20 percent wider than the diameter of the arm. Cuffs that are too narrow give falsely high readings, while cuffs that are too wide will give falsely low readings.

agents. The test end of the paper strip is dipped in freshly voided urine, or the woman is instructed to pass the end of the strip through a stream of urine. The test strip is then read by comparing it with a color chart.

Ordinarily neither protein nor glucose is found in normal urine. The presence of protein may result from contamination by vaginal secretions, especially during the third trimester. For this reason, a clean-catch urine specimen is preferred. Proteinuria, however, may also indicate urinary tract infection or preeclampsia and therefore is a finding which deserves careful attention.

Glucosuria may be a normal result of the physiologic alterations in glomerular filtration rate and renal threshold. Persistent positive findings or large amounts of glucosuria may suggest a need for more precise evaluation of the woman for gestational diabetes mellitus.

Reagent strips for testing ketonuria may be used when indicated as in the woman who is losing weight or failing to gain weight or in the diabetic woman.

5. *Obtain necessary assessment and/or intervention by consultants.*

The mechanisms for carrying out this part of the visit will be largely determined by the type of health care facility, as well as the individual client needs. For example, in the office practice of an obstetrician the woman is most likely to consult with the physician at each visit. In this circumstance it is frequently the physician who collects most of the subjective and objective data and the nurse may play a relatively minor role. In other situations the physician may see the client on alternate visits or perhaps not until near term. The nurse may request the physician to make an assessment because of data she has collected which warrant medical evaluation. Many different arrangements of health care practice are in use.

In addition to medical consultation, it may be desirable to seek the expertise of nutritionists, social workers, childbirth educators, counselors, or others to help with a particular problem or client need.

6. *Validate or modify plan of care.*

Based on the information exchanged and the judgments made during the visit the plan of care should either be determined accurate and workable or modified to suit changing circumstances. It seems obvious that the woman herself, and frequently other family members, must have an active role in formulating any care plan. She is usually the best judge of what will be likely to be helpful and workable for her and her family.

7. *Pursue appropriate teaching and counseling.*

Although teaching and counseling activities are likely to be interspersed throughout the antepartum visit, it is usually profitable to schedule some time during each visit for the client and nurse to sit down together in consultation. The client should be dressed, and both she and the nurse seated comfortably before the discussion begins. It may be desirable for other family members and/or professionals to be present on some occasions.

Questions and concerns which require more than a couple of minutes to resolve should be dealt with at this time. In addition to incidental teaching which answers particular client questions, the nurse will also need to do some anticipatory teaching. She will wish to anticipate with the woman the physical and emotional changes she may encounter, preparation of older children for the new baby, the challenges inherent in the woman's own role change, and many other topics.

GENERAL HEALTH DURING PREGNANCY

Grooming and Hygiene

Pregnancy is a time of rapid and dramatic physical changes which require the woman to make continual adjustments in her self-image. With a little attention to herself she can feel, as well as look, more feminine and attractive.

The excretory function of the skin is enhanced during pregnancy, resulting in increased perspiration. The skin and hair may become more oily, and more frequent bathing and shampooing may be necessary. Some women find it helpful to use a shampoo especially designed for oily hair and to adopt a hair style that is easy to manage.

Tub baths are permitted throughout pregnancy. During the latter weeks of gestation, however, the woman's physical clumsiness may make it more difficult to negotiate the climb in and out of the tub. At this time she may find it easier to shower unless someone is available to help her up out of the water. Baths tend to be quite relaxing and may be good therapy for tired muscles, backache, or insomnia. Bath oils, powders, and lotions are often a treat which makes a woman smell nice and feel special, and they need not be expensive.

If a chloasma or "mask of pregnancy" appears, the woman may wish to experiment with various makeup foundations if she finds it unattractive.

Maternity fashions range from bathing suits to evening gowns. These clothes can be quite costly, but with a little care and effort the expectant mother can be well-dressed on a very modest budget. Since maternity clothes almost never get worn out, friends or relatives of the same size are a good source of hand-me-downs. Garage sales and second-hand clothing stores are other inexpensive places to acquire a wardrobe. If the woman sews, she will find that maternity clothes are quick and easy to make. Since they require little fitting, even beginning seamstresses can produce very attractive garments.

It is wise to select fabrics that are washable. If the pregnancy occurs during warm weather, cotton or other absorbent materials are more comfortable. This is particularly true for undergarments.

Some women may find it desirable to wear a maternity girdle to support the enlarging uterus. This is particularly true of the woman who has flaccid abdominal musculature which gives poor natural support to the uterus. These women often get considerable relief from backaches and pressure symptoms when a girdle is worn, since it lifts some of the weight of the heavy uterus from the blood vessels and ligaments. The girdle worn before pregnancy, regardless of how large, will not be satisfactory during pregnancy. It will become uncomfortable, and may even be harmful, as it tends to push the uterus down into the pelvis, causing backache and cramps in the legs.

A brassiere which gives good support to the breasts is advisable. Most women will require a larger size during pregnancy to accommodate the normal growth of the breasts. If the woman is planning to breast-feed she may wish to purchase a nursing bra which she can continue to use after the baby is born.

Any clothing which restricts circulation should be avoided, especially during pregnancy. As the woman gains weight, garments which fit properly before pregnancy may become too tight. Bras, panties, and knee socks are common offenders. Of course, garters should never be worn as they are especially apt to retard circulation, thus favoring development of varicosities and muscle cramps.

Shoes that are comfortable, provide firm foot support, and promote good posture and balance are advisable for everyone, including pregnant women. This does not mean that they must be unattractive or that frivolous shoes shouldn't be worn for some occasions. However, as the woman's center of gravity shifts due to the increasing weight of the uterus, she will find it more difficult to maintain her balance in very high-heeled or platform-soled shoes.

Pregnancy is ordinarily a period of well-being for a woman. If she gives herself a little special care, she will increase her self-confidence in her appearance and will look happy and pretty.

Care of Breasts and Nipples

The importance of a well-fitting bra has already been mentioned. In addition, if the woman is planning to breast-feed, some preparation of the breasts and nipples during pregnancy is advisable.

Toughening the nipples for the abrasive and stretching action of sucking during breast-feeding has been given much consideration. Some authors have recommended the avoidance of soap on the nipples during pregnancy and lactation. This is felt to prevent drying and cracking by promoting the natural protective mechanisms of the body. Normally, dead cells form a protective covering for the nipples, while copious secretions of the sebaceous and sweat glands keep the skin pliable and maintain a normal acid condition. Frequent washing with soap tends to remove all these substances.

Ointments may inhibit evaporation of perspiration and cause the skin to become soft and tender, although lanolin is sometimes recommended.

Gentle rubbing of the woman's clothing is often an effective way to toughen the nipples. The mother may either omit wearing her brassiere for a few hours each day, or if the brassiere has flaps, such as on a type used for nursing, the flaps may be left down for a few hours. Friction from drying with a rough towel is still another way to gradually toughen the nipples for nursing.

Some authorities have recommended manual expression of colostrum during the last month of pregnancy as a way of facilitating lactation. Milk then comes in earlier after birth and the discomfort due to engorgement is usually avoided. Other writers, however, discourage this practice in the belief that the colostrum is wasted and the infant does not get the advantage of the immune substances it contains. More research is needed to determine if there is a unique advantage of colostrum over breast milk as well as to establish the efficacy of antepartum expression of colostrum.

Exercise

Exercise is beneficial to health as it improves circulation, enhances appetite and digestion of food, provides better bowel function, promotes restful sleep, and gives diversion from routine responsibilities. Walking is particularly recommended. Many physically active women continue to swim, jog, or play tennis well into their pregnancies. For the more sedentary woman, however, pregnancy is probably not a good time to embark upon a strenuous physical fitness program.

Both the active and the sedentary woman should avoid fatigue and should stop exercising when she begins to feel tired. Moderation is the best watchword.

A change in balance with advancing pregnancy and the increased mobility of the pelvic joints may limit the pregnant woman's physical ability to continue some of her normal sports activities, at least in the latter weeks of pregnancy.

Rest and Relaxation

Pregnant women tire easily, and every effort should be made to prevent undue fatigue. As the abdomen increases in size and weight, the body's center of gravity changes, and the pregnant woman is required to make a constant though unconscious effort to stand upright. Frequent rest periods are needed by all pregnant women, but are even more necessary for those with poor body alignment than for those who have good posture. Accordingly, the expectant mother may need rest frequently during the day, for 10 to 15 minutes at a time, in order to avoid needless fatigue. She should work and exercise in short periods, sitting or lying down if possible when tired. Many times some rest can be obtained by doing all work that can possibly be done in a sitting rather than a standing position.

If a woman is having trouble resting, it is often useful for the nurse to review a typical day with her in detail so they can plan together how to organize rest and work more efficiently. Sometimes the woman must adjust to less exacting standards of housekeeping in order to rest. Another woman may need help in setting limits for her preschool children to save herself steps. The woman who works outside her home may need suggestions for relaxation techniques and positions in order to get maximum benefit from her work breaks. (See Figure 9-3.)

Sitting can be fatiguing unless the hips are

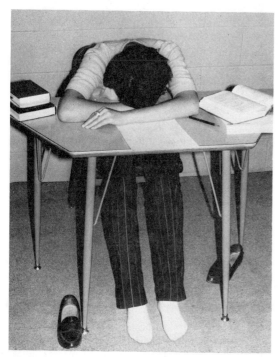

Figure 9-3. Relaxing at desk, with all muscles loose and limp, and feet flat on the floor.

well back in the seat of a chair that gives adequate support to the back. The seat must not be so deep, however, that there is pressure under the knees and thus on the veins. The feet should rest on the floor or on a stool of suitable height, or a pillow. Sitting with the legs elevated on a stool, or pillow, will ensure rest as well as relieve a strain on varicosities and decrease swelling of the feet and legs (Fig. 9-4). For the position to be restful the knees should be in slight flexion, and the footstool slightly lower than the chair to avoid pressure in the groins. Often a rocking chair, or a straight chair, with armrests and good back support, of a height that allows the feet to rest easily on the floor, is very comfortable for rest.

Fatigue can often be reduced by good posture and by taking care to avoid strain at work. Standing tall reduces stress. Changing position frequently is helpful. Stooping and lifting should be avoided whenever possible, but if they are

necessary, the woman should bend at the hips or knees, keeping the back straight.

Since eight hours' sleep is usually considered necessary for the average person, the pregnant woman cannot expect to be comfortable with less. For good rest a comfortable position should be assumed, preferably on a bed with a firm mattress to prevent back strain.

In early pregnancy lying flat on the back with a pillow under the head and under the knees may be very comfortable. Clothing should be loose, and muscles should be allowed to become loose and limp. Slow abdominal breathing is conducive to relaxation and may help to induce sleep. Later in pregnancy when the abdomen enlarges, it usually becomes necessary for the mother to lie on her side with the hips partially rotated to allow the abdomen to rest on the bed. It may be necessary to use a pillow for support to the upper leg. All joints should be bent slightly to prevent muscle tenseness. With conscious effort all of the skeletal muscles can be relaxed in this position.

Recreation is important to the expectant mother's pleasure and relaxation. It is advisable for her to continue most of her recreational ac-

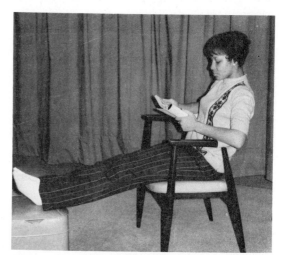

Figure 9-4. Relaxing in a chair with hips well back in the chair, adequate support to the back (not visible here), and legs elevated to relieve strain on varicosities and decrease swelling of feet.

tivities during pregnancy, with limitations as necessary to avoid fatigue.

Sexuality

The desire for sexual expression may vary widely from one woman to the next and even from time to time during pregnancy for the same woman. There may be increased desire as the woman has a new awareness of her body and feels increasingly close to the man whose child she carries. At other times or in other women, this same body awareness may make intercourse repugnant to her. Still others have a fear of harming the baby.

Typically there is slight decrease in sexual tension during the first trimester because of fatigue and, perhaps, nausea. During the second trimester increasing pelvic congestion tends to heighten the woman's sexual desire; interest in sex may exceed that of her nonpregnant state. Again in the third trimester her interest in coitus declines as the fetus grows more demanding of her energy. In addition, her physical size makes positioning awkward. The penis thrusting against the "immovable object" of the fetal presenting part may be uncomfortable for both partners.

The man, too, varies in his sexual response to his pregnant partner. He may have diminishing sexual interest as pregnancy progresses because of the woman's swollen body and the fear of hurting her or the baby. Nurturant and protective feelings toward the woman may become dominant.

Couples should be aware that these changes in feelings are common. They are less likely to become confused and distressed by fluctuations in interest in sexual activity if they are able to anticipate it as a normal happening.

Adjustment to sexuality during pregnancy depends on the strength of the couple's total relationship, their maturity, culture, marital status, and feelings about this pregnancy. A couple with a stable, loving relationship who are able to communicate feelings to each other will adapt to each other more easily. They will be more apt to see sexual behavior as only one form of intimacy.

Coital positions may need to be altered at various times throughout gestation to provide greater comfort. During the first trimester breast tenderness may require avoiding direct pressure on the breasts, while in the third trimester the markedly enlarged uterus is clearly in the way of the traditional male-superior position. Many pregnant couples find the side-by-side, rear entry, or female-superior positions preferable. Coitus is necessarily gentler in these positions as well.

In the last trimester of pregnancy the woman may experience a single orgasmic contraction lasting as long as a minute rather than the rhythmic, multiple contractions of the nonpregnant state. She may also have some cramps or a backache following orgasm resulting from the pelvic congestion. This is usually relieved by a back rub.

At the same time the woman's desire for coitus may be declining she ordinarily has an increasing need for physical closeness and cuddling. Kissing, hugging, and caressing are important ways of expressing love and affection.

There are no medically valid reasons for prohibiting sexual intercourse during a normal pregnancy. Certain complications or risk factors, however, may make restrictions necessary. These include threatened abortion, ruptured membranes, vaginal bleeding, and premature labor that has been stopped pharmacologically.

The Use of Drugs During Pregnancy

A single evening of television viewing is sufficent evidence that this is indeed a "drug culture." No human malady, however great or small, need be suffered if the drug commercials are to be believed. Pregnant women, no less than others, ingest a variety of drugs both prescribed and over-the-counter. For most of these drugs the effects on the fetus are unknown.

The dramatic tragedy of thalidomide-induced congenital anomalies raised the consciousness of the public as well as professionals to the risks inherent in medications taken during pregnancy. It is to be hoped that the result of this increased awareness will be a reluctance to prescribe or to take any but the most essential drugs during gestation.

In order for a drug to be teratogenic certain conditions must be met. First, the drug must cross the placenta and reach the fetus in concentrations sufficient to cause damage. It is generally believed that most drugs cross the placenta. The concentration achieved in the fetal bloodstream depends on a variety of factors. Probably, in most instances, there is an equilibration across the placenta so that the concentration in the fetus approximates that in the mother. In some cases the fetal concentration may be elevated because of the inability of the immature fetal liver to break down the drug or the immature fetal kidney to excrete it.

Second, the drug must reach the fetus at a critical time for the development of a particular organ or structure. Different structures are vulnerable to damage at different times depending on when in embryonic or fetal life they are undergoing maximum differentiation (Fig. 9-5). In general, the first trimester is the period of greatest danger from malformation-inducing agents. Since the woman is unaware of her pregnancy for at least some part of this critical first trimester, there is a convincing argument for all women who are at risk to become pregnant to avoid taking drugs whenever possible.

Finally, the drug must reach a susceptible host. The effects of drugs are species-specific, e.g., that which causes malformations in mice may be safe for rats, or that which is safe for monkeys may cause anomalies in human beings. This complicates the testing of drugs for safe use

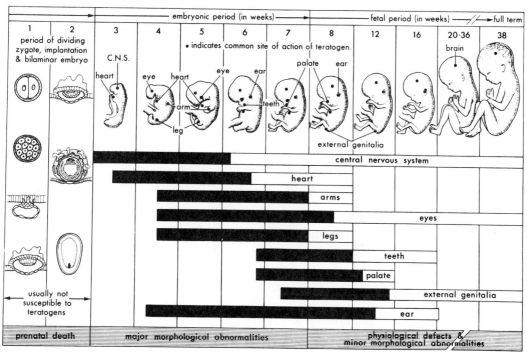

Figure 9-5. Schematic illustration of the sensitive or critical periods in human development. Dark bars denote highly sensitive periods; white bars indicate stages that are less sensitive to teratogens. [*Reproduced with permission from Keith L. Moore,* Before We Are Born, *revised reprint, W. B. Saunders Co., Philadelphia, Pa., 1977.*]

Table 9-1. List of Some of the Drugs Taken During Pregnancy and Their Effect on the Fetus or Newborn*

Drug	Fetal or Neonatal Effect
Thiazides	Electrolyte imbalance, thrombo-cytopenia with possible neonatal bleeding
Meclizine (Bonamine, Antivert)	? Cleft lip and palate
Thalidomide	Multiple malformation syndrome (phocomelia, eye and ear defects, cardiac and GU anomalies)
Valium	? Cleft lip and palate, hypothermia
Tetracyclines	Teeth discoloration, hypoplasia of enamel, inhibition of bone growth
Oral progestins, androgens, estrogens	Masculinization of fetus, advanced bone age with later growth failure
Diethylstilbestrol (DES)	Vaginal adenocarcinoma in childhood and adolescence
Corticosteroids	? Cleft palate ? Anencephaly
Radioactive iodine (^{131}I)	Thyroid cancer, hypothyroidism, cretinism, chromosomal damage
Dicumerol	Fetal or neonatal hemorrhage
Coumadin	Fetal or neonatal hemorrhage Hypoplastic nasal structure
Heparin	Does *not* cross placenta
Tolbutamide (Orinase)	Thrombocytopenia in newborn, multiple congenital anomalies
Chlorpropamide (Diabinese)	? Multiple anomalies, severe neonatal hypoglycemia, stillbirths
Reserpine	Nasal congestion with possible respiratory obstruction, hypothermia
Salicylates	Neonatal bleeding (hypoprothrom-binemia)
Narcotic addiction	Sterility, abortion

Morphine
   Heroin
   Methadone
   Meperidine (Demerol)
	Intrauterine withdrawal (increased fetal activity, seizure, death)
	Respiratory depression at birth
	Intrauterine growth retardation
	Neonatal withdrawal syndrome (tremor, salivation, yawning, sneezing, pyrexia, sweating, vomiting, diarrhea, irritable screaming, seizures, coma, death)
	Behavioral dysfunction

Table 9-1. (continued)

Drug	Fetal or Neonatal Effect
Dilantin	Cleft lip and palate, congenital heart disease, neonatal hemorrhage
Alcohol (chronic use)	Fetal alcohol syndrome, respiratory depression at birth, intrauterine growth retardation, neonatal withdrawal
Lead	CNS deficit, mental retardation, intrauterine growth retardation, failure to thrive (infants)
Amphetamines	Neonatal withdrawal, ? congenital heart disease, biliary atresia
Ergonovine maleate (Ergotrate)	Poland's syndrome (multiple anomalies)
Sulfonamides	Kernicterus
Smoking	Intrauterine growth retardation

*Where the effects are suspected but not proven a question mark is used to denote the uncertainty of the research.

in human beings. Individuals, as well as species, differ in their susceptibility to drug effects because of their varying genetic makeup. Furthermore, there appears to be a specificity of certain drugs for certain organs or systems. Thus a particular drug may cause a cleft palate but does not interfere with cardiac development even if taken at the critical time for differentiation of the heart and circulatory system. Another drug may affect only limb development or kidney development.

Drugs taken during pregnancy may exert their effects in several different ways. They may cause lethal damage and thus result in a spontaneous abortion or, less commonly, a stillbirth. Developing organs may be affected so that the infant is born with congenital malformations. Other drugs may adversely affect the neonatal adjustment, e.g., aspirin, which is associated with neonatal hemorrhage, and thiazide diuretics, which cause neonatal electrolyte imbalances and thrombocytopenia. The effects of some drugs may not be evident until later on in the life of the child. An example of this is the occurrence of adenocarcinoma of the vagina in young girls whose mothers took diethylstilbestrol (DES) during their pregnancies.

Women should be advised not to take any medication prescribed prior to pregnancy until they have checked with their physician. Whenever possible they should avoid taking all drugs, whether prescribed or not, during pregnancy. Obviously, there are occasions when drugs must be taken because of maternal illness or obstetric complications. Whenever such an occasion arises there should be a deliberate evaluation of the balance between the therapeutic good to be achieved and the risk to the fetus. Such a pause for judgment will eliminate casual prescription writing.

Although the effect of many commonly used drugs is not known, problems with some have been identified. Table 9-1 gives a partial list of drugs which may be administered during pregnancy and the effects on the fetus and newborn.

Alcohol is the most frequently abused drug in

the United States among all age groups including teenagers. In addition to the social and nutritional problems arising from excessive drinking, there is a pattern of malformations in infants born to women with chronic alcoholism. This pattern, called the "fetal alcohol syndrome" (FAS), is characterized by a variety of malformations, the chief of which are craniofacial anomalies and mental and growth retardation. Unlike the malnourished fetus whose weight is too little for his length, the fetus with FAS is unusually short for his weight. Furthermore, the infants continue to show a failure to thrive independent of their postnatal environment. Women who are chronic alcoholics have a 30 to 50 percent risk of having an infant with FAS.

What about the nonalcoholic who drinks beer, wine, or spirits on occasion? At this time information is sketchy and inconclusive. Evidence favors the position that the amount of alcohol is significant so that the more that is consumed the greater the risk. As with most drugs, the first trimester appears to be the most critical period. The best advice for pregnant women appears to be either not to drink at all or to do so in moderation. A glass of wine with dinner or a single cocktail at a party is probably safe, but getting "high" or drunk is risky. In addition, many pregnant women find they are more sensitive to the effects of alcohol than when they are not pregnant. It is wise to proceed with caution.

Cigarette smoking has been clearly demonstrated to increase the risk of various pulmonary and cardiovascular diseases. Smoking during pregnancy is associated with a significant increase in low-birthweight (small-for-gestational-age) babies. The mechanism for retarding fetal growth is subject to some debate. Some feel it is the vasoconstricting effect of the nicotine, while others implicate the increased blood levels of carbon monoxide which reduces the oxygen-carrying capacity of maternal blood. As in the case of alcohol, amounts appear significant, with heavy smokers having the greatest risk for small infants. Some researchers have suggested that even though the infants are small they may not be subject to the same risks as infants who are small for other reasons and that catch-up growth is rapid during the first year of life. Regardless of the severity of the fetal risk it is a good health teaching practice to encourage the pregnant woman to stop or cut down her smoking if possible.

Employment

Women comprise an increasingly large proportion of the labor force, and many pregnant women continue to work through much of pregnancy for personal satisfaction as well as financial reward. If a few important considerations are borne in mind, there is no reason why a healthy woman cannot be employed throughout gestation if she wishes.

The work environment should, of course, be safe not only for the woman but also for her developing fetus. Severe physical strain, such as heavy lifting, is to be avoided, as are prolonged periods of sitting or standing still. Women should not work around ionizing radiation or chemical hazards. Industries will often consider reassignment of work for the pregnant woman, which will permit continued employment.

As gestation progresses the expectant mother will tire more easily and may need an extra rest period if possible. She is likely to find herself more fatigued after work and less able to keep up with her accustomed activities at home. The husband who is sensitive to her energy limitations will be able to do much to help her with household chores and, at the same time, provide her with the increasing nurturance she needs as she approaches term.

Women often find as they enter the third trimester that their interest in their job declines somewhat. This is a normal response to the increasing inner awareness of pregnancy. Some women, however, find this very disturbing and feel that it is a weakness of which they should be ashamed. Often they can be helped to see that their introversion is a natural result of doing something as important as making a baby and that their pregnancy is a celebration of their total womanhood.

For the woman who plans to return to work soon after the birth of her baby preparations should begin during pregnancy. Nurses can expect to be called upon for sharing of information about day care, breast feeding while working, and so on.

Care of the Teeth

The teeth require the same good care during pregnancy that they do at all times. The old wives' tale that the mother will lose a tooth for each baby has no basis in fact. The fetus does not drain the calcium from the mother's teeth! However, nausea, acid regurgitation, ptyalism (excessive salivation), and changing dietary habits may contribute to cavity formation during pregnancy.

Dental work is rarely contraindicated, but the dentist should be aware of the pregnancy before choosing drugs or anesthetic agents. The second trimester is the best time for dental work, since the woman feels well and is not too heavy to sit still for a while. X-rays for dental diagnosis should be postponed until the second half of pregnancy if not until after delivery. As always, a lead apron should be employed to cover the abdomen during the x-ray procedure.

During pregnancy the gums may have a greater tendency to bleed as a result of increased estrogen levels. At times they may appear red and swollen. Use of a softer bristled toothbrush will usually help.

Travel

As with many other details of antepartum care, the advisability of travel is determined by the mother's condition. Her tendency to nausea, the length of the trip, the ease with which it may be made, and whether or not she has had, or been threatened with, an abortion or premature labor are considered. The expectant mother may be advised to avoid travel in the early months of pregnancy if there is a tendency to abortion, and at any time if she tends to have premature labor. Travel is inadvisable during the last month of pregnancy because labor may begin early. The availability of quality medical care en route and at the destination is also a factor for consideration.

A trip should be made as comfortably and smoothly as possible. When the woman is traveling by car, frequent rest periods are recommended to stretch her legs and promote circulation. Similarly, during a plane trip the woman should occasionally walk up and down the aisle. Modern commercial airlines with their pressurized cabins and availability of oxygen do not pose any threat to the pregnant woman or her fetus.

Before plans are made for a major trip it is wise to seek consultation with the physician whenever practical.

Preparations for the Baby

All of pregnancy is, by its very nature, a physical and psychological preparation for having a baby. During the last weeks of gestation this preparation takes on the outward characteristics of making the home ready to receive the new family member. A room, or area within a room, is designated as "the baby's" and a crib or bassinet is installed. Clothes, toys, and other infant paraphernalia are acquired through gifts or purchase. If there are other children in the family these preparations can be one way of helping them realize that a baby is coming and allows them to participate in the fun of anticipation.

The types and amount of baby equipment and clothing is largely dependent upon the parents' preferences and financial resources. The availability of laundry facilities is also an important factor to consider. It is wise to bear in mind that young infants grow rapidly so a large wardrobe for any one age is not very practical.

Some parents, because of their cultural backgrounds, may consider it bad luck to purchase baby clothes prior to birth. Other parents, particularly those who have had a previous stillbirth or neonatal death, may prefer to wait until they are sure the baby is healthy.

In addition to acquiring furniture and other

possessions for the baby, a number of decisions are ordinarily made during the late weeks of pregnancy. Tentative names are agreed upon and a choice is made between bottle- and breast-feeding. This is also the appropriate time to choose a physician to care for the baby. Whenever possible the parents should meet and talk with this physician prior to delivery.

About three weeks before her due date the woman should organize her belongings that she plans to take to the hospital or maternity home. In addition to her own clothes and toilet articles it is a good idea to pack the baby's going home clothes. Arrangements should be completed for the care of older children.

The last few weeks before delivery can be very wearing on the whole family as they wonder each day if today will be THE day. The woman becomes exquisitely sensitive to her body as she awaits the first sign of beginning labor. Family and friends tease, "When are you going to have that baby?" Social interactions as well as her ponderous abdomen increase her readiness to end the pregnancy and begin the next phase of motherhood.

COMMON DISCOMFORTS DURING PREGNANCY

Many minor disturbances may cause the pregnant woman discomfort. Although they are not serious in themselves, the mother's comfort is increased by alleviation of these disturbances. Often the nurse can anticipate the development of symptoms with the client and help her acquire self-management strategies either to prevent or treat them herself. When any symptom is severe or persists over time, medical intervention is indicated.

Gastrointestinal Symptoms

Nausea and vomiting are probably the most common disturbances of pregnancy, occurring in about 50 percent of expectant mothers. The symptoms vary from the slightest feeling of nausea when the woman first raises her head in the morning to persistent and frequent vomiting, which then assumes grave proportions and is termed "pernicious vomiting." Although even the slightest nausea may be due to certain organic changes in the body, emotional factors probably also exert an influence. Nausea may very likely be due to a state of tension. Some emotional tension may well be expected, even when a pregnancy is greatly desired, since certain adjustments must always be made. In addition to nausea the woman may also complain of a "bad taste" in her mouth.

Nausea and vomiting will usually disappear at the end of the first trimester, probably at a time when certain adjustments, both physical and emotional, have been made. It can often be relieved earlier by certain preventive measures. Adequate rest and relaxation will often help to reduce tension and may therefore be stressed as a preventive measure for nausea. Certain dietary measures, explained below, often give relief.

Nausea and/or vomiting of pregnancy may occur at any time during the day, but since it appears most frequently in the early morning, as soon as the woman gets up, it is commonly called "morning sickness." This early-morning nausea is often relieved by eating two or three crackers or a piece of toast, with nothing to drink, immediately on awakening, then lying quietly in bed for 20 to 30 minutes, and thereafter arising and eating a light breakfast.

Another very common time of day for nausea to occur is in the late afternoon or early evening, around the supper hour. This is often a somewhat hectic time of day when young children are irritable and hungry, adults are returning home tired from a day's work, and a meal must be prepared in the midst of some confusion. Using plan-ahead and cook-ahead foods is one way of distributing some of this stress more evenly throughout the day. The woman who is employed outside the home will often feel better if she comes home and has a light snack and a short rest before rushing into dinner preparations. Many other strategies can be developed in consultation with women who will know what will fit in with their family life styles.

If the nausea occurs at other times during the day, it is advisable for the expectant mother to eat six small meals a day rather than three large ones in an attempt to keep some food in the stomach at all times. The nausea seems to be worse when the stomach is empty than when it contains some food. Foods that are largely carbohydrate, do not have a strong odor, and are of extremes of temperature, either very hot or very cold, give the most relief. It may also be well to take liquids and solids separately instead of taking both at the same meal. Fried or greasy foods should be avoided.

If it is known that nausea occurs at a certain time of day, the expectant mother should eat 30 minutes earlier; she should be given specific instructions concerning the best times for eating and the kinds of food she should have, as well as assurance that she will obtain relief. Lying flat and very quiet for a short time after meals, or whenever there is the slightest premonitory symptom, will frequently prevent or relieve nausea.

Antihistamines, tranquilizers, or anti-motion sickness drugs should be used sparingly. However, when nausea is severe enough to interfere with usual activities or when maternal nutrition is affected, drug therapy becomes necessary.

Heartburn, so called, is experienced by many pregnant women. It is caused by a bubbling back of stomach contents into the esophagus and is usually described as a burning sensation first in the stomach and then rising into the throat. It may be prevented, as a rule, by substituting frequent small meals for the usual three larger ones. If frequent small meals do not give relief, the physician may recommend an antacid preparation such as aluminum hydroxide, magnesium trisilicate, or magnesium hydroxide (Amphojel, Gelusil, Maalox, milk of magnesia) alone or in combination, preferably as a liquid, to be taken at the time of the burning sensation. The nurse may caution the patient against mixing the antacid with citrus fruit juice for palatability, since

the acidity of the juice immediately inactivates the antacid. A common custom of taking baking soda in a glass of water for relief of heartburn is contraindicated during pregnancy because of the possibility of retention of sodium and subsequent edema.

Distress, a vague and ill-defined form of discomfort, occurs after eating. It may be neither heartburn nor pain, but resembles both and makes the mother very uncomfortable. It is more likely to occur in the person who eats rapidly, does not chew food thoroughly, or eats more at one time than the stomach can hold comfortably. Small amounts of food taken slowly and masticated thoroughly may prevent distress.

Flatulence may or may not be associated with heartburn. It is fairly common and rather uncomfortable. It is usually due to bacterial action in the intestines, which results in the formation of gas. Hypochlorhydria during pregnancy and deceased motility of the entire gastrointestinal tract retard normal peristalsis, and gas sometimes accumulates to a very uncomfortable extent. A daily bowel movement is important in prevention and relief of flatulence. Foods that form gas should be excluded from the diet. The chief offenders are parsnips, beans, the cabbage family, corn, fried foods, pastry, and very sweet desserts.

Constipation may become a problem during pregnancy especially for the woman who ordinarily has a tendency toward constipation. Relaxation of the smooth muscle tone of the bowel during pregnancy is considered the major cause of constipation. Impaired tone of the stretched abdominal muscles may be a contributing factor.

Management of constipation is the same whether or not it accompanies pregnancy. Prevention is the best treatment. The diet should contain adequate amounts of fresh fruits, coarse vegetables, whole-grain breads and cereals, and abundant fluids. Exercise is also beneficial. A regular time for defecation should be established and action upon the desire for defecation should be prompt. When trying to have a bowel movement the woman should sit comfortably back on the commode seat with her feet flat on the floor or supported on a low step. This is the best posture for efficient muscle action.

Laxatives and cathartics should be taken only if prescribed by the physician. Dioctyl sodium sulfosuccinate (Colace, Doxinate) is a commonly used drug because it is bland, nonirritating, and nonlaxative; it acts as a fecal softener through its detergent action. Pericolace, a combination stool softener and mild stimulant laxative, may be prescribed for its gentle peristaltic stimulation.

Irritant cathartics and enemas are to be avoided during pregnancy unless all other treatment has been ineffective. Mineral oil is contraindicated as it inhibits the absorption of fat-soluble vitamins.

Pressure Symptoms

Under the general heading of pressure symptoms are several kinds of discomfort resulting from pressure of the enlarging uterus on the veins returning from the lower part of the body, thus interfering with the return flow of blood. This pressure is likely to be greatly increased if lumbar lordosis and tilting forward of the pelvis are marked. As both the cause and relief of these symptoms are associated with the force of gravity, methods of prevention are apparent. In general, the heavy abdomen may be supported by a properly fitting girdle if the abdominal muscles are not strong enough to give good support, and the mother should keep off her feet as much as possible and elevate the swollen part. Support of the heavy abdomen not only gives relief but will often prevent the occurrence of pressure symptoms.

The most common pressure symptoms are swollen feet, varicose veins, hemorrhoids, cramps in the legs, and shortness of breath. Although they may appear at any time during the latter half of pregnancy, they grow progressively worse as pregnancy advances. If the mother is alarmed over the appearance of these symptoms her fears may be allayed by the explanation that such conditions are neither unusual nor serious.

Swelling of the feet is very common during pregnancy, and sometimes there is also swelling of the hands. The edema may be confined to the back of the ankles, or it may extend up the legs to the thighs and may even include the vulva. This edema is considered a physiologic occurrence resulting from mechanical interference with venous return and other circulatory modifications of pregnancy. (See Chapter 6, page 131.)

When the edema is slight it may not be particularly uncomfortable. Some women, however, find they are unable to wear their shoes and are quite miserable. For these women efforts should be made to increase fluid mobilization and reduce edema. Lying down in a lateral position favors venous return from the lower extremities and is thus most likely to effect a decrease in fluid retention. This explains the common occurrence of nocturia during the latter weeks of pregnancy. Sitting with the feet resting on a chair or footstool will also give some relief and, at times, is more practical than lying down. For the woman who is employed, elevation of the feet for 10–15 minutes several times a day may considerably increase her comfort.

Dietary salt restriction is not indicated for the edema of pregnancy, since sodium retention is not an etiologic factor in its development. Sodium intake is necessary to maintain normal maternal and fetal electrolyte balance.

While using the above harmless and clearly indicated measures for patient comfort, the nurse must be keenly aware of the fact that, although edema of the feet, legs, and vulva may be of solely mechanical origin, it is also a sign of toxemia. Any swelling should prompt further investigation.

Varicose veins are not peculiar to pregnancy, but are among the pressure symptoms that frequently accompany pregnancy during the later months, particularly among women who have borne children. The superficial veins in the legs will often be equal to the tension put on them the first time, but will not tolerate the repeated strain during subsequent pregnancies. The distention of the veins is not serious as a rule but may be very uncomfortable. Aching of the legs is a common symptom even when the veins are not visible. Pain coupled with their appearance sometimes has an adverse effect on the mother's feeling of well-being. Varicose veins may occur in the vulva, although they are usually confined to the legs.

Varicose veins are most likely to develop when the mother must stand for long periods of time or sit with her legs dependent. One preventive measure is to sit down with the feet elevated. If the woman will keep in mind that she should sit with her feet elevated whenever possible, she will find many instances in which she can do this while doing daily work that she might ordinarily do standing up. If it is necessary for her to remain on her feet for the major part of the day, moving about, which improves circulation in the veins of the legs, is better than standing still. When the legs are moved, as in walking, circulation is improved by the massaging action of the muscles close to the veins. Tight bands such as those often found on knee socks or round garters interfere with return circulation and should never be worn.

Relief from the discomfort caused by varicose veins is obtained as a rule by keeping off the feet, and particularly by elevating them, as well as by use of elastic hose or bandages. When a woman finds it difficult or nearly impossible to sit or lie down for any length of time, she may accomplish a great deal in a short time by lying flat on the bed with her legs elevated 45 degrees, resting them on a footstool (Fig. 9-6).

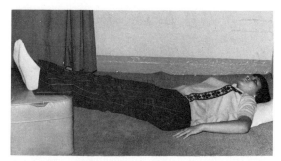

Figure 9-6. Resting the legs on a footstool for 5 to 10 minutes during the day as necessary for comfort and at night before going to sleep. This position promotes good circulation in the legs, reducing discomfort from varicose veins, edema, and leg cramps and fatigue.

This position, maintained for 5 to 10 minutes, three or four times a day, by promoting drainage of the veins, will usually help reduce varicose veins and decrease aching of the legs. Elevation of the legs to an angle of more than 45 degrees may compress the veins in the groin and interfere with venous return from the legs.

In addition to proper posture, elastic stockings or spiral elastic bandages will give relief and help to prevent the veins from growing larger. They should be put on before getting up in the morning or after the legs have been elevated for a few minutes so that the veins are relatively empty at the time they are applied. Elastic stockings offer an advantage over the bandages in ease of application and appearance. When an elastic bandage is used, it is applied spirally with firm, even pressure, starting with a few turns over the foot to secure it and leaving the heel uncovered. The bandage is carried up the leg to a point above the highest swollen vessels.

Engorged veins in the vulva may be relieved by lying flat and elevating the hips, or by adopting the elevated Sims' position for a few moments several times a day.

Hemorrhoids are varicose veins that protrude from the rectum, but unlike those in the legs, they are extremely painful. They may also itch and bleed. Since the straining incident to constipation may cause these engorged veins to prolapse, this condition constitutes one reason for preventing constipation. A pregnant woman who has a daily evacuation is less likely to have hemorrhoids. Hard stools and straining increase the tendency.

For relief of discomfort from hemorrhoids, the first measure often is to push them back gently into the rectum. The mother can usually do this herself, quite satisfactorily, after lubricating her fingers with petroleum jelly or cold cream. Lying down, with the hips elevated on a pillow, and application of an ice bag or cold compresses to the anus will usually give relief. When the condition is severe, the physician may prescribe medicated ointments, lotions, or suppositories. Operation is rarely resorted to during pregnancy because there is marked improvement after delivery. The hemorrhoids are usually worse during the first few days after delivery, but as a rule they disappear a short time after removal of the pressure previously made by the enlarging uterus.

Cramps in the legs, numbness, or tingling may be the result of overstretching of muscles and fascia, or they may be due to circulatory impairment in the muscles due to pressure of the large, heavy uterus on the pelvic veins. Muscular tetany, resulting in leg cramps, is sometimes caused by depression of available serum calcium, due to excess phosphorus in the blood, as explained on page 183. The cramps may be very severe. They are most likely to occur while the woman is at rest.

Relief is usually obtained by standing up. The cramps may also be relieved by extending the cramped leg, flexing the ankle, and forcibly pushing the forefoot upward, with the toes pointing toward the knee (Fig. 14-8, p. 314). If cramps occur during labor, or at any other time when the mother cannot get onto her feet readily, this latter method is one the nurse can employ. Sometimes the mother will be able to feel the cramped muscle and will automatically begin to massage it to relieve the cramping. Application of a hot-water bottle often gives comfort.

As the baby's head descends into the pelvis, the expectant mother may experience *pain in the thighs* and *aching of the perineum.* There is also *increased urinary frequency* due to the pressure on the bladder.

Shortness of breath, due to crowding of the diaphragm, is sometimes very troublesome toward the end of pregnancy. As is apparent, this is due to the upward and not downward pressure of the uterus. It is aggravated by the mother's lying down and relieved by her sitting up, preferably in a straight chair, or by being well propped up on pillows while lying down. In addition, pregnant women appear to be prone to shortness of breath as a result of an increased sensitivity of the respiratory center to the carbon dioxide content of the blood. That is, inspiration will be triggered at a lower PCO_2 level

than when she is not pregnant. (See Chapter 6, page 136.)

Whenever breathlessness seems particularly troublesome, it can be relieved by lying on the back with the arms extended above the head and resting on the bed. Since this position stretches the thoracic cavity to its maximum, even normal breathing will allow for expansion of all available lung tissue, and breathlessness is relieved. When relief has been obtained by remaining in this position for a few minutes, and especially if this is done before sleep at night, it will soon be possible to change to the side position and relax, without experiencing much difficulty in resting. Intercostal breathing may also give some relief.

When the baby sinks in the pelvis, the breathlessness and constant sense of pressure of the uterus under the ribs are relieved. Shortness of breath may be a symptom of cardiac disease, especially if it occurs before the uterus has enlarged enough to cause pressure.

Supine hypotensive syndrome may cause dizziness and a faint feeling during the latter part of pregnancy. The inferior vena cava may be compressed by pressure of the heavy pregnant uterus when the mother lies on her back (Fig. 9-7). Venous return to the heart is then diminished. The effect of pressure on the inferior vena cava may be so severe that the cardiac output is markedly decreased and hypotension becomes serious. An immediate change of position to the left side is important for the mother's and fetus' well-being as well as for the mother's comfort. A mother is likely to recognize that a change of position relieves her faintness. If distress occurs during an examination or a treatment she must be permitted to change position immediately.

Round Ligament Pain

As the uterus grows, the round ligaments are necessarily stretched. This stretching may cause abdominal pain and tenderness. Other causes of abdominal pain should be ruled out whenever a woman presents with this complaint. However, round ligament stretching is probably the most

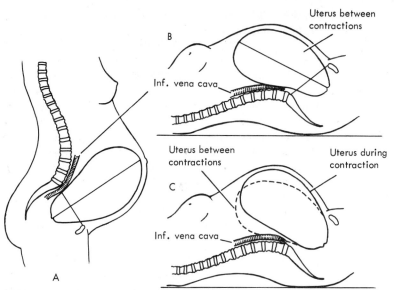

Figure 9-7. Position of the uterus in relation to the pelvis, spine, and inferior vena cava. *A.* Relation of the uterine axis to the axis of the inlet in the erect position. *B.* Changes in these axes when the gravida is supine. Note the compression of the inferior vena cava by the heavy gravid uterus. *C.* Position of the uterus between contractions and during contractions. The coordinated effects of the uterine ligaments pull the uterus anteriorly, thus eliminating compression of the vena cava. [*Reproduced with permission from John J. Bonica,* Principles and Practice of Obstetric Analgesia and Anesthesia, *Vol. 1,* Fundamental Considerations. *F. A. Davis, Philadelphia, Pa., 1967, p. 32.*]

likely explanation. Rest and a change of position will usually provide relief.

Backache

Backache is a common complaint in pregnancy due to the muscular fatigue and strain that accompany poor body balance. Backache and various other discomforts, including varicosities and swelling of the feet and ankles, may be due to faulty body alignment.

During pregnancy the normal amount of lordosis is increased in an effort to balance the body. It becomes severe if the abdominal muscles are relaxed and in poor tone before pregnancy, which allows for marked protrusion of the abdomen as the uterus enlarges. This causes a great increase in the forward tilt of the pelvis and an increased strain at the sacroiliac joints.

With this increased lordosis there is an increase in kyphosis of the dorsal spine and a forward protrusion of the head and neck. This is followed by more stretching and thinning of the abdominal muscles and shortening of the long muscles of the back. Backache is a common result of all of these changes. Since each pregnancy causes further stretching and loss of muscle tone, disturbances are more numerous in women who have borne several children.

A woman who has achieved good body alignment as a young girl will not experience much discomfort from the added strain of pregnancy. If body alignment is not good, every effort must be made to improve the posture, beginning early in pregnancy. Good alignment means that the body does not slump, that there are no marked spinal curvatures, and that the forward tilt of the pelvis is minimal. The feet are not unduly flattened or spread at the forefoot. The uterine enlargement is upward rather than forward. The abdomen does not protrude forward to a marked degree, but rather is full nearest the xiphoid.

Exercises, improvement of posture, and abdominal supports aid in the prevention of backache. Squatting, tailor sitting, and pelvic rock help to relieve discomfort. When stooping or bending is necessary, the bending should take place at the hips and knees while the back is kept straight. Squatting, with the back straight and the feet in broad stance and turned slightly outward, is easier and more comfortable than stooping. This position can be used many times a day, especially when it is necessary to open low drawers, pick articles up from the floor, or care for a child. Picking up a toddler is much easier from a squatting than a stooping position. By squatting the mother not only avoids back strain but actually practices an exercise which prepares her muscles for the position she will assume on the delivery table.

Tailor sitting may relieve backache and can be used during some daily routines such as sewing or talking on the telephone, and also prepares for the delivery position (Fig. 9-8A, B).

Pelvic rocking is another exercise which can be used during the daily routine of work as the woman stands at a sink washing dishes or at a table performing other tasks. Pelvic rocking helps to relieve abdominal pressure and low backache during pregnancy and also low backache during labor. Pelvic rocking can be done while standing (Fig. 9-9A, B), sitting, lying down (Fig. 9-10A, B), or leaning on both knees and both hands (all fours). Some persons believe that doing pelvic rocking on all fours may put too much strain on the back and they do not recommend it. However, a kneeling position may be comfortable when it is necessary to do something at ground level.

Discomfort of backache can also be prevented or relieved by proper arrangement of household appliances. They should be at a working level that makes it possible to keep the arms in a comfortable position and the back straight, with all bending taking place from the hips alone. All working material should be near enough to avoid undue stretching and reaching, and twist-

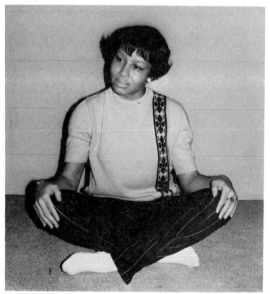

Figure 9-8. **A.** Normal tailor-sitting, which may be used during some daily household routines.

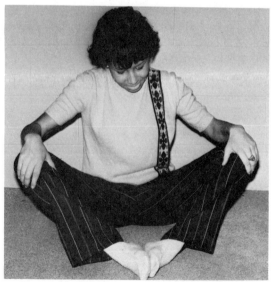

B. The woman is pressing on her knees to stretch the muscles of her thighs. Such pressure will prepare the muscles for the position on the delivery table.

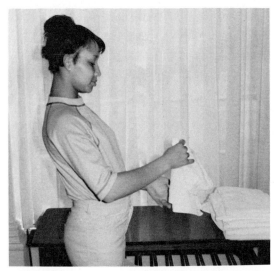

Figure 9-9. **A.** One movement of the pelvic rock is shown while the woman is standing at a table folding linen. Her lower back is arched in as her shoulders are thrown back. This movement rocks the pelvis forward.

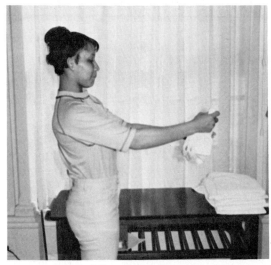

B. Immediately following the forward rock shown in Figure 9-9A, the woman rocks her pelvis backward by reversing her position and standing up straight. Changing her posture back and forth will rock her pelvis by tilting it forward and backward. During pelvic rocking the feet should be kept together, and the feet and shoulders should remain in the same vertical plane.

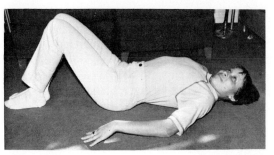

Figure 9-10. **A.** The pelvic rock done in the recumbent position. While lying on her back, with her legs bent, and her feet flat on the floor, the woman tips her pelvis forward by arching her lower back.

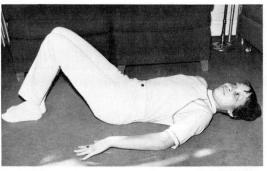

B. Following the movement shown in Figure 9-10A, the woman rocks her pelvis backward by flattening her lower back against the floor. The pelvic rock may be repeated several times at any one time and used several times daily.

ing of the body. Ironing boards and work tables should be raised or lowered as necessary, whenever possible. Blocks can often be used to raise working surfaces. When working areas cannot be lowered, it may be possible to use footstools to raise the worker to a comfortable level. There are many ways in which the home can be arranged to minimize fatigue and strain.

A waddling gait is frequently seen late in pregnancy owing to an instability of the joints. This is the result of relaxation of the sacroiliac joints and the symphysis pubis which normally occurs in pregnancy. Severe backache may accompany this condition, especially if the relaxation is marked and if considerable lumbar lordosis is present.

Fatigue

Many women experience marked fatigue and lassitude early in pregnancy. They require many more hours of sleep during this time than they normally do. This feeling of great fatigue usually disappears by the end of the third month of pregnancy, but tiredness is likely to reappear during the last month.

Insomnia

Insomnia is not uncommon late in pregnancy. It is sometimes difficult for the woman to find a comfortable position in bed because of her large and cumbersome body. Fetal activity is often vigorous and disturbing—a small jabbing fist or foot can be quite uncomfortable. Furthermore, as labor and delivery become more imminent the excitement and anticipation of birth may make it hard to relax and "turn off" her mind for sleeping. Dreams about labor and the baby may be more frequent and are sometimes frightening. The woman may rise in the morning feeling very little more refreshed than when she went to bed.

There are a variety of measures which the woman can try which may promote relaxation and sleep. Some of these are a warm drink or warm bath at bedtime or reading some light material in bed. A backrub with a soothing lotion relieves backache and tired muscles and promotes relaxation. It also serves to satisfy a couple's need for touching and closeness. Relaxation techniques learned in prenatal classes are as beneficial now as during labor and may be used with great success. Lying on the side and using small pillows or rolled towels to support the heavy abdomen and upper leg will usually permit greater muscle relaxation. It is often helpful to concentrate on having every part of the body limp and then to make a conscious effort to have each inspiration and expiration exactly the same length and depth.

Periods of rest and sleep during the day become important during these last weeks of pregnancy in order to compensate for loss of sleep during the night.

Vaginal Discharge

Vaginal discharge is normally greatly increased during the latter months of pregnancy. Ordinarily the moderately profuse yellowish or whitish discharge has no particular significance, although it may be annoying. Douching should be avoided during pregnancy except when specifically ordered by the physician, because the normal vaginal secretions have excellent antiseptic properties. In addition to regular bathing, the vulva may be rinsed with warm water after each voiding to minimize the accumulation of the sticky secretions in the pubic hair. Cotton panties or those lined with a cotton-lined crotch are usually more comfortable because they are more absorbent and permit better circulation of air to the body.

Some patients have an abnormally profuse discharge and may be distressed by persistent itching and burning. Such symptoms may be due to *Trichomonas vaginalis* vaginitis, to a yeast infection, to a gonorrheal infection, or to a nonspecific bacterial infection.

Trichomonas vaginalis, an actively motile, flagellate parasite, may produce a profuse, irritating, foamy secretion, yellowish green in color, and of an unpleasant odor. This discharge is very irritating to the vagina and the external genitalia and causes intense itching. It may cause symptoms anytime, but they frequently flare up during pregnancy. The specific cure for this condition is metronidazole (Flagyl). It rapidly passes through the placenta and enters the fetal circulation. Its effects on fetal development are not definitely known. It is thus contraindicated during the first trimester of pregnancy. Use later is apparently not harmful but may be restricted if possible. The drug is excreted in breast milk. Its effect on the newborn is not known.

Yeast infection, caused by *Candida (Monilia) albicans,* also often flares up during pregnancy because the increased glycogen content of the vaginal epithelium is conducive to its growth. It produces a profuse white, watery, curdy discharge which is very irritating to the vagina and external genitalia. This infection is treated by nystatin (Mycostatin), an antibiotic against fungi. Mycostatin is usually administered in the form of vaginal tablets, but may also be used orally in conjunction with vaginal treatment. Application of 2 percent aqueous solution of methylrosaniline chloride (gentian violet) to the vaginal mucous membrane is occasionally used as treatment.

The presence or absence of symptoms will often determine if treatment is given for vaginal discharge. Sometimes douches seem indicated for excessive vaginal secretion. Douches are prescribed by the physician. Several important precautions are necessary with douching during pregnancy to prevent high fluid pressure and possible entry of air or fluid into the uterus. Hand bulb syringes should never be used. The douche bag should be held no higher than 2 feet above the level of the hips, and the douche nozzle should not be inserted more than 3 in. These are safe precautions in douching at any time, but should be particularly observed during pregnancy.

A *gonorrheal infection* is always treated, regardless of symptoms, both to protect the baby's eyes in its passage through the birth canal and to protect the mother from the infection ascending through the uterine cavity and up to the fallopian tubes after delivery. This infection can successfully be treated with penicillin.

Smears of the vaginal discharge, to be examined for the gonococcus especially and also for the presence of yeast or trichomonas, often are taken routinely at the first or an early prenatal visit. If there is reason to suspect a gonorrheal infection, a culture may be of more diagnostic value, since the organism cannot always be demonstrated on a smear when the infection has reached a chronic stage. If the appearance of the discharge suggests a trichomonas infection, a diagnosis can easily be made by the hanging drop method.

Itching

Itching of the skin is a fairly common discomfort. Several factors contribute to this annoying symptom. The increased excretory function of the skin may result in the elimination of irritating substances by the skin glands. There is also a stretching of the skin due to weight gain, the growing uterus, and fluid which is held in the skin. The breasts, abdomen, and palms of the hands are commonly affected areas, although itching may be generalized to the entire body. Since the discomfort is more difficult to ignore when people and activities are not available for distraction, rest and sleep may be inhibited. It may be hard to relax and fall asleep due to the itching and some women will scratch themselves in their sleep even to the point of causing bleeding.

Bathing in tepid, rather than hot, water and adding sodium bicarbonate (baking soda) to the bath water are soothing measures. Lotions and oils are often helpful and rubbing them on the uncomfortable area is a constructive alternative to scratching. Sometimes changing soaps or reducing the use of soap to a minimum will provide relief. Blotting dry after a bath rather than rubbing with the towel will reduce stimulation of the skin and is less likely to produce itching. Loose, nonrestrictive clothing is more comfortable and not so apt to induce itching.

Some women complain of discomfort caused by the stretching of the skin over the enlarged abdomen, which becomes so tense it feels as though it might break. There is a very old and still current belief that this sensation may be relieved by rubbing the abdomen with an oil or an ointment, and that such oiling will increase the elasticity not only of the superficial layers of the skin but of the deeper layers as well, and by this means striae may be prevented. Since striae are caused by a combination of hormonal "priming" of the connective tissue and the particular genetic make up of the individual, there appears to be no basis in fact for this belief. However, if such oiling increases the woman's physical and/or mental comfort there is no reason why she should not do it.

A study of all the minor discomforts and complications of pregnancy could lead one to believe that this is indeed a disastrous nine months. It is important to bear in mind that for most women pregnancy is a time of joy and physical well-being. The few discomforts any one woman has are amenable to correction or relief with good health care practices. Many of them are preventable. Nursing during this phase of the life cycle can be highly satisfying to the practitoner who directs her management toward health maintenance and health promotion.

PRENATAL CLASSES

The needs of the pregnant woman and her family for information and education can be met in a variety of ways. It has been emphasized that a portion of each antepartum visit should be set aside for consultation between nurse and client. In addition there are many books, films, and television programs available to the pregnant family to answer their questions. Throughout history, perhaps the most common source of childbirth education has been conversations with other women. Another, somewhat more formal means of education, is the prenatal class.

Although it cannot be expected that all couples or all women will be interested in participating in a childbirth education program, prenatal classes are a needed community resource. Such classes are organized under a variety of auspices, depending on the community. They may be sponsored by the public health agency, a voluntary health organization such as the Red Cross, the family life department of a junior college or univeristy, or the local hospital. In some instances, groups of interested individuals or parents have formed organizations for the specific purpose of offering childbirth education programs.

The format of the classes and their content is determined by the philosophy and objectives of the sponsoring group. Some groups concentrate almost entirely on preparation for labor and delivery, while others may include material on the physical changes of pregnancy or infant care. For some courses there is a scheduled series of meetings which a group of people enroll in and the group remains the same throughout the series. Other classes may be ongoing and people move in and out of the group at irregular times. Some classes utilize a lecture presentation and may invite guest speakers for different topics. For example, a nutritionist may discuss diet or a physician may explain obstetric anesthesia. Other classes use a group discussion format, usually directed by a group facilitator. Instead of having clearly defined content, the interests of the group members may determine what is covered during the class. Often a portion of the class is set aside for demonstration and practice of breathing and relaxation techniques.

Ideally, the teacher would identify the particular interests and learning needs of the group and adapt the class to meet these needs. Unfortunately this is not always practical. In larger communities this may be solved in part by having several different kinds of classes with differing philosophies available from which couples can choose.

Regardless of the underlying philosophy or emphasis of the prenatal classes, all have as their overall objectives to dispel errors and myths about pregnancy and childbearing; to replace those errors with accurate information; and to teach some physical and/or mental skills which will improve their ability to cope with labor and delivery and, sometimes, with early parenting. To meet these objectives content is usually presented in the following areas:

1. Physical changes of pregnancy
2. Emotional changes of pregnancy
3. Nutrition
4. Breathing and relaxation exercises
5. Mechanisms of labor and delivery
6. Early baby care

A visit to the hospital is frequently arranged to acquaint couples with the maternity unit. This tour is usually conducted by a member of the perinatal nursing staff who can explain hospital procedures and answer questions about policies and customs. Options which the couple may wish to consider should be discussed if any are available. For example, the woman may be able to choose to labor and deliver in the same room, to have or not have fetal monitoring in the absence of any risk indicators, or to choose early discharge within 8 to 24 hours after delivery. Such discussion should not replace consultation with the woman's physician, but it does provide valuable information at a time and location where the rooms and monitors can be seen and some of their mystique dispelled.

A growing trend in prenatal education is the inclusion of an increasing amount of information relative to parenting. Some groups are extending their classes into the postpartum period or are forming new groups of young parents to help them deal with the issues of child rearing.

In large families older children learn child care by practicing on their youngest siblings and the younger children practice on their nieces and nephews as their older siblings begin their own families. In the modern, smaller family such opportunities do not exist as often. When young couples become parents their own mothers and other older women relatives are quite likely to be employed and unavailable to help with baby care and to act as role models. In addition, couples today tend to form isolated nuclear families which may be quite distant from the extended family, geographically as well as psychologically. Thus, the support structure, as well as the sanctions of the kinship group are often missing. It is in an attempt to fill this gap that postpartum parent groups are being formed. The school system, too, in response to this need is increasing the sophistication and usefulness of the family life education courses being offered to young people.

The timing of classes during pregnancy depends to some extent on the length of the series of classes and their availability in the community as well as the couples' own schedule. Generally speaking, these classes should be arranged toward the end of the second trimester, which will permit completion by the thirty-sixth week of gestation. By this time the fetus is quite active, the woman looks pregnant, and is feeling well. She has adapted to her pregnancy and is now ready to consider preparation for the reality of labor and delivery and an infant. Whenever possible the father should participate in the classes. He will gain needed information first hand and obtain the support necessary to facilitate the assumption of his new role. Some classes have one session for men only, so there is an opportunity to share feelings, doubts, and concerns without "feeling dumb" in front of the women.

RELAXATION TECHNIQUES, POSITIONS, AND EXERCISES

Physical preparation of the mother for childbirth, through instruction in relaxation techniques, rest positions, and exercises, is one of the objectives of parents' classes. This preparation is designed to help the pregnant woman minimize stress by improving her posture, developing an ability to relax and improve rest, practicing specific exercises for neuromuscular control and breathing response during labor, and learning methods useful in postpartum restoration of the body. Fathers are taught how to assist the woman with antepartum conditioning, with the practice of exercises, and about the

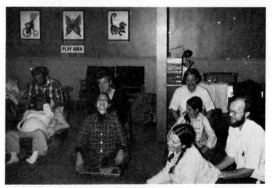

Figure 9-11. A group of expectant parents practicing relaxation and breathing exercises in preparation for labor and delivery.

techniques of coaching these exercises during labor. Since men, as well as women, are subject to stress and physical tension, it is to be supposed that the relaxation responses would be equally beneficial to them. (See Figure 9-11.)

The notion of deliberate physical conditioning for childbirth is a phenomenon of a technologic civilization where muscular activity is largely foreign to more sedentary occupations and birth is removed from the everyday experience.

The late Dr. Grantly Dick Read, a London obstetrician, originated the idea that pain during labor was caused by fear. He published his first book on the influence of fear on the course of labor in 1933 under the title *Natural Childbirth*. According to Dr. Read, women can be prepared for a natural physiologic labor unaccompanied by fear and tenseness when they learn to regard childbirth as a natural process. With education and preparation the patient knows what to expect because she has learned the physiology of pregnancy, labor, and delivery, and she understands how to assist herself during the various phases of labor. By natural childbirth Dr. Read meant labor and delivery uninhibited by physical, chemical, or psychologic factors and a labor that was not accompanied by great discomfort.

Dr. Read contended that to achieve natural childbirth the fear–tension–pain syndrome must be broken. This triad has considerable influence on the course of labor. Tension increases with fear, and tension may cause muscle spasms and increase pain. Tension not only interferes with cervical dilation, but also causes involuntary spasm of abdominal and back muscles, resulting in pain. With an understanding of labor and of the means of relaxation during labor, fear and apprehension are reduced, tension is lessened, and pain is decreased.

The Read method is sometimes called the psychophysical method of preparation. In this method, the mother is taught how to release muscle tension and how to relax all her muscles completely at her will. Slow abdominal breathing is practiced for use during contractions of much of the first stage of labor and is helpful in precluding painful spasms of the abdominal

muscles. Rapid chest breathing is learned for use toward the end of labor if abdominal breathing becomes difficult at that time. The mother is encouraged to practice complete relaxation and abdominal breathing daily to achieve an increasingly greater ability to do so and to become so adept that it can be done at will and under stress.

As the Read method of preparation for childbirth was becoming established, another method was devised, known as the psychoprophylactic or Lamaze method. Its author, Dr. Fernand Lamaze accepted Dr. Read's theory that women often have been negatively conditioned to expect pain in childbirth; therefore, education to expunge previous negative impressions of childbirth is an important part of the program. Its major difference is in the method of preparation for labor. Lamaze joined Read's theory to the Russian psychoprophylactic system, based on Pavlovian neurodynamics, using conditioned responses to uterine contractions.

The positive conditioning of the Lamaze method is accomplished through training in chest-breathing and relaxation techniques, which will become a specific response to uterine contractions, i.e., a conditioned reflex which prevents or diminishes the painful sensations arising from the contracting uterus. In this intensive training program the woman, who must be strongly motivated, is taught several specific levels of chest breathing, and she must learn with which kind of respiratory response, or level of chest breathing, she should react to the different phases of labor. Lamaze's chest-breathing method, as compared to Read's abdominal breathing, is considered easier and more comfortable throughout labor. The various levels of breathing and their use are described in detail on pages 309–12 and in Figure 14-4, page 310.

Expectant parents are taught that preparation-for-childbirth exercises are not designed to produce a painless childbirth, but rather to help them participate actively in the delivery of their baby. Preparation does not preclude use of analgesia, but it often reduces the amount necessary. Some women will not require medication.

They are told that pain-relieving medication is available when it is indicated or desired. They are also taught that obstetric intervention, such as forceps delivery, may become necessary for delivery, and that the physician will make this decision according to the best interest of mother and baby.

Essentially each preparation-for-childbirth program stems from the Read or the Lamaze method, although there are variations in technique. However, all programs make the effort to erase previous negative impressions of pregnancy, labor, and delivery and plan to recondition the couple toward acceptance of a healthy positive attitude. Physical exercises to improve the woman's general well-being are usually included. Instruction in respiratory and relaxation techniques are designed to help the woman reduce her perception of pain arising from the uterine contractions and to participate actively in her labor and delivery.

MATERNAL DEVELOPMENT DURING PREGNANCY

Pregnancy is a developmental event. This is self-evident from the point of view of the fetus. The entire gestational period is uniquely designed for the most dramatic and concentrated period of growth and development in human life. But for the pregnant woman, the mother, it is also a developmental and maturational period. It has already been seen that physiologically the changes are enormous. Virtually every organ and system undergoes substantial growth and development as well as functional modifications. In addition, it is a time of identity reformulation and reordering of interpersonal relationships. As her body changes in contour and appearance she asks herself, "Who am I?" The woman becoming a mother necessitates the man becoming a father, their parents becoming grandparents.

Crisis theory categorizes life changes or challenges according to whether they are developmental or situational. Developmental crises may be thought of as normative events, those which are expected and/or inevitable, such as parent-

hood, departure of children from the parental home, physical decline, and death. Situational or nonnormative crises are categorized as unexpected events, such as mental retardation, illness, alcoholism, and divorce. An event qualifies as a crisis when it creates a situation for which the usual behavior patterns or coping patterns of a person or family are inadequate.

Although pregnancy is a biologically normal event, it is an exceptional one in the life of a woman and her family and, as such, requires a shift in the organization of values and roles. These characteristics have led several authors to describe pregnancy within the framework of crisis theory as a maturational or developmental crisis. This crisis acts as an impetus to a lengthy period of adaptation and reorganization, often necessitating the development of new coping mechanisms, acquisition of new knowledge and skills, and modification of interpersonal relationships.

How each woman works through the crisis of pregnancy will be largely determined by her own style as well as the culture in which she lives. There is, however, an increasing belief in the theory that her "work" can be described by certain developmental tasks common across cultures. Deutsch, Bibring, Caplan, Tanner, and Rubin have described various tasks or goals to be achieved by the woman during the nine months of her pregnancy. These tasks are briefly summarized as follows:

1. Acceptance of pregnancy as a symbiosis with the fetus and then moving toward acceptance of the infant as an individual distinct from herself in preparation for the physical separation of delivery.
2. Ensuring acceptance of the child she bears by her significant others (Rubin, 1975).
3. Seeking safe passage for herself and her child through pregnancy, labor, and delivery (Rubin, 1975).
4. Adoption of the mother role.

Erik Erikson and other developmental theorists have postulated that each life stage has certain tasks which can be most efficiently accomplished given the age, social and psychologic development, and other parameters of that stage. They have suggested further that failure to master the developmental tasks of any given stage interferes with the ability to meet successfully the challenges of the stage to follow. In colloquial terms this can be stated as "you must crawl before you can walk."

The tasks of pregnancy can be regarded as a special case of Erikson's developmental stage theory. These tasks are the particular way in which a woman works out the stage of Generativity vs. Stagnation during that very circumscribed time defined by the conception and delivery of an infant. She works at the tasks simultaneously, weaving them all tapestry-fashion throughout gestation. One or the other of the tasks may assume dominance for an individual woman, and, for all women, there appears to be a shifting dominance of tasks from trimester to trimester as pregnancy progresses. The woman must achieve some resolution of each task for each of her pregnancies.

Trimester I

If a single word could be chosen to characterize the first trimester of pregnancy it would be ambivalence. Regardless of how planned and how desired the pregnancy, the awareness of the fact that conception has indeed occurred causes the expectant mother to doubt the wisdom of her choice. Another time—any other time—might have been better. She realizes a certain loss of control over her body and, indeed, her whole destiny. If the option of abortion is set aside, the woman finds herself embarked upon a course from which there is no escape except through the trial of labor and birth. Following that she is a mother forever. Added to that is her feeling of physical ambivalence. Her symptoms are primarily of absence of menstruation rather than the presence or addition of anything. She is tired, she may be nauseated. She is not ill but she doesn't feel well, either.

During this first trimester the woman seeks confirmation of her pregnancy and reassurance that she can bear a child. She wants—and needs—an expert opinion that what she believes is true, that she is healthy and that the pregnancy is "good." This is the goal of the first antepartum visit to the physician.

In addition to accepting herself as pregnant, the woman must ensure acceptance of her pregnancy by those who are important to her. This appears to be the most crucial of the tasks, since its successful accomplishment secures the support necessary for the woman as she becomes a mother. It seems to give her the energy for her other tasks, yet it differs from the other tasks in that it is bound to social interaction, whereas most of the remaining tasks are internal.

The family adjusts to the notion of pregnancy by asking if this is a suitable state for my wife? my daughter? my mother? The husband sees his lover becoming a mother and all the memories of Mother are evoked. He realizes that if she is a mother he must be a father and his role readjustment begins. The child is acutely aware of the sexual implications of pregnancy for the mother he has heretofore considered asexual. The grandparents-to-be relive their own pregnancies and are struck with the implications of mortality/immortality inherent in another generation. As pregnancy progresses all of these bonds within the family will have to be reordered to admit a new member.

By around 16 weeks of gestation most women have resolved the ambivalence of rejecting/accepting and have incorporated the idea of self-as-pregnant-woman. This psychologic acceptance of pregnancy is analogous to physical implantation. If the blastocyst does not attach firmly to the uterine wall, development stops and the pregnancy is aborted. Similarly, if the pregnancy is not psychologically accepted, the development of attachment to the child stagnates and the mother–child relationship may be aborted.

Trimester II

As the second trimester begins, the physical changes which are occurring hasten the resolution of ambivalence. The woman has increasing energy, her nausea is gone, she begins to acquire a pregnant figure. She feels good and has a sense of well-being. Then quickening occurs. This event makes the woman acutely conscious of a presence within. She says she has felt Life. At first she regards the infant as part of herself. Gradually, throughout the rest of gestation, the infant becomes a reality that is within her but is not her. She must achieve this attitude in order to bear the idea of birth, physical separation. This shift in attitude is achieved in interaction with the fetus and in a rich fantasy life. She pokes her tummy to get the infant to poke back. She places her husband's hand on her belly so he, too, can feel. She describes the infant as sleeping or active. She attributes intention to him. "He just kicks at bedtime to keep me awake." She dreams and daydreams how he will be: boy or girl, blue eyes or brown, curly hair or bald, and, most of all, normal or abnormal.

As she begins increasingly to regard the infant as a reality apart from herself the pregnant woman begins to consider her role as a mother. She must sort out for herself what being a mother means and what the cost/benefit balance is for her. This is closely wrapped up with the idea of self-identity—Who am I? The pregnant woman is assisted in her ability to rework old problems and come up with better solutions and a clearer identity by the characteristic shift in personality equilibrium which occurs as a phenomenon of pregnancy. This is most evident to the observer in the extraordinary openness and talkativeness of pregnant women. Thus it appears pregnancy offers women a unique and valuable maturational opportunity.

Exploration of what motherhood is all about is accomplished primarily through the woman's relationship with her own mother. It is not unusual to find an increase in frequency of visits, letters, and telephone calls between a mother and her pregnant daughter. For women who have not had a close relationship with their mothers there is often an attempt at reconciliation.

Because of the intense work of accepting the infant and adapting to her role change, the pregnant woman has a characteristic introversion and passivity. This change begins with the second trimester and gradually increases until around the seventh or eighth month (30–35 weeks). Her most essential reality is within. All her relationships and interests become reordered. Only those relationships and interests which are essential to her in this situation of being pregnant are compatible with her inner world.

The woman, as well as her family, is often confused by this change from her former outgoing, giving self. She is now often preoccupied and wishes to be given to rather than to give. She is increasingly dependent and looks for much love and attention, gifts of time and self to her. Fathers feel shut out from a world they cannot fully share or even understand. As with all creative work, every energy is directed inward as the woman struggles to make both a baby and a mother.

Pregnant women are notorious for their emotional lability. Partly from preoccupation, partly from hormonal changes, and partly from realization of the impact of pregnancy the woman becomes increasingly sensitive and irritable. She is equally likely to laugh uproariously at something which no one else regards as funny and to burst into tears without knowing why.

During the second trimester the pregnant woman develops an interest in learning about herself and her baby. This is the time most women seek out prenatal classes, read books, and talk with other pregnant women. She is definitely pregnant but not yet close enough to labor for it to be an imminent threat, so it is a "safe" time to gather all the information that she can. When labor does become imminent she will be armed with knowledge and skills to master it safely.

Trimester III

During the last weeks of pregnancy the expectant mother hastens to complete all the tasks. Physically she is now great and clumsy; she tires more easily, has difficulty adjusting to

Table 9-2. Summary of the Antepartum Period*

Weeks Gestation	Physical Signs and Symptoms	Characteristic Behaviors	Maternal Tasks—In Order of Usual Dominance	Suggested Interventions
0–16	Amenorrhea Fatigue Nausea; vomiting Breast tenderness and growth Frequent urination	Ambivalence Seeks medical supervision and confirmation of pregnancy Tells selected close persons re pregnancy Mood swings from depression →euphoria	Acceptance of pregnancy Seeks acceptance of pregnancy by significant others Seeks safe passage—first for herself, then for her infant	Confirm pregnancy History and physical exam—risk assessment Diet history and instruction Help to talk out and resolve ambivalence Anticipatory guidance/teaching (include family) related to —drugs —radiation —embryology —individual signs and symptoms —reportable signs of possible complications —normality of her mood swings
16–30	Quickening "Pregnant figure" ↑Energy Feeling of well-being Round ligament pain	Wears maternity clothes Tells the world Interested in learning about birth and babies—reads books, seeks out and questions friends and family, attends classes ↑Talkativeness ↑Dependency as time goes on Begins examining relationship with own mother	Acceptance of infant Seeks acceptance of infant by significant others Adoption of mother role Seeks safe passage but in more abstract, general way than in other trimesters	On-going assessment of maternal/fetal status —FHR —fundal height —urine tests —B/P —nutrition Give to woman—time, knowledge, pamphlets, etc. Anticipatory guidance/teaching (include family) related to —libido changes —mood swings —dependency —introversion —reportable signs of possible complications

30–40	Dependent edema	↑Introversion	Safe passage for self and infant through labor and delivery	Continue physical assessment at more frequent intervals
	Pressure in lower abdomen	↑Dependency (craves attention and tenderness)	Ensuring acceptance of infant by significant others	Reassure—give ego support for attractiveness and self-worth
	Frequent urination	May ↓ interest in genital sex	Acceptance of infant as individual apart from herself	Anticipatory guidance/teaching (include family) related to
	Round ligament pain	Intensifies study of labor and delivery	Adoption of the mother role	—signs and symptoms of labor
	Backache	↑Vulnerability		—environmental modification for coming infant and to provide rest for mother
	Insomnia	Prepares nursery—buys baby things		—fulfilling maternal dependency needs
	Clumsiness	Decides on feeding method		—early infancy, especially developing parent/child attachment (help them verbalize mental picture of baby and concepts of selves as parents)
	Fatigue			

*It is well to remember that women and pregnancies differ, and, while an outline may serve as a useful overview and guide, the nurse should assess each client individually. Health care during pregnancy should be a cooperative endeavor between the clients and the professionals with the client taking an active role in planning and decision making.

her new body boundaries, and is uncomfortable. She begins to be tired of pregnancy but is still hesitant about delivery. The fluttering of her infant within has become vigorous intrusive kicks. She has an increasing sense of vulnerability, exhibited by preoccupation with locks on the door, cautioning others to drive carefully, and avoiding running, bumping children. The physical discomforts and increasing burden of the pregnancy serve to instill a psychologic readiness for labor and delivery in spite of the threats.

As evidence that she has accepted the infant as separate from herself, she makes decisions about his care, how she will feed him, what his name will be. Acceptance of the infant by others in the family assumes crucial importance. There must be a place for him when he comes—a physical niche in the house and, more importantly, an emotional niche in the hearts of his family. Rejection of the child now is a rejection of the woman herself. She must have approval of the product she is preparing. To promote this she spends much time with her children describing how it will be to have a baby in the family. She urges participation of her husband in name selection, nursery furnishings, and preparation for and participation in the labor and delivery itself.

As desperately as the woman wants her husband to want the baby, he wants the wife back he feels he has lost to the child. If they love each other enough and are open to sharing and communication of feelings, both will get their wishes and the child will come into a richer home.

The end of pregnancy comes at last. The woman has moved through 40 weeks of growing into motherhood. Through an intricate intertwining of physical changes and psychologic work she has accepted first the pregnant state and then the fact of a child. She has sought help to assure her own health and the intactness of her child and has prepared herself and her loved ones to accept a new family member. Finally she returns full circle to the ambivalence of the first trimester. She hates the pregnancy, wants the child, but fears birth. Her behavior in labor will appear as a telescoping of the emotions and behaviors of the entire pregnancy. It is as if she makes an intense summary of the whole process of baby-making so that she is ready to begin the next step in mothering. If the work has gone well, particularly if she has established a secure support system for herself and her child, she is most likely to have continued success as a woman and as a parent.

Implications for Therapeutic Intervention With Families

The implications of this framework of emotional change and maternal tasks for therapeutic intervention with families during childbearing are considerable. Three suggested applications will be discussed briefly here as illustrations.

1. *As an organizing framework for antepartum teaching.*

The concept of maternal tasks could effectively serve as a guide for organizing classes for expectant parents. Not only content but also timing and methodology are suggested. For example, infant care activities and how-to's might well be appropriate for the third trimester when the woman is beginning to perceive the infant as an individual separate from herself. The same content is likely to be met with indifference earlier in pregnancy because it is not synchronous with the woman's own agenda at that time. In contrast, information about her own body and how it works would be more suitably approached early in gestation when her concerns for "safe passage" are principally self-centered.

2. *Anticipatory guidance in self-understanding.*

Knowing that pregnancy is commonly greeted with marked ambivalence under the best of circumstances can do much to reduce the guilt of a woman who finds herself with these feelings. Similarly, if she can be helped to recognize and understand in herself the increasing dependency, mood swings, and other emotions as features of pregnancy that are as normal as increasing uterine size, then she will find her feelings less confusing and disturbing. An interesting observation is the conflicting effect of these emotions of pregnancy and the current feminist movement. Young women who think of themselves as independent, assertive, and "liberated," find the feelings of pregnancy incongruent with their self-image and may well need help to resolve this dissonance.

3. *Anticipatory guidance for significant others.*

Persons who live with pregnant women often describe them as "different people" than when they are not pregnant. A man may be confused and/or threatened by his wife's changing sexual response, for example. If he is clued to expect that her sense of vulnerability and introversion as well as her physical contours may cause a loss of interest in conventional sexual expression, a potential area of conflict may be avoided. At the same time the couple may be helped to explore alternate methods of expressing love and affection and the woman's increased need for tenderness and attention can be pointed out. The pregnant woman's alarming tendency to cry for "no reason" and to laugh at jokes which are not funny can cause consternation for both partners, especially if their relationship was not securely developed prior to conception. Understanding that such mood swings and inappropriate affect stem from the intensive psychologic work can help them cope together enjoyably with "crazy pregnant women."

Table 9-2 summarizes the physical findings, frequent behaviors, and maternal tasks by trimester. Suggested nursing interventions are indicated as a guide. It must always be remembered that each woman, each family, and each pregnancy is unique.

BIBLIOGRAPHY

Adams, Bert N., *The Family: A Sociological Interpretation.* Rand McNally, Chicago, Ill., 1975.

Aguilera, Donna C., Messick, Janice M., and Farrell, Marlene S., *Crisis Intervention.* Mosby, St. Louis, Mo., 1970.

American Journal of Nursing: Programmed Instruction, Correcting common erros in blood pressure measurement, 65:133–166, 1965.

Benedek, Therese, The psychology of pregnancy, in *Parenthood, Its Psychology and Psychopathology,* edited by E. James Anthony and Therese Benedek. Little, Brown, Boston, Mass., 1970.

Benton, Barbara D. A., Stilbestrol and vaginal cancer, *Am. J. Nurs.* 74:900–901 (May) 1974.

Bibring, Grete, A study of the psychological process in pregnancy and of the earliest mother–child relationship, *Psychoanalytic Study of the Child,* Vol. XVI, 1961.

———, Some considerations of the psychological processes in pregnancy, *Psychoanalytic Study of the Child,* Vol. XIV, 1959.

Burch, George E., and DePasquale, Nicholas P., *Primer of Clinical Measurement of Blood Pressure.* Mosby, St. Louis, Mo., 1962.

Caplan, Gerald, *An Approach to Community Mental Health.* Grune and Stratton, New York, 1961.

Clark, Ann (ed.), *Maturational Crisis of Childbearing.* University of Hawaii Press, Honolulu, 1971.

Coleman, Arthur, and Coleman, Libby, Pregnancy as an Altered State of Consciousness, *Birth Family J.* 1:7–11 (Winter) 1973–74.

David, Miriam L., and Doyle, Elaine, First trimester pregnancy, *Am. J. Nurs.* 76:1945–1948 (Dec.) 1976.

Derthick, Nancy, Sexuality in pregnancy and the puerperium, *Birth Family J.* 1:5–9 (Fall) 1974.

Deutsch, Helene, *The Psychology of Women: Motherhood.* Bantam Books, New York, 1973.

Doust, Bruce D., Role of ultrasound in obstetrics and gynecology, *Hosp. Pract.* 9:143–153 (Oct.) 1973.

Erikson, Erik, The eight stages of man, in *Childhood and Society,* by Eric Erikson. Basic Books, New York, 1956.

Erickson, Margarita, Catz, Charlotte S., and Yaffe, Sumner J., Drugs and pregnancy, *Clin. Obstet. Gynecol.* 16:199–224 (Mar.) 1973.

Farber, Bernard, Crisis and the revision of commitments, in *Family: Organization and Interaction,* edited by Bernard Farber. Chandler Publishing Co., San Francisco, Calif. 1964.

Farris, Lorene Sanders, Approaches to caring for the American Indian maternity patient, *MCN,* 1:82–87 (Mar.–Apr.) 1976.

Forfar, John O., Drugs that cause birth defects, *Contemp. Ob/Gyn* 4:61–65 (July) 1974.

Green, Marvin, Alston, Frances K., and Rich, Herbert, Prenatal exposure to narcotics—What is the risk of long-term damage to the central nervous system? *Pediatr. Ann.* 4:78–87 (July) 1975.

Greenhill, J. P., and Friedman, Emanuel A., *Biological Principles and Modern Practice of Obstetrics.* Saunders, Philadelphia, Pa., 1974.

Goldman, Allen S., Influence of hormones on sex differentiation, *Contemp. Ob/Gyn* 3:69–80 (Jan.) 1974.

Goodlin, Robert C., Can sex in pregnancy harm the fetus? *Contemp. Ob/Gyn,* 8:21–26, 1976.

Hawkins, Margherita Modica, Fitting a prenatal education program into the crowded inner city clinic, *MCN* 1:226–230 (Jul./Aug.) 1976.

Heardman, Helen, *Relaxation and Exercise for Natural Childbirth,* 3rd ed., revised and reedited by Maria Ebner. Livingstone, Edinburgh and London, 1966.

Hill, Reubin, An integrated approach to the study of families, in *Crisis Intervention: Selected Readings,* edited by Howard J. Parad. Family Service Association of America, New York, 1965.

Hanson, James W. *et al.,* Fetal alcohol syndrome, *JAMA* 235:1458–1460 (Apr. 5) 1976.

Hobbs, Daniel F., Jr., and Cole, Sue Peck, Transition to parenthood: A decade replication, *J. Marriage Family* 38:723–732 (Nov.) 1976.

Horsley, Stephan, Psychological management of the pre-natal period, in *Modern Pespectives in Psycho-Obstetrics,* edited by John G. Howells. Brunner/Mazel, New York, 1972.

Holt, Jacqueline Rose, The crisis of expectant fatherhood, *Am. J. Nurs.* 76:1436–1439 (Sept.) 1976.

Hytten, Frank E., and Leitch, Isabella, *The Physiology of Human Pregnancy,* 2nd ed. Blackwell Scientific Publications, Oxford, 1972.

Jessner, Lucia, Weigert, Edith, and Foy, James L., Development of parental attitudes during pregnancy, in *Parenthood, Its Psychology and Psychopathology,* edited by E. James Anthony and Therese Benedek. Little, Brown, Boston, Mass., 1970.

Karmel, Marjorie, *Thank You, Dr. Lamaze.* Lippincott, Philadelphia, Pa., 1959.

Lancour, Jane, How to avoid pitfalls in measuring blood pressure, *Am. J. Nurs.* 76:773–775 (May) 1976.

LeMasters, E. E., Parenthood as a crisis, in *Crisis Intervention: Selected Readings,* edited by Howard J. Parad. Family Service Association of America, New York, 1970.

Luke, Barbara, Maternal alcoholism and fetal alcohol syndrome, *Am. J. Nurs.,* 77:1924–1926 (Dec.) 1977.

MacGillivray, I., Rose, G. A., and Rowe, B., Blood pressure survey in pregnancy, *Clin. Sci.* 37:395–407, 1969.

Meister, Susan Blanch, Charting a family's developmental status—For intervention and for the record, *MCN,* 2:43–48 (Jan./Feb.) 1977.

Mirkin, Bernard L., Effects of drugs on the fetus and neonate, *Postgrad. Med.* 47:91–95 (Jan.) 1970.

Mulvihill, John J. *et al.,* Fetal alcohol syndrome: Seven new cases, *Am. J. Obstet. Gynecol.* 125:937–941 (Aug. 1) 1976.

Nabatoff, Robert A., and Pincus, Joseph A., Management of varicose veins during pregnancy, *Obstet. Gynecol.* 36:928–934 (Dec.) 1970.

Nishimura, Hideo, and Janimura, Takaski, *Clinical Aspects of the Teratogenicity of Drugs.* American Elsevier, New York, 1976.

Pillari, Vincent T., Special problems and management of the pregnant drug addict, *Pediatr. Ann.* 4:11–21 (July) 1975.

Read, Grantly Dick, *Childbirth Without Fear,* 2nd rev. ed. Dell, New York, 1959.

Reid, Duncan E., Ryan, Kenneth J., and Benirschke, Kurt, *Principles and Management of Human Reproduction,* Saunders, Philadelphia, Pa., 1972.

Ringquist, Mary Ann, Psychologic stress in the last 3 months of pregnancy" in *Current Practice in Obstetric and Gynecologic Nursing,* edited by Leota K. McNall and Janet T. Galeener. Mosby, St. Louis, Mo., 1976.

Rubin, Reva, Maternal tasks in pregnancy, *Matern. Child Nurs. J.* 4:143–153, 1975.

Sameroff, Arnold, Psychological needs of the mother in early mother–infant interactions, in *Neonatology,* edited by Gordon B. Avery. Lippincott, Philadelphia, Pa., 1975.

Sandstrom, B., Adjustments of the circulation to orthostatic reaction and physical exercise during the first trimester of pregnancy, *Acta Obstet. Gynecol. Scand.* 53:1, 1974.

Shapiro, Samuel *et al.,* Perinatal mortality and birth weight in relation to aspirin taken during pregnancy, *Lancet* 7974:1375–1376 (June 26) 1976.

Slone, Dennis *et al.*, Aspirin and congenital malformations, *Lancet* 7974:1373–1375 (June 26) 1976.

Streissguth, Ann Pytkowicz, Maternal drinking and the outcome of pregnancy: Implications for child mental health, *Am. J. Orthopsychiatry*, 47:422–431 (July) 1977.

Sumner, Georgina, Giving expectant parents the help they need: The ABC of prenatal education, *MCN*, 1:220–225 (Jul./Aug.) 1976.

Tanner, Leonide M., Developmental tasks of pregnancy, in *Current Concepts in Clinical Nursing*, Vol. 2, edited by Betty S. Bergersen *et al.* Mosby, St. Louis, Mo., 1969, pp. 292–297.

Vellay, Pierre *et al.*, *Childbirth Without Pain*, translated from the French by Denise Lloyd. Dutton, New York, 1959.

Zalor, Marianne K., Sexual counseling for pregnant couples, *MCN*, 1:176–181 (May–June) 1976.

Part Three

Intrapartum Care

10

Obstetric Anatomy of Mother and Baby— The Passage and the Passenger

The mechanical factors concerned with the birth process are often referred to as the "powers, passenger, and passage." The "powers" which force the baby through the birth canal are supplied by contractions of the uterine muscle and the muscles of the abdomen; the "passenger" is the baby who must travel through the "passage," the mother's pelvis. In order to anticipate whether or not the passage (pelvis) can be expected to accommodate the passenger (baby), the physician obtains as much information as possible about their relationship before the onset of labor. Such information forms a basis for prognosis concerning the ease or difficulty with which the approaching delivery is likely to be accomplished. The passage and the passenger are described below; the powers and the movement of the passenger through the passage are described in Chapter 12.

THE MOTHER'S PELVIS

The pelvic canal (birth canal) is the passage through which the baby moves during birth; its size and shape are therefore very important factors in the mechanism of labor. Slight disproportion between the size of the baby's head and the size of the pelvis may delay the progress of delivery; greater disproportion may make birth through the pelvis very difficult or impossible. Knowledge of the structure and size of the mother's pelvis is important to an understanding of the mechanism by which the baby passes through the birth canal.

Anatomy of the Pelvis

Four bones enter into the construction of the pelvis: the two hipbones, or innominate bones, which form the sides and the front, and the sacrum and the coccyx, which complete it in back. These bones come into close contact at four joints and are firmly held together by ligaments. The four places of articulation are the symphysis pubis, the two sacroiliac joints, and the sacrococcygeal joint (Fig. 10-1).

The *hipbones* (*innominate bones*), symmetrically placed on each side, are broad, flaring, and scoop-shaped. Each hipbone consists of three main parts: the ilium, ischium, and pubis. Although these parts are firmly welded together in the adult, they are usually described separately.

The *ilium* is the broad, fanlike, upper part of the hipbone. The upper anterior prominence of this bone, which may be felt as the foremost angle of the hipbone, is the *anterior superior iliac spine*, and the margin that extends backward from this point is termed the *iliac crest* (Fig. 10-1). The anterior superior iliac spines and the iliac crests have sometimes been used in making measurements of the pelvis.

The *ischium* is the heavy bone below the ilium which forms the lower part of the hipbone. Its lower end terminates posteriorly in a rough protuberance. It is on these lower projections, known as the *ischial tuberosities* (Fig. 10-1), that the body rests when in a sitting position. The ischial tuberosities serve as landmarks in making pelvic measurements. A sharp process, known as the *ischial spine*, arises from the posterior border of the ischium and juts into the pelvic cavity (Fig. 10-1). The ischial spines are important in obstetrics because the distance between the spines is the shortest diameter of the pelvic cavity. The spines can be palpated during a vaginal or rectal examination and are used as landmarks to determine the descent of the baby's head into the birth canal.

The *pubis* is the part of the hipbone that forms the front of the pelvis. The two pubic bones are united in the median line by heavy cartilage and ligaments to form a joint that is called the *symphysis pubis* (Fig. 10-1). The descending rami of the pubic bones form a rounded arch under which the baby's head passes as it emerges from the birth canal (Fig. 10-1).

The sacrum and coccyx, which form the back of the pelvic girdle, are the terminal parts of the vertebral column. The *sacrum* is a wedge-shaped bone formed by the fusion of five vertebrae, which become progressively smaller in size from above downward. The upper anterior portion of the body of the first sacral vertebra projects forward toward the pelvic cavity. This projection, known as the *promontory of the sacrum*, can be felt on vaginal examination and serves as an important landmark in making pelvic measurements (Fig. 10-1). The inner surface of the sacrum is relatively smooth and has both a vertical and a lateral concavity. The sacrum is joined at each side to the hipbones by means of cartilage and strong ligaments. These areas of articulation are called the *sacroiliac joints* (Fig. 10-1). The coccyx, which also has a triangular shape, makes up the terminal part of the vertebral column. It extends downward and forward from the lower margin of the sacrum to which it is joined by an intervertebral disk or by partial or complete fusion with the last sacral

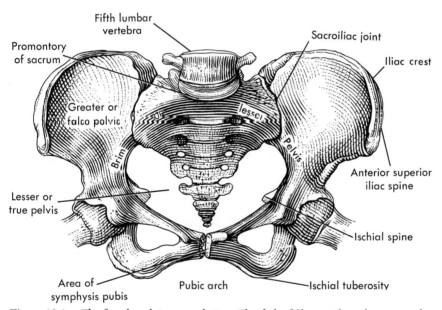

Figure 10-1. The female pelvis, ventral view. The disk of fibrocartilage that unites the pubic bones is not shown in order that the end of the coccyx may be seen. [*Modified from D. Kimber, C. Gray, C. Stackpole, and L. Leavell,* Anatomy and Physiology, *14th ed. Macmillan Publishing Co., Inc., New York, 1961.*]

vertebra. This articulation, known as the *sacro-coccygeal joint*, usually permits backward movement of the coccyx during passage of the baby through the birth canal, but the coccyx may be immovable because of partial or complete fusion of the bones at the joint.

Although the pelvis is a rigid, bony structure, there is slight movement at the places where the bones articulate. Movement is somewhat increased during pregnancy owing to relaxation and softening of the ligaments and cartilages. Such changes permit a limited amount of motion in these joints. An ovarian hormone, termed *relaxin*, promotes this relaxation.

Divisions of the Bony Pelvis

The pelvic cavity is divided into two parts, the *false pelvis* and the *true pelvis*, by a slight constriction known as the *brim of the true pelvis* or the *linea terminalis* (Fig. 10-1). With the person in the upright position the pelvis is tilted forward and the plane of this brim is not horizontal, but rather slopes up and back from the symphysis pubis to the promontory of the sacrum. The sacral promontory is about 4 in. higher than the upper border of the symphysis pubis. Since the pelvis is swung on the heads of the femurs, the relation of the pelvis to the entire body differs in the sitting and standing positions. When a woman stands upright, the plane of the brim, and thus also of the inlet of the true pelvis, is at a 50- to 60-degree angle with the horizontal. There may be considerable variation in this position, which is called the *inclination of the pelvis*.

The False Pelvis

The false pelvis (pelvis major, greater pelvis) is the shallow, expanded portion above the brim or linea terminalis (Fig. 10-1). Its walls are formed by the lumbar vertebrae behind, the fanlike flare of the ilium on each side, and the lower portion of the abdominal wall in the front. It serves as a support to the abdominal viscera. The false pelvis has little obstetric importance. However, it supports the enlarged uterus dur-

ing pregnancy, and acts as a funnel to direct the baby's head into the true pelvis below.

The True Pelvis

The true pelvis (pelvis minor, lesser pelvis) is an irregularly shaped, bottomless basin which lies below the pelvic brim (Fig. 10-1). Its bony walls are more complete than those of the false pelvis. They are formed by the sacrum, the coccyx, and the lower portion of the hipbones. The true pelvis is of great obstetric importance since it constitutes the passage through which the baby must be forced during birth by the "powers" of uterine and abdominal muscle contractions. It is with this portion of the pelvis, its size and shape and the relationship of the baby's head to its cavity, that the remainder of this chapter is concerned. The position of the baby's head within this cavity will be considered in the following chapter.

THE PELVIC INLET The *inlet*, or *superior strait*, is the upper boundary of the true pelvis (Fig. 10-1). It is at this plane that the fetal head enters the birth canal. The inlet is bounded by the upper margins of the pubic bones in front, the linea terminalis (brim) on the sides, and the body of the first sacral vertebra (promontory of the sacrum) in the back. The inlet may be almost round in shape, or its anteroposterior diameter may be shortened by the promontory of the sacrum, which gives it a blunt, heart-shaped outline (Fig. 10-2).

Four diameters of the inlet are usually described: the anteroposterior, the transverse, and the right and left oblique diameters (Fig. 10-2). The *anteroposterior diameter*, the distance from the symphysis pubis to the sacrum, is the shortest of the inlet measurements and thus the most important. Three different measurements of this diameter may be distinguished, depending on the specific point on the symphysis pubis from which the distance to the sacrum is measured. These diameters are the true conjugate, the obstetric conjugate, and the diagonal conjugate. The *true conjugate*, which is the distance from the top of the symphysis pubis to the middle of

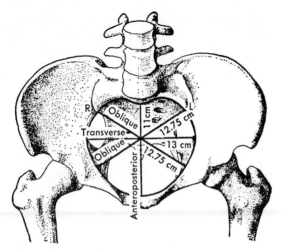

Figure 10-2. Diagram of the pelvic inlet, seen from above, showing important diameters.

the promontory of the sacrum, normally measures 11 cm or slightly more. The distance between the inner surface of the symphysis pubis and the sacral promontory, the *obstetric conjugate,* is a few millimeters shorter than the true conjugate. It is, therefore, the shortest inlet diameter through which the baby's head must pass as it descends into the birth canal. The *diagonal conjugate,* the distance from the lower margin of the symphysis pubis to the sacral promontory, is from 1.5 to 2 cm longer than the true conjugate, depending on the height of the symphysis pubis (Fig. 10-7). In a pelvis of normal size the diagonal conjugate is approximately 12.5 cm long.

The diagonal conjugate is the only diameter of the inlet that can be measured without the use of x-ray. Knowledge of its length is very important in estimating the anteroposterior inlet diameter, a distance that may be shortened in several types of abnormal pelves. Clinical measurement of this diameter is made during an early prenatal examination.

The *transverse diameter* is the greatest width of the inlet (Fig. 10-2). It lies at right angles to the true conjugate and is the greatest diameter between the linea terminalis on each side of the inlet. This diameter measures 13 cm or slightly

less, depending on the shape of the inlet. The two diagonal diameters, which are the distance from each sacroiliac joint to a point of the pelvic inlet diagonally across from that joint, are known as the *right* or *left oblique diameter,* respectively, according to the starting point of the measurement (Fig. 10-2). These diameters normally measure about 12.75 cm.

The baby's head usually enters the pelvis with the suboccipitobregmatic diameter lying parallel to the transverse or one of the oblique diameters because these are longer than the anteroposterior diameter. It is very important, however, that all measurements are within normal limits. If the anteroposterior diameter or the transverse diameter, or both of these distances, are short, the inlet may be too constricted for a full-term baby's head to enter.

In summary, the pelvic inlet is a bony ring capable of very little expansion. Hence, if it is greatly decreased in size, the inlet may form an absolute barrier to the passenger. Inadequacy of the anteroposterior diameter of the inlet, the *obstetric conjugate,* is the commonest form of inlet contraction. This diameter can be measured directly by x-ray technique, but is estimated clinically by determination of the diagonal conjugate.

THE PELVIC CAVITY   The cavity of the true pelvis, the area between the inlet and the outlet, is a curved canal. The posterior wall of this canal, which is the sacrum, measures approximately 12 cm in length as compared with the shorter anterior wall, formed by the symphysis pubis, which is from 4.5 to 5 cm long. Because of this difference in length between the anterior and posterior walls of the pelvis, the part of the baby's head that lies toward the sacrum traverses a longer distance in its passage through the pelvis than the part that lies under the symphysis pubis (Fig. 10-3).

The caliber of the canal varies at different levels. The narrowest area, called the *plane of least pelvic dimensions* or the *midpelvic plane,* is of particular importance because it is small, and if in addition it becomes contracted, the baby's

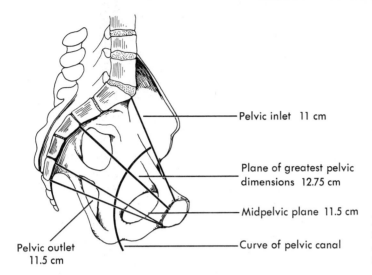

Pelvic inlet 11 cm

Plane of greatest pelvic
dimensions 12.75 cm

Midpelvic plane 11.5 cm

Curve of pelvic canal

Pelvic outlet
11.5 cm

Figure 10-3. Diagram of sagittal section of the true pelvis showing the curve of the pelvic canal and some important pelvic diameters.

head may be arrested at this point. If significant contraction exists at this level, further descent of the passenger may be impossible. The midpelvic plane passes from the lower margin of the symphysis pubis, through the area between the ischial spines, to the sacrum (Fig. 10-3). The *anteroposterior diameter* of the midpelvis measures 11.5 cm. The average *transverse (interspinous) diameter of the midpelvis,* which is the distance between the ischial spines, is 10.5 cm (Fig. 10-4). Diameters of the midpelvis can-

not be measured clinically but can be estimated from the outlet measurements described below.

The curve in the pelvic canal begins rather sharply at the midpelvic plane, and it is at this place that the axis of the birth canal changes. As the baby's head passes through the birth canal, it descends in a straight line until it reaches the level of the ischial spines and then curves forward toward the pelvic outlet (Fig. 10-3).

In thinking of the midpelvic plane, it is well to remember that the posterior circumference is partly formed by the pliable uterosacral ligaments. Hence, significant midplane (midpelvic) contraction may be a less absolute barrier to descent of the baby than would a comparable degree of inlet contraction.

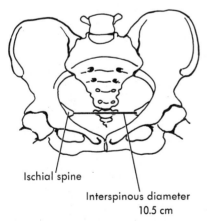

Ischial spine

Interspinous diameter
10.5 cm

Figure 10-4. Diagram of ischial spines jutting into the pelvic cavity, as seen from above, showing the transverse (interspinous) diameter of the midpelvis.

THE PELVIC OUTLET The *outlet,* or *inferior strait,* is the lower boundary of the true pelvis. It is in this area that the fetal head emerges from the birth canal. The outlet has a diamond-shaped appearance or one that resembles two triangles with their bases placed against each other. The base of each triangle is the imaginary line between the ischial tuberosities. The apex of the anterior triangle is at the lower margin of the symphysis pubis and that of the posterior triangle at the tip of the sacrum.

The three diameters of the outlet commonly

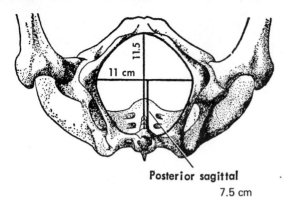

Posterior sagittal

7.5 cm

Figure 10-5. Diagram of the pelvic outlet, seen from below, showing important diameters.

described are the anteroposterior, the transverse (intertuberous), and the posterior sagittal (Fig. 10-5). The *anteroposterior diameter* extends from the middle of the lower margin of the symphysis pubis to the tip of the sacrum (Fig. 10-5). Measured to the tip of the coccyx, the length of the diameter is 9.5 cm, but the baby's head usually pushes the coccyx back as the head passes through the birth canal and the diameter is extended to the lower end of the sacrum. The measurement of the anteroposterior diameter is therefore usually considered to be approximately 11.5 cm, which is the distance from the middle of the lower margin of the symphysis pubis to the end of the sacrum. The anteroposterior diameter is the longest diameter of the outlet. When the baby's head emerges from the pelvic canal, the long diameter of his head (occipitofrontal) is parallel to the long diameter of the outlet (anteroposterior).

The *transverse diameter* of the outlet (biischial, intertuberous) is the distance between the inner edges of the ischial tuberosities; it measures 11.0 cm (Figs. 10-5 and 10-8). This is the most important measurement of the outlet because it is the shortest diameter through which the baby must pass as he emerges from the pelvic canal. The ischial tuberosities come closer together with narrowing of the pubic arch. Therefore, the narrower the pubic arch, the shorter the intertuberous diameter will be.

Since this is true, it becomes apparent that the shorter the intertuberous diameter is, the less the available space for the baby's head to pass directly under the symphysis pubis. Whenever the head must stem itself lower down along the pubic arch in passing through the outlet, the distance between the intertuberous diameter and the tip of the sacrum becomes very important. This is known as the *posterior sagittal diameter*. It is the distance from the midpoint of an imaginary line between the ischial tuberosities to the tip of the sacrum; this distance normally measures 7.5 cm (Fig. 10-5).

Isolated outlet contraction (in the absence of associated midplane contraction) is quite rare. The outlet measurements just described will give a fair estimate of such associated midplane narrowing.

Passage of the Fetal Head through the Pelvis

From the above description of the pelvis, it is apparent that the long diameter of the pelvic outlet, the anteroposterior, lies at a right angle, or nearly so, to the long diameter of the inlet, the transverse. The baby's head must rotate in making its descent through this bony canal. When the head enters the pelvis, its long diameter (suboccipitobregmatic) conforms to one of the long diameters of the inlet, either transverse or oblique; during descent the head turns so that its long diameter lies anteroposteriorly, in conformity to the long diameter of the outlet, through which it emerges from the pelvis.

The canal through which the baby must pass resembles a bent cylinder, with the posterior wall (sacrum) nearly three times the length of the anterior wall (symphysis pubis), making it necessary for that portion of the baby's head that lies posteriorly to travel a longer distance than the part that lies anteriorly (Fig. 10-3). It is apparent therefore that the structure of the pelvis makes it necessary for the baby's head not only to rotate in its passage through the birth canal, but also to describe an arc. This twisting and curving of the birth canal must be appreciated to understand the mechanism of labor, which is described on pages 270–74.

PELVIMETRY

Measurements of the pelvis are an important part of a complete examination during pregnancy. They are made for the purpose of estimating as accurately as possible the size of the passage through which the "passenger" must advance during labor. Since the measurements of the mother's pelvis are one important factor in determining the ease or difficulty with which the baby will move through the birth canal, the physician considers it essential to obtain as much information as possible about the size and shape of the pelvis before the onset of labor. Measurements of the bony pelvis can be made clinically and by the use of x-ray.

Although the size and configuration of the pelvis have a great influence on the progress of labor, several other factors determine whether or not the baby can be delivered through the pelvic canal. The physician will consider these other factors along with pelvic size as he plans for the management of labor. Quite obviously,

the size of the fetal head is one such factor. As will be explained in the following chapters, the position in which the baby enters the birth canal, the moldability of the baby's head, and the force of the uterine contractions will also affect the course of labor.

Clinical Pelvimetry

Clinical pelvimetry is the measurement of distances between certain points on the pelvis with a pair of calipers, termed a pelvimeter (Fig. 10-6), or with the hand. Clinical pelvimetry does not permit measurement of all pelvic diameters, but it usually gives sufficient information about the size of the pelvis for assessment of its adequacy for delivery of the baby through the birth canal. Clinical measurements are often made early in pregnancy, at the woman's first or second visit to the physician, at other times they are postponed until somewhat later in pregnancy. Doubtful findings are usually rechecked by a repeated examination later in pregnancy.

Table 10-1.   Average Measurements of Diameters of the Female Pelvis

Diameter	Average Length in Centimeters*
Inlet measurements	
True conjugate	11
Obstetric conjugate	10.6
Diagonal conjugate	12.5
Transverse	13
Oblique (right and left)	12.75
Midpelvic measurements	
Anteroposterior	11.5
Interspinous (transverse)	10.5
Outlet measurements	
Anteroposterior	11.5
Intertuberous (transverse)	11
Posterior sagittal	7.5

*All measurements represent average figures.

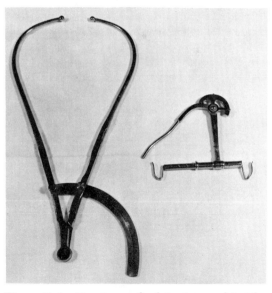

Figure 10-6.   Two types of pelvimeters used in taking pelvic measurements. *Left,* Martin's; *right,* Thoms'.

Internal Measurements

PELVIC INLET MEASUREMENTS   The single important diameter of the pelvic inlet that can be measured clinically is the diagonal conjugate. This measurement is made with the patient in the lithotomy position. The first two fingers of the examiner's hand are introduced into the vagina until the tip of the second finger touches the promontory of the sacrum (Fig. 10-7). The point at which the lower margin of the symphysis pubis rests on the forefinger is then marked by the nail of the index finger of the other hand, and the fingers in the vagina are withdrawn. The nail of the index finger, which is used as the marker, is held firmly in place until the distance between it and the tip of the second finger (the finger that touched the sacral promontory) is measured. This distance is the length of the diagonal conjugate, which normally measures 12.5 cm. The diameter of the true conjugate is then estimated by subtracting 1.5 to 2.5 cm from the measurement of the diagonal conjugate.

It may be difficult to reach the promontory of the sacrum during the early months of pegnancy because of tightness of the vaginal tissues and ri-gidity of the perineum. Measurement of the diagonal conjugate is therefore sometimes deferred until the middle part of pregnancy, when these tissues stretch more easily. Measurement of the diagonal conjugate may be somewhat uncomfortable for the patient and requires reassurance by the physician and the nurse.

MIDPELVIC MEASUREMENTS   There is no satisfactory manual or instrumental method of measuring the midpelvis; measurements can be obtained only by x-ray. However, an approximate but useful estimate of the space in the midpelvis may be obtained by vaginal examination. The ischial spines, which project into the region of the midpelvis (Fig. 10-4), are readily felt during a vaginal (or rectal) examination. Although the distance between these spines cannot be measured clinically, their bluntness or prominence can be estimated. The slope of the side walls of the pelvis, the curve of the sacrum, and the width of the sacrosciatic notch can also be palpated during vaginal examination.

A midpelvic contraction may be suspected if the ischial spines are prominent, if the side walls of the pelvis converge, or if the sacrosciatic notch feels narrow. A contraction of the mid-

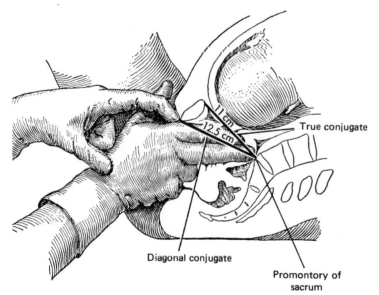

True conjugate

Diagonal conjugate

Promontory of sacrum

Figure 10-7. Diagram showing method of measuring the diagonal conjugate in order to estimate the length of the true conjugate.

pelvis may also be suspected when the inter-tuberous measurement (transverse diameter of the outlet) is 8.5 cm or less, because the distance between the ischial spines is usually small whenever the space between the ischial tuberosities is decreased.

PELVIC OUTLET MEASUREMENTS Measurements of the pelvic outlet are also made with the patient in the lithotomy position. In addition to making measurements, the coccyx is examined for mobility at this time, and the general contour of the pelvic outlet is ascertained. The shape of the subpubic arch is outlined by palpation of the bony sides of the outlet from the symphysis pubis down to the ischial tuberosities. When the thumbs of each hand are placed along the descending portion of the pubic bone on each side of the pelvis, the angle at which these bones come together can be observed. Information about the width of the pubic arch is very valuable in making an estimate of the adequacy of the outlet and hence, indirectly, of the midpelvis. A narrow arch, which is typical of a male pelvis, is almost always associated with other characteristics of a masculine-type pelvis.

In addition to estimation of the width of the pubic arch, distances between points are also measured. The distance between the inner, lower aspect of the ischial tuberosities, the intertuberous diameter, which is the most important measurement of the outlet, is measured with a pelvimeter (Fig. 10-8) or with the examiner's hand. When the examiner uses the hand to make this measurement, he presses three or four knuckles of one hand between the ischial tuberosities and measures the distance across the portion of the hand that fits into this space. The average measurement between the ischial tuberosities is 11 cm.

The posterior sagittal diameter, a distance that has special importance when the intertuberous diameter is short, is obtained by measuring, with a pelvimeter, the distance from the midpoint between the ischial tuberosities to the tip of the sacrum. This distance is normally an average of 7.5 cm in length.

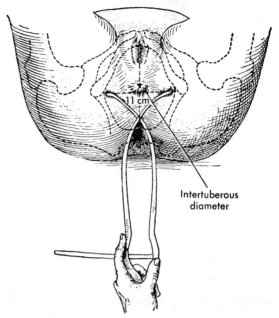

Figure 10-8. Diagram showing method of measuring the transverse diameter of the outlet (intertuberous diameter).

X-ray Pelvimetry

X-ray technique may be used to measure the diameters of the pelvis that cannot be measured clinically and at the same time to recheck measurements that have been obtained with the pelvimeter and the hand. If the x-ray is taken late in pregnancy or during labor, it not only aids in determining pelvic size and shape, but also provides valuable information about the relationship of the baby (presentation, position, and station) to the maternal pelvis (Figs. 10-9 and 10-10).

X-ray examinations are a valuable diagnostic aid in pregnancy, but because they increase, albeit slightly, the radiation exposure on *two* individuals, they are used only when clinical examination indicates that additional information is essential. Although diagnostic x-rays have some slight effect on any exposed body cells (somatic effect), the major concern in their use during pregnancy is the effect on reproductive cells

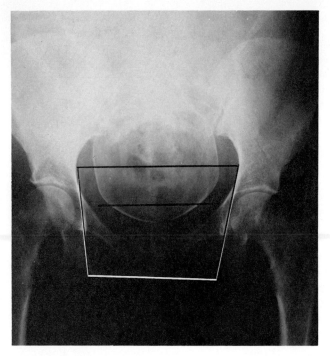

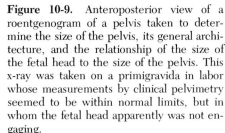

Figure 10-9. Anteroposterior view of a roentgenogram of a pelvis taken to determine the size of the pelvis, its general architecture, and the relationship of the size of the fetal head to the size of the pelvis. This x-ray was taken on a primigravida in labor whose measurements by clinical pelvimetry seemed to be within normal limits, but in whom the fetal head apparently was not engaging.

The horizontal dark lines on the film designate the diameters measured. The uppermost horizontal line indicates the transverse diameter of the inlet, which measured 12.2 cm. The center horizontal line runs between the ischial spines and measures the transverse diameter of the midpelvis; this measured 10.1 cm. The lowermost horizontal line lies between the ischial tuberosities and thus measures the transverse diameter of the pelvic outlet; this was found to be 10.2 cm. (After the distances had been measured on the film, a correction factor was applied to make adjustment for magnification and other technical considerations.)

This x-ray shows the presentation to be cephalic with the occiput anterior. The back lies anteriorly and slightly to the right. The fetal head is small compared to the size of the pelvis.

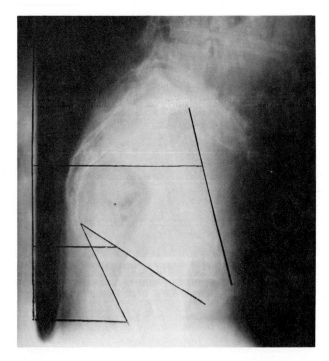

Figure 10-10. Lateral view roentgenogram of the pelvis shown in Figure 10-9. This x-ray was taken with the patient in an upright position and shows that the fetal head is engaged just within the pelvis. The oblique dark lines designate the diameters measured. The anterior line is the AP diameter of the pelvic inlet which measured 13.1 cm; the center line indicates the AP diameter of the midpelvis which measured 10.7 cm; and the posterior line shows the posterior sagittal diameter which measured 7.8 cm. (These measurements are the readings after application of the correction factor.)

The conclusion that was drawn from the x-rays shown in Figures 10-9 and 10-10 was that the pelvic diameters are adequate for the size of this baby and that there is no apparent reason for difficulty in delivery due to disproportion between the fetal head and the bony pelvis.

(genetic effect). The genetic effect of radiation on reproductive cells may be cumulative from the time of conception through the reproductive years. Deleterious or harmful mutations may be produced which are then passed on to the next generation. Pelvic x-rays are in the gonadal region, and when taken during pregnancy they involve two persons, a mother in the reproductive years and a very young individual, the fetus. The gonads of both the mother and the fetus are exposed to a certain amount of radiation, and in addition, the fetus receives radiation to other parts of his body.

To keep radiation exposure to a minimum, the physician will carefully evaluate the need for an x-ray and then take all precautions possible in the technique and method of taking the films, precautions that keep the exposure as low as possible. Whenever justifiable, an x-ray examination is postponed until after onset of labor. The baby is then well beyond the period during which the x-ray may have a deleterious effect on his somatic development. Also, the x-ray serves several purposes; it provides information about fetal size, maturity, position, and development in addition to size of pelvis.

X-ray pelvimetry, if necessary, is ordinarily done only as indicated sometime during the course of labor. It becomes imperative in conditions such as suspected disproportion between the fetal head and the pelvis; abnormal presentation and position; suspected abnormal fetal development; and prolonged or arrested labor. In the hope that x-ray pelvimetry may prove unnecessary, physicians await labor before obtaining films on a woman with a pelvis of questionable size. For example, descent of the fetal head with the beginning of labor might terminate fears regarding the adequacy of the pelvic inlet.

Whenever a patient in labor must have an x-ray, it is highly desirable that a nurse accompany her to the x-ray room. The patient and her husband are often worried and frightened, and the reassurance of a nurse is of great comfort to them. The mother is usually uncomfortable from her labor, which sometimes has continued for hours, and both parents will be concerned over its outcome and the safety of mother and baby. The nurse can help to interpret the purpose of the x-rays and the general overall procedure in taking the films. The nurse can also be of considerable assistance in helping the patient move into the proper positions for the films (views from several positions may be necessary), and she should remain in the room, close to the patient, until all is in readiness for taking the films. In most instances the patient can be left alone during the short interval required for taking the x-ray, and, if possible, the nurse should leave the room because she too must keep her total radiation dosage to a minimum. If the occasional patient requires assistance from the nurse in maintaining a position, or for some other reason, lead-lined aprons are available for the nurse's protection. The nurse must observe labor carefully while the patient is in the x-ray department and while en route. She must be prepared to notify the physician immediately at the appearance of signs of imminent delivery or threatened uterine rupture and also be prepared to handle other emergencies.

Variations in Pelvic Size and Shape

There are many variations in size and shape of pelves. Variations in shape are found in pelves of normal size as well as in pelves with one or more abnormal dimensions. Each variation in a pelvis of normal size, as well as in one that is contracted, has some effect on the mechanism of labor. A number of factors exert an influence on pelvic form; racial characteristics, general body build, nutritional diseases (especially rickets), developmental defects, and disease or injury of the spine, the pelvic bones, and the lower extremities—all may alter the size and contour of the pelvis.

A general classification, based on pelvic shape, describes four main types of pelves; these are termed (1) gynecoid, feminine-type, inlet nearly round or blunt heart-shaped; (2) android, masculine-type, inlet wedge-shaped; (3) anthropoid, apelike, inlet oval-shaped from front to back; and (4) platypelloid, flat, inlet oval-shaped transversely. This general classification is based on contour and size of the pelvic inlet, gynecoid pelves including most of those with normal measurements. In addition to this general classification according to form, abnormal pelves are also described according to type of contraction. Description of a pelvis according to contraction does not exclude its classification according to one of the four main types.

A pelvis is considered contracted when one or more of its diameters are shortened enough to interfere with the normal mechanism of labor, but not necessarily sufficiently contracted to prevent delivery of the baby through the birth canal. Delivery may be, and frequently is, accomplished through a pelvis that is not normal in size or shape. The size and moldability of the baby's head may be a determining factor. A small pelvis may permit spontaneous delivery of a small baby, but may be inadequate for passage of a full-sized baby, while a woman with a normal pelvis may have an extremely difficult labor with an unusually large baby. The outcome depends on whether or not the passage is large enough for the particular baby involved.

The types of pelvic contraction are inlet contraction, midpelvic contraction, outlet contraction, and any combination of the three. Solitary outlet contraction is unusual. Contracted pelves may be described by terms such as generally contracted, flat, funnel, rachitic, and a number of others applied to less common varieties of contraction. The terms are often self-explanatory. A flat pelvis is contracted anteroposteriorly, mainly at the inlet. Rickets is a common cause of a flat pelvis. A funnel pelvis is one in which the pelvic cavity becomes smaller from inlet toward outlet; such a contraction may be chiefly at the pelvic outlet, but a contraction of the midpelvic region is often associated with an outlet contraction. A generally contracted pelvis is one in which all diameters are small. When contractions exist in more than one region, a combination of terms may be used to describe the contraction; an example is the term "generally contracted funnel pelvis." The management and the progress of labor and delivery in a pa-tient with a contracted pelvis are described in Chapter 16.

THE BABY'S HEAD

The fetal head is the most important part of the body from the standpoint of passage through the birth canal. The head is the largest and least malleable part of the body; it is also the part that ordinarily passes through the birth canal first. The process of labor is essentially a series of adaptations of the size, shape, and position of the fetal skull to the size and shape of the maternal pelvis—an adaptation of the "passenger" to the "passage." Since the pelvis is quite rigid and inflexible, adjustment must be made by the fetal head, which is moldable because of incomplete ossification and bone fusion at this age. If the head passes through the pelvis safely, the rest of the delivery will usually be accomplished with comparative ease, unless the baby is excessive in size. A marked disproportion between the diameters of the head and the pelvis, or limited moldability of the head, constitutes a serious complication, which will be described later as a complication of labor (Chapter 16).

Bones of the Skull

A baby's skull is proportionately larger than other parts of his body; the face forms a relatively small part of the head. The major portion of the head, the dome or vaultlike structure, which forms the top, sides, and back of the head, is made up of separate and as yet ununited bones—two *frontal*, two *parietal*, two *temporal*, and the *occipital* bone. The bones are separate structures with membranous tissues between their margins. The membranous tissues between the bones are called *sutures,* and the irregular membranous areas at the intersection of two or more sutures are called *fontanels.*

Sutures and Fontanels

The sutures are named and situated as follows: the *frontal* lies between the two frontal bones; the *sagittal* extends anteroposteriorly between the parietal bones; the *coronal* lies between the frontal bones and the anterior margin of the parietals, while the *lambdoidal* suture separates the posterior margins of the parietals from the upper margin of the occipital bone (Fig. 10-11). These sutures can be palpated on vaginal, and sometimes rectal, examination.

There are two fontanels of obstetric significance. The *anterior*, or *large*, *fontanel*, also called the *bregma*, is located at the meeting of the coronal suture from each side, the sagittal suture, and the frontal suture (Fig. 10-11). It is diamond- or lozenge-shaped, is about 3 cm in diameter, and is usually not obliterated during labor. The *posterior*, or *small*, *fontanel* is a triangular space at the intersection of the sagittal suture and the lambdoidal sutures (Fig. 10-11).

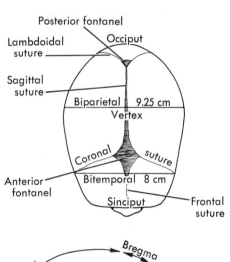

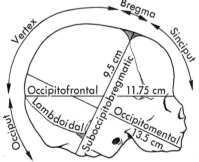

Figure 10-11. Top and size views of fetal skull, giving average length of important diameters.

This space may be obliterated as the surrounding bony margins approach each other during labor.

The sutures and fontanels are of great diagnostic value during labor because some can be outlined during a rectal or vaginal examination after the cervix has thinned and dilated. Correct recognition of these sutures and fontanels will determine the fetal position. The fontanels are differentiated from one another by their size and also by the number of suture lines that enter the space.

Areas of the Skull

The skull is divided into four areas that are designated as the occiput, the vertex, the bregma, and the sinciput (brow). The *occiput* is the region behind the small fontanel and is named from the bone that forms it; the *vertex* lies between the two fontanels and extends on each side of the head to the protuberances of the parietal bones; the *bregma* is the area of the large fontanel; and the *sinciput* (brow) is the area in front of the large fontanel and is formed by the frontal bone (Fig. 10-11). Terms used to describe presentation and position of a fetus indicate the relationship that exists between an area of the fetal skull and an area of the mother's pelvis.

Diameters and Circumferences

Information about the normal shape and average size of a newborn baby's head is important from the standpoint of the relationship between the measurements of the head and the measurements of the bony canal through which the head will pass during birth. The diameters that are usually described and their normal size are as follows (Fig. 10-11):

1. The *occipitofrontal diameter* (abbreviation, OF), measured from the bridge of the nose to the occipital protuberance, is 11.75 to 12 cm.

2. The *biparietal diameter* (BP) is the greatest transverse diameter, being the distance between the parietal protuberances, and measures 9.25 cm.
3. The *bitemporal diameter* (BT) is the greatest distance between the temporal bones and measures 8 cm.
4. The *occipitomental diameter* (OM) is the longest diameter. It extends from the point of the chin to the most prominent part of the occiput and measures 13.5 cm.
5. The *suboccipitobregmatic diameter* (SOB), measured from the undersurface of the occiput, where it joins the neck, to the center of the anterior fontanel, is 9.5 cm.

The *greatest circumference* of the fetal head is at the plane of the occipitofrontal diameter and measures 34.5 cm (13.8 in.). The *smallest circumference* is at the plane of the suboccipitobregmatic diameter and measures 32 cm (12.8 in.). With a normally flexed fetal head, this is the circumference that must traverse the birth canal. Until the baby weighs approximately 4500 gm (10 lb) the circumference of the head is greater than the body circumference at the shoulders. The size of the shoulders is therefore not likely to present a problem during delivery unless the baby has developed to excessive size and the circumference at the shoulders has become greater than the circumference of the head. Even then, the size of the shoulders may not cause difficulty if their firmness does not interfere with a certain amount of compression in their passage through the pelvis.

The measurements given above, like all of those which it is possible to give, only represent averages taken from a large number of term babies. Individual variations will be found among normal babies. For example, the size of the baby is affected by race. Black babies average a smaller size than those of the white race. As might be expected, the size of the parents is likely to be reflected in the size of their infants; parents of large stature tend to have large babies.

Molding

The fact that the skull is made up of separate bones, with soft membranous spaces interposed between them, permits its being compressed and changed in shape to a considerable extent as it passes through the birth canal. In this process, called molding, opposing margins of bones meet, or overlap to such a degree that the shape of the head changes and certain diameters are appreciably diminished (Fig. 17-6A, page 442). Such change permits passage of the baby's head through a relatively narrow canal. Moldability varies greatly, however, and the difference in the degree of compressibility of heads of approximately the same size may determine the difference between an easy and a difficult birth, or even the impossibility of passage through the birth canal. A newborn baby's head may be so distorted and elongated by the molding process that its abnormal appearance gives the parents great concern; the nurse can be quite confident, however, in giving them assurance that the head will assume its normal outline in a few days.

BIBLIOGRAPHY

Danforth, David N. (ed.), *Obstetrics and Gynecology*, 3rd ed. Harper and Row, New York, 1977.

Francis, Carl C., *The Human Pelvis*. Mosby, St. Louis, Mo., 1952.

Friedman, Emanuel A., *Labor, Clinical Evaluation and Management*. Meredith Publishing Co., Des Moines, Iowa, 1967.

Greenhill, J. P., and Friedman, Emanuel A., *Biological Principles and Modern Practice of Obstetrics*. Saunders, Philadelphia, Pa., 1974.

Oxorn, Harry, and Foote, William R., *Human Labor and Birth*, 3rd ed. Appleton-Century-Crofts, New York, 1975.

Pritchard, Jack A., and MacDonald, Paul C., *Williams Obstetrics*, 15th ed. Appleton-Century-Crofts, New York, 1975.

Reid, Duncan E., Ryan, Kenneth J., and Benirschke, Kurt, *Principles and Management of Human Reproduction*. Saunders, Philadelphia, Pa., 1972.

11

Presentation and Position of the Fetus

Knowledge of the exact relationship of the baby's position to the mother's pelvis is important in management of labor and delivery. Examinations are made during the latter part of pregnancy to determine this relationship and to estimate the baby's size. Further examinations are made at the onset of labor to confirm previous findings or discover changes and, at intervals during labor, to ascertain if the baby's progress through the birth canal is satisfactory. The baby's position in relation to the mother's pelvis is described as lie, presentation, and position of the fetus. This relationship is determined by abdominal palpation and rectal and vaginal examination, and sometimes by x-ray.

FETOPELVIC RELATIONSHIPS

During the latter months of pregnancy the fetus is curved and folded upon itself into an ovoid mass which corresponds to the shape of the uterine cavity. In this position it occupies the smallest possible space. The relationship of the various parts of the baby's body to one another, the posture assumed *in utero*, is called the baby's *attitude*. The usual intrauterine posture, or characteristic attitude, is with the back flexed; the head bent forward, with the chin close to the chest; arms crossed on the chest; thighs flexed on the abdomen; and knees bent. The umbilical cord lies in the space between the upper and lower extremities. With a few exceptions, the long axis of the fetus is parallel to the long axis of the mother, and most frequently the head is downward (Fig. 11-1). Although the fetus moves about and changes its position during the early part of pregnancy, it is less likely to alter its relation to the mother's body during the tenth lunar month and quite unlikely to do so after the onset of labor.

Lie of the Fetus

Lie is the term employed to indicate the relationship of the longitudinal axis of the baby to the longitudinal axis of the mother. The lie may be either longitudinal or transverse. In a *longitudinal lie*, the long axis of the baby's body is parallel to the long axis of the mother's body. In the *transverse lie*, the longitudinal axis of the baby's body is at right angles to the longitudinal axis of the mother's body.

Presenting Part and Presentation

The terms "presenting part" and "presentation" are used to designate the part of the baby's body that lies closest to, or has entered, the true pelvis. The part of the body that is lowermost is called the *presenting part*.

The *presentation* of the baby is named after the presenting part and is therefore a phrase used to describe the fetus in terms of its lowermost part. In longitudinal lies the head or the breech (buttocks) will be the lowermost portion

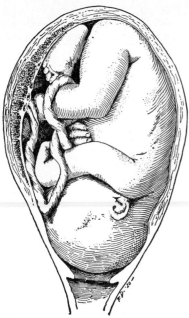

Figure 11-1. Most common attitude of fetus in uterine cavity at term.

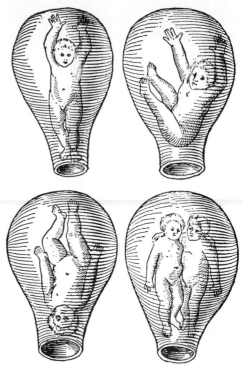

Figure 11-2. Illustrations from the first textbook on obstetrics, Roesslin's "Rosengarten," 1513, showing a former concept of fetal positions *in utero*.

of the baby and thus the presenting part. When the head is lowermost (presenting part), it is termed a *cephalic* presentation (Fig. 11-3), and when the breech is downward (presenting part), it is called *breech* presentation (Fig. 11-4). In transverse lie the shoulder is usually closest to the pelvic inlet (presenting part), and it is termed a *shoulder* presentation (Fig. 11-5). Well over 99 percent of all lies are longitudinal. A transverse lie is a serious obstetric complication.

Cephalic presentations are further divided into two main types, vertex and face presentation, and two transitory types, sincipital and brow presentation. These terms define more specifically the area of the baby's head that becomes the presenting part. The degree of flexion that the baby's head assumes in relation to his own body determines the area of the head that will be lowermost. The posture usually assumed is one in which the head is sharply flexed with the chin near the chest; the vertex is then lowermost in the pelvis, making a *vertex presentation* (Fig. 11-3). Occasionally the head is

sharply extended with the occiput nearly touching the back and the face lowermost; this is called a *face presentation* (Fig. 11-5).

The fetal head may assume a position intermediate between sharp flexion and sharp extension; when it is partly flexed, the large fontanel is the lowermost part making a *bregma* or a *sincipital presentation;* and when it is partly extended, the brow becomes the presenting part, making a *brow presentation* (Fig. 11-5). Sincipital and brow presentations are usually transient; the head either flexes or extends more completely as labor progresses, and the presentation changes to vertex or face, the vertex being far more common. Cephalic presentation occurs in over 96 percent of longitudinal lies; the ratio of vertex presentation to face is over 300 to 1.

Breech presentations are also described in several varieties according to the position of the baby's lower extremities in relation to his body. The baby's legs may be in the position that they characteristically assume *in utero* with the thighs flexed on the abdomen and the legs flexed on the thighs (squatting position); the buttocks and the feet then present, and the term *complete breech* or *full breech presentation* is used (Fig. 11-4). Often the legs are extended so that they lie against the anterior trunk with the feet touching the face; in this position only the buttocks present, and the term *frank breech presentation* is applied (Fig. 11-5). In another variety, *incomplete breech presentation,* one or both feet or knees have prolapsed so that they are lower than the buttocks and become the presenting part (Fig. 11-5). When only one foot presents, the other leg assumes the position that it would take in either a complete or frank breech presentation. An incomplete breech presentation may be of two types, a *footling presentation,* either *single* or *double,* or a *knee presentation.* Breech presentation occurs in about 3.5 percent of deliveries, and the frank breech is the most frequent variety.

Presentation does not become fully established until the presenting part has entered the pelvic inlet, and it may therefore change during the latter part of pregnancy, most frequently changing from breech to cephalic. The possibility of change lessens, however, as the end of pregnancy approaches.

Position

After the lie and presentation of the fetus have been established by the examiner, the relationship of the presenting part to the mother's pelvis is defined more specifically. This is done by stating the *position* of the baby. The term "position," as used here, means the relation that an arbitrarily chosen point on the presenting part of the baby bears to a specific part of the mother's pelvis. The arbitrary points designated for describing the baby's position are the occiput in a vertex presentation; the chin (mentum) in a face presentation; the sacrum in all varieties of breech presentations; and the scapula in a shoulder presentation. For purposes of stating quite precisely the relationship of the arbitrarily chosen point (occiput, chin, or sacrum) to the mother's pelvis, the pelvis is divided into six segments—an anterior, transverse, and posterior segment on the right side, and an anterior, transverse, the posterior segment on the left

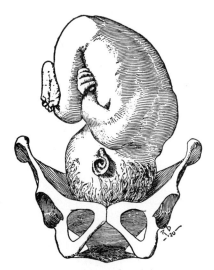

Figure 11-3. Attitude of fetus in vertex presentation.

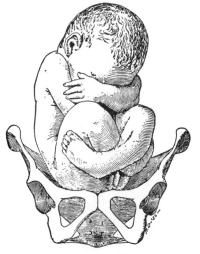

Figure 11-4. Attitude of fetus in complete or full breech presentation.

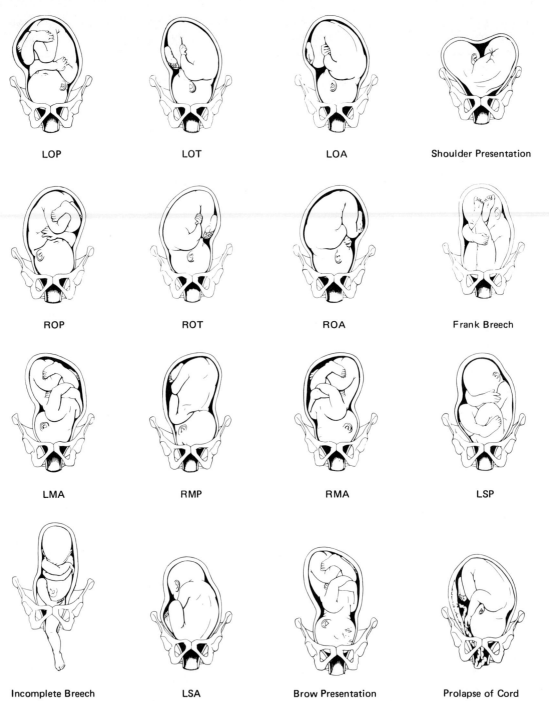

LOP   LOT   LOA   Shoulder Presentation

ROP   ROT   ROA   Frank Breech

LMA   RMP   RMA   LSP

Incomplete Breech   LSA   Brow Presentation   Prolapse of Cord

Figure 11-5. Categories of presentation. [*Reprinted with permission from* Obstetrical Presentation and Position, *Ross Clinical Education Aid #18, Ross Laboratories, Columbus, Ohio.*]

side. The occiput, the chin, or the sacrum may occupy any one of these six segments, thus making it possible to describe six positions for each presentation (Figs. 11-6, 11-7, and 11-8).

When the baby is so positioned in the uterus that his head is lowermost and flexed, with his chin resting on his chest, the vertex is the presenting part, and the occiput is the arbitrarily chosen point. If the occiput is found to be lying in the left anterior segment of the mother's pelvis, the position is occiput left anterior. However, in general usage, the right or left side is usually specified first when position is stated, and the position described above is called a left occiput anterior instead of an occiput left anterior.

Positions are usually expressed in abbreviations, determined by the first letter of each word; the left occiput anterior position is therefore usually stated as an LOA position. When the occiput is turned *directly* toward the mother's left side, neither to the front nor the back, the position is a left occiput transverse, or LOT, and when it lies in the left posterior segment of the pelvis, the position is left occiput posterior, or LOP. As there are three corresponding segments on the right side of the pelvis, anterior, transverse, and posterior, there are six possible positions for the baby to occupy in the vertex presentation (Figs. 11-5 and 11-6). The names and abbreviations of these positions are shown in Table 11-1. Similarly, there is a possibility of six face positions (Fig. 11-7) and six breech positions (Fig. 11-8). When the chin (mentum) rests in the left anterior segment of the mother's pelvis, the position is left mentum anterior, or LMA. When the breech presents and the sacrum is in that relation, the position is left sacrum anterior, or LSA (Figs. 11-5 and 11-8).

In a shoulder presentation (transverse lie) there are only four positions, since the shoulder is either anterior or posterior on the right or the left side of the mother's pelvis (Fig. 11-5). The scapula (of the presenting shoulder) is usually chosen as the point of direction; sometimes the acromion process is chosen.

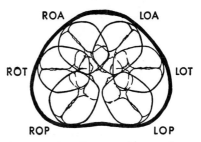

Figure 11-6. Diagram showing the six possible positions of a vertex presentation, as seen when looking at the pelvis from below.

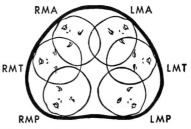

Figure 11-7. Diagram showing the six possible positions in a face presentation, as seen when looking at the pelvis from below.

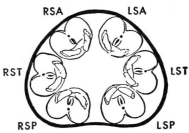

Figure 11-8. Diagram showing the six possible positions in a breech presentation, as seen when looking at the pelvis from below.

The baby's position may change frequently before engagement of the presenting part. His back may be toward one side of the mother's body on one day and toward the other side on another day. After the presenting part becomes engaged in the pelvis, positional changes are in a narrower range, taking place from one segment to another on the same side of the pelvis.

Internal rotation of the head (in the pelvis), one of the movements in the mechanism of labor, described on pages 270–74, brings about a change in position whereby the anteroposterior diameter of the head comes to lie in the anteroposterior diameter of the pelvic outlet; this change is necessary for the head to emerge from the pelvis. The rotation is usually such that the occiput comes to lie directly behind the symphysis pubis; the position is then described as *direct occiput anterior, direct OA*. Sometimes the head turns so that the occiput lies in the hollow of the sacrum; this is known as *direct occiput posterior, direct OP*.

Table 11-1. Categories of Lie, Presentation, and Position of the Baby *in Utero*

Lie	*Presentation*		*Position and Abbreviation*			
Longitudinal	Cephalic	Vertex	Left occiput anterior	LOA	Right occiput anterior	ROA
			Left occiput tranverse	LOT	Right occiput transverse	ROT
			Left occiput posterior	LOP	Right occiput posterior	ROP
		Face	Left mentum anterior	LMA	Right mentum anterior	RMA
			Left mentum transverse	LMT	Right mentum transverse	RMT
			Left mentum posterior	LMP	Right mentum posterior	RMP
		Sincipital	....			
		Brow	....			
	Breech	Complete (full) breech	Left sacrum anterior	LSA	Right sacrum anterior	RSA
		Frank breech	Left sacrum transverse	LST	Right sacrum transverse	RST
		Incomplete breech	Left sacrum posterior	LSP	Right sacrum posterior	RSP
		Footling Single Double Knee				
Transverse	Shoulder		Left scapula anterior	LScA	Right scapula anterior	RScA
			Left scapula posterior	LScP	Right scapula posterior	RScP

Some positions are more common than others at the onset of labor. Since a vertex presentation occurs in the majority of cases, the occiput position is most common. The head enters the pelvis with the occiput in a transverse position more frequently than in an anterior or posterior position and is directed toward the left side of the mother's pelvis more frequently than toward the right side.

ENGAGEMENT AND STATION

Engagement of the Presenting Part

Engagement means that the presenting part of the fetus has descended into the mother's pelvis to the level where its widest diameter has passed through the pelvic inlet. In cephalic presentation the widest diameter is the biparietal, and in breech presentation it is the intertrochanteric. Engagement of the head thus means that the baby has descended into the pelvis to a level where the biparietal plane (the greatest transverse diameter) of the head has passed through the pelvic inlet. Engagement of the head is evidence that the pelvic inlet is large enough to accommodate the fetal head. Engagement does not provide information about the relationship between the size of the head and the remainder of the pelvic canal (the midpelvis and the pelvic outlet).

Engagement may be gradual or quite sudden. In the majority of women in their first pregnancy, engagement takes place before the onset of labor; many times it occurs somewhere around two weeks before labor begins and at times even earlier. In women who have previously had children, engagement generally does not take place until the onset of labor. The baby does not sink into the pelvis as readily as in a first pregnancy because the multigravida is likely to have more relaxed abdominal muscles and there is less downward pressure on the baby.

In certain abnormalities, or in disproportion between the baby's head and the mother's pel-vis, engagement of the head may not take place until after labor is well established, or possibly not at all. An unengaged head at the beginning of labor in a primigravida is not necessarily indicative of disproportion between the baby's head and the mother's pelvis, but close observation for such a possibility is considered essential.

Engagement is ascertained by abdominal palpation and by vaginal or rectal examination. From abdominal examination, engagement is determined by palpation of the presenting part of the baby for the degree of its descent into the pelvis. In vertex presentation, this is ascertained from the part of the baby's head that can be felt when the examiner's hands are placed on each side of the lower abdomen and the fingers are pushed downward toward the pelvis. If the lower part of the head can be palpated with the fingers, it is not engaged; if it cannot be felt, it is probably engaged.

On vaginal or rectal examination, engagement is determined by the relationship of the lowermost part of the presenting part of the fetus to the level of the ischial spines. In vertex presentation, the head is engaged when its lowest part is at or below the level of the ischial spines, unless it is markedly elongated due to molding of the bones or swelling of the scalp. If unusual elongation is suspected, an x-ray is ordinarily indicated to establish the relationship between the fetal head and the pelvis.

In breech presentation, engagement of the breech has taken place when the bitrochanteric diameter has passed through the inlet of the pelvis. The breech is less likely to engage prior to the onset of labor than is the fetal head, but descent of the breech ordinarily progresses well during active labor. Estimation of degree of descent is likely to be more difficult in breech than in vertex presentation. X-ray facilitates diagnosis when there is doubt. Since the breech is smaller than the head, its engagement does not have the same significance concerning size of the pelvic inlet as does engagement of the head. Descent of the breech in the pelvis is important to the progress of labor.

Station of the Presenting Part

The station of the presenting part is the degree to which it has descended into the pelvis. A method of describing station is to state the distance (in centimeters) between the lowermost level of the presenting part and the level of the ischial spines. The most dependent area of the presenting part may be at the level of the spines or above them or below them.

The relationship between the presenting part and the ischial spines is determined by vaginal or rectal examination; the soft rectovaginal wall readily permits palpation through it on rectal examination. In the examination, the most dependent portion of the presenting part (usually the top of the baby's head) is located first; next the side walls of the pelvis are palpated to find the ischial spines, and an imaginary line is drawn between them; then the vertical distance (up or down) between this imaginary line and the most dependent portion of the presenting part is estimated in centimeters.

The station (degree of descent) is stated in numerical terms. The line between the ischial spines is called a zero station, any distance above the line is called a minus station, and any distance below the line is called a plus station. When the lowest level of the presenting part is on the level of the line between the ischial spines, the presenting part is said to be at zero station (or at the spines); when it is above the line, it is said to be at −1 (1 cm above), −2 (2 cm above), or −3 (3 cm above) station; and when it is below the line, it is described as at +1 (1 cm below), +2 (2 cm below), or +3 (3 cm below) station (Table 11-2).

Certain general terms, other than numbers, may be used to describe degree of engagement. A presenting part that is not engaged is said to be *high;* it may be further described as floating or as fixed in the inlet. Both of these stations can be determined by abdominal palpation. When palpation reveals the presenting part to be freely movable above the pelvic inlet, it is described as *floating;* when it is entering the pelvis, as *dipping* or entering; and when it is no longer movable, but not yet low enough to be engaged, it is described as *fixed in the inlet.* When the head has descended to the place where the biparietal plane has passed through the pelvic inlet, the term *engaged* is used, and when the presenting part is well below the level of the ischial spines, it is said to be *low.* If the presenting part is sufficiently low to push on the pelvic floor, the degree of descent may be described by the term *on the pelvic floor,* and when it has descended so far that it distends the perineum, the term *bulging of the perineum* is used. This last usually occurs only toward the end of labor.

Accurate information about the degree to

Table 11-2. Correlation of Terms Used to Describe Descent of the Presenting Part into the Pelvis

Broad Terms	Specific Terms	Station
Presenting part high	Floating	−4
	Dipping	−3
		−2
	Fixed, but not engaged	−1
	Engaged	Ischial spine >—0—< Ischial spine
		+1
Presenting part low		+2
	On the pelvic floor	+3
	Bulging of the perineum	+4

which the presenting part has descended at the beginning of labor, and about the rate of descent during labor, is necessary in evaluation of progress of labor. Descent may occur prior to labor, during dilatation of the cervix (first stage of labor), during the second stage of labor, or, gradually, at all these times; this is explained more completely in Chapter 12. Degree of descent is determined each time the woman is examined during the latter part of pregnancy and during labor.

DIAGNOSIS OF PRESENTATION AND POSITION

Presentation and position of the baby are ascertained by means of abdominal palpation, vaginal examination, and x-ray.

Abdominal Palpation

Palpation of the baby's body through the mother's abdominal wall is ordinarily possible during the latter months of pregnancy because the uterine and abdominal muscles are so stretched and thinned that the various parts of the baby's body may be felt through them. Abdominal palpation is the most useful method of making a diagnosis of presentation and position in the latter part of pregnancy; it can also be used for the same purpose during labor, if it is performed in the intervals between uterine contractions. Palpation is sometimes difficult with hydramnios, and it may be impossible in very obese patients. Abdominal palpation is also used to obtain other important information. It is one means of determining the distance to which the presenting part has descended into the pelvis. If the head has not descended, it may be possible to detect disproportion between the fetal head and the pelvic inlet by ascertaining whether or not the head overrides the symphysis pubis when it is pressed toward the inlet. Palpation is also used to make a rough estimate of the baby's size.

Abdominal palpation is a method that is readily available to the nurse for determination of presentation and position. During this examination the client should lie flat on her back with her knees slightly flexed. The bladder should be empty for comfort and for ease of palpation. Successful results require that pressure be applied to the abdomen with firmness and evenness, but this must be done gently. Cold hands, or quick, jabbing motions with the fingers, will usually stimulate the muscles lying beneath them to contract, thus somewhat obscuring the outline of the baby. Such movements are also uncomfortable for the woman, whereas firm, even pressure, started gently, with warm hands, ordinarily does not cause discomfort. Abdominal palpation should be performed in a systematic manner. One such system, described below, consists of four maneuvers, often called the maneuvers of Leopold.

Before beginning the maneuvers of Leopold, the general contour of the uterus should be observed and outlined, to determine if the baby's body is parallel or transverse to the mother's body. As noted above, the baby's body is usually parallel to the mother's, and the presentation is either cephalic or breech. With this much information, the examinations described below are made to ascertain presentation and position more exactly.

First Maneuver (Figs. 11-9 and 11-13)

The purpose of the first maneuver is to determine what is in the fundus; this is usually either the breech or the head. Facing the client the nurse gently applies the entire tactile surface of the fingers of both hands to the upper part of the abdomen, on opposite sides and somewhat curved around the fundus of the uterus. The outline of the pole of the fetus that occupies the fundus may be palpated. If the head is uppermost, it will be felt as a hard, round object which is movable, or *ballottable*, between the two hands, and if it is the breech, it will be felt as a softer, less movable, less regularly shaped body.

Second Maneuver (Figs. 11-10 and 11-13)

Having determined whether the breech or the head is in the fundus, the next step is to locate the baby's back and small parts in their relation to the right and left side of the mother. This is accomplished, while still facing the woman, by sliding the hands down to a slightly lower position on the sides of the abdomen. Firm, even pressure is made with the entire palmar surface of both hands. The back is felt as a smooth, hard surface under the palm and fingers of one hand, and it offers a resistance that prevents the hand from being pressed in as deeply as the hand on the opposite side. The small parts (hands, feet, elbows, knees) are felt as irregular knobs or lumps under the hand on the side opposite from the back.

At the same time that the fetal back is palpated, the nurse should note whether it is in the anterior or lateral portion of the right or left side of the abdomen. This information will be valuable in determining the relationship of the presenting part to the anterior, transverse, or posterior segment of the mother's pelvis.

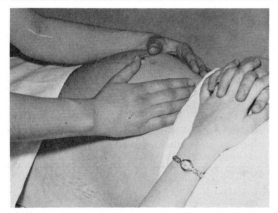

Figure 11-9. First maneuver in abdominal palpation to discover position of fetus.

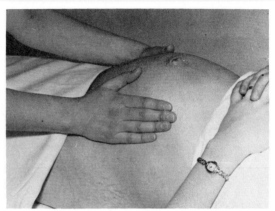

Figure 11-10. Second maneuver in abdominal palpation.

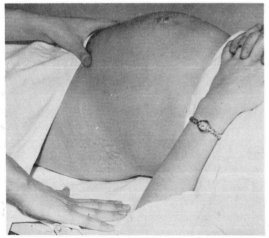

Figure 11-11. Third maneuver in abdominal palpation.

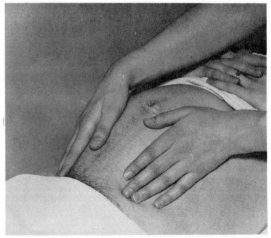

Figure 11-12. Fourth maneuver in abdominal palpation.

Third Maneuver (Figs. 11-11 and 11-13)

The third maneuver confirms the impression gained by the first maneuver as to which fetal pole is directed toward the pelvis and also indicates whether the presenting part is floating or has entered the pelvis. The thumb and fingers of one hand are spread as widely as possible, applied to the abdomen just above the symphysis pubis, and then brought together to grasp the part of the fetus that lies between them.

Either head or breech may be identified; the head gives the sensation of a hard, round mass at the lower fetal pole. If engaged, the presenting part may be difficult to palpate because it has descended so deeply into the pelvis. If the lower pole is movable, engagement has not occurred; if the lower pole is fixed, it may be engaged or merely entering the pelvic inlet.

Fourth Maneuver (Figs. 11-12 and 11-13)

The fourth maneuver is of particular value after the presenting part has become engaged. The nurse faces the woman's feet and places the tips of the fingers of each hand on each side of the midline of the lower abdomen. Deep pressure is then made in a downward and slightly inward direction—toward the pelvic inlet—with somewhat of a gliding motion that moves the skin on the lower abdomen downward along with the fingers. With the head presenting, the fingers on one side may be arrested in their downward progress by the cephalic prominence, the most marked protrusion of the baby's head, while the fingers on the other side may descend farther. A cephalic prominence felt on the same side as the small parts is the brow; this gives evidence that the head is flexed, that the vertex is lowermost in the pelvis, and thus that the pre-

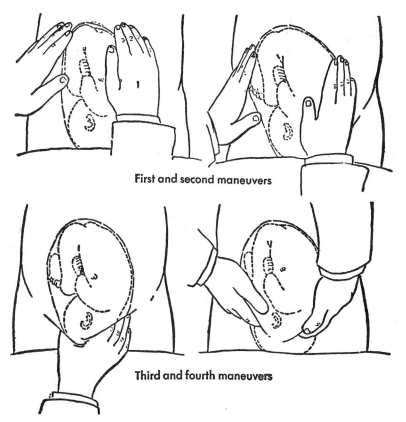

First and second maneuvers

Third and fourth maneuvers

Figure 11-13. Diagram showing relation of examiner's hands to fetus in the four maneuvers in abdominal palpation.

sentation is vertex. A cephalic prominence on the same side as the baby's back is the occiput; the head is then extended and the face is downward, making a face presentation.

The fourth maneuver helps to determine how far the presenting part has descended into the pelvis. When the cephalic prominence is readily palpable, the head is not engaged. After engagement it becomes quite difficult to feel the cephalic prominence.

Vaginal Examination

When a vaginal (or a rectal) examination is done during pregnancy, while the cervix is still closed, the presenting part of the fetus must be palpated through the lower uterine segment. This makes identification of landmarks difficult and the findings concerning presentation and position may add little to those obtained by abdominal palpation. However, from vaginal examination, information concerning the station of the presenting part, the softness and length of the cervix, and the pelvic configuration can be ascertained.

During labor, when the cervix has thinned and dilated, a vaginal (or a rectal) examination provides valuable information about presentation, position, and station of the baby, as well as information about cervical effacement and dilation. The presenting part is more easily palpated through a dilated cervix and landmarks can often be differentiated. In a vertex presentation, a diagnosis of position is made by feeling the sutures and fontanels of the baby's head and determining from them which segment of the pelvis is occupied by the occiput. In a face presentation, the features of the face are differentiated; and in a breech presentation, the buttocks and the sacrum are palpated for their placement in the pelvis. Fairly accurate determinations can often be made by rectal examination, but when there is a question of cephalopelvic relationship or of an abnormal presentation, or when there is doubt about the findings of a rectal examination, a vaginal examination is essential. Findings on vaginal examination are usually more reliable than those on rectal examination, since the cervix and the fetal landmarks are palpated directly rather than through several layers of maternal tissue. In general, rectal examinations are now obsolete and are ordinarily replaced by vaginal examinations. Details of performing a vaginal examination, one that nurses frequently make, are presented on pages 335–37.

X-ray

Presentation, position, and station of the baby can be visualized by an abdominal x-ray. This method of diagnosis is sometimes used when abdominal palpation of the fetus is difficult or impossible for some reason (for example, obesity) or when the information gained by vaginal examination during labor is uncertain (Figs. 11-14 and 11-15). X-ray is often used to gain additional information when the baby is found to be in a markedly abnormal position. When x-ray pelvimetry is required to determine whether disproportion exists between the mother's pelvis and the baby's head, fetal presentation, position, and station can also be determined from the pelvimetry films. An x-ray is of value in making an accurate diagnosis when there is a question of multiple pregnancy; it is an aid in estimating the size and development of the fetus; and it may show the existence of fetal abnormalities.

AUSCULTATION OF THE FETAL HEART

The fetal heart is auscultated when abdominal palpation is done, and preceding and following other examinations. The fetal heart is heard through a stethoscope placed against the mother's abdomen (Fig. 11-16).

The sounds of the heartbeat are usually transmitted through the convex surface of the fetus that lies closest to the uterine wall; in vertex and breech presentations this is the back, and in face presentation it is the thorax. The area of the mother's abdomen in which the fetal heart is heard best depends on the position of the baby and the degree of descent into the pelvis. In

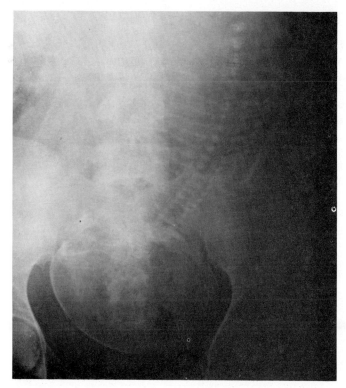

Figure 11-14. An x-ray taken on a woman who was believed to be close to term. It had previously been determined that a cesarean section was indicated, but since the gestational age was not definitely known and palpation of the abdomen was difficult, a roentgenogram seemed indicated to determine fetal size and position.

This x-ray shows a single well-developed fetal skeleton with the head presenting at the inlet and with the back lying to the left and anteriorly. The fetal size and skeletal development correspond to those of the last month of gestation. There is no evidence of fetal skeletal abnormalities.

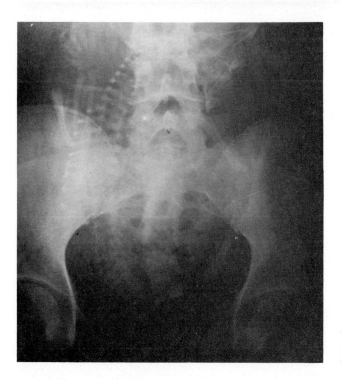

Figure 11-15. This roentgenogram shows a well-developed fetus in a frank breech presentation with the sacrum to the right and anterior.

cephalic presentations the heart is usually heard best below the umbilicus; this may be very low, close to the pelvic region, if the head is deeply engaged. In breech presentation the heart is usually heard best at, or above, the level of the umbilicus. When the occiput occupies the anterior segment of the mother's pelvis, the fetal heart is generally heard best near the midline of the mother's abdomen; when the occiput is in the transverse segment of the pelvis, the heart is heard farther toward the mother's side; and when in the posterior segment, the heartbeat is heard far toward the mother's back. Location of the maximal fetal heart sound sometimes reinforces the findings of presentation and position by palpation.

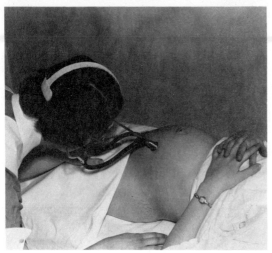

Figure 11-16. Auscultation of the fetal heart.

BIBLIOGRAPHY

Danforth, David N. (ed.), *Obstetrics and Gynecology,* 3rd ed. Harper and Row, New York, 1977.

Francis, Carl C., *The Human Pelvis.* Mosby, St. Louis, Mo., 1952.

Friedman, Emanuel A., *Labor, Clinical Evaluation and Management.* Meredith Publishing Co., Des Moines, Iowa, 1967.

Greenhill, J. P., and Friedman, Emanuel A., *Biological Principles and Modern Practice of Obstetrics.* Saunders, Philadelphia, Pa., 1974.

Oxorn, Harry, and Foote, William R., *Human Labor and Birth,* 3rd ed. Appleton-Century-Crofts, New York, 1975.

Pritchard, Jack A., and MacDonald, Paul C., *Williams Obstetrics,* 15th ed. Appleton-Century-Crofts, New York, 1975.

Reid, Duncan E., Ryan, Kenneth J., and Benirschke, Kurt, *Principles and Management of Human Reproduction.* Saunders, Philadelphia, Pa., 1972.

12

The Clinical Course and Mechanism of Labor and Delivery

The series of processes that consist of rhythmic uterine muscle contractions that lead to progressive effacement and dilatation of the cervix and descent of the presenting part, with eventual expulsion of the baby and the other products of conception, is known as *labor*. The actual birth of the baby is called the *delivery*. Ordinarily labor occurs near the end of the tenth lunar month, at which time pregancy is said to be *at term*.

At term the pregnant uterus is a thin-walled, muscular sac containing the mature fetus, the placenta to which the fetus is connected by the umbilical cord, and the amniotic fluid, which surrounds the fetus. The fetus and fluid are contained in the sac formed by the amniotic and chorionic membranes. The average fetus at term is about 49.4 cm (19½ in.) long and weighs about 3300 gm (7¼ lb).

Somewhere near term, contractions of the uterine muscle become forceful enough to expel the products of conception, the series of processes being called labor. Sometimes pregnancy ends prior to term; when this occurs *after* the baby has reached the period of viability (about the twenty-sixth week of pregnancy), but *before* the end of the thirty-sixth week of gestation, the term *premature labor* is used. From the end of the thirty-sixth week to term the fetus and hence the labor may be considered as term.

The course of labor is dependent on many variables, each differing not only from one woman to another, but also in successive labors of the same woman. A typical course of labor may be outlined as described below, with the understanding that any given labor may differ markedly from this prototype.

At the onset of labor the uterine contractions are weak and infrequent, being anywhere from 10 to 30 minutes apart. As labor progresses, the contractions become more forceful and more frequent until the interval between them is approximately two to three minutes. These involuntary uterine contractions dilate the cervix until it is large enough to permit the baby to pass through; then with the aid of voluntary contractions of the abdominal muscles, the uterine contractions move the baby down through the birth canal. Finally the placenta is separated from the uterine wall and expelled.

The three factors—powers, passenger, and passage—concerned with the process by which the baby is born have been discussed previously. The passage, the passenger, and their interrelationship have been described in Chapters 10 and 11. The present chapter will describe in detail the powers—those forces that move the passenger through the passage—as well as the mechanism by which such passage takes place.

LABOR

Cause of Labor

The cause of the onset of labor is not definitely known. Many theories have been advanced to explain why the muscular contractions, which have occurred painlessly and without expulsive force throughout pregnancy, finally become effective at approximately the end of the tenth month of pregnancy. It is also not known why some labors occur before and others after the expected date.

Labor appears to be the result of a combination of factors, which include fetal control, steroid hormone changes, production of prostaglandins, oxytocin stimulation, and uterine muscle changes. It appears that all these factors play some role, and that labor is the result of a combination of interrelated physiologic changes, particularly endocrine changes, but all factors are not necessarily essential at any one time.

From evidence to date it is thought that at some appropriate time, determined by the fetus, the fetal pituitary gland secretes increasing amounts of ACTH and oxytocin. Fetal ACTH is believed to stimulate the adrenal to increased activity, and fetal oxytocin is thought to cross the placenta and add to the action of maternal oxytocin. Evidence of the influence of the fetal endocrine system is not certain, but is inferred from observations of prolonged pregnancies associated with fetal pituitary and adrenal abnormalities.

ACTH, and possibly fetal prolactin, stimulate the fetal adrenal to secrete increasing amounts of cortisol, which precipitates a series of events that initiate labor and also promote fetal lung maturation.

Steroid hormone changes that take place near the end of pregnancy include a decrease in progesterone production (progesterone withdrawal), which allows increased uterine muscle excitability, and an increase in estrogen production, which enhances rhythmic uterine contractions and their responsiveness to oxytocin. These changes in production of steroids by the placenta appear to be the result of increased fetal adrenal gland activity—utilization of progesterone and increased production of estrogen precursors.

Prostaglandins, which stimulate uterine contractions, increase significantly in amniotic fluid during labor and may thus have a considerable influence on the initiation of labor.

The myometrium becomes more excitable and contractile with increasing volume as pregnancy progresses, and it is known that the uterus becomes more responsive to oxytocin with advancing pregnancy. Although definite evidence is lacking, it is assumed that oxytocin plays a role in the initiation of labor.

Although the exact processes are obviously not known, changes in endocrine relationships appear to stimulate the onset of labor. Some of these changes begin to appear several weeks before labor begins.

Stages of Labor

The process of labor is divided into three periods or stages:

First stage or stage of dilatation—begins with the onset of regular contractions and ends with complete dilatation of the cervix.

Second stage or stage of expulsion—begins with complete dilatation of the cervix and ends with complete delivery of the baby.

Third stage or placental stage—begins immediately after the baby is born and ends when the placenta is delivered.

The Forces of Labor

The forces of labor are muscular contractions, primarily of the uterine muscle and secondarily of the abdominal muscles. Uterine muscle contractions effect all the changes during the first stage of labor, which lead to complete effacement and dilatation of the cervix. The secondary force of abdominal muscle contractions is effective only after the cervix has been completely dilated and at that time is ordinarily added to the primary force.

Duration of Labor

The duration of normal labor may vary from an extremely short time, comprising only a few contractions, up to approximately 24 hours. Although there is wide variation, the average length of first labors is approximately 14 hours. This is an average figure; some primiparous labors will be considerably shorter and some much longer. When the 14 hours are divided according to the duration of each stage, the length may be as follows: first stage, 12½ hours; second stage, 80 minutes; and third stage, 10 minutes. Subsequent labors average about 8 hours in length, with a first stage of a little over 7 hours, a second stage of 30 minutes, and a third stage of 10 minutes.

The duration of labor depends in part on the effectiveness of the powers—the strength and frequency of the uterine contractions—and in part on the amount of resistance that must be overcome as the baby accommodates to the bony pelvis while the soft tissues stretch to permit passage of the baby. The longer labor in primigravidas as compared with multigravidas is due chiefly to the greater resistance offered by the cervix, by the soft parts of the vagina and pelvic floor, and by the perineum.

Premonitory Signs of Labor

Sometimes labor seems to start suddenly, but often signs of its approach appear several hours, a day, or even a week or more before its actual onset. In general, these signs are lightening, false labor pains, changes in the cervix, show, and rupture of the membranes. The woman herself can be aware of all of these signs with the exception of changes in the cervix, which may be noted by the physician when he performs a vaginal examination. Lightening and sporadic false labor pains may occur at any time during the last weeks of pregnancy, and the nearness of labor cannot be closely judged from these signs. The appearance of bloody show and rupture of the membranes are better evidence of imminent labor. In some instances the woman is not aware of any premonitory signs of labor; in other instances she has noticed most, or all, of the signs.

Lightening

Lightening is the descent of the uterus downward and forward, which takes place when the presenting part descends into the pelvis far enough to become fixed, and often deep enough to become engaged. With descent of the uterus, the top of the fundus settles to the level that it had reached at about the eighth month of pregnancy (Fig. 7-4, page 166), and the lower part of the abdomen becomes more prominent. As with engagement, lightening may come about gradually or quite suddenly, and it is more common in women with good abdominal muscle tone. Primigravidas are much more likely to experience lightening than multigravidas.

The woman is aware of the occurrence of lightening, which she often speaks of as "dropping" of the baby, through a lowering of her waistline and through relief of pressure in the upper abdomen but increased pressure in the pelvic region. She usually breathes more comfortably after this change in abdominal contour, but, at the same time, may have cramps in her legs, more difficulty walking, frequent micturition, and pressure in the rectum.

The time at which lightening takes place may vary from a few weeks to a few days before the onset of labor. In multigravidas lightening may not occur before labor. Lightening is a sign of approaching labor, but because of the variable time of its appearance it is not very useful in predicting the onset of labor. As a rule, lightening is evidence that the fetal head will not be too large for the pelvic inlet.

False Labor Pains

Contractions which may be more or less regular and may become quite uncomfortable, but which subside without effecting dilatation of the cervix, are termed *false labor*. This occurs more often in the multigravida than in the primigravida. In false labor, the painless uterine contractions, called *Braxton-Hicks contractions*, which may have been present throughout pregnancy, become painful, similar to true labor contractions. These moderately painful contractions often occur at night and then subside toward morning.

The appearance of false labor pains usually indicates that true labor is imminent, but sometimes false labor contractions recur for days before true labor begins, and they may even recur intermittently for three to four weeks before the onset of labor. It is difficult to distinguish false labor from true labor, and the woman may enter the hospital thinking that she is in labor.

This is a disappointing, and may be an embarrassing, experience for her. Sometimes a woman is admitted to the hospital for a second or even a third time in false instead of true labor. She will need considerable assurance that false labor is not uncommon and that she does not need to be apologetic for being unable to distinguish false from true labor contractions.

False labor may be suspected when the contractions occur irregularly, when they do not appear with increasing frequency, and when their intensity does not increase. The discomfort from false labor contractions is usually located in the abdomen instead of beginning in the back, as with true labor contractions, and it is generally not intensified, and may be lessened, with activity. *The major differentiating feature is that the cervix does not change appreciably in thickness and does not dilate during false labor, while in true labor the cervix becomes progressively thinner and dilatation takes place.*

Changes in the Cervix

As labor approaches, the cervix, which during pregnancy has been long, relatively firm, and closed, usually becomes softer and shorter and sometimes slightly dilated. It may have become very short, almost completely obliterated, by the time labor begins, and the diameter of the external os may have increased in size to a measurement of 1 to 2 cm.

Show

A tenacious mucoid vaginal discharge may appear shortly before the onset of labor. This may be pinkish in color or it may be slightly blood streaked. The discharge is known as the *show* or *bloody show,* or it may be termed *expulsion of the mucous plug.* This mucus, secreted by the cervical glands, has accumulated in the cervical canal during pregnancy, where it served to close the opening leading to the uterine cavity. As the cervix shortens and the canal enlarges toward the end of pregnancy or at the onset of labor, the mucous plug is expelled from the canal and discharged from the vagina. Sometimes some of the superficial mucosa of the cervical canal is expelled with the mucous plug. The slight oozing that accompanies this separation results in the blood streaking.

Labor ordinarily begins 24 to 48 hours after the mucous plug or show appears. However, the mucous plug may not be observed until the onset of labor, and blood streaking may not appear until labor has been in progress for several hours. Bloody show usually increases in amount as the cervix continues to thin and dilate during labor; a rather sudden and marked increase is often indicative of the approaching end of the first stage of labor. Bloody show and any increase in amount must be distinguished from true bleeding, since any bleeding, either before or during labor, that amounts to more than blood-streaked mucus is abnormal and serious and requires special attention (see pages 633–40)

Rupture of the Membranes

The fetal membranes containing the amniotic fluid that surrounds the baby (the *bag of waters*) may break at any time before or during labor, or they may remain intact until the physician ruptures them some time during the course of labor. Rupture before onset of labor is called *premature rupture of the membranes.* The break in the membranes usually occurs in the portion of the sac that lies over the cervical opening.

Rupture of the membranes is manifested by escape of clear fluid from the vagina. The amount of fluid that drains out at the time of rupture varies from a trickle to a gush and is often dependent on the point of rupture and the position of the presenting part. If the break in the membranes is small or high, there may be only an occasional trickle of fluid, and the woman may believe she is having urinary incontinence. If the break is more complete, the fluid in front of the presenting part may come in a gush and in an amount so large that it saturates the mother's clothing. Thereafter fluid continues to drain, especially with uterine contractions. The amount depends somewhat on the snugness with which the presenting part fits against the cervix.

During instructions given to the expectant mother in the antepartum period, she is told what to expect if the membranes rupture and is also instructed to notify her physician of the occurrence. The physician often wishes the client to be admitted to the hospital and to remain in bed. There is some possibility of prolapse of the umbilical cord through the cervix at the time of rupture, especially if the presentation of the baby is abnormal, or if the presenting part is not well down in the pelvis (Fig. 16-3, page 394). The chance of intrauterine infection increases when the barrier of intact fetal membranes is broken. Women sometimes fear that a "dry labor"—one in which the membranes rupture early—will make labor prolonged or difficult, but such fear is unfounded since amniotic fluid continues to be produced until delivery, and hence the condition does not exist.

Labor may begin soon after rupture of the membranes. If it does not begin spontaneously in a few hours, and if the fetus is mature enough for extrauterine survival, labor is induced to attempt to effect delivery within 24 hours.

In most instances there is little question about the integrity of the membranes, because amniotic fluid can be observed draining from the vagina at intervals and sometimes flakes of vernix caseosa can be seen in the fluid. In some instances, however, fluid is not seen draining, and the question arises of whether or not the membranes are ruptured. Sometimes the moisture on a perineal pad can be differentiated from urine by its odor. The odor of urine is quite readily recognized. The characteristic odor of amniotic fluid is often recognized by persons experienced in caring for maternity patients.

A test for the acidity or alkalinity of the vaginal secretion may be helpful in making a diagnosis of intact or ruptured membranes. The diagnosis is based on the fact that the pH of normal vaginal secretions ranges from 4.5 to 5.5, and the pH of amniotic fluid is usually from 7.0 to 7.5. A simple and fairly reliable chemical test used for this purpose is the phenaphthazine (Nitrazine) test. To make the test, a sterile cotton-tipped applicator is inserted into the vagina or into the pool of fluid in the posterior fornix during a sterile speculum examination, the wet cotton tip of the applicator is applied to a test paper impregnated with Nitrazine, and the change in color of the test paper is compared with a color chart. When the color change on the Nitrazine test paper indicates that the pH of the vaginal secretion being tested is 6.5 or above, it is assumed that amniotic fluid is present and that the membranes are ruptured, and when the pH is 6.0 or below, the membranes are considered to be intact. The information obtained by this test may be misleading if the amount of amniotic fluid present is too small to alter the pH of the vaginal secretion, or if blood (bloody show), which is alkaline, changes the indicator paper sufficiently to give an alkaline reading.

Sometimes the membranes can be felt bulging if a sterile vaginal examination is done, or fluid may be observed draining from the cervix during a sterile speculum examination.

The vaginal fluid may also be placed on a glass slide, allowed to dry, and examined microscopically for ferning. Ferning is normally absent in late pregnancy, but reappears with rupture of the membranes due to the sodium chloride present in the fluid. Blood and vaginal secretions invalidate this test, just as they do the Nitrazine test.

Microscopic examination of the vaginal fluid may also be done. It is placed on a slide, stained, and examined for evidence of fetal squamous cells, which are exfoliated into the amniotic fluid, and also for vernix and lanugo.

Presence of such cells is positive proof of a break in the membranes.

CLINICAL COURSE OF NORMAL LABOR

In the following description of a normal labor, it will be assumed that the fetus is a vertex presentation, the position rotating spontaneously from LOT to OA.

First Stage (Stage of Dilatation)

The first stage of labor is called the stage of dilatation, because it is during this period that the cervix is completely effaced and dilated. The "powers" during the first stage are the uterine muscle contractions, transmitted by the pressure of the bag of waters or the presenting part against the cervix (Fig. 12-1). The major resistive force during this time is the cervix, which must be dilated. The birth canal, a major resistive force in the second stage of labor, also offers some resistance during the first stage.

The time at which the first stage actually begins is sometimes difficult to determine, particularly when the woman has had false labor before the onset of true labor contractions. The onset of labor is often marked by a dull, low backache and a feeling of tightness in the abdomen. Soon the woman becomes conscious of the uterine contractions through intermittent dragging pains which may be felt first in the back and then in the lower part of the abdomen and possibly in the thighs. Early labor may be similar to menstrual cramps. Bloody show may be coincident with these early contractions. The beginning of regular uterine contractions, as perceived by the patient, is accepted as the start of labor by some physicians. Others consider the definitive time of onset of labor as the time at which the cervix begins to dilate.

Characteristics of Uterine Contractions

Contractions of the uterine muscle are *intermittent;* the periods of relaxation between contractions are longer than the periods of contrac-

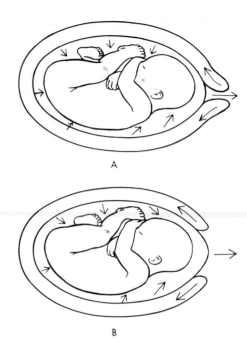

A

B

Figure 12-1. Effect of uterine contractions, resulting in effacement and dilatation of the cervix. A. Cervix is long and closed. B. Cervix is effaced and dilating and the "bag of waters" is bulging.

The arrows within the uterine cavity show the effect of the uterine contractions in producing hydrostatic pressure, which assists in dilating the cervix, the area of least resistance. When the membranes have ruptured, the presenting part of the fetus is pushed against the cervix instead of the bag of waters.

The arrows in the cervical tissue show the cervix being pulled up by the uterine contractions. This retraction of the cervical tissue during contractions is the main factor in effacement and dilatation of the cervix.

tion. The intervals of relaxation provide the mother with rest; give rest to the uterine muscle, which has a great amount of work to accomplish; and allow adequate circulation in the uterine blood vessels, important to fetal oxygenation, through adequate placental function.

Contractions of the uterine muscle are *involuntary* and cannot be controlled by the will of the patient.

After labor is established, contractions usually occur with *regularity*. At the beginning of labor, contractions are mild and cause little discomfort, may occur at 10- to 20-minute intervals, and last from 15 to 30 seconds. As labor progresses, the contractions gradually increase in intensity, increase in frequency until they recur every 3 to 4 minutes, and increase in length until each contraction lasts from 50 to 75 seconds or even longer. Occasionally weak contractions are interspersed with strong ones.

As the contractions *increase in intensity*, they become increasingly forceful and *painful* and are therefore frequently called labor pains. The discomfort of a contraction generally begins in the back and then moves slowly forward to the abdomen and sometimes down into the thighs. The pain is usually most severe in the abdominal region, but some women feel most of the discomfort in their back instead of their abdomen throughout the entire labor. Generally the woman is comfortable between contractions. Until they become frequent she will usually feel able, and in fact may prefer, to be up, but if she is on her feet when a contraction begins, she will usually seek relief by assuming a characteristic leaning position or by sitting down until it has subsided. Late in labor she may not be entirely free of discomfort between contractions. Such discomfort is probably due to increasing pressure in the pelvis as the baby is pushed downward.

During each uterine contraction there is a *period of increasing intensity* (this is the longest period), *a period of full intensity*, and a *period of decreasing intensity* (Fig. 12-2). The woman usually does not experience discomfort during the early part of the increasing-intensity period or during the latter part of the decreasing-intensity period. An examiner, placing a hand on the woman's abdomen, can feel the uterus becom-

ing firm as a contraction begins, very hard at the acme of the contraction, and decreasing in firmness as the contraction subsides. An experienced observer may feel the beginning of a contraction before the woman experiences discomfort and may continue to feel the contraction for a short time after the woman's discomfort subsides.

Although the above description of uterine contractions is typical, many variants occur. Some women, for example, notice only mild to moderate discomfort even at the period of full intensity of contractions.

Measurement of Intrauterine Pressure

Measurement of intrauterine pressure can give information about the strength of uterine contractions that cannot be obtained by the usual clinical observations. Measurements have shown that intrauterine pressure at the peak of a normal contraction reaches from 35 to 60 mmHg above a normal baseline tone. There is a normal resting basal tone in the uterine muscle between contractions of 5 to 10 mmHg. Then as the uterus contracts the pressure on the amniotic fluid, the intrauterine pressure, rises considerably above this baseline tone. Measurements of the baseline pressure and of the uterine contraction pressure can be made by means of a catheter inserted into the uterine cavity and attached to a recording device (Figs. 14-13, page 323 and 14-14, page 324).

At the beginning of labor the intrauterine pressure may be no higher than 25 mmHg, exclusive of tonus. There is usually a gradual increase in strength of contractions until pressures of 50 to 60 mmHg, exclusive of tonus, are reached toward the end of labor. The Braxton-Hicks contractions of pregnancy may reach an

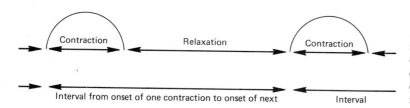

Figure 12-2. Diagram showing increasing, full, and decreasing intensity of uterine contractions, and the interval of relaxation of the uterine muscle.

intrauterine pressure of 20 to 40 mmHg during the last two to three weeks, causing them to be painful.

The exact duration and strength of a contraction cannot be determined precisely without a recording device. For many normal labors, however, clinical evaluation of uterine contractions is adequate for determination of their normalcy.

If thickness and tone of the abdominal wall do not interfere with easy palpation of the uterus, a uterine contraction may be felt by an experienced observer when the amniotic fluid pressure is up to 20 mmHg. The woman ordinarily does not feel the contraction until the pressure reaches about 25 mmHg. When intrauterine pressure reaches 40 mmHg during a contraction, the uterine wall feels very firm and it is too hard to indent. Strength of contractions or amount of pressure must be closely observed during labor, especially when contractions are stimulated, in order to guard against abnormal pressures.

To summarize characteristics of uterine contractions:

1. Uterine contractions during well-established, active labor normally occur about every 3 minutes, last for 50 to 60 seconds, and create an intrauterine pressure of approximately 50 mmHg, exclusive of resting tonus of the uterine muscle.
2. Normal resting baseline tone, or tonus, of the uterine muscle between contractions is 5 to 10 mmHg.
3. There is normally a gradual progressive increase in frequency and intensity of uterine contractions from late pregnancy, through labor, and through delivery.
4. Braxton-Hicks contractions are usually of low amplitude, between 10 and 20 mmHg, but may reach an intrauterine pressure of 20 to 40 mmHg during the latter part of pregnancy, becoming painful.
5. As labor progresses the intensity of the uterine contractions also progresses, from an average intrauterine pressure of 30 mmHg, exclusive of tonus, in early labor to an average of 50 mmHg, exclusive of tonus, in advanced labor, and rising much higher, up to 100 mmHg, during periods of "bearing down" in the second stage.
6. Uterine contractions may be perceived by abdominal palpation when intrauterine pressure reaches 20 mmHg, about 10 mmHg above normal tonus. The uterus feels firm and is too hard to indent at a pressure of 40 mmHg.
7. The woman ordinarily does not perceive pain until the intrauterine pressure reaches 25 mmHg, approximately 15 mmHg above normal tonus.

Changes in the Uterus

Contractions of the uterine muscle bring about changes in the position and shape of the uterus. They cause the uterus to become differentiated into an upper and a lower portion, and they obliterate the cervix. The uterus lies close to the vertebral column when it is relaxed, but during each contraction it is pulled forward against the abdominal wall (Fig. 9-7C, page 209). Such a change in position brings the long axis of the uterus into line with the direction of the birth canal. As contractions progress, the uterus becomes longer and somewhat narrower, and the baby's body becomes a little straighter. With straightening of the body, one pole of the baby pushes against the fundus, and the other pole, usually the head, is pushed farther down into the pelvis. These changes become more marked in the second stage. As lengthening of the uterus is taking place in the first stage, the lower uterine segment and the cervix are pulled upward, an important factor in obliteration of the cervix.

As labor continues, the uterus becomes differentiated into two distinct portions—an upper contractile portion, which becomes thicker as labor advances, and a lower passive portion (the lower uterine segment), which, together with the cervix, becomes thinner and more expanded as labor progresses. This lower uterine portion and the cervix form the fibromuscular canal through which the baby passes as it is pushed out of the uterus. The boundary line between the thickening upper uterine segment and the thinning lower segment becomes quite well defined by a ridge on the inner uterine surface. This ridge or ring is called the *physiologic retraction ring*. It may become pronounced in obstructed labor and is then pathologic (see pages 391–92).

Cervical Effacement and Dilatation

Cervical effacement and cervical dilatation are the major changes of the first stage of labor. *Cervical effacement* is the process by which the cervical canal is progressively shortened to a stage of complete obliteration. During this process, the cervical canal changes from a structure that is from 1 to 2 cm long to one that is so short that a canal no longer exists; all that remains is a circular opening surrounded by very thin tissue, which is often described as "paper-thin." *Cervical dilatation* is the process by which the external os of the cervix enlarges from an orifice that is only a few millimeters in diameter to one that is large enough to permit the baby's head to pass through it (approximately 10 cm) (Fig. 12-1).

Effacement occurs as contractions of the uterine muscle pull the fibers of the cervix closest to the internal os into the lower uterine segment. As the cervix gradually becomes a part of the lower uterine segment in this pulling-up process, it becomes increasingly shorter. The shortening process begins at the internal os, which grows wider, and the cervical canal takes on a funnel-shaped appearance. The funnel becomes increasingly broader at the top and shallower in depth as more and more of the cervix is taken up, until finally only a thin edge of cervix is left at the external os (Fig. 12-3, No. I, No. II, and No. III). As changes take place in the cervix, the mucous plug may be expelled.

Often the cervix has become partly effaced,

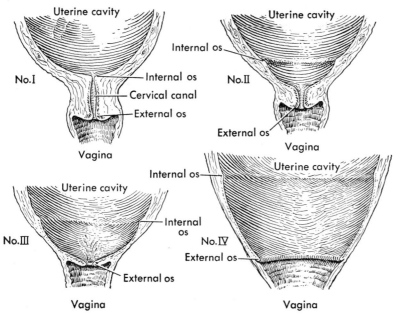

Figure 12-3. Diagrams showing progress in effacement and dilatation of the cervix during labor. No. I. Cervix long and closed. No. II. Internal os is widened, cervical canal is funnel-shaped, and the cervix is shorter. No. III. Effacement is complete, with a thin edge of cervix at the external os; dilatation is just beginning. No. IV. Cervical dilatation is complete.

and in some instances somewhat dilated, during the last weeks of pregnancy as the result of Braxton-Hicks contractions or false labor contractions. Ordinarily labor proceeds more quickly when the cervix is thin and slightly open at the beginning of labor than when it is long and closed at its onset.

After the cervical canal has become completely obliterated and is continuous with the lower uterine segment, dilatation of the external os takes place (Fig. 12-3, No. III and No. IV).

Several factors may be involved in bringing about cervical dilatation. Pressure exerted on the cervix by the bag of waters, sometimes called hydrostatic pressure of the bag of waters, or pressure from the presenting part apparently has considerable effect. Pressure is placed on the amniotic fluid with each uterine contraction; this pressure is distributed equally in all directions and puts considerable tension on the cervix, which is the point of least resistance. In addition, the uterine contractions force the fetal membranes that lie over the cervical canal, and some of the amniotic fluid, into the canal, and the bulging bag of waters, sometimes called the *fore waters,* acts as a dilator (Fig. 12-1). The fetal membranes in the area of the lower uterine segment become loosened from their attachment to underlying tissues early in labor. Such loosening allows the bag of waters to slide into the cervical opening quite freely during contractions. When the membranes rupture before or early in labor, the presenting part of the baby is forced against the cervix during contractions instead of the bag of waters.

In the primigravida the external os of the cervix may be closed or barely admit one fingertip at the beginning of labor, but with subsequent pregnancies the os is usually open enough to allow one fingertip to pass through easily (2 cm dilatation) at the onset of labor.

During the first stage of labor, dilatation of the cervix progresses from a very small opening to complete dilatation, the external os being large enough to permit the baby's head to pass (Fig. 12-3). For the full-term baby this usually means progressive dilatation until the diameter of the os measures approximately 10 cm. In the course of this stretching process the cervix may sustain tiny tears from which blood oozes and tinges the vaginal discharge. The blood-tinged vaginal discharge may appear at the very onset of labor or at any time during the period of dilatation. This oozing of blood, as well as that which may take place when the cervical mucous plug separates, is known as bloody show. The oozing usually increases rather suddenly as the dilatation gets close to completion.

The time required for complete dilatation is usually considerably longer in the primigravida than in the multigravida, whose cervical tissues do not offer as much resistance because of previous dilatation and who may begin labor with the external os slightly dilated. The longer time required for cervical dilatation in the primigravidous woman is the major reason for a longer first stage in a first labor than in subsequent labors.

Descent of the baby in the pelvis ordinarily takes place in the second stage of labor, but it may begin in the first stage. If descent accompanies dilatation, the woman may note increasing, persistent desire to empty the bowels and bladder, because of pressure on these two organs by the presenting part. Also, she may vomit when the cervix becomes nearly or completely dilated, a nervous reflex not wholly understood.

To *ascertain the amount of effacement and dilatation* the cervix is palpated for consistency, length, and size of the external os. Palpation is done by vaginal examination or possibly through the rectovaginal septum by rectal examination. In stating effacement from the findings of the examination, the cervix may be described as long, partly effaced, thin, or obliterated. Its consistency may also be described at this time in terms such as firm or soft. Another method of describing the degree of effacement is to estimate the length of the cervix in centimeters and to state the length in numerical terms, such as 1.5 cm, or 1.0 cm, or 0.5 cm long; when the cervix is very short and cannot be measured by this method, it is said to be paper-thin or obliterated.

For amount of cervical dilatation, an estimate is made of the diameter of the external os. This estimated measurement is stated in centimeters, and the cervix is said to be 2, 3, 4, or more, up to 10, cm dilated. Sometimes, when the os has reached a diameter of approximately 9 cm, the dilatation is described as "a rim of cervix remaining." When a rim of cervix can no longer be felt surrounding the baby's head, dilatation is full or complete. For delivery of a full-term baby the diameter of the cervical opening then measures approximately 10 cm.

The Transition Phase of the First Stage

This latter part of the first stage of labor, during which rapid changes leading to the second stage take place, may be called the *transition phase* (the transition from the first to the second stage of labor). This phase begins when the cervical os has reached a dilatation of 7 or 8 cm and ends with complete dilatation of the cervix. Progress through the transition phase can be expected to occur fairly quickly. This phase is characterized by a decided increase in the degree or intensity of the signs and symptoms of the first stage—in the strength and frequency of uterine contractions, sometimes in the amount of bloody show, and in the amount of pressure in the pelvis caused by descent of the presenting part.

Pattern of Cervical Dilatation

Cervical dilatation in either a primigravida or a multigravida is slow at first, taking much longer for the first half of dilatation than for the latter half. The average pattern of progress of the first stage of labor in primigravidas, a pattern of progress in cervical dilatation plotted against time elapsed in labor, is shown in Figure 12-4. This pattern, or graphic analysis of labor, sometimes called the Friedman labor graph, divides labor into a latent phase and an active phase, and further subdivides the active phase into an acceleration phase, a phase of maximum slope, and a deceleration phase. In a normal labor each of these phases has a characteristic pattern of progress.

The *latent* phase extends from the onset of labor to a point where the curve begins a definite upward trend. During this phase uterine contractions become well established; the cervix thins, making cervical effacement the major change of this phase; and the cervix dilates between 2 and 3 cm. The latent phase may take a number of hours, because considerable time usually elapses between the beginning of true

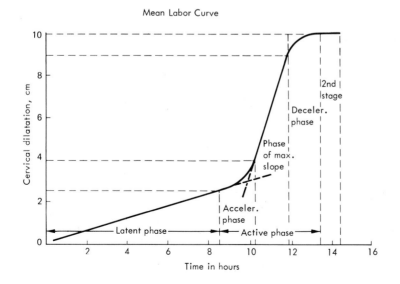

Mean Labor Curve

Figure 12-4. Average labor pattern for nulliparas showing the several phases, obtained by means of plotting cervical dilatation estimates against elapsed time in labor. See text, pages 267–68, for discussion. [*Reprinted with permission from Emanuel A. Friedman: "Use of Labor Pattern as a Management Guide,"* Hosp. Topics *46:58* (Aug.) *1968.*]

labor and the onset of good progress in dilatation. The latent phase in primigravidas averages 8.6 hours and normally does not exceed 20 hours; in multigravidas this phase averages 5.3 hours and usually does not exceed 14 hours.

The *active* phase of labor begins when the curve of estimated cervical dilatation starts a sharp upward trend and ends with complete cervical dilatation. Dilatation now progresses more rapidly. There is an initial period of acceleration when dilatation progresses from 2.5 or 3.0 to 4 cm; a phase of maximum slope between 4 and 9 cm, during which the cervix dilates most rapidly; and a deceleration phase, when dilatation slows somewhat as complete dilatation approaches.

In a normal labor in primigravidas, the slope of active phase of cervical dilatation averages 3.0 cm/hour and is not less than 1.2 cm/hour. In multigravidas, dilatation in the active phase normally proceeds at an average of 5.7 cm/hour and is seldom less than 1.5 cm/hour. At about 9 cm dilatation a deceleration or slowing in dilatation is likely to appear and progress may lag somewhat.

It is apparent from the above description and from Figure 12-4 that the latter half of the first stage of labor in primigravidas may require less than one third as much time as the first half.

In multigravidas the latent phase of labor is slow and may normally be from five to six hours long. The active phase is short, lasting only a few hours and sometimes being completed within one hour. Acceleration of progress in dilatation is usually rapid in multigravidas and the phase of maximum slope is fast. The lag in dilatation at 9 cm may not be apparent in multigravidas, since the deceleration phase may last only minutes. It is apparent that advance in labor in a multigravida is ordinarily rapid after 4 cm of cervical dilatation and that complete dilatation can be expected very soon after the cervix reaches 6 cm dilatation. See Figure 16-1, page 387.

Although the first stage of labor is called the stage of dilatation, only a small part of this period is actually concerned with rapid productive cervical dilatation. There is a long period of time from onset of labor to active dilatation. Some cervical dilatation may have occurred before labor began and a small additional amount takes place during the latent and acceleration phases (up to about 4 cm) but almost all of the dilatation occurs during the relatively short phase of maximum slope.

When the beginning of labor is accepted as the time of onset of regular contractions, the early hours, which may be many, may be considered a preparatory period to active cervical dilatation. This preparatory phase then consists of all of the time from the beginning of regular contractions perceived by the woman through the latent phase and sometimes to the end of the acceleration phase.

Second Stage (Stage of Expulsion)

The second stage of labor is termed the stage of expulsion because it is during this period that the forces of labor move the baby through the birth canal and effect his birth. The "powers" during this stage arise from two sources—contractions of the uterine muscle as in the first stage and now, additionally, voluntary contractions of the abdominal muscles. Resistance to these powers comes from the birth canal, to which the baby's head must accommodate, and the muscles and fascia of the pelvic floor.

If the membranes have not ruptured prior to this time, they frequently rupture at the beginning of the second stage, and the presenting part may suddenly descend somewhat farther in the pelvis. Rupture of the membranes is manifested by a sudden gush of that part of the fluid which is below the baby. Rupture usually occurs at the height of a contraction. After rupture, a little fluid may escape with each contraction. Sometimes the membranes retain their integrity until artificially ruptured to allow for birth of the baby. Very infrequently, the membranes remain intact during birth and the baby is born surrounded by them. In rare instances the baby's head is surrounded by the fetal membranes or covered with a portion thereof at birth. When this happens he is said to be born with a *caul;* a superstitious belief is that this will bring him good luck. In this rare instance, the membranous covering must be removed immediately so that the baby can breathe.

Second-stage uterine contractions are regular at two- to three-minute intervals; they last from 50 to 90 seconds and are very forceful. Intraabdominal pressure, created by strong contractions of the abdominal muscles, is added to intrauterine pressure during the second stage to move the baby through the birth canal.

Contractions of Abdominal Muscles

Contractions of the abdominal muscles are a very important force in expulsion of the baby, but their power must be exerted at the same time that the uterine muscle is contracting. Either one of these forces—uterine muscle contractions or abdominal muscle contractions—when applied alone is only moderately effective. Applied simultaneously they are highly efficient in expulsion.

Contractions of the abdominal muscles are controlled voluntarily at first. The woman is able to increase their power by taking a deep breath, closing her lips, holding her breath, bracing her feet, pulling against something with her hands, and straining with all her might—"bearing down." Such action contracts the abdominal muscles and forces the diaphragm down; this increases intraabdominal pressure and thus pressure on the uterus. The bearing-down action is similar to that involved in the process of defecation, but must be greatly intensified to be effective in moving the baby through the birth canal.

During the second stage, the woman is instructed to add the secondary force of abdominal muscles by contracting them and pushing downward as long as each uterine contraction persists. "Bearing down" superimposes 50 or more mmHg pressure on the intrauterine pressure of a contraction. This brings the total pressure up to 100 or more mmHg, depending upon the strength of the contraction and the ability of the woman to apply abdominal muscle pressure.

As the second stage progresses, especially when the head reaches the perineal floor, the bearing-down process becomes virtually involuntary; there is then an intense urge to push. Under normal conditions, the baby descends a little farther through the birth canal with each simultaneous uterine contraction and bearing-down effort.

Birth of the Baby

The vagina and perineum have been prepared for the tremendous amount of stretching that is necessary to allow for passage of the baby. Changes that have taken place are hypertrophy and increased fluid content of tissues and an increased vascularity of these structures. The changes are most marked in the levator ani muscles, which must be stretched considerably, and in the perineal body, which is changed from a thick, wedge-shaped mass of tissue to a very thin structure as the baby passes through the birth canal.

When the baby descends in the birth canal and the presenting part comes well down in the vagina, the perineum begins to bulge, and soon the presenting part becomes visible at the vaginal opening. With each contraction the perineum becomes more distended. The vaginal opening is stretched to an ever-greater diameter, changing from a small, narrow opening to one that is first ovoid in shape and finally wide and round (Fig. 12-5). With each expulsive effort more of the presentimg part becomes visible. The presenting part advances with each contraction, slips back a little as the contraction subsides, but progresses somewhat farther with the next contraction. When the head has advanced so far that its widest diameter (the biparietal area) is encircled by the vaginal opening, it is said to be *crowning* (Fig. 12-5). After crowning occurs, the head does not recede between contractions, and the baby is soon delivered.

By the time the head crowns, the perineum has become very thin and very tense; it may be so stretched that it tears downward from the vaginal opening unless it is incised by the physi-

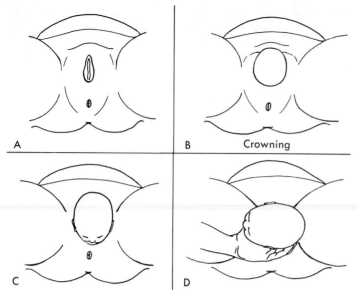

Figure 12-5. Birth of the head. [*Adapted from Anita M. Jones, A Manual for Teaching Midwives. U.S. Department of Labor (Now U.S. Department of Health, Education, and Welfare), Children's Bureau, Washington, D.C., 1939.*]

cian to enlarge the opening. The pressure of the head often distends the anus at this time so that the anterior rectal wall can be seen through it.

The head is born during the one or two contractions that occur after crowning. The perineum retracts under the baby's chin as soon as the head is born (Fig. 12-5). After the birth of the head, with the next one or two contractions, the rest of the body is delivered. As soon as the baby is born, the amniotic fluid that was behind the baby's body drains out of the vagina in a steady stream or with a gush and may be followed by a small amount of blood.

The mother puts forth tremendous efforts during the second stage of labor. The strong, frequent uterine contractions allow for only very short intervals of rest, and her exertion in forcefully contracting her abdominal muscles may cause her to perspire freely and to become very flushed. The second stage ends with a great sense of relief following birth of the baby.

Like the first stage, the second stage of labor requires a longer time for completion in the primigravida than in the multigravida. During this stage, the resistance of the pelvic floor and of the perineum slows progress in the primigravida; after these tissues have once been stretched, their resistance is overcome more easily. Sometimes only a few contractions are necessary to complete the second stage in the multigravida.

Mechanism of Labor

The *mechanism of labor* is defined as the sequence of passive movements of the presenting part that permits passage through the birth canal. It is the adjustment that the passenger makes to the passage. The majority of positional changes comprising the mechanism of labor consist of twisting and curving movements of the fetal head, by which it is adapted to the size and shape of the maternal pelvis. Again in the following discussion, a normal vertex position will be assumed.

The long diameter of the baby's head first conforms to one of the long diameters of the inlet (Fig. 10-2, page 232) and then turns so that the length of the head is lying anteroposterior in conformity to the long diameter of the outlet (Fig. 10-5, page 234). The head must also flex in its passage through the pelvic canal so that its smallest circumference presents, and later it must extend to emerge from the canal. As the head descends and rotates, it also describes an arc, because the posterior wall of the pelvis, consisting of the sacrum and coccyx, is about three times as deep as the anterior wall formed by the symphysis pubis (Fig. 10-3, page 233). That part of the baby's head which passes along the posterior wall must therefore travel three times as far in a given time as the part which moves downward under the short symphysis pubis.

The several movements of the baby's head as it accommodates to the birth canal during its passage through the canal are described as engagement, descent, flexion, internal rotation, extension, and external rotation. The mechanism of expulsion of the rest of the body consists of rotation and birth of the shoulders, which takes place immediately after delivery of the head, and rapid birth of the rest of the body.

Although the movements of the head are usually described separately, they do not take place independently; descent takes place during other movements, and several others may also occur simultaneously. Most of the movements occur during the second stage of labor, but those of descent and flexion begin before or soon after the onset of labor and continue to a slight degree during the first stage.

ENGAGEMENT   Engagement (described on page 249) is the mechanism by which the fetal head enters the pelvis. This movement takes place prior to labor or early in labor and is the beginning of the movement of descent. In this first movement of accommodation of the fetal head to the pelvis, the head enters the pelvis with its long diameter, the suboccipitobregmatic or at times the occipitofrontal, conforming to one of the long diameters of the inlet, frequently the transverse diameter but also one or the other of the obliques.

DESCENT   Descent begins with engagement and continues until the baby is delivered (Fig. 12-6). It is therefore a movement that occurs simultaneously with the others. If the head is already engaged and deep in the pelvis at the onset of labor, there may be very little or no fur-

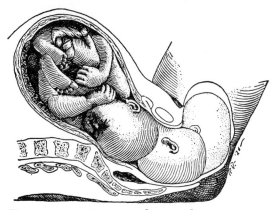

Figure 12-6.   Diagram indicating descent, flexion, internal rotation, and extension of the baby's head during birth.

ther descent until the cervix is fully dilated. If the head is not in the pelvis at the onset of labor, descent begins in the first stage at the time at which the head engages.

FLEXION   In the normal fetal posture (attitude) during the latter part of pregnancy the head is flexed to some degree. When the head descends into and through the pelvis, it becomes more flexed as it meets with resistance; the chin comes closer toward the thorax, and the occiput becomes the lowermost part (Fig. 11-3, page 245). In extreme flexion the head is in a position whereby its smallest circumference is presented to the birth canal. In marked flexion the suboccipitobregmatic diameter, 9.5 cm, is substituted for the occipitofrontal diameter, 11.75 cm, of a less flexed head. (See Fig. 10-11, page 241, for diameters of fetal head.) Flexion therefore reduces the diameters of the fetal head that are presented in the birth canal.

The point at which extreme flexion takes place varies. If the pelvic inlet is somewhat small for the size of the fetal head, marked flexion may be necessary before the head can engage in the pelvis. If the head has entered the pelvic inlet with only moderate flexion, further movement of the chin toward the thorax usually takes place when the head meets the resistance of the pelvic floor, but sometimes earlier, occurring when the head is pushed against the cervix or against the walls of the pelvis.

INTERNAL ROTATION The fetal head, which entered the pelvis with its long diameter (suboccipitobregmatic or sometimes occipitofrontal) conforming to one of the long diameters of the inlet, must rotate in the pelvic canal before it can emerge from the outlet. The long diameter of the head must conform to the long diameter of the outlet before birth can take place; the sagittal suture then occupies the anteroposterior diameter of the outlet (Fig. 12-6). Rotation takes place sometime during the descent which follows engagement. It often occurs before the head reaches the pelvic floor, but sometimes not until the head meets the resistance of those tissues. As the head is pushed downward, the structure of the midpelvis, the resistance of the muscles and fascia of the pelvic floor, and the groovelike shape that the floor assumes when it is depressed bring about rotation.

When the head rotates, it usually turns in the direction that will bring the occiput toward the symphysis pubis. In some instances, however, when the occiput occupies one of the posterior segments of the pelvis, the head moves in a direction that will bring the occiput toward the sacrum. The distance that the head must rotate will depend on the position in which it entered the pelvis. When the head enters the pelvis with its anteroposterior diameter conforming to the transverse diameter of the inlet, the sagittal suture lies at right angles to the anteroposterior diameter of the outlet. For the head then to occupy a position in which the sagittal suture will conform to the anteroposterior diameter of the outlet and the occiput to lie behind the symphysis pubis, the head must rotate through an arc of 90 degrees (Fig. 12-7).

When the head enters the pelvis with its anteroposterior diameter conforming to one of the oblique diameters of the inlet, the occiput may occupy either the anterior or the posterior segment of the right side of the mother's pelvis or the anterior or posterior segment of the left

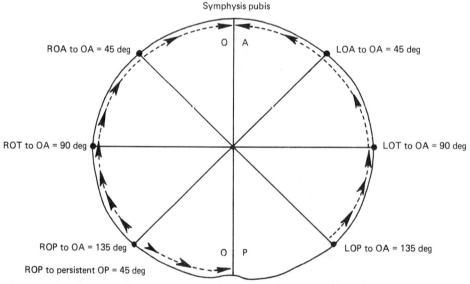

Figure 12-7. Diagram illustrating degree of rotation of the fetal head in the pelvis from an occiput anterior, transverse, or posterior position to a direct occiput anterior, and from a right occiput posterior position to a direct occiput posterior, becoming a persistent occiput posterior position. The heavy dots in the illustration indicate the position occupied by the occiput. The arrows show the direction of rotation. See text for detailed explanation.

side. When the occiput occupies either of the anterior segments of the pelvis, it rotates 45 degrees to reach the symphysis pubis; from the posterior segments of the pelvis it must rotate 135 degrees to lie underneath the symphysis (Fig. 12-7). Since rotation from the posterior segment of the pelvis is through a greater arc, internal rotation takes longer from the posterior position than from the transverse or anterior position.

Occasionally, when the occiput occupies the posterior segment of the pelvis, it rotates toward the hollow of the sacrum instead of anteriorly toward the symphysis pubis, becoming then a "persistent occiput posterior" (Fig. 12-7). When the head is delivered with the occiput posterior (the face upward), the perineum is distended more than usual during delivery, and a deep incision of the perineal tissues is often necessary. Occasionally the head fails to rotate from the transverse position; this condition is called deep transverse arrest. These failures of normal rotation and their management are described on pages 392–93.

EXTENSION   Extension takes place following internal rotation. The head, which is greatly flexed as it reaches the pelvic floor, must be extended to be born. This is essential because the vaginal opening is directed upward and a flexed head would only be forced down against the pelvic floor where it could not be delivered.

As the head is pushed down by the contractions, the resistance of the pelvic floor pushes it forward and toward the vaginal opening, thereby bringing about extension. The occiput passes under the symphysis pubis and appears at the distended vaginal outlet while the face passes down the posterior wall and along the floor of the pelvis (Fig. 12-6). The base of the occiput comes to lie firmly against the lower margin of the symphysis pubis, where it remains and acts as a point around which the head pivots until the entire head is born. With continuing pressure from the rapidly succeeding contractions, extension of the head increases as it pivots around the symphysis pubis; the occiput rises in

front of the symphysis, and the face moves farther downward and forward. More and more of the occiput becomes visible at the vaginal opening, and with continuing extension of the head the bregma appears over the anterior margin of the perineum; then the brow, eyes, nose, mouth, and chin appear in turn; soon the entire head is born (Fig. 12-5). The baby's head then drops forward in relation to its own body, with its chin resting very close to the mother's anal region.

EXTERNAL ROTATION   A few moments after birth of the head, the neck, which became somewhat twisted during internal rotation of the head, untwists. In so doing the occiput rotates toward either the mother's right or left thigh, the direction depending on fetal position before birth (Fig. 12-5). In this movement, sometimes called *restitution*, the occiput resumes the relationship it bore to the pelvis before internal rotation. The head then turns somewhat more to-

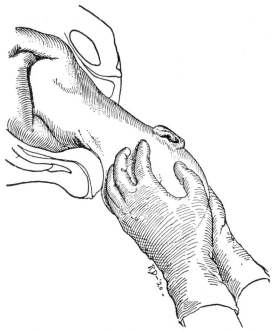

Figure 12-8. *Gentle* downward traction is sometimes made to impinge the anterior shoulder under the symphysis pubis.

ward the right or left when the baby's shoulders, which enter the pelvis in a transverse position, rotate to the anteroposterior position, with one shoulder near the symphysis pubis and the other shoulder resting on the perineum (Fig. 12-8). As the shoulders rotate internally, the head, which is on the outside, rotates externally.

EXPULSION *Delivery of the shoulders* takes place quickly after external rotation of the head. Almost immediately the anterior shoulder becomes fixed under the symphysis pubis; very soon the posterior shoulder is delivered over the perineum by pivoting upward; and promptly thereafter the anterior shoulder follows (Figs. 12-8 and 12-9). Sometimes the anterior shoulder delivers first. After the shoulders are delivered, *expulsion of the rest of the body* is rapid. A definite mechanism is not necessary for birth of the rest of the baby, which is smaller than the head and shoulders, but the body follows the upward curve of the lower part of the birth canal.

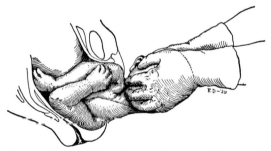

Figure 12-9. Lifting the head during delivery of posterior shoulder.

Pattern of Descent of the Fetus

As with the pattern of cervical dilatation, the pattern of descent of the presenting part of the fetus may be divided into a latent phase and an active phase, with a slow beginning of active phase, and a later phase of maximum slope (Fig. 12-10). Until cervical dilatation enters the phase of maximum slope, there is essentially no downward movement of the presenting part of the fetus from its station at the onset of labor. After

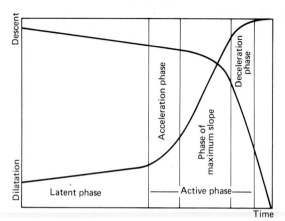

Figure 12-10. Graphic display of the normal patterns of cervical dilatation and descent of the presenting part showing the characteristic phases of the first stage. [*Reprinted with permission from Emanuel A. Friedman, "Patterns of Labor as Indicators of Risk," Clin. Obstet. Gynecol. 16:172–183 (Mar.) 1973, p. 176.*]

such a latent phase, descent slowly begins its active phase during the phase of maximum slope of cervical dilatation.

Descent reaches its maximum slope at the same time that the dilatation curve begins the deceleration phase. Thus, when dilatation of the cervix is nearly complete the presenting part begins its descent through the pelvis in a fairly rapid, progressive manner. The phase of deceleration of labor is thus a combination of progressive cervical dilatation, although somewhat slower, and beginning of rapid descent.

Descent of the presenting part of the fetus continues its steady downward movement to the end of the second stage of labor, normally proceeding in an uninterrupted linear descent until it reaches the perineum and thereafter is delivered from the birth canal. In continuing its steady downward movement the presenting part adjusts to the pelvis according to the cardinal movements of the mechanism of labor.

The slope of descent, without complicating factors, averages 1.6 cm/hour in primigravidas and is normally greater than 1.0 cm/hour. In multigravidas it averages 5.4 cm/hour and is normally greater than 2.1 cm/hour.

Evaluation of the Labor Pattern

To determine if labor is progressing satisfactorily and within the wide variation that is possible in normal labors, it is very helpful to examine the progress of each woman in labor according to the normal curves of dilatation and descent. Figure 12-10 shows the cervical dilatation and the descent curves as they interrelate in a normal labor.

Labor curves can easily be constructed for each woman in labor, using a graph as shown in Figure 12-11. As the progress of labor is recorded, a pattern of progress of cervical dilatation and progress of descent of the presenting part evolves. From observation of these patterns a fairly objective evaluation of the progress of labor can be made. If abnormal patterns in any of the phases of labor develop, they can be recognized early and managed as described in Chapter 16.

Third Stage (Placental Stage)

The third stage of labor, called the placental stage because the placenta is delivered during this period, is made up of two phases—the phase of placental separation and the phase of placental expulsion.

At the beginning of the third stage, the

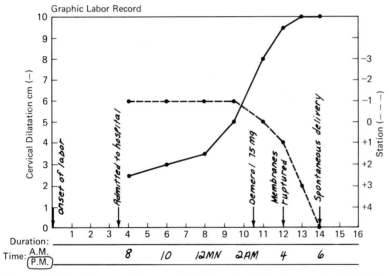

Figure 12-11. Representative graphic labor record showing cervical dilatation and descent patterns as they evolved, taken from a patient's hospital chart. [*Reprinted with permission from Emanuel A. Friedman, "Patterns of Labor as Indicators of Risk," Clin. Obstet. Gynecol. 16:172–173 (Mar.) 1973, p. 175.*]

Using a square-ruled graph paper, the hours of labor are written across the paper horizontally, numbers are written along the left side in ascending order to represent centimeters of cervical dilatation, and numbers are written along the right side in descending order to denote station of the present part.

The onset of labor is recorded as the time of onset of regular uterine contractions as perceived by the woman herself. Each examination for cervical dilatation and station of the present part is recorded on the appropriate line along with the time of the examination. As each recording is joined to the previous notation, a pattern of cervical dilatation and descent of the presenting part evolves.

uterus, which contracted down as its contents were diminishing during the birth of the baby, is a firm mass above a collapsed lower uterine segment and is quite freely movable in the abdominal cavity. Its walls are considerably thicker than they were earlier in labor, and it has so decreased in size that the top of the fundus lies slightly below the umbilicus. Its cavity now contains only the placenta and the fetal membranes.

Placental Separation

Contractions of the uterine muscle continue at three- to four-minute intervals as in the first and second stages, but with minimal or no discomfort; they can be felt by an examiner palpating the uterus through the abdominal wall. On palpation of the uterus one may note a perceptible change in shape with contraction and relaxation. While the placenta is attached, the uterus assumes a globular shape during a contraction and a flattened (discoid) shape during relaxation; after the placenta is separated, its shape is globular also during relaxation. A persistent globular shape is therefore a sign of placental separation.

With the sudden decrease in the overall size of the uterus as the baby is born, there is a corresponding decrease in the surface area at the site of placental attachment. With this decrease in size, the placenta becomes considerably thicker, but being a noncontractile organ, it cannot completely accommodate itself to the decreased area of its place of attachment. It begins to fold up and is literally squeezed off the uterine wall. Separation usually takes place in the first few minutes of the third stage; it may occur as soon as the baby is born or may take place during the next few contractions of the uterine muscle.

Placental separation takes place in the spongy layer of the decidua, and a portion of the decidua is expelled with the placenta. Detachment usually begins at the center of the placenta, but sometimes it starts at its edges (Fig. 12-12). Some bleeding accompanies separation. When detachment begins at the center of the placenta and progresses to its margins, blood collects in the space behind the placenta and generally does not appear until the placenta is expelled. When separation starts at the edges, there may be a continuous trickling of blood throughout the third stage.

The fetal membranes and the decidua vera are also unable to accommodate to the decreased uterine size; they become thicker, but cannot completely adjust themselves, and their separation begins. Separation of the membranes is completed by traction of the placenta. As the placenta slides out of the uterus, the membranes, which are continuous with it, are dragged along and are peeled from the inner surface of the uterus.

Placental Expulsion

After the placenta is separated, the continuing uterine contractions push it out of the upper cavity into the relaxed lower uterine segment or into the upper portion of the vagina. As it slides into the lower segment, it fills this cavity, which has been collapsed, and pushes the fundus upward. After expulsion of the placenta from the upper segment, the uterine muscle contracts firmly and the cavity of the fundus becomes very small. Uterine contractions do not effect further expulsion of the placenta. It lies in the lower uterine segment or the vagina as a foreign body until additional pressure is applied to it, either by abdominal muscle contractions, as in the second stage of labor, or by manual means.

The placenta can be delivered by bearing-down efforts of the mother, which increase intraabdominal pressure, but this method may take considerable time or may be impossible if the mother is under the influence of analgesia or anesthesia. Its expulsion from the lower uterine segment or the vagina is therefore usually completed manually. To some extent the length of the third stage varies according to the time that elapses before effort is made to express the placenta. When the physician expresses the placenta, he places his hand over the fundus of the uterus and makes downward pressure on it; the uterus in turn places pressure on the placenta

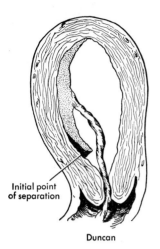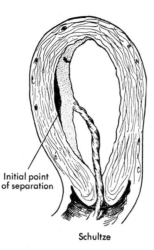

Initial point of separation

Initial point of separation

Duncan

Schultze

Figure 12-12. Diagrams showing the Duncan and Schultze mechanisms of placental separation and extrusion.

and pushes it out of the vagina. The fetal membranes, because of their attachment to the placenta, follow immediately.

Signs of Placental Separation and Expulsion from the Upper Uterine Segment

Four signs generally make their appearance when the placenta has separated and dropped into the lower uterine segment. The uterus changes from a discoid to a *globular shape* when the placenta separates; this shape *persists* during relaxation as well as during contraction. There is usually *bleeding from the vagina* with separation; this may come with a gush if the placenta has separated from its center first, or it may appear as a continuous trickling when separation begins at the edges. As the placenta sinks into the lower uterine segment or into the vagina, the *fundus rises* up to or above the umbilicus, and the *umbilical cord*, which is protruding from the vagina, becomes *limp* and *advances* several inches.

Mechanism of Extrusion of the Placenta

As the placenta is delivered, it appears at the vaginal outlet with either the fetal or the maternal surface foremost. In the most common method, known as the *Schultze mechanism,* the placenta becomes inverted on itself, and the

glistening fetal surface appears at the vaginal outlet first. There is ordinarily little bleeding before the placenta is extruded; blood from the placental site collects behind the placenta and follows immediately after its expulsion (Fig. 12-12). Less frequently, the placenta descends sideways and presents at the vaginal outlet with its roughened maternal surface; this is called the *Duncan mechanism.* It is usually acompanied by slight but continuous bleeding during the third stage (Fig. 12-12).

Contraction of Uterine Muscle Following Third Stage.

The uterus continues contracting as separation and expulsion of the placenta take place. It becomes a solid mass of muscle that lies below the level of the umbilicus; its walls are thick and lie so close to each other that they practically obliterate the cavity (Fig. 12-13 and 12-14). The tightly contracted muscle fibers constrict the large blood vessels that were opened up at the placental site with separation of the placenta, and they control bleeding by acting as ligatures. Inadequate muscle contraction results in excessive bleeding (described under the heading "Postpartum Hemorrhage" on pages 692–96).

A certain amount of bleeding takes place from the placental site during the third stage of labor

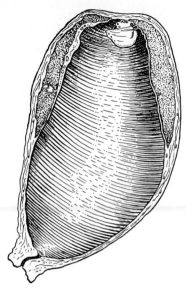

Figure 12-13. Longitudinal section through uterus showing thinness of uterine wall before expulsion of fetus, contrasting sharply with thickened wall in Figure 12-14—twin placentas are still adherent in upper segment. [*Drawing of photograph of specimen in the obstetrical laboratory, Johns Hopkins Hospital.*]

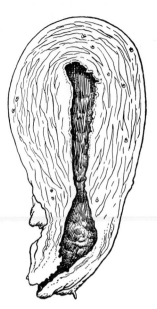

Figure 12-14. Longitudinal section through uterus, immediately after delivery, showing marked thickening of wall as a result of muscular contraction. [*Drawing of photograph of specimen in the obstetrical laboratory, Johns Hopkins Hospital.*]

even when muscle contraction is excellent; the amount varies from 50 to 200 ml (1.7 to 7 oz). In addition, there is some bleeding from an episiotomy. The total amount of blood lost in the third stage if often from 200 to 300 ml (7 to 10 oz).

The necessary continuous observation of the mother during the first hour or longer after delivery for excessive bleeding and for systemic reactions to the stress of labor is described on pages 378–81. After the completion of labor, which is an exhausting experience, the mother is in great need of rest. Unless labor has been short, she is very tired physically and, in addition, has been under considerable emotional strain. At the same time, however, she is promptly wide awake, exhilarated by the birth of the baby and the feeling of relief that the labor is finished, and she is not immediately aware of her exhaustion.

The mother also has a great need to see and hold her baby immediately after birth. She should be given this opportunity just as soon as possible so that mother and baby can begin to form a close attachment to each other in this first very early period after birth.

After seeing and holding her baby and visiting with her husband she may be ready for rest and sleep.

BIBLIOGRAPHY

Caldeyro-Barcia, Roberto, and Poserio, Juan J., Physiology of the uterine contraction, *Clin. Obstet. Gynecol.* 3:386–408 (June) 1960.
———, *et al.*, Effect of position changes on the intensity and frequency of uterine contractions during labor, *Am. J. Obstet. Gynecol.* 80:284–290 (Aug.) 1960.
Danforth, David N. (ed.), *Obstetrics and Gynecology*, 3rd ed. Harper and Row, New York, 1977.
Friedman, Emanuel A., Patterns of labor as indicators of risk, *Clin. Obstet. Gynecol.* 16:172–183 (Mar.) 1973.
———, The functional divisions of labor, *Am. J. Obstet. Gynecol.* 109:274–280 (Jan. 15) 1971.

————, An objective method of evaluating labor, *Hosp. Pract.* 5:82–87 (July) 1970.

————, Use of labor pattern as a management guide, *Hosp. Topics* 46:57–59 (Aug.) 1968.

Greenhill, J. P., and Friedman, Emanuel A., *Biological Principles and Modern Practice of Obstetrics.* Saunders, Philadelphia, Pa., 1974.

Martin, Joseph E., and Pauerstein, Carl J., The initiation of labor, in *Clinical Anesthesia. Parturition and Perinatology,* edited by Gertie F. Marx. Davis, Philadelphia, Pa., 1973, pp. 51–69.

Oxorn, Harry, and Foote, William, *Human Labor and Birth,* 3rd ed. Appleton-Century-Crofts, New York, 1975.

Pritchard, Jack A., and MacDonald, Paul C., *Williams Obstetrics,* 15th ed. Appleton-Century-Crofts, New York, 1975.

Reid, Duncan E., Ryan, Kenneth J., and Benirschke, Kurt. *Principles and Management of Human Reproduction.* Saunders, Philadelphia, Pa., 1972.

Speroff, Leon, What initiates labor, *Contemp. Ob/Gyn* 7:113–121 (May) 1976.

Vorherr, Helmuth, Disorders of uterine function during pregnancy, labor, and puerperium, in *Pathophysiology of Gestation,* edited by Nicholas S. Assali. Academic Press, New York, 1972, pp. 145–268.

13

Analgesia and Anesthesia During Labor and Delivery

Anesthesia was introduced into obstetric practice in 1847 by Sir James Y. Simpson of Scotland, who first used ether, and later chloroform. Its use in the United States was subsequently introduced by Dr. Walter Channing of Boston. In the early days the use of anesthesia for delivery was greeted with a storm of protest, from both the clergy and the laity, because of their belief that pain relief of women in childbirth was contrary to the teachings of the Bible.

In the majority of cases today some agent is used to lessen the discomfort of labor and delivery. Since the first introduction of anesthesia for delivery, many different drugs have been used for analgesia, amnesia, and anesthesia during both labor and delivery. Some methods of pain relief have had deleterious effects on mother and/or baby. Judicious use of drugs, carefully chosen for the individual woman and the existing conditions, will give considerable relief of discomfort, with comparative safety for both mother and baby. Since there is no single satisfactory method of analgesia or anesthesia during labor and delivery, the drug chosen and its method of administration is that which appears to be best suited for the specific situation.

In recent years, several different methods of preparation for childbirth, all with basic similarities but also with some marked differences, have

been introduced. The amount of analgesia and anesthesia necessary to relieve discomfort is often considerably reduced for mothers who are physically and psychologically prepared for labor. Some of these mothers do not require pain-relieving drugs.

Analgesia and anesthesia during labor and delivery present special problems not encountered in the nonpregnant individual. During pregnancy, two persons, mother and baby, must always be considered. Every systemic drug can be expected to cross the placenta and influence the fetus. Slight maternal hypoxia, having little or no effect on the mother, may have an untoward effect on the baby. Similarly, if maternal hypotension follows administration of a drug, it may adversely affect the fetus. The influence of the drug on uterine contractions requires consideration. Planned preparation for anesthesia, such as withholding food and fluids for an ample period of time prior to its administration, is often not possible in obstetric clients.

Methods used to relieve discomforts of labor and delivery are primarily psychologic and physical preparation for labor, administration of drugs that have a systemic effect, and use of conduction or nerve-block techniques.

Education-for-childbirth programs prepare mothers for labor by helping them understand its physical and emotional aspects and by teaching controlled relaxation and breathing techniques that may be used during labor and delivery. The prepared mother is less distressed by the pain of labor than the mother who is unprepared. She is better able to cope with the discomfort of labor than the woman who is fearful and anxious, and she is less concerned with the various phenomena of labor because she knows what to anticipate.

Preparation for childbirth does not preclude use of analgesia and anesthesia. The need for medication is minimized, however, when the mother is trained how to respond to contractions and when she has support and guidance in her efforts from an interested and skilled person.

Emotional support during labor can also help alleviate discomfort in mothers unprepared for labor. Often they can be assisted with proper breathing during contractions through instructions given at the moment. Such help is likely to reduce their need for pain-relieving medications.

Hypnosis is occasionally used to reduce use of drugs and anesthesia during childbirth. With adequate time for preparation and a receptive client, this method allows some women on whom it is used to go through labor and delivery without analgesia or with only a minimal amount of medication. Hypnosis has limited application. It is time consuming, it requires special training in its use, and some women are poor risks for hypnosis.

ANALGESIC, SEDATIVE, AND AMNESIC DRUGS

Drugs with a systemic effect are administered to the majority of women in labor to reduce the discomfort of uterine contractions. Since systemic drugs readily pass through the placenta, their effect on the fetus is always an important consideration. The kind of drug, its dosage, and time of administration are determined by the mother's physical condition, the baby's maturity and general condition, and the progress of labor.

Particular caution is used when labor is premature.

Pain cannot be completely eliminated with systemic drugs, but the mother can usually be made reasonably comfortable.

Analgesic Drugs

One of the synthetic narcotic drugs is often given during labor. Among those commonly used are meperidine (Demerol), alphaprodine (Nisentil), anileridine (Leritine), and pentazocaine (Talwin).

Demerol has been widely used. It resembles morphine as an analgesic and atropine as an antispasmodic. Less potent and depressing than morphine, in therapeutic doses, it also has a relatively shorter action, with slight sedative effects. It is administered intramuscularly in a dose of 50 to 100 mg.

Nisentil is closely related to Demerol, but its action is more rapid and of shorter duration. It is used in doses of 20 to 40 mg. Leritine is also closely related to Demerol, but with considerably greater potency. Its sedative effect seems to be less. It is given intramuscularly in a dose of 25 to 50 mg. Its respiratory depressant effect, as compared to morphine and meperidine, appears to be the same in depth, but shorter in duration in the mother. It appears, however, to have a greater depressant effect on the newborn than meperidine. Talwin, used in dosage of 30 or 40 mg, appears to provide good analgesia but does not appear to be significantly different from meperidine in either providing analgesia for the mother or resulting in depression in the newborn.

A narcotic drug is often given when the mother is making definite progress in labor, having reached 4- or 5-cm cervical dilatation. If it is possible to predict the rapidity of labor, a narcotic is usually given at least two and preferably three hours before the anticipated time of delivery. After administration, the mother's discomfort is considerably reduced in degree, but she usually continues to be aware of some pain, especially at the height of a contraction. She usually rests well between contractions for two or more hours. In a long labor the drug may be repeated after several hours.

Barbiturates

A short-acting barbiturate, pentobarbital (Nembutal) or secobarbital (Seconal), may be given during labor for its sedative and hypnotic effects. If used, it is usually given early in labor to relieve tension and permit relaxation, to provide rest, and to produce sleep. The usual dose of Nembutal or Seconal ranges from 100 to 200 mg, given orally or intramuscularly.

Barbiturates do not provide analgesia. When pain increases, a narcotic is usually administered. Barbiturates alone in the presence of severe pain may cause restlessness and excitement, sometimes extreme.

Tranquilizing Drugs

Some of the phenothiazine derivatives are used during labor for their tranquilizing effect. They are sometimes used alone, but often as an adjunct to an analgesic. Hydroxyzine hydrochloride (Atarax, Vistaril) is widely used. Among other phenothiazine derivatives used during labor for their sedative and tranquilizing actions are propiomazine hydrochloride (Largon) and promethazine hydrochloride (Phenergan). Diazepam (Valium) is another tranquilizer that is sometimes used as an adjunct in obstetric analgesia. It is both a sedative and a muscle relaxant and may therefore be used as an anticonvulsant for preeclampsia–eclampsia treatment. As with other tranquilizers, when used along with an analgesic drug, the dosage of the analgesic can be considerably reduced.

A tranquilizing drug is sometimes given early in labor if the client is tense and apprehensive. At other times it is given to augment an analgesic drug. The tranquilizers markedly enhance the sedative action of narcotics and barbiturates. The dosage of a narcotic or a barbiturate is, therefore, decreased by one half when it is used in conjunction with a tranquilizer.

Scopolamine

Scopolamine may be used in combination with an analgesic drug, but it is currently used infrequently. Dosage is usually 0.3 mg (1/200 gr).

Scopolamine, if used, is given for its amnesic effect. A usual effect of scopolamine is drowsiness, but in women who have pain it may produce excitement and restlessness. The mother rests and often sleeps between contractions, but may become restless and excited during a contraction. She may complain bitterly of pain during contractions, but after delivery usually has little recollection of discomfort. A restless mother must have someone with her constantly. The excitement the drug causes in the presence of pain contraindicates its use alone or in women who have not had a good effect from an analgesic.

Preparation and Observation of Client Receiving Medication

To obtain maximum effect of a drug, the mother is psychically prepared by being told she is being given something for pain relief. She is made as comfortable as possible physically by a change of pads and bed linens, and she is helped to a comfortable position. An environment conducive to relaxation is important. The room is darkened, unnecessary noise is excluded, and the temperature of the room is adjusted to the mother's comfort. She should remain in bed after receiving medication.

The mother's vital signs and the fetal heart are checked before a drug is given and carefully observed after administration. For evidence of respiratory depression the mother's respirations are counted for 30 seconds when she is not having a contraction. Capillary refill time may be observed by pressure on the forehead or the nailbeds to check for cardiovascular depression. If a mother's reaction to a drug is excitement and restlessness, she must have someone with her continuously. In addition, side rails are used to help prevent injury from a fall.

Progress of labor is carefully observed after a drug for pain relief is administered. Labor may be slowed, but often it progresses rapidly. After medication the mother feels less pain to strong contractions and her reactions are less dependable in determining the progress of labor.

INHALATION ANALGESIA AND ANESTHESIA

Inhalation anesthetics relieve pain by general depression of the nervous system. Among those used are nitrous oxide, cyclopropane, ether, halothane, and methoxyflurane. In obstetrics one of these agents is sometimes used during the latter part of the first stage of labor to produce analgesia and during the second stage either to anesthetize the mother for delivery or to provide analgesia during contractions. The latter means that the agent is given with each contraction, but consciousness is maintained. Many volatile anesthetics produce analgesia before loss of consciousness, but nitrous oxide and methoxyflurane are the most satisfactory for intermittent use, to relieve pain with each contraction.

Nitrous oxide and oxygen may be used to produce analgesia with each contraction during the second stage of labor. This is given as soon as the mother begins to have a contraction. She is relieved of pain, but remains conscious. Occasionally this method of analgesia is begun late in the first stage.

High concentrations of the gas may be required to produce analgesia. It must be carefully administered to avoid hypoxia in the fetus. Its concentration is varied, as indicated by the reactions of the baby and the strength and duration of the contractions, but is never increased to a level whereby the woman becomes cyanotic. Properly administered, it may be used for analgesia over a rather long period of time during the second stage of labor without reducing contractions and without danger to mother or baby.

During second-stage contractions the mother is asked to take two or three deep breaths of the nitrous oxide and oxygen mixture and with her lungs full to hold her breath and bear down as long as possible. If the contraction is long, she takes another deep breath and bears down a second or even a third time. As soon as the contraction begins to subside, pure oxygen is given to get as much as possible to the baby. Nitrous oxide may be used as an analgesic agent up to or even during actual delivery. During delivery of the fetal head the analgesia may be deepened with the mixture or may be augmented with another agent. Nitrous oxide will not produce deep anesthesia.

Cyclopropane is frequently used as an anesthetic for operative deliveries. It may also be used to augment nitrous oxide for delivery of the baby's head, because a much higher concentration of oxygen can then be given. It is not used for intermittent pain relief because of its explosive nature, which makes frequent removal of the mask a potential explosion hazard.

Ether is sometimes used, mainly for continuous anesthesia, as in operative deliveries. It gives good muscle relaxation. It is not very satisfactory for analgesia because it takes effect so slowly that the mother may not get its maximum effect at the height of her contractions. It is unpleasant to her because of its irritation to the respiratory passages.

Ether has a wider margin of safety than most of the anesthetic agents. It can be administered by an open-drop method with a cylinder fitting quite snugly over the mother's mouth and nose. It also is irritating to the skin, and petroleum jelly may be applied to the face for protection. The eyes may be protected by covering them. With administration of ether the chin may drop because of relaxation, and it is supported to prevent obstruction of the airway.

Methoxyflurane (Pentrane) is a potent inhalation anesthetic agent. It may be used for analgesia during the later part of the first stage of labor and during bearing-down contractions and delivery of the baby in the second stage. It is also sufficiently effective for general anesthesia for vaginal delivery. Pentrane must be used with caution to avoid unnecessary depths of anesthesia which may lead to maternal hypotension and infant respiratory depression. Administration of a light concentration of the anesthetic is ordinarily sufficient for use in obstetrics.

Methoxyflurane is a clear, colorless volatile liquid. It is nonflammable and nonexplosive and it is chemically stable to light and moisture. Its fruity odor is nonirritating to the majority of women.

Self-Administration

Methoxyflurane may be used as a self-administered analgesic. With the use of a small portable inhaler, the mother holds a mask lightly over her mouth and nose during uterine contractions and breathes in room air mixed with the anesthetic vapor. In preparing the inhaler care must be taken that it is not filled to a level that will permit overflow of the Pentrane liquid and accidental introduction into the mother's eyes. A dial on the inhaler can be adjusted to regulate the concentration of the anesthetic vapor. There is some cumulative effect of Pentrane in the body and the dial on the inhaler may need to be adjusted downward during prolonged use, in order to reduce the concentration of the anesthetic vapor.

A number of precautions must be observed when a client uses Pentrane. She must never be left alone. She must be watched so that she does not prop the hand that is holding the mask, which would prevent the mask from falling away if she loses consciousness. To avoid producing unwanted anesthesia it is imperative that no one holds the mask for her. The mother often requests assistance, because of her discomfort. It is difficult for the nurse to refuse, but she must do so, with a brief explanation that only the mother may use the inhaler. The mother's vital signs must be closely observed, particularly noting a decrease in blood pressure and slow or shallow respirations, which are indications of need to decrease dosage. Pentrane persists in the body between contractions. This may result in drowsiness, but with analgesic concentrations of the agent it should not lead to un-

responsiveness. When the mother is finished with use of the vaporizer it must be emptied of any remaining liquid.

Pentrane may be used for anesthesia by an adequately informed individual thoroughly familiar with the anesthetic and its properties. When it is used as an anesthetic, analgesia may persist after consciousness has returned.

Trichloroethylene (Trilene, Trimar) is a volatile liquid inhalation anesthetic that produces prompt analgesia. It has often been used as a self-administered inhalation analgesic for relief of discomfort from labor contractions during the latter part of the first stage of labor and during second-stage contractions and delivery of the baby. With the increasing popularity of Pentrane for analgesia during the latter part of labor Trilene is currently used less frequently.

Self-administration of Trilene for analgesia demands precautions similar to those described above for Pentrane administration. For obstetric analgesia the setting of the inhaler for regulation of the potency of the vapor that the woman can inhale is adjusted according to her reaction, but is usually not increased much above midway between the minimum and maximum settings.

With analgesic concentrations there is usually no loss of consciousness, but the mother may experience slight dizziness, tingling, and numbness. Her vital signs must be closely observed. Early signs that she is obtaining too much Trilene are rapid respirations and an irregular pulse.

Trichloroethylene should be stored in closed containers and away from light. The unused amount in the inhaler must be discarded each day to prevent any possibility of danger from the decomposition products that result from oxidation.

Trilene is never used in a closed circuit with soda lime. A chemical reaction between these two substances produces a compound that is extremely toxic, especially to the nervous system. Trilene is slowly released from the body. The possibility that the Trilene that the mother absorbed is being very slowly eliminated and its incompatibility with soda lime make it dangerous to use a closed circuit for any inhalation anesthesia following use of Trilene.

Complications

Inhalation anesthetics reach the baby through the placenta. Depression in the baby is proportional to the depth and duration of the mother's anesthesia.

Vomiting with aspiration of food or fluid into the lungs is a formidable threat with inhalation anesthesia. Since the onset of labor cannot be predicted, food and fluids have not been withheld as for general surgery. Solid food is not offered a mother during labor, and frequently fluid is withheld. However, she may have food in her stomach even when ample time has elapsed since her last meal, because emptying of the stomach is considerably prolonged and may even stop completely during labor.

Even when the stomach is empty of food, gastric juices may collect during prolonged labor and fasting. In addition, analgesic drugs will retard stomach emptying time, and anxiety and pain may contribute to retention of food and fluids. All women in labor must, therefore, be considered as having a full stomach.

Suction should always be available in the delivery room, and endotracheal intubation should be used for all obstetric clients receiving general anesthesia. The delivery table should be easily adjustable for quick change to a Trendelenburg position.

Atropine or scopolamine may be administered before inhalation anesthesia to suppress secretions in the respiratory passages.

If aspiration of stomach contents should occur there is danger of obstruction of the tracheobronchial tree by food particles which then leads to atelectasis, and there is danger of a chemical pneumonitis from the very acid gastric secretions which have a pH of 2.5 or less. This fluid is extremely irritating to the bronchial lining and results in pulmonary edema, a fulminating pneumonitis, cyanosis and hypoxia, and profound hypotension and shock.

If aspiration should occur, treatment includes aspiration of all foreign material through the endotracheal tube and bronchoscopy if necessary, administration of oxygen, and assisted positive pressure ventilation with 100 percent oxygen. Also, large doses of parenteral corticosteroids, such as hydrocortisone, may be administered to combat the inflammatory reaction in the bronchopulmonary tree, and antibiotics may be given to combat secondary infection.

With the use of all inhalation anesthetic agents, every known precaution must be taken to prevent explosions.[1]

During use of any analgesic or anesthetic agent it is important to guard against a prevalent tendency to talk freely while the mother is losing consciousness. A mother may be distressed by hearing, or partly hearing, a conversation not intended for her, which takes place in her hearing while she is partly anesthetized.

The obstetric nurse should never become involved with administration of an inhalation agent for analgesia. These are dangerous agents, and two patients are always involved. In the absence of a person skilled in administration of analgesia, the nurse can assist the mother by remaining with her and reassuring her.

REGIONAL ANALGESIA AND ANESTHESIA

In regional anesthesia the nerves that carry sensations from the uterus and the pelvic region to the spinal cord are blocked. Included in

---

[1] Many precautions must be observed if explosion of anesthetic agents is to be prevented. The nurse must help to eliminate sparks from static electricity and from electrical equipment. Safety regulations that will especially concern the nurse are that (1) all delivery room personnel are required to wear cotton (never wool or synthetic textile) clothing; (2) conductive shoes are worn and tested each time; (3) wool blankets are not used in the delivery room; (4) only conductive rubber material is used on the delivery table and anesthesia equipment; (5) anesthesia equipment is not touched while anesthesia is in progress; (6) all appliances are grounded; and (7) all electrical appliances are kept in good repair. (Further information may be obtained from *Flammable Anesthetics Code 1962.* National Fire Protection Association, Boston, Mass., 1962.)

methods of producing regional anesthesia are pudendal nerve block, spinal anesthesia, saddle block, caudal anesthesia, lumbar epidural block, and paracervical nerve block (Fig. 13-1). Among agents used for regional anesthesia are procaine (Novocaine), lidocaine (Xylocaine), mepivacaine (Carbocaine), and bupivacaine (Marcaine). These agents cross the placenta and may produce an adverse effect in the fetus. Since the maternal blood level is a significant determinant of the amount of a drug that reaches the fetus, the lowest effective amount of the drug that will provide adequate analgesia is used.

Pudendal Nerve Block

A pudendal block is local infiltration of the pudendal nerves, with one of the local anesthetic agents. Blocking of the pudendal nerves

provides anesthesia of the perineum and vulva and is used for episiotomy, delivery, and repair of the perineum. It does not relieve the pain of uterine contractions, and the mother may need an analgesic, such as Pentrane or nitrous oxide, for pain relief during delivery. A pudendal block does not interfere with uterine contractions, and the mother continues with her expulsive efforts. It relaxes the perineal muscles, thus reducing the resistance of these muscles. This method of anesthesia does not ordinarily affect the baby.

A pudendal block is done after the mother has been prepared and draped for delivery. The obstetrician carries out the procedure. A 20-ml syringe and a no. 20 gauge needle, 10 to 12½ cm (4 to 5 in.) long, are used for injection of the anesthetic. The injection is made in the area just below and beyond the ischial spines. The needle

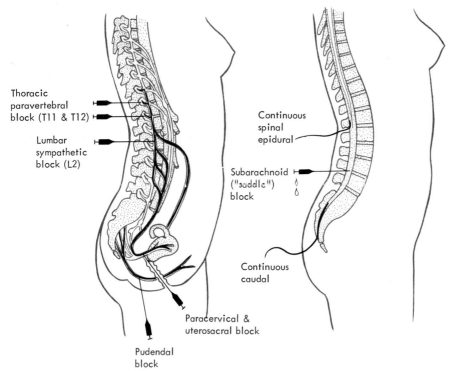

Thoracic paravertebral block (T11 & T12)

Lumbar sympathetic block (L2)

Continuous spinal epidural

Subarachnoid ("saddle") block

Continuous caudal

Paracervical & uterosacral block

Pudendal block

Figure 13-1. A schematic diagram depicting the most important regional anesthetic techniques used to control the pain of parturition. [*Reproduced from John J. Bonica, "an Atlas on Mechanisms and Pathways of Pain in Labor,"* What's New, *No. 217, Abbott Laboratories, Abbott Park, North Chicago, Ill., Figure 6.*]

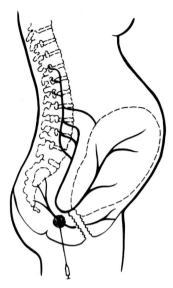

Figure 13-2. Schema of site of pudendal nerve block. Nerves to uterus are not involved with use of this technique. [*Reproduced with permission from John J. Bonica,* Principles and Practice of Obstetric Analgesia and Anesthesia, *Vol. 1. F. A. Davis Co., Philadelphia, Pa., 1967, p. 492.*]

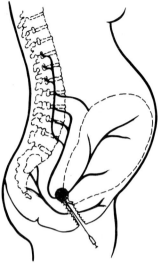

Figure 13-3. Schematic diagram showing sensory (pain) pathways concerned with parturition and the site of interruption when using paracervical block. The pathways from the uterus, including the cervix, are interrupted, thus relieving pain during the first stage of labor. (Compare with Figure 13-2.) [*Reproduced with permission from John J. Bonica,* Principles and Practice of Obstetric Analgesia and Anesthesia, *Vol. 1. F. A. Davis Co., Philadelphia, Pa., 1967, p. 512.*]

is inserted either through the perineum or through the vagina while the physician is palpating the ischial spine with his finger and guiding the needle. A metal or plastic needle guide may be used for transvaginal infiltration. The nerve on each side is blocked separately (Fig. 13-2). Sometimes a nerve block is unsuccessful.

Paracervical and Uterosacral Block

A paracervical block is an infiltration of a local anesthetic agent into the pelvic plexus, through which the nerves which supply the uterus, vagina, bladder, and rectum are distributed. Blocking of these nerves provides relief of pain from uterine contractions and cervical dilatation. It does not block the pudendal nerve and thus does not relieve perineal pain during delivery. Perineal pain is interrupted by the additional use of a pudendal block at the time of delivery.

The anesthetic agent is injected into the paracervical tissues just above each lateral fornix.

This places the medication along the base of the broad ligaments and the lateral walls of the lower uterine segment, blocking the pain pathways from the uterus (Fig. 13-3). The block is usually given after the onset of the active phase of labor, at 4 to 6 cm cervical dilatation, depending upon when the mother experiences moderate to severe pain with her contractions.

Briefly the technique of the procedure consists of locating landmarks, and, with the use of a needle guide that permits the needle to protrude from its tip, injecting medication into each lateral fornix. Aspiration for blood is made before and during injection to avoid intravascular administration. The block is made first on one side, and after one or two contractions, the opposite side is injected. Any of the local anesthetic agents may be used.

Relief of pain in an effective block is quick, within three to five minutes, and lasts from one to two hours depending upon the type and concentration of the anesthetic agent. When the block "wears off," pain returns quite abruptly. For good relief of pain by a block of pain pathways through the pelvic plexus, the block may need to be repeated one or more times, depending on the duration of labor. The technique of the block becomes more difficult and the hazard to the fetus is increased when cervical dilation reaches 8 cm or more and the fetal head is below a +2 station.

Some physicians use a continuous paracervical block, starting at approximately 3 cm dilatation. A plastic catheter, which may have a needle fixed to the end, is left in place. Medication is injected as necessary for the mother's comfort, but not without prior careful check of the position of the catheter. The possibility of the needle moving is a hazard and addition of medication is thus not a function of the nurse, unless she is specifically trained in the technique. With the marketing of bupivacaine, a more recently developed long-acting local anesthetic, the use of the continuous method may be decreased or discontinued.

Fetal bradycardia is a relatively common accompaniment of paracervical block, since absorption of the anesthetic may result in high fetal blood levels. Although the bradycardia is usually transitory, in many cases it may be a serious complication. All local anesthetics are myocardial depressants, and reactions will depend on dosage, rate of absorption, and client response. The FHR must be very carefully monitored every five to ten minutes until assurance that it is remaining stable. With detection of fetal bradycardia a FHR monitor should be placed to assess more carefully the pattern of the fetal heart rate. It is highly desirable to have a FHR monitor in place prior to injection of the anesthetic agent. The mother's vital signs and general reaction are also checked for any signs of maternal systemic reaction.

Spinal Anesthesia

With this method, anesthesia of the operative area is produced by injection of one of the local anesthetic agents into the subarachnoid space. Either a single injection or a continuous method may be used. For obstetric clients, spinal anesthesia is usually used only for cesarean sections.

With the mother on her side, a spinal needle is inserted into the subarachnoid space through the third or fourth lumbar interspace. For a single injection the anesthetic agent is usually dissolved in a few milliliters of spinal fluid, injected, and the needle removed. This anesthesia lasts for approximately an hour. For the continuous method a small plastic catheter is passed through the needle, taped into place, and injections of the solution are made in small doses until the preferred anesthetic level is reached. After surgery has been started, repeated small doses are given as necessary to maintain adequate anesthesia.

Saddle Block (Low Spinal)

This is a spinal anesthetic, differing from the one described above in that the drug is localized in the conus of the dural sac. Addition of glucose to the anesthetic agent, which makes it heavy, facilitates its localization. Saddle block anesthesia is of relatively short duration. It is not ordinarily used for relief of labor pains, but for delivery only. It is administered when delivery is anticipated within approximately an hour.

The mother must be in a sitting position for a saddle block. This position is distressing to her at this advanced stage of labor. The nurse must do all she can to provide adequate support for the mother to lean on while in the sitting position and to give reassurance during the procedure.

The anesthetic agent is injected through a spinal needle inserted into the subarachnoid space through a lumbar interspace (Fig. 13-1). The woman remains sitting for approximately 30 seconds; the time must be accurate but varies with the drugs used. At exactly the proper time, following injection, she is placed on her back with her head on a pillow to keep her neck sharply flexed. Anesthesia occurs in that area of the body which would ordinarily come in contact with a saddle while riding horseback; from this it derives its name. The leg and thigh muscles and the abdominal muscles are not greatly affected by the anesthesia.

Caudal Analgesia and Anesthesia

With this method analgesia and anesthesia of the pelvic region are obtained by injection of one of the local anesthetic agents into the caudal space, which is the area within the sacrum at the lowermost part of the bony spinal canal. A dural sac separates this space from the spinal cord. A number of sacral nerves emerge from the dural sac and pass through this space. By filling the canal with an anesthetic solution, the pain sense of these nerves is abolished, and anesthesia is produced in the pelvic region supplied by these nerves.

The anesthetic solution is placed into the caudal canal through a spinal needle inserted through a foramen present at the lower end of the sacrum (Fig. 13-1). The patient is in a Sims' or knee–chest position during the procedure. After insertion of the needle attempts are made at aspiration to ascertain that the dura has not been pierced. If spinal fluid is obtained, the procedure is discontinued since a large injection of medication into the spinal canal is very dangerous. For anesthesia of short duration a single injection of anesthetic solution is made. When the analgesia is to be of long or indefinite duration, termed continuous caudal anesthesia, a polyethylene tube or a specially designed malleable needle is left in place for further injections.

A continuous caudal block provides analgesia during labor and anesthesia for delivery. It may be started when the mother is in active labor, having reached approximately 4 cm cervical dilatation. Analgesia is usually present in 5 to 15 minutes or at least in 30 minutes following injection. If analgesia is satisfactory, sensations are lost in the pelvic region and the pain of uterine contractions is relieved. The lower extremities become tingly and motor weakness develops. Supplemental injections are given as frequently

as indicated by the mother's reactions; these may be necessary approximately every 40 to 60 minutes. Caudal analgesia may be continued for several hours or longer.

When successfully administered, this method gives relief of pain without great inhibitions of the uterine contractions and gives good perineal relaxation. Since the anal sphincter also relaxes, the bowel should be empty. The drug, as with paracervical block, may cause a transient bradycardia in the fetus.

Lumbar Epidural Block

An epidural block is a method of obtaining anesthesia by injection of a local anesthetic agent into the epidural space. As with an injection into the caudal space, the anesthetic agent is placed outside of the dura, but in this procedure it is placed higher in the spinal canal, being injected in the lumbar region. The spinal nerves, as they leave the spinal cord to emerge from the vertebral column, traverse the epidural space. The nerves that pass through the area in which the anesthetic agent has been deposited are blocked by the drug.

With the mother lying on her side and her head and knees flexed toward her chest, a needle is inserted through one of the intervertebral spaces in the lumbar region until it reaches the epidural space (Fig. 13-1). This space is identified by a loss of resistance to insertion of the needle. It is possible to insert the needle beyond the space and puncture the dura. With the point of the needle in the epidural space, a small polyethylene tube is inserted through the needle and beyond it for a few centimeters. The needle is then withdrawn over the tubing, leaving the catheter in place. The catheter is taped to the mother's back, with the distal end left accessible for subsequent injections of the anesthetic agent.

For analgesia during labor an epidural block is usually done when the mother is in active labor, having reached a cervical dilatation of 3 or 4 cm. After the initial dose, medication is injected at intervals as required for pain relief, usually every one-half to one hour. For anesthesia for delivery, the dose of medication is increased over that used during labor.

The mother has relief of pain from uterine contractions in about 5 to 10 minutes after the initial injection. She also feels tingling and numbness of her feet. Blood pressure may fall and she must be carefully observed for evidence of hypotension and the need to take measures to combat it. (Treatment is described below.) Blood pressure is very closely checked, especially after the initial dose of medication, after any increase in dose, and after moving the mother to the delivery room. At these times it may be checked every two or three minutes.

Both caudal block and epidural block are specialized procedures. Technical difficulties and possible complications make it essential that they be performed by a trained and experienced individual.

During continuous analgesia with either epidural block or caudal block, the mother is not left alone. After the initial dose of medication has been given and untoward effects have not occurred, the nurse may be responsible for continued observation of the mother.

The blood pressure must be checked frequently. Untoward reactions reported by the mother, such as faintness, dizziness, nausea, and pounding of the heart, are reported to the physician immediately. The mother is observed for respiratory difficulty, pallor, weak pulse, and cold sweats.

The fetal heart is checked frequently, preferably monitored continuously. Since the mother is unaware of her contractions, frequency and strength of contractions are observed by abdominal palpation or preferably by electronic monitoring of both uterine contractions and fetal heart beat.

The mother's ability to void is greatly lessened with this type of analgesia. Her bladder must be observed for fullness and catheterization done as necessary. She is requested to empty her bladder before analgesia is begun.

For delivery the mother often needs to be in-structed when to bear down, since she does not feel strong contractions or the urge to push. The incidence of operative deliveries is increased, but perineal resistance to delivery is lessened, since both types of anesthesia give relaxation of perineal muscles.

Complications

The problems that are common to some or all methods of conduction anesthesia are management of hypotension, prevention of infection, and management of postspinal headache.

Hypotension may develop following any method of spinal anesthesia. When sympathetic nerve fibers are blocked by the anesthetic agent there is loss of vasoconstrictor ability in the affected vessels, and as a result, blood tends to pool in the peripheral vessels, venous return to the heart is decreased, cardiac output decreases, and the systemic blood pressure falls.

Autonomic blocking produces a more marked response, a greater degree of hypotension, in the pregnant than in the nonpregnant individual. The hypotension and circulatory alterations in pregnancy are related to venous pooling in the legs produced by the autonomic block. The increased capacity and the high pressure in the veins of the legs in pregnancy tend to favor a very large amount of venous pooling, especially when the sympathetic tone is blocked and vascular tone is practically nil. If a supine position is permitted, thereby aggravating the pooling even more, the problem of hypotension may become very serious.

A drop in systolic blood pressure to below 100 mmHg is considered hypotension in the pregnant woman, and while she could probably tolerate a lower systolic pressure very well, uterine blood flow is likely to be too low for adequate fetal oxygenation. The blood pressure must therefore be monitored very closely, and measures for combating a serious fall in pressure must be immediately available.

Administration of intravenous fluids with a large bore needle always precedes a spinal or epidural block. This provides a means of giving fluids rapidly, and drugs if indicated, should hypotension develop. Some physicians recommend administration of up to 1000 ml of fluids prior to the block if time permits. Such prehydration helps to increase the blood volume to counteract the effects of peripheral vasodilation.

The mother is kept in a lateral recumbent position whenever possible to optimize return of blood from the lower extremities and avoid the hypotension that may develop due to pressure of the heavy uterus on the inferior vena cava. When a supine position must be used, as for a cesarean section, the uterus is displaced to the left. This can be done by placing a hand on the right flank, under the uterus as much as possible, and pushing the uterus to the left and upward, lifting it off the inferior vena cava.

Should maternal hypotension develop, immediate counteractive steps would include turning the mother to a lateral position or displacing the uterus to the left, increasing the rate of the intravenous infusion to expand blood volume rapidly and returning pooled blood to the circulation. The mother's legs should be elevated to a 90 degree angle immediately to drain the pooled blood that has accumulated due to the changes in the circulatory system during pregnancy and the epidural block. A moderate Trendelenburg position, with a pillow under the head, may be necessary if there is concern that cerebral circulation may not be adequate.

If the blood pressure is not promptly restored, administration of 100 percent oxygen by face mask may improve maternal and, concomitantly, fetal oxygenation. Oxygen is often administered during delivery to patients under regional anesthesia.

Vasopressors are used conservatively, only after other methods do not prove effective quickly. Placental circulation may be seriously decreased by the vasoconstrictive effect of drugs and present a further hazard to the fetus. When vasopressors have been used, ergonovine or methylergonovine should not be used after delivery because of the danger of a combination of these drugs causing severe hypertension in the mother.

It is necessary to be always prepared for severe hypotension; therefore, resuscitation equipment with airways, endotracheal tubes, laryngoscope, suction apparatus, oxygen, and vasopressors should be immediately available whenever a spinal block is being done.

Infection of the epidural or subarachnoid space is serious, since the body does not easily combat infection in this area. All equipment, including polyvinyl catheters and the ampuls of drugs, must be sterile. Autoclaving of ampuls or vials sterilizes the outside of the containers, making them easier to handle without chance of contamination of other supplies. Unused plastic catheters are discarded because reautoclaving them causes brittleness. The patient's skin is carefully prepared for the procedure. Sterile gloves are always worn. For continuous analgesia the site of the catheter insertion is covered with a sterile occlusive dressing while the catheter is in place.

Some women have a headache following a conduction anesthesia that involves entering the dura. It is believed to be caused by leakage of spinal fluid through the puncture hole with resultant decrease in cerebrospinal fluid volume and pressure, causing traction on pain-sensitive tissues. A headache is less likely to develop when it has been possible to use a small needle and to make only one puncture.

For treatment of headache the mother is kept quiet, and a recumbent position may be ordered for the first 12 to 24 hours following delivery if she has had a spinal anesthetic involving dural puncture, since headache is aggravated when the head is elevated. Hydration therapy is initiated to hasten replacement of fluid; the mother is urged to drink large quantities of fluid frequently, raising her intake to 3000 to 4000 ml per day. Analgesics are given as necessary to relieve discomfort of headache. In persistent severe cases an epidural infiltration may be effective.

EFFECT OF ANALGESIA AND ANESTHESIA ON THE NEWBORN

Analgesic and anesthetic agents cross the placenta from mother to fetus. Accordingly it can be assumed that the fetus will receive some of the drug that is given to the mother, regardless of route of administration. Transfer of drugs across the placenta can be very rapid, sometimes reaching appreciable concentration in the fetus within minutes of administration to mother. The drug effect on the infant is often dependent on dose and time of administration before birth.

There are, however, other factors that influence the effect of maternal medication. A drug may be modified in the course of its passage by either the placenta or the fetus and may affect fetal function by its influence on placental function. Conditions such as acidosis and asphyxia may alter the influence of a drug on the fetus or the newborn. The kidney of the newborn cannot excrete easily, and there may be difficulty in conjugation of a drug by the liver in the early days of life. A vareity of other factors may have an influence.

Placental transfer of narcotic drugs is rapid, especially if the drug is given intravenously as is done on occasion. Dose and time of administration are important factors in neonatal depression; the most potent effect from an average dose given intramuscularly appears to be between 1 and 3 hours. There does not, however, appear to be an absolute pattern of drug influence on the fetus. Plasma levels of drugs may not be representative of drug concentration in the central nervous system. Acidosis and hypoxia may contribute to adverse effects.

Tranquilizing drugs cross the placenta rapidly. Studies on diazepam have shown that this drug crosses the placenta very rapidly, and after equilibrium is attained the concentration of the drug is higher in the fetal than in the maternal blood for up to more than 24 hours. Fetal tissue levels of diazepam peak one hour after a maternal dose. The fetal brain is one of the areas in which the drug localizes in a high concentration

and from which it clears slowly. Neither the fetus nor the newborn can metabolize diazepam easily. It is retained for some time, its effects persisting for as long as one week after delivery.

Newborns with diazepam in their tissues, when mothers have had relatively large doses, have been observed to have hypotonia and apneic spells. They may be lethargic, feed poorly, and make poor metabolic responses to cold. Small maternal doses have not appeared to exert a serious adverse influence on the newborn, but any baby exposed to diazepam prenatally must be carefully observed. Diazepam is one of the drugs that may be used in management of preeclampsia either prior to or during labor.

Barbiturates transfer to the fetus easily and rapidly, but they are not readily excreted by the newborn. These drugs can depress newborn infants for several days and result in decreased attentiveness and in poor suck and ability to take food.

Inhalation anesthetics cross the placenta readily and they will quickly equilibrate between the maternal and fetal circulation. The newborn may therefore be depressed at birth, depending upon the depth and duration of the anesthesia. Someone must be available to resuscitate the baby promptly and expertly as indicated by his condition.

Inhalation anesthetics undergo little or no biotransformation, and whatever amount of drug is in the newborn at birth must be exhaled by the baby after birth. The rapidity with which the infant clears the anesthetic agent will depend on how well his respiratory system functions. If the baby is depressed from the anesthetic at birth and has slow and shallow breathing, clearance of the anesthetic will be slow.

Local anesthetic injections by any route—epidural, paracervical, pudendal, or local infiltration—are quickly taken up by the maternal bloodstream. These drugs cross the placenta rapidly and appear in the fetal bloodstream soon after administration, and since fetal blood is relatively more acidotic than maternal blood, the concentration of a local anesthetic in the fetus can exceed that of the mother at equilibrium due to some trapping of the drug. This has raised the question of the wisdom of prolonged epidural block with high-risk infants, especially with some of the drugs available. There are differences in passage of local anesthetic agents; e.g., there is evidence that bupivacaine does not cross the placenta as readily as some of the other drugs used, and it is cleared from the blood of the newborn very rapidly compared to other local anesthetics.

Fetal bradycardia is the most frequent and serious complication of regional obstetric anesthesia, being most apparent in paracervical block. Its onset is often between 10 and 15 minutes, and it usually lasts 15 minutes or less. Even when bradycardia is of short duration it must be considered a sign of fetal distress, which results in some hypoxia and perhaps acidosis. It can induce significant changes in acid–base balance in the fetus.

There is concern that some of the local anesthetics may compete with bilirubin for albumin binding and, in displacing the bilirubin, may predispose the neonate to kernicterus. Local anesthetic agents may also cause discernible changes in neurobehavioral responses during the first hours after birth.

Until recently, the Apgar score was the most commonly used index of the influences of medications and the stress of birth on an infant. This score gives an evaluation of the function of the respiratory and circulatory systems and of the lower centers of the nervous system—tone and reflex irritability. It reflects the condition of the baby immediately after the stress of birth, but does not evaluate the subtle effect of drugs on the infant's nervous system.

Within recent years tests of neurologic function and of the behavioral state of the baby have been used in evaluation of the influence of analgesic and anesthetic drugs. These tests have shown that the Apgar score serves as a rough guide for evaluation of the well-being of the newborn, but it should be supplemented by assessment of the baby's neurologic ability.

Newborns are not necessarily able to function to their best capabilities when the Apgar score has been good at birth and when their blood gases quickly return to normal. These two methods of evaluation do not show the more subtle effects that analgesia may have had on the infant. A baby may have an excellent Apgar score and remain alert and active for 15 to 30 minutes or so after birth and then become relatively unresponsive and remain so for hours. The stimulation of birth and the change in environment keeps the baby alert for a time, but then the effects of the medication are noticeable. The baby then may make little effort in spontaneous movements, his heart rate and respirations may be slow, his ability to clear mucus is poor, and his suck is poor. He may remain neurologically depressed from the drug for hours or even days.

Brackbill and colleagues found that habituation to a repetitive sound stimulus was delayed in infants with obstetric premedication, and also that their ability to respond was slowed. They write:

The results of the present study indicate not only that obstetric premedication affects neonatal functioning but also that it affects these functions differentially. The most potent effect is on the infant's ability to stop responding when the exigencies of the situation demand this. . . . Phrased differently, response inhibition is that function most sensitive or vulnerable to premedication effects. The next most potent effect of premedication is on the infant's ability to respond. Within this broad category, one may distinguish even further between premedication effects on externally elicited responses and on spontaneously emitted responses, the first of these functions apparently being more sensitive to premedication effects. . . .

All in all, the psychophysiologic effects of premedication may be described as follows. The greater the environmental demands on the infant and the more complex the action required of him to cope with these demands, the greater the difference in quality of performance among infants in terms of their perinatal premedication history.[2]

[2] Y. Brackbill, J. Kane, R. L. Manniello, and D. Abramson, Obstetric premedication and infant outcome, *Am. J. Obstet. Gynecol.* 118:382–383, (Feb. 1) 1974.

From various studies it appears that babies whose mothers have received medication in labor may show differences in alertness and responsiveness from those who have not had medication. For example, babies whose mothers received analgesia are often less responsive, less alert, more difficult to arouse, irritable, slower to feed well, and have poor suck and decreased visual attentiveness.

Concern has been expressed that early mother–infant relationships may be adversely affected by depressant drugs and especially that this effect may come at a critical imprinting time. A depressed infant, and sometimes a depressed mother, may not be able to respond appropriately to carry out normal mother–infant interactions. The baby's responsiveness to his mother's voice, to her efforts to alert him or to soothe him, and his response to attempts to feed him may be impeded.

V. Dubowitz writes:

It is only by this careful assessment of the neonate that accurate evaluation of possible deleterious effects of drugs in labour can be made. Thus it is quite possible that an hypnotic drug given to the mother in labour, with no apparent influence on the Apgar scoring of the infant, may nevertheless cause marked depression of the infant's higher nervous function, with a resultant state of irritability and poor rousability with consequent difficulties in consoling the infant, and associated feeding difficulties. In turn, this may seriously affect the early mother-infant interrelationship and bonding and could well be a predisposing factor to later problems in the management of the infant.[3]

It appears that to assure minimal influence of maternal medication on the newborn's ability to function well neurologically, every effort must be made to use only a minimum well-controlled amount of maternal analgesia during labor and delivery.

[3] V. Dubowitz, Neurological fragility in the newborn: Influence of medication in labour, *Br. J. Anaesth.* 47:1007 (Sept.) 1975.

FACTORS DETERMINING CHOICE OF ANESTHESIA

Many factors are considered in selecting anesthesia for an individual client. No one method is preferable. Among factors considered are existing complications of pregnancy, such as antepartum bleeding, toxemias, diabetes, or heart disease; presentation and position of the baby, such as breech; maturity of the baby; the time the mother last ate; the availability of an anesthesiologist; the mother's desire to participate in the delivery; and the mother's request, if possible. Although it is not always desirable for the mother to determine the type of anesthesia, her objection to a particular method is an important consideration. When not contraindicated, regional anesthesia may be chosen over inhalation because of the mother's desire to be awake and to participate as much as possible in the birth and the desire of both parents for the father to be with his wife during labor and delivery.

Although aspiration of vomitus by the mother is more likely to occur with inhalation anesthesia than with other kinds, inhalation may be the method of choice in some cases. Among reasons for its use is the relaxation that it will provide for a delivery in which good relaxation is necessary. It may be more quickly administered than conduction anesthesia when the need for immediate delivery arises. The duration and depth of inhalation anesthesia are easily controlled. With the relatively light amount of anesthesia required for many deliveries, the inhalation method may present little or no problem of fetal depression, although the threat of maternal aspiration is always present.

Regional anesthesia reduces danger of maternal aspiration of food and fluid and, when used for analgesia during labor, eliminates use of narcotic drugs. However, regional anesthesia is sometimes contraindicated. It is not used in cases of obstetric hemorrhage because of the hypotension that often accompanies conduction anesthesia. Spine deformities in the mother are another contraindication to its use. It has also been advised that paracervical block should be contraindicated in prematurity, in the presence of preexisting fetal distress, and in the presence of uteroplacental insufficiency.

Finally, to quote Dr. William Kruel:

Liberal does of T.L.C. (tender loving care) should be given by the obstetrician and his nursing staff. Depression does not accompany its use. Excessive doses are difficult if not impossible to administer. T.L.C. saves on drugs.[4]

BIBLIOGRAPHY

Ahokas, Robert A., and Dilts, P. V. Jr., Assessing narcotics and their antagonists, *Contemp. Ob/Gyn* 5:55–59 (June) 1975.

Bonica, John J., *Principles and Practice of Obstetric Analgesia and Anesthesia*, Vol. I. Davis, Philadelphia, Pa., 1967.

Bowes, Watson A., Jr., Brackbill, Yvonne, Conway, Esther, and Steinschneider, Alfred, The effects of obstetrical medication on fetus and infant, *Monogr. Soc. Res. Child Dev.* Serial No. 137, Vol. 37, No. 4 (June) 1970.

Brackbill, Y., Kane, J., Manniello, R. L., and Abramson, D., Obstetric premedication and infant outcome, *Am. J. Obstet. Gynecol.* 118:377–385 (Feb. 1) 1974.

Brazelton, T. Berry, Effect of prenatal drugs on the behavior of the neonate, *Am. J. Psychiatry* 126 II:1261–1266 (Mar.) 1970.

Brown, Walter U., Jr., Bell, George C., and Alper, Milton H., Acidosis, local anesthetics, and the newborn, *Obstet. Gynecol.* 48:27–34 (July) 1976.

Caton, Donald, Obstetric anesthesia and concepts of placental transport: A historical review of the nineteenth century, *Anesthesiology* 46:132–137 (Feb.) 1977.

Clark, Richard B., Analgesia during labor: Effect on the fetus and neonate, in *Clinical Anesthesia. Parturition and Perinatology*, Vol. 10/2, edited by Gertie F. Marx. Davis, Philadelphia, Pa. 1973, pp. 140–155.

Cree, Jean E., Meyer, Joseph, and Haily, David M., Diazepam in labour: Its metabolism and effect on the clinical condition and thermogenesis of the newborn, *Br. Med. J.* 4:251–255 (Nov. 3) 1973.

Desmond, Murdina M., Obstetric medication and infant behavior, *Anesthesiology* 40:111–113 (Feb.) 1974.

Dilts, P. V. Jr., Pharmacology in labor and delivery, *Contemp. Ob/Gyn* 5:67, 71, and 72 (Apr.) 1975.

Dubowitz, V., *Neurological fragility in the newborn: Influence of medication in labour*, Br. J. Anaesth. 47:1005–1010 (Sept.) 1975.

Finster, Mieczyslaw, and Mark, Lester C., Thiobarbiturates in obstetric anesthesia, in *Clinical Anesthesia. Parturition and Perinatology*, Vol. 10/2, edited by Gertie F. Marx. Davis, Philadelphia, Pa., 1973, pp. 164–172.

Fishburne, John I. Jr., Local anesthetics in obstetrics, *Contemp. Ob/Gyn* 6:101–105 (Oct.) 1975; 7:15 (Feb.) 1976.

Gottschalk, William, Regional anesthesia. Spinal, lumbar epidural, and caudal anesthesia, *Obstet. Gynecol. Annu.* 3:377–405, 1974.

———, Principles of obstetric anesthesia, *Obstet. Gynecol. Annu.* I:193–218, 1972.

Grad, Rae Krohn, and Woodside, Jack, Obstetrical analgesics and anesthesia, *Am. J. Nurs.* 77:242–245 (Feb.) 1977.

Greiss, Frank C., Jr., Obstetric anesthesia, *Am. J. Nurs.* 71:67–69 (Jan.) 1971.

James, Francis M., Inhalation anesthetics, *Contemp. Ob/Gyn* 5:73–76 (Apr.) 1975.

Kruel, William, A current concept of anesthesia for obstetrical delivery, *Wis. Med. J.* 68:196 (May) 1969.

Levinson, Gershon, and Shnider, Sol M., Placental transfer of local anesthetics: Clinical implications, in *Clinical Anesthesia. Parturition and Perinatology*, Vol. 10/2, edited by Gertie F. Marx. Davis, Philadelphia, Pa., 1973, pp. 173–185.

Scanlon, John W. *et al.*, Neurobehavioral responses and drug concentrations in newborns after maternal epidural anesthesia with bupivacaine, *Anesthesiology* 45:400–405 (Oct.) 1976.

Sherline, Donald M., The barbiturates, the phenothiazines, and diazepam, *Contemp. Ob/Gyn* 6:77–80 (July) 1975.

[4]William Kruel, Mother and child—Labor and analgesia, *Wis. Med. J.* 68:120 (Feb.) 1969.

Shnider, Sol M., *Obstetrical Anesthesia, Current Concepts and Practice.* Williams and Wilkins, Baltimore, Md., 1974.

————, and Moya, Frank (eds.), *The Anesthesiologist, Mother, and Newborn.* Williams and Wilkins, Baltimore, Md., 1974.

Thiery, Michel, and Vroman, Stefaan, Paracervical block analgesia during labor, *Am. J. Obstet. Gynecol.* 113:988–1036 (Aug. 1) 1972.

Thoms, Herbert, Anesthésie á la reine, *Am. J. Obstet. Gynecol.* 40:340–346 (Aug.) 1940.

Tronick, Edward *et al.,* Regional obstetric anesthesia and newborn behavior: Effects over the first ten days of life, *Pediatrics* 58:94–100 (July) 1976.

14

Clinical Management During Labor

A nurse who attends women during labor and delivery should possess extraordinary skills in the physiologic/technical dimensions of care as well as warmth and sensitivity to the breadth and depth of human emotional response. She must be able to make rapid judgments and employ the latest technology in an emergency situation. Yet she must also know when not to intervene in nature's own process but to be calm, reassuring, and create a milieu where the woman and her family can give birth joyfully.

The nurse's knowledge and skill are very important to a safe outcome of labor for both mother and baby. She is often responsible for a large part of the mother's care during the first stage of labor and for preparation and adequacy of supplies and assistance to the physician throughout labor and delivery. To a considerable degree the safety of the mother and baby depends on the nurse's continuous close observation; her alertness in early recognition and immediate reporting to the physician of abnormal signs and symptoms; and her ability to make a good judgment and take prompt action as indicated when complications arise. The nurse must also be able to determine the mother's physical and emotional needs through a sometimes long and tedious labor and to meet these needs through individualized care. In addition, she must have competence in the technical skills that are necessary for safe and satisfactory conduct of labor and delivery.

The nurse's attitude in caring for a mother in labor will depend on her appreciation of the emotional stress and physical discomfort that the woman in labor experiences; her understanding of the importance of this event to the family and their deep emotional involvement; and her desire and ability to meet the needs of the mother and her family according to each individual's particular needs.

The sympathetic insight that constantly underlies effective nursing care in all situations is necessary in the fullest sense during this crucial time of labor. The woman in labor experiences some of the most poignant of human emotions, including awe, expectancy, doubt, uncertainty, or dread, and in some cases fear, amounting almost to terror. Throughout the intense emotional experience the mother is also having pain which may become harder and harder to bear and often leads to a feeling of exhaustion. Great emotional stress—fear, worry, apprehension—increases the discomforts of labor, may affect its course, and sometimes impedes its progress.

Encouragement and reassurance from an understanding nurse can have a marked influence in lessening the emotional stress and the physical discomforts of labor. The nurse makes every effort to understand each person's reactions and behavior, accept each one's right to her own feelings and responses, show a kindly understanding, and develop a sensitivity to the manner in which she can best meet the mother's needs. The nurse's sincere appreciation of the mother's great emotional and trying physical experience, and her acceptance of the woman's behavior, should be conveyed to her client. She must give the mother an opportunity to discuss her feelings, ask questions, and express her fears, and provide encouragement and constant reassurance in a manner that shows an unhurried and friendly interest in the particular person to whom she is giving care.

Labor is an occasion of paramount importance to the family as well as to the woman herself. Family members or other support persons have varying emotional reactions and behavior. As in her care of the mother, the nurse must make every possible effort to understand and accept the feelings of family members and to meet their needs in a friendly and dignified manner. Many times the husband is the only family member in the labor room, but others may be nearby. At no time must either the mother or her family be allowed to feel that the labor is being taken lightly or as a matter of course among many others. The nurse must show by her conduct that each is considered a very important event in itself.

FIRST STAGE (STAGE OF DILATATION)

The onset of labor is usually gradual, as described in Chapter 12, and in the majority of labors there is accordingly ample time for unhurried attention, unless complications develop requiring immediate attention.

Admission to the Hospital

The expectant mother usually enters the hospital in the early part of the first stage of labor, carrying out the instructions that she was given during the antepartum period. Early admission means less discomfort in traveling, less mental anxiety, and more time to prepare for delivery without haste. At the time of admission to the hospital the mother may, therefore, be having regular contractions at 5- to 10-minute intervals, or at times more frequently; she may be having a bloody show; and her membranes may have

ruptured. Sometimes labor is far advanced and delivery is imminent. At other times the mother enters the hospital before active labor has begun, having been directed by her physician to go to the hospital because of rupture of membranes, or for observation of signs such as slight bleeding, which may signify the possibility of complications.

As soon as the woman enters the birth room the nurse should greet her pleasantly and with a reassuring attitude. As quickly as possible an admitting assessment should be made upon which to base the beginning plan of nursing care (see Figure 14-1).

Ideally, every woman would be cared for during labor by a nurse familiar to her from antepartum care who would already know her history, personality, and family circumstances. Such a situation, however, is extremely rare in the current health care system. Nevertheless, the alert, thoughtful nurse can observe many behavioral clues simply from seeing the woman enter the room. She will notice a face relaxed and confident or contorted with pain; hands relaxed at her side, clenched and white-knuckled, or clutching her abdomen or her husband's arm. The woman's eyes, dilated and searching, may indicate fear and anxiety. How she talks and what she talks about may provide information about her apprehension and also about the stage of her labor (see page 306).

Because hospitalization, as well as labor, may be a new and strange experience for her, the nurse should make an effort to orient the mother and her family to the personnel and environment. Depending on the mother's comfort and the rapidity of the progress of her labor, this may be limited to a few seconds of introduction to the nurse herself and the immediate labor room or may include a more extensive tour of the hospital unit.

As the nurse introduces the woman to her labor room, she obtains the following information in a conversational manner: when the contractions began, how frequently they are occurring, approximately how long they last; whether or not the membranes have ruptured; if

NAME _____ L.M.P. _____ E.D.C._____

DOCTOR _____ HOSPITAL _____

MOTHER'S BIRTH DATE _____ DATE OF ADMISSION _____

ADMISSION WEIGHT _____ TIME OF ADMISSION _____ A.M. / P.M.

ONSET OF LABOR: DATE _____ TIME _____ NOT IN LABOR

TIME SCORING COMPLETED _____ A.M. / P.M.

A BASELINE DATA:

e.g. Age 35+ . . . 1 ☑

Age 35+ . . . . 1 ☐	
40+ . . . . 2 ☐	
Para 0 . . . . 1 ☐	
6+ . . . . 2 ☐	
Interval Less Than 2 Yrs . . . . 1 ☐	
Obesity 200 Lb+ . . . . 1 ☐	
Diabetes Mild-Moderate . . . . 2 ☐	
Severe . . . . 3 ☐	
Chronic Renal Disease . . . . 1 ☐	
with Diminished Renal Function . . . . 3 ☐	
Preexisting Hypertension	
140+/90+ . . . . 1 ☐	
160+/110+ . . . . 2 ☐	

PREVIOUS OBSTETRICAL HISTORY:

Abortion . . . . ☐
Stillbirth . . . . ☐
Neonatal Death . . . . ☐
Surviving Premature Infant . . . . ☐
Antepartum Hemorrhage . . . . ☐
Toxemia . . . . ☐
Mid-Forceps Delivery . . . . ☐
Cesarean Section . . . . ☐
Major Congenital Anomaly . . . . ☐
Baby 10 Lb + ... ☐
  One Instance of Above . . . . 1 ☐
  Two or More Instances of Above . . . . 2 ☐

RH Isoimmunized Mother . . . . 2 ☐
+ History of Erythroblastosis . . . . 3 ☐

B PRESENT PREGNANCY

e.g. Hydramnios . . . 3 ☑

Bleeding, Before 20 Weeks
  Alone . . . . 1 ☐
  With Pain . . . . 2 ☐

Bleeding, After 20 Weeks
  Ceased . . . . 1 ☐
  Continues . . . . 2 ☐
  With Pain . . . . 3 ☐
  With Hypotension . . . . 3 ☐

Spontaneous Premature
  Rupture of Membranes . . . . 1 ☐
  Latent Period 24 Hr + ... 2 ☐

Anemia 8 to 10 gm . . . . 1 ☐
  Less than 8 gm . . . . 2 ☐

No Prenatal Care . . . . 2 ☐
  1 to 3 Prenatal Visits . . . . 1 ☐

Toxemia Mild Moderate . . . . 1 ☐
  Severe . . . . 3 ☐

Hydramnios (Single Fetus) . . . . 3 ☐

Multiple Pregnancy . . . . 2 ☐

Abnormal Glucose Tolerance . . . . 1 ☐

  Decreasing Insulin Requirement . . . . 3 ☐

  Maternal Diabetic Acidosis . . . . 3 ☐

Maternal Pyrexia . . . . 1 ☐
Pyrexia + FHR Greater than 160 . . . . 2 ☐

RH Negative
  With Antibody Titer . . . . 2 ☐
  With Amniotic Fluid Liley Zone 111 . . . . 3 ☐

C GESTATIONAL AGE (at time of scoring):

e.g. 29-32 Wks . . . 3 ☑

28 Wks or under . . . . 4 ☐
29-32 Wks . . . . 3 ☐
33-35 Wks . . . . 2 ☐

36-37 Wks . . . . 1 ☐
38-41 Wks . . . . 0 ☐
42 Wks . . . . 1 ☐
43 Wks OR More . . . . 2 ☐

PRESENTATION AT TIME OF ADMISSION _____
ASSESSED BY RECTAL/VAGINAL/ABDOMINAL EXAM

TOTAL SCORE
PARTS A. B. C. _____

CERVICAL DILATATION AT TIME OF ADMISSION _____ CM
ASSESSED BY RECTAL/VAGINAL/ABDOMINAL EXAM

PROTEINURIA: YES ☐   NO ☐

A score of 4 or more marks a high-risk pregnancy, as does any presentation other than vertex.

If the score is 4 or more, the patient's physician should be notified immediately.

Figure 14-1.   One example of an admitting history/risk assessment form for use in the intrapartum setting.

there has been any bleeding; the expected date of confinement; and the number of pregnancies and the number of children the mother has had. This information is recorded accurately and concisely on the nurse's record on the client's chart. The number of pregnancies, including miscarriages, and the number of children previously delivered may be recorded as gravida and para—gravida referring to the number of pregnancies including the present one and para referring to the number of previous pregnancies that have continued to the period of viability, including any stillborn infants. An example of recording gravida and para is given on page 169.

The antepartum course and medical history should be reviewed. In most instances a copy of the antepartum record from the physician's office or clinic should be available in the hospital for this purpose. The information from this record can be validated with the client, compared with the various findings on admission, and used to plan further care.

Weight of the mother is measured, compared to previous weights, and recorded, unless it seems necessary to put her to bed immediately. Conditions such as vaginal bleeding, ruptured membranes, and contractions severe enough and close enough to make delivery seem imminent require immediate bed rest. A urine specimen is collected, and the nurse tests the urine for protein and records. Temperature, pulse rate, respiratory rate, and blood pressure reading are taken and recorded as a part of the nurse's admission procedure. The fetal heart is auscultated and the rate recorded. During admission the nurse should observe uterine contractions for frequency and palpate the mother's abdomen to make her own observation of the strength and duration of contractions. The nurse also makes a vaginal examination if such is the policy of the institution. Depending on the rapidity with which labor is progressing, the nurse notifies the physician before or after she has completed admission of the mother and reports her findings to him.

In some institutional settings the physician also examines the woman's labor status. He also makes an evaluation of the cardiac and respiratory systems and of other body systems included in a physical examination, and includes abdominal palpation, auscultation of the fetal heart, and vaginal examination. The physician may order certain laboratory studies.

In addition to the critical physical data discussed above, the nurse should discover the kind of preparation, if any, made by the couple for labor and delivery, their knowledge of the course of labor and use of breathing techniques, and their expectations for care. One person may wish to know as little as possible and be "knocked out" with drugs as soon as she can, while another may refuse all medication and want to know all about everything. Some couples may prefer periods of time alone, while the constant presence of a nurse is helpful to others. Plans for whether the father or other support person will remain in the room during examinations and procedures and for his (her) presence in the delivery room should be clarified early to avoid unpleasantness or last minute rushes. Particular desires for a delivery position other than the traditional lithotomy, immediate breastfeeding, or any other details which may make the labor and birth experience more satisfactory for the family should be ascertained as early as possible. Nurses and physicians should begin to recognize that these things are proper for the clients themselves to decide unless a true complication warrants intervention. When an effort has been made to establish a relationship of mutual respect and trust, emergency interventions will usually be accepted without question, provided explanations are given as soon as is practical after the event.

Physical and Emotional Needs

The sequence of the different aspects of nursing care during the first stage of labor as presented under the headings "Physical and Emotional Needs" and "Observations During Labor" is not in order of priority. Such an order would be impossible to give, since each labor is different and each mother's response varies. The rapidity of labor and the condition of the mother and baby will sometimes determine priorities. At other times, the mother's reaction to labor will indicate the area of care that needs early attention. Some aspects of the care described below can be met simultaneously. The nurse can provide emotional support through reassurance and her attitude and manner even while she is hurriedly preparing for an imminent delivery or meeting an emergency situation. In each such instance, she must use good judgment in making a decision of the best sequence of the various aspects of care important to the woman in labor.

Measures to Prevent Infection

Prevention of infection is an important part of planning for the care of the mother in labor. One of the first and foremost precautions is careful hand washing before and after giving care or handling equipment. Thorough washing at the beginning of the day with a liquid soap or detergent containing a bactericidal agent is an important safeguard. For a continuing bacteriostatic effect, one of the antibacterial preparations such as green soap containing G-11 or pHisoHex is often used exclusively for hand washing in the labor and delivery room area.

Uniforms worn by personnel caring for women in labor should not be worn outside of the labor and delivery unit. The attire of personnel is frequently a "scrub dress," provided by the hospital. A cap that covers the hair is also usually required for the delivery room.

Personnel in the labor unit must be free of all signs of infection. Anyone with evidence of upper respiratory infection, skin lesions, diarrhea or gastrointestinal upset, or any infectious disease should be excluded. Anyone having recently cared for a person with an infection must also be excluded from care of the woman in labor.

To prevent contamination from other patients, each mother must have her own personal equipment—bedpan, wash basin, and emesis basin. Each mother is carefully observed for possible signs of infection at the time of admission and also during labor; such signs are reported to the physician at once. If a mother has an infection or develops one, arrangements for isolation must be made immediately.

Preparation of the Mother

Preparation of the Vulva

In the past it was routine to shave the suprapubic region, vulva, inner surface of the thighs, and anal region prior to delivery. It was believed by many physicians that removal of the hair allowed for more adequate skin preparation in the delivery room, easier perineal repair, and better cleansing of the perineal area during the postpartum period. Research has not supported this position, however. On the contrary, there is some evidence that shaving may even increase the risk of infection as a result of nicks and abrasions which provide a portal of entry for organisms.[1,2] The current trend is to limit shaving, removing only the hair from the area between the lower labia to just past the anus. The safest procedure is to omit shaving altogether and clip the hairs from the perineum with scissors if necessary to facilitate episiotomy repair.

Some high-risk intrapartum patients and those scheduled for cesarean section still have the abdomen and perineum shaved in anticipation of surgery. This shaving procedure will be easier to carry out and less uncomfortable for the mother if it is done early rather than in the rush of an emergency situation.

The nurse washes her hands carefully before starting the procedure, to prevent contamination of the perineal area from an outside source. The equipment that is used (basin and razor) are sterile. A liquid soap or detergent containing pHisoHex or another bacterial agent, and a safety razor are used. The mother lies on her back during the shaving, and she should be

[1] R. C. Burchell, Predelivery removal of pubic hair, *Obstet. Gynecol.* 24:272–273 (Aug.) 1964.
[2] H. I. Kantor, *et al.*, Value of shaving the pudendal–perineal area in delivery preparation, *Obstet. Gynecol.* 25:509–512 (April) 1965.

adequately draped and screened to minimize embarrassment. The area is well lathered with the soap or detergent, using a gauze sponge or cotton ball. The skin is held taut, and the hair is shaved off with short, even strokes of the razor in a downward direction. Care must be taken to avoid contamination of the vagina. This care includes precautions against soap solution or loose hair entering the vaginal opening and against return of sponges and razors to the vulvar area after they have touched the anal region. Preparation of the vulva is done with sufficient care to assure removal of all hair and also removal of smegma, which may have acumulated in the folds between the labia. A good light facilitates preparation. Loose hair is quite easily wiped off with dry gauze or gauze moistened with the soap or detergent solution. Sometimes the vulva is washed with warm water after shaving, but if a nonirritating antiseptic solution is used, it may be left on the skin for its continuing bacteriostatic effect.

After complete preparation of the vulvar area, the mother is asked to turn to her side for shaving of the anal region. All other areas should be completely finished before preparation of the anal region is begun to avoid returning to a cleaner area after the anal region is touched. The entire preparation is done as quickly as possible. The mother may become very uncomfortable due to the position she must assume; she may also become faint while on her back. It is often necessary to stop the procedure temporar-

ily during contractions for the comfort of the mother. She may find it necessary to turn to her side during a contraction. Faintness is usually relieved if the mother temporarily assumes a side position to relieve hypotension.

Enema

An enema is usually ordered by the physician, to be given fairly early in labor, unless the client's obstetric history or examination contraindicates such stimulation. An enema is given for one or more of several reasons—it helps to stimulate uterine contractions; it removes fecal material from the rectum which may, especially if present in large amounts, interfere with descent of the fetal head and also possibly interfere with adequate examination (Fig. 14-2); and it lessens the possibility of expulsion of fecal material during delivery, with subsequent contamination of the field.

The major contraindication to an enema in labor is vaginal bleeding. In addition, when the fetal head has descended deep into the pelvis and is exerting pressure on the rectum, the mother may have considerable difficulty in expelling an enema. To avoid expulsion of fluid and liquid fecal material during the delivery, the enema is sometimes omitted when the head is low, since it is easier to remove solid fecal material from the field during delivery than the fluid of an enema. An enema may also be omitted if labor is progressing rapidly, to avoid the

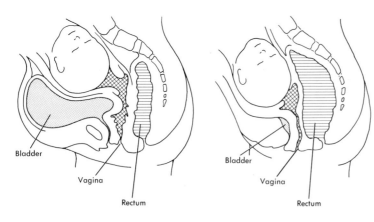

Figure 14-2. Relation of full bladder and full bowel to position of baby's head. [*Reproduced from Anita M. Jones,* A Manual for Teaching Midwives. *U.S. Department of Labor (now U.S. Department of Health, Education, and Welfare), Children's Bureau, Washington, D.C., 1939.*]

possibility of the baby being born during expulsion of the enema.

Some women will have several bowel movements or even diarrhea during early labor as a result of the increased parasympathetic activity as well as the excitement of beginning the long-awaited labor. For this reason, it is wise to obtain information from the woman on admission concerning recent bowel function and, perhaps, even to do a rectal examination. If the bowel is empty an enema is unnecessary.

A common solution used for the enema is warm tap water. A small enema is sufficient, usually 250–500 ml to empty the lower bowel of fecal material. Saline or sodium bicarbonate enemas are not used during pregnancy; if absorption takes place, the sodium content in the body may be increased above a desirable amount. Prepackaged, disposable enemas of hypertonic solution, such as Fleet are quite satisfactory and more comfortable for the mother than large quantities of tap water. Sometimes a suppository is used to stimulate a bowel movement instead of an enema.

The mother may expel the enema on the toilet unless complications require bed rest. In all cases of labor, the mother must have at hand a means of calling for assistance, and the nurse must be near and readily available. The fetal heart should be checked after expulsion of the enema has been completed.

Activity

The findings during the admission assessment of the mother will determine whether she is to remain in bed during her entire labor or is to be allowed activity out of bed. Among the indications for complete bed rest are faulty presentation and position of the baby; complications of pregnancy, particularly vaginal bleeding; and advanced labor. Bed rest is often necessary when the membranes are ruptured, being indicated when the presenting part is high because of the possibility of prolapse of the umbilical cord. When the head is low in the pelvis, the mother may be out of bed with ruptured membranes during the first part of her labor. If the membranes rupture while the mother is out of bed, the nurse should help her into bed immediately, check the fetal heart rate, and perform a vaginal examination to check the station and position of the presenting part and make sure that prolapse of the cord has not occurred. The attending physician should be notified at once of this change in the mother's condition. Another indication for placing a mother at complete bed rest is the administration of a sedative or analgesic drug. Many mothers will not present conditions that require bed rest and may therefore be out of bed as they desire.

Since contractions are infrequent and mild at first, the mother may prefer to be up and about much of the time in the early part of the first stage, particularly during the daytime. Some mothers tend to stay in bed too much during the first stage and are advised to be out of bed, since being on their feet often promotes their comfort, and activity may make the contractions more regular and efficient. However, the mother must be cautioned against tiring herself and should, therefore, sit or lie down often enough and long enough to avoid fatigue. When labor begins at night, it is often advisable for the mother to stay in bed and try to sleep as much as possible until morning. Even though her sleep is disturbed by the contractions, she will be less tired in the morning than if she had gotten up.

Position

When the laboring woman is in bed she may assume any position she finds comfortable. The supine position should be avoided, however, because of the risk of vena caval compression by the heavy uterus, which can result in decreased cardiac output and diminished blood flow to the placenta and fetus. This risk as well as strain on her back can be prevented by elevating the head of the bed 30 to 40 degrees when the mother is on her back. The side position may be most comfortable when she obtains relief of back discomfort from strong pressure applied to the lower back by her husband or the nurse during contractions. Some mothers find sitting up straight on the edge of the bed with their feet on a chair most comfortable if they have considerable discomfort in their back during contractions. Sitting tailor fashion on the bed with the head of the bed rolled all the way up so she can periodically lean back to rest is also comfortable for many women.

Dr. Roberto Caldeyro-Barcia and others make the following comments from findings in the great majority of cases they included in a study on "Effect of Position Changes on the Intensity and Frequency of Uterine Contractions During Labor":

. . . when the patient lies on the side (right or left), uterine contractions have a greater intensity and a lower frequency than when the patient lies on the back.

The uterine tonus is higher in the dorsal position, possibly because when the patient lies on her side the frequency diminishes and there is thus more time for completing relaxation of the uterus. This factor is particularly significant in cases of too frequent contractions, where the tonus is likely to be elevated. . . . Excessive contractility and tonus in the patient who is supine may be lessened by turning her to the side, which represents a useful clinical application of these observations.

With the patient on her side, the contractions appear to be better coordinated than when the patient is supine. This is particularly true in prelabor. . . .[3]

The mechanisms by which the changes of position of the patient have such important effects on uterine contractility are completely unknown.

The characteristics of the contractions suggest that those produced when the patient lies on her side should be more efficient for the progress of labor than those produced when the patient is on her back.[4]

[3] Roberto Caldeyro-Barcia, Luis Noriega-Guerra, Luis A. Cibils, Hermogenes Alvarez, Juan J. Poseiro, Serafin V. Pose, Yamandu Sica-Blanco, Carlos Mendez-Bauer, Carlos Fielitz, and Venus H. Gonzalez-Panizza, Effect of position changes on the intensity and frequency of uterine contractions during labor, *Am. J. Obstet. Gynecol.* 80:285 (Aug.) 1960.
[4] *Ibid.*, p. 288.

Food and Fluids

Opinions vary concerning the amount and kind of fluids and nourishment allowed or offered during labor, and the nurse should obtain an order from the physician before offering fluid or nourishment. Digestion is slowed or ceases during labor, and the stomach does not empty well. Food in undigested form may be retained in the stomach for 12 hours, or even much longer. Sometimes gastric dilatation develops, and the mother may have a large amount of food and fluid in her stomach when she is ready for delivery. If a general anesthetic must be administered when food has recently been ingested or when the stomach is full, there is great danger of aspiration of vomitus. Solid food is therefore, generally, not given during labor.

Women in labor rarely desire food and are not uncomfortable without it; some do not retain it because of vomiting. Sometimes clear liquids such as water, tea, clear broth, ginger ale, or other soft drinks are offered in small amounts as desired by the mother during early labor unless progress appears to be rapid. These liquids are given to supply her with fluid and with some nourishment for the exhausting effort of labor. Hard candy, ice chips, and popsicles are also used to relieve the dry, unpleasant taste in the mouth and to supply some fluid and calories. At other times all oral food and fluid are withheld throughout the entire labor; an empty stomach is preferred because many emergencies in the intrapartum period are not predictable.

Fluid intake during labor is recorded. If the mother is not allowed fluid orally, takes little, or vomits all that has been taken, or if labor is prolonged, fluid may be administered parenterally. An intravenous infusion of a liter of fluid may be given every 8 to 12 hours in order to furnish the calories used during labor and to prevent hypoglycemia and dehydration.

Care of the Urinary Bladder

The mother should be encouraged to void frequently, at least every two to three hours, during labor. It is sometimes easier for her to empty her bladder if she voids before it becomes distended. If she is unable to void and if her bladder becomes distended, the physician will usually wish to have her catheterized. Bladder distention is fairly common during labor, and in extreme cases the bladder may extend to the umbilicus. The bladder is drawn up in front of the lower uterine segment during pregnancy and thereby becomes an abdominal organ; with such placement, distention is easily visible and palpable, except in very obese women, and the nurse should watch the lower abdomen for bladder distention (Fig. 14-3). The volume of urine voided is also observed.

A distended bladder may retard labor by interfering with descent of the baby's head (Fig. 14-2) and by reflex inhibition of uterine contractions. A full bladder increases the mother's discomfort, and the bladder itself may be traumatized when distended. Trauma may predispose to postpartum urinary retention and cystitis.

If catheterization is necessary, a few special precautions must be observed. Care is taken that solutions used to clean the area around the urethral orifice, prior to insertion of the catheter, do not enter the vagina. This can be prevented by using sponges moistened just enough

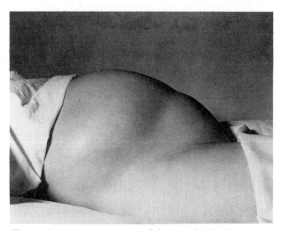

Figure 14-3. A woman in labor with the lower abdomen showing a distended bladder. The bladder becomes an abdominal organ during pregnancy, and distention is easily visible and palpable.

to clean, but not soaked with an excess amount of solution. To minimize discomfort and possible trauma, especially if the baby's head is pressing against the urethra, a small (no larger than no. 14 French), flexible catheter is used, and the catheter is well lubricated with a water-soluble lubricating jelly so that it will slide in easily. The catheter is inserted between contractions, since pressure from the fetal head against the urethra is less at that time than during a contraction, and the mother has less discomfort from the procedure when it is performed between contractions.

The urinary output during labor is recorded. This may have special significance if the patient has a toxemia of pregnancy or shows signs of an impending toxemia.

Emotional Support

The woman in labor needs a sympathetic, understanding person with her almost constantly— one who communicates a personal interest in her through both words and actions. Providing reassurance and emotional support is a very important aspect of a nurse's care of the mother in labor. It is often impossible for the nurse to stay with the mother constantly, but she can contribute a great deal to the mother's comfort during frequent, short intervals at the bedside if that time is used effectively. Evidence of interest, sympathy, and understanding from the nurse and the illusion that the nurse is not hurried will be comforting to the mother. There are many ways in which the nurse's interest in the mother can be conveyed to her; the nurse must decide how best to do this in the individual situation. Complete concentration on the mother during the interim of time that the nurse is with her is important. Giving physical care—washing the face, giving a back rub, or changing bed linen— provides not only bodily comfort, but also demonstrates an interest in the mother. If the nurse works easily and avoids quick, bustling movements she is less likely to give the impression that she is hurried. When the nurse cannot remain with the mother for more than short intervals, it is helpful to know that the nurse will not be far away and will be back soon. The mother needs to have the feeling that she may call the nurse frequently without apology or concern that she is asking for undue attention. The nurse must always give the mother an adequate explanation of how to use the signal system and make sure that the signal is within easy reach.

Explanation of the reasons for various aspects of care and interpretation of normal occurrences during labor, which the mother may not understand and which may cause her alarm, will do much to dispel anxiety and fear. The mother will wish to have frequent reassurance that she is making progress and that she is cooperating and conducting herself well. The woman in labor is very alert to her environment. She is acutely aware of the tone of voice, facial expression, disinterest, or false enthusiasm of those around her, but also responds just as readily to genuine interest. Conversations outside of the labor room are easily overheard and may be misinterpreted; the attitude and conduct of everyone in the labor room area are, therefore, important.

In providing for the mother's emotional needs, the nurse recognizes the importance of the husband's role in giving his wife emotional support and relieving her anxiety. He may be her primary source of support—sometimes by actively assisting her with relaxation and sometimes by sitting at her bedside without active participation in her care. Each couple can best decide for themselves the most desirable way the husband can help relieve his wife's discomfort and anxiety. Sometimes the husband has attended preparation-for-childbirth classes with his wife and has learned how he can assist her to use to best advantage the breathing and relaxation techniques she learned and how he can help to relieve her back discomfort. Some husbands do not know what they can do and appreciate suggestions from the nurse. In certain instances, the husband's presence without active participation in easing discomfort seems most desirable to both him and his wife, and in still other instances his presence in the waiting room, with only brief periods in the labor room, is preferred by both. The nurse must be sensitive to the desires of both and provide an opportunity for the husband to give support to his wife in the way that seems best to both of them.

Throughout labor the nurse should be aware of the expected behaviors of the laboring woman. To the experienced labor-room nurse, these behaviors may be as accurate an indication of the progress of labor as cervical dilatation.

Early in labor the woman is likely to be quite excited that labor has begun. Contractions are milder and easier to control. If she is at home the woman will usually go about her work, stopping to time contractions or to breathe through the contraction if necessary. In the hospital she may be up and about, walking around, visiting with her family, watching TV, or playing cards. She is usually talkative, interested in her surroundings and in other women in labor. As the active phase of labor begins (about 4 cm cervical dilatation), more energy is required to cope with the work of labor. The woman puts aside her cards or TV and will usually either go to bed or find a comfortable place to sit. She verbalizes in single sentences and tends to talk only about things necessary for her comfort and work. She may ask for medication, direct someone where to rub her back, request to have her face wiped with a cool cloth. Between contractions she may seem to doze; her eyes are often closed to shut out the environment.

During transition (7–10 cm cervical dilatation) the contractions are most painful. In addition, discomfort from pressure of the descending presenting part may make it difficult for the woman to tell when contractions are starting and stopping. She tends not to talk at all unless absolutely necessary and then in short phrases or single words. She may cry out with the pain of contractions and frustration that labor will never end. She may become nauseated, her legs may shake uncontrollably, and she is often irritable, restless, and does not want to be touched. Constant attendance by the nurse is essential to help the woman cope with this phase of labor and to help the family understand her behavior.

The second stage of labor is characterized by egocentrism and extreme concentration on the physical task of delivery. Between pushing efforts the woman often becomes amnesic and seems unaware of her surroundings. Even though apparently oblivious to what is happening around her, she is often able to recall events with precise accuracy after delivery. For this reason, personnel must be careful not to say anything which could alarm her unnecessarily or speak or act in a way which implies lack of respect for her and the birth taking place.

As soon as the baby is born a dramatic change occurs in most women. Now there is great interest in the baby and the father. Drowsiness and introversion are replaced by euphoria, talkativeness, and a happy fatigue.

Just as the physiologic events of labor vary from one woman to the next, so the behavioral responses may vary. In particular, the woman who has epidural anesthesia during labor will not manifest the behaviors described above for the second half of labor. Therefore, the nurse will need to rely more heavily on physical findings to judge the progress of labor, and will need to provide different kinds of support for the woman and her family. To provide emotional support during labor to women with a variety of needs and a variety of reactions to labor, the nurse must be very sensitive to each situation and plan her care accordingly. This is an aspect of care which challenges her ability, but also one which will provide satisfaction to her as well as to her patients.

Personal Hygiene

Restlessness, perspiration, vaginal discharge, and drainage of amniotic fluid add to the physical discomforts of labor. Sometimes so much of the mother's and the nurse's attention is directed toward alleviating the discomfort of the contractions that there may be less awareness of these physical discomforts than under less trying circumstances. However, attention to personal hygiene will give physical comfort. The presence of the nurse, and her demonstration of personal interest while she is giving physical care, will at the same time provide emotional support. Washing the mother's face and hands, combing her hair, changing moist and wrinkled gown and bed linen, and an occasional sponge bath, or a shower if the mother is allowed out of bed, are important aspects of nursing care during labor.

If the physician's orders permit the mother to be out of bed, a warm shower is refreshing. The nurse must remain with the mother while she takes a shower and assist her as much as possible. Provision should be made for the mother to sit down when she has a contraction while in the shower by placing a chair close to the shower stall or by putting a metal stool, covered with a quilted pad, in the shower stall.

The mother's mouth may become very dry and uncomfortable as a result of vomiting or lack of fluids or both. Provision for mouth rinses, ice chips if permitted, and cream to dry lips will give some relief.

Care of the Vulva

The vulva and perineal area require special attention during labor because of the relatively large amount of vaginal discharge and because precautions are necessary to prevent contamination of the area. The vulva is wiped free of discharge after examinations and after voiding and is washed with soap and water whenever indicated to prevent accumulation of discharge and its drying on the skin. This vaginal discharge is a tenacious mucus; it is uncomfortable as it dries and is then very difficult to remove. Care must be taken that solutions used in cleaning the vulva do not enter the vagina. The nurse must wash her hands before giving care.

The mother is ordinarily not permitted to wear a perineal pad during labor, except as necessary when she is up and walking about. The perineal pad is apt to slide back and forth, and in so doing, the portion of the pad that touched the anal region will come in contact with the vaginal orifice. A sterile, disposable, absorbent pad is kept under the mother's hips to absorb the bloody mucous discharge and the amniotic fluid that drains from the vagina. This pad is changed frequently. The pad should be handled in such a way that the side that will be placed next to the mother is not touched with the hands.

Breathing and Relaxation Techniques

The woman who has attended preparation-for-childbirth classes needs considerable support and encouragement to use successfully the breathing and relaxation techniques that she has learned. Even the mother who is well prepared for labor may become confused and forget while she is under the emotional and physical stress of labor, and need frequent reminders. An important part of a mother's success in using the methods she learned is the support provided her during labor. She needs assistance from a person who understands the physical and psychologic aspects of labor and who can provide an environment conducive to the application of the techniques she has learned.

Since different education-for-childbirth programs vary in the techniques taught and may make changes in some of the techniques from time to time, the nurse should be knowledgeable about the methods currently taught in her geographic area. The nurse should then learn from the mother her specific preparation for labor and her expectations of herself and of others. With such knowledge the nurse can support the mother in her response to uterine contractions in the way she desires. The husband or the nurse, who understands the mother's preparation, is able to give her the necessary encouragement and coaching. Under stress she is likely to need frequent reminders in spite of long hours of practice. The nurse's evidence of a sincere interest in the mother is important in giving her support.

The husband often encourages and coaches his wife throughout most or all of the labor and delivery. He has often attended the training sessions with her and assisted her in practicing the techniques that are taught. In addition, the husband can often relieve his wife of other worries and concerns that may increase tension. The husband is with his wife during labor as much as is possible and as is mutually agreeable to both.

Mothers prepared for abdominal breathing during labor may have trained to take long slow deep abdominal breaths or some variation of abdominal breathing. One modification is the use of several slow abdominal breaths during each contraction instead of only one or possibly two long breaths. Another variation combines raising of the abdominal wall with chest breathing. It consists of raising of the abdominal wall with an inhalation at the beginning of a contraction, holding the abdominal wall up while continuing with slow deep chest breathing during the contraction, and then slowly lowering the abdominal wall at the end of the contraction. Lifting of the abdominal wall during most of the contraction permits the uterus to push forward during the contraction without resistance from a tense abdominal wall. It also precludes painful spasms of tense abdominal wall muscles.

Mothers trained in abdominal breathing have also learned how to release muscle tension and relax muscles at will. While the mother concentrates on abdominal breathing, she will plan to relax the rest of her body, lying quietly, with hands limp and face muscles relaxed.

Conscious effort at relaxation is probably not necessary in early labor, while contractions are mild. The mother is aware of her contractions at this time and she may be somewhat apprehensive, but she is also often pleased that labor has begun. During this early stage the mother will probably wish to visit, read, and walk about.

As contractions become uncomfortable, relaxation and abdominal breathing during contractions are started. This effort will require considerable concentration on the part of the mother and careful coaching by the nurse or the husband. As the contractions increase in frequency, intensity, and length, more and more concentration is necessary to achieve relaxation, and every effort must be made to help the mother. She has become very serious by this time, is often quite tired, and perhaps is anxious. Her need to have someone remain with her becomes greater than it has previously been. The nurse should watch the mother for signs of tenseness, such as tightening of the facial muscles and clenching of the hands, and remind her to relax these muscles. It may be comforting to the mother to be able to hold someone's hand, but this should not be a squeezing grip and again may necessitate a reminder not to tense muscles. The nurse can do much to help the mother get rest between contractions by encouraging her to rest as much as possible during such intervals, but without making a conscious effort to relax at these times. Abdominal breathing may be continued in the intervals between contractions, but at a faster rate than during contractions.

Toward the end of the first stage of labor—during the transition phase—when dilatation is almost complete, the contractions become more intense, and the mother may become very tired and discouraged. She may become quite restless and may show an increasing amnesia between contractions so that she seems to be unaware of happenings around her. She becomes very warm and may wish to have the room quite cool.

Mothers who do abdominal breathing during the first part of labor usually find it is difficult or impossible by the time the transition phase of labor arrives. The mother ordinarily changes to chest breathing at this time, and she must increase her efforts to relax.

Although it may not have been necessary or possible for the nurse to stay with the mother at all times during the early part of labor, especially if she has been relaxing well and if she has felt free to call someone whenever she wished, it does become important for the nurse to be with her during the period of transition. The mother needs frequent reassurance that this period, which is the most uncomfortable part of her labor, usually does not last long and that she will feel better as soon as the cervix is completely dilated, at which time she may begin bearing down. For an uninformed mother such explanation is especially important since she may assume that her discomfort will become

progressively worse and she may become very discouraged.

Mothers prepared according to the Lamaze method have learned several levels of intercostal breathing and have practiced exercises for neuromuscular release. The mother has learned to do rapid shallow breathing with full intensity and concentration. She will use chest breathing during each uterine contraction, changing the level to an increasing intensity with the progress of labor (Figure 14-4A, B, C, D, E). She has also learned to concentrate actively on relaxing quickly the muscles that are not involved when a certain group of muscles is contracted. She now uses this learning to release other muscles while the uterine muscle is contracting and also to relax between contractions. The mother consciously relaxes the rest of her body at the same time that she responds to a contraction with controlled breathing. She actively participates in her labor with a conditioned response to each uterine contraction. During each contraction she concentrates intently on the level of breathing appropriate to the progress of labor and on relaxation of the muscles not involved in labor. With this conditioned response and concentration on a specific method, the mother blocks out the painful sensations of the contractions.

During the early first stage of labor, when contractions are mild, intense concentration on breathing and relaxation is ordinarily not necessary. The mother will, however, ordinarily begin her breathing techniques. Slow deep chest breathing is used during the contractions of early labor. Conscious release of muscles during and between contractions is also begun.

The mother makes a change to slow, even pant breathing when slow chest breathing no longer gives comfort or good control. This is usually necessary as soon as contractions increase in intensity and is likely to be at approximately 4 cm of cervical dilatation. Beginning now the mother must give her full concentration to good response to the contractions. Back pressure and massage during contractions may be helpful. A wet washcloth to her face is cooling and comforting (Fig. 14-5). Frequent emptying

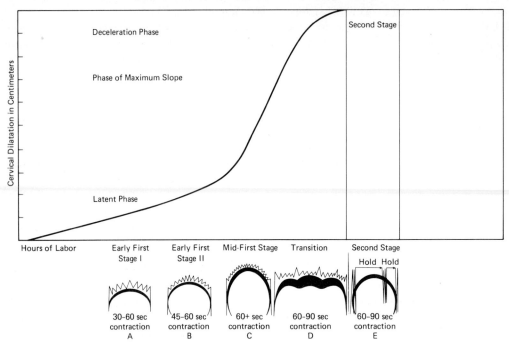

Figure 14-4. Diagrams of Lamaze breathing techniques shown against a Friedman curve to illustrate the appropriate time during labor for each type of breathing.

A. Early first stage breathing is used from onset of true labor to approximately 4 cm dilatation. Slow chest breathing is used during each contraction in the earliest part of the first stage of labor. The mother may be able to do her breathing through the early contractions as slowly as six to nine breaths per minute. It is likely that this slow chest breathing will be started at home, before admission to the hospital.

B. As the uterine contractions become closer and longer, the mother changes to slow pant breathing when she finds that slow chest breathing no longer gives comfort and control

C. During the mid first stage, which lasts from approximately 4 to 7 cm dilatation, the mother must give full concentration to her breathing during contractions. She may begin this phase of labor by using slow, even, pant breathing and continue with it until she feels the need for faster breathing over the peak of her contractions. She then changes to accelerated-decelerated breathing. She uses rapid, but light and shallow, chest breathing, which she accelerates in pace toward and over the peak of the contraction and decelerates in pace as the contraction begins to wane.

D. A pant-blow technique of breathing is used during the transition phase of labor. After taking a cleansing breath, the mother does rapid, shallow panting. Between each 4, 5, or 6 pants she blows her breath out forcefully. She continues the pant-blow breathing throughout the contraction and at the end of the contraction takes another cleansing breath.

The cleansing breath is important before and after each contraction and is thus used with the breathing in each part of the illustrations of Figure 14-4.

E. During the second stage of labor the mother takes two deep breaths at the beginning of the contraction, takes a third deep breath and holds it, and pushes as long as she can hold that breath. When necessary to take another breath she again takes two deep breaths, takes a third deep breath and holds, and pushes until the contraction ends. She then takes a cleansing breath, leans back, and relaxes. [*Figures 14-4* A, B, C, D, *and* E *courtesy of Dr. Sandra O'Leary, R.N., Instructor in Parentcraft, member of American Society for Psychoprophylaxis in Obstetrics, Inc.*]

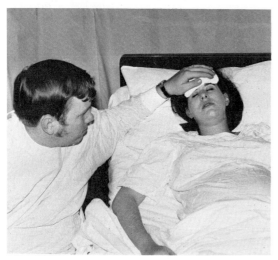

Figure 14-5. The husband is encouraging and coaching his wife during labor, and is providing physical comfort. The mother appears to be giving full concentration to slow, even, pant breathing and to relaxation of the muscles that are not involved in labor.

of the bladder avoids discomfort from its fullness.

When the mother feels the need for faster breathing during the peak of each contraction, she makes a change from slow pant breathing to accelerated and decelerated breathing. She then uses rapid, but light and shallow, chest breathing, which she accelerates and decelerates in pace with the duration and intensity of each contraction. The mother accelerates her breathing toward and over the peak of the contraction and when the contraction begins to wane she decelerates the pace of her breathing. It is helpful to the mother if her husband or another person tells her when 15, 30, and 45 seconds have passed (Fig. 14-6). Intense concentration and active participation with each contraction take a great deal of effort, especially if the contractions come in close succession. The mother may begin to feel tired and become discouraged, and needs encouragement to continue in her efforts. It is helpful to the mother to have someone check her for muscle release as well as for breathing techniques. It is important that her

breathing remain shallow and superficial to avoid hyperventilation.

During the transition phase of labor the mother may change to a rapid, light, pant-blow breathing. She blows her breath out forcefully at intervals while doing shallow panting during each contraction. This is the most difficult phase of her labor. The mother may feel irritable and she may be uncomfortable from leg cramps, nausea, chills, and perspiration. She may feel a vague sense of loss of control. She needs encouragement and reminders that she will soon be ready to push with her contractions. Complete relaxation between contractions is very important at this time. Concentration on breathing and relaxation will be most effective if distractions are kept to a minimum.

Hyperventilation may become a problem with rapid breathing if the breathing is not shallow enough or if panting is prolonged. Hyperventilation increases the loss of carbon dioxide and leads to a respiratory alkalosis and the appearance of symptoms. The mother may feel tingling

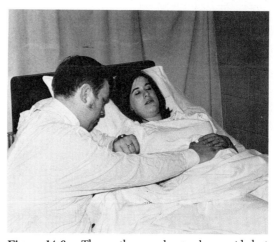

Figure 14-6. The mother accelerates her rapid, but light shallow chest breathing toward and over the peak of her contraction and then decelerates the pace of her breathing when her contraction begins to wane. Her husband is assisting her in determining when the peak of the contraction has passed and is also checking her for muscle release. Note that the mother's left hand appears relaxed.

and numbness in her hands and feet and may develop carpopedal spasms. Possible adverse effects of maternal alkalosis on the fetus are being investigated.

The effects of hyperventilation can be overcome by having the mother slow the rate of her breathing and hold her breath for a few moments or rebreathe air in a paper bag. The prepared mother will ordinarily keep her breathing sufficiently shallow and she has usually been instructed in management if she notes symptoms of hyperventilation. She may, however, overanticipate the necessity for rapid breathing and need reminders to slow the rate of breathing if it becomes very rapid, or a suggestion to keep her breathing very shallow. When an untrained mother breathes with hyperventilation she is likely to become distressed by both the symptoms and her lack of understanding of their cause. She needs explanation to relieve her concern and needs instructions in proper breathing. Since some trained mothers have difficulty in using rapid shallow breathing effectively and some become fatigued with the method, changes in respiratory techniques, with substitution of a slower breathing for the very rapid breaths, have been made in some education-for-childbirth classes.

Most methods of preparation for childbirth recommend that the mother take a deep breath in and out at the start of each contraction, before beginning the series of shallower breaths used during the contraction. They also recommend that she take a deep inhalation at the end of a contraction and then let her breath out slowly and relax as with a sigh. The deep inhalation and slow exhalation used at the beginning and the end of each contraction are often called a complete breath or a cleansing breath. The slow deep breath provides for a good exchange of oxygen and carbon dioxide before and after the shallower breathing that is done during the contraction. It may also be useful in overcoming hyperventilation. In addition, a complete or cleansing breath at the end of a contraction helps the mother to define for herself that the contraction has ended and it provides a good beginning for the relaxation between contractions.

Mothers prepared by the Lamaze method may use light rhythmic massage (effleurage) over the lower abdomen in conjunction with their controlled breathing. This may be done by the mother herself or by her husband or the nurse. The massage is used as an aid in relaxing the abdominal muscles during contractions.

The need for analgesia is minimized when the mother has been prepared for labor and when she has the support of a skilled person. However, its use need not be eliminated during either the first or second stage of labor. The mother should know that she may ask for pain relief if she feels she needs it, or medication may be offered when the person caring for her observes signs suggesting the need for analgesia. Use of medication for pain relief and for relaxation does not mean failure in carrying out a preparation-for-childbirth program.

Some women are not prepared for labor. The unprepared mother is likely to be very anxious and tense and will need a great deal of support, assistance with relaxation, and detailed explanation of what is taking place as labor proceeds. She will, however, respond to the reassurance of a calm, sympathetic, and understanding nurse and can often be given considerable assistance with relaxation by instructions and suggestions that seem indicated at the moment. Instructions and frequent reminders to breathe slowly and deeply during each contraction, will be very helpful to her. When she is concentrating on slow, deep breathing she is less likely to tense other muscles in her body than when she takes short, quick breaths or holds her breath at intervals.

Administration of Drugs

Drugs that have a tranquilizing effect are often used during labor to relieve anxiety and apprehension, and analgesic drugs are frequently administered to reduce pain. These drugs are another means of reducing the discomfort of labor. They are more completely described in Chapter 13. The time of administration, the kind of drug used, and the dosage are determined by the physician, but the observations of the nurse caring for the client will be useful to him in his decision. The nurse informs the physician of the mother's request for pain relief and keeps him informed of her own observations of the mother's reactions to labor.

Since all drugs given to the mother affect the fetus as well, a general dictum is that the less medication given during labor the better. It should also be remembered, however, that an anxious mother in severe pain who is having difficulty coping with contractions may also distress her fetus. Increased maternal epinephrine produced in response to anxiety, can reduce uterine blood flow; therefore, the progress of labor may actually be impeded by severe anxiety. A carefully chosen analgesic and/or tranquilizer, when coupled with appropriate nursing support, is often sufficient to enable the woman to relax, get some rest, and regain control of her labor.

In general, intravenous administration of analgesics is desirable, providing faster relief at lower dosages. This also permits greater accuracy in predicting effects on the fetus, since it is not necessary to account for variability in the rate of muscular absorption. The administration should be timed to permit a sufficient interval for the placenta to clear the drug from fetal circulation prior to delivery.

After administration of a drug, it is important that the nurse provide an environment conducive to relaxation. The mother is made as comfortable as possible for a period of rest by suggesting that she attempt to void first, a change of bed linen, and assistance into the most comfortable position. The fetal heart is auscultated before the drug is administered, and the mother's pulse, respiration, and blood pressure are checked. The mother is usually informed that she is being given medication for rest and is urged to relax as much as possible in order to obtain maximum benefit from the drug. The room should be quiet and its temperature adjusted to the mother's comfort; most mothers wish to have the room quite cool.

After administration of a drug, the nurse must watch the mother and baby carefully. The mother is watched for respiratory depression. Careful observation of strength and frequency of contractions is necessary; labor may be slowed or it may progress rapidly. It may be difficult to decide from the mother's reactions when the second stage is reached, and close observation for signs of progress in labor is important. If a drug that causes excitement is given, the mother must be watched every moment to prevent her from injuring herself. The fetal heart tones are checked frequently.

Discomfort from Pressure

Pressure of the baby's head on pelvic structures—nerves, ligaments, and organs—may cause discomfort, sometimes severe, in the lower back, the pelvis, and the legs.

Low backache, over the lumbosacral region, may be experienced with each contraction, or it may be continuously present, with exacerbation during contractions. In some labors, pain in the lower back causes more discomfort throughout labor than the abdominal pain that accompanies each uterine contraction. Massage of the lower back with the palm of a hand, in the form of firm back rubbing, mainly pressure, may give relief. This massage may be done by the husband or by the nurse (Fig. 14-7). A small pillow placed under the lumbar region, if the mother is on her back, may give some comfort.

Cramps in the legs, especially if the baby's head is low in the pelvis, may be a source of discomfort in labor. These cramps usually cause excruciating pain and require immediate attention; they may return at frequent intervals. Relief is obtained by elevating and extending the leg, making pressure on the knee to keep the leg straight, flexing the foot, and forcibly pushing the forefoot as far as possible toward the knee

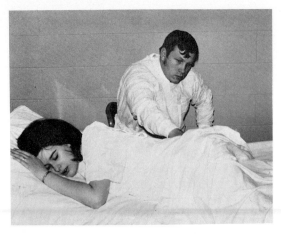

Figure 14-7. This woman's husband is putting very hard pressure over her lumbosacral area during contractions to provide relief from back pain.

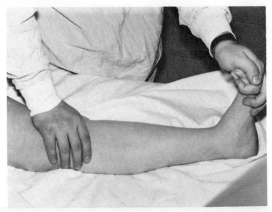

Figure 14-8. A leg cramp may be relieved by counterpressure on the foot. The leg is kept straight by pressure on the knee and the foot is flexed by forcibly pushing the forefoot toward the knee.

(Fig. 14-8). Stepping on the foot and walking about relieve muscle cramps if the mother is able to be up.

Pressure on the rectum, if the baby's head has descended low in the pelvis, is another source of discomfort, sometimes through a considerable part of labor. This pressure may prompt the mother to ask for the bedpan frequently, only to find that she cannot use it. Use of the bedpan often and unnecessarily is tiring; its frequent use may be reduced if the nurse gives the mother an adequate explanation for this constant feeling of a desire to empty her bowel. Since pressure on the rectum is often a sign of imminent delivery, especially if it appears late in labor, the nurse must assure herself of the stage to which labor has progressed when the mother complains of this pressure.

Occasionally, when the head is deeply engaged, there is so much *pressure low in the pelvis* that the mother has a certain amount of *involuntary bearing down* with contractions before dilatation of the cervix is complete. Such effort usually cannot be controlled, but the mother should be advised against any voluntary effort to bear down during the first stage. Voluntary effort at this time does not hasten labor,

uses energy unnecessarily, and may possibly cause edema of the cervix and small cervical tears. Pant-blow breathing during contractions may reduce the urge to push down.

OBSERVATIONS DURING LABOR

Important functions of the nurse caring for a woman in labor are (1) careful observation of the mother and the baby for their reactions to the stress of labor, and for early signs of complications that may affect their welfare, and (2) close observation of the progress of labor.

Observations of the Condition of the Mother

Temperature

The mother's temperature is taken every four hours unless prolonged labor or fever indicates that more frequent observation, along with other vital signs, is desirable. Normal labor has relatively little effect on the mother's temperature, and it should be expected to remain within normal limits. A rise to 37.6°C (99.6°F), or above, should be reported to the physician and is an indication for frequent checking.

Pulse and Respiration

The mother's pulse and respiration change relatively little during normal labor, except possibly during a contraction. The pulse and respiration are observed every hour; any increase is reported to the physician and indicates the need for more frequent observation. A pulse rate of 100 beats per minute is generally considered the upper limit of normal.

Blood Pressure

The mother's blood pressure is checked on admission to the hospital and every two to four hours thereafter, unless more frequent observation is indicated by elevation prior to or at the time of admission, or by the presence of other signs of toxemia or impending toxemia. It is best to obtain the blood pressure reading between contractions because there may be an increase from 5 to 10 mmHg during a contraction.

Frequent checking of blood pressure, as often as every 15 to 30 minutes, may be necessary if it is elevated. The doctor should be notified of an increase to 140 mmHg systolic and 90 diastolic, or sooner if the blood pressure was low on admission and appears to be steadily rising. Although the urinary output should be carefully recorded at all times, it must be particularly noted when the blood pressure is elevated.

Intake and Output

The importance of close observation of fluid intake and urinary output has been described on pages 304–305.

Headache

A headache during labor may be an indication that toxemia is developing. The blood pressure should be checked if a headache develops and both observations reported to the physician.

Vaginal Bleeding

Bleeding from the vagina, other than bloody show, however slight, necessitates immediate report to the doctor. Vaginal bleeding can usually be distinguished from bloody show by the character of the drainage. The show is a mucoid material containing a small amount of blood, whereas bleeding which is due to other causes appears as a trickle, or as a gush of bright red blood not mixed with mucus. At times it is difficult to determine the difference between bloody show and vaginal bleeding. If the nurse has any questions, she must bring it to the physician's attention.

Other Observations

The nurse must be alert to many other signs of impending danger and report all abnormal behavior so that treatment can be instituted early. Among some of the other signs that may indicate development of complications are dizziness, visual disturbances, frequent vomiting, epigastric pain, abnormally long and hard contractions or rigidity of the uterus, extreme sensitivity of the lower abdomen or constant abdominal pain, and undue restlessness.

Observation of the Condition of the Fetus

The second intrapartum client, the fetus, is more difficult to assess than the laboring woman. Most of the usual means of physical examination are unavailable to the nurse, since the fetus cannot be directly inspected, palpated, or manipulated.

The stress of uterine contractions poses a potential threat to every fetus. Fortunately, the vast majority are healthy and possess sufficient reserve to withstand labor with no ill effects. For the benefit of the few who cannot readily tolerate labor, however, the nurse must maintain a high index of suspicion and carefully monitor each fetus throughout the intrapartum period.

Because the chances of fetal distress are greater in high-risk pregnancies, the first step in fetal assessment is careful attention to the maternal history and the antepartum course of events. This is accomplished on admission to the labor suite by interview with the mother and review of the antepartum record (see page 298). Additional information about fetal presentation and position as well as a very crude estimate of fetal size can be obtained by palpation of the maternal abdomen (Leopold's maneuvers). Vaginal examinations give further evidence of presentation, position, and station of the presenting part. Other studies of a chemical or electronic nature may have been done during pregnancy or may be done during labor. Studies such as L/S ratio and ultrasound scans are discussed in Chapter 21.

While all clinical data must be considered in relationship to the total situation, the single most informative parameter of fetal well-being during labor is the fetal heart rate. For this reason observation of the fetal heart rate is an important responsibility of the nurse caring for a woman and fetus in labor. The rate must be counted often and recorded each time it is counted. It is essential that the nurse recognize abnormalities in rate so that prompt medical consultation may be obtained when necessary.

Patterns of Fetal Heart Rate

The normal range of fetal heart rate (FHR) is 120 to 160 beats per minute. Although the rate differs in different babies, it usually remains constant within a small variation of less than 10 beats per minute in an individual baby. If the heart rate has been carefully noted throughout gestation, the antepartal rate should provide a reasonably reliable baseline against which to compare the intrapartum values.

The uterine contractions of labor cause a transient reduction or arrest in maternal blood flow through the placenta. A healthy fetus will have enough oxygen reserve to sustain him during this time and no change in baseline heart rate will occur. In addition, the contractions compress the fetal head and body, and circulation through the umbilical cord can be occluded during a contraction if the cord is in a position where it receives pressure. The fetus may respond to these stresses of labor with a momentary slowing of the heart during some of the contractions, but then it quickly resumes the baseline rate. *Brief* arrests in maternal blood flow through the placenta and *short* periods of pressure do not appear to affect the fetus adversely, especially if the interval between contractions permits a complete recovery.

Abnormalities in the pregnancy; strong, long, very frequent contractions; or failure of the uterus to relax completely between contractions are likely to interfere with adequate fetal–maternal exchange in the placenta. Under such conditions the reduction in exchange of oxygen and carbon dioxide between fetal and maternal blood results in fetal hypoxia, hypercapnia, and metabolic disturbances, resulting in acidosis, all of which cause fetal distress. The fetus responds to distress with adaptive reactions in his circulatory system and his heart rate in an attempt to protect his vital organs and to restore his placental exchange to normal. Reactions to inadequate exchange manifest themselves in changes in normal FHR patterns. These changes may be manifested as alterations in the baseline rate or as periodic changes occurring in relation to uterine contractions.

Baseline Fetal Heart Rate

Baseline fetal heart rate is defined as the heart rate when the woman is not in labor or the rate between periodic changes during labor. In the absence of periodic changes (i.e., in normal labor), it is simply the level of the heart rate in beats per minute. Any rise or drop in baseline which persists for more than 10 minutes is regarded as a change to a new baseline.

A baseline FHR above 160 beats per minute is designated as *tachycardia* and is frequently associated with fetal immaturity and/or maternal fever. Tachycardia is often the first response of the fetus to hypoxia and, as such, should be regarded as an early sign of fetal distress.

A baseline FHR below 120 beats per minute is designated as *bradycardia*. Persistent bradycardia may be associated with congenital heart anomalies or, when accompanied by periodic changes in FHR, fetal distress and neonatal depression.

In addition to determining the level of the

baseline FHR, which can be readily accomplished using a fetoscope, continuous FHR monitors permit an evaluation of the *beat-to-beat variability* in the baseline. The level of the baseline, as well as the various periodic changes which may occur, is determined by a physiologic control mechanism which consists of interacting cardioaccelerator and cardiodecelerator reflexes. This interaction is dynamic rather than static, as the reflexes respond to each other and to other physiologic stimuli. As these accelerator and decelerator reflexes attempt to achieve balance, momentary fluctuations occur about the FHR baseline. These beat-to-beat fluctuations are considered to be a sign of a well-developed and well-functioning neurologic system. Maternal medications such as narcotics, tranquilizers, magnesium sulfate, or other central nervous system depressants will temporarily reduce or eliminate baseline variability. In the absence of maternal medication, loss of baseline variability must be regarded as an ominous sign of fetal acidosis, especially if it is accompanied by periodic decelerations. (See Figure 14-9.)

Periodic Fetal Heart Rate Changes

Periodic changes in fetal heart rate occur in relation to uterine contractions. These alterations may be either accelerations or, more commonly, decelerations. They are transitory departures from the baseline level followed by a return to the baseline after a short interval. Accelerations may occur in association with contractions as the fetus attempts to compensate for the temporarily decreased placental blood flow, or they may occur as a response to fetal activity. (See discussion of FAD, Chapter 21, page 621). Tactile stimulation of the fetus during vaginal examinations or by the contracting myometrium during contractions may also produce FHR accelerations. Accelerations which recur with each contraction may result from isolated compression of the umbilical vein and may precede the development of variable decelerations. Accelera-

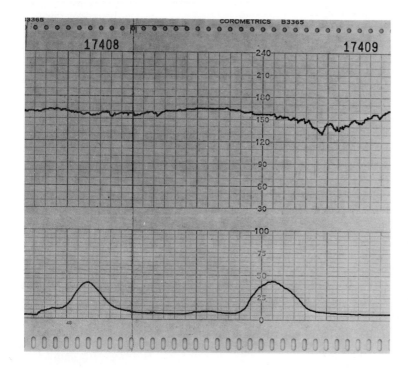

Figure 14-9. Fetal monitor tracing showing loss of variability in the baseline fetal heart rate. Compare this almost smooth baseline with that seen on the tracing in Figure 14-17. A *late deceleration* can be seen in conjunction with the second uterine contraction.

tions of 10–15 beats per minute occurring late in the contraction cycle and accompanied by loss of beat-to-beat variability are ominous signs of fetal distress and frequently evolve into late decelerations.

Decelerations are classified according to the *shape* of the deceleration curve. Some decelerations are of uniform shape and reflect the shape of the uterine contraction curve, while others are of variable shape and have little or no correlation with the shape of the uterine contraction. FHR deceleration patterns may be further classified according to the *time relationship* between the onset of the uterine contraction and onset of the deceleration.

The classification according to the time relationship is as follows.

EARLY DECELERATION Early deceleration has its onset early in the contraction cycle, reaches its lowest point at the time of the acme (peak) of the contraction, and has generally returned to the baseline by the end of the contraction. The degree of deceleration is usually proportional to the amplitude (intensity) of the contraction, although the heart rate rarely falls below 110–115 beats per minute. (See Figure 14-10.)

Early decelerations are thought to be caused mainly by compression of the fetal head, which results in increased intracranial pressure and decreased cerebral blood flow. The resulting local hypoxia stimulates the vagus nerve and produces a transient rise in vagal tone, which slows the heart rate. Early decelerations occur only in vertex presentations and are rare before 6 to 7 cm cervical dilatation. They are more common when the membranes are ruptured.

Even though cerebral hypoxia is one feature of the pathophysiology of early decelerations, these episodes are brief and appear to be well tolerated by the fetus. They are considered innocuous and are not associated with neonatal depression. Their clinical significance results from the need to differentiate them from late decelerations, which are similar in shape but occur at a different time in the contraction cycle and represent fetal distress.

LATE DECELERATION The late deceleration, like the early deceleration, is of uniform shape. Unlike the early deceleration it has its onset later in the contraction cycle, reaches its lowest point well after the acme of the contraction and may not begin recovery until after the contraction has subsided. (See Figure 14-10.)

Late decelerations are a sign of fetal hypoxia resulting from a reduction in maternal blood flow through the intervillous space during a contraction. There is a lag between the height of the contraction and the late deceleration, reflecting the fact that intervillous blood flow and, consequently, oxygen transfer to the fetus decreases as the contraction becomes more severe. In addition, some oxygen continues to be available to the fetus from oxyhemoglobin. In consequence, there is a lag in the fall in fetal PO_2 below a critical level.

Any condition in which there is a reduction in fetal–maternal exchange in the placenta is likely to result in late decelerations. Among such conditions are complications associated with reduced placental blood flow; placental pathology; maternal hypotension, which decreases placental perfusion; and strong frequent contractions which do not permit sufficient time to overcome the effects of the transient hypoxia of a contraction before the next one begins. Late decelerations which have a smooth curve and a smooth baseline (loss of variability) are indicative of a severely, and often chronically, asphyxiated fetus. These are most characteristic of the fetus from a high-risk pregnancy in which there is long-standing maternal or placental pathology. More acute impairment of fetal–maternal exchange usually produces late decelerations with no loss of heart rate variability or even with some increase in variability. Among these conditions are maternal hypotension resulting from supine position or conduction anesthesia and uterine hyperactivity. If the underlying cause can be recognized rapidly and corrected, these fetuses will usually recover quickly.

Late decelerations are frequently preceded and accompanied by a baseline tachycardia. These changes in fetal heart rate during distress

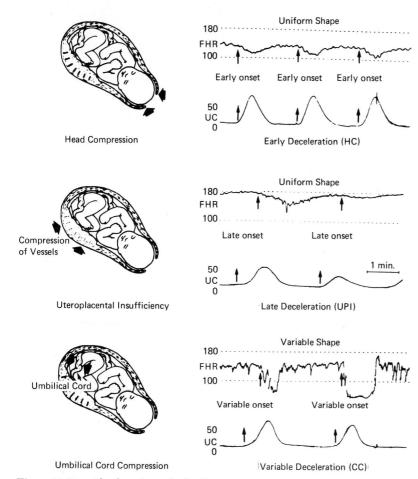

Figure 14-10. The three periodic fetal heart rate patterns.

The early deceleration pattern is thought to be due to fetal head compression. It is of *uniform shape*, reflects the shape of the associated intrauterine pressure curve, and has its onset *early* in the contracting phase of the uterus. Hence, it has been labeled "early deceleration." HC = head compression, UC = uterine contraction.

The late deceleration pattern is thought to be due to acute uteroplacental insufficiency as the result of decreased intervillous space blood flow during uterine contractions. It is also of *uniform shape* and reflects the shape of the associated intrauterine pressure curve. In this case, however, in contradistinction to the uniform FHR early deceleration pattern (above), its onset occurs *late* in the contracting phase of the uterus. Hence, it has been labeled "late deceleration." This FHR deceleration pattern is considered indicative of uteroplacental insufficiency. UPI = uteroplacental insufficiency.

The variable deceleration pattern is thought to be due to umbilical cord occlusion. It is of *variable shape*, does not reflect the shape of the associated intrauterine pressure curve, and its onset occurs at a variable time during the contracting phase of the uterus. CC = cord compression. [*Reproduced with permission from Edward H. G. Hon,* An Introduction to Fetal Heart Rate Monitoring. Corometrics Medical Systems, Inc., North Haven, Conn., 1973.]

are brought about by a decrease in the fetal oxygen supply, the retention of carbon dioxide, and the metabolic acidosis that results from inadequate oxygenation. When the fetus is deprived of adequate oxygen, glucose is incompletely metabolized. Lactic acid and other organic acids are produced instead of the carbon dioxide and water that would result from complete metabolism of glucose. This leads to an accumulation of lactic acid and a lowering of the pH of the blood. Hypoxia, hypercapnia, and metabolic acidosis are assumed to elicit a rise in the sympathetic tone of the fetus. This rise in sympathetic tone causes a persistent increase in the basal heart rate. With the rapid fetal heartbeat there is a greater flow of blood through the placenta, which tends to increase exchange between mother and baby and may thus improve the condition of the fetus.

The increase that has taken place in sympathetic tone also causes vasoconstriction of the skin, muscles, lungs, and visceral organs. Such vasoconstriction results in a decreased blood flow to organs not immediately essential and an increased flow to the brain and the heart. This redistribution in circulation protects the organs that are vital to survival of the fetus by supplying them with the available oxygen. The pulmonary vasoconstriction that occurs at this time, although tolerated satisfactorily by the fetus, may show a detrimental effect later. It is likely to initiate an adverse change in the lungs, which may lead to respiratory distress after birth.

Late decelerations that appear during distress reflect a temporary increase in vagal tone, resulting from the transient increase in fetal hypoxia during strong uterine contractions. A deceleration soon after the acme of a uterine contraction helps to conserve cardiac reserve. Each uterine contraction reduces and virtually stops circulation through the intervillous space. A large blood flow through the chorionic villi at this time would require a considerable amount of energy without improvement in the fetal condition. After the contraction has ended and the blood flow in the intervillous space resumes, bringing a fresh supply of blood to the placenta,

the fetal heart returns to the rapid rate. The fetal heart is thus rapid when the benefits of fetal–maternal exchange in the placenta are best and slow when exchange would be poor. Although late decelerations are a sign of fetal distress, they are apparently also a mechanism for saving cardiac energy during that interval following the height of a contraction, when the expenditure of energy demanded by a rapid rate would not net good results.

VARIABLE DECELERATION   The variable deceleration is well named, since it varies in almost every respect from the early and late decelerations. It is variable in its shape, not reflecting the uterine contraction curve; in its time relationship to the contraction cycle; in its magnitude and configuration; and even in its occurrence with successive contractions. The sides of the curve tend to sharp slopes, and the shape usually resembles a V or a squared U. (See Figure 14-10.)

Variable decelerations are the result of umbilical cord compression. As the umbilical vessels are occluded, the flow of oxygenated blood to the heart and thence to the head and upper trunk is decreased. In its place acidotic blood from the inferior vena cava flows through the foramen ovale and into cephalic circulation. This acidotic blood produces a strong vagal stimulation, which lowers the heart rate. A healthy fetus will usually tolerate variable decelerations that do not exceed 30 to 45 seconds witout distress. Decelerations lasting 1 minute or longer may produce distress even in the healthy fetus. Signs of fetal distress are similar to those discussed above: first an increase in baseline rate, followed by loss of baseline variability. Another finding suggestive of fetal distress is a brief acceleration of the heart rate immediately before and after the deceleration (see Figure 14-11).

Occasionally variable decelerations may occur between contractions presumably because of maternal or fetal movement which compresses the cord.

When variable decelerations are prolonged, preparations should be made for immediate de-

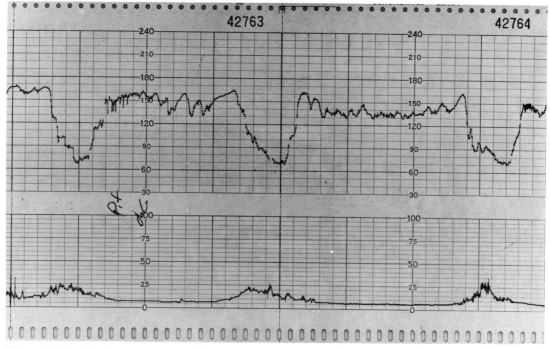

Figure 14-11. Fetal monitor tracing showing variable decelerations. These decelerations occur with each contraction, although the contractions are mild (amplitude less than 25 mmHg). Note the slight acceleration of the baseline heart rate immediately before and after each deceleration. The notation in panel 42763 indicates that the Pitocin being used to augment the labor was discontinued.

livery while efforts are being made to correct the fetal heart rate pattern. Such efforts include maternal position change, Trendelenburg or knee–chest position, upward displacement of the fetal head, and administration of oxygen.

See Figure 14-12 for a summary of the patterns of heart rate changes described above.

Methods of Monitoring the Fetal Heart Rate

The fetal heart rate may be counted with a fetoscope or with an electronic fetal heart monitoring device (see Figure 14-13). The patterns described above have been studied by simultaneous recordings of FHR and uterine contractions. When such an electronic device is available, it should be used for continuous monitoring of the fetal heart whenever conditions that may endanger the fetus are present or are likely to develop. When electronic monitor-

ing equipment is not available or its use is not indicated, the fetal heart should be auscultated with a fetoscope or Doppler unit. (See Figure 14-19).

Continuous Electronic FHR Monitoring

There are two principal methods of continuous FHR monitoring in current use: external or indirect and internal or direct. The external, or indirect, method utilizes ultrahigh-frequency sound waves to detect FHR. A transducer which both sends and receives ultrasound signals is applied to the maternal abdomen in the area where the loudest fetal heart sounds can be heard with a fetoscope. The transducer is "sealed" to the skin with a contact gel and held in place by an elastic belt. The beam of ultrasound waves is thus directed through maternal and fetal tissues where it is deflected by the

---

CLASSIFICATION OF
FETAL HEART RATE PATTERNS

I. **Baseline FHR** is observed in the absence of periodic FHR changes. Baseline FHR assessment consists of the determination of the FHR level in beats per minute (bpm) and FHR variability.

  A. *FHR level* may be categorized as follows:

    1. Marked bradycardia — 99 or fewer bpm
    2. Mild bradycardia — 100–119 bpm
    3. Normal — 120–160 bpm
    4. Mild tachycardia — 161–180 bpm
    5. Marked tachycardia — 180 or more bpm

  B. *FHR variability:* The fluctuations in beat-to-beat FHR are normally 6–10 bpm.

II. **Periodic FHR** is related to uterine contractions (UC). The response to uterine contractions may be categorized as follows:

  A. *No change:* The FHR maintains same characteristics as in the preceding baseline FHR.

  B. *Acceleration:* The FHR increases in response to uterine contractions.

  C. *Deceleration:* The FHR decreases in response to uterine contractions. Decelerations may be divided into three categories or patterns:

    1. Uniform patterns — reflect shape of uterine contractions and are usually repetitive.
      a. Early deceleration (head compression)
      b. Late deceleration (uteroplacental insufficiency)
    2. Variable patterns (cord compression) — have a variable time of onset, variable waveform and may be nonrepetitive.
    3. Combined or mixed patterns — may be difficult to define and exhibit characteristics of any of the above patterns.

Figure 14-12. Classification of fetal heart rate patterns. [*Adapted from* ACOG Technical Bulletin No. 32, *American College of Obstetricians and Gynecologists, 1974.*]

movement of the fetal heart walls or valves. The deflected waves, which are of a different frequency, are received by the transducer. The difference between the transmitted and received frequencies is known as the *Doppler signal*. The greater the velocity of the target (in this case, the greater the fetal heart rate), the greater the signal received by the transducer. The monitor processes the Doppler signal and

prints the heart rate on a graphic record (see Figure 14-14).

External monitoring is a noninvasive procedure which can be done with the fetal membranes intact. It is widely used for antepartum monitoring (Chapter 21, pages 618–21 and for intrapartum screening. It does, however, lack the precision of the internal methods. In particular, it cannot be used to assess baseline variability since machine-produced "noise" or a faulty signal may be the cause of marked variability regardless of the true state of the fetus. In addition, an active fetus or a mother who is restless during her labor may necessitate continual adjustment of the transducer, and, in some cases, a satisfactory tracing is impossible to obtain even with great patience.

The internal, or direct, method is the most reliable, but the most invasive, way of monitoring FHR. A stainless steel spiral electrode is inserted into the fetal scalp where it picks up the electrical impulse from the fetal QRS complex (Fig. 14-15). Like the ultrasound signal this is processed by the monitor and instantaneously printed on a graphic record (see Figure 14-14).

The major disadvantage of the internal method is that the fetal membranes must be ruptured in order to apply the electrode. Because the electrode penetrates the fetal skin there is also a risk of infection to the electrode site as well as a risk of intrauterine infection as a result of the manipulations required to anchor the fetal electrode. In a large number of cases, however, there has not appeared to be any significant increase in either maternal or fetal morbidity resulting from use of the internal monitor. The quality of the tracings is not affected by maternal or fetal activity. Although the application of the monitor is uncomfortable for the mother, once it is in place she is frequently more comfortable and has greater freedom of movement than the woman being monitored externally.

In order to evaluate periodic patterns of fetal heart rate, it is necessary to monitor uterine contractions simultaneously. When external fetal

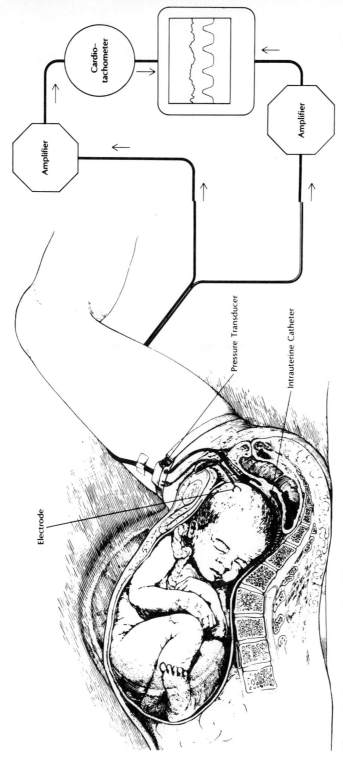

Figure 14-13. System developed for direct monitoring of fetal heart activity. A clip electrode is seen attached to the fetal scalp. Currently a special screw electrode is used and is attached to the fetal presenting part by means of a guide tube. The FECG thus obtained is fed to an amplifier and signal conditioning circuit. An instantaneous cardiotachometer measures the interval between FECGs and plots a continuous FHR graph; its output is displayed on one channel of a two-channel oscillograph. Intrauterine pressures are obtained from a catheter inserted into lower part of uterus and attached to a transducer in the leg plate. Transducer's output is amplified and displayed beneath the FHR record on the oscillograph. [*Reproduced with permission from Eduard H. G. Hon, "Direct Monitoring of the Fetal Heart," Hosp. Pract., 5:91–97 (Sept.) 1970.*]

323

heart rate monitoring is being done, a tocodyna-mometer or uterine transducer is secured in place over the uterine fundus by a belt which encircles the maternal abdomen. (See Figure 21-7, page 620.) A pressure-sensitive button on the tocodynamometer receives the pressure from the contracting uterus much as the nurse's fingers feel the pressure. This "push" on the button is converted to an electrical signal which may be printed out on chart paper. This external monitoring gives accurate information about the frequency and duration of the contractions but does *not* monitor amplitude (intensity) of contractions or baseline tone of the uterus. See Figure 14-14 for diagram of printout of uterine contractions.

In situations where it is important to evaluate baseline tone and amplitude of the contractions (for example, during oxytocin stimulation of labor) or when a fetal electrode is being applied, an internal catheter system is used. After the fetal membranes have been ruptured, a small, fluid-filled, open-ended catheter is inserted through the vagina into the amniotic cavity. The opposite end of the catheter is then connected to a strain gauge which sends out an electrical signal proportional to the pressure exerted on it. During a contraction the pressure in the uterus increases and then returns to the baseline as the contraction subsides. In order to measure intrauterine pressure accurately the strain gauge should be located at the same height as the presumed height of the intrauterine catheter tip. A plug of meconium or vernix or an air bubble or leak in the system may result in inaccurate recordings. (See Figure 14-13 for internal catheter system set-up.)

Figures 14-16 and 14-17 show monitor tracings of hypotonic and hypertonic uterine function. These abnormal uterine contraction patterns are discussed on page 390.

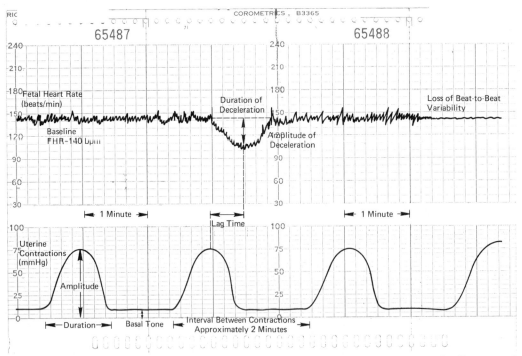

Figure 14-14. Diagram of fetal monitor tracing showing terms commonly used in "reading" FHR and uterine contraction tracings.

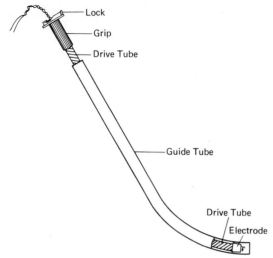

Figure 14-15. Spiral electrode for direct fetal heart rate monitoring. The guide tube is inserted transvaginally and the drive tube advanced until the spiral electrode rests against the fetal head. The lock is then released and the electrode attached to the fetal scalp by turning the drive tube clockwise. Once the electrode is secured the drive and guide tubes are removed, leaving the wires which are connected to a leg plate attached to the mother's thigh.

Nursing Care of the Monitored Client

Fetal monitors have been hailed as both a great blessing and a great curse. There are those who believe every fetus should be monitored throughout labor in order to detect and treat the least sign of distress very early. Others maintain that, since labor is a physiologic process, very few fetuses will encounter conditions which would place them at risk and thus justify the use of a monitor. Regardless of the opinion held by any one practitioner, one thing is certain: the use of electronic monitoring is *not* a substitute for the skilled, personal care and support which each laboring woman deserves. In the few reported studies of client response to monitoring, nearly all of the negative responses were related to attitudes of personnel and procedures surrounding the monitoring rather than to the monitoring itself.

During pregnancy couples should receive in

formation about monitors and the local customs for their use as a part of their overall preparation for labor. If a monitor is to be applied during labor, the woman and her husband should be advised of this and their approval secured prior to assembling the equipment. Except in emergency situations, a brief lesson on monitors should be given, allowing the couple opportunity to closely examine the equipment. This is particularly important when a fetal electrode is to be applied. No parent relishes the idea of having a piece of steel screwed into her baby's head! However, when they have seen the electrode and been reassured that it only penetrates the skin about 1 mm, they will be much more comfortable.

Once the monitor is in place and operating many parents are fascinated by seeing the tracing of their baby's heart. If the husband is coaching his wife in breathing and relaxation, he will find the uterine contraction tracing very helpful in knowing when to cue her for the cleansing breath at the beginning and end of a contraction.

All labor room personnel must carefully train themselves never to enter a labor room and look first at the monitor tracing before acknowledging the presence of the woman. Certainly the worst offense is to enter, check the tracing, and leave, as if no patient were there at all. The laboring woman and her fetus must remain the central focus with the monitor only one adjunct to quality care.

Finally, it should be noted that the monitor tracings are only as useful as the expertise of the human practitioners makes them. Unless there are skilled nurses and physicians available to interpret the FHR patterns and take appropriate action, monitors are of no value.

A summary of interventions appropriate for various FHR findings is contained in Figure 14-18.

Ausculation of the Fetal Heart

When continuous FHR monitoring is not employed, the fetal heart should be ausculated and the rate counted using a fetoscope or Doppler

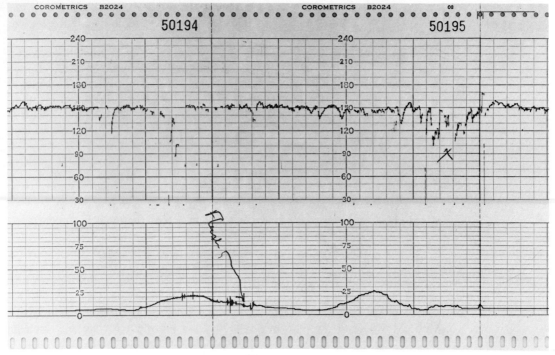

Figure 14-16. Fetal monitor tracing showing *hypo*tonic uterine function. This woman remained at 5 cm cervical dilatation for more than two hours with infrequent contractions of low amplitude. Following oxytocin augmentation labor proceeded normally to a spontaneous vaginal delivery of a healthy daughter. Note the occurrence of a FHR deceleration following the second contraction.

unit. (See Figure 14-19.) The fetal heart rate should be counted and recorded at least every hour during very early labor, every half hour or more frequently after acceleration of labor begins, and every 15 minutes after approximately 4 or 5 cm of cervical dilatation. In the presence of complications, especially when there is a possibility of some detachment of the placenta or interference with good blood perfusion of the placenta, the fetal heart should be observed very frequently—every 5 to 10 to 15 minutes, depending upon the situation. Frequent observation is necessary when contractions are strong and close together and during induction of labor. During the second stage, the fetal heart is observed after each contraction. The fetal heart should be observed immediately after the membranes rupture and during the next two or three contractions. Careful check is also important during the first few contractions that follow regional anesthesia.

To count the fetal heart rate with a stethoscope, the bell is placed over the area of the mother's abdomen where the heartbeat can be heard best. The place of maximum intensity of the heart sound is found by moving the stethoscope until that point is located. The fetal heart can be heard with an ordinary stethoscope, but when it is used, the bell is frequently held firmly in place with rubber bands to reduce sounds made by the fingers as they hold the bell. The heart sounds are generally heard more clearly with a head stethoscope because the heart tone is augmented by bone conduction of sound through the headpiece of the stethoscope (Fig. 11-16, page 256). The fetal heart can be heard as a double sound. It may be heard as somewhat muffled and far away and is often de-

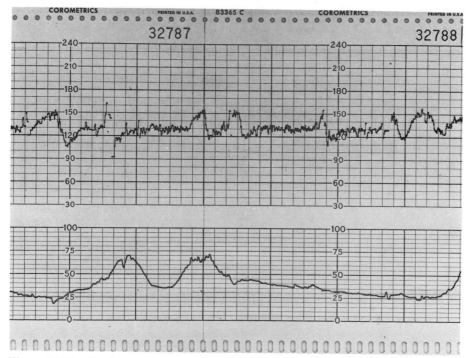

Figure 14-17. Fetal monitor tracing showing *hyper*tonic uterine function. Note the coupling of contractions and the basal tone above 25 mmHg. This pattern is most likely to be seen when intravenous oxytocin is being administered. The FHR shows a pattern of frequent, short accelerations from the baseline of 130 bpm.

scribed as sounding like the ticking of a watch under a pillow.

The maternal pulse may be mistaken for the fetal heartbeat, especially during auscultation of the lower abdomen. The pulsation in the aorta may be loud, or the *uterine souffle*, a soft blowing sound made by blood passing through the greatly enlarged uterine vessels, may be heard. These sounds are synchronous with the mother's pulse. A slower than expected FHR should alert the nurse to the possibility that she is hearing the mother's pulse, but when in doubt, she should place a finger on the mother's radial pulse while she listens to the fetal heartbeat. She will be able to differentiate the fetal heartbeat from the maternal pulse by the difference in rate.

Another sound sometimes heard while listening to the fetal heart is a whistling sound, known as the *fetal* or *funic souffle*, but this is synchronous with the fetal heartbeat. This sound is due to a rush of blood through the umbilical vessels, which may be audible when the vessels are subjected to tension or pressure.

There are now several ultrasound stethoscopes on the market which permit easier, more accurate location of the fetal heart and counting of its rate. They frequently permit auscultation of the heart throughout the contraction cycle, which is rarely possible with a conventional fetoscope. In addition, the heart rate can usually be counted while the mother is lying on her side or sitting up. In obstetric units where no equipment is available for continuous electronic monitoring such an ultrasound stethoscope is an essential aid to accurate fetal assessment.

To recognize the pattern of the fetal heart rate correctly, the beats must be counted over a period of one to several minutes, depending upon conditions. To obtain an accurate basal rate, the fetal heartbeat is counted between contractions for at least two, and preferably four, consecutive 15-second periods, or for two consecutive 15-second periods, short rest, and again two consecutive 15-second periods. Since uterine contractions should not normally affect the fetal heart rate, it should ordinarily not be necessary to wait for 15 to 30 seconds after a contraction ends before beginning a count. However, it may be advantageous to listen to the fetal heartbeat at the end of a contraction and again later in the interval between contrac-

FHR PATTERN	CHARACTERISTICS	UNDERLYING PATHOPHYSIOLOGY	THERAPEUTIC INTERVENTION
Baseline Changes			
Tachycardia	Baseline over 180 bpm or a rise of 10% of previous baseline	Mild fetal hypoxia Maternal fever Maternal tachycardia Fetal neurologic immaturity	Monitor maternal vital signs Change maternal position Continue to watch closely
Bradycardia	Baseline under 120 bpm or a drop of 10% of previous baseline	Congenital heart abnormalities Fetal distress (when accompanied by periodic changes)	Inform neonatal personnel Change maternal position Administer oxygen to mother Prepare for immediate delivery
Loss of variability	Smooth baseline as recorded by *internal* fetal monitor	Maternal medication Fetal acidosis (especially if accompanied by late decelerations) Fetal neurologic immaturity	Note time and dose of medication on record See "late decelerations" below
Periodic Changes			
Early deceleration	Uniform shaped dip Onset, maximal fall, and recovery coincides with onset, peak, and end of contraction	Head compression	Distinguish from late deceleration Observe mother for progress in labor as these are usually indicative of cervical dilatation of 6-7 cm or more
Late deceleration	Uniform shaped dip Onset coincides with peak of contraction with recovery occurring at the end of after the end of the contraction	Uteroplacental insufficiency	Correct underlying cause; e.g.; supine hypotension — change maternal position conduction anesthesia — elevate legs, increase hydration with I.V. fluids, apply elastic stockings or leg wraps uterine hyperactivity — reduce or discontinue dosage of oxytocin Left lateral position during labor Administer oxygen to mother Fetal scalp sampling Be prepared for operative delivery if fetal condition warrants
Variable deceleration	Variably shaped dip Usually shaped like a V or a squared U May occur any time during contraction cycle May be nonrepetitive	Cord compression	Change maternal position If severe, lasting more than one minute — attempt upward displacement of presenting part; help mother into knee-chest or Trendelenburg position; prepare for immediate delivery if pattern does not improve Administer oxygen to mother

Figure 14-18.   Summary of FHR patterns, their underlying pathophysiology, and suggested interventions.

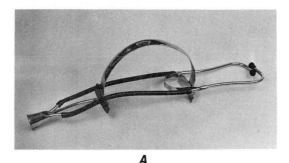

A

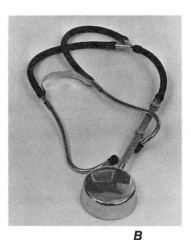

B

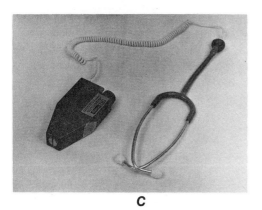

C

Figure 14-19. *A.* DeLee-Hillis fetoscope with head piece to provide bone conduction to enhance hearing of fetal heart tones. *B.* Leff stethoscope with large, weighted bell to amplify fetal heart tones. Frequently used in delivery rooms since the bell can be placed beneath sterile drapes. *C.* Ultrasound stethoscope which utilizes Doppler effect to count fetal heart rate.

tions. Normally the rate should be approximately the same at each count. If a distinct difference is noted in the two counting periods, a deceleration pattern must be considered. Then the count obtained one minute after a contraction ends would be the basal rate, since recovery from a dip should have taken place. The average of the counts made between contractions, excluding any count that may signify a dip, is the basal fetal heart rate.

The basal FHR can be expected to remain the same throughout labor, if conditions permit adequate fetal-maternal exchange in the placenta. There is not a normal increase in rate as labor advances. The rhythmic oscillations normally present in the fetal heart rate are usually not perceived by auscultation when their amplitude is under 10 beats per minute. If the amplitude of these oscillations is greater, they may be noted as an irregularity in the heartbeat rhythm.

A rise in basal FHR during labor, one that remains persistently high, must be considered an early sign of fetal distress. If this occurs, it is important to count the heart rate through entire cycles of before, during, and following contractions, to observe if late decelerations are also present. Even when the basal rate remains constant, an occasional count of an entire cycle is useful to assure that the fetal heart rate does not change markedly as the result of a contraction. Late decelerations can be recognized as a slow fall in rate beginning after the peak of a contraction and a slow recovery after a minimum rate has been reached. Early decelerations are not likely to be noted on clinical auscultation, since they occur at a time when extreme tenseness of the uterine muscle may make the heartbeat indistinct. If an early deceleration is heard, it is noted as a very rapid, brief reduction in rate, which probably cannot be estimated in actual count because of its short duration.

It may be difficult to hear the fetal heart during contractions, especially at their height, when the uterus is very tense, and it may also be difficult for the mother to lie quietly during contractions. However, it is very important to count the fetal heartbeat over a period of time, especially when the basal rate is not within normal range. It is advisable to have the mother assume the most comfortable position that she can find, but one which will also permit the nurse to listen to the fetal heartbeat where the sounds can be heard well. Since a side position is often fairly comfortable and also desirable during labor, the mother may be requested to lie on the side opposite from where the maximum heart sound is heard, except when she needs a change of position. Use of a Doppler (ultrasound) stethoscope is preferred to the conventional fetoscope for this purpose.

When the fetal heartbeat is indistinct, or not audible, during contractions, it should be possible to recognize a high basal heart rate and a late deceleration if auscultation is done during the entire periods between two or more contractions. Since the fall in fetal heart rate of a late deceleration begins after the peak of a contraction and reaches a minimum rate 30 to 50 seconds later, the minimum rate is probably lowest as the contraction is ending, or after it has stopped. A slow rate, if present, should therefore be noticeable if auscultation is started as soon as the contraction begins to wane. Since recovery of the basal rate is also slow and may not be reached until a minute or more after the con-

traction has ceased, continuing auscultation until the next contraction is important. It is only by auscultation during the entire interim from the waning of one contraction to the beginning of the next contraction that observation can be made of continuous rapid rate with no sign of a dip, or of evidence of a dip and recovery to a rapid rate, or of failure of recovery from a dip. Counting must be continued through at least 20 consecutive 15-second periods and each count recorded in its time relationship to a contraction (Fig. 14-20). The changes in fetal heart rate in late deceleration may not be perceived if the rate is not recorded in this way.

Since late decelerations extend into the periods between contractions, it is apparent that intermittent or single auscultations of the fetal heartbeat between contractions would not give a true picture of the heart rate pattern. The high rate of a tachycardia and the lowest rate of a late deceleration may both fall within the normal range of a fetal heart rate, between approximately 120 and 160 beats per minute. Spot checks of the fetal heartbeat would not necessarily find the rate abnormal even when the serious pattern of tachycardia and late decelerations were present. For example, a rate of 124 per minute, obtained shortly after a contraction had

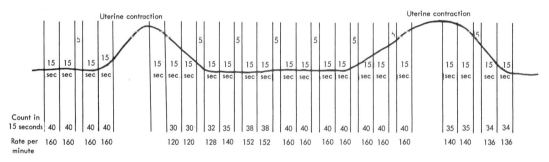

Figure 14-20. Clinical auscultation of the fetal heart rate. Count of the heart rate is begun as soon as a contraction begins to wane and is continued until the next contraction begins to reach its height, or through the entire succeeding contraction if the mother is not too uncomfortable. The count is made in consecutive 15-second periods, with 5-second intervals between each two counts for rest and recording. A total of at least 20 consecutive 15-second counts should be made. The rate per minute for each count is recorded and the pattern of the heart rate in relation to the uterine contractions noted. In this example the perceived drop of 40 beats per minute after the acme of the contraction, from the previous basal rate of 160 should be considered a late deceleration. A return to the previous basal rate of 160 indicates that the amplitude of the dip was 40 beats per minute. The lag time in this example was at least 30 seconds, and probably 45 seconds, in length.

ceased, would appear to be within a normal range of a fetal heart rate when it might actually be the low rate of a late deceleration if the basal rate was as high as 160 beats per minute.

To recapitulate, the correct method of checking the fetal heart rate and recognizing its pattern is to obtain the basal heart rate by counting for two or more 15-second periods between contractions or between dips, if present. The basal rate should be obtained as early in labor as possible. If the basal rate rises during labor, the heartbeat should be counted either through entire cycles of before, during, and at least two minutes following a contraction, or through entire periods between contractions. A slow rate of late deceleration with recovery to a rapid rate can be recognized in this way, or if recovery does not take place, a persistent bradycardia will be evident.

Treatment of Fetal Distress

Early recognition of an abnormal fetal heart rate pattern often permits treatment before the condition of the fetus becomes serious. Some measures can readily be instituted and they frequently modify or eliminate the cause of the distress. Among such actions are change in maternal position, correction of maternal hypotension, decrease in uterine activity when an oxytocic is used for stimulation of labor, and administration of oxygen to the mother.

Maternal Position Change

Change of maternal position may have the effect of correcting one of several different possible causes of interference with good circulation to the fetus or to the placenta. A change of position may relieve pressure on the umbilical cord during uterine contractions, and a change from a supine to a side position may remove pressure of the uterus from the large blood vessels in the abdomen.

The *umbilical cord may be in a position where it becomes compressed* between the fetus and the uterine wall or the maternal pelvis during contractions. Interference with good circulation through the umbilical cord is likely to result in a fetal heart rate pattern associated with distress. Dips in fetal heart rate due to umbilical cord compression may occur at variable times in relation to the associated uterine contractions. Sometimes the dips begin early in a contraction and sometimes later, and they may be of variable duration. Very frequently a change in the mother's position will redistribute pressure points and modify or alleviate pressure on the umbilical cord during contractions.

A pregnant woman at or near term may develop hypotension while lying in the supine position. While the woman is on her back the heavy uterus may press on the inferior vena cava and interfere with venous return to the heart. The impaired venous return results in reduced cardiac output and consequently a fall in arterial pressure. As a result, exchange of oxygen and carbon dioxide between maternal and fetal blood is reduced and the fetus is likely to begin to show signs of distress.

Hypotension resulting from pressure on the inferior vena cava can usually be remedied by having the mother change to a side position. Although it may not be readily determined if a mother's supine position is a cause of distress to either mother or fetus, a change to a side position is advocated if signs of difficulty appear. Previous occurrence of a hypotensive syndrome in a mother during the latter part of her pregnancy suggests that it is not advisable for her to lie on her back at any time during labor. Actually a side position is recommended for all women in labor.

It may not be possible at first to determine the cause of an abnormal fetal heart rate pattern. Initially, however, it is important to change the mother's position as soon as an abnormal fetal heart rate pattern appears. Change in maternal position may ordinarily be carried out easily and it can usually be instituted immediately.

Correction of Maternal Hypotension

Maternal hypotension interferes with good perfusion of blood through the placenta and may result in reduced exchange of blood gases and other materials between maternal and fetal blood. Restoration of good maternal arterial pressure is essential to increasing the blood flow through the intervillous space and consequently adequate transfer of materials across the membranes.

Corrective measures for hypotension include elevation of the legs and rapid administration of intravenous fluids. A side position corrects the supine hypotensive syndrome. When spinal anesthesia is used, careful observation of blood pressure and readiness to combat hypotension is important to the fetus as well as the mother. The nurse should not wait for the physician to arrive to carry out corrective measures for hypotension. She should quickly change the mother's position, elevate the foot of the bed, and begin administration of intravenous fluids.

Decreased Stimulation of Uterine Contractions

Strong uterine contractions decrease, and virtually stop, blood flow through the intervillous space, at least during their greatest contracting phase. If the contractions are long, there may be considerable impairment in transfer of oxygen and carbon dioxide across the placenta. When the contractions are also frequent, the relaxation intervals between them may be too short for the fetus to be able to recover adequately from the previous impairment of transfer of blood gases. The length of these intervals of relaxation is significant since fresh oxygenated blood is circulated through the intervillous space to meet the needs of the fetus.

Stimulation of uterine muscle contractions with an oxytocic is the leading cause of strong, long, frequent contractions. Occasionally unusually strong contractions develop in a spontaneous labor.

Abnormally strong, frequent contractions accompanying oxytocin stimulation can ordinarily be avoided. Careful regulation of the amount of the medication will usually keep the contractions within physiologic limits. If contractions become abnormal, the nurse should immediately decrease or terminate the oxytocin. A de-

crease in length and frequency of contractions will usually provide sufficient time for fresh blood to circulate through the intervillous space in the interval between the stresses of contractions. This will permit adequate transfer of oxygen and carbon dioxide between mother and fetus.

Administration of Oxygen

Administration of oxygen to the mother will increase the maternal blood oxygen tension, often increase transfer of oxygen to the fetus, and may help to keep the oxygen tension of the fetal blood above a critical level. Administration of oxygen to the mother when the fetus is distressed has often been found to reduce the incidence of late deceleration. Oxygen may be used effectively for a sudden episode of fetal difficulty, while preparation is made for other treatments.

Administration of Glucose

Partial asphyxia causes rapid mobilization of glucose, and if the fetus does not receive an adequate amount of glucose from his mother, his own glycogen stores may become depleted. Since glucose readily passes across the placenta from mother to fetus, administration of intravenous glucose to the mother will assure that she is not becoming hypoglycemic and that glucose will be readily available to the fetus as he needs it.

Delivery of the Baby

An abnormal fetal heart rate pattern may develop as a result of a combination of causes. The presence of one complication may exaggerate the effects of another. As an example, severe uterine contractions may contribute to the effects of decreased blood flow through the placenta from another cause, such as maternal hypotension or decreased functional capacity of the placenta.

Corrective measures for fetal distress will be effective in a large number of patients. If the fetus has not been severely affected, his condition may return to normal when the cause of his distress is removed. If an abnormal fetal heart rate pattern persists after institution of therapeutic measures, it is likely that the physician will make the decision that labor should be terminated by operative delivery.

Passage of Meconium

Passage of meconium *in utero* is a sign of fetal distress. The bowel shows increased peristalsis during hypoxia and its contents are likely to be expelled. The fetus may expel meconium during any period of distress, either during the latter part of pregnancy or during labor. As meconium escapes from the bowel it mixes with the amniotic fluid, giving the fluid a yellowish-green or dark-green color. The discolored fluid is described as *meconium-stained amniotic fluid.*

Meconium-stained amniotic fluid can be recognized through intact membranes, if the fluid is observed through an amnioscope, introduced through the cervix. Amnioscopic examinations may be carried out in some circumstances during pregnancy if the fetus is likely to be at risk. However, under most circumstances passage of meconium is not observed until the membranes rupture and the amniotic fluid begins to drain. The meconium may appear as a thick, tarry material draining from the vagina, or it may be well mixed with the amniotic fluid. The color of the fluid is likely to be dark when the meconium staining is of recent origin; it becomes more yellow than green if the meconium was passed several days or weeks earlier.

Meconium-stained fluid should be considered a sign of previous fetal hypoxia and a warning signal that the condition of the fetus may worsen. Its appearance should be immediately reported to the physician. The fetus should be carefully protected against undue stress and closely observed during the remainder of labor. Excessive fetal movements are occasionally noted in association with meconium passage and are considered further evidence of fetal difficulty.

Meconium is expelled under normal as well as abnormal circumstances when the breech is the presenting part. Uterine contractions apply considerable pressure on the baby's abdomen and meconium is easily forced out of the bowel by this pressure. Although fetal hypoxia may be present, passage of meconium during labor when the breech is presenting is not a clue to the fetus' condition; other observations must be relied on for evidence of fetal distress.

The presence of meconium-stained amniotic fluid should be reported to the nursery staff as soon as it is noted and arrangements made for pediatric attendance at delivery. In addition to the risk of a depressed or asphyxiated neonate, meconium aspiration is a serious threat to the infant (see page 792).

Fetal Blood Analysis

Examination of blood taken from the scalp may serve as an important additional factor in the physician's evaluation of the fetus and in making a decision if operative delivery is indicated. Almost any disturbance that affects the fetus results in acidosis. Since the range of pH in which body cells can function in a normal manner is very small, a fall in the pH of the fetal blood is a serious risk to him. Analysis of the fetus' blood for acid–base balance, when facilities are available to carry out the procedure, may be used to obtain valuable information about the reactions of the fetus to the stresses of pregnancy and labor. Analyses of blood aid in identifying fetuses with intrauterine asphyxia and also those who have clinical signs of distress but no evidence of acidosis. Such analyses may be helpful in determining when immediate delivery is indicated.

Usual indications for fetal blood sampling are pregnancies associated with a high risk of hypoxia, such as diabetes and toxemia, and abnormalities in fetal heart rate and rhythm and passage of meconium. Fetal acidosis is usually associated with the typical pattern of high basal fetal heart rate and late decelerations. This pattern is related to depression of the newborn.

A sample of fetal blood for analysis is obtained by collection of a few drops of capillary blood from the fetal scalp. An instrument for making a very small incision in the skin of the scalp is inserted through the cervical canal after the membranes are ruptured. A few minims of blood are collected from the small scalp puncture wound into a heparinized capillary tube. The puncture site usually bleeds very little. The pH of the blood is immediately determined. Repeated samples are usually collected as labor advances, especially when the fetus is at risk or shows signs of distress. The blood may be analyzed for changes in PCO_2 and base excess or deficit as well as for level of pH.

A pH of less than 7.2 is evidence of fetal distress and when accompanied by other signs of inadequate placental exchange of blood gases indicates that the baby is likely to be distressed at birth. If the fetus' condition does not improve with treatment for hypoxia and acidosis, immediate delivery may be necessary.

Fetal scalp blood may also be used to type and crossmatch the Rh($-$)-sensitized infant for immediate extrauterine exchange transfusion.

OBSERVATIONS OF THE PROGRESS OF LABOR

Observation of Uterine Contractions

The *frequency, duration,* and *strength of the uterine contractions* should be carefully observed by the nurse. The woman and her husband may be asked to help time the contractions for short intervals, and they frequently do so without request. Their observations are very useful, but the nurse must make her own evaluation of contractions at frequent intervals. The mother's and the nurse's evaluation of contractions are not always in complete agreement. The mother may not feel discomfort at the beginning and at the end of the contraction, and its actual duration may be longer than the period of her discomfort; or she may continue to have discomfort, due to pressure, after the contraction has ended and therefore believe that it lasted longer than it actually did. An estimate of the strength of the contraction by the mother's reaction may

also not be completely reliable because of the differences in reaction by different women to contractions of approximately the same intensity.

To make her own observations of uterine contractions, the nurse places her hand lightly on the mother's abdomen, over the fundus of the uterus, and gently palpates, with her fingers, changes in uterine muscle tone. With experience she can learn to detect the beginning of a muscle contraction, feel its maximum firmness when the uterus seems to "stand up" and become hard, and perceive when the muscle is again relaxed. The nurse should stay with the mother long enough at any one time to observe several contractions in order to note the general pattern. It is important for her to ascertain that the uterine muscle relaxes completely in the intervals between the contractions.

The *length of the contraction* is the time interval between the first sensation of tightening of the muscle and its subsequent complete relaxation—this may differ from the time during which the mother feels discomfort. The

Interval	Beginning of Contraction	Duration of Contraction
3 min.	7¹²	50 seconds
4 min.	7¹⁵	60 "
4 min.	7¹⁹	60 "
3 min.	7²³	50 "
3 min.	7²⁶	50 "
4 min.	7²⁹	50 "
	7³³	60 "

Figure 14-21. A record of the length and interval between uterine contractions. The frequency with which contractions occur is timed from the beginning of one contraction to the beginning of the next. When contractions are timed at various intervals during labor, a chart similar to the above may be kept at the woman's bedside. The frequency and length of the contractions are recorded for short periods of time. This aids the nurse in accurately recording her observations of the contractions on the woman's record. This chart shows that the woman had contractions of 50 to 60 seconds' duration occurring every three to four minutes.

frequency of the contractions is the time interval from the beginning of one contraction to the beginning of the next; it is not the time that elapses between the end of one contraction and the beginning of the following one (Fig. 14-21). The *strength of the contractions* can be estimated by the firmness of the uterine muscle. A weak contraction is one in which the uterine muscle becomes firm, but not hard; the contraction is also generally short, around 30 seconds' duration. A moderate contraction is usually longer, around 45 seconds' duration, and the uterine muscle becomes moderately firm. A strong contraction generally lasts around 60 seconds, and the uterus becomes very hard. During a hard contraction the examining fingers cannot indent the uterus, whereas some indentation is possible with weaker contractions.

Palpation of the abdomen for evaluation of uterine contractions must be done gently and with a minimum amount of manipulation. The examining hand need not be moved about on the abdomen from one area to another, and frequent efforts to indent the uterus are not necessary. The mother's abdomen is often very tender and manipulation adds to her discomfort.

Among the many factors that affect the progress of labor, the force of the uterine contractions exerts an important influence. Labor can be expected to progress steadily, and sometimes rapidly, when the uterine contractions are strong, last approximately 60 seconds, and recur at three- to four-minute intervals, unless the resistance of the soft tissues is great or the relationship of the baby to the mother's pelvis makes passage difficult.

Uterine contractions may also be continuously monitored by a tocodynamometer or by an intrauterine catheter as described on page 324.

Examinations to Determine Progress of Labor

Abdominal Palpation

At an early examination of the mother after the beginning of labor, the abdomen is palpated, according to the description on pages 251-54 for diagnosis of presentation, position, and engagement of fetus. Abdominal examination may be repeated later in labor for further observation of position of the fetus and for descent of the presenting part, and the findings of the examination may be correlated with those obtained by rectal or vaginal examination. Abdominal examination must be made between contractions.

Vaginal Examination

Vaginal examinations are frequently employed methods of determining the progress of labor. Progress is ascertained by palpation of the cervix for degree of effacement and dilatation and of the fetal presenting part for station and position. The examination is made when the mother is admitted to the hospital in labor and is repeated at intervals during labor, perhaps only once but often several times.

To some extent, the progress of labor can be followed by the other observations enumerated in this section on "Observations of Progress of Labor." Vaginal examination is used to confirm the judgment that labor is progressing, concluded from other signs, and is performed whenever necessary to determine more definitely the amount of progress that has been made. The frequency of examinations varies considerably in individual situations and is somewhat determined by the reliance that can be placed on other signs of progress. Since the examinations are not entirely without danger of infection to the birth canal and are also disturbing to the woman, they are not repeated more often than seems essential.

When a vaginal examination is to be performed, the nurse should explain the procedure, assist the mother to a position on her back, ask her to flex her knees, and drape her in such a manner that she will be covered, but with the perineal area exposed. The nurse provides a sterile glove and lubricant and remains with the mother during the examination to provide support and to encourage her to relax her muscles during the examination when it is being done by the physician (Fig. 14-22).

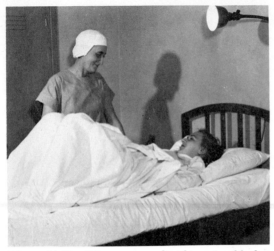

Figure 14-22. Woman covered with a cotton blanket awaiting an examination to determine progress of cervical effacement and dilatation and station and position of the fetus. The drape can be removed as much as necessary to expose the perineal area sufficiently for the examination. The nurse is available to coach the mother with the appropriate breathing and relaxation techniques during a physician's examination.

For some examinations, such as questionable cephalopelvic disproportion, abnormal presentation, questionable placenta previa, and further evaluation of the pelvis, a lithotomy position is used during the vaginal examination. Because such examinations cannot be done satisfactorily with the woman on her bed, she is placed on an examining table or the delivery table where better positioning and better preparation can be done.

VAGINAL EXAMINATION BY THE NURSE   The nurse herself often performs vaginal examinations. Such findings, added to the nurse's other observations, increase her information concerning the progress of labor. To become skillful in using vaginal examinations as a means of determining progress, the nurse must have many opportunities to perform the examination and at first needs assistance in interpreting the findings.

To proceed with a vaginal examination, two fingers of a gloved hand are lubricated and introduced into the vagina. The cervix, the presenting part, and the ischial spines are palpated directly for the following information: the consistency, effacement, and dilatation of the cervix; the station of the presenting part; and the position of the baby (Fig. 14-23).

During palpation of the cervix, its opening is felt as a depression with a surrounding circular ridge. The *amount of cervical dilatation* is determined by palpating this depression and estimating its diameter in centimeters (Fig. 14-23). The *amount of cervical effacement* is determined by palpation of the thickness of the ridge around the depression (Fig. 12-3). See pages 265–67 for a more complete description of cervical effacement and dilatation. The *consistency*

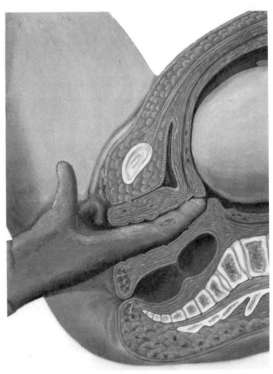

Figure 14-23. Diagram showing method of ascertaining cervical effacement and dilatation, station of the fetal head, and position of the fetus by means of a vaginal examination. The examining finger palpates the cervix, the fetal head, and the ischial spines.

of the cervix is also noted at this time; a cervix that is soft usually thins and dilates faster than one that is still firm. Sometimes *information about the integrity of the membranes* is obtained during this examination. If the membranes are intact, they are sometimes felt bulging through the cervical opening, especially during a contraction; if the membranes are ruptured, amniotic fluid may drain out of the vagina during a contraction.

The *station,* or degree of descent, is ascertained by touching the fetal head, feeling for the ischial spines on the side walls of the pelvis, and correlating the level of the head to the level of the ischial spines. The stations of the head are described on pages 250–51 and in Table 11-2 on page 250.

It may be possible to determine the *position of the baby* on vaginal examination if the cervix is quite well dilated. When the vertex is presenting, the sagittal suture can usually be felt through the cervical opening, and if dilatation is advanced, the suture can sometimes be followed to a fontanel. By feeling some portion of the landmarks of the fetal head it may be possible to determine the placement of the occiput. Correlation of the direction of the sagittal suture with those of an abdominal examination may be helpful in diagnosing the position. The positions assumed by the fetal head are described on page 245 and its sutures and fontanels on page 240.

Overlapping of sutures due to marked molding of the head may interfere with differentiation of landmarks. Sometimes the soft tissues of the baby's head become very edematous during labor, making palpation of the underlying structures difficult or impossible.

The nurse must be aware of contraindications to a vaginal examination, which include *vaginal bleeding, however slight,* and abnormal findings upon abdominal palpation, such as a transverse presentation.

Vaginal examinations may be made either during or between contractions. An examination made between contractions reveals the amount of cervical dilatation and effacement and descent of the head when the cervix and the head are not under pressure of a contraction. An examination performed during a contraction shows the maximum amount of thinning and stretching of the cervix and descent of the head under the influence of a contraction. There may be some recession in cervical effacement and dilatation after each contraction, but the cervix does not completely return to its state before the contraction began. Each contraction makes some change; toward the end of labor this change may be rapid.

Signs of the Transition Phase

The appearance of the transition phase is evidence that the first stage will soon be completed. This phase may be recognized by changes in the mother's behavior and by an increase in the intensity of contractions and an increase of pressure in the pelvis made by the presenting part. The contractions become intense and frequent and are sometimes so close together that they seem almost continuous. Pressure on the rectum increases and cramps in the legs and buttocks may begin or become more marked. The back and abdomen often become sore to touch. This discomfort may be so marked that the mother requests the nurse not to touch her abdomen to palpate uterine contractions, and when palpation is necessary, it must be done very lightly. The mother may have nausea and sometimes emesis at this time.

The mother's entire mien grows more serious during the transition phase. Relaxation becomes more difficult, and she may have trembling of her legs which she may find difficult or impossible to control. The mother may feel irritable at this time, and she may become restless. Signs of amnesia to varying degrees may also appear.

Signs of Approach or Onset of Second Stage

Rupture of the Membranes

The membranes may break at any time before or during labor, but when rupture occurs after the mother has been in labor for several hours it may be an indication that the cervix is completely dilated. The station and position of the presenting part may change when the membranes rupture, and there is some possibility of prolapse of the umbilical cord with the gush of fluid, if the presenting part is still high in the pelvis at the time of rupture (Fig. 16-3, page 394). The nurse should instruct the mother to notify her at once if she feels a sudden gush of fluid from the vagina. The amount of fluid that escapes will depend on the point of rupture and the position of the presenting part; it may vary from a small amount that soaks only a portion of the pad under the mother to a quantity that completely saturates the lower bedding. After rupture has occurred, some fluid will escape with each contraction. Rupture of the membranes should be reported to the physician promptly. The fetal heart should be checked immediately for rate and rhythm, and a vaginal examination is usually made at once to determine the condition of the cervix and the station and position of the presenting part. The color of the amniotic fluid is observed and evidence of staining with meconium reported to the physician.

Increase in Bloody Show

Increasing bloody show, resulting from tiny lacerations in the cervix, is a good indication that labor is progressing well and that the cervix is steadily dilating. There may be considerable increase in bloody show toward the end of the first stage. This bloody mucoid discharge must be distinguished from bright red blood, which is abnormal during labor.

Nausea and Vomiting

Sudden appearance of nausea and vomiting, if it has not been present throughout labor, is often a sign that the first stage has ended. The nurse must also realize that complications such as toxemia may first present this way.

Pressure on the Rectum

At the end of the first stage of labor the mother usually has an almost continuous desire to empty her bowels, because of pressure made on the rectum by the presenting part as it descends more deeply into the pelvis. This descent frequently takes place when the cervix becomes completely dilated, and if pressure has not been present in early labor and then rather suddenly appears, it may be a sign that the second stage has been reached. In addition to rectal pressure, cramps in the buttocks, thighs, and legs may also begin.

Involuntary Bearing Down

When the mother begins to bear down involuntarily with contractions, the second stage of labor has probably begun. Whenever there is bearing down, the perineum must be inspected for bulging at the height of the contraction.

Deep Grunting Sounds

The appearance of deep grunting sounds during contractions, in contrast to earlier utterances of a sharp and complaining nature often signifies that the second stage has begun. The grunting sound may appear very suddenly and may be so distinct from earlier sounds that this sign of second-stage labor is unmistakable, at least to the experienced obstetric nurse.

The Mother's Feeling That She Is Ready to Deliver

When the mother, especially the multigravida, says that her "baby is coming" she is usually correct, regardless of the findings of a recent rectal or vaginal examination, even if it was performed only a few minutes earlier. Such a remark must not be ignored. Although a very recent examination revealed little cervical dilatation, it is important to realize that the cervix can dilate very rapidly, and the mother's observation demands further investigation.

Bulging of the Perineum

Bulging of the perineum is always a sign that delivery is imminent.

Close observation of the mother is necessary

to allow adequate time to prepare for delivery. If the mother is to be taken to a delivery room for birth, the time at which she is moved will depend on how soon the birth of the baby is anticipated. The intensity of uterine contractions, the station and position of the presenting part, and previous progress are considered in making this judgment.

The primigravida is usually taken to the delivery room when the cervix has become completely dilated, if the head is low and in an anterior position. If the head has not descended to the perineal floor or has not rotated anteriorly, the mother may remain in her bed in the labor room during the early part of the second stage of labor. She is encouraged to bear down with contractions and is closely observed for advancement of the presenting part.

The multigravida, who ordinarily completes the latter part of the first stage of labor and all of the second stage quite rapidly, is often taken to the delivery room when the cervix is 7 to 8 cm dilated. If her progress is rapid, there may not be adequate time for complete preparation if it is not begun before the second stage. On the other hand, if there is reason to expect that delivery of the multigravida will be delayed, preparation for the birth may not be started before complete dilatation of the cervix has been reached.

The nurse caring for the mother in active labor must be alert to the possibility of rapidly changing conditions. When a multigravida who is having strong contractions suddenly shows signs of second-stage labor, rapid delivery can usually be anticipated. If the mother's membranes rupture, if she feels sudden pressure on her rectum, and if she begins to have involuntary bearing down, the nurse must notify the physician immediately and also quickly prepare for delivery. The nurse must also appreciate that in some instances conditions are favorable in the primigravida for rapid completion of the latter part of the first stage and of the entire second stage of labor. In such case, labor in the primigravida may be quite similar to that of a multigravida.

SECOND STAGE (STAGE OF EXPULSION)

The second stage of labor is shorter and more intense than the first stage. The uterine contractions are stronger, more frequent, and more expulsive, and the baby steadily descends through the birth canal. The mother must not be allowed out of bed during this stage, and she must be attended at all times by someone who is capable of recognizing any change in condition. Vigilance in observing the progress of labor, and in watching both mother and baby for signs of complications, is of extreme importance.

Care of the Mother

Most of the care that was given in the first stage of labor is continued during the second stage. Close observation of the progress of labor, and observation for unfavorable signs are of extreme importance. The mother needs continuing emotional support, she may need coaching in making the best use of expulsive efforts to deliver the baby, and she needs relief from discomfort insofar as possible. She needs a person capable of giving expert care with her at all times.

Amniotomy (Artificial Rupture of the Membranes)

If the fetal membranes do not rupture spontaneously at complete dilatation of the cervix, they are ruptured artificially at the beginning of the second stage, since they may now retard progress of labor. Under conditions favorable for the onset of labor and with the presenting part low in the pelvis, an amniotomy may be performed before labor begins, being used as a method of induction of labor. At other times, the membranes are ruptured at varying times during the first stage of labor, either after labor is established or after cervical dilatation is progressing well.

In performing the amniotomy, precautions are taken to prevent contamination of the vagina, and close observation is made of its effects on the labor and the fetus. The mother's vulva is washed with an antiseptic solution. The physician prepares his hands and puts on sterile gloves. A sterile forceps, frequently an Allis clamp, or a sharp hook, is introduced into the vagina to rupture the membranes, which are usually quite tense. The break is made between uterine contractions. Sometimes only the forceps is introduced into the vagina to grasp the membranes and break them; at other times the physician performs a vaginal examination and inserts the instrument while two fingers of one hand are in the vagina touching the membranes. The physician may hold his fingers in the vagina while some of the amniotic fluid drains out and then note the change that may take place in the position of the presenting part. As following spontaneous rupture, the rate of the fetal heart is observed and recorded immediately following artificial rupture of the membranes, and the color and characteristics of the fluid are observed and recorded.

Pushing with Uterine Contractions

During the second stage the force of intraabdominal pressure is added to intrauterine pressure to move the baby through the birth canal. This force is exerted through bearing-down efforts at the time that the uterine muscle is contracting. Bearing down is discouraged before the cervix is completely dilated, but is advised as soon as the second stage begins.

Bearing down is reflex and spontaneous during the second stage, and as labor advances it becomes a very strong impulse. Occasionally a mother does not use this reflex advantageously during the early part of the second stage, and coaching is helpful. The nurse is often the person who explains to the mother what she should do and gives her encouragement to put forth her best effort. Mothers who have attended preparation-for-childbirth classes have had instructions in pushing; they need support in their efforts.

Good breathing technique, contraction of abdominal muscles, and relaxation of the peri-

neum are important for effective pushing. As the contraction begins, the mother takes two deep breaths in and out and then takes a third deep breath and holds it, and pushes from her waist down, using her abdominal muscles, for as long as she can hold that breath. While holding her breath the mother should tighten her abdominal muscles and relax her perineum as she pushes toward the vaginal opening. If one holding breath does not take a mother through a contraction she lets out her breath, takes two deep breaths in and out, inhales a third deep breath and holds and pushes again (Fig. 14-4E). Each push should be as long and sustained as possible, since a long, continued effort is much more effective than short, grunting attempts. If the mother opens her mouth and lets her breath out or utters sounds, she fails to use her contraction to the best advantage.

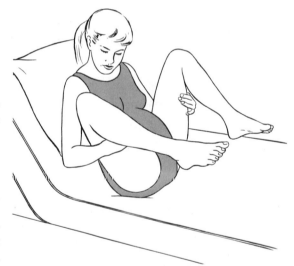

Figure 14-24. Pushing position. The position and breath-holding in this illustration have been practiced during pregnancy, but *without* actual pushing, as is done during the second stage of labor. The stretch afforded by the pushing position, without simultaneous use of the breath-holding pattern, may give a mother some relief from middle backache during the antepartum period if she wishes to use the pushing position for that purpose. [*Modified from Maternity Center Association,* Preparation for Childbearing, *4th ed., revised, New York, 1973, p. 34.*]

The effect of bearing down is increased if the mother is in a good position for pushing and if she pulls on something with her hands. If she is on her bed the head of the bed should be rolled up. On the delivery table it is helpful if the mother has two pillows under her head and shoulders and if the nurse or her husband holds her up. While pushing, immediately after taking the holding breath, the mother should put her chin on her chest, round her shoulders, put her elbows out, bend her knees and separate her legs, and pull with her arms while grasping behind her knees or on the hand grips on the delivery table (Fig. 14-24). In this position she can

PHASE OF LABOR	MECHANISMS OF LABOR	RESPONSES OF PATIENT	NURSING INTERVENTIONS
Latent Phase			

0-2 or 3 cm	Cervical effacement
	Slow dilatation (duration:
	  primigravida—8 hr;
	  multigravida—3 to 5 hr)
		Surge of energy and excitement
		Talkative, outgoing
		Easily distracted from contractions
		Anxiety is low and promotes learning
			Orient to hospital environment and personnel
			Assess history and physical status
			Assess attitudes, past experiences, expectations
			Teach about labor
			Practice breathing and relaxation techniques

2-3-4 cm	Effacement completed
	Slight acceleration of rate of dilatation
		Becomes quieter; settles into rhythm of of contractions
		Breathes with contractions
		May grimace, squeeze hands
		Less easily distracted but still interested in surroundings
			Teaching still appropriate but should be specific to immediate needs
			Reemphasize relaxation; purpose of contractions
			Monitor physical status:
			  Vital signs including FHR
			  Voiding
			  Amount and character of vaginal discharge
			  Warmth and comfort
			  Oral hygiene

Active Phase			

5-6-7 cm	Period of most rapid dilatation
	  Dilatation for primigravida should be at least 1.2 cm/hr; for multigravida at least 1.5 cm/hr
		Serious, talks only in short sentences or phrases; cries out in pain
		Focused on self and her pain
		Restless, tossing body about during contractions
		Regression and increasing dependency
		Own resources may not be adequate to cope with contractions
			Anticipate needs:
			  Sponge face
			  Keep bed clean and dry
			  Care for dry, cracked mouth
			  Check bladder for fullness
			Stay at bedside working through each contraction with patient; praise woman's efforts, point out progress
			Reinforce supportive efforts of the father
			Use touch to soothe, relax, comfort
			Check FHR q 15 min, B/P q 30 min
			Observe for hyperventilation
			May need analgesia to enhance coping

8-9-10 cm	Slight deceleration in rate of dilatation around 8-9 cm Descent of presenting part	Maximum concentration needed to cope with contractions May be nonverbal except for moans, single words, cries for help Nausea, occasional vomiting Legs shake uncontrollably Back pain and perineal pressure often continuous; can't distinguish beginning and end of contractions	Continue physical and supportive care as above Use palpation or uterine contraction monitor to help patient define contractions and rest periods Observe perineum for bulging

Second Stage	Expulsion of fetus	Becomes exhausted by great physical effort
		May be amnesic between contractions
		May become aggressive: hitting, scratching, vulgar language
		Panic that she will rip apart
			Direct pushing efforts with father for each contraction
			Provide comfort measures and facilitate rest between contractions:
			  Cool cloth to face
			  Keep perineum clean and dry
			  Environment quiet
			Encourage efforts; point out progress
			Explain preparations being made for delivery
			Check FHR with each contraction
			Help with panting for delivery of head and shoulders

Third Stage	Expulsion of placenta	Relief, fatigue, euphoria Cries with relief and joy Talkative Focused on baby and husband; keenly aware of people and things in environment	Congratulate Initiate contact with infant Coach in relaxation for delivery of placenta and perineal repair

Figure 14-25.   Summary of observations and nursing care during labor.

lean on her diaphragm, tighten her abdominal muscles, and push toward the vaginal opening. It is important that the mother relaxes her perineum and her legs as she pushes.

Rest between pushes is important, and the mother is urged to relax as much as possible between contractions. When the contraction is over the mother should let out her breath, lean back, take a deep breath and sigh it out, and try to relax all over. Every minute between contractions should be used for rest.

Although the contractions of the second stage are very strong, the mother usually feels less discomfort than she did during the latter part of the first stage. With bearing down, she generally feels that she is accomplishing something and making progress in the delivery of her baby. She should be given assurance that she is doing well and that her efforts are advancing the baby. Sometimes it is necessary to urge her to make greater effort through encouragement and advice in how to increase the force of her pushing.

As the second stage progresses the father is able to see first the bulging of the perineum and then the top of the baby's head as it comes further down the birth canal with each contraction. This visible sign of progress is not only encouraging and exciting for him but enables him to effectively urge the mother on through the last few difficult moments of labor.

The birth of the baby and immediate postdelivery care of mother and infant is discussed in Chapter 15.

Figure 14-25 gives a summary of the physiologic and psychologic changes during labor and appropriate nursing interventions for each stage and phase of labor.

BIBLIOGRAPHY

Affonso, Dyanne, Assessment of pain during labor, in *Current Concepts in Clinical Nursing*, Vol. IV, edited by Edith H. Anderson *et al.* Mosby, St. Louis, Mo., 1973, pp. 187–193.

Anderson, Sandra F., Childbirth as a pathological process: An American perspective, *MCN* 2:240–253 (July–Aug.) 1977.

Arms, Suzanne, *Immaculate Deception, A New Look at Women and Childbirth in America.* Houghton Mifflin, Boston, Mass., 1975.

Buten, Judith Ann, A philosophy of labor and delivery nursing, in *Current Concepts in Clinical Nursing*, Vol. IV, edited by Edith H. Anderson *et al.* Mosby, St. Louis, Mo., 1973.

Caldeyro-Barcia, Roberto *et al.*, Effect of position changes on the intensity and frequency of uterine contractions during labor, *Am. J. Obstet. Gynecol.* 80:284–290 (August) 1960.

Case, Lynda L., Ultrasound monitoring of mother and fetus, *Am. J. Nurs.* 72:725–727 (April) 1972.

Chassie, Marilyn Bache, Supporting the laboring couple, *Current Practice in Obstetric and Gynecologic Nursing*, Vol. I, edited by Leota K. MacNall and Janet T. Galeener. Mosby, St. Louis, Mo., 1976.

Cogan, Rosemary, Pain and hyperventilation with fast panting, slow panting, and "He" breathing during labor, *Birth Family J.* 4:59–64 (Summer) 1977.

———, and Edmunds, Evelyn, The unkindest cut? *Contemp. Ob/Gyn* 9:55–62 (April) 1977.

Contemporary Ob/Gyn, How LAC-USC detects the distressed fetus 1:12–32 passim, 1973.

Flynn, Anna, and Kelly, John, Continuous fetal monitoring in the ambulant patient in labor, *Br. Med. J.* 2:842–844, 1976.

Freeman, Roger, and Barden, Tom P., Interpreting labor tracings, *Contemp. Ob/Gyn* Monthly continuing series beginning April 1976.

Friedman, Emanuel A., Patterns of labor as indicators of risk, *Clin. Obstet. Gynecol.* 16:172–283 (March) 1973.

———, The functional divisions of labor, *Am. J. Obstet. Gynecol.* 109:274–280 (Jan. 15) 1971.

———, *et al.*, Dysfunctional labor XII: Long-term effects on the infant, *Am. J. Obstet. Gynecol.* 127:779–782 (April 1) 1977.

Grad, Rae Krohn, and Woodside, Jack, Obstetric analgesics and anesthesia: Methods of relief for the patient in labor, *Am. J. Nurs.* 77:242–245 (Feb.) 1977.

Haire, Doris, *The Cultural Warping of Childbirth.* International Childbirth Education Association, Milwaukee, Wisconsin, 1972.

Hobel, Calvin J., Problem-oriented risk assessment during labor, *Contemp. Ob/Gyn* 8:120–128 (Aug.) 1976.

——, *et al.*, Prenatal and intrapartum high-risk screening, *Am. J. Obstet. Gynecol.* 117:1–9 (Sept. 1) 1974.

Hon, Edward H., Biophysical intrapartal fetal monitoring, *Clin. Perinatol.* 1:149–160 (March) 1974.

——, *An Introduction to Fetal Heart Rate Monitoring.* Harty Press, New Haven, Conn., 1971.

Huprich, Patricia A., Assisting the couple through Lamaze labor and delivery, *MCN* 2:245–253 (July–Aug.) 1977.

James, L. Stanley, Fetal blood sampling, *Clin. Perinatol.* 1:141–148 (March) 1974.

Kopp, Lois, M., Ordeal or ideal—The second stage of labor, *Am. J. Nurs.* 71:1140–1143 (June) 1971.

Landry, Karen E., and Kilpatrick, Darla M., Why shave a mother before she gives birth? *MCN* 2:189–190 (May–June) 1977.

Lasater, Carol, Electronic monitoring of mother and fetus, *Am. J. Nurs.* 72:728–730 (April) 1972.

Luckner, Kleia Raubitschek, Fetal heart rate monitoring; The nurse's role as facilitator, in *Current Concepts in Clinical Nursing*, Vol. IV, edited by Edith H. Anderson *et al.* Mosby, St. Louis, Mo., 1973.

Mahan, Charles S., When patients ask about "gentle birth," *Contemp. Ob/Gyn* 5:51–55 (April) 1976.

Milic, Ann M. B., and Adamsons, Karlis, Fetal blood sampling, *Am. J. Nurs.* 68:2149–2152 (Oct.) 1968.

Miller, F. C. *et al.*, Hyperventilation during labor, *Am. J. Obstet. Gynecol.* 120:489–495 (Oct. 15) 1974.

O'Gureck, Joan E. *et al.*, A practical classification of fetal heart rate patterns, *Obstet. Gynecol.* 40:354–361 (Sept.) 1972.

Parer, J. T., and Dulock, Helen L. (eds.), Intrapartum evaluation of the fetus, *JOGN Nurs.* 5(5 Suppl.):35–80S (Sept.–Oct.) 1976.

Phillips, Celeste R., The essence of birth without violence, *MCN* 1:162–163 (May–June) 1976.

Quilligan, Edward J., The obstetric intensive care unit, *Hosp. Pract.* 7:61–69 (June) 1972.

Rice, Gail Taylor, Recognition and treatment of intrapartal fetal distress, *JOGN Nurs.* 1:15–22 (Aug.) 1972.

Ritchie, C. Ann H., and Swanson, Lee Ann B., Childbirth outside the hospital—The resurgence of home and clinic deliveries, *MCN* 1:372–377 (Nov.–Dec.) 1976.

Rovinsky, Joseph H., Symposium: Managing breech presentation, *Contemp. Ob/Gyn* 2:73–114 passim (Nov.) 1973.

Russin, Ann Woolbert, O'Gureck, Joan E., and Ronx, Jacques F., Electronic monitoring of the fetus, *Am. J. Nurs.* 74:1294–1299 (July) 1974.

Sasmor, Jeanette L., Castor, Constance R., and Hassid, Patricia, The childbirth team during labor, *Am. J. Nurs.* 73:444–447 (March) 1973.

Scott, J. R., and Rose, N. B., Effect of psychoprophylaxis (Lamaze preparation) on labor and delivery in primiparas, *N. Engl. J. Med.* 294:1205–1207 (May 27) 1976.

Smith, Barbara A., Priori, Robert M., and Stern, Mona K., The transition phase of labor *Am. J. Nurs.* 73:448–450 (March) 1973.

Stewart, Elizabeth, To lessen pain—Relaxation and rhythmic breathing, *Am. J. Nurs.* 76:958–959 (June) 1976.

Turbeville, Jane S., Nurse's role in intrapartum care, *Hosp. Topics* 50:85–88; 103 (June) 1972.

Tyron, Phyllis A., Assessing the progress of labor through observation of patients' behavior, *Nurs. Clin. North Am.* 3:315–326 (June) 1968.

Ueland, Kurt, and Hansen, J., Maternal cardiovascular dynamics. Part 2. Posture and uterine contractions, *Am. J. Obstet. Gynecol.* 103:1–7 (Jan. 1) 1969.

Whitson, Betty Jo, Hartley, Lucy M., and Wolford, Helen G., Complemental nursing, *Am. J. Nurs.* 77:984–988 (June) 1977.

Wisconsin Medical Society, Division on Maternal and Child Welfare, Pitocin: An alert to complications, *Wisc. Med. J.* 73:33 (Aug.) 1974.

Wood, Carl, Scalp blood pH in assessing fetal well-being, *Contemp. Ob/Gyn* 5:87–93 (Jan.) 1975.

15

Clinical Management
During Delivery

Care of the mother and fetus during the first stage of labor has been described in Chapter 14. This chapter deals with the actual delivery of the baby (second stage of labor), delivery of the placenta (third stage of labor), and the immediate care of both mother and baby after the birth.

The second and third stages of labor may take place in the same room as the first stage, or the mother may be moved to another room known as the birth room or delivery room. The place of birth may depend in part on the preference of the mother and in part on the normalcy of labor and expectations for a normal birth.

When a delivery room is used, the mother is transferred from her bed to the delivery table during either the latter part of the first stage or the early part of the second stage of labor, depending on her parity and progress of labor. Final preparation for delivery may be made immediately after this transfer, or after a variable period of bearing down with contractions, depending on the imminence of the birth. Efforts are made to allow sufficient time, thus avoiding hasty or inadequate preparation, and yet not to complete the preparation too far in advance of the actual delivery. When preparation is made too early, the mother's legs may be in stirrups an undue length of time; this may lead to muscle soreness, sluggish leg circulation, and venous thrombosis. Early preparation also leaves sterile supplies uncovered for a long time, which increases danger of contamination.

It is desirable for the same nurse who cared for the mother during labor to care for her also during delivery. This nurse will be a familiar person in a strange environment, and communication between the nurse and the parents will probably have been well established. If the father will be with his wife during delivery it is also desirable that he accompany her to the delivery room at the time this transfer is made.

THE DELIVERY ROOM

All or a considerable part of the second stage of labor, and also all of the third stage, are conducted in the delivery room. There are many similarities between a delivery room and an operating room. Maintenance of aseptic technique to prevent infection is the same in both. An adequate amount of equipment for the management of complicated as well as normal cases, for administration of anesthesia, and for meeting all emergencies is equally important in both areas.

Prevention of Infection

The woman in labor is very susceptible to infection brought to her from without. Personnel in the delivery room must be dressed in clean cotton uniforms that have not been worn outside the labor and delivery room area. A cap must be worn to keep loose hair from falling on the sterile field, and a mask to prevent droplet infection from the mouth and nose. Both mouth and nose must be well covered, and the mask must be changed at least every hour, and preferably every one-half hour, but a mask will not be sufficient protection if any of the attendants has a bacterial respiratory infection. No one with an infection of any type should attend the woman in labor. Only personnel directly concerned with the delivery should be permitted in the delivery room, and then only when in proper operating room attire. The delivery room is used only for obstetric clients. Frequent hand washing is important. A soap or detergent that contains hexachlorophene (G-11) or another bacteriostatic agent is usually preferred to other soaps.

Everything that touches the perineal region or that is used directly for the delivery—gloves, gowns, instruments, draping sheets, towels, and gauze—must be sterile. Preparation of the hands, gowning, and gloving of persons who directly assist with the delivery is similar to preparation for assisting with an operation.

Equipment

Much of the equipment in the delivery room is similar to that of the operating room; some is different because of the special purpose for which the delivery room is used.

Gloves, gowns, drapes, and many of the instruments and suture equipment are similar to those of an operating room. Some equipment, such as obstetric forceps, is special for the purpose of delivery.

The delivery table usually consists of two adjoining sections which can easily be separated; it is equipped with stirrups and with hand grips; and it is adjustable to various heights and positions. The mother is often put in the lithotomy position, with her legs in stirrups, for the delivery, and the lower half of the table is rolled under the main section for easier access to the perineal area.

Anesthesia machines and anesthetic agents and supplies are the same as those used in the operating room.

Equipment must be available for adequate care of the baby. This includes a heated crib or incubator and warmed blanket; an umbilical cord clamp; identification material; silver nitrate solution or penicillin for the eyes; and aspiration, oxygen, and intubation equipment in case the baby needs resuscitation.

Equipment and supplies for administration of intravenous fluids, for blood transfusion, and for drugs that may be necessary to meet an emergency must be available. Other essential equipment consists of suction devices for both mother and baby and an oxygen supply for both. Emergency call lights or signals and facilities for adequate lighting and for adequate temperature control are important. Mechanical devices must be checked frequently for proper function.

Since most deliveries are normal and only a small amount of supplies are used, much of the equipment mentioned above will be used infrequently. It is prepared to be available and in readiness for the less common complicated deliveries and the emergencies that may arise.

OBSERVATIONS

Observations of the Mother

Frequency of making observations and the vigilance in watching for changes must be increased during the second stage because of the increased rapidity and stress of labor. The uterine contractions are observed closely. The monitor is watched carefully, or the abdomen is palpated for frequency, duration, and strength of contractions, and also to ascertain that the uterine muscle relaxes well between contractions. The abdominal contour during contractions is observed to make certain that the uterus is contracting evenly.

The perineum is inspected during bearing down for bulging or for appearance of the presenting part, and also for abnormal vaginal discharge, such as bleeding and expulsion of meconium. Before the baby's head can be seen at the vaginal outlet, or its advance noted by bulging, the stage of its descent is sometimes ascertained by palpating through the perineum, the fingers of a gloved hand pressing upward on one side of the vulva.

The mother's vital signs, with the exception of temperature, are checked frequently. The pulse and blood pressure are taken every 5 to 10 minutes.

Muscle cramps in the legs may be a source of discomfort and will need immediate attention (see Fig. 14-8, page 314). The uncomfortable feeling of perspiration on the face may be relieved by wiping the face frequently and by applying a cool, moist cloth to the forehead. Discomfort caused by dryness of the mouth and lips may be relieved by moistening the lips with a wet cloth.

Observations of the Fetus

The reactions of the fetus must be very carefully observed throughout the second stage of labor. As in the first stage, this is done by close observation of the monitor or by auscultation of the fetal heart and by watching for expulsion of meconium. Fetal distress may be brought about by an interference with its oxygen supply. Heart rate pattern is watched very carefully and checked every five minutes, or following each contraction, during the entire second stage, until the baby is born.

Oxygen administered to the mother may satisfactorily treat the fetus if signs of hypoxia appear and thereby prevent respiratory depression at birth. This treatment may be beneficial when the fetus is deprived of an adequate oxygen supply from such causes as a low concentration of oxygen with an anesthetic agent, obstruction in the maternal respiratory tract, respiratory depression due to drugs, a failing maternal circulatory system, placental separation, or pressure on the umbilical cord during contractions. With signs of fetal hypoxia high concentration of oxygen may be administered to the mother between, as well as during, contractions while awaiting spontaneous delivery, or while preparation is being made for an operative delivery.

PUSHING WITH CONTRACTIONS

Pushing with contractions, as described on page 340, is continued throughout the second stage of labor. Pushing on the delivery table is facilitated by a semipropped position, with back curved and head forward. The mother's head and shoulders can be supported by raising the head of the delivery table or with extra pillows. If her legs are not in stirrups, she can flex her thighs toward her abdomen and grasp her thighs or her legs just below the knees while she pushes.

The father usually supports the mother's back as she pushes and coaches her in breathing and in relaxation between contractions.

PREPARATION FOR DELIVERY

Traditionally the lithotomy position has been used for delivery and the mother's legs are put in stirrups when the delivery is imminent. Sometimes the mother is delivered with her knees bent and her feet resting on the foot end of the delivery table. Many physicians prefer the lithotomy position for easier access to the perineal area and for readiness in the event that an operative delivery becomes necessary as an emergency measure.

When the lithotomy position is used care must be taken to prevent a strain on the ligaments of the pelvis during positioning of the legs in stirrups. They must not be separated too widely, and one leg should not be placed higher than the other. It is important that both legs are elevated together and placed into the stirrups at the same time. The legs or thighs should not be permitted to press against the bars holding the stirrups. The legs are strapped to the stirrups immediately after being placed there, to avoid the danger of the mother's moving a leg out of the stirrup. They must never be unstrapped after the delivery until the very moment that they are to be put down on the table, since the mother may be partly under the influence of an anesthetic and unexpectedly move her legs. When the legs are taken out of the stirrups they must be moved gently and both should be lowered to the bed at the same time. Such movement will lessen ligamentous and muscle strain and prevent any sudden change in circulation and blood pressure.

The mother's arms are restrained to prevent her from accidentally touching the sterile field. She needs an explanation of the purpose of the restraints.

The perineal region is regarded as the field of a major surgical operation and is prepared accordingly. Preparation consists of thorough washing of the skin of the lower abdomen, inner aspect of the thighs, vulva, and anal region to make it as clean as possible. During preparation, precautions are taken to avoid bringing bacteria to the mother and also carrying bacteria from her own skin to the vagina and thus permitting entry to the uterine cavity. All materials used for this preparation are sterile, and the nurse wears cap and mask and sterile gloves.

A fairly typical method of preparation for delivery, or sterile vaginal examination, is as follows. The mother's legs are positioned in stirrups, and she is covered with a sheet according to the extent of area to be prepared. The mother should be protected from embarrassment of unnecessary exposure at all times during labor.

The field which is to be prepared for examination or delivery must be uncovered, and a certain amount of exposure is unavoidable, but there are many ways in which the nurse may show her consideration for the mother and she will appreciate this effort.

The lower half of the delivery table should not be removed until everything is in readiness for skin preparation and draping. The mother should never be left alone for a moment without careful observation of the perineum after the lower portion of the table has been removed.

The nurse washes her hands and arms using soap or detergent containing a bactericidal agent, puts on a pair of sterile gloves, and then prepares the skin. Firm, even movements are made for washing the perineal region, using soap or detergent containing an appropriate bactericidal agent. These movements are repeated a sufficient number of times to clean the skin well, removing all blood and mucus. Each sponge is used only once, being discarded after approaching the anal region, or after stroking away from the vaginal opening in any direction. Washing is done from the center outward to avoid carrying material from surrounding areas to the vaginal outlet. The vaginal orifice is covered with a dry cotton ball while the surrounding skin area is prepared, to prevent solutions from entering the vagina. After the perineal area

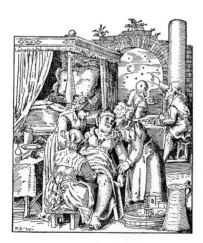 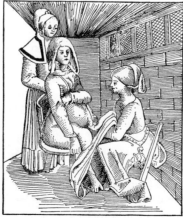

Figure 15-1. Old prints illustrating early ideas of suitable methods of making examinations and conducting deliveries, furnishing contrast with present-day methods. Concern seems to be divided between the patient and the signs of the zodiac in the picture at left.

is washed it is rinsed with sterile water, and other antiseptic solutions may then be poured over or sprayed on the skin. If fluid is poured over the vulvar region, it is not allowed to run into the vagina from the surrounding skin.

After skin preparation, as much of the prepared area as possible is covered with sterile drapes. The gloves used for preparation are considered contaminated. A sterile gown and a fresh pair of sterile gloves should be put on before sterile linen and other supplies are handled. Sterile leggings are placed over the mother's legs and as deeply into the groin as possible, and sterile sheets are placed under her buttocks and over her abdomen. Commercially packaged sterile drapes of a waterproof paper, which are disposable after use, are ordinarily used.

Since skin can only be cleaned, not sterilized, care is taken to avoid touching the vulva and surrounding skin insofar as possible during examination and delivery. Special precautions are taken against touching the anal region with sterile gloved hands. Whenever draping sheets or towels become wet from amniotic fluid and blood, they must be considered contaminated from the skin underneath; wet drapes are therefore not touched, and if possible they are replaced with dry ones. Instruments, towels, and sponges that are ordinarily used for a normal delivery are arranged on a table that has been covered with a sterile draping sheet.

An area on which the baby may be placed, for immediate care after birth, is arranged. For this, a warmed incubator or crib may be covered with a sterile sheet. Sufficient padding with sterile blankets or towels over the area where the baby will be placed is provided to protect him and to keep the area under him sterile. The baby's skin is wet, and inadequate layers of draping sheet will become moist throughout and unsterile from the table underneath.

While the above preparations are being made, the physician prepares his hands and arms as for surgery and puts on a sterile gown and gloves for the delivery. If a local anesthetic or a pudendal block is planned, the physician injects an anesthetic drug into the vulvar and perineal tissues after the preparation and draping. If the mother has not recently emptied her bladder the physician may catheterize her at this time. The perineum is kept clean while awaiting the birth of the baby by sponging in a downward direction, with cotton balls soaked in an antiseptic solution. Amniotic fluid and bloody mucus may drain from the vagina. Also particles of fecal material are sometimes expelled while the mother is bearing down, because of the pressure that is exerted on her rectum by the baby's head.

BIRTH OF THE BABY

Delivery of the Baby's Head

The physician controls delivery of the baby's head to prevent its rapid and forceful expulsion at the height of a contraction. Uncontrolled, forceful extrusion of the head may result in a deep tear in the perineal tissues and may also be injurious to the baby because of a sudden change of pressure on his head. Sometimes, when the perineum has offered considerable resistance to the head, the resistance is suddenly overcome; one contraction may then force the head out of the vagina. If the head is not yet well extended, force against the perineal body instead of upward toward the vaginal opening increases the possibility of a deep perineal tear. Delivery of the head is therefore controlled so that it emerges from the birth canal slowly and in good extension. The head is often delivered between contractions, the time at which control is easiest.

To control delivery, the physician places his hand on the baby's head, after it begins to distend the perineum and separate the labia and holds it in such a position as to be able to control its progress if this becomes necessary. While placing pressure on the occiput, the physician may also apply upward pressure on the brow through the perineum, a method termed *Ritgen's maneuver*. For this maneuver the physician covers his fingers with sterile toweling and, after the head has descended far enough to distend the vulva with its parietal bosses, places the fingers of one hand directly behind the anal region, or directly before it in a modified procedure, and makes upward pressure through the perineum while the other hand is held in readiness to restrain progress of the head should the vulvar resistance be overcome suddenly.

With restraint on the occiput, and sometimes upward pressure on the baby's chin, delivery of the head is slow and controlled in a manner favoring extension (see Figs. 15-2, 15-3, 15-4, and 15-5 for appearance, advance, and birth of head during normal delivery).

The mother may be asked to pant during the last few contractions before the birth of the

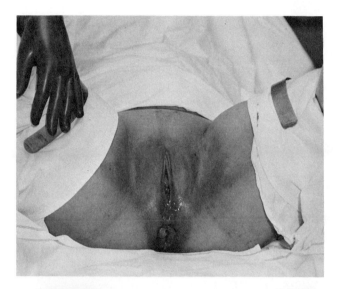

Figure 15-2. The baby's head is appearing at the vulva at the height of a contraction; separation of the labia is beginning.

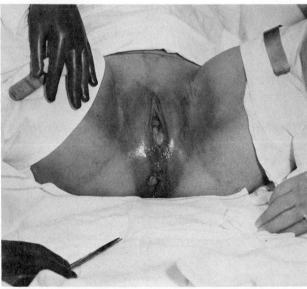

Figure 15-3. Advance of the head is indicated by distention of the vulva and perineum.

head, after crowning occurs, so that bearing down, which is involuntary, and the resultant intraabdominal pressure will be considerably reduced, preventing rapid advancement of the head. The head may then be allowed to advance slowly during a uterine contraction, or the physician may deliver it after the contraction has ceased. For delivery between contractions a certain amount of pressure is necessary. This pressure may be applied from above by asking the mother to bear down, this time without a simultaneous uterine contraction; or an assistant may exert a small amount of pressure on the uterine fundus.

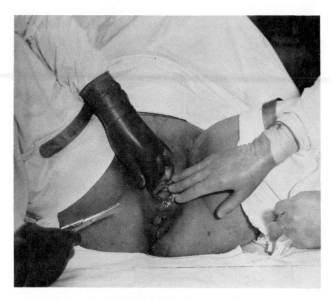

Figure 15-4.   Preparation for an episiotomy during a contraction. Note that the perineum has become quite thin and that the anus has begun to distend.

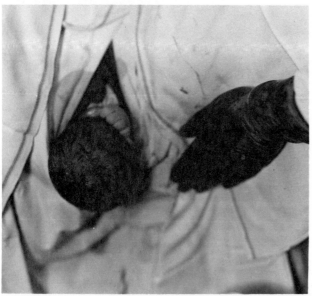

Figure 15-5.   The head has been born, and external rotation toward the right has taken place. In this delivery a hand has prolapsed alongside the head; this is not ordinarily the case.

Episiotomy (Perineal Incision) and Perineal Laceration

Lacerations are occasionally prevented, and often limited in extent, by skillful delivery of the baby, but in spite of the most careful efforts, tears of some degree will occur in most primigravidas and in many multigravidas unless an episiotomy (incision of the perineum) is done. A laceration may be no larger than a nick in the vaginal *mucous* membrane, it may extend down into the perineal body to any degree, or it may extend entirely through the perineal body and through the rectal sphincter. Perineal lacerations are very likely to occur when the perineal tissues are rigid and do not stretch well, or when they are friable; when the baby is delivered rapidly; when the baby is large; when a small pelvic outlet does not permit the head to fit closely against the symphysis pubis; and when delivery takes place from an abnormal presentation or position. Lacerations are usually described as being of first, second, or third degree, according to their extent.

A *first-degree laceration* is one that extends only through the fourchet, the vaginal mucous membrane, and the skin at the anterior margin of the perineum, without involving any of the muscles.

A *second-degree laceration* is one that involves the muscles of the perineal body. It extends down into the perineal body to varying degrees, sometimes to the rectal sphincter, but not through it. Such a tear usually extends upward into the vagina on one or both sides, making a triangular injury.

A *third-degree laceration* extends entirely through the perineal body and through the rectal sphincter and sometimes up the anterior wall of the rectum. This variety is often called a *complete tear*, in contradistinction to those of first and second degree, which are incomplete. A third-degree tear occurs infrequently. When the laceration extends up the anterior wall of the rectum, the term *fourth-degree laceration* is sometimes used to designate the extent of involvement.

Some times *lacerations* occur in the *labia* or *around the urethra*. These may be only slight abrasions, or they may be deep enough to bleed freely.

Episiotomy (Perineotomy)

An episiotomy, which is an incision through the perineal body, is very frequently performed, shortly before the baby's head is born, to facilitate delivery by enlarging the vaginal orifice. The major purposes of an episiotomy are (1) to spare the muscles of the perineal floor from undue stretching and bruising, and (2) to prevent prolonged pressure of the baby's head against the perineum. An episiotomy will also prevent the frequently unavoidable tears of the perineum, and substitute repair of a cleancut incision for an irregular tear. It is especially useful in cases of rigid perineum, when rapid delivery is necessary, when laceration seems inevitable, when presentation and position of the baby are abnormal, and when the baby is premature.

An episiotimy incision starts at the posterior margin of the vaginal opening and either may be made directly in the midline down to the sphincter ani muscle, called a *midline* or *median episiotomy*, or made at a 45-degree angle to either side, termed a *mediolateral episiotomy*. A bluntpointed scissors is used to make the incision, which is ordinarily performed at the height of a contraction, while the perineum is stretched (Fig. 15-4). For the comfort of the mother, analgesia is ordinarily used when the incision is made. Analgesia may be obtained from a regional anesthetic previously administered or from an inhalation anesthetic if such is being used for analgesia during contractions. The episiotomy is usually performed when the baby's head is low enough to distend the perineum and apply some pressure to the incision. Generally it is done before undue stretching has occurred, but not so early as to allow for excessive blood loss while awaiting the birth of the baby.

The decision as to whether to make a midline or a mediolateral incision will depend on a number of factors. The midline incision is easy to repair, heals well, and probably heals with less discomfort to the mother than the mediolateral, but there is danger of extension through the sphincter muscle if further tearing occurs. Extension of a mediolateral episiotomy does not injure the sphincter muscles, and it may therefore be employed when the baby is large or when his presentation or position is unusual. Many physicians favor the midline incision in most cases, preferring to incise the sphincter ani if a laceration appears imminent.

Palpation for Umbilical Cord Around the Baby's Neck

Immediately after birth of the baby's head, the physician palpates around the baby's neck to determine whether or not loops of umbilical cord surround it. At times one or more loops of cord do encircle the baby's neck, and they may be so tight that the vessels become constricted. If these coils of cord are fairly loose they may be slipped over the head, but if they are tight the cord is clamped and cut immediately.

Delivery of the Shoulders and Body

The baby's shoulders appear at the vulva as soon as external rotation of the head has taken place, and they are usually born spontaneously. However, it may be necessary to hold the baby's head between the two hands and make gentle downward traction to guide the anterior shoulder under the symphysis pubis, then lift the head upward to deliver the posterior shoulder, and downward again to deliver the anterior shoulder (Figs. 15-6, and 12-8 and 12-9 on pages 273 and 274). At times it is easier to deliver the anterior shoulder first. After delivery of the shoulders the rest of the body usually follows easily.

Manipulations to deliver the shoulders and body must be gentle to avoid injury to the brachial plexus or the clavicle or the nerves of the arm. Any necessary traction is made moderately and only in the direction of the long axis of the baby to avoid bending his neck on his body, which may result in excessive stretching of the brachial plexus. The fingers are not placed in the axillae to aid delivery, since this may put undue pressure on the nerves of the arms.

If force is necessary for delivery of the shoulders or for extrusion of the body, it is applied from above, by bearing-down efforts of the mother, or by suprapubic pressure made by an assistant.

As soon as the body is delivered the baby is held head downward for postural drainage of

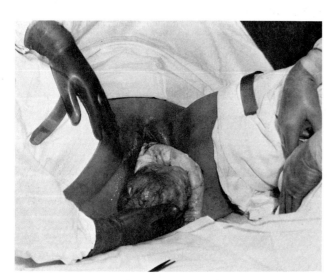

Figure 15-6. The anterior shoulder has been delivered. Birth of the rest of the body follows quickly.

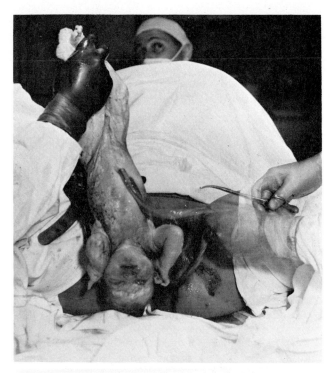

Figure 15-7. The baby is held with his head dependent for postural drainage of lung water and secretions in the respiratory tract. The physician is ready to clamp and cut the umbilical cord after respirations are initiated, unless need for immediate resuscitation is apparent. The baby will probably be placed on a level with the mother's body (the placenta) before the cord is clamped.

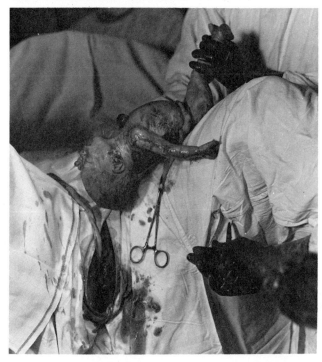

Figure 15-8. The umbilical cord has been severed, and the baby is moved to an incubator for further care.

secretions and to decrease the risk of lung water syndrome (Fig. 15-7). After the baby cries, or sooner if in distress, he is placed on a level with his mother's body and his umbilical cord is clamped and cut. The baby is then moved to a warmed incubator for further care (Fig. 15-8).

CARE OF THE BABY IMMEDIATELY AFTER BIRTH

Establishing Respirations

The newborn requires prompt attention to ascertain that he begins breathing almost at once, or to give him aid that will assist him in establishing adequate respirations. The lungs must immediately take over the respiratory function of the placenta, which, until birth, has served as the organ through which gas exchange has taken place.

Respirations are established within one minute after birth in most normal babies; many take their first breath within a few seconds and often cry vigorously as soon as they are born. A strong cry shortly after birth is evidence that the respiratory system has begun functioning well. Some babies, however, have a delay in onset of respirations, or they make respiratory movements shortly after birth but do not sustain these. With these infants resuscitative efforts must be taken immediately to prevent asphyxia, which progresses rapidly if untreated, and which may result in damage to brain cells or in death of the infant. Resuscitation should be done by the most experienced health team member present. Each nurse should be skilled in the techniques and should take prompt positive action if the physician is not immediately available.

Clearing the Air Passages

Fluid and mucus, and sometimes blood, meconium, and vernix, may be present in the baby's mouth, nose, and pharynx at birth; it is of the utmost importance that he does not aspirate this material with his first inspiration. A baby who has not become asphyxiated during a nor-

mal labor and birth process will probably not aspirate with inspiration. An asphyxiated baby is likely to aspirate the secretions that are present in his mouth and oropharynx when he takes his first breath.

To permit secretions to drain by gravity from the pharynx, postural drainage should be instituted immediately after birth. The baby is held in a position with his head dependent and his neck extended, before he takes his first breath, if possible, so that he does not draw foreign material into the trachea and lungs (Fig. 15-11A). Sometimes a baby gasps before the body is completely delivered and before he can be held head down but postural drainage is instituted as quickly as possible.

Some physicians use a rubber bulb syringe (Fig. 15-9) to remove excess mucus from the mouth and nose as soon as the baby's head is delivered, or they wait until immediately after delivery of the entire body, or they use suction at both times, after birth of the head and again after delivery of the body. When suction is

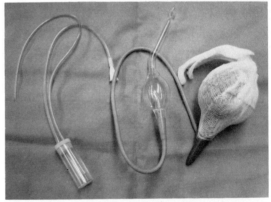

Figure 15-9. Equipment that may be used to remove secretions from the baby's mouth, nose, and throat.

Right, soft rubber bulb syringe. A piece of gauze placed around the syringe prevents slipping when it is handled with gloves.

Middle, a soft rubber catheter, size no. 12 or 14 French, attached to a glass mucous trap.

Left, a plastic catheter with mucous trap. The mucous trap may be used to send the mucus to the laboratory for culture. The unit is disposable.

used, the mouth is aspirated first, since stimulation of the nose may cause the baby to gasp and aspirate secretions from the mouth. The initial suction of the mouth with the bulb syringe may induce coughing and gagging and facilitate the baby's own efforts to clear fluid and mucus.

Suction on a catheter may also be used to aspirate the mouth, pharynx, and nose. A disposable polyvinyl catheter attached to mechanical suction or to a DeLee mucous trap on which the operator makes suction (Fig. 15-9) may be used. The catheter may be more effective than the bulb syringe because it reaches farther down into the throat.

For further suctioning, the baby is provided with warmth and put in the supine position with head lowered. To permit the baby's airway to extend and straighten, his head is slightly extended by placing a hand or a pad under his shoulders to elevate them. The baby's jaw is brought forward to lift his tongue from the posterior pharynx. The suction catheter is placed as far back as possible into the baby's throat, and suction is made on the mouthpiece of the mucous trap (Fig. 15-11B, C). The position of the catheter is changed frequently. The nose may also be aspirated.

Suctioning must be gentle to prevent injury to mucous membranes, and all should be brief —less than a minute is recommended. Unless suctioning is brief the baby may hold his breath and develop laryngeal spasm during stimulation of his pharynx. Prolonged suction may also cause severe bradycardia and cardiac arrythmia, complications that may result from vagal stimulation and lack of adequate oxygen.

Gastric suction is also sometimes done, but it is ordinarily delayed until respirations are established. Early gastric suction may also cause bradycardia and cardiac arrythmia.

Maintenance of Body Temperature

The baby is born into a room many degrees cooler than his body, and he will begin to lose body heat immediately. From the moment of birth he must be kept warm to minimize the metabolic demands that are produced when he tries to increase his heat production to maintain his body temperature. A sterile blanket should be in readiness to cover the baby at birth. He should then be quickly dried with a warm towel to reduce heat loss from evaporation of amniotic fluid from his body. The wet blanket should be replaced by a warm dry one. When the blanket is prewarmed the baby does not need to warm it with his own body heat.

To provide warm surroundings the baby should then immediately be placed in a delivery room incubator warmed to 97 to 98°F (36.1 to 36.7°C) or preferably one with an overhead radiant heater (Fig. 15-10). Care such as identification and eye treatment can be carried out in the incubator. A radiant heater over the incubator will provide warmth while the baby is receiving care. If a source of radiant heat is not available, blankets around the baby will reduce radiation of heat from the baby's body to the cold tables and walls of the delivery room. If inhalation anesthesia is used, it is essential that any source of radiant heat or lamp is either properly grounded or is used outside of the delivery room.

Immediate Appraisal of the Newborn

Appraisal of the newborn should begin the moment the baby is born. He should be carefully observed for the time of his first gasp, his first cry, and the beginning of sustained respirations, and a record made. The nurse usually has the responsibility of making these observations. Many babies take their first gasp and begin crying within seconds after birth. It is therefore important to note the time of birth on a clock with a second hand so that the time of the first gasp, first cry, and sustained respirations can be recorded in the exact number of seconds that they appear following birth.

Most hospitals use a scoring system, devised by Dr. Virginia Apgar in 1952, for making a clinical evaluation of the baby's condition at one minute after birth and again at 5 minutes and perhaps at 10 minutes.

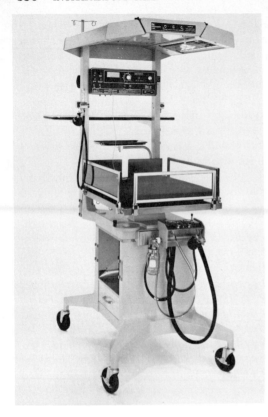

Figure 15-10. An incubator that is called a Neonatal Intensive Care Center, Deluxe Model. This "open incubator" provides an overhead radiant heater, of major importance in supplying warmth to the baby, and also provides ample space for personnel to work and care for the baby while he remains under the radiant heater. The incubator has equipment for aspiration of secretions and for administration of oxygen at either atmospheric or variable positive pressures. A normally breathing, as well as a distressed baby, will benefit from the protection that the heater of this incubator provides against loss of body heat to the cool environment as he receives delivery room care. [*Photograph courtesy of Ohio Medical Products (Division of Airco, Inc.), 3030 Airco Drive, Madison, Wisconsin 53707.*]

The Apgar Scoring System

In the Apgar scoring method five vital signs—heart rate, respiratory effort, muscle tone, reflex irritability, and color—are observed at exactly one minute after complete birth of the baby, irrespective of delivery of the placenta. Each sign is evaluated according to the degree to which it is present and is give a score of 0, 1, or 2 (Table 15-1). The five scores, one given to each of the five signs, are added together for a total score. It has a possibility of ranging from 0 to 10. An infant in excellent condition could receive the maximum score of 10, and a baby in poor condition would receive a very low total score, possibly even 0.

All signs do not have equal importance, and they are not individually independent. Color is the least important sign and the first to change,

and the heartbeat is the most important and the last to be absent. When all signs are not present they disappear in the following order: color, respirations, muscle tone, reflex irritability, heartbeat.

Scoring is done by one of the persons in the delivery room who observes the baby during the first minute after birth; the nurse may be requested to make the observations and scoring. Scoring does not interfere with other care and can be done while the baby is receiving other necessary attention. It may take time for the nurse to become confident in her ability to do the scoring, and she may want confirmation from another person until she has had experience. Two observers do not necessarily obtain the same total score, but variations should not be wide.

Scoring has been found to be easiest when a

Table 15-1. Apgar Scoring System*

Sign	0	1	2
Heart rate	Not detectable	Slow (below 100)	Over 100
Respiratory effort	Absent	Slow, irregular	Good, crying
Muscle tone	Flaccid	Some flexion of extremities	Active motion
Reflex irritability 1. Response to slap on sole of foot	No response	Grimace	Cry
2. Response to catheter in nostril (tested after oropharynx is clear)	No response	Grimace	Cough or sneeze
Color	Blue, pale	Body pink, extremities blue	Completely pink

*Scoring chart arranged according to information from Dr. Virginia Apgar.

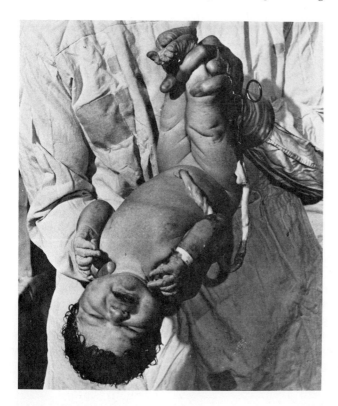

Figure 15-11. Recommended equipment and procedures. [*Reproduced from* Resuscitation of the Newborn Infant, *published by the American Academy of Pediatrics, Evanston, Ill., 1958, pp. 23 and 24.*] **A.** Method of holding infant at time of delivery.

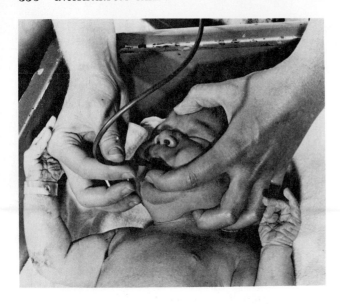

Figure 15-11 (*Cont.*)
    B. Simple method of suctioning pharynx.

decision is made quickly, between 55 and 60 seconds after birth of the baby. For this reason careful timing of birth on a clock with a second hand is important. The person doing the scoring may find it helpful to make a quick survey of the baby's general appearance and decide in which order to observe the signs. If the baby cried immediately at birth, the observer may wish to check the respirations and color first. If the baby seems mildly depressed and respirations are absent at this time, the last three signs to disappear—muscle tone, reflex irritability, and heartbeat—can quickly be checked. If the baby seems severely depressed, concentration on the last two signs to disappear—heartbeat and reflex irritability—is important.

HEART RATE   The heart rate is the most important sign. It may be checked by observing pulsation in the umbilical cord at its juncture with the abdominal wall, by feeling the pulsation in the cord, or by auscultation of the heart with a stethoscope (Fig. 15-11 C). A heart rate under 100 beats per minute is a sign of serious asphyxia and indicates resuscitation is necessary. If bradycardia is present, the other signs will be absent or present in only a minimal degree. If

the heart rate increases during resuscitation, the prognosis is generally good; failure to increase during ventilation is a grave sign or an indication of ineffective resuscitation efforts.

RESPIRATORY EFFORT   Respiratory effort is the second important sign. The vigorous baby should have respirations well established within one minute. He usually cries lustily at birth and continues to breathe well. The baby whose breathing is shallow, slow, and irregular and who has only a weak cry is considered to be having some difficulty. Apnea requires early treatment.

MUSCLE TONE   Muscle tone is scored according to the amount of flexion of the extremities and their resistance to extension. A term baby with excellent muscle tone keeps his arms and legs flexed, resists efforts to extend them, and has good movement of all extremities. If tone is only moderate, the baby appears sleepy, he is not active, and he does not keep his extremities flexed consistently. Poor muscle tone indicates that the baby has a low blood and tissue pH and that he is asphyxiated. A baby without tone is very limp and unresponsive.

REFLEX IRRITABILITY The reflex irritability sign is often tested by a slap on the sole of the baby's foot. The vigorous baby responds to this stimulation with a cry. If his response is not good he will only grimace, and if he is quite depressed he will not respond.

As an alternative method, reflex response may be tested by placing the tip of the catheter that was used to clear the pharynx of mucus just inside the nose. This method is not easily used before the baby has been moved to a table away from the field of delivery and may therefore not be the method of choice when clamping of the umbilical cord is delayed. A vigorous baby responds with a cough or sneeze when the catheter is placed just inside the nose. The less vigorous one responds with only a grimace, and the depressed baby does not respond. Lack of response indicates that the nervous system is depressed.

COLOR Color is the least important sign. Most babies, even when vigorous, do not become completely pink in one minute. All babies have some cyanosis at birth, and one to three minutes usually elapse, even in the healthy baby, before the entire body is pink. Vigorous babies that receive a score of 2 for all other signs, may therefore have only a score of 1 for color, because their extremities may still be blue at one minute after birth. For this reason, even the baby in excellent condition often has a score of less than 10. If the baby's entire body is blue or pale at the end of one minute his score for color is 0.

GROUPING ACCORDING TO SCORE The baby may be placed into one of three broad clinical groups according to the score he receives. Vigorous infants score from 7 to 10. These infants usually cry within a few seconds after birth. They generally do not require treatment. Infants in the depressed group score 4, 5, or 6, and may require some resuscitative measures to improve their condition. They have good heart rate and reflex irritability, but do not make satisfactory respiratory effort, their color is cyanotic, and their muscle tone may not be good. Infants in the severely depressed group score from 0 through 3; these babies require immediate resuscitation.

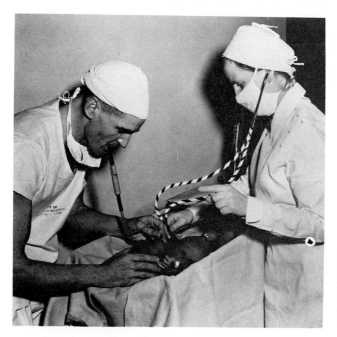

Figure 15-11 (*Cont.*)
  C. Method of indicating silently heart rate of infant. A slow heart rate usually indicates inadequate oxygenation of baby and need for assisted ventilation or treatment of shock. Rubber catheter and DeLee glass trap may be useful in aspirating stomach contents.

RESUSCITATION

The baby who does not breathe at birth will have a rapid (1) decrease in blood PO_2 (decrease in concentration of oxygen in the blood), (2) rise in blood PCO_2 (in carbon dioxide concentration in the blood), and (3) fall in pH of blood and tissues. The PO_2 falls to a very low level, approaching zero, in one minute. Carbon dioxide continues to accumulate and the PCO_2 can rise to a very high level in three to four minutes. When adequate oxygen is not available, glucose is incompletely metabolized to lactic acid instead of being completely metabolized to carbon dioxide and water. Liberation of this lactic acid into the bloodstream and the accumulation of carbon dioxide results in a rapid fall in pH. Acidosis and lack of oxygen interfere with the normal function of body cells and both must be corrected early. Unless resuscitative measures are instituted quickly, the baby's heartbeat will decrease in rate and heart action will soon stop.

If the baby does not breathe almost immediately after birth, ventilation of the lungs must be started at once to prevent or reverse sharp changes in the baby's physiologic condition. Ventilation of the lungs is used to reoxygenate the blood, remove carbon dioxide, and raise the pH by removal of carbon dioxide and restoration of complete glucose metabolism. Most babies who do not breathe within one minute after birth need only a few inflations of the lungs to initiate spontaneous breathing. A severely depressed baby may need ventilation for minutes or even hours. Ventilation is continued until the baby has sustained respirations.

The condition of the baby at birth is related to the degree of hypoxia or asphyxia before birth. A baby who has not suffered hypoxia, caused by antepartum complications or the labor and delivery process, is likely to require very little assistance or none with breathing. Babies with a severe depression, usually caused by asphyxia prior to birth, require that resuscitation be started immediately, without waiting to ascertain the one minute Apgar score. The heart should immediately be auscultated for evidence of its action; poor muscle tone indicates a serious condition. The longer ventilation of the lungs is delayed, the longer is the delay before spontaneous breathing will begin. Anesthetic agents administered to the mother may increase the baby's difficulty in spontaneous breathing. Cooling of the infant increases the rapidity of fall in pH. Cooling along with asphyxia can produce an almost irreversible condition within a few minutes.

Resuscitative measures include first making certain that the airway is clear, administration of oxygen, intermittent positive pressure ventilation to expand the lungs, and sometimes infusion of a base to help restore the pH of the

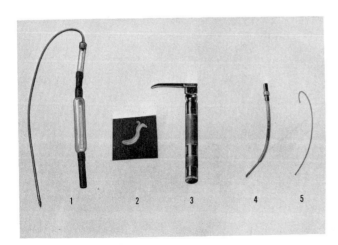

Figure 15-11 (*Cont.*)

D. Essential equipment for resuscitation. *1.* Two-holed Rausch rubber catheter (size 12) and DeLee glass trap. *2.* Berman plastic pharyngeal airway. *3.* Pencil-handle laryngoscope with premature blade. *4.* Cole endotracheal catheter (sizes 10, 12, and 14). *5.* Malleable wire stylet.

baby's blood. Methods of resuscitation are described below. In general, resuscitation should begin with the measures that are the least vigorous, and, if those are not effective, move to the more aggressive ones.

If the baby is breathing, but not with regularity, suction of the mouth and oropharynx and administration of oxygen may be sufficient treatment to improve his respiratory function. Sometimes sensory stimulation, such as a slap to the soles of the baby's feet, and oxygen flow with a mask against the face may stimulate respiration. If these measures are not quickly effective, or if the baby is not breathing, suction and positive pressure ventilation with a bag and mask or tracheal intubation as well as administration of oxygen become necessary. If the baby is obviously unresponsive at birth, no time can be lost in ventilation of the lungs.

Very important to resuscitation is to anticipate a problem and to be ready for it. Personnel and equipment for resuscitation must be ready at all times, so that the baby can be given aid immediately, even when difficulty is not expected. Someone in the delivery room should always be assigned to be responsible for assisting the baby in case he has difficulty breathing.

Clearing the Air Passages and Provision of Warmth

Clearing the air passages and providing warmth are essential to all babies and surely cannot be omitted in care of the baby with respiratory difficulty. This has been discussed under "Resuscitation" above. The need for clearing of the air passages before attempting ventilation is rather obvious, but the need for warmth is just as great.

Maintenance of body temperature is critical because cooling causes increased consumption of oxygen and glucose, both of which are essential for the energy that the brain and other cells need, and cooling quickly leads to acidosis and acid–base disturbance. The baby with respiratory difficulty may not have enough oxygen available to meet the even greater metabolic demands that are created by the stress of chilling.

A baby in need of resuscitation sometimes cannot be as carefully protected as recommended, but every effort must be made to keep him warm. Whenever possible resuscitative procedures should be carried out under a radiant heater. When this cannot be done the baby should be covered with warm blankets as much as circumstances permit.

Sensory Stimulation

If the airway is clear, a mildly to moderately depressed baby often can be stimulated to take deep breaths, and to cry, by rubbing his back, flicking the soles of his feet or flicking a finger against his heels several times. This method may already have been used to check reflex response, but may be repeated for stimulation. More vigorous methods, such as forcibly spanking the buttocks, slapping the back, or compressing the chest, are ineffective, waste valuable time, and may be injurious.

Oxygen

As a first measure oxygen administered by a mask held next to the baby's face will increase the oxygen he inspires during his first breaths. Increased oxygen to the brain may improve respirations. The baby's respirations, tone, reflexes, and heart rate are closely observed while oxygen is administered. If he does not breathe adequately within a minute or two or if his heart rate drops or does not improve if already low within 15–30 seconds with administration of oxygen, other treatment is usually started to prevent increasing asphyxia.

Ventilation

Mask and Bag Inflation

A mask and anesthesia bag may be used to administer oxygen in 100 percent concentration. The mask is held snugly over the baby's face, his head is tilted back slightly, his chin is held up and forward, and oxygen is administered by intermittent pressure on the bag (Fig. 15-11G). Ventilation is begun with a light squeeze on the bag and thereafter the squeeze is regulated according to chest movements. Careful observation for amount of chest expansion is essential. It may be necessary to apply increasing pressure on the bag at first and then to decrease pressure when the lungs open. Ventilation is carried out at 55 to 60 times per minute. An oropharyngeal airway may be put in place prior to ventilation to hold the tongue away from the posterior pharynx so that it does not obstruct the airway. It is important to know the capabilities of the resuscitation bag used, as some, especially self-inflating ones, will only deliver 40 percent oxygen and may not deliver any without compression. Oxygen may pass into the baby's stomach and gentle pressure on the baby's abdomen may be necessary to deflate the stomach. If bag and mask ventilation continues more than 5 minutes, a nasogastric tube should be passed to provide for stomach decompression.

With effective ventilation the baby's chest should soon aerate well, his color should improve rapidly, and his heart rate should quickly reach a normal rate.

Direct Laryngoscopy and Tracheal Intubation

If the baby does not quickly improve with the use of mask and bag and oxygen, a laryngoscope is introduced to visualize the larynx, suction is used to clear the larynx and trachea, and a tube is inserted into the trachea to be used for inflation of the lungs. For the severely depressed baby (Apgar score 0, 1, 2, or 3), the laryngoscope is ordinarily used immediately, without first using the methods described above.

A pencil-handle laryngoscope with a premature blade is used to visualize the larynx (Fig. 15-11E). For its insertion the baby is placed on his back on a firm surface; his head is positioned over a towel so that it will be extended, with the chin pointing slightly upward; and the baby's head is kept in a straight line with his body. After insertion of the laryngoscope, suction may be made with a catheter to remove mucus, blood, meconium, or vernix (Fig. 15-12), or an endotracheal tube may be inserted and suction made through it. The laryngoscope is removed and the endotracheal tube is left in place until respirations are established.

Clearing the trachea may be sufficient to stimulate respirations, which is evident when the

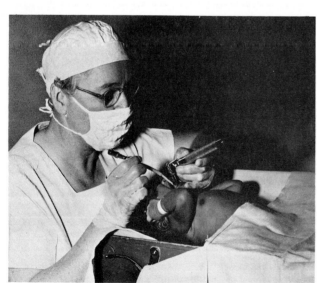

Figure 15-11 (*Cont.*)
E. Method of introducing endotracheal tube. Note folded towel under shoulders, extension of the head, laryngoscope held in left hand, tube in right hand; slot in laryngoscope is for vision. Tube introduced at right corner of mouth.

baby makes a gasping sound. If respirations do not begin, the lungs are inflated through the endotracheal tube by one of several methods, until the baby gasps and breathes.

The physician may breathe into the endotracheal tube a few times, using short breaths that cause the baby's chest to rise gently. He may use air from the room before each breath into the tube or put a tube from which oxygen is flowing freely into his mouth to increase the amount of oxygen delivered to the baby (Fig. 15-11F). Intermittent pressure on an anesthesia bag, attached to the endotracheal tube with an adaptor, may be used to inflate the lungs and

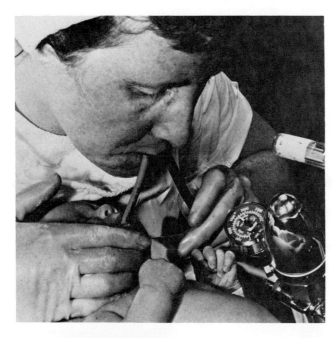

Figure 15-11 (*Cont.*)
F. Method of inflating lungs with oxygen-enriched air. Tube with oxygen is in operator's mouth. Inflation should be with short and sharp breaths, using only the volume of air in the operator's mouth.

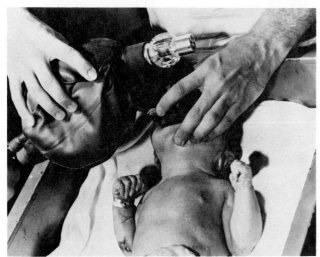

Figure 15-11 (*Cont.*)
G. Equipment for inflating lungs with small mask and bag. Short, sharp inflation is given by squeezing bag with hand. Entry of air into lungs is checked with stethoscope. If no air is heard, intubation is obligatory.

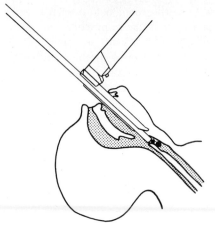

Figure 15-12. Quick, brief suction through laryngoscope to remove foreign material in respiratory tract. [*Adapted from* Resuscitation of the Newborn, *rev. ed. Smith Kline & French Laboratories, Philadelphia, Pa., 1963.*]

deliver oxygen, or a respirator may be used to deliver oxygen, under controlled pressure, into the endotracheal tube.

Use of Respirator

A positive pressure respirator may be used for artificial ventilation if ventilatory support is still needed after the initial resuscitative efforts. The respirator is set for the desired resuscitative pressure. Pressures of 15 to 20 cm of water are usually safe when carefully applied, but brief pressures as high as 30 cm or more water pressure may be necessary at first to expand the alveoli. Oxygen is administered by controlled intermittent pressure. The lungs deflate between each application of pressure by their elastic recoil. The intermittent positive pressure thus inflates the lungs, supplies oxygen, and removes carbon dioxide.

Inflation, by any method, is used for the shortest time and with the lowest pressure that is effective. A few inflations may be sufficient, or repetition for several minutes or occasionally several hours may be necessary before spontaneous respirations are well established. Required pressures and tidal volumes change

rapidly during the first minutes of ventilation. Use of a method or machine that permits easy adjustment to the necessary change is important. Movements of the chest are observed during inflation. If the stomach rises, the tracheal tube is in the esophagus; its position must be changed. The endotracheal tube is removed when respirations are well established, usually after the baby has taken several spontaneous breaths. Sometimes it must be kept in place for a longer period until there is assurance that respirations are sustained.

Mouth-to-Mouth Inflation

Mouth-to-mouth breathing may be used instead of a bag and mask if equipment is not immediately available. Equipment is not necessary for mouth-to-mouth breathing, and it is therefore a method always available in an emergency.

To do mouth-to-mouth breathing, the baby is placed on his back on a firm surface, and the operator places his mouth directly over the baby's mouth and nose or over two or three layers of clean gauze first put over the baby's face, if gauze is readily available. The baby's nose and mouth must be covered with the operator's mouth, or if the nose is not covered it must be held closed so that air will not come out through it. The baby's head should be tilted back slightly and the lower jaw should be pushed forward so that the chin juts out; this lifts the tongue and raises it from the posterior pharynx, where it may obstruct the air passage. Air is breathed into the baby at a rate of 35 to 40 times per minute. The breaths into the baby must be gentle so that his lungs are not injured. The breaths should be no more vigorous than the person's normal breathing; only the air in his mouth, not his lungs, is used. The operator should look for chest expansion; a small amount of chest movement is sufficient to indicate that the procedure is being performed vigorously enough.

While carrying out mouth-to-mouth breathing, the individual should take in a breath of room air before each breath into the baby or, if oxygen is available, take in a breath of oxygen from a tube attached to the oxygen supply; this increases the amount of oxygen that is delivered to the baby. Room air or oxygen will dilute the carbon dioxide present in the operator's mouth at the end of his own expiration. A depressed baby already has acidosis; additional carbon dioxide may increase it and therefore should be limited as much as possible.

Since air breathed into the baby's mouth and nose may enter either his lungs or stomach, the individual's hand should put slight pressure over the baby's epigastrium to prevent his stomach from being filled with air. The elastic recoil of the baby's lungs will usually deflate them, but expiration will be favored by slight pressure on the baby's chest.

Mouth-to-mouth breathing is sometimes disapproved of because of danger of infection. Its ready availability however, and its effectiveness may make it the best procedure in certain instances. Antibiotics may be administered after use of this method.

External Cardiac Massage

Closed chest cardiac massage is initiated when a heart rate is not detectable and does not return with three or four insufflations. With cardiac massage the heart is manually compressed and artificial circulation is maintained. As the heart is compressed between the chest wall and the vertebral column blood is forced into the arteries. Relaxation of pressure allows the heart to fill with venous blood. When combined with proper ventilation manual heart compression is often able to maintain sufficient blood pressure to keep the heart and brain adequately oxygenated until the heart can begin beating by itself.

To perform external cardiac message the baby's sternum is rhythmically compressed at the rate of 100 to 120 times per minute while artificial ventilation is also given. The baby is placed in the supine position on a firm surface. The index and middle fingers of the operator's hand are pressed sharply against the *middle* third of the baby's sternum to a depth of ½ to ¾ inch at the rate of 100 to 120 times per min-

ute. The heart beat is coordinated with the ventilation at a ratio of 3 cardiac massages to 1 ventilation—3 heartbeats, pause for 1 ventilation, 3 heartbeats, pause for 1 ventilation, and so on. The two procedures should not be performed simultaneously because the pressure applied during cardiac massage may injure a lung that has just been inflated. The pressure for cardiac massage is best applied against the middle third of the sternum, since pressure against the lower third is less effective and limits movement of the liver. The peripheral pulses are monitored for evidence of adequate perfusion of the peripheral vessels.

An alternate method of cardiac massage is for the operator to place his hands around the baby's chest with the fingertips to the baby's back and the thumbs touching over the sternum. The middle third of the sternum is compressed vigorously with the thumbs. This technique is more applicable if the baby should for some reason be kept in the lateral position. The two-finger technique, however, has the advantage of being carried out successfully with one hand, leaving the other free to palpate the temporal or femoral pulses.

Ventilation must be maintained during the time that compression of the heart is carried out. Cardiac compression and ventilation are continued until a regular heartbeat is discerned. Massage is stopped briefly every 30 seconds for observation of signs of spontaneous heartbeat. As soon as a rhythmic beat can readily be heard massage is discontinued.

Use of Epinephrine

Epinephrine may be used in conjunction with cardiac compression to stimulate the heart if other methods fail to produce a cardiovascular response. It may be administered intracardiac or intravenously. Care must be used in preparing the minute dose of 0.05 to 0.1 mg from the concentrated standard solution. A standard epinephrine ampul (1:1000) contains 1 mg/ml or 1000 μg. This 1-ml ampul is diluted to 10 ml with saline or 5 percent glucose, making a 1:10,000 dilution. A dosage of 0.1 ml/kg of a

1:10,000 solution may be ordered. If a more dilute solution is desired, 9 ml of the 1:10,000 solution are discarded and the remaining 1 ml is again diluted to 10 ml, making a 1:100,000 dilution.

Administration of a Base

If asphyxia is severe, intravenous infusion of a base will help to restore the blood pH. An Apgar score below 2 at 1 minute, below 3 at 3 minutes, and below 5 at 5 minutes suggests need for a base. With asphyxia the pulmonary arterioles constrict, resistance to blood flow is high, and less blood reaches the alveolar cells. Also, the ductus arteriosus does not close or it opens again, permitting blood to be shunted past the lungs. The pulmonary arterioles and the ductus arteriosus are sensitive to blood Po_2 and pH. Ventilation of the lungs will supply oxygen and if the blood Po_2 can be raised in this way the pulmonary arterioles will respond with reduced resistance. However, dilatation of the pulmonary arterioles is also dependent upon a blood pH above the level of 7.2.

In severe asphyxia the blood pH is low and must be raised for good lung response to oxygenation. Removal of carbon dioxide by ventilation will improve the pH somewhat, but when the pH is very low, administration of a base may be important in treatment. Initially sodium bicarbonate or tris (hydroxymethyl) aminomethane (THAM) may be given intravenously over a two- to five-minute period into one of the vessels of the umbilical cord to raise the pH to a level at which the lungs will respond by arteriolar dilatation to take up the oxygen that is being administered by ventilation. Initial dose of sodium bicarbonate is 2–4 mEq/kg diluted with an equal amount of sterile water or saline. Dilution of the base before injection is essential. After the initial injection the base may be continued by slow intravenous drip.

Since sodium bicarbonate breaks down to carbon dioxide, good ventilation is essential when sodium bicarbonate is used. Ventilation is also very useful in reducing acidosis by removal of carbon dioxide from the body.

Administration of Glucose

Intravenous glucose, 5 or 10 percent, will provide a source of energy for the baby whose stores may quickly be depleted. The glucose is important to assure that the baby's metabolic requirements, which are likely to be increased with this stress, will be adequately met. Glucose administeration is begun as soon as other emergency measures permit.

Drugs

The use of drugs in addition to the resuscitative measures described above is very limited. If the baby's depression is believed to be due to a narcotic administered to the mother during labor, a *narcotic antagonist*, such as nalorphine (Nalline) or levallorphan (Lorfan) or naloxane (Narcan), may be administered after the air passages have been cleared and the lungs have been ventilated. These drugs reduce the respiratory depression and other side effects of morphine and its derivatives, but have no effect in lessening depression caused by other drugs, such as barbiturates, or by anesthetics.

Nalline, Narcan, and Lorfan may be administered intramuscularly or by injection into the umbilical vein. If the baby's circulation is satisfactory, the effect from intramuscular injection becomes apparent in a few minutes. The usual neonatal Nalline dose is 0.1 to 0.2 mg; Nalline is available in this dosage in 1-ml ampuls. The dosage of Lorfan for the newborn is 0.05 mg. Lorfan is presently not available in dosages smaller than 1 mg in 1-ml ampuls; it must therefore be diluted to be measured in proper amount for administration. The dosage of Narcan is 0.1 mg/kg of body weight. Narcotic antagonists may be administered to the mother 5 to 15 minutes prior to delivery, if depression of the baby from a drug administered to the mother is anticipated. Since a narcotic antagonist is a depressant of itself, the baby must be closely observed for such effect after its administration. Narcan is becoming the drug of preference for the newborn because it does not depress respiration or cause sedation and would not do harm by such action if the baby's depression was not narcotic-induced.

Stimulants

Most stimulants, including such drugs as alphalobeline, pentylenetetrazol (Metrazol), and nikethamide (Coramine), are considered potentially dangerous to a depressed baby. In the infant, the margin between therapeutic dose and toxic dose of stimulants is often very narrow. Such drugs are only considered on rare occasions. Use of epinephrine has been discussed.

Evaluation of Circulatory Status

A baby with asphyxia may have hypovolemia and hypotension. If the baby has a low circulating blood volume he will have inadequate perfusion of some organs and will develop shock. The baby is likely to appear pale and "shocky." Poor capillary filling may be noted when an area of skin is blanched by firm pressure and return of color is slow. The extremities may be cold and the pulses may be weak, especially the radial and posterior tibial pulses. Other early signs are a low arterial or central venous pressure, and metabolic acidosis. Blood pressure should be monitored frequently on an asphyxiated infant by doppler or from the umbilical artery. Tachycardia may or may not be present. Anemia may or may not be present initially but will appear later.

When shock is present, treatment must be started early. For initial blood volume expansion, albumin, 1 gm/kg of body weight, diluted 1:4, may be used. After this the baby's response is evaluated and a determination of further therapy is made. For severe hypovolemia and for babies with severe asphyxia, administration of plasma or whole blood may be indicated for circulatory support. Some of the initial effects of the sodium bicarbonate administered for acidosis may result from its effect as a volume expander as well as from the correction of pH.

Subsequent Observations

An Apgar score should be done on all babies at five minutes after birth, but such evaluation of a baby who required resuscitation is absolutely essential. A baby with a low score at one minute after birth should soon have a higher score if he responds well to resuscitation. If the baby's score has not reached 8 at five minutes of age, another scoring is indicated at ten minutes and perhaps more frequently.

For any baby who received a high Apgar score at one minute of age, a second scoring at five minutes is also indicated. A baby with a high score at one minute usually does not drop to a lower one, but he also needs further close observation because his condition may change rapidly, especially if he has obstructing material in the trachea, or if he is under the influence of drugs administered to the mother.

It is important to make an accurate record of the time of each Apgar score on a baby. Scoring at specific times assures regular observation of a baby during his early period of life and greatly increases the likelihood of identifying a baby in distress. All other behavior of the baby must be closely observed and described. Respiratory effort, movement of the chest, rate of respirations, heart rate, and color are valuable observations. Frequency and lustiness of cry, whether spontaneous or stimulated, should be recorded. Muscle tone and activity must be closely observed, since a baby with poor tone, who lies in a flaccid position, may require treatment for acidosis.

Continuous close observation in the nursery is mandatory for any baby who has required resuscitation or who has become chilled.

Care of the Umbilical Cord

The umbilical cord is compressed a few inches from the baby's abdominal wall with two hemostatic clamps and cut between the clamps. The placental end of the cord is placed on the mother's abdomen until the placenta is expressed, to prevent its contamination from contact with the mother's anal region (Fig. 15-8). The clamp is left on the placental end of the cord until the placenta is expelled, because of the possibility of another baby in the uterus and the danger of serious blood loss from that baby through the open cord.

The umbilical cord may be clamped immediately after the baby's birth, or clamping may be postponed for a few minutes, until pulsation in the umbilical cord ceases. A short delay in clamping of the cord permits the amount of blood which flows between the placenta and the baby to stabilize. Blood is pushed from the baby to the placenta as he passes through the birth canal, flows back quickly and overcompensates, and then some returns to the placenta and begins to stabilize. Holding the baby at the level of the perineum permits good equalization of the blood between baby and placenta. Delay in clamping of the cord until his respirations are established also provides a reservoir for the lung fluid which is quickly removed from the baby's lungs by his circulatory system. Clamping of the cord may be necessary early when the umbilical cord is snugly around the baby's neck and when resuscitation must be instituted immediately. It may be desirable when the mother is deeply anesthetized to avoid further anesthesia to the baby, or when complications, such as hemolytic disease, are anticipated. The time of clamping is determined for the individual baby.

The umbilical cord stump is ligated close to the baby's abdomen with a small plastic or metal clamp or a cord tie, and the hemostat is removed. Several kinds of umbilical cord clamps are available. They are ordinarily left on the cord for 12 to 24 hours and removed when the umbilical cord vessels are crushed and thrombosed.

If a ligature of bobbin is used to ligate the cord, it must be strong and heavy enough to be noncutting. It is tied tightly, in a square knot that will not slip and permit bleeding, about an inch from the baby's abdominal wall. If the ligature is applied slowly and at interrupted intervals, the Wharton's jelly in the cord is squeezed out from under the ligature, and the blood vessels will be constricted better than with one rapid pull on the tie. When the Wharton's jelly is not squeezed out, it may escape later and the cord will then retract, leaving the tie loose, with subsequent bleeding. It is considered a safe precaution to bend the cord back on itself and tie it a second time with the same ligature, as the danger of hemorrhage from a loosely tied cord is serious.

The blood vessels are clearly visible at the ends of the moist freshly cut umbilical cord. The two arteries can be seen as two small vessels of equal size and the umbilical vein as a larger vessel. Examination for the number of vessels in the umbilical cord and a record of the findings are recommended. Babies with only one umbilical artery are reported to have a higher incidence of congenital anomalies, especially renal and gastrointestinal. A finding of only two umbilical vessels serves as an alert for a search for other anomalies in the baby.

A dressing is not applied to the umbilical cord stump, but it and the surrounding area must be kept clean to prevent infection. Precautions consist of careful handwashing prior to care, keeping moisture around the cord to a minimum, and application of 60 percent alcohol or other antiseptic several times a day (see p. 456).

Care of the Eyes

The baby's eyes may become infected during birth if gonococci are present in the birth canal, but proper care of the eyes at birth will prevent almost all cases of ophthalmia neonatorum. A germicide properly dropped into the eyes soon after birth will kill any organisms that are present.

The Credé method, named for and made famous by the Viennese obstetrician who introduced it in 1881, was to drop from a glass rod a single drop of nitrate of silver, 2 percent, into each eye immediately after birth. The routine use of this prophylaxis reduced the occurrence of ophthalmia in Credé's clinics from 10 to 1 percent among the newborn babies. Later the strength of silver nitrate was reduced to 1 percent and was made mandatory in many countries.

Since penicillin is highly gonococcocidal, its use has often been recommended as a prophylactic agent against ophthalmia neonatorum, and it is being used as a preventive treatment. Its efficiency is good, but it, as well as silver nitrate, has certain disadvantages. Penicillin sensitivity, although rare, may occur and there is the possibility of infection with an antibiotic-resistant strain of gonococcus. Some physicians,

therefore, do not wish to abandon the silver nitrate treatment.

A prophylactic treatment against ophthalmia neonatorum is required by law or regulation in most states in this country; in a number of them the silver nitrate method is specified.

Before instillation of drops or ointment into the eyes, the outer surface of each eyelid is wiped from the nose outward with a sterile cotton ball moistened with sterile water to remove mucus, blood, and vernix.

For instillation of silver nitrate, wax ampuls containing a 1 percent solution are supplied by state health departments. This is an important safety factor since danger of accidental use of a

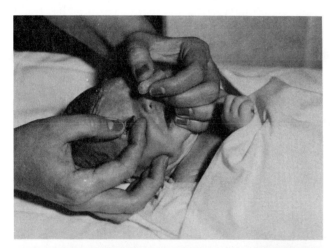

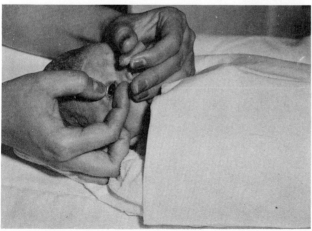

Figure 15-13. Placing drops of a 1 percent silver nitrate solution into the conjunctival sac for prevention of ophthalmia neonatorum.

Top: The eyelids are not sufficiently separated, and there is danger of dropping the medication directly on the cornea, where it may cause trauma and injury.

Bottom: The eyelids have been separated sufficiently to permit placing the medication on the lower eyelid or into the conjunctival sac.

stronger solution is eliminated. The ampuls are hermetically sealed, so that the solution does not deteriorate rapidly, as does a more exposed solution in a dropper bottle. They should, however, be protected from exposure to light. They also eliminate danger of evaporation and subsequent increase in concentration of solution. Each ampul contains sufficient solution for treatment of one baby. To use the ampul, one end is pierced with a sterile pin, allowing the solution to be squeezed out one drop at a time.

For instillation of silver nitrate, the lower lid is pulled downward as far as possible and 2 drops of a 1 percent solution of silver nitrate are placed into the conjunctival sac (Fig. 15-13). After the lid is released, the solution will spread over the entire conjunctiva. Care must be taken not to drop the medication directly on the cornea, where it may cause trauma and injury. Excess solution that squeezes out of the eye when the lids are closed should be wiped off. If it is not removed, it causes a brown or black discoloration of the skin around the eyes that must wear off and that concerns the parents until it disappears.

The silver drops may be left *in situ* without further treatment, or the eyes may be irrigated one to two minutes after the instillation, using warm *sterile* water or warm physiologic salt solution and a soft bulb syringe. The irrigation will wash out excess silver nitrate and form a precipitate with the remainder when saline is used. Care must be taken that the silver nitrate is not washed out of the eyes so soon after instillation that it does not have time to be effective.

When penicillin is used as a prophylactic agent against ophthalmia neonatorum, it is either administered intramuscularly or instilled into the eyes as drops or as a penicillin ophthalmic ointment. To prevent penicillin solution or ointment from becoming inactive it must be kept refrigerated and not used beyond the expiration date.

Prophylactic treatment of the eyes has traditionally been carried out as soon as possible after birth and before the baby leaves the delivery room. From studies of mother–infant bonding it appears advisable to postpone this treatment for about an hour so as not to interfere with the baby's quiet and alert eye contact with his mother. Such contact between mother and baby seems to trigger important maternal attachment responses to her baby during the very sensitive period following birth.

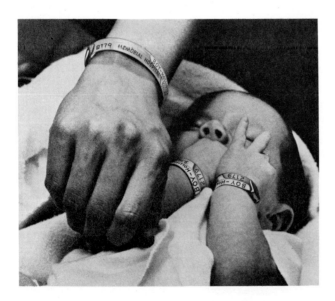

Figure 15-14. Correlated Mother/Baby Ident-A-Band® bracelets available from Hollister Incorporated, 211 East Chicago Avenue, Chicago, Illinois 60611. With this newborn identification system three joined bands bearing identical numbers and inserts for recording of other identical identifying information can easily be separated and applied to mother and baby before they leave the delivery room. One band is placed on the mother's wrist and two bands are applied to the baby. [*Photo courtesy of Hollister Incorporated.*]

Eye treatment is best postponed to early care of the baby in the nursery, when the same procedure that has been described above may be carried out after the mother has had initial contact with her infant.

Identification

Every baby must be properly identified *before the infant and the mother are transferred from the delivery room.* Identification bands with identical numbers for both baby's and mother's wrists or bands fastened to the baby's wrist and ankle are frequently used (Fig. 15-14). Minimum identifying information on the bands includes the baby's sex and surname, the mother's given name, and the date and time of birth. Other identifying information such as the name of the physician may also be added. The nurse preparing the identification bands should have another person check the information with her as additional certainty against error.

The identification band is checked each time the baby is taken to the mother or moved from his bassinet for any reason. The mother is shown the identification and is instructed to check it each time the baby is brought to her. The baby is discharged without removal of identification unless he is wearing two identical bands, in which case one is removed and attached to the infant's record.

A footprint, which is a permanent means of identification, should also be made and filed with the hospital records (Fig. 15-15). In some states footprinting is mandatory. The footprint does not replace other more readily observable methods of identification, but is used as a supplemental means in case doubt arises concerning a baby's identity. This is especially important after the baby leaves the hospital. The print is made on a form that contains other identifying data, similar to that on the identification band, and also the mother's fingerprint.

If taken carefully, a footprint is positive identification, because the arrangement of the ridges on the fingers, toes, palms, and soles is unique to each individual. These ridges are present at birth; they begin forming in the fetus about the fourth month; and they do not change during the individual's lifetime.

The footprint should be made in the delivery room whenever possible. A print of the mother's

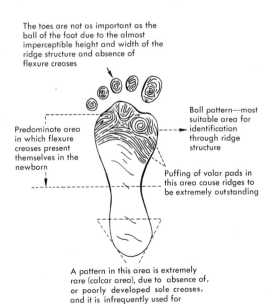

The toes are not as important as the ball of the foot due to the almost imperceptible height and width of the ridge structure and absence of flexure creases

Ball pattern—most suitable area for identification through ridge structure

Predominate area in which flexure creases present themselves in the newborn

Puffing of volar pads in this area cause ridges to be extremely outstanding

A pattern in this area is extremely rare (calcar area), due to absence of, or poorly developed sole creases, and it is infrequently used for identification purposes

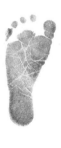

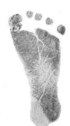

Figure 15-15. Footprint identification pointers. [*Reprinted with permission from* Footprinting Pointers and Procedures. *Bureau of Maternal and Child Health, New York State Department of Health, Albany, N.Y.*]

finger, on the same record as the baby's foot-print, is also made at this time. In some hospitals a baby's palmprint or fingerprint is taken instead of a footprint; these are somewhat more difficult to make.

Ridges in a baby's skin are fine, and the footprint must be made with great care to be legible. Smudging of prints or heavy inking that fills in the skin ridges makes the print illegible and useless.

To make a print of the baby's foot, the nurse should study the instructions for the particular material she will use. Instructions that apply to all methods are as follows. The baby's foot is wiped clean and dry, and lint is brushed off. A thin film of printer's ink is applied to the foot, care being taken that the ink is not so heavy that it fills the ridges of the skin. The foot is then pressed firmly on the paper on which the print is to be recorded. Excessive pressure is avoided, and both paper and foot must be held firmly to prevent smudging. The ball of the foot is the best area for identification of ridge detail, and efforts should be made to get this area as clear as possible (Fig. 15-15). The print is examined immediately with a magnifying glass. If the nurse is able to recognize some ridge detail, the print can be considered legible; if not, it must be redone.

Photographs of babies' ears are being studied for their value as permanent identification. Size, form, and configuration of the ear are unique to each individual, and changes during growth are apparently minute.

Inspection for Abnormalities

Before the baby is taken from the delivery room physician and nurse inspect him for abnormalities, especially those which may not be apparent immediately, such as supernumerary digits, clubfoot, hypospadias, imperforate anus, and birthmarks. They again observe the baby's color and general behavior to determine if he needs special attention such as incubator care or oxygen.

Protection from Chilling, Trauma, and Infection

Warmth, gentle handling, and cleanliness are imperative throughout the entire regimen of a baby's care. Until birth his existence was completely dependent on his mother, but immediately after birth he must establish independent functions of respiration and changes in circulation. He must also begin existence in surroundings that are very different from the protective and unchanging environment of his mother's body.

One of the most immediate environmental changes for the baby is temperature. The delivery room is many degrees cooler than the very warm habitat from which he has just emerged. Body warmth is a valuable aid in helping to establish normal functions, so every effort is taken to prevent undue cooling.

To protect the baby against infection, all equipment used for his care is sterilized, if it can withstand sterilization, or is kept as clean as possible. It is important that persons caring for the baby wash their hands before giving care.

The baby is protected from trauma by gentle handling during all care, especially removal of mucus, stimulation of respirations, and treatment of the eyes.

Baptism

The Roman Catholic Church teaches that no child can reach heaven without being baptized. Parents who are Roman Catholic wish to have their baby baptized if it is in danger of death. If time permits, a priest should be called to administer baptism. If there is not sufficient time, the nurse or the physician should perform the baptism. Baptism is conferred by pouring ordinary water on the child's forehead while saying the words: "I baptize you in the name of the Father and of the Son and of the Holy Spirit." It is necessary for validity that the person performing the baptism have the intention of doing what the Roman Catholic Church wishes. The

Church teaches that every fetus and embryo should be baptized if possible. When it is doubtful that the subject is capable of receiving baptism, conditional baptism is administered with the form: "If you are capable of receiving baptism, I baptize you in the name of the Father and of the Son and of the Holy Spirit."[1]

Most Protestants observe infant baptism. Those who practice this rite usually desire to have their baby baptized if his condition is serious. The physician or nurse should, therefore, consult with the parents to determine their wishes regarding their baby's baptism, and arrange to call a minister of their faith. If time does not permit calling a minister, an emergency baptism may be performed by anyone else. If time does not permit for consulting with the parents regarding their baby's baptism, the physician or nurse should baptize the baby, since many Protestant parents consider this rite very important and desire to have it done. The baptism is administered by pouring water, usually with the palm of the hand, over the child's head, and at the same time saying the words: "I baptize thee (or you) in the name of the Father and of the Son and of the Holy Ghost." If time permits, the Lord's Prayer and/or Apostles' Creed may also be spoken; however, these are not essential to the rite of baptism.

Early Contact of Baby with Mother

Every effort must be made to permit the mother to see and touch her baby as soon as possible after birth, especially if the baby is well, alert, and responsive. A sensitive period in mother- and father-infant attachment in the early minutes and hours of life make early mother-infant contact important to later development.

Facilitating the mother's opportunity to touch and explore her baby should be at her pace. She

[1] Rev. Edward J. Hayes, Rev. Paul J. Hayes, and Dorothy Ellen Kelly, *Moral Principles of Nursing*. Macmillan, New York, 1964, pp. 179ff.

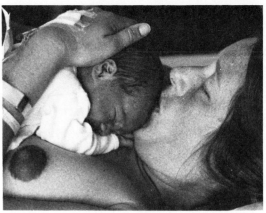

Figure 15-16. Mother cuddling her baby a few minutes after birth. The intravenous infusion is firmly anchored so that it does not inhibit maternal–infant interaction. [*Photograph courtesy of Dr. and Mrs. Daniel Wikler.*]

may wish only a very short period of contact at first because of fatigue and preoccupation with other events. A short time, or perhaps a longer time, later she will wish to have more contact, or she may wish to hold the baby for a longer time from the beginning (Fig. 15-16). It is important for persons caring for the mother to avoid comments that may inhibit her own expression of what she wishes to do and how she feels. It is not helpful to the mother who says she is disappointed that she did not have a boy to remind her that she should be happy to have a healthy baby regardless of sex. A better response would be, "Boys are nice, but sometimes things don't come out as we hoped." One should not add to this, "but girls are just fine." When the father is in the delivery room he also has the opportunity to have early contact with his baby (Fig. 15-17).

There ordinarily does not need to be concern over the baby becoming chilled while he is with his mother. As the mother holds him in her arms she provides some body warmth. The mother's later contact with her baby in the recovery room can be in a warmer room and sometimes a portable warmer can be used.

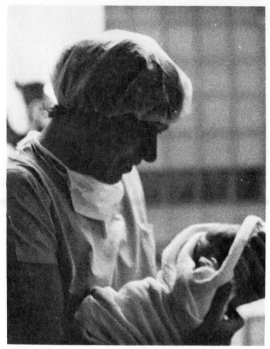

Figure 15-17. The father takes his turn inspecting his newly born infant in the delivery room. He is wearing a scrub suit for his participation in the birth. [*Photograph courtesy of Dr. and Mrs. Daniel Wikler.*]

The opportunity for early parent–infant contact as parents wish it without needing to conform to hospital practices is an important reason why they choose home birth or birth at an alternative birth center.

THIRD STAGE (PLACENTAL STAGE)

The third stage of labor and the hour immediately following delivery of the placenta are, at times, hazardous to the mother. This period requires careful management because of the great danger of hemorrhage.

Delivery of the Placenta

Immediately after the birth of the baby, the physician palpates the uterus for placental sepa-ration or requests the nurse to do so and to keep him informed concerning its size and consistency. The uterus can readily be felt through the mother's abdominal wall. The nurse may place a hand on the mother's abdomen and gently palpate the fundus, noting its consistency, and its height in relation to the level of the mother's umbilicus.

Since the placenta may descend very quickly into the lower uterine segment or into the vagina, the nurse also watches for and reports the signs of this occurrence—a rise in the abdomen of the uterine fundus, an increase in the amount of umbilical cord protruding from the vagina, and a trickling or a spurt of blood from the vagina. The nurse palpates the uterus for the above signs, watching very carefully that the uterus does not relax and enlarge (balloon out) from bleeding into the uterine cavity.

After the placenta has separated, pressure is exerted on it from above to effect its delivery. The physician first ascertains that the uterus is firmly contracted; he may use massage to stimulate contraction of the muscle, and then he exerts firm but gentle, steady, downward pressure on the fundus in the direction of the pelvic inlet (Fig. 15-18). In this manner pressure is ex-

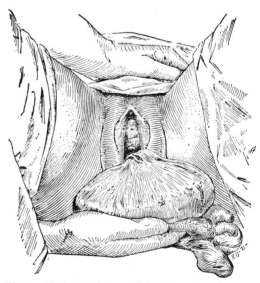

Figure 15-18. Delivery of the placenta.

erted on the placenta with the fundus. The umbilical cord may be used to guide the placenta out of the vagina, but traction on it is avoided. Sometimes the mother is asked to apply the pressure by bearing down, but such efforts are frequently not practicable at this time. In either case, the uterus must be firm before pressure is applied to avoid inversion of the uterus, which involves prolapse of the uterine fundus, through the cervix, into the vagina. This is a grave obstetric accident.

The physician holds his hand or a basin just below the vaginal outlet to receive the placenta and supports it close to the vulva to prevent sudden tension on the membranes and possible tearing of the membranes before their separation from the uterine wall is complete (Fig. 15-18). The membranes are then slowly peeled from the inner surface of the uterus by gentle traction. They are extracted by pulling the placenta gradually away from the vulva, or by turning the placenta over several times to twist the membranes, or by alternately grasping them with a forceps and applying gentle traction (Fig. 15-19). The latter method is especially useful if the membranes have torn away from the placenta.

The placenta and membranes are examined immediately to see if the cotyledons of the placenta fit together and if the membranes are complete. If fragments of either break off and remain in the uterus, they prevent its firm contraction and thus may be a cause of postpartum hemorrhage. It is to prevent tearing that only gentle pressure and traction are used in expressing the placenta and withdrawing the membranes. The use of force is more likely to leave small particles adherent to the uterine wall. After inspection, the placenta is placed in a receptacle for disposal. Sometimes the physician orders a laboratory examination of the placenta. In addition to inspection of the placenta, some physicians routinely palpate the inside of the uterus to assess for complete placental delivery.

If a placental fragment has remained in the uterus, although small and causing no immediate bleeding, it is manually removed at once because of the possibility of causing bleeding at a later time. Occasionally separation of the placenta is delayed, or spontaneous separation does not take place, or the placenta separates, but is retained in the uterus. Several attempts at simple expression may be necessary before the placenta is expelled, with intervals of waiting and careful observation for bleeding between such efforts. Manual removal becomes necessary when the placenta does not separate or when it cannot be expressed following its separation (see page 413).

With delivery of the placenta there is a gush

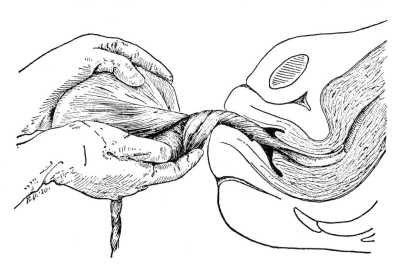

Figure 15-19. Twisting the membranes while withdrawing them from the uterus.

of the blood that collected behind it during its separation. The amount varies considerably, frequently between 50 and 200 ml. The amount of blood behind the placenta is, to a large extent, determined by how firmly the uterine muscle fibers contracted as the placenta separated and also by the length of time that elapsed between its separation and its expulsion. The bleeding usually subsides quickly. The blood vessels, which are as large as a lead pencil, are closed by involuntary contraction of the network of uterine muscle fibers in which they are enmeshed, and which are sometimes referred to as "living ligatures." If the bleeding continues, contraction of the muscle fibers is stimulated by massage and by oxytocic drugs.

The uterus should be a firm, hard mass after delivery of the placenta and should remain so; this is evidence of strong muscle contraction. For a variable period of time a hand is kept on the mother's abdomen to palpate the fundus continuously to ascertain that it remains firmly contracted and, if relaxation occurs, to detect this immediately. As soon as relaxation of the muscle is discerned, the uterus is firmly grasped through the abdominal wall and massaged gently until the muscle contracts. If the uterus has not spontaneously risen upward in the abdomen following the pressure that was placed on it to expel the placenta, it may be necessary to pull it up before it can be grasped for massage. The uterus is freely movable at this time and can usually be moved upward if the fingers of both hands are placed against the lower abdominal wall, just above the pubic bones, and pressed inward and upward so that they make pressure against the lower part of the uterus and lift it up.

Oxytocic Drugs

Drugs with an oxytocic[2] action are often given after delivery of the placenta to stimulate contraction of uterine muscle fibers; they are some-

[2] Oxytocic means rapid parturition. An oxytocic is an agent that promotes the rapidity of labor.

times given during or immediately after delivery of the baby's body. The drugs used for this purpose are an oxytocic alkaloid of ergot, natural or synthetic, and the oxytocic principle of the posterior pituitary hormone in synthetic form.

Ergonovine maleate is the principal oxytocic alkaloid of ergot, a fungus that grows on rye and other grains. A term frequently used as a synonym for ergonovine is Ergotrate, a trade name for the drug. Ergonovine is a powerful stimulant to uterine muscle contraction and exerts an effect that may last for hours. The contraction of the uterine muscle is sustained after administration of the drug and is a valuable aid in control of postpartum bleeding.

Ergonovine may be administered orally or parenterally. It is prepared in tablet form in doses of 0.2 mg ($^1/_{320}$ gr) for oral administration and in 1-ml ampuls containing 0.2 mg ($^1/_{320}$ gr) dissolved in water for injection intramuscularly or intravenously. The usual amount of ergonovine administered at one time by any route is 0.2 mg. The uterine muscle contracts quickly, within a very few minutes after an intramuscular injection, and even within 5 to 10 minutes after oral administration, since the drug is readily absorbed from the gastrointestinal tract. The oral route of administration is used after the mother is permitted to take fluids. Ergonovine is generally contraindicated in women who have hypertension, particularly when it is caused by toxemia. The nurse should check the blood pressure before she gives this drug.

A synthetic derivative of ergonovine, methylergonovine maleate (Methergine), is often used in place of ergonovine. It is also prepared in 0.2-mg ($^1/_{320}$-gr) doses and may also be administered by either the oral or parenteral routes.

Ergot preparations are being used less and less as a routine postpartum medication. Intravenous administration of a 0.2 mg dose (1-ml ampul) as a rapid injection is inadvisable. It may cause severe hypertension due to serious cerebral vasospasm.

Oxytocin, the oxytocic principle of the posterior pituiatry hormone, also produces marked contractions of the uterine muscle. Unlike the long-sustained contraction produced by ergonovine, these contractions last for only 5 to 10 minutes, after which there are intermittent periods of muscle relaxation. The periods of rhythmic contractions of the uterine muscle are very strong, however.

Posterior pituitary extract contains two hormones, oxytocin (Pitocin), with strong oxytocic properties, and vasopressin (Pitressin), with marked vasopressor and antidiuretic properties. The pressor and antidiuretic principle is undesirable because hypertension and water retention are common problems in pregnancy; for this reason the oxytocic principle alone is administered in preference to the entire posterior pituitary extract. Oxytocin is produced synthetically, and the synthetic hormone (Pitocin or Syntocinon) is now used in place of the natural hormone.

Oxytocin is prepared in an aqueous solution for injection containing 10 USP units in 1 ml of solution; it is available in 0.5- and 1-ml ampuls and is administered intramuscularly or intravenously; it has no value by the oral route. When given intramuscularly after delivery, the usual dosage is 10 units. Oxytocin is not administered in such a large dose in a single intravenous injection. When it is given intravenously, 10 or more units are diluted in 500 to 1000 ml of 5 percent dextrose in Ringer's lactate or in water, and it is administered as an intravenous infusion, since a large single dose intravenously may produce a profound hypotension. In addition to postpartum administration, intravenous infusion of oxytocin is also used for induction of labor, but it then is administered with extreme caution (more dilute, very lowly) because of danger of violent uterine contractions (see pages 397–400).

When oxytocics are administered intramuscularly following delivery, they are often most easily given into the deltoid muscle because position of the mother and draping sheets interfere with using other areas. It is important to use a needle at least 2.5 cm (1 in.) in length in order to reach the muscular tissue of the arm.

The area should be thoroughly massaged for quick absorption.

The time of administration of an oxytocic drug in relation to delivery of the baby or delivery of the placenta varies with the preference of the physician. Some physicians give an oxytocic at the time the baby's body is being delivered or immediately thereafter (before the end of the third stage of labor), and sometimes repeat an oxytocic at the end of the third stage; others object to the administration of any oxytocics before delivery of the placenta. When an oxytocic is used during or immediately after the birth of the baby, it is done in an effort to deliver the placenta quickly and thereby reduce blood loss. The incidence of retained placenta and its manual removal is higher when oxytocic drugs are administered before its delivery than when they are withheld until the end of the third stage.

The nurse who is responsible for preparing the drugs, and probably for their administration, must have a clear understanding of which oxytocic the physician wants given and of when the drug is to be administered—after delivery of one shoulder, after delivery of both shoulders, after birth of the body, or after delivery of the placenta. Timing is particularly important, and the nurse must have the drug and other necessary equipment prepared in advance so that it will be possible to administer the drug at exactly the time that the physician orders it. Certain unusual deliveries, such as breech delivery or twin pregnancy, may alter the plan for the time of administration that is followed in normal cases. In general it seems advisable to wait with administration of an oxytocic until after delivery of the placenta.

If the uterine muscle does not contract well after the administration of an oxytocic drug, an intravenous infusion of oxytocin is commonly started.

Repair of the Perineum

An episiotomy or a laceration is repaired either in the interval between the delivery of the baby and expulsion of the placenta or after delivery of the placenta. Some physicians prefer to wait until the end of the third stage of labor before the repair is begun in order to deliver the placenta as soon as it has separated and also to avoid placing tension on the repaired area if exploration of the uterus is necessary. Bleeding from the wound is kept to a minimum by placing pressure against the edges of the wound with sterile gauze until it can be sutured. Other physicians prefer to do the repair while waiting for the placenta to separate. It may be necessary to interrupt the repair temporarily to deliver the placenta when its separation has taken place.

Regardless of when the repair is done, the physician, an assistant, or frequently the nurse, must palpate the uterus for size and consistency during the time that the physician is doing the repair. If the placenta is not delivered, observation is made for signs of placental separation and its expulsion into the lower uterine segment and for evidence of any enlargement of the uterus from bleeding into the cavity. If the placenta has been delivered, observation is made to ascertain that the uterus remains firmly contracted. When the nurse is responsible for making the observations she informs the physician immediately of changes in uterine size and consistency.

The cervix is frequently inspected for lacerations and is repaired if indicated. Cervical inspection is made before the perineum is repaired. Additional information on cervical lacerations is given on page 414.

In the repair of an episiotomy or a laceration, the structures of the perineum—vaginal mucosa, levator ani muscle, fasica, and skin—are anatomically approximated. Chromic catgut sutures varying in size from no. 00 to no. 0000 are frequently used; these are put in place with a round needle with either a taper or a cutting edge. Anesthesia, usually regional, is used during the repair. If regional anesthesia was used for delivery, it is frequently still effective.

If a tear has been sustained around the urethra, the repair is made with thin, nontraumatic needles and fine catgut, size 000 or smaller, since the tissue in this area is thin and tears easily. Following this repair, an indwelling catheter may be placed into the bladder for a day or two to prevent trauma or tension on the sutured area, which may accompany a catheterization should the mother be unable to void.

FOURTH STAGE OF LABOR (IMMEDIATE POSTPARTUM PERIOD)

Although the puerperium is considered to begin following delivery of the placenta, the immediate postpartum period is so closely associated with the process of labor that it is included with the care of the patient in labor. The mother is still in the delivery room at the beginning of this immediate postpartum period, and when moved from the delivery room she needs continuous observation for a variable period of time, to prevent complications that may result from labor and delivery.

Labor is ordinarily divided into three stages, as previously described on page 258, but from time to time obstetricians have referred to the immediate postpartum period as a fourth stage of labor.

The duration of the fourth stage of labor is variable. It has long been customary to consider the first hour post partum as a special period during which the mother needs continuous observation. This one hour of close observation is sufficient for most mothers, but often the events of labor and delivery make one hour an inadequate time for recovery from labor. The immediate postpartum period, or "fourth stage of labor," should therefore be considered as that interim of time after delivery of the placenta that is necessary to assure that the mother is reacting satisfactorily to the stress of birth, that the uterus is remaining firmly contracted, and that vaginal bleeding is not excessive.

After delivery and repair of the episiotomy, the vulva is cleaned of blood with sterile cotton balls; the thighs and buttocks are dried; a sterile pad is applied to the perineum or placed under the buttocks; and the mother is moved to a clean bed. The mother is usually tired and often cold at the conclusion of labor and she may have a shaking chill. The reason for the chill is not known. It may be in part a nervous reaction or in part may be due to vasomotor changes. Although this chill is not serious, the mother is nonetheless uncomfortable and should be warmly covered. A warmed, cotton blanket cover usually adds to the comfort of all women immediately following delivery.

Many hospitals have a postpartum recovery room to which the mother is moved following delivery, for close observation until there is assurance that immediate complications are not likely to develop. Recovery room care includes observation of vital signs, of contraction of the uterus, and of the amount of vaginal bleeding.

The mother's vital signs are checked immediately after delivery and at least every 15 minutes during the immediate postpartum period; deviations from a normal range require more frequent checking, sometimes every five minutes. A marked rise or fall in blood pressure and/or pulse rate are reported immediately to the physician. A toxemia of pregnancy may cause the blood pressure to rise immediately post partum even when it has not been unduly elevated during labor. Blood loss during delivery may result in rising pulse and respiratory rate and a lowering of blood pressure. Response to drugs may affect the vital signs. Existing cardiac or respiratory disease may influence vital signs. Headache, dizziness, and persistent nausea and vomiting are also reported.

To detect early uterine muscle relaxation, the nurse keeps a hand on the mother's abdomen to palpate the fundus for at least one hour after delivery, and longer if indicated by previously existing conditions. During this period, sometimes referred to as "the placental hour," the consistency, the size, and the height of the uterus are observed (Fig. 15-20). As long as the uterus is felt as a firm, round mass below the umbilicus, its irregularly arranged muscle fibers are contracted around the blood vessels and will prevent excessive blood loss. If the fundus feels soft and boggy, its muscle fibers are relaxed, constrictions are accordingly somewhat released from the open vessels, and serious bleeding may occur unless these fibers are stimulated to contract again. The uterine muscle may suddenly relax and a severe hemorrhage may occur very quickly.

Observation of the size and height of the

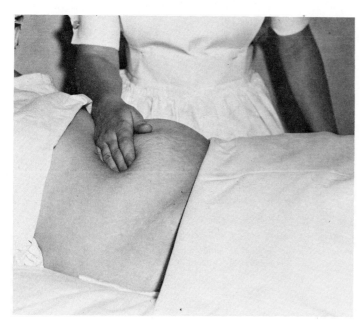

Figure 15-20. The nurse palpates the fundus very frequently after delivery of the placenta to observe the consistency, size, and height of the uterus. This is an essential safeguard against hemorrhage due to uterine muscle relaxation.

fundus as well as its consistency is essential, because blood can be retained in the uterus with the muscle fairly well contracted around the blood clot. Consistency of the muscle may then be misleading, but an enlarged uterus high in the abdomen, above the umbilicus, will be indicative of excessive bleeding within the uterus.

If the uterus relaxes or rises in the abdomen, it should be grasped through the abdominal wall and massaged vigorously until it contracts. The fundus should be grasped by the entire hand, with the thumb curved across the anterior surface and the fingers directed deep into the abdomen, behind it, or it may be held between the two hands—one to give support and the other to massage (Fig. 15-21). Rubbing the top of the fundus with the fingers is usually not sufficient stimulation. Massage is discontinued as soon as the uterus has contracted, but vigilance in observation for further relaxation is essential. The physician is notified of departures from normal uterine consistency and size.

Palpation and gentle massage of the uterus, just sufficient to expel clots from the vagina if present, may be carried out every 15 minutes or so for the first hour or two, but vigorous massage should not be used unless the uterus relaxes. Massage may cause uterine muscle fatigue; this fatigue then predisposes to relaxation. Unnecessary massage makes the mother uncomfortable, the uterus being sensitive to manipulation after delivery.

If there has been no relaxation of the uterine muscle during the first hour after delivery of the placenta, there is usually no great danger of hemorrhage. The mother may then be made comfortable in any position she desires and left to rest, but the nurse must still return frequently to check on the consistency of the uterus and the amount of vaginal bleeding.

The mother should be taught how and where to palpate her uterus, what it should feel like when firmly contracted, and how to massage it. She can then assist in making observations.

The perineal pad must be inspected frequently to discover excessive external bleeding. Although the uterus remains firm and is probably not a source of excessive blood loss, bleeding may originate from the cervix or vaginal wall and appear on the perineal pad. Saturation of more than one or two perineal pads with blood during the first hour is considered excessive. A small continuous drizzle of

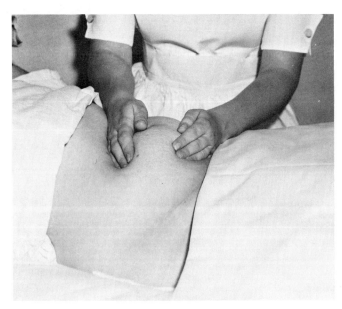

Figure 15-21. Grasping the uterus through the abdominal wall and massaging vigorously to stimulate contraction of the muscle.

blood from the vagina can soon become a serious blood loss and it must be observed as closely as larger gushes. It is also important to look for pooling of blood under the buttocks. Such evidence of bleeding may be missed unless the nurse frequently examines the pad under the woman's hips.

Intravenous fluids begun during labor or delivery are likely to be continued for a variable period of time in the recovery room. Sometimes oxytocin has been added to the intravenous fluids to aid in uterine muscle contraction.

The mother usually has great thirst following delivery, due to restriction of fluids in the later part of labor and loss of fluid in the effort that is exerted during labor and delivery. Unless nausea is present, she will wish to have large amounts of water to drink. Ordinarily fluids are not contraindicated, and, unless there is a reason for withholding them, the nurse should give the mother cold water, or other liquids, as soon as she wishes and in the quantity she desires.

The mother may be exhausted and tense after delivery. She may have generalized discomfort and perineal pain. To ensure rest and relaxation, she may wish to have an analgesic drug when she returns from the delivery room. If the mother is then made as comfortable as possible by a change of perineal pads, proper amount of covering, comfortable position, and a quiet, well-ventilated room she will be able to rest.

Many mothers expect to sleep immediately, but may find that sleep is not possible for several hours and sometimes not for 8 to 12 hours, because of the physical and nervous exhaustion and the excitement that follows the birth of the baby. The nurse should explain this to the mother and advise her that if sleep is not possible she should try to lie quietly and get as much rest as she can.

The mother remains in the recovery room from one to several hours, being moved to the postpartum unit when the fundus remains firm, vaginal bleeding is not excessive, and vital signs are stable.

Mother and baby are often moved from the delivery room together, unless this is contrain-

dicated by the condition of either, frequently with the mother holding the baby in her arms. The father accompanies them from the delivery room. The baby may remain with the mother for a time depending upon his condition and provisions for keeping him warm or he may be taken to the nursery where he is weighed, wrapped in warm blankets, and placed in a warmed bassinet. Depending upon the alertness of the baby and the mother, the baby may be taken back to the parents for another get-acquainted visit while the mother is in the recovery room.

EMERGENCY DELIVERY BY THE NURSE

It sometimes happens that labor progresses with unexpected rapidity, and the nurse is confronted with the emergency of being alone with the mother during part or all of the delivery.

When the baby is making such rapid descent that the nurse expects it may be born before the physician's arrival, she may be able to slow labor somewhat by instructing the mother to open her mouth, breathe deeply, and try not to bear down during contractions. Such instructions must be repeated continuously during each contraction because of the mother's almost uncontrollable desire to bear down. Exerting force to delay birth is very dangerous from the standpoint of injuring the baby and causing it to have marked hypoxia, and the nurse is never justified in forcibly holding back the baby's head.

The nurse must not leave the mother alone—not even for a moment—when delivery is imminent. The baby may be born very suddenly while she is away. It is also very frightening to the mother to be left alone, even if the birth does not occur immediately. Someone else—another employee or a relative—can usually summon the physician.

The mother will be frightened, and it is important to reassure her as much as possible. She will be able to cooperate better if she has confidence that she is receiving adequate care until the physician arrives. Calmness of the nurse is essential to the mother's reassurance.

To assist with the delivery, the nurse should put on a pair of sterile rubber gloves or cover her hand with a sterile towel, whichever is more easily available, and apply moderate pressure to the baby's head as it is advancing with contractions, not with the intent of retarding delivery, but to prevent a rapid, unassisted birth. It is rapid distention of the perineum that causes lacerations; also sudden expulsion of the baby's head at the height of a contraction may cause injury to his brain. As the scalp appears at the introitus, the nurse should apply pressure to the head during contractions to prevent its sudden expulsion and to keep it well extended by pressing it up toward the symphysis pubis so that the perineum is not unduly and rapidly stretched. The head should be allowed to progress a little farther with each contraction. After the brow is visible, pressure is gradually released and the head allowed to emerge, or the mother may be asked to bear down between contractions to deliver the head between, rather than with, the force of uterine contractions.

The nurse should remember that there is no need for haste in delivery of the head, since a slow delivery is less dangerous to both the mother and the baby than rapid expulsion. If the membranes have not ruptured when the head is born, they must be broken immediately to minimize aspiration of fluid. Blood and mucus should quickly be wiped from the baby's mouth and nose when the head is delivered. After the head is born, it drops down toward the mother's rectum, and external rotation takes place.

The shoulders will usually be born spontaneously with the next contraction, or the mother may be asked to bear down to deliver them. Occasionally the shoulders are not delivered in a reasonable time and some assistance is given. To assist in delivery of the shoulders, the baby's head may be held between both hands, and with a gentle downward motion the anterior shoulder can be brought under the symphysis pubis, and then with a gentle upward motion the posterior shoulder may be delivered. The

rest of the body follows easily. All manipulation must be very gentle to prevent injury to the baby's neck or arms.

The baby should immediately be held with his head dependent; additional mucus and fluid should be cleared from his air passages. Respirations and cry are usually spontaneous in this type of delivery, but if the baby does not breathe immediately, he should be stimulated by flicking the soles of his feet.

After delivery of the baby, the nurse's hand should be placed on the mother's abdomen to palpate the uterus for size and consistency and to make certain that she is not bleeding. If the uterus remains firm, there is no necessity for delivering the placenta before the physician's arrival. If it appears necessary to deliver the placenta, the nurse should make certain that the fundus is firm and then ask the mother to bear down to expel it from the vagina. If the mother's efforts do not deliver the placenta, the nurse may make gentle downward pressure on the fundus with her hand on the mother's abdomen. The nurse should support the placenta on her hand as it is expelled. After delivery of the placenta, the uterus must remain firm; it should be carefully observed and massaged when necessary. If massage is not successful in producing uterine contractions and bleeding persists, the nurse should use additional treatment measures if available. Administration of oxytocin 10 IU intramuscularly stimulates muscle contraction, and use of appropriate intravenous fluids, such as dextrose 5 percent in Ringer's lactate solution, helps to maintain an adequate blood volume. It is advisable whenever possible for the nurse to have prior clarification of actions she may take in emergency situations.

There is no reason for haste to cut and tie the umbilical cord even if the placenta is separated soon after the baby is born. Bleeding does not occur through the surface of the placenta. An intact umbilical cord prohibits moving the baby any distance, but if he is well covered, he will be sufficiently warm until there is time to give him further attention. After his breathing is well established, he does not need other care immediately; the nurse can attend to matters that may be more urgent. When sterile equipment can be obtained, the umbilical cord is wiped with an antiseptic solution and clamped and cut under conditions that are as clean as possible.

When the nurse must manage an emergency delivery until the physician arrives, she will need to do whatever is necessary to protect mother and baby, but she should not do more than the emergency demands, allowing delivery to proceed normally insofar as possible and with minimal assistance.

Precipitate Delivery

Sometimes delivery has taken place before the physician or nurse arrives. Such an unassisted delivery is termed a *precipitate delivery.* Immediate attention must be given to the baby to prevent him from aspirating fluid in his attempts to breathe as he lies in the amniotic fluid that escapes after delivery. He must be picked up immediately and held head dependent for postural drainage. There will be no time for hand washing otherwise recommended prior to handling a baby. As soon as the baby's breathing is established, the mother is observed for evidence of excessive uterine bleeding, and care of mother and baby is continued as outlined above.

Delivery Outside the Hospital

In the event of an emergency delivery in a home or elsewhere outside of the hospital, the cleanest area possible should be selected for the birth of the baby. When delivery is imminent, the mother should remove clothing that may interfere with the birth and lie on her back with her knees drawn up. If possible, something should be put under the mother's hips for protection—a clean towel or cloth or plastic or newspaper if available.

The person who will assist at the delivery should wash her hands thoroughly, preferably under running water, if circumstances permit. If

in addition, an antiseptic agent such as alcohol or pHisoHex is available, it may be applied to the hands and allowed to dry. The mother must be cautioned against touching the vaginal opening. As a reminder to keep her hands away from the perineal area, she may be instructed to clasp her hands over her chest, or to grasp her knees.

After the baby's birth and establishment of respirations he may be placed on his mother's abdomen, on his side, with his head down. Such a position promotes drainage of mucus. His mother's body will provide warmth and, in addition, he should be covered to reduce loss of body heat.

If mother and baby are to be transported to a hospital immediately, the placenta may be delivered through the mother's bearing-down efforts or it may remain in the lower uterine segment or vagina and be delivered later. It is important for the nurse to keep the uterus firm to prevent excessive bleeding.

Under unusual circumstances, when the mother cannot receive medical care for some hours, the umbilical cord may be cut and clamped after urgent matters have been given attention. Tape or narrow strips of white cloth and scissors may be boiled for this purpose. If possible, the cord should be cleaned before it is cut, especially if an antiseptic such as alcohol is available. Since there is danger of infection through the open end of an umbilical cord if it is cared for with unclean equipment, it is best to leave the cord intact until much later if there is assurance that better facilities will then be available.

The baby must be kept warm by wrapping him in blankets and placing him in his mother's arms. If the baby has mucus, postural drainage can be instituted by positioning him with his head toward one side. Unless contraindicated by either the baby's or mother's condition the baby may be put to breast. As soon as the placenta has been delivered sucking at the breast stimulates the uterine muscle to contract.

If there is any possibility of separation of mother and baby, as in a disaster, identification of the baby by some means is very important.

BIBLIOGRAPHY

Abramson, Harold (ed.), *Resuscitation of the New-born Infant: and Related Emergency Procedures in the Perinatal Care Nursery,* 3rd ed. Mosby, St. Louis, Mo., 1973.

Apgar, Virginia, The newborn (Apgar) scoring system, reflections and advice, *Pediatr. Clin. North Am.* 13:645–650 (Aug.) 1966.

Auld, Peter A. M., Resuscitation of the newborn infant, *Am. J. Nurs.* 74:68–70 (Jan.) 1974.

Bancalari, Eduardo, Resuscitation of the newborn, *Postgrad. Med.* 57:89–92 (Mar.) 1975.

Behrman, R. E., James, L. S., Klaus, M., Nelson, N., and Oliver, T.; Treatment of the asphyxiated newborn infant, *J. Pediatr.* 74:981–988 (June) 1969.

Brenner, William E., The oxytocics: Action and clinical indications, *Contemp. Ob/Gyn* 7:125–132 (Jan.) 1976.

Buten, Ann Judith, A philosophy of labor and delivery nursing, in *Current Concepts in Clinical Nursing,* Vol. 4, edited by Edith H. Anderson *et al.* Mosby, St. Louis, Mo., 1973, pp. 179–186.

Clark, J. Michael, Brown, Zane A., and Jung, August L., Resuscitation equipment board for nurseries and delivery rooms, *JAMA* 236:2427–2428 (Nov. 22) 1976.

Clausen, Joy, The fourth stage of labor, in *Maternity Nursing Today,* 2nd ed., edited by Joy P. Clausen *et al.* McGraw-Hill, New York, 1977, pp. 498–523.

Committee on the Fetus and Newborn, *Resuscitation of the Newborn Infant.* American Academy of Pediatrics, Inc., Evanston, Ill., 1958.

Contemporary Ob/Gyn, Rise in home births a fact: So are physicians' fears of possible dangers, 7:67–69, passim (Apr.) 1976.

Danforth, David N. (ed.), *Obstetrics and Gynecology,* 3rd ed. Harper and Row, New York, 1977.

Evans, James A., Fundamentals of infant resuscitation, *Int. Anesthesiol. Clin.* 11:141–161 (Summer) 1973.

Friedman, Emanuel A., Failure to progress in labor—Evaluation and management, *Contemp. Ob/Gyn* 4:41–47 (Dec.) 1974.

———, Patterns of labor as indicators of risk, *Clin. Obstet. Gynecol.* 16:172–183 (Mar.) 1973.

———, The functional divisions of labor, *Am. J. Obstet. Gynecol.* 109:274–280 (Jan. 15) 1971.

Green, Josephine M., Emergency care of the obstetric patient, *Nurs. Outlook,* 6:694–696 (Dec.) 1958.

Greenberg, Martin, and Morris, Norman, Engrossment: The newborn's impact upon the father, *Nurs. Digest* 4:19–22 (Jan.–Feb.) 1976. (See Judd reference.) Original article condensed and reprinted from *Am. J. Orthopsychiatry* 44:520–531 (July) 1974.

Greenhill, J. P., and Friedman, Emanuel A., *Biological Principles and Modern Practice of Obstetrics.* Saunders, Philadelphia, Pa., 1974.

Gregory, George A., Resuscitation of the newborn, *Anesthesiology* 43:225–237 (Aug.) 1975.

Hales, D. J., Lozoff, B., Sosa, R., and Kennell, J. H., Defining the limits of the sensitive period, *Dev. Med. Child Neurol.* 19:454–461 (Aug.) 1977.

Hogan, Aileen, Bomb born babies, *Public Health Nurs.* 43:383–385 (July) 1951.

Hoover, J. Edgar, The newborn's footprints, *Hospitals* 33(II):38–41; 118 (Nov. 16) 1959.

James, L. Stanley, Onset of breathing and resuscitation, *Pediatr. Clin. North Am.* 13:621–634 (Aug.) 1966.

Judd, Judy M., Nursing implications, *Nurs. Digest* 4:19–22, 1976. (See Greenberg and Morris reference.)

Klaus, Marshall H., Kennell, John H., Plumb, Nancy, and Zuehlke, Steven, Human maternal behavior at the first contact with her young, *Pediatrics* 46:187–192 (Aug.) 1970.

Kopp, Lois M. Ordeal or ideal—The second stage of labor, *Am. J. Nurs.* 71:1140–1143 (June) 1971.

Littlefield, Vivian, The third stage of labor, in *Maternity Nursing Today,* 2nd ed., edited by Joy P. Clausen *et al.* McGraw-Hill, New York, 1977, pp. 476–497.

Mahan, Charles S., When patients ask about "gentle birth," *Contemp. Ob/Gyn* 7:51–54 (Apr.) 1976.

New York State Department of Health, *Footprinting Pointers and Procedures.* Bureau of Maternal and Child Health, State of New York Department of Health, Albany, N.Y.

Ormsby, Hugh L., Prophylaxis of ophthalmia neonatorum, *Am. J. Nurs.* 57:1174–1175 (Sept.) 1957.

Oxorn, Harry, and Foote, William R., *Human Labor and Birth,* 3rd ed. Appleton-Century-Crofts, New York, 1975.

Phillips, Celeste R., The essence of birth without violence, *MCN* 1:162–163 (May/June) 1976.

————, Neonatal heat loss in heated cribs vs. mothers arms, *JOGN* 3:11–15 (Nov.–Dec.) 1974.

Pritchard, Jack A., and MacDonald, Paul C., *Williams Obstetrics,* 15th ed. Appleton-Century-Crofts, New York, 1975.

Regester, Arianne Schrodel, The second stage of labor, in *Maternity Nursing Today,* 2nd ed., edited by Joy P. Clausen *et al.* McGraw.Hill, New York, 1977, pp. 452–475.

Reid, Duncan E., Ryan, Kenneth J., and Benirschke, Kurt, *Principles and Management of Human Reproduction.* Saunders, Philadelphia, Pa., 1972.

Rising, Sharon Schindler, The fourth stage of labor. Family integration, *Am. J. Nurs.* 74:870–874 (May) 1974.

Roberts, Joyce E., Suctioning the newborn, *Am. J. Nurs.* 73:63–65 (Jan.) 1973.

Robson, Kenneth S., The role of eye-to-eye contact in maternal–child attachment, *J. Child Psychol. Psychiatry* 8:13–25 (May) 1967.

Scanlon, John W., How is the baby?: The Apgar score revisited, *Clin. Pediatr.* 12:61–67 (Feb.) 1973.

Smith, Kline and French Laboratories, Resuscitation of the new born, a medical motion picture, Philadelphia, Pa., 1963 revision.

16

Complications of Labor; Obstetric Operations

Labor and delivery do not always proceed in the normal manner described in Chapter 12. Abnormalities may develop in any of the three stages.

A difficult labor is termed *dystocia*. This is a slow or complicated labor and/or delivery resulting from an abnormality in the mechanical factors involved in the birth process. It may be caused by deviations from normal of the powers, or of the passenger, or of the passage. Included among such abnormalities are poor uterine muscle action, uncommon fetal presentation and position, and pelvic contraction. Less frequent are excessive size of the fetus, certain fetal abnormalities, poor abdominal muscle contractions, abnormalities of the pelvic organs, and overdistention of the uterus from such conditions as multiple pregnancy or hydramnios, which decrease the efficiency of uterine contractions. Any condition that interferes with the normal mechanical processes of labor may make labor and delivery difficult. The cause may be unknown.

Sometimes labor with associated abnormalities, although prolonged, terminates spontaneously. At other times operative interference is necessary.

ABNORMAL UTERINE MUSCLE CONTRACTIONS

Prolonged or Arrested Labor

In the past, labor was considered prolonged when it continued for more than 24 hours after the onset of regular uterine contractions. Such a definition is very broad, has only a single criterion, does not define the time at which a problem arises, and may include women who actually have a normal labor pattern in all but the latent phase. A current method of defining abnormal labor and recognizing one that is prolonged is to compare each phase of the labor to an established normal labor curve.

Many problems arise when labor is prolonged. The incidence of perinatal morbidity and mortality is increased. The mother is vulnerable to intrauterine infection and to postpartum hemorrhage; she becomes fatigued and exhausted and may become dehydrated. Intravenous fluids can supply minimum fluid requirements, but the woman does not receive adequate food or rest during a long labor. The fetus is subjected to prolonged stress from uterine contractions, and there is increased likelihood of infection in the baby, with intact as well as with ruptured membranes.

A graphic analysis of each labor will help the professional to recognize undue prolongation of labor in any of its phases, so that appropriate treatment can be given early. It is advisable to record the time and the findings of each observation of cervical dilatation and station of the presenting part on a graph as shown in Figure 12-11, page 275. The professional can then compare the particular labor curve with a normal curve to evaluate the labor in progress and appraise its normalcy or deviation in one or more of the specific dilatational or descent phases.

Labor may be prolonged or arrested in any one of the cervical dilatational phases of labor or in the fetal descent pattern (Figs. 16-1 and 16-2). Six specific dysfunctional labor patterns may be defined; these are described below. Each pattern is an independent entity, which may appear individually or in combination with any of the other patterns in a given labor.

Prolonged Latent Phase of Cervical Dilatation

The latent phase of cervical dilatation is ordinarily considered prolonged when it exceeds 20 hours in the primigravida and 14 hours in the multigravida. A prolonged latent phase has often been called primary dysfunctional labor. The ac-

celeration phase may also be prolonged and can be considered along with a long latent phase, since it is often affected by the same causative factors (Fig. 16-1).

Among the causes of a prolonged beginning phase of labor are false labor, a long firm cervix which is not prepared by the softening and shortening that usually occur prior to onset of labor and thus has to be accomplished during the latent phase, dysfunction of uterine contractions, and excessive sedation early in labor.

When the latent or acceleration phases of labor are prolonged, the patient becomes very tired before active labor begins. A period of rest for the exhausted patient, as well as for the

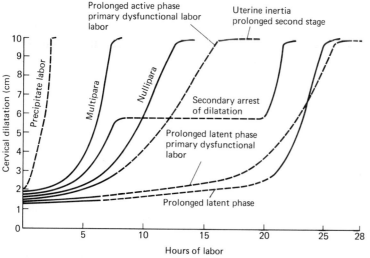

Figure 16-1. Normal and abnormal labor curves as diagrammed in the time relationship of cervical dilatation and progression of first and second stages of labor. The duration of labor and its pattern is different in primigravidas and multiparas. The multiparas have definite advantages through previous labor experience: they display better coordinated and stronger uterine activity, faster cervical dilatation, and an easier and more rapid expulsion of the fetus through the birth canal. The net result is a shorter duration of labor by an average of 4–8 hours as compared to primigravidas. In precipitate labor the first and second stage may be very short and inseparable; in these cases the child may be born within a few minutes by a few uterine contractions.

Prolonged or arrested labor patterns in the cervical dilatational phases of labor are prolonged latent phase, prolonged active phase, prolonged deceleration phase, and secondary arrest of dilatation. [*Reproduced with permission from Nicholas S. Assali (ed.),* Pathophysiology of Gestation, *Vol. I.* Maternal Disorders. *Academic Press, New York, 1972, p. 191.*]

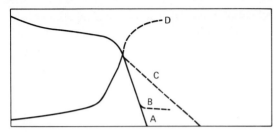

Figure 16-2. Abnormal patterns of descent of the presenting part during labor according to Friedman's graphic labor patterns. *A.* Normal descent pattern. *B.* Arrest of descent. *C.* Prolonged descent. *D.* Prolonged deceleration. Prolonged deceleration, a part of the cervical dilatation pattern, is shown with abnormal descent pattern because of its close relationship to abnormal progress of the presenting part through the pelvis.

uterine muscle, is often beneficial. Medication for pain is administered in sufficient dosage to give relief, good rest, and sleep if possible. During or after a period of rest most labors advance into the active phase with a normal pattern and subsequently are followed by vaginal delivery. Some women awaken not in labor, indicating that they were in false labor. In a small number of cases the labor pattern may remain unchanged. If oxytocin stimulation of uterine contractions is not contraindicated, it may be used when progress of labor does not improve after therapeutic rest.

The prognosis for a prolonged latent phase is usually good for vaginal delivery and the fetus is usually not at risk.

Prolonged Active Phase of Cervical Dilatation

The active cervical dilatation phase is considered prolonged if cervical dilatation during the phase of maximum slope does not progress at 1.2 cm or more per hour in a primigravida or 1.5 cm or more per hour in a multigravida (Fig. 16-1).

Prolonged Descent of the Presenting Part

The descent phase of labor, which reaches its maximum slope toward the end of the first stage of labor (concurrent with the deceleration phase of cervical dilatation) is prolonged when the slope of descent does not progress at at least 1 cm per hour in primigravidas and 2 cm per hour in multigravidas (Fig. 16-2).

Discussion of Prolonged Active Phase and Prolonged Descent

Prolonged active phase dilatation and prolonged descent are considered together here because of certain similarities. The cause is often not known, although cephalopelvic disproportion is present in 28 percent of these cases. Sometimes malposition of the fetus, excessive sedation of the mother, and early conduction anesthesia slow the labor.

To determine the possible cause of a long active phase of cervical dilatation or a prolonged descent phase, and the appropriate treatment, the mother's pelvis and the baby's position are reexamined. A sterile vaginal examination is done to ascertain the condition of the cervix, to determine the presentation and position of the baby, and to reevaluate the size and configuration of the pelvis. X-ray pelvimetry may be done to measure the pelvis accurately, determine the exact fetal position, and evaluate the cephalopelvic relationship.

If a cephalopelvic disproportion exists, a cesarean section is done to deliver the baby. If neither disproportion between the fetus and the mother's pelvis nor fetal malposition is detected, physical and emotional supportive measures are indicated, and conservative management is recommended. Dilatation and descent may proceed slowly, followed by vaginal delivery, or if labor continues without progress a cesarean section may yet become necessary.

Intravenous fluids are used during a prolonged labor to prevent dehydration, provide glucose, and maintain a good electrolyte balance. Sedation and analgesia rarely inhibit normal progress of the active phase of dilatation as is so often evident in the latent phase, but with abnormally slow progress sedation can diminish advancement even more.

Sometimes during the course of a long labor an amniotomy may be done with the anticipation of improving contractions. An amniotomy is carefully considered since it may not prove helpful and it may lead to complications arising from premature rupture of the membranes.

Stimulation of contractions with oxytocin by intravenous drip may be used if there are no contraindications. (See pages 397–400 for use of oxytocin drip.) Oxytocin is not used if it cannot be anticipated that the baby will pass through the birth canal easily, or if the uterus is overdistended. Oxytocin may be administered for a few hours, discontinued for a period of rest, and then resumed.

Risk to mother and fetus from the delivery following prolonged active phase of dilatation or prolonged descent of presenting part is not significantly increased if management is conservative, if labor progress continues, and if delivery is spontaneous or by low forceps. Difficult forceps delivery increases risk to the fetus considerably. Prolonged labor, however, does increase the risk of infection to mother and fetus.

Prolonged Deceleration Phase of Dilatation

The deceleration phase of dilatation is prolonged when it exceeds 3 hours in a primigravida and 1 hour in a multigravida. Although the deceleration phase is a part of the cervical dilatation pattern, a prolongation of this phase is closely related to abnormal descent of the presenting part through the pelvis. It is an arrest pattern.

Secondary Arrest of Dilatation

An arrest in dilatation during the phase of maximum slope is diagnosed by documenting that there has been no progress in cervical dilatation for over a period of 2 hours or longer (Fig. 16-1).

Arrest of Descent

Arrest of descent is diagnosed when there is an arrest in the descent pattern, usually in the second stage, for at least 1 hour (Fig. 16-2).

Discussion of Prolonged Deceleration, Secondary Arrest, and Arrest of Descent

Cephalopelvic disproportion must be suspected in prolonged deceleration, secondary arrest, and arrest of descent. A pattern of arrest is often the first sign of disproportion and constitutes a warning. Other associated factors in arrest are fetal malpositions, excessive sedation, and conduction anesthesia in conjunction with other inhibitory factors. Evaluation for cephalopelvic disproportion and fetal position is essential whenever an arrest pattern develops.

If cephalopelvic disproportion is discovered, termination of labor by cesarean section as soon as possible is indicated.

If disproportion is not evident, continuation of labor is usually permitted. Therapeutic rest may be indicated for the woman who is becoming exhausted. Later, if there are no contraindications, stimulation with oxytocin may be instituted. Most women will respond to this stimulation with progress in dilatation and descent. Occasionally progress is not good or fetal distress occurs and a cesarean section will still be indicated.

Risk to the fetus is considerably increased with arrest patterns and therefore requires early diagnosis and careful management.

Nursing Care

Nursing care of a mother during prolonged labor includes providing physical comfort, giving reassurance, and making observation of untoward effects. The mother often becomes anxious, discouraged, and frequently irritable, especially when she is tired. She needs much encouragement and is often less anxious when someone is with her. Constant nursing care by a calm, reassuring person should be provided if the mother wishes it. Reduction of tension may increase effectiveness of contractions. Frequent baths, back rubs, fresh linen, and changes of position are refreshing and add to the mother's general comfort. If she may be out of bed, a shower and fresh bed linen often help her to relax and rest more comfortably. When an analgesic is given, provision for good ventilation and a quiet environment promotes rest.

The mother is observed for signs of exhaustion, dehydration, and acidosis. Her vital signs are checked frequently. The fetal heart is closely observed. Deviations from normal are reported to the physician immediately.

When the uterus has not contracted well in the first or second stage of labor, a similar action can be expected in the third stage. It is necessary to watch for ineffective uterine contraction after delivery and be ready to give treatment if bleeding becomes excessive.

Abnormal Uterine Action

Abnormal uterine muscle contractions may be characterized as hypotonic or hypertonic.

Hypotonic contractions are short, irregular, infrequent, and often without much discomfort, with one or more of the following features in evidence: less than 15 mmHg intrauterine pressure, duration of less than 40 seconds, and more than 3 minutes between contractions. The contractions may occur farther and farther apart and become very irregular. The uterus is easily indented even at the acme of a contraction, and the contractions are ineffective in promoting progress of labor.

Hypotonic contractions are most likely to occur in the active phase of dilatation or in the second stage, usually after labor has been in progress for awhile; then labor is slowed or arrested. Hypotonic contractions may be a protection against labor continuing with strong contractions when there is some degree of cephalopelvic disproportion or an abnormality of fetal position. Other causes of hypotonic contractions are uterine overdistension and persistent OP position of the fetal head toward the end of labor.

Evaluation of the pelvis, the fetal position, and the relationship of the fetal head to the pelvis are made when hypotonic labor develops to rule out abnormalities. If none is found the hypotonic labor is usually successfully treated by stimulation of the contractions with oxytocin, sometimes interspersed with periods of rest.

Hypertonic contractions occur frequently and are cramplike; they are regular, strong, and painful, but ineffectual in producing anything more than minor progress in the labor. In hypertonic dysfunction the uterine muscle usually maintains a greater than normal tonus, but the contractions themselves are of poor quality.

Duration of the contractions varies from 50 seconds back to 10 seconds and up to 70 seconds, their intensity varies from 20 to 40 mmHg, and their frequency varies from 2 to 3 to 5 minutes. The contractions are erratic in all respects. They are clinically more painful than palpation of the uterus would indicate, and they can quickly cause maternal exhaustion. They are also likely to lead to early fetal distress because of inadequate relaxation between contractions.

Hypertonic contractions are most likely to occur in the latent phase of labor. As with hypotonic labor, hypertonic contractions may develop with cephalopelvic disproportion or abnormal fetal position. It is important to look for such underlying problems.

The initial treatment of hypertonicity usually consists of rest by stopping the abnormal contractions and the pain with morphine. The pain appears to aggravate the dysfunction and should be relieved. The medication is not likely to have adverse effects on the fetus because there is time for it to be eliminated before labor ends. If there is no underlying obstructive problem, normal labor often ensues after a period of good rest.

Occasionally the hypertonic uterine contractions do not convert to normal after rest. At that time contractions may be stimulated with oxytocin in the hope that they will become normal; however, the drug must be administered with even greater caution—considerably smaller dosage—than normally used in stimulation of labor. The mother must be carefully observed for any evidence of tetanic contractions. The fetus must be monitored assiduously for signs of distress.

With either type of abnormal uterine contraction, hypotonic or hypertonic, a cesarean section will be performed if abnormalities in pelvic size or fetal position are discovered, or if labor does not change and progress normally, or if fetal distress develops.

Precipitate Labor and Delivery

An abnormally rapid, intense labor in which cervical dilatation occurs quickly and descent of the presenting part is rapid is termed a precipitate labor. This should be distinguished from a "precipitate delivery" which usually refers to a rapid delivery over an unprepared and unsterile field.

In precipitate labor the uterine contractions are unusually strong and frequent and in addition there may be little resistance from the maternal soft parts. The uterine contractions cause the cervix to dilate very rapidly and also move the baby through the birth canal very quickly. Often the abdominal muscles also contract very strongly and thus assist in rapid delivery.

Precipitate labor has been defined as a labor of 2 to 4 hours in duration. The rate of cervical dilatation in the active phase is greater than 5 cm per hour in primigravidas and greater than 10 cm per hour in multigravidas (Fig. 16-1).

Precipitate labor may be injurious to both mother and baby. Trauma to both may be a serious problem and hypoxia of the fetus may occur because of the rapidly occurring uterine contractions.

For precipitate delivery the fetal head should be controlled and guided over the perineum to prevent traumatic damage to the fetal head and the mother's perineum. No attempt, however, should be made to delay the delivery forcibly.

Tetanic Contractions

A patient has a tetanic contraction of the uterus when it stays contracted continuously, instead of relaxing at regular intervals. This condition usually occurs with overstimulation of the uterus with an oxytocic or it may be found in prolonged labor, due to a mechanical obstruc-

tion to advancement of the baby. These contractions are very painful. There is danger of asphyxia of the baby due to interference with placental circulation and of rupture of the uterus. Oxytocin, if being given, is promptly discontinued. An obstructed labor is ended as soon as it can safely be accomplished.

Pathologic Retraction Ring or Bandl's Ring

Normally there is a physiologic retraction ring between the upper and lower uterine segments during labor. In an obstructed labor this may become more pronounced and thus pathologic. An excessive amount of thinning of the lower uterine segment develops, and the upper segment becomes thicker and more tightly contracted than normal. The retraction ring rises to, or nearly to, the level of the umbilicus. It can be seen as a depression across the abdomen. The mother may have intense pain above the symphysis pubis. There is considerable danger of rupture of the uterus when a pathologic retraction ring develops. A cesarean section is done because the obstruction does not permit descent of the baby.

Ruptured Uterus

A ruptured uterus is a splitting of the uterine wall at some point that has become thinned or weakened and is unable to stand the strain of further stretching or the force of uterine contractions. It is accompanied by an extrusion of all or a part of the uterine contents into the abdominal cavity. Spontaneous rupture of a normal uterus is a rare accident, and usually occurs only in obstructed labors and with improper use of oxytocics. A multiparous, aging uterus is more prone to rupture than that of a primigravida. Even a slightly obstructed labor, possibly due to a large baby, may be serious in a woman who has had many children. Rupture of the uterus at the site of a scar from a previous cesarean section sometimes occurs because of a weakened wall.

In obstructed labors the lower uterine segment becomes thinner and thinner as the contractions pull the retraction ring higher. Finally the lower segment becomes tetanic, the contraction ring becomes very prominent, and the pulse becomes rapid. A patient in whom there is some possibility of obstructed labor must be carefully observed for ballooning out of the lower uterine segment or rising up of a retraction ring. These signs and pain above the symphysis pubis are premonitory signs of rupture of the uterus. If they appear, prompt termination of labor is necessary.

A common sign of rupture is sudden and acute abdominal pain during a contraction, which the patient describes as being unlike anything she has ever felt and as though "something had given way" inside of her. With complete rupture there is immediate cessation of labor pains because the torn uterus no longer contracts. Bleeding takes place internally, and sometimes also through the vagina. The patient soon shows signs of shock. Her face becomes pale and drawn and covered with perspiration; her pulse is weak and rapid; she appears exhausted and may complain of chilly sensations and air hunger. On abdominal palpation the contracted uterus, partly or entirely empty, may be felt as a hard mass alongside the fetus. In some cases there is an incomplete rupture. Blood loss is then slower and signs of shock may be delayed. Labor may continue.

Pain and abdominal tenderness are always present with rupture, incomplete as well as complete. These signs should lead to the suspicion that rupture may have occurred. It may be possible to institute treatment before shock develops. First a laparotomy is done to remove the baby, usually followed by a hysterectomy. Occasionally the laceration in the uterus is sutured, but it may be subject to rupture in a subsequent pregnancy. Blood transfusions are given to overcome shock and to replace the blood loss. Antibiotics are administered to prevent infection, to which the traumatized tissues are very susceptible.

A ruptured uterus is a grave accident. The baby usually dies due to placental separation. The maternal mortality rate is high. Early diagnosis, immediate treatment, blood transfusions, and antibiotics should improve maternal prognosis.

ABNORMAL PRESENTATION, POSITION, AND DEVELOPMENT OF THE FETUS

Variation in labor, with prolongation in the active phase of dilatation or in descent of the presenting part or frequently in both, is likely when the fetal position is one of the less common varieties. Excessive size of the fetus influences labor. Occasionally an abnormal development of the fetus complicates labor and delivery.

Occiput Posterior Position

Labor is usually prolonged when the vertex presents with the occiput in the posterior portion of the pelvis, the occiput posterior position. The mechanism of labor is the same as that described for vertex presentation (pages 270–74) except that the occiput must rotate a longer distance to reach the symphysis pubis. When the occiput is in the anterior portion of the mother's pelvis, it rotates only 45 degrees to reach the symphysis pubis, while the distance is 135 degrees from the posterior position (Fig. 12-7, page 272). Internal rotation of an occiput posterior occasionally takes place as the head is descending, but often not until the vertex reaches the pelvic floor. The longer distance of rotation prolongs the second stage of labor.

In some cases the occiput rotates to a posterior position so that it lies directly over the sacrum instead of under the symphysis pubis. This is termed a *direct occiput posterior position*. During delivery from this position the part of the head near the large fontanel fixes itself under the symphysis pubis, and the head becomes more and more flexed until the occiput slips over the perineum. Spontaneous delivery occurs in many instances, but the second stage is prolonged. An episiotomy is made deeper than with the direct occiput anterior position since a larger diameter of the head distends the vulva during delivery.

In a small number of cases the occiput does not rotate, a condition termed *persistent occiput posterior*. In others rotation is incomplete with the head arrested when it reaches the transverse position. This is designated a *deep transverse arrest*.

With enough time, complete rotation of the head and spontaneous delivery often take place from an occiput posterior position. If the head is arrested and little or no progress is made, rotation may be completed manually or with the aid of forceps. Then forceps is used to deliver the head. The head may be delivered as a direct occiput posterior, or it may be rotated to an anterior position for delivery provided this can be accomplished quite readily.

Breech Presentation

Breech presentation may alter the normal course of labor and complicate delivery. Labor and delivery in breech presentation are described on pages 407–410, later in this chapter.

Face Presentation

In face presentation the head is in extension as it descends into the pelvis instead of the usual position of flexion. Here the occiput points toward the back, and the face enters the pelvis first (Fig. 11-5, page 246). Diagnosis by palpation is sometimes difficult, and an x-ray may be necessary to establish it. X-ray pelvimetry is important to evaluate the pelvic size, a common influence on the method of delivery. Face presentations are rare, but the perinatal mortality rate is increased in this abnormal presentation.

Spontaneous delivery cannot occur unless the chin rotates anteriorly so that it lies under the symphysis pubis. This rotation may not occur until late in labor. When the chin lies anteriorly, the neck can slip around the short symphysis pubis without difficulty. If the chin lies

posteriorly, the neck is too short to allow the chin to travel the relatively long distance along the anterior surface of the sacrum. Delivery is impossible without a change in position, unless the baby is small enough to allow the shoulders to enter the pelvis also. When the chin lies posteriorly, spontaneous rotation to the anterior position often takes place after the face reaches the pelvic floor. If this does not occur, a cesarean section is performed. A cesarean section is considered preferable whenever any condition indicates that a vaginal delivery will be difficult or traumatic.

During delivery of the head, after the chin has rotated anteriorly, the mouth appears at the vaginal opening, the chin stems against the symphysis pubis, and the head flexes so that the nose, eyes, brow, and finally the occiput slip over the perineum. The face usually becomes edematous due to effusion of serum under the skin during labor, and the skull becomes markedly molded.

Transverse Lie

In a transverse lie the longitudinal axis of the fetus lies at right angles to the longitudinal axis of the mother, and a shoulder is usually over the pelvic inlet. This is called a shoulder presentation (Fig. 11-5, page 246). Delivery is impossible in this position unless the baby is very small. If labor progresses with the baby presenting transversely, the shoulder usually becomes wedged in the pelvis and the arm frequently prolapses into the vagina. If hard uterine contractions continue, a thinning and even rupture of the lower uterine segment may occur. Fortunately a transverse presentation occurs in only a small percentage of all cases.

Spontaneous version to a longitudinal presentation occasionally occurs after onset of labor; otherwise, a cesarean section is done.

In a primigravida a transverse lie is suggestive of a pelvic contraction. If x-ray pelvimetry shows a contracted pelvis, a cesarean section is performed before onset of labor. If the pelvis is of normal size, the cesarean section may be delayed until the onset of labor on the chance that the lie may change.

A transverse lie is frequently associated with placenta previa. This complication will determine the time at which a cesarean section is performed.

Excessive Size of Fetus

The relationship between the size of the baby and the size of the pelvis is one determining factor between an easy and a difficult delivery. A slight disproportion may delay progress, and a greater one make delivery through the birth canal difficult or impossible. The baby's head must always accommodate to the mother's pelvis. With some degree of cephalopelvic disproportion, considerable molding of the head may be necessary, and this may prolong labor.

When a baby develops to excessive size, the chance of a prolonged or difficult labor increases. His head is not only larger, but also less moldable, than that of an average-sized baby. With average pelvic measurements, the baby's size usually presents no problem until he reaches a weight of 4500 gm (10 lb).

After the baby reaches a size of 4500 gm (10 lb), the size of the shoulder girdle may also complicate delivery. The circumference at the shoulders may then be greater than the circumference of the head, and they may not compress easily due to firmness.

Occasionally malformations of the fetus resulting in an enlargement of a part of the body may make delivery difficult.

PROLAPSE OF THE UMBILICAL CORD

The umbilical cord may prolapse into the cervical canal alongside the presenting part (occult prolapse) or through the cervix into the vagina and occasionally may protrude from the vagina. This complication can occur when the presenting part of the fetus does not fit firmly against the pelvic inlet (Fig. 16-3). It occurs most frequently when the membranes rupture while

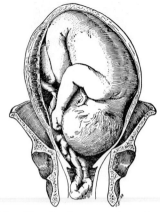

Figure 16-3. Showing how a prolapsed cord may be pressed between the baby's head and the pelvic bones, resulting in interference with circulation between the baby and the placenta.

the presenting part is still above the pelvic inlet or with abnormal presentations, such as a footling presentation. Diagnosis is made by palpation of the umbilical cord below or alongside the presenting part on vaginal examination, or seeing the cord outside the vagina.

Prolapse of the cord endangers the life of the fetus through interference with its circulation. The great likelihood that the cord will be compressed between the presenting part of the fetus and the pelvic wall requires that treatment be instituted immediately. The condition is often first suspected by the nurse because of notation of a slowed fetal heart rate due to cord compression. Preferably the presenting part is first elevated up off the umbilical cord by either the knee–chest position or manually with the examiner's hand. The patient is then promptly moved to the cesarean section room and placed on the operating table in marked Trendelenburg position. If this position is insufficient to relieve cord compression during contractions, the examiner's hand must be used to prevent the compression. Direct manipulation of the cord should be avoided.

On diagnosis of a prolapsed cord the mother should quickly be placed in a position to relieve or minimize pressure of the presenting part on the cord. Either a knee–chest or an *exaggerated*

Trendelenburg position is used. Many hospital beds are easily adjustable for lowering the head and raising the foot end. If this cannot be done, the foot of the bed is elevated as high as possible on a chair, stool, or blocks. If a physician is not immediately available, the nurse must take the prompt action described above to relieve cord compression and to prepare for delivery. *Someone else* should notify the physician, leaving the nurse available to manage the patient. If delivery does not appear imminent, the nurse should instruct others to make all preparation for cesarean section so that there will be no delays in treatment when the physician arrives.

When an umbilical cord has prolapsed, the baby is delivered as quickly as possible. Time is very important. If the cervix is already completely dilated, immediate delivery through the birth canal may be possible. If the cervix is not completely dilated or if vaginal delivery would be delayed because of the possibility of some disproportion, a cesarean section is performed as quickly as possible. Haste in preparation for the cesarean section is of utmost importance. During this preparation the physician may keep the fetal presenting part up from the umbilical cord by pressure applied to it from below through the vagina. Oxygen is given to the mother. The FHR is checked continuously.

DYSTOCIA CAUSED BY PELVIC CONTRACTION

The size and configuration of the bony birth canal influence the progress of labor. Shortening of one or more of the pelvic diameters or variations in the shape of a pelvis of normal size alter the normal mechanism of labor to some degree. Labor may then be prolonged in the first stage by slow cervical dilatation and in the second stage by the longer time required for molding of the fetal head, or delivery through the birth canal may be impossible.

The size and moldability of the baby's head may determine if delivery through a pelvis with some degree of contraction is possible. The outcome depends on the size of the passage in relation to the size of the passenger. For this reason in two women with pelves of the same size and shape one will have a spontaneous delivery and the other require a cesarean section. The former has a relatively small baby which can pass through her pelvis; the second woman's baby is too large, or his head is not sufficiently moldable, for passage through the pelvis.

In some cases the pelvic measurements taken during the antepartum period determine a significant pelvic contraction and suggest that delivery should be by the abdominal route. A cesarean section is then planned before the onset of labor.

Pelvic contractions are usually classified into four groups: inlet contraction, midpelvic contraction, outlet contraction, and combinations of inlet, mid, and outlet contractions. As the baby's head passes through the birth canal, it may be arrested at any one of the divisions of the pelvis.

Inlet Contraction

If contraction at the pelvic inlet is pronounced, a cesarean section for delivery of the baby is planned in advance. If contraction is mild or borderline, the decision may rest on the relationship of the size of the baby's head to the size of the pelvis at the time of labor.

Engagement of the fetal head is evidence that the pelvic inlet is large enough to accommodate it. Before engagement, evidence of disproportion can sometimes be determined by grasping the head through the abdominal wall, pressing it toward the inlet, and checking for overriding of the head over the symphysis pubis. An x-ray with the patient in a standing position gives information on the relationship between the size of the fetal head and the size of the pelvis. Taken during labor it often demonstrates if the head is engaging.

A *trial of labor* may be given in cases of borderline inlet contraction. The patient is allowed to have labor for several hours to determine if an uncomplicated vaginal delivery can be anticipated. Engagement may take place after labor is well established. If labor does not progress satisfactorily, with engagement of the head, during a few hours of fairly strong contractions of about 50 mmHg intrauterine pressure, 50 seconds duration, occurring approximately every 3 minutes, a cesarean section is done.

Midpelvic Contraction

Midpelvic contraction usually prolongs labor. The uterine contractions must push the fetal head through an area that is shortened more than normal, and this takes time. After the biparietal diameter has passed the midpelvic area and the head is on the perineum, delivery may progress rapidly and spontaneously, or forceps may be used to complete it. Midpelvic contraction may cause a transverse arrest of the head.

Outlet Contraction

When the pelvic outlet is contracted, the pubic arch is narrowed. The baby's head does not fit closely to the pubic arch and cannot emerge from the birth canal directly under the symphysis pubis. The head must occupy more of the posterior part of the outlet (the posterior triangle) as it emerges from the birth canal. The degree to which a contracted outlet causes dystocia depends on the posterior sagittal diameter as well as on the intertuberous measurement. When both measurements are decreased, dystocia is most likely to result.

Midpelvic contraction often accompanies outlet contraction and may add to or be the major cause of dystocia. In midpelvic contraction as in outlet contraction the head occupies the posterior portion of the pelvis in its passage. In the midpelvis the uterosacral ligaments, which partly form its posterior circumference, are often pliable enough to permit passage through a pelvis contracted between the ischial spines. At the outlet the apex of the posterior triangle is located at the tip of the sacrum, but there are no bony sides, and the perineum will distend to permit room for passage in most cases. Because

of a certain degree of pliability of soft tissue at both the midpelvis and the pelvic outlet, narrowing in these areas does not present the absolute barrier to the baby's passage that narrowing at the pelvic inlet may present. The pelvic inlet is a bony ring which is incapable of expansion, as compared with some degree of flexibility of the midpelvis and the outlet.

Pelvic outlet contraction increases the necessity for forceps deliveries. Since the occiput cannot emerge directly under the symphysis pubis, the perineum is consequently distended more than in delivery through a normal-sized outlet. A deep episiotomy is usually necessary to facilitate delivery and may be made in a mediolateral direction to prevent tearing through the anal sphincter.

INDUCTION OF LABOR

Artificial termination of pregnancy may be accomplished by cesarean section or by induction of labor. A cesarean section is used only when termination of pregnancy is urgent for medical or obstetric complications and an induction is contraindicated or conditions for its success are unfavorable.

Labor may be induced for obstetric or medical complications of pregnancy, or it may be an elective procedure. Among common indications for induction are premature rupture of the membranes and toxemias of pregnancy, diabetes, and other conditions with associated placental insufficiency.

When the membranes rupture before onset of labor in a term pregnancy and contractions do not begin within a few hours, induction with oxytocin is started.

An elective induction is one that is done at the option of the physician and the patient when it is not indicated by medical or obstetric conditions. Sometimes an elective induction is done to assure that the patient is in the hospital if she has a history of rapid labors. At other times there is anxiety about the distance the patient must travel to reach the hospital after labor begins or concern about being able to arrange for care of children on short notice.

Oxytocin may be used to stimulate uterine contractions when a patient develops uterine inertia some time during the course of labor. This is termed *stimulation of labor* rather than induction of labor.

Certain conditions are necessary for a successful induction. The cervix should show some of the changes that normally take place shortly before labor. It should be soft and partly effaced, and the canal should be open sufficiently to admit one finger. The baby's head should be fixed in the pelvis.

Induction of labor is contraindicated when there are contraindications to spontaneous labor. This would include previous cesarean section and known cephalopelvic disproportion. Certain complications such as an abnormal fetal presentation and overdistention of the uterus require especially close supervision by the obstetrician if stimulation of uterine contractions is to be carried out. Some cases of antepartum bleeding are contraindications to induction of labor.

Two methods are used commonly for induction of labor. One is to administer a very dilute solution of oxytocin intravenously. The other method is artificial rupture of the membranes. Either of these procedures may be used separately or may be used together. A warm enema may be given before an induction is started, not only to clean the bowel, but also for its stimulating effect on the uterus.

Amniotomy

Artificial rupture of the membranes is carried out in the hospital. During a vaginal examination the physician loosens the membranes from their uterine attachment in the region of the cervix with a finger inserted through the cervix. Then he nicks the membranes, allowing amniotic fluid to escape. Sometimes stripping of the membranes from the lower uterine segment alone will initiate labor within a day or two; this may be done in outpatient status and used when there is no urgency for delivery. When the membranes are artificially ruptured to induce labor, the procedure may be carried out before oxytocin is started, or after labor is in progress with the use of oxytocin. Sometimes no further immediate treatment is given after rupture of the membranes, with the anticipation that this method alone will cause onset of labor in a few hours. Membranes are not ruptured if there is risk of prolapsed cord. The fetal heart is checked immediately after an amniotomy and closely observed thereafter.

When an amniotomy is done a time limit is set—a commitment to deliver the baby within 24 hours or preferably less. This presents a problem if labor does not begin and may necessitate delivery by cesarean section. Early amniotomy is therefore reserved for those women who are very likely to go into labor or who must be delivered for medical reasons even if labor does not occur.

Prior to the amniotomy the procedure should be explained to the woman so that she understands how it will feel and how it will affect her labor. Whenever possible she should participate in the decision regarding rupture of the membranes.

Use of Oxytocin

When oxytocin is used it is usually administered by intravenous drip in a very dilute solution. From 5 to 10 units of oxytocin (Pitocin or Syntocinon) are added to 1000 ml of appropriate intravenous solution. Sometimes a lesser amount of oxytocin is used, giving a more dilute solution and making control of administration easier. The intravenous bottle must be well labeled with the name of the drug, the amount added, and the date and time of addition of the drug. The dosage of oxytocin administered from the mixture can be calculated from the amount of drug added to the amount of intravenous solution. Oxytocin 10 IU equals 10,000 milliunits (mU). When 10 IU (10,000 mU) of the drug are added to 1000 ml of fluid each milliliter of the mixture contains 10 mU of oxytocin. The oxytocin dosage used during induction of labor is spoken of as number of milliunits given per minute. The amount of oxytocin administered per minute is regulated by the number of milliliters of solution given per minute.

Administration of oxytocin is the responsibility of the physician. Oxytocin is a dangerous drug when used before delivery, and the nurse must not take full responsibility for giving it. A nurse skilled in care of labor patients and well informed about the implications of the use of oxytocin for stimulation of labor usually collaborates with the physician in monitoring maternal and fetal responses and making sure that the woman is never left alone.

Oxytocin induction may be administered by a very slow intravenous drip, with careful regulation of the number of drops per minute, or by use of a continuous infusion pump. An infusion pump is highly preferable to the drip method, since it gives assurance of a constant rate. The fluctuations in rate that are permitted by the drip method may be especially dangerous when the uterus is very responsive to the drug.

When the oxytocin infusion is first started, it is given very slowly to test the patient's sensitivity to the drug. Then the flow may be gradually increased at 15- to 30-minute intervals to obtain the desired response in strength and frequency of uterine contractions. A professional palpates the uterus continuously while the flow is regu-

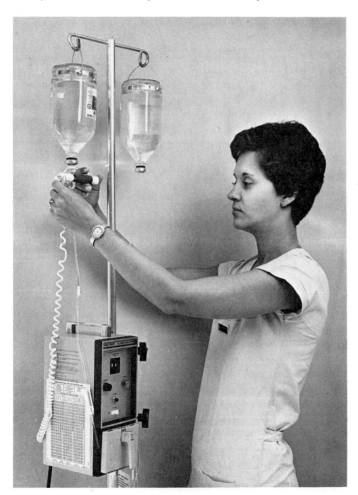

Figure 16-4. A continuous intravenous infusion pump, a precision instrument, which may be set at variable speeds to deliver exact volumes of fluid intravenously. An exact dose of oxytocin can be given within an exact time interval. It is apparent that calculations for various settings of the dial for delivery of different amounts of oxytocin as milliunits per minute have been attached to the machine.

lated. The induction is started with no more than 1 to 2 mU of oxytocin per minute or possibly only 0.5 mU. As the rate of flow is increased it is also done slowly. Five to 10 mU per minute is often enough to stimulate good contractions; sometimes the dosage is increased somewhat more. As labor progresses the flow may again be decreased, or the oxytocin may be discontinued when labor is well established. One method of changing dosage of oxytocin is to double the dose each time it is increased, going from 1 mU to 2 mU, then to 4 mU, and then to 8 mU. In decreasing the dosage it may be halved with each change, unless there is indication for immediately stopping the medication.

The rate of oxytocin administration is regulated according to the response of the uterine muscle. It is given at a rate that will produce effective uterine contractions of about 50 mmHg pressure, lasting 40 to 50 seconds, occurring about every 3 minutes. Contractions should not occur more than every 2 minutes, since there must be time for adequate relaxation between contractions to avoid fetal distress. Contractions should not be greater than 60 to 70 mmHg pressure; sometimes even less than 50 mmHg will bring about cervical dilatation. Contractions should not be longer than 60 seconds duration; a longer contraction comes close to what might be considered tetanic.

When oxytocin is used for enhancement of labor the uterus may be very sensitive and responsive to the drug. Only a small dose of the drug may be necessary to produce effective contractions. A two-bottle setup is desirable for oxytocin administration. This makes it possible to discontinue and restart the oxytocin drip readily without removing the intravenous needle. The intravenous solution without medication is given while the oxytocin solution is clamped off.

Uterine contractions begin almost immediately after an oxytocin drip is started, but these early contractions are not true labor contractions. Later the contractions become more efficient contractions. Sometimes an induction is unsuccessful. If true labor does not start after several hours, or sometimes as long as 8 to 10

hours, the induction is discontinued. It may be restarted the following day. In some cases, such as the presence of diabetes or toxemia, when early delivery is indicated, an induction may be started before the cervix is well effaced. If unsuccessful, it may be repeated on several successive days to soften and efface the cervix and finally induce labor.

Careful observation of uterine contractions during oxytocin administration is absolutely essential. Tetanic contractions can develop. Severe and prolonged contractions could result in uterine rupture, premature separation of the placenta, and fetal hypoxia. When any danger signs appear, the oxytocin should be discontinued immediately. A hemostat should be at the patient's bedside for quick clamping of the intravenous tubing. Violent, prolonged contractions may on rare occasions need to be countered by ether anesthesia.

Although the nurse does not take the major responsibility for oxytocin administration, she usually assists with observation of the patient. The uterus is carefully observed for frequency and duration of contractions and for relaxation between contractions. The fetal heart is checked approximately every 15 minutes or more frequently if indicated. A change in rate or rhythm is reported immediately. The mother's blood pressure and pulse are checked every 15 minutes or oftener. Either a rise or fall in blood pressure or a rapid pulse is reported at once. Progression of labor and any unusual physical phenomena must be closely observed. When the drip method is used the rate of flow of the oxytocin solution is carefully watched by counting the number of drops per minute at frequent intervals. Although the flow has been carefully regulated, it may accidentally increase in speed when the patient moves her arm or if the clamp on the tubing loosens.

If continuous electronic fetal heart rate monitoring and intrauterine pressure recording equipment are available, they are used to check uterine response to oxytocin. Careful and continuous clinical evaluation of uterine muscle response and fetal reaction to induction may be satisfactory with an uncomplicated pregnancy. Clinical evaluation is necessary for all patients when monitoring equipment is not available, but use of continuous electronic monitoring is highly desirable for all high-risk pregnancies.

When an oxytocin infusion has been used to induce labor, it may be slowed or discontinued during delivery and restarted after the placenta is expelled. It is then administered more rapidly than prior to delivery. Given after delivery oxytocin aids in control of postpartum bleeding through stimulating the uterine muscle to contract.

Oxytocin is sometimes administered intranasally or transbuccally. When it is administered intranasally, a cotton pledget saturated with 10 units (15 minims) of oxytocin is placed against the inferior turbinate bone. The oxytocin absorbs slowly through the mucous membrane of the nose, and the effect of the drug can be stopped quickly, by removing the nasal pack, if the uterine contractions become too hard and too long.

With transbuccal administration the oxytocin is given by placing oxytocic linquets into the parabuccal space adjacent to the upper molars or under the tongue at approximately 30-minute intervals. In the event of an adverse reaction the tablets must be promptly removed and the mouth thoroughly washed, since particles of the partially dissolved tablets may remain in the mouth.

Nasal and buccal methods of administration of oxytocin are less precise and less predictable than the intravenous route. Intramuscular injection, another method by which the drug is effective, should *not* be used for induction of labor since the drug cannot be removed in case of an untoward reaction, and its effect continues until it is completely absorbed.

Administration of oxytocin by the intravenous route is safer than any other method. Intravenously the dosage can be carefully regulated and promptly discontinued. The effect of the drug does not linger because oxytocin is rapidly inactivated and excreted. For these reasons intravenous administration of oxytocin should replace all other methods.

Other Uterine Stimulants

Sparteine sulfate (Tocasamine), a plant alkaloid, is an oxytocic agent that has been used for induction or stimulation of labor. Sparteine, which is given intramuscularly, does not assure constant and precise control and is not as safe as early experience with the drug appeared to indicate.

Alkaloids of ergot are not used for induction of labor. They create contractions of a hypertonic or sustained nature or of an inappropriate frequency and do not permit adequate relaxation of the uterine muscle.

Prostaglandins are also effective uterine stimulants which may find increasing utilization in obstetrics.

SUMMARY

In summary, careful monitoring is absolutely essential during induction of labor. The physician or a properly instructed substitute must be with the patient constantly, and the physician must be immediately available to deal with any emergency that may arise. Inappropriate uterine muscle stimulation, which results in contractions more frequent than every two minutes and of very intense strength, or uterine tetany, leads to fetal hypoxia and may also endanger the mother.

Midtrimester Termination of Pregnancy

Hypertonic Saline Induction of Labor

Intraamniotic instillation of hypertonic saline solution may be used for termination of an early pregnancy, after the fourteenth week of gestation, and for induction of labor after intrauterine fetal death.

Instillation of the solution is a sterile procedure; the abdomen is prepared with iodine and all equipment is sterile. The bladder is emptied just prior to injection of the solution to lower its level as much as possible. The abdominal wall at the site of injection is locally anesthetized. A long spinal needle is inserted through the abdominal wall and the uterine wall into the amniotic cavity. As much amniotic fluid as possible is removed, varying from 100 to 250 ml, depending upon gestational age. Thereafter an equal volume of 20 percent sodium chloride is injected, *very slowly* at first, at approximately 1 ml per minute. Before the needle is withdrawn it may be flushed with normal saline solution to minimize the possibility of peritoneal spill of hypertonic solution. Pain is minimal, except for some feeling of fullness and cramping, and for discomfort when the needle penetrates the peritoneum. Vital signs are checked every 15 minutes after the injection until assurance of stability.

A saline induction is a relatively safe procedure but serious complications can occur. One of the greatest dangers is inadvertent intravascular injection of the solution. It is for this reason that the injection of the hypertonic solution is made very slowly at first. With intravascular injection of hypertonic sodium chloride a hypernatremia, with severe dehydration and increased intravascular volume, can become evident in 1 minute. The patient must be closely observed for sudden sensations of heat, increased pulse rate, flushed face, dry mouth, ringing in the ears, and severe headache. If symptoms occur, the injection is stopped immediately and intravenous 5 percent dextrose in water is quickly administered to prevent cerebral dehydration. Hypernatremia would be especially dangerous for a patient with cardiovascular or renal disease.

A spill of hypertonic saline solution into the peritoneal cavity as the needle is withdrawn, or leakage into the peritoneal cavity through the fallopian tubes during labor, may cause hypernatremia by drawing fluid from the serum and the extracellular tissues.

Injection of hypertonic sodium chloride into the bladder can occur when the bladder is very close to the site of injection. The bladder must be empty and the uterine fundus must be high enough for easy accessibility of the amniotic cavity. Amniocentesis and injection cannot be done before the fundus has reached a height of 14 weeks gestation and it may be postponed for another two or three weeks. In case of bladder injection immediate irrigation of the bladder is necessary.

Labor may begin spontaneously within several hours after an intraamniotic saline induction, but there is no certainty that it will begin for days. Cramping may occur and a small amount of amniotic fluid may drain from the vagina during the next several hours. To hasten delivery of the fetus, an induction with intravenous oxytocin is usually begun 6 to 12 hours after the sodium chloride injection if labor has not started.

Induction of labor is carried out with a larger dose of oxytocin in the intravenous fluid and more rapid administration than with an induction of a term pregnancy, and it does not require the constant supervision of the physician. The small uterus, with a much thicker muscular wall, and the dead fetus, do not pose the complications of induction of a term pregnancy.

The labor usually causes considerable discomfort. The patient is not prepared as for normal labor and she does not anticipate it with the same feeling of accomplishment. Medication is administered quite freely to relieve pain, at least to some degree, but timing of medication is important, since labor could also cease with its early administration.

Delivery of the fetus is usually imminent when the patient feels rectal pressure, usually at 4- to 5-cm cervical dilatation. Pushing down is usually necessary for delivery. The placenta may be expelled along with the fetus or it may be retained for 1 to 2 hours longer. Careful observation for excessive bleeding is essential during placental retention. Sometimes a retained placenta must be surgically removed. Blood for transfusion should be available.

If large doses of oxytocin are used to induce labor and are administered rapidly and for a prolonged period, the antidiuretic property of the oxytocic may cause water retention. Prevention of water intoxication is usually possible by limiting the dosage of oxytocin to 45 mU per minute or less and by use of fluids with electrolytes. The nurse should observe the patient for any signs of water intoxication, which include edema, drowsiness, confusion, decreased urinary output, and headache. Cerebral edema is a serious consequence of water intoxication. A careful record of urinary output during induction of labor will reveal oliguria early in any developing problem. Treatment of water retention may be by discontinuation of oxytocin and fluids and permitting unhampered time for excretion of fluid, or by administration of fluids with electrolytes, but without oxytocin. Excretion of the excess accumulated fluid in the body is evidence of improvement.

Prostaglandin Intraamniotic Injection

Injection of prostaglandin ($PGF_{2\alpha}$) into the amniotic cavity (or sometimes urea injection) is replacing use of hypertonic saline in a number of cases. Prostaglandin use does not carry the risks of hypertonic saline—hypernatremia, changes in coagulation factors, renal and cardiac problems, and fluid overload. Prostaglandin use, however, is contraindicated for patients with respiratory problems such as asthma because it causes constriction of the bronchial musculature, and is also contraindicated when hypertension is present.

Prostaglandin is injected into the amniotic cavity similar to the procedure for hypertonic saline, except that the amniotic fluid is not first removed. The first milliliter of $PGF_{2\alpha}$ is injected very slowly over a five-minute period to observe for adverse reactions. If no side effects appear the remainder is injected over another five-minute period. The half-life of prostaglandin is very short and recovery from any adverse effects may be quite rapid if administration is stopped. The prostaglandin may be administered in one

dose, with a repeat of a smaller amount in 24 hours if abortion has not occurred, or it may be given in two 25 mg doses, six hours apart. Prostaglandin injection may be followed by oxytocin induction if action is delayed.

Contractions usually begin within the first half hour after injection of $PGF_{2\alpha}$ and abortion often takes place within 24 hours or at least within 36 hours. Overall, the induction–abortion interval has been found to be shorter with $PGF_{2\alpha}$ than with saline. According to a large study conducted by the World Health Organization, comparing the effects of intraamniotic $PGF_{2\alpha}$ and hypertonic saline, the success rate was found to be significantly higher in the first 48 hours when $PGF_{2\alpha}$ was used. The unpleasant side effects of nausea, vomiting, and diarrhea were more frequently a problem with prostaglandin but were within acceptable limits.[1]

Patient Teaching

A detailed explanation to the patient of what to anticipate of the abortion procedure is important. She should be told about management of the injection procedure, the latent process before labor, the induction with oxytocin, and the labor. The patient needs ample time to get her questions answered. She needs physical care and emotional support from the nurse during the entire process. A trusting relationship with the nurse will help the patient to cope with the fears and pain of delivery, and the crisis she must deal with in resolving her feelings regarding the abortion.

Patients who are Rh negative are given RhoGam following delivery to avoid sensitization.

[1] *British Medical Journal*, Comparison of intra-amniotic prostaglandin F$_{2\alpha}$ and hypertonic saline for induction of second-trimester abortion. International multicentre study by the Task Force on the Use of Prostaglandins for the Regulation of Fertility of the World Health Organization's Expanded Programme on Research, Development, and Research Training in Human Reproduction. 1:1373–1376 (June 5) 1976.

OBSTETRIC OPERATIONS

Forceps Delivery

The obstetric forceps is an instrument used to extract the baby's head in certain conditions where progress is arrested and which may result in dangers, immediate or remote, to the mother and/or baby. The forceps is a valuable instrument in obstetrics. Before its invention the only operative method of delivering a live baby was by version and extraction, and in these cases the fetal death rate was high. Prior to the advent of forceps, the obstetric instruments in use were designed for the destruction of the baby in utero. Use of forceps may be hazardous, however, and this method of delivery is carried out only when all conditions for proper application are fulfilled.

The forceps was devised and first used in great secrecy, early in the seventeenth century in England, by a Dr. Chamberlen, who jealously guarded all information relating to his invention from everyone but members of his own family. There were several doctors in the Chamberlen family who practiced obstetrics and who used the forceps, but knowledge concerning the nature of the instrument and methods of using it was not shared with physicians outside of that family until the beginning of the eighteenth century. Since that time the use of forceps has been widely extended, and the original Chamberlen instrument has been so modified and improved

that now there are a large number and variety in existence and in use (Fig. 16-5). Over 600 kinds, varying in size and shape, have been designed. The type of forceps is not as important as its application and use. Each physician usually becomes accustomed to one or two kinds and uses them almost exclusively.

The forceps consists of two parts, designated as the right and left blade according to the side of the pelvis in which it lies when it is applied to the baby's head. Each blade is curved outward to fit around the baby's head and curved upward to correspond to the axis of the mother's pelvis. These are known as the cephalic and pelvic curves (Fig. 16-5). A few blades are solid, but most are fenestrated. Since the left blade always fits to the left side of the mother's pelvis and the right blade to the right side, one can distinguish the right from the left blade by articulating the blades and holding them before the vulva to visualize the forceps in position.

There are two groups of indications for use of forceps: those relating to the condition of the baby and those relating to the mother. Indications for their use in the interests of the baby are signs of fetal distress, as manifested by a change in the rate or rhythm of the fetal heartbeat. Fetal hypoxia may be due to many causes, including analgesia or anesthesia, premature separation of the placenta, pressure on the umbilical cord, and prolonged pressure of the head on the pelvic floor. Proper use of forceps is be-

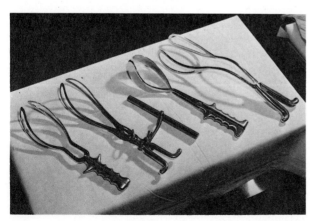

Figure 16-5. Several kinds of obstetric forceps. *Left to right:* Simpson; Tarnier, with axis traction attachment; McLean–Tucker; Piper, for delivery of the aftercoming head in breech extraction.

lieved to reduce incidence of intracranial bleeding in the baby, resulting from a long, hard labor.

The most frequent indication for the use of forceps is poor progress of the fetal head through the birth canal. This slow progress may be due to poor contractions of the uterine and abdominal muscles, great resistance of the perineal muscles, or failure of the head to rotate. Other maternal indications are severe toxemia, heart disease, pulmonary disease, and exhaustion. Low forceps delivery in these conditions alleviates some of the exertion of the second stage of labor.

Forceps operations are usually designated as *low, mid,* or *high,* corresponding to the level to which the head has descended into the pelvis when the forceps is applied.

Low forceps operation is application of the blades after the baby's skull has reached the perineal floor, has rotated so that the sagittal suture is anteroposterior, and the head has become visible. This type of forceps delivery is relatively easy and is attended by little danger to mother or baby.

Midforceps operation is application of the blades after the lowermost part of the skull is at or below the level of the ischial spines, but has not descended or rotated sufficiently to meet the criteria for low forceps. A midforceps delivery is more difficult and more serious than a low forceps delivery.

High forceps operation is application of the forceps before engagement of the head. This operation is no longer used, having only historical interest. A cesarean section is now performed when the fetal head does not engage.

Many forceps operations are *elective low forceps.* The procedure is elective as distinguished from indicated when the physician elects to use forceps to deliver the baby when immediate delivery is not absolutely necessary. In these cases spontaneous delivery could be expected to take place in approximately 15 minutes. The forceps is used to relieve the mother of the strain of the last part of the second stage of labor and to relieve the cerebral tissues of the baby from pressure against the perineum. The criteria for a low forceps must be met. Only gentle traction is necessary, and the delivery is performed easily and with safety.

Before applying forceps the physician satisfies himself that all conditions are favorable. The cervix must be completely dilated to prevent

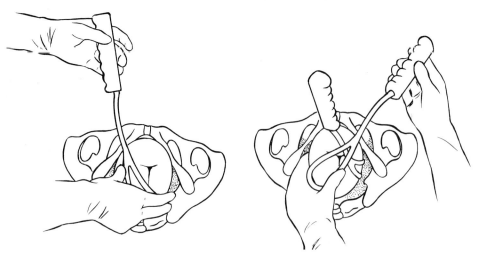

Figure 16-6. Low forceps extraction showing application of blades. [*Reproduced with permission from J. Robert Willson, Clayton T. Beecham, and Elsie Reid Carrington,* Obstetrics and Gynecology, *5th ed. The C. V. Mosby Co., St. Louis, Mo., 1975, p. 508.*]

severe lacerations and bleeding. There must be no considerable disproportion between the size of the head and the pelvis because extraction would then be dangerous to both mother and baby. The head must be engaged, the position of the baby's head must be known for proper application of the forceps, and the membranes must be ruptured. The head must not be so large or so small that the forceps will not grasp it securely.

The patient is catheterized before a forceps operation to facilitate delivery and prevent trauma to the bladder.

The physician lubricates his gloves for the vaginal examination performed prior to application of the forceps and lubricates the blades for ease of insertion. An antiseptic solution or a sterile liquid soap solution may be used for lu-

brication. A lubricant squeezed from a tube is not used because of the small opening and the inadequate protection from the cover on the tube against contamination of the lubricant.

The forceps blades are applied directly to the sides of the baby's head with the fenestra of the blades over the parietal bosses. A hand in the vagina guides the blades into proper position. The blades are applied separately (Fig. 16-6). After both are in place, the handles are locked; these close easily when application of the blades is accurate. An episiotomy is usually performed, either before or after application of the forceps. The fetal heart is observed continuously during a forceps delivery.

The forceps is used mainly for traction to deliver the head, but sometimes it is also used to rotate it. Rotation takes place with traction

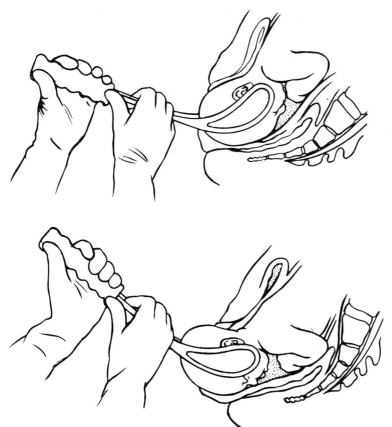

Figure 16-7. Low forceps, extraction of the head. The traction force is downward as well as outward until the occiput appears beneath the pubic arch. The handles are then raised to extend the head over the perineum. [*Reproduced with permission from J. Robert Willson, Clayton T. Beecham, and Elsie Reid Carrington*, Obstetrics and Gynecology, *5th ed. The C. V. Mosby Co., St. Louis, Mo., 1975, p. 509.*]

unless the position is occiput posterior or occiput transverse. In those cases the physician may either rotate the head manually before application of the forceps or perform a forceps rotation of the head.

In a forceps delivery, nature is imitated as much as possible. Gentle intermittent traction, with as little force as necessary to advance the head, is made in the direction of the axis of the pelvis (Fig. 16-7). Traction is applied with the arms flexed and the elbows close to the thorax so that body weight is not used in the pull. The head is allowed to recede in the intervals between each application of traction, as it does in a spontaneous delivery. The head is delivered slowly enough to allow time for the perineum to stretch. The head may be delivered completely with the forceps, or the blades may be removed after the head is well advanced and the delivery completed by the modified Ritgen's maneuver. Each forceps blade is removed separately and gently to prevent injury to the baby's ears.

A midforceps operation may become necessary when progress of the fetal head through the birth canal is arrested. The sagittal suture is usually in an oblique or transverse position. To apply the forceps to the sides of the head, the physician locates the posterior ear for application of the first blade. The second blade is applied opposite the first one. Traction alone may rotate the head, but rotation with the forceps may be necessary. Difficult midforceps extractions are done less and less in favor of cesarean sections to avoid maternal and/or fetal trauma.

For delivery of the head from an occiput posterior position it may be possible to rotate the head manually to a transverse position before the forceps is applied. If the head cannot be manually rotated, it may be delivered, with forceps, in a direct occiput posterior position, or it may be rotated anteriorly with the forceps. When forceps is used for anterior rotation, the pelvic curve of the forceps is pointed downward after the rotation. This necessitates removal of the blades and reapplication. This double application of the blades is termed a *Scanzoni maneuver*.

Unless there are indications for immediate delivery, a forceps delivery is usually not performed until the mother has been in second-stage labor for a variable period of time. Uterine contractions and bearing-down efforts will usually advance the head and perhaps rotate it, making a forceps delivery less complicated. The forceps is applied after the head has advanced satisfactorily for easy delivery, or when progress slows considerably or ceases.

All operative deliveries are potentially dangerous, but the danger is reduced to a minimum with proper indications and technique. A forceps delivery is often essential to prevent or minimize danger to mother and/or baby.

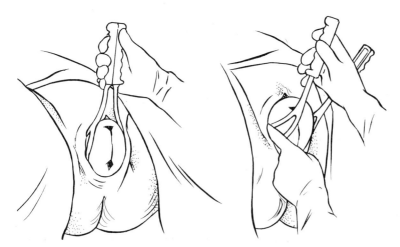

Figure 16-8. Low forceps extraction showing completion of delivery of the head and removal of forceps. [*Reproduced with permission from J. Robert Willson, Clayton J. Beecham, and Elsie Reid Carrington, Obstetrics and Gynecology, 5th ed., The C. V. Mosby Co., St. Louis, Mo., 1975, p. 510.*]

Breech Extraction

Labor is usually longer in breech presentation than in vertex presentation. The membranes frequently rupture early, and the breech does not make a good dilating wedge. The incidence of prolapse of the umbilical cord is higher than in a vertex presentation, and the fetal heart must be observed frequently throughout labor. If continuous electronic fetal heart monitoring equipment is available it is used.

Meconium is often expelled during labor, due to downward pressure of the contracting uterus on the fetus, but this does not have the same significance that it does in a head presentation. If the membranes are ruptured, meconium is seen draining from the vagina. Bed rest and constant watchfulness throughout labor are important.

If the presentation is a footling, one or both feet may prolapse through the vagina as labor progresses. This does not necessarily mean that birth is imminent. The patient is often not ready for delivery when the feet appear. They may prolapse when the cervix has dilated sufficiently to allow them to pass through, although not yet dilated enough to allow the largest part of the baby to be born.

In breech presentation, delivery is complicated by the larger part of the baby being born last, whereas in vertex presentations the larger part of the baby, the head, is born first, and the rest of the body follows quickly. In breech presentation the head does not have time to mold, since it must pass through the birth canal quickly. It is often even slightly widened because it has been flattened somewhat in utero by pressure from the fundus. The possibility of cephalopelvic disproportion is carefully considered before labor, and x-ray pelvimetry is obtained when it is suspected. Sometimes delivery by cesarean section is indicated.

In most cases of breech presentation, particularly in primigravidas, it is necessary to assist the natural forces in delivery of the baby. Occasionally delivery is spontaneous. When it is assisted, it is termed a *breech extraction*. This

may be either partial or total depending on how far the baby has been delivered spontaneously before traction is made to complete the delivery (Fig. 16-9). This procedure was probably the earliest obstetric operation performed.

For delivery, a lithotomy position, with the woman's buttocks over the end of the table, is used to facilitate ease of manipulation. Preparation for delivery is made early so that extraction is possible as soon as indicated. After appearance of the umbilicus the fetal heartbeat may show evidence of interference with circulation in the umbilical cord. The cord may be pressed between the fetal head and the pelvic bones. There is a possibility of placental separation after the uterus is partly emptied. The fetal heart rate must be watched very closely throughout the second stage of labor.

In the majority of cases assistance is given after the body has been delivered spontaneously as far as the umbilicus. If there is interference with umbilical cord pulsation, complete delivery

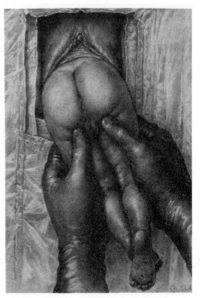

Figure 16-9. Breech extraction; traction upon the thighs. Sterile towel not illustrated. [*Reproduced with permission from Jack A. Pritchard and Paul C. MacDonald,* Williams Obstetrics, *15th ed. Appleton-Century-Crofts, New York, 1976, p. 890.*]

of the head is not necessarily rapid, but the head is delivered far enough to permit access of air to the baby's mouth so that pulmonary respiration can be established. The body is held upward to favor drainage of mucus and amniotic fluid from the respiratory tract, and mucus is wiped from the baby's mouth.

When the baby's body is born to the umbilicus, his feet or legs are grasped by a towel, to prevent the hands from slipping, and downward traction is made on the body until the lower halves of the scapulas are outside the vulva. During this procedure gentle pressure may be made on the uterus to keep the baby's head flexed and to help in delivery.

The shoulders are delivered after one of the

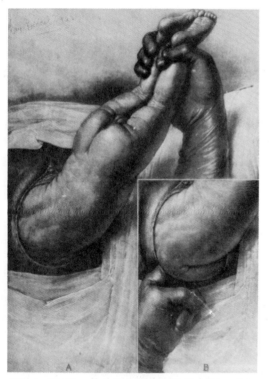

Figure 16-10. Breech extraction. *A.* Upward traction to effect delivery of posterior shoulder. *B.* Freeing posterior arm. [*Reproduced with permission from Jack A. Pritchard and Paul C. MacDonald,* Williams Obstetrics, *15th ed. Appleton-Century-Crofts, New York, 1976, p. 892.*]

axillae has appeared. When the arms remain flexed, this is relatively easy. The body is drawn upward toward the mother's groin to deliver the posterior shoulder and bent down to deliver the anterior one (Fig. 16-10). The arms usually follow spontaneously after each shoulder is delivered. However, if the arms are extended above the baby's head, the physician introduces his hand into the vagina and sweeps each down across the chest. Unless the physician's fingers reach the elbow and are used as splints, fractures of the humerus or clavicle may occur during delivery of the extended arms. Very occasionally the arm lies around the baby's neck; this is termed a *nuchal arm.* Delivery of the arm then becomes more difficult.

After delivery of the shoulders and arms the body rotates spontaneously or is rotated manually so that the back is directed upward in line with the mother's abdomen. The head is then in position to be delivered. Delivery is usually completed by what is known as *Mauriceau's maneuver,* which consists of keeping the baby's head flexed with one hand, while his body is supported on the physician's arm (Figs. 16-11 and 16-12). Downward traction is then made with the other hand, which is placed over the baby's shoulders. At this juncture, delivery is facilitated by an assistant making carefully controlled suprapubic pressure. After the occiput appears beneath the symphysis pubis, the body is lifted upward, and the mouth, nose, forehead, and entire head are born (Fig. 16-12). Often the after-coming head is delivered by Piper forceps, rather than by means of Mauriceau's maneuver, and the nurse should be prepared for this possibility by having the forceps ready. If rotation of the head is impossible, it becomes necessary to deliver it from the occiput posterior position, but care is taken by the physician to avoid this position if possible.

Occasionally, due to some condition dangerous to the mother or the baby, extraction becomes necessary before the breech has been delivered spontaneously. In these cases the physician introduces his hand into the vagina, grasps the feet, and brings them down with traction, or hooks his fingers into the baby's groins and makes downward traction. Pressure on the mother's abdomen supplements traction on the baby's body. Delivery in this manner is difficult, especially when the breech is high. The cervix must be examined for complete dilatation before attempts at extraction are made; otherwise deep cervical lacerations result. Complete anesthesia for good relaxation is usually necessary. A deep episiotomy is often made to decrease the resistance from the pelvic soft parts as much as possible.

Breech extraction is not very dangerous for the mother, but the fetal and neonatal mortality

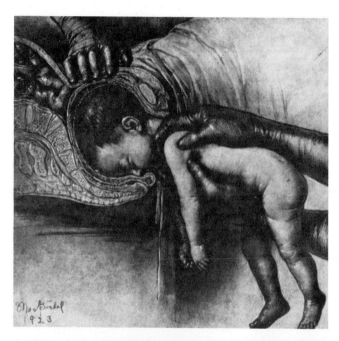

Figure 16-11. Breech extraction. Suprapubic pressure and horizontal traction have caused the head to enter the pelvis. Mauriceau's maneuver. [*Reproduced with permission from Jack A. Pritchard and Paul C. MacDonald,* Williams Obstetrics, *15th ed. Appleton-Century-Crofts, New York, 1976, p. 894.*]

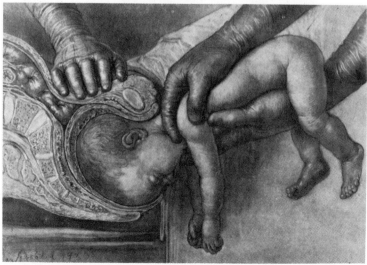

Figure 16-12. Breech extraction. Mauriceau's maneuver, upward traction. [*Reproduced with permission from Jack A. Pritchard and Paul C. MacDonald,* Williams Obstetrics, *15th ed. Appleton-Century Crofts, New York, 1976, p. 894.*]

are higher than with cephalic presentation. Part of the increased mortality is due to a higher incidence of breech presentation in premature labors and in pregnancies where other complications already exist. Babies delivered by breech extraction have an increased chance of intracranial hemorrhage. Fractures of the humerus and clavicle cannot always be avoided, but are usually not serious. Overstretching of the neck or too much pressure on the bracial plexus may be followed by paralysis of the arm, which must be carefully treated in the postnatal period. A hematoma of the sternocleidomastoid muscle may occasionally occur, but usually disappears spontaneously. Adding to the complications of breech deliveries is an increased necessity for aggressive resuscitative management over that ordinarily required by many of the babies who present with the vertex. Delay in adequate resuscitation increases neonatal loss. For these reasons it is increasingly common for breech presentation to be regarded as an indication for cesarean section. This is especially true if the mother is a primigravida.

Version

By version is meant the turning of the baby within the uterus so that the part which was presenting at the pelvic inlet is replaced by another part. Its purpose is to facilitate delivery. Version is used infrequently in the present day. Cesarean section has replaced version as a method of managing the complications for which the procedure was once used.

In *external cephalic version* the baby is turned, by manipulation through the external abdominal wall, from a breech presentation or transverse lie to a cephalic presentation. This procedure may be attempted in the last weeks of pregnancy or in early labor, unless there are definite contraindications. There is a tendency for the baby to return to its original position after the version has been done.

A *podalic version* is one in which the baby's feet are grasped and pulled through the cervix. It is followed by a breech extraction. For this procedure the physician introduces a hand into the uterine cavity after the cervix is completely dilated and grasps one or both feet of the baby before rupture of the membranes if they are still intact. Podalic version may occasionally be used for delivery of a second baby in a twin pregnancy when that baby is in an abnormal position or when birth is delayed and immediate delivery is urgent.

Cesarean Section

A cesarean section is an operation by which the baby is delivered through an incision in the abdominal and uterine walls. It is sometimes believed that the operation was named for Julius Caesar, who was supposedly delivered by this method, but this seems improbable. The operation was almost always fatal in those days, and, moreover, as the uterine wall was not sutured after the baby was extracted, a woman was not likely to have other children afterward even if she did live. Caesar's mother had several children after he was born. Another explanation for the name is that during the reign of Numa Pompillius (715–672 BC), a law, initially called royal law and later called Caesar's law, was passed, which required that the abdomen be opened and the baby extracted in every case in which a woman died late in pregnancy, as one means of increasing the population. Thus it is apparent that a cesarean operation on a woman who has just died is a very ancient procedure.

Cesarean sections have become progressively safer, and the incidence of this operation has increased in recent years. Cesarean sections have a higher maternal and fetal mortality rate than normal deliveries, but when complications exist, the operation is often safer for mother and baby than a difficult vaginal delivery. In some cases, such as in the presence of antepartum bleeding, a cesarean section may be necessary for survival of the baby and sometimes of the mother. Obstetric or medical complications that make surgery essential may be an important contributing factor to its increased hazard for mother and baby.

Indications for a primary cesarean section are

dystocia, antepartum bleeding, fetal distress, breech in a primigravida, some cases of toxemia, and certain medical complications. The most common primary indication is dystocia, usually due to cephalopelvic disproportion. There may be more than one indication in the same patient.

The most frequent reason for cesarean sections is a previous cesarean. These are termed repeat cesarean sections. Cesarean sections have been repeated 10, or possibly more, times in the same patient, but because of some danger of a weakened uterine wall, the physician may advise the patient not to have more than three pregnancies when cesarean section is the only method by which she can safely be delivered.

One delivery by cesarean section does not necessarily mean that all of the following deliveries must be by the same route. If the first operation was performed because of a contracted pelvis, subsequent pregnancies will necessarily be terminated similarly. If it was performed because of toxemia or antepartum bleeding and if the postoperative course was uncomplicated, a vaginal delivery may be considered for subsequent pregnancies, unless there is some possibility of dystocia or the uterus is greatly distended. Whether or not the patient had a previous vaginal delivery will be considered in making this decision. However, the patient should be in a hospital and under constant observation as soon as labor begins. Everything must be in readiness for an emergency operative delivery if indications arise. Tenderness over the former operative site and any evidence of bulging of the area are danger signals. A number of physicians believe that "once a cesarean, always a cesarean" is a good rule to follow to avoid danger of uterine rupture.

The time for a cesarean section varies with its indication. Sometimes it can be planned for a specific date; at other times it is an emergency procedure. When it is an elective procedure, termed an elective cesarean section, the time for the operation is planned in advance. A fetal lung maturity study should be done prior to surgery. The operation is often scheduled from one to two weeks before the expected date of delivery, depending on assessment of maturity of the fetus. This gives the baby the advantage of reaching maturity before birth and yet often makes is possible to perform the operation before labor starts. Some patients will begin labor before the planned date, and the operation must then be performed as an emergency so that labor does not progress too long. Common reasons for an elective procedure are repeat cesarean section or significant pelvic contraction.

Sometimes a cesarean section is performed when a trial of labor has proved a cephalopelvic disproportion. For antepartum bleeding it is usually an emergency operation and often must be done before term, resulting in delivery of a premature baby. For any emergency cesarean section speed in preparation of the patient and of the room for operation is important.

Another reason for an emergency cesarean section is appearance of ominous fetal distress during labor before the cervix is sufficiently dilated to permit vaginal delivery. Fetal distress is a term that may cover several conditions that suggest that the fetus will be in jeopardy if delivery is delayed. Persistent changes in rate and rhythm of the fetal heart which include tachycardia, late decelerations, severe bradycardia, or loss of beat to beat variability are considered serious changes that require early delivery, especially if they do not respond to treatment.

There are several types of cesarean section. These are commonly known as the classical; the low segment or low cervical, which may be intra- or extraperitoneal; and the cesarean hysterectomy. The low segment operation is usually considered the procedure of choice. Among other reasons, the danger of postoperative infection is decreased, and the probability of rupture of the scar in a subsequent pregnancy is much less. At times, however, a classical operation is considered best, as in cases of placenta previa, or when adhesions near the lower segment make an operation in that area difficult.

In the *classical* operation the abdomen is opened in the midline between the umbilicus and symphysis pubis, a packing may be placed around the uterus to keep amniotic fluid and blood out of the abdominal cavity, and an incision is made through the anterior wall of the uterus. It may be necessary to displace the placenta if it lies anteriorly. A hand is inserted into the uterine cavity, and the baby is grasped by the feet and extracted. The cord is cut after respirations are initiated if the baby's status is good. Ergonovine or an oxytocin preparation is given as the baby is delivered to aid in contracting the uterine muscle, and the placenta and membranes are removed immediately. An experienced assistant gives further attention to the baby. The uterine and abdominal walls are then approximated with sutures.

In the *low segment cesarean section*, after the abdomen is opened the bladder is separated from the uterus, the lower uterine segment and upper part of the cervix are exposed, and an incision is made in the lower part of the uterus, behind the bladder, instead of through the fundus. This incision may be either longitudinal or transverse. The baby's head is delivered either by applying forceps to the head or by lifting it out of the incision with the hand while pressure is applied to the fundus. After closure the uterine incision in this operation is outside the peritoneal cavity.

In a *cesarean hysterectomy*, the abdomen and uterus are incised, and the baby and placenta are extracted. Then a hysterectomy is performed, often for a diseased uterus, such as fibroids, or for a defective scar from previous cesarean sections.

When a woman dies undelivered during the latter months of pregnancy, a cesarean section is often performed immediately after death with the hope of saving the baby. This is termed a *postmortem cesarean section*.

Preoperative Preparation

Preparation of a patient for a cesarean section is similar to preparation for any abdominal operation. In addition, arrangements are made for immediate care of the baby.

Ideally the patient is admitted to the hospital 24 hours before surgery so that she may rest and be prepared as for any other operation. This is often possible for an elective procedure. Typing and crossmatching for blood transfusion are always done before surgery. Skin preparation and withholding of food and fluids are the same as for other abdominal surgery. For bowel preparation an enema may be given the evening before surgery.

An indwelling catheter is inserted into the bladder before surgery. It is left open and draining to keep the bladder empty during the operation. Insertion of the catheter may be the responsibility of the nurse, and she must be certain that the bladder is empty. The fetal heart rate is checked before surgery and during preparation, since maternal hypotension resulting from the supine position may cause fetal hypoxia.

Preoperative medication is ordinarily scopolamine or atropine. A narcotic drug may narcotize the baby, and if used at all it is given to the mother after the baby has been delivered.

The anesthetic may be either inhalation or spinal anesthesia or local infiltration of the operative field. All preparation, including skin cleaning and draping, is done before the anesthesia is begun so that the time between its administration and delivery of the baby is short. However, undue haste to effect the delivery after anesthesia is begun is not warranted.

Preoperative teaching should include an explanation of all the preparations which will be made prior to the anesthesia so the mother does not become alarmed that surgery will be begun before she is anesthetized. It is helpful for her to have someone she knows with her to reassure and explain events to her. Ideally, this person would be her husband.

Equipment for care of the baby and an incubator with an overhead radiant heater are prepared. An experienced person is available to care for the baby, to help him establish breathing, and to clamp the umbilical cord. This allows the surgeon and his assistant to continue with the operation. When the baby's breathing is well established, he is taken to the nursery for further care and observation.

Ergonovine and/or oxytocin preparation is administered just as the baby is born. It may be necessary to repeat these oxytocics later during the operation to control uterine bleeding. The nurse should have these medications ready to give immediately as ordered. Intravenous fluids are given during the operation, and blood for transfusion is available to be used as necessary.

Postoperative Care

Care of a patient after a cesarean section includes both postoperative and postpartum care. Since the patient has had an anesthetic and an abdominal operation, she must have the same care as for any patient after abdominal surgery. She must be closely watched until she has recovered from the anesthetic. Vital signs are carefully checked at frequent intervals.

Parenteral fluids are administered on the day of operation, but may not be necessary the following day. The patient has had very little manipulation of the bowel during surgery and is ready to take food and fluids early. Many physicians permit her to drink water as soon as she recovers from nausea, take solid food in 24 hours, and resume a regular diet as soon as she can tolerate it.

Gas pains and abdominal distention are often minimal, but if they cause discomfort, a rectal tube and heat to the abdomen will usually give relief. Occasionally such serious complications as ileus and acute dilatation of the stomach occur. These are treated as quickly as possible. The nurse must be alert to any signs of their development. Vomiting and abdominal distention should be reported to the physician.

The patient's position may be any comfortable one and should be changed frequently. Ordinarily she is out of bed the evening of surgery and continues progressive ambulation thereafter. The indwelling catheter in the bladder may be connected to a drainage bottle and left in place for a day. In most instances the patient has no difficulty voiding after its removal.

Postpartum hemorrhage must be guarded against, just as after vaginal delivery. The abdominal dressing may make it difficult or impossible to palpate the fundus without disturbing the wound, but the blood pressure reading, the pulse rate, and the amount of vaginal bleeding will help determine whether or not there is excessive intrauterine bleeding. If the dressing is not high, the abdomen may be palpated above it to determine if the fundus is above or below the umbilicus. Care of the perineum and the breasts is the same as for any postpartum patient as outlined in Chapter 20.

OTHER COMPLICATIONS

Retention of the Placenta

Retention of the placenta means failure of expulsion within one-half hour after delivery of the baby. In most cases of retained placenta the uterine contractions have apparently not been sufficiently strong to separate it from the uterine wall. In some instances adhesions between the placenta and the uterus interfere with separation. Sometimes the placenta is retained after separation by contraction of the uterus below the placenta.

Improved methods of obstetric care have minimized the former dangers of manual removal of the placenta. Consequently, the present tendency is to proceed with its removal as soon as it becomes apparent that the placenta cannot be easily expressed by downward pressure on the fundus and before blood loss becomes excessive. Delay in removal for more than 5 to 10 minutes is now uncommon.

For manual removal of the placenta, rigid aseptic technique is essential. The physician may change into another pair of sterile gloves. Sometimes the external genitalia are again cleaned with an antiseptic solution, and fresh sterile draping sheets are put on. With one hand inserted into the uterus and the other hand grasping the fundus through the abdominal wall, the physician peels the placenta from its attachment to the uterus. It is inspected carefully to make certain that fragments have not been left behind. Oxytocic drugs are given after the placenta has been removed. Blood transfusion may be necessary if blood loss exceeds normal.

Cervical Lacerations

Small lacerations of the cervix almost always accompany delivery, but heal rapidly and without complications. These lacerations change the shape of the cervix so that it is no longer round as in a nullipara. Sometimes tears of the cervix are deep; they may even extend into the vagina or into the lower uterine segment. Extensive tears are most likely to occur during operative deliveries, especially if delivery is attempted before the cervix is fully dilated. A violent labor and precipitous delivery may result in cervical lacerations. Profuse bleeding accompanies deep lacerations.

Whenever bleeding during or after the third stage of labor is excessive and the fundus remains well contracted, lacerations of the cervix or vaginal wall are suspected. The cervix and vagina are very flabby following delivery, and direct inspection around the entire circumference of the cervix is necessary to discover and repair lacerations. For an examination of the cervix the vaginal walls are separated by retractors, and the cervix is brought into view by grasping the cervical lips with an ovum or sponge forceps and applying traction. Sometimes downward pressure is also made on the fundus. Forceps with teeth cannot be used to grasp the cervix because the tissues are very vascular and friable. If lacerations are found, the bleeding is controlled by approximating the lacerated edges of the cervix or vaginal wall with sutures.

To detect lacerations which may bleed later, many physicians inspect the cervix after all deliveries; others examine it only after operative deliveries unless otherwise indicated; still others inspect it only when indicated by a difficult delivery or by bleeding that is apparently not originating from the uterus.

BIBLIOGRAPHY

Berk, Howard, Complications of intrauterine instillation of saline for abortion, *Contemporary Ob/Gyn* 2:11–13, 1973.

Bock, Johannes E., and Wiese, J., Prolapse of the umbilical cord, *Acta Obstet. Gynecol. Scand.* 51:303–308, 1972.

Brant, H. A., and Lewis, B. V., Prolapse of the umbilical cord, *Lancet* ii:1443–1445 (Dec. 31) 1966.

Brenner, William E., The oxytoxics: Action and clinical indications, *Contemp. Ob/Gyn* 7:125–132 (Jan.) 1976.

———, Bruce, R. D., and Hendricks, C. H., The characteristics and perils of breech presentation, *Am. J. Obstet. Gynecol.* 118:700–712 (Mar. 1) 1974.

British Medical Journal, Induction of labour, 6012:729–730 (Mar. 27) 1976.

———, Fetal damage from breech birth, 5964:158–159 (Apr. 26) 1975.

Burnett, Lonnie S., Wentz, Anne Colston, and King, Theodore M., Methodology in premature pregnancy termination. Part II, *Obstet. Gynecol. Surv.* 29.6 (Jan.) 1974.

Cetrulo, Curtis L., Freeman, Roger K., and Knuppel, Robert A., Minimizing the risk of twin delivery, *Contemp. Ob/Gyn* 9:47–51 (Feb.) 1977.

Cibils, Luis A., Enhancement and induction of labor, in *Risks in the Practice of Modern Obstetrics,* edited by Silvio Aladjem. Mosby, St. Louis, Mo., 1972, Chapter 6, pp. 126–153.

Cronenwett, Linda R., and Choyce, Janice M., Saline abortion, *Am. J. Nurs.* 71:1754–1757 (Sept.) 1971.

Danforth, David N. (ed.), *Obstetrics and Gynecology,* 3rd ed. Harper and Row, New York, 1977.

Diddle, A. W., Semmer, J. R., and Slowey, J. F., Cesarean section: Changing philosophy, *Postgrad. Med.* 53:160–165 (Mar.) 1973.

Friedman, Emanuel A., Failure to progress in labor-evaluation and management, *Contemp. Ob/Gyn* 4:41–47 (Dec.) 1974.

———, Patterns of labor as indicators of risk, *Clin. Obstet. Gynecol.* 16:172–183 (Mar.) 1973.

Greenhill, J. P., and Friedman, Emanuel A., *Biological Principles and Modern Practice of Obstetrics.* Saunders, Philadelphia, Pa., 1974.

Klein, Theodore, and O'Leary, James A., Rupture of the gravid uterus, *J. Reprod. Med.* 6:43–47 (May) 1971.

Laufe, Leonard E., *Obstetric Forceps,* Harper and Row, New York, 1968.

Melody, George F., Guide to forceps delivery, *Hosp. Med.* 6:7–27 (July) 1970.

Obstetrical and Gynecological Survey, Neonatal mortality of breech deliveries with or without forceps to the aftercoming head, 31:289–290 (Apr.) 1976.

Oxorn, Harry, and Foote, William R., *Human Labor and Birth,* 3rd ed. Appleton-Century-Crofts, New York, 1975.

Phillips, Robert D., and Freeman, Malcolm, The management of the persistent occiput posterior position, *Obstet. Gynecol.* 43:171–177 (Feb.) 1974.

Pritchard, Jack A., and MacDonald, Paul C., *Williams Obstetrics,* 15th ed. Appleton-Century-Crofts, New York, 1975.

Ranney, Brooks, and Stanage, W. F., Advantages of local anesthesia for cesarean section, *Obstet. Gynecol.* 45:163–167 (Feb.) 1975.

Reid, Duncan E., Ryan, Kenneth J., and Benirschke, Kurt. *Principles and Management of Human Reproduction.* Saunders, Philadelphia, Pa., 1972.

Rovinksy, Joseph J. (moderator), Symposium. Managing breech presentation, *Contemp. Ob/Gyn* 2:73–114 passim (Nov.) 1973.

———, Miller, Jay A., and Kaplan, Solomon, Management of breech presentation at term, *Am. J. Obstet. Gynecol.* 115:497–513 (Feb. 15) 1973.

Speroff, Leon (moderator), Symposium. A report on prostaglandins for abortion, *Contemp. Ob/Gyn* 2:83–108 passim (Dec.) 1973.

Vorherr, Helmuth, Disorders of uterine function during pregnancy, labor, and puerperium, in *Pathophysiology of Gestation,* edited by Nicholas S. Assali. Academic Press, New York, 1972, pp. 145–268.

Wisconsin Medical Society, Division of Maternal and Child Welfare, Pitocin: An alert to complications, *Wis. Med. J.* 73:33 (Aug.) 1974.

Part Four

The Postpartum Family

17

Characteristics of the Newborn

The nurse, to be able to fulfill her role in caring for a newborn, needs an understanding of the baby's development at birth, the many adaptive changes that he must of necessity make to adjust to extrauterine life, and his needs during the adjustment period. The characteristics and physiology of newborns, mature and immature, and those born with deviations from intrauterine growth will be described in the following chapters. Insofar as feasible, the nurse's functions in the care of these infants will be described, but the nurse must determine the details of nursing care for the individual baby through an evaluation of his specific needs.

The first four-week period after birth is usually designated as the *neonatal,* or newborn, period, although its chief characteristics pertain to the first two weeks of postnatal life. During this period the baby makes the physiologic adjustments necessary for the change from intrauterine to extrauterine life. The most drastic changes occur at the moment of birth, and many other important ones take place during the first day or two of life. Then adjustments continue at a somewhat slower rate, mostly during the first two weeks, but some are not complete for a month or more. The greatest mortality rate of any period in infancy and childhood occurs during the neonatal period. The incidence of morbidity is also high, especially during the first few days. In recognition of the unique dangers in-herent in the first four weeks of life, students of obstetrics and pediatrics, of growth and development, and of biostatistics give them separate and important consideration.

At the time of birth a baby makes the most abrupt and complete changes in his environment and physiologic functions that he will make in his entire life. In a favorable intrauterine environment the fetus is supplied with the necessities for his development and survival. He is kept at an optimal and even temperature and is protected from exertion and injury. At birth the baby suddenly emerges from a very protective environment into one that is vastly different. He must immediately begin life as an independent being who needs first and foremost to establish pulmonary ventilation and marked circulatory changes.

Many adaptive changes are necessary to extrauterine life, but those of the respiratory and circulatory systems are of first importance and must be rapid and radical. Changes in function of all other body systems can then be established more slowly.

The hazards that the newborn may be presented with at birth and during his adjustment to extrauterine life must be anticipated and minimized if his optimum possibilities are to be realized. Care must be directed toward providing him with conditions that are most favorable to normal function, with minimal stress.

THE RESPIRATORY SYSTEM

The respiratory system must function immediately after birth if life is to be maintained. Loss of the placenta, through which gas exchange has taken place until birth, necessitates immediate and radical changes to permit the lungs to take over this function. Pulmonary ventilation must begin immediately after birth, and a marked increase in pulmonary circulation must also quickly take place.

Adequate maturation of the lungs is essential to extrauterine life. Of all the body organs, the stage of maturation of the lungs at birth is most crucial, since viability is not possible until the lungs are structurally developed to a degree of maturity sufficient to permit maintenance of good lung expansion and adequate exchange of gases. Development of the lungs rarely reaches an adequacy that will permit sufficient function to sustain life before the fetus is at least 26 weeks old.

Structural Development of the Lungs

Structurally the lungs are in a continuous stage of development during fetal life and into childhood. Bronchi and canals first appear and thereafter the potential air spaces develop. These air spaces which eventually become alveoli begin as small buds off the bronchi, grow in size, and later begin indentations and a thinning of their walls. During this progressive development of air spaces, the vascular portion of the lungs also develops more completely, with an ever-increasing number of capillaries extending toward and coming into close contact with the air spaces.

Beginning with the twenty-fourth week of fetal life, the air spaces of the lungs, the terminal air sacs, appear as saccules. As the saccules continue to develop, their membranes become thinner, and blood vessels grow closer to the membranes. By the twenty-sixth week of fetal life the thinness of the saccular membranes and the nearness of the blood vessels may be sufficient to maintain life if the baby is born at this

time. Until then the lung capillaries and the saccular membrane are not developed for exchange of gas. Up to the thirtieth week the fetal lung remains structurally immature, and there is little or no reserve for maintenance of extrauterine life if any condition develops that reduces optimum function. Beginning with the thirtieth week the reserve is better and the baby is able to increase his ventilation to some extent should it become necessary.

Between the thirtieth and thirty-sixth week of fetal life, the saccules of the lung become increasingly indented, changing in structure from saccules to alveoli. The enlarging surface area of the air spaces, resulting from indentation, and the increase in number of blood vessels close to the alveoli give the lung more reserve and increases a baby's ability to maintain extrauterine life.

After the thirty-sixth week of fetal life, the air spaces of the lungs are true alveoli and the lungs of a baby born at this time are structurally ready to function as well as those of a full-term baby. Lung development continues after birth, with alveoli increasing in number up to the age of eight years. Only one eighth to one sixth of the adult number of alveoli are present at birth, but the capacity for pulmonary gas exchange is very adequate in relation to body weight.

Lung Fluid

The fetal lung produces a considerable amount of fluid during the latter half of intrauterine development. This secretion is produced continuously and fills the fetal lung with fluid, partially expanding the air spaces. In addition, some of the fluid drains out of the lung into the amniotic fluid and some is swallowed. From 80 to 110 ml of fluid are present in the respiratory passages of a normal term fetus at birth. This must be removed to provide for adequate movement of air in and out of the lungs. Some of the lung fluid, approximately one third, is squeezed out of the lungs during normal birth as the baby's chest is compressed in his passage through the birth canal. When the chest walls return to their normal position with release from the birth canal, their recoil draws air into the lungs to replace the fluid that was squeezed out. The remainder of the fluid is drawn back into the lungs with the first breath and is then absorbed into the blood stream through the pulmonary capillaries and the pulmonary lymphatics. It is not known how quickly the fluid in the alveoli is absorbed, but under normal circumstances it is probably rapid. In a full-term, healthy baby the lungs may be cleared by the time the baby has taken a few breaths, or at least within the first hour after birth.

Babies who are immature and those who have had a complicated antenatal or delivery course may have a delay in clearing of their lung fluid. An immature baby does not have the lymphatics developed as well as a full-term infant and thus may have a decreased rate of fluid absorption from the lungs. Sometimes the birth process does not compress the chest walls and very little or no fluid is pushed out of the lungs. This is likely in delivery of a very small baby through the birth canal and in birth by cesarean section. If the baby is asphyxiated at birth, having poor lung expansion, the pulmonary vascular resistance may be high, resulting in a decreased volume of blood flowing through the lungs and a delay in removal of fluid.

Pulmonary Surfactant

A surface-active material, called pulmonary surfactant, normally lines the alveoli of the lungs. Surfactant has the properties of changing surface tension as the surface area changes and of achieving a very low surface tension when the surface area becomes small. Surface tension between any two moist surfaces is normally strong and would be high between the moist alveolar surfaces without the presence of this surface tension-reducing material. For effective respiratory function in the newborn, it is thus essential not only that the potential air spaces of the lungs are developed to the stage at which inflation is possible, but also that the surface-active alveolar lining has been produced.

Surfactant is a substance produced by the alveolar lining cells of adults and infants and is secreted out onto the surface of the alveoli, forming a lining film. It is a complex of proteins and lipids, a lipoprotein, of which lecithin, a very important natural emulsifying agent, is a significant surface-active component. The time of appearance of surfactant in the fetal lung is somewhat uncertain, but it is probably present to some degree beginning at about the twenty-third week of development and perhaps sooner. It is thereafter produced in increasing quantity and is usually present in sufficient amount for adequate lung function by the thirtieth week and in some infants enough may be present earlier.

See pages 612–13 for discussion of lecithin/sphingomyelin (L/S) ratio, where production of surfactant in the fetal lungs and measurement of its presence is described.

Pulmonary surfactant, owing to its property of reducing the cohesive force between the moist surfaces of the alveoli, is necessary to maintenance of good lung expansion. An absence or a deficiency in this surface-active film causes the surface tension at the air–fluid interface in the alveoli to be high and to become even higher as they retract during expiration. The result of this increasing surface tension is considerable retraction of the alveoli with each expiration. Such retraction greatly reduces the residual air that is ordinarily retained in the lungs at the end of expiration, and the lungs collapse more than they normally should with each expiration. This then requires greater than normal effort with the next inspiration in order to again fill the lungs, and each breath may require as much effort as the first breath of life.

Pulmonary surfactant not only has the property of achieving a low surface tension as the alveolar surfaces come closer together during expiration, but also of creating a constantly changing surface tension in each alveolus as its area changes. This has the effect of equalizing the pressure in alveoli of various sizes and preventing flow of air from one alveolus into another. It thereby prevents collapse of some alveoli and overdistention of others (Fig. 17-1).

Without surfactant and under the usual forces of surface tension, the collapsing force of the air and fluid interface in small alveoli is greater than in large ones. The collapsing force in the curved moist alveoli is determined by their size. Without surfactant this collapsing pressure increases as the radius of the curved surface decreases. A small alveolus with half the radius of a large one will have twice as much collapsing pressure in it as the large one. When two or

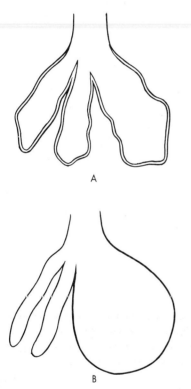

A

B

Figure 17-1. *A.* An alveolar lining film of a surface-active material, called pulmonary surfactant, is present. This keeps the surface tension in different-sized alveoli equal and prevents passage of air from a small alveolus to a larger interconnected alveolus. *B.* Without surfactant, the smaller alveoli, with the largest collapsing pressure, have emptied into the larger alveolus, which had a lower collapsing pressure, causing it to become overdistended. The result is atelectasis due to collapsed alveoli and interconnected overdistended ones.

more alveoli are interconnected, the smaller alveolus with the largest collapsing pressure is likely to empty into the larger alveolus, which has a lower collapsing pressure. The small alveolus will then collapse and the large aveolus will become distended (Fig. 17-1). With inhalations the large alveoli may receive some of the air that might have entered the small alveoli if they were not collapsed. The result of this process is areas of atelectasis due to collapsed alveoli and other areas of distended alveoli.

Surfactant has the property of bringing about a rapid variation in surface tension as the surface area changes. Specifically, it produces a decreasing surface tension as an area becomes smaller and an increasing surface tension as an area becomes larger. With a pulmonary surfactant film, as the surface area of an alveolus becomes smaller during expiration and the surfactant is compressed, it becomes more active and reduces the surface tension in the alveolus to a very low level. Then as the area of the alveolus becomes larger with expansion on inspiration and the surfactant is stretched, the surface tension in the alveolus becomes higher. Such increased surface tension tends to limit the extent to which alveoli become inflated, enhances their recoil, and prevents their overdistention. Due to these changes in surface tension, brought about by pulmonary surfactant, the small alveoli, in which the film has produced a very low surface tension, will not deflate into the larger ones, where the surface-active film has caused the surface tension to be higher, and the alveoli will not completely collapse as they become very small on expiration.

In summary, pulmonary surfactant acts to stabilize respirations and to prevent atelectasis. This lining, which has the property of achieving a very low surface tension when compressed, prevents complete collapse of the alveoli with each expiration. Some residual air is then retained in the lungs at the end of expiration and they do not need to be reopened with each new breath. The property of surfactant to change surface tension as the area changes, creating very low surface tension in small alveoli and higher surface tension in larger alveoli, keeps the pressure in alveoli of different sizes equal. This averts passage of air from small to large alveoli and thereby prevents collapse of some alveoli and overdistention of others.

Fetal Breathing Movements

Fetal breathing movements *in utero* have been reported from time to time over the past 75 years, but most often they were disregarded or explained on the basis of some unusual stimulus. In the past it was felt that respiratory-like movements did not appear to be present to prepare the respiratory system for function after birth. However, there is now reason to believe that the respiratory system does have practice before it must suddenly begin to function with considerable competence.

With the use of ultrasound equipment fetal breathing movements can be observed. These movements have been detected as early as 11 weeks gestation, but until the twentieth week they are very irregular; thereafter, the movements appear with more consistency. Occasionally respiratory movements are seen through the mother's abdominal wall.

Fetal breathing movements have been noted to be present 55 to 90 percent of the time. They involve both the diaphragm and the intercostal muscles; they are episodic and irregular, varying in depth and rate; and they are associated with rapid eye movements later in gestation. Rate varies from 30 to 70 times per minute. Diurnal variations in fetal breathing have been detected in direct relation to maternal blood glucose levels and fetal blood glucose concentration.[1]

Hypoglycemia and mild hypoxia will diminish or abolish fetal respiratory movements. Hypercapnia increases the movements. Gasping may occur in the fetus, especially during severe hypoxia and acidosis, and may cause the fetus, or the infant at the time of birth, to aspirate amniotic fluid.

Notation that fetal breathing becomes abnormal during labor when pH and Po. are decreasing suggests that observations of fetal breathing movements may be useful in the future as an indicator of fetal well-being.

Respirations

The exact mechanism by which onset of respiration is initiated is not certain. Sensory stimuli and chemical changes appear to exert an influence. It appears that the asphyxia normally present to varying degrees in all infants at birth is very important in initiation of the first breath in babies free of organic or physiologic dysfunction. Chemical changes in the blood—a lowered oxygen level, an increase in the carbon dioxide level, and a lowered pH—resulting from a brief period of asphyxia during delivery stimulate the respiratory center. However, if breathing is delayed for some reason, the asphyxia increases and may then depress instead of stimulate the respiratory center and resuscitation may be necessary. Also, the physical stimulation of the birth process and sudden change in the baby's environment (cold, touch, noise, pain, lights) may offer a stimulus to him to take his first breath. Boddy and Dawes say that if it is accepted that fetal breathing movements are normally present, an important question now is why breathing becomes continuous postnatally instead of remaining episodic as before birth.[2]

A normal healthy baby, who is not depressed by medications administered to the mother or by the process of delivery, will have respiration established within one minute after birth, often taking his first breath within a few seconds after he is born. A lusty cry usually accompanies establishment of respiration. The baby's first breath may require forceful contraction of the inspiratory muscles, mainly of the diaphragm, to overcome the fluid in the airways and the surface tension in the alveoli. Aeration of the lungs is rapid, however, occurring largely with the

[1] K. Boddy and G. S. Dawes, Fetal breathing, *Br. Med. Bull.* 31:3–7 (Jan.) 1975.

[2] K. Boddy and G. S. Dawes, Fetal breathing, *Br. Med. Bull.* 31:3–7 (Jan.) 1975.

first breath, and continuing respiratory effort is normally not great.

The baby who begins to breathe normally immediately after birth will quickly overcome the effects of the transient asphyxia that normally develops during the birth process. With good oxygenation and excretion of carbon dioxide through the lungs, the oxygen tension rapidly rises to normal, the carbon dioxide tension quickly decreases, and the acid–base balance returns to relatively normal limits in the first hours of life. A delay in return to normal values is likely if the baby is asphyxiated at birth or if he becomes chilled after birth.

Respirations in the newborn should be quiet, accompanied by neither dyspnea or cyanosis. The color of the baby's body is somewhat cyanotic at birth, but normally it becomes pink within a few minutes and remains so. Cyanosis of the hands and feet, and circumoral cyanosis, may persist for an hour or two, but thereafter these parts of the body should also be pink. Sluggish peripheral circulation or low body temperature may account for these areas of cyanosis.

The average respiratory rate is approximately 40 per minute. Breathing of the normal infant is regular in rhythm and without chest retraction, although the baby may on occasion normally have short periods of irregularity in rhythm, momentary periods of apnea, and slight signs of retraction. Periodic breathing is common in prematures. A rate increase to over 60 or a decrease below 30 per minute may be serious, especially in the presence of other difficulty. Rate and rhythm of respirations are normally easily altered by stimuli and may vary with activity. Normal variations in respiratory function in the early hours of life are described on pages 492 and 493.

Respiratory movements of the newborn are carried out by the diaphragm and the abdominal muscles. There is very little thoracic movement. Pressure against the diaphragm from abdominal organs, especially if the baby has been placed in a position with his head and shoulders lower than the rest of his body, may limit excursion and cause the respirations to be shallow and rapid. If such positioning is used for drainage of mucus, careful observation is necessary to note if it interferes with the baby's respiratory movements and then to find for him the position of easiest respirations.

A newborn may have mucus in his nose, mouth, and oropharynx and may spit up or vomit stomach contents during the early hours of postnatal life. This mucus or fluid may cause episodes of gagging and occasionally choking and the baby may need assistance to clear the respiratory tract.

Mucus is cleared from the baby's upper respiratory tract by suction. A soft bulb syringe removes mucus from the mouth effectively. When the mucus is far back, suction on a catheter may be indicated, since the catheter can be placed farther back in the throat than the bulb syringe. Deep suction, however, should be avoided, especially in the first five minutes of life because of vagal stimulation possibly causing cardiac arrhythmia. The mouth must always be cleared first, as stimulation of the nares may cause a reflex gasp and aspiration of oropharyngeal contents.

The Nose

The newborn's nose is small, shallow, and narrow; the openings into the nasal cavity are small. A delicate nasal mucous membrane causes the baby to sneeze vigorously and frequently, which helps to clear the tiny passages. Clear nasal passages are very important to the newborn because he normally breathes through his nose. Breathing through the mouth is very difficult for a baby, and nasal obstruction will cause considerable distress.

THE CIRCULATORY SYSTEM

At birth, when the placental circulation ceases and the baby's oxygen and carbon dioxide exchange must take place through the lungs, his pattern of circulation must change from a fetal to an adult type. Shifts in the circulatory system include a manyfold increase in pulmonary circulation, cessation of blood flow through the umbilical vessels and the placenta, and closure of the ductus arteriosus, the foramen ovale, and the ductus venosus. With cessation of the placental circulation, about 100 cm (40 in.) of low-resistance vascular channels are removed. Elimination of this low-resistance circuit causes a marked rise in the systemic vascular resistance. This rise takes place at the same time that the pulmonary vascular resistance is dropping. This results in orientation of pressure and pathways of circulation to the adult type.

Changes in the circulatory system occur abruptly at birth, but all are not immediately complete. There is a short period of time, up to a day or two after birth, during which a small amount of blood may continue to flow through the ductus arteriosus and the foramen ovale, or, if these vessels have closed, they can reopen during this period, reversing some of the changes previously made. Since the circulation during this time of conversion from a fetal to an adult circulation has characteristics that are peculiar to it alone, being neither a fetal nor an adult pattern, it may be called a period of *transitional circulation*. The transition to an adult pattern of circulation in the normal term infant is usually complete in a few days, when functional closure of the fetal structures becomes quite effective. Anatomic occlusion of fetal vessels is not complete for weeks or months, but functional closure is adequate to produce the necessary changes.

Changes in Pulmonary Blood Flow and Closure of the Ductus Arteriosus

It will be recalled that in fetal circulation a vessel termed the ductus arteriosus connects the pulmonary artery to the aorta (Fig. 5–9, page 107). Before birth, only about 10 per cent of the blood that flows into the pulmonary artery passes through the lungs; the remainder bypasses the lungs by flowing into the ductus arteriosus and then directly into the aorta. Immediately after birth, when gas exchange must take place through the lungs, a great increase in pulmonary blood flow becomes essential. A marked alteration in circulation is quickly brought about *through changes in the lungs themselves*, in which resistance to blood flow is markedly lowered when the blood vessels dilate with aeration, and *through constriction of the ductus arteriosus*. With these changes all of the blood pumped into the pulmonary artery will very soon be conveyed to the lungs for exchange of gases instead of being shunted in considerable amount through the ductus arteriosus.

The ductus arteriosus constricts within a few minutes after birth but functional closure is not immediately complete and a very small amount of blood may normally flow through this vessel for a few hours or a few days. This shunting of blood may follow the fetal pattern (from pulmonary artery to aorta) or it may take place in the opposite direction. Since the vessel is patent, blood flow from the aorta to the pulmonary artery (the reverse of fetal circulation) is temporarily possible. This takes place while the resistances of the pulmonary and systemic circulations are in transition. Shunting may thus take place in either direction, or it may at times be in both directions. With good ventilation, normal blood oxygen tension, and normal pH, the ductus arteriosus continues to constrict and shunting soon ceases.

Normal progression of the circulatory changes following birth may be slowed or interrupted by asphyxia and by alterations in normal acid-base balance. The ductus arteriosus responds to hypoxia and a reduced blood oxygen tension with a delay in closure, or a reopening of the vessel if it has already constricted. The pulmonary blood vessels are sensitive to changes in alveolar or arterial oxygen and carbon dioxide tension and to acidosis, but in contrast to the ductus arteriosus they are likely to constrict with a lowered blood Po_2 and pH. Constriction of the vessels reduces the pulmonary blood flow and the possibility of good gas exchange. A return to some of the features of a fetal type of circulation—increased pulmonary vascular resistance, decreased blood flow through the lungs, and consequently considerable shunting of blood from the pulmonary artery through the ductus arteriosus—may reach a dangerous degree and make oxygenation difficult. The respiratory and circulatory systems are so intimately associated in function that a deficiency in the function of one readily interferes with good function of the other.

Closure of the Foramen Ovale

The foramen ovale, the direct opening between the right and left atria of the heart, closes quickly after birth, but, similar to the ductus arteriosus, some shunting of blood may occur for the first few hours or few days. Closure of the foramen ovale is largely due to pressure changes in the atria. Pressure in the left atrium is raised when the marked increase in pulmonary blood flow after birth brings about a large increase in venous return to the left atrium and a rise in systemic resistance is brought about by cessation of placental circulation.

Pressure in the right atrium is lowered after birth. Aeration of the lungs decreases the pulmonary resistance and thus the pressure in the right atrium, and removal of the placental circulation decreases the amount of blood flowing through the inferior vena cava to the right atrium. With these changes in atrial pressures, the pressure in the left atrium is greater than that in the right and the valve over the foramen ovale closes. Blood that formerly passes from the right to the left atrium, through the foramen ovale (Fig. 5-9, page 107), now moves into the right ventricle, and from there to the lungs to be aerated.

If at any time during the transitional period of circulatory adjustment the right atrial pressure is raised or the left atrial pressure falls, there may be some reopening of the foramen ovale and a shunting of blood from right to left atrium. A small shunt may persist for a few hours or a day after birth without significant consequences. Greater shunting reduces effective cardiac function and oxygenation of blood. Asphyxia may cause a serious right to left shunt which may ap-

pear together with a shunt through the ductus arteriosus.

The Placenta, Umbilical Cord Vessels, and Ductus Venosus

Circulation through the placenta is usually interrupted by clamping of the umbilical cord, but even without clamping this circulation would soon stop. The umbilical vessels constrict very soon after birth and the cord ceases to pulsate in five to ten minutes. The ductus venosus, the connecting vessel between the umbilical vein and the inferior vena cava, is sealed off after birth by the closing of a sphincter at the umbilical end. Although these vessels are constricted soon after birth, the umbilical vessels and ductus venosus are sufficiently patent for the first four to five days to permit insertion of a small polyethylene tube when this is necessary for treatments such as infusion of fluids, frequent sampling of blood gases, and exchange blood transfusion. Final anatomic closure of these vessels occurs some days or weeks after birth.

The blood flow between the placenta and the baby reaches an equilibrium when a few minutes elapse between birth and the clamping of the umbilical cord, or if clamping is delayed until pulsation of the cord has ceased. If the cord is clamped before the equilibrium, the blood volume of the baby must be increased or decreased depending upon the amount of blood that is in the baby and in the placenta at the moment of clamping. The baby's blood volume is increased by 30 to 50 ml and the number of red blood cells are increased if the baby is held lower than the placenta before the cord is clamped. At present it is not certain if there is any value to the baby in an increased amount of blood, or if he may be at a disadvantage with an additional amount. Owing to the low-resistance placental reservoir, absorption of lung water by the pulmonary veins is enhanced if cord clamping can be delayed until the baby has taken his first breath.

Heart

The heart is relatively large at birth, is higher in the chest, and is in a more horizontal position than it is later in life. Its rate of growth slows after birth.

Transitory heart murmurs, which disappear in a few days and usually do not have pathologic significance, are heard in some newborn infants. Some of these murmurs are evidence of delayed closure of the fetal openings which ceased functioning at birth, the murmur being caused by leakage of blood through channels that have not yet been completely obliterated. Conversely, significant murmurs may not be present immediately after birth.

The peripheral circulation of the newborn is somewhat sluggish. The hands and feet may therefore be somewhat cyanotic for an hour or two after birth. Peripheral circulation is often not sufficient to keep the baby's hands and feet as warm as the rest of his body, and circulatory instability may cause the skin to have a mottled appearance when exposed to air.

Variability in pulse rate is characteristic of the newborn. The pulse rate is affected by stimuli and is therefore under less environmental influence when counted during sleep. It is usually rapid, with an average of 120 to 140 beats per minute. It may increase to 180 beats per minute with crying or other activity and may drop to between 80 and 90 during sleep. Irregularity of rhythm of the pulse may follow the same pattern as that of the respiratory system—when the respirations are slow, the pulse may be slow, and when the respirations become rapid, the pulse may also become rapid. However, a persistent rate above 160 or below 110 may be indicative of problems.

Blood Pressure

Until recent development of an ultrasonic technique, blood pressure in the newborn was measured by an auscultation, palpation, or color change (flush) method. These methods are somewhat difficult to use in the newborn and are not precise. The conventional auscultation method is unreliable because the arteries of small babies seldom produce audible Korotoff sounds, and the palpation and flush methods are only estimates of when the arterial walls open. The newer ultrasound (Doppler) method detects systole and diastole accurately, is more reliable, and is as simple to use as the conventional method with the stethoscope. It can detect very weak impulses and pick up sounds where the sphygmomanometer is unable to detect any blood flow. One other method of obtaining blood pressure measurements is by direct recording through an arterial catheter; this may be used in conditions in which a baby's illness requires an arterial catheter to be in place for checking of blood gases or for therapy. Good correlation has been shown between pressures obtained by the Doppler method and by intraarterial catheter.

A baby's normal blood pressure varies somewhat with his size and age. For example, the baby weighing under 2000 gm (4 lb 7 oz) normally has a somewhat lower blood pressure than the over 3000 gm (6 lb 10 oz) baby. A baby 10 days old normally has a higher blood pressure than he had at birth. Also the blood pressure is somewhat higher in the popliteal artery than in the brachial artery. From a study on blood pressures in neonates, using the Doppler method, Hernandez, Meyer, and Goldring defined values for well, normal infants in the first week after birth as follows: [3]

Normal blood pressure:
  Brachial artery pressure ranges from 46/20 mmHg (−2 SD) to 96/69 mmHg (+2 SD), with a mean value of 71/49 mmHg.
  Popliteal artery pressure ranges from 58/37 mmHg (−2 SD) to 103/72 mmHg (+ SD), with a mean value of 80/55 mmHg.
Hypertension, using two standard deviations above the mean as a definition, means a

[3] Antonio Hernandez, David A Meyer, and David Goldring, Blood pressure in neonates. *Contemp. Ob/Gyn* 5:34–37 (Mar.) 1975.

systolic pressure higher than 96 mmHg in the brachial artery or 103 mmHg in the popliteal artery.

Hypotension. using two standard deviations below the mean as a definition, means a systolic pressure below 46 mmHg in the brachial artery or 58 mmHg in the popliteal artery.

For measurement of blood pressure the baby must be quiet, since activity will raise the blood pressure, and the cuff must be of proper size, covering about two thirds of the upper arm, or two thirds of the thigh if the latter is used as the site of measurement, and the bladder of the cuff should completely encircle the arm or leg. The pressure should be obtained at about heart level.

With the Doppler ultrasonic-sphygmomanometer method the sphygmomanometer cuff is wrapped snuggly around the limb and held in place by a strip of adhesive tape. The transducer, a substitute for the stethoscope, is placed under the cuff and applied to the skin directly over the brachial or popliteal artery where the Doppler signal is heard most clearly in the headphones. This sensor emits ultrasonic pulses when the arterial wall opens or closes under the inflated cuff. It yields Doppler shift signals that are converted to sound. With the cuff and transducer in position, the cuff is inflated to 20 to 30 mmHg above the expected systolic pressure and then slowly deflated. The systolic pressure is heard when the cuff is sufficiently deflated to permit motion of the arterial wall. Between the systolic and diastolic pressures two signals, produced by the pulsating artery, are heard per cardiac cycle. At the diastolic pressure these signals merge and are heard as a change from a loud, sharp sound to a softer, muffled sound.

If the Doppler method of measuring blood pressure is not available, the color change (flush) method may be used. With the flush method the cuff is wrapped around an extremity either just above the wrist or just above the ankle, the extremity below the cuff is squeezed to blanch the distal area, the manometer is pumped to 120 to 140 mmHg, and the manometer gauge is then allowed to fall 5 mmHg/second, allowing perfusion of the extremity to take place. The pressure reading is noted at the time the extremity flushes, and the reading is recorded as the approximate mean diastolic–systolic pressure. If the reading is above 60 mmHg or below 30 the procedure is repeated on a different extremity to rule out error or confirm finding.

The Blood

Erythrocytes and Hemoglobin

The infant is born with a large number of red blood cells, approximately 5,000,000 per cubic mm of blood, with a range from 4,000,000 to 6,000,000. The hemoglobin level at birth is high, measuring from 14 to 19 gm per 100 ml of blood. The newborn also has a high hematocrit, ranging from 48 to 60 mm/100 ml of blood. This extra number of red blood cells and high hemoglobin level, which are carryovers of fetal life, were necessary to provide an adequate amount of oxygen *in utero;* after birth such large numbers apparently do not need to be produced.

There is a slight increase in the red blood cells and hemoglobin concentration in the first hours of life, probably due to a readjustment in blood volume, with very little change during the first week in both full-term and premature babies. During the next several weeks there is a progressive decline in mean hemoglobin values, greater in the premature than in the full-term baby.

The blood cell count and hemoglobin concentration are higher in blood obtained from a capillary source (heel puncture) than from a venous source (venipuncture) during the first few days of life; by the end of the first week the readings become similar.

During the first week an infant of more than 34 weeks gestation is anemic if he has a hemoglobin level of 13.0 gm or less in a venous sample and less than 14.5 gm/100 ml of blood in a capillary sample. The baby has polycythemia and may have problems with blood hyperviscosity and sluggish circulation when the hemoglobin is 22.0 gm/100 ml or more or the hematocrit is 65 percent or greater in a venous sample. See page 814.

Immature Cells

From 1 to 5 percent of the red blood cells present at birth are *nucleated;* a number over 10 percent is considered abnormal. These immature cells arise from the extramedullary blood-forming centers—liver, spleen, and lymph nodes—which function in the fetus in addition to the bone marrow. Shortly after birth the bone marrow entirely takes over the function of hematopoiesis. These nucleated red blood cells decrease rapidly during extrauterine life and disappear within a few days. The reticulocyte count is also elevated at birth, to 3 percent or slightly above, but with a decrease in erythropoietic activity drops quite abruptly to 0.5 to 1 percent during the first week.

In time of emergency the extramedullary blood-building sites must function, and the liver, spleen, and lymph nodes may become enlarged.

White Blood Cells

The range in normal variations in total number of white blood cells present during the newborn period is wide, making it difficult to determine if a count is significantly abnormal. A leukocytosis, with a count varying from 9,000 to 30,000 cells per microliter, is present at birth. Polymorphonuclear cells make up a large part of the total white cell count at birth and a number of these cells are immature. There is a fairly rapid fall in total count, with a considerable decrease apparent in a few days, the total count reaching a mean value of approximately 12,000 cells per microliter at the end of one week. There is also a shift in the type of cells. The number of polymorphonuclear neutrophils decreases rapidly, and the lymphocytes increase progressively, until they predominate at the end of a week.

Anemia

Most infants are at risk of developing an anemia during the early months of postnatal life. Erythropoiesis is very slow or virtually ceases for six to eight weeks after birth, red blood cells break down as their life span ends, and the circulatory system of the infant expands with growth. As a result anemia is a common occurrence. A decrease in hemoglobin concentration and erythrocyte count occurs until a low point is reached at the age of three months, with the red blood cells reduced to between 3,700,000 to 3,400,000 per mm^3, the hemoglobin level to 11 gm per 100 ml of blood, and the hematocrit to 33 percent. This drop in hemoglobin and erythrocytes is often termed *physiologic anemia* of the newborn. The above readings are considered normal for physiologic anemia, but any drop below these levels raises concern for anemia in the infant. After the third month of life a slow gradual rise in the number of red blood cells and in the hemoglobin level takes place, provided sufficient iron is available to build up the blood level.

Much of the iron that is released by red cell destruction stays in the body and is very valuable as a source of iron during the early months. When hematopoiesis resumes, this iron is used for replacement of erythrocytes. The amount of the red cell mass at the time of birth will determine the amount of iron obtained from cell breakdown. If the initial red cell count and hemoglobin level are low, the baby is at risk of iron-deficiency anemia unless he is given supplemental iron beginning in the early newborn period, when he ordinarily would not receive iron from his food. The value of feeding iron-supplemented formula or milk to infants is now emphasized as a preventive measure against iron-deficiency anemia in infants. Iron supplementation is discussed on pages 547–48.

Physiologic Jaundice (Icterus Neonatorum)

An elevated bilirubin content in the blood causes a slight, but visible, degree of jaundice of the skin, and sometimes of the sclera, in the early days of life in about 50 percent of newborns. Jaundice becomes visible in varying degrees on the second or third day of life, sometimes as early as 36 hours; it increases for a few days, begins to decrease by the sixth or seventh day, and has usually disappeared by the fourteenth day. In prematures, the increase in serum bilirubin is generally slower and over a longer period of time, and it tends to rise higher.

The slight degree of jaundice so common in newborns has been called physiologic jaundice because of the transient limitation in the baby's capacity to metabolize and excrete bilirubin in the first few days of life. There is, however, some uncertainty regarding use of the term "physiologic." A serum bilirubin concentration within a so-called physiologic range may be pathologic under some circumstances, especially in the sick baby or the premature baby. Therefore, it is always important to evaluate the jaundice for a physiologic or a possible pathologic cause and for its effect on the infant.

The pigment in the serum and the tissues that causes the physiologic jaundice in the newborn is unconjugated, indirect-reacting bilirubin, which cannot be excreted into the bile or through the kidneys because it is fat-soluble. The unconjugated bilirubin combines with albumin and is transported to the liver where the action of the enzyme glucuronyl transferase causes the free bilirubin molecule to conjugate with a glucuronide radical, resulting in a conjugated, direct-reacting, water-soluble bilirubin glucuronide that can be excreted through the biliary tree into the gastrointestinal tract and through the kidneys (Fig. 17-2).

The mechanism by which bilirubin is converted to a water-soluble excretable form is not well developed in the immediate newborn period. The fetus is limited in his capacity to conjugate bilirubin to a glucuronide and also to excrete it from liver cells. Relatively little bilirubin enters the intestines of the fetus. The fetus does not need, in fact cannot utilize, the postnatal route of bilirubin excretion. The major pathway of elimination in the fetus is via the placenta, and the bilirubin must be in the unconjugated form to cross the placenta.

With advancing gestational age there is a gradual increase in the capacity of the fetus to metabolize bilirubin according to the adult pathway. However, since the fetus must continue to use the placental route of elimination, his capacity to conjugate and excrete the water-soluble form remains limited until late in gestation. At birth, he must quickly convert from a fetal to an adult pattern of bilirubin metabolism. Gestational age and the degree to which the fetus has developed an adult pattern will therefore influence the degree to which the newborn will show jaundice.

The major source of bilirubin in the body is from the degradation of red blood cells. There is a considerable increase in the rate of bilirubin production in the newborn over that of the adult because he has a higher circulating red blood cell volume per kilogram of weight than the adult, and his red cells also have a shorter mean life span. The more immature the baby the greater the likelihood of an increased rate of hemoglobin degradation.

The bilirubin load on the liver may also be increased by intestinal reabsorption. The newborn probably reabsorbs a significantly larger amount of unconjugated bilirubin than does the adult by way of an enterohepatic circulation of bilirubin. This reabsorption may be due to the absence of bacterial flora and the increased activity of a deconjugating enzyme, β-glucuronidase, in the intestine. As a result, conjugated bilirubin, which has been excreted into the bowel and cannot be reabsorbed in that form, is converted back to unconjugated bilirubin, which is lipid-soluble and reabsorbable by the intestinal mucosa. The bilirubin is thus recycled and increases the load on the liver (Fig. 17-2). The fetus has a high concentration of β-glucuronidose in the intestine and this reabsorption of unconjugated bilirubin, which is useful in the fetus for placental excretion, carries over to the early newborn period when it adds to the load on the liver.

In summary, the increase in serum bilirubin,

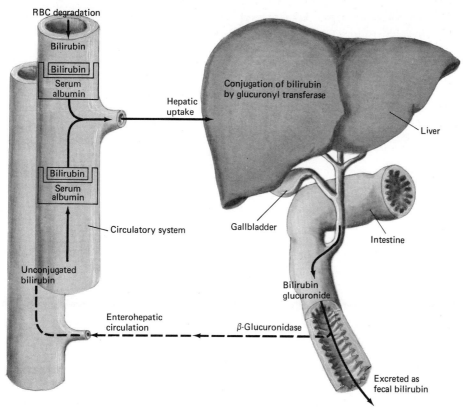

Figure 17-2. Neonatal bilirubin metabolism. See text for a more complete explanation.

which produces physiologic jaundice results from (1) a temporary impairment in the ability of the liver to clear bilirubin from the plasma, and (2) an increased load of bilirubin on the liver cells. The decrease in the ability of the liver to clear bilirubin from the plasma in the early neonatal period is the result of several factors: defective uptake in the early days of the newborn, a deficiency in the activity of the enzyme glucuronyl transferase at birth, and possibly a deficiency in excretion if the bilirubin load becomes large.

Clinical evidence of jaundice becomes apparent at total serum bilirubin levels of 5–7 mg/100 ml. In full-term babies the total serum bilirubin reaches a mean peak of about 6 mg/100 ml by 48 to 72 hours and then decreases to below 2 mg/100 ml by two weeks of age. In premature

infants a peak in the bilirubin level is reached on the fourth or fifth day. The total serum level has a mean value of 10–12 mg/100 ml in prematures, and the level declines more slowly than in the full-term baby. Clinical evidence of jaundice disappears by the end of the two weeks in the premature.

The following are general criteria of physiologic jaundice:

1. Clinical jaundice does not appear until after the first 24 hours of life.
2. Total serum bilirubin concentration does not exceed 12 mg/100 ml. (A laboratory report of total serum bilirubin includes both the direct and indirect fractions.)
3. Direct serum bilirubin concentration does not exceed 1–2 mg/100 ml. (This is a sepa-

rate report from the total bilirubin. Accumulation of conjugated direct-reacting bilirubin is never considered physiologic.)

4. Daily increments in total serum bilirubin concentration do not exceed 5 mg/100 ml-24 hours.
5. The baby does not show signs of illness.
6. Clinical jaundice does not persist for more than one week in a full-term infant or two weeks in a premature.

When bilirubin levels are higher than stated in the above criteria, or jaundice appears earlier or lasts longer than stated, a search for causes other than physiologic is indicated.

Transitory Coagulation Defects

Newborns manifest a transitory deficiency in blood coagulation between the second and fifth postnatal days. This transitory deficiency results from a temporary decrease following birth in substances important in blood coagulation, factors produced in the liver under the influence of vitamin K. Intestinal synthesis of vitamin K is not established during the first few days of life, when bacterial flora in the intestinal tract that are important in synthesis of this vitamin are not yet present.

Blood coagulation returns to normal spontaneously after several days. However, the transitory defect in coagulation is often minimized or prevented by administration of vitamin K_1 to the baby on the day of birth.

Vitamin K_1 is often administered as a single dose of 0.5 to 1.0 mg soon after birth. It is given intramuscularly. Sometimes the dose is repeated in two or three days. Excessive amounts of vitamin K (over 5 mg) may be harmful, predisposing to hyperbilirubinemia. Some physicians recommend administration of vitamin K_1 to all infants; others order it for premature babies and babies born following difficult labor and delivery. Sometimes vitamin K_1 is not administered at birth, but is used later, during one of the first few days of life, if a tendency to bleed appears.

BODY TEMPERATURE AND HEAT PRODUCTION

The growing fetus produces heat which he must dissipate. Under normal conditions the temperature of the fetus is approximately 0.5°C (0.9°F) above that of the mother, and the fetus gives up heat to the mother to maintain a steady body temperature. Most of this heat exchange takes place between fetal and maternal blood via the placenta. Some heat may also be conducted to the amniotic fluid and to surrounding maternal tissues. Although a baby's body temperature at birth is 0.5°C higher than the mother's, under the usual environmental conditions in the delivery room his body temperature may fall quickly after he is born unless special precautions are taken to protect him against heat loss. These precautions include providing the baby with a thermal environment which prevents heat loss from the body, conserving physical energy expenditures needed to maintain warmth, and avoiding the serious effects of the increase in metabolism that becomes necessary when the body must produce a large amount of heat. The premature or small baby is in greater danger of the potential consequences of cooling than is the full-term, normal-sized infant.

Loss of Body Heat

The newborn baby loses body heat by evaporation, conduction, convection, and radiation. *Evaporation* can account for a large heat loss immediately after birth, when the baby's entire body is wet with amniotic fluid. Evaporation of this moisture removes heat from his body and rapidly lowers his temperature. In addition to evaporation, the baby may lose body heat to the cool environment of the delivery room by convection, conduction, and radiation, as described below.

Unless the baby is adequately protected, his body temperature may fall to 94°F (34.4°C) or even as low as 92°F (33.3°C) as the amniotic fluid evaporates and heat is lost to the cool room. The skin temperature falls more rapidly than the deep body temperature (core temperature, ascertained by taking a rectal temperature), and may drop to 93°F (33.9°C) or 92°F (33.3°C) in 15 minutes. As heat from the inner body is conducted to the outside, the core temperature also falls but at a somewhat slower rate than the skin temperature. Immediately after birth the skin temperature can fall as much as 0.5°F (0.3°C) per minute, especially in the premature, and the body temperature as much as 0.3°F (0.1°C) per minute. The calculated heat loss with such a temperature drop is approximately 100 calories per pound per minute. Considering that an ounce of milk provides 20 calories, a loss of each 100 calories is equivalent to the calories that would be provided by 5 oz. of milk.

The fall in body temperature at birth indicates that the baby's heat production is not sufficient to make up for heat loss in the immediate period after birth. The baby's heat production will quickly increase upon exposure to cold, but it may take many hours before the body temperature returns to normal unless the baby's heat loss is halted and he is placed in a heat-retaining environment.

Heat loss by ways other than evaporation must be considered both in the immediate period in the delivery room and also at a later time in the nursery. Since heat is transferred from one object to another, flowing from a warm body to a cooler one, the baby may lose heat by *convection* to the cool air in the delivery room and by *conduction* to the cool sheet or blanket on which he may be placed for clamping of his umbilical cord, stimulation of breathing, and sometimes identification and eye care. This heat loss is also significant if the baby is placed into blankets or an incubator that have not previously been warmed. When clothing and blankets are cool, heat will flow from the baby's body to the cool sheets or clothing, warming them.

As soon as the baby is dressed and placed into a warm nursery or into an incubator that is warm, heat loss by convection and conduction may become negligible. Clothing and covers help to insulate the baby and warm dry surfaces will not conduct heat away from his body.

Loss of body heat by *radiation* may account for a considerable amount of a baby's total heat loss. While loss of heat by convection is to the surrounding air and loss by conduction is through transfer of heat directly to the material touching the baby, radiation loss is to solid objects at a greater distance. Radiant heat given off by the baby's warm body travels through the air to the cooler objects in the room, where it is absorbed. Radiant heat loss may continue during the days following birth, especially from an unclothed baby in an incubator. An incubator alone does not necessarily provide a constant thermal environment.

A baby's body temperature will vary in an incubator which is maintained at a constant temperature as conditions outside of the incubator change, or if his temperature does not change he is changing his metabolism for production of heat. When a window or an outside wall of a nursery becomes cooled at night, the baby's temperature will either drop or his heat production must be greatly accelerated to maintain a normal temperature. The baby radiates heat from his body, through the air in the incubator, to the walls of the incubator, which are profoundly affected by the temperature of the windows or walls of the nursery. A warm incubator will provide comfort to the baby, but it does not protect him against variations in the environment outside of the incubator.

A baby's temperature may rise to above normal when a source of heat in close proximity to the incubator, such as a radiator or sunshine through a window, warms the environment considerably. It may be necessary to move the incubator from such a source of radiant heat or to lower the incubator temperature to prevent overheating of the baby.

Production of Body Heat

The newborn is capable of increasing his heat production a considerable amount when he is cool and is thereby able to compensate for some or all of the heat loss from his body. A baby is able to generate heat (1) by shivering, (2) by metabolism of brown fat, and (3) by increasing his general metabolism. A baby with hypoxia or increased P_{CO_2} or under the influence of drugs will encounter difficulty in regenerating body heat.

An immediate way of generating heat is by *shivering*, and a newborn can quickly begin to increase his heat production in this way. He shivers when he is cold. A baby's shivering may not be as apparent as shivering is in an adult, but he shows increased muscular activity, restlessness, crying, and at times intermittent shivering may be noticeable. A large baby is better able to produce heat by shivering than a small baby, since he has a larger amount of muscle available for this increased activity.

Metabolism of brown fat is an important source of heat production in the newborn. Brown fat is a unique kind of adipose tissue, which functions to produce heat under the stress of cooling. Each cell of brown fat has many small droplets of fat, in contrast to the single, much larger fat vacuole in cells of normal white adipose tissue. Brown fat has a rich nerve and blood supply. Its fat is quite easily metabolized and when it is used to produce heat, the cells may become partially or completely depleted of fat.

The newborn has a significant accumulation of brown fat. It is found in the interscapular region, in the posterior triangle of the neck, and in the axillae. When the baby is cooled, his autonomic nervous systems stimulates the brown fat deposits to metabolize this fat, which produces heat. A baby who has a good accumulation of brown fat will, under cold stress, have a warmer skin temperature between the shoulders and over the nape of the neck than he does over other parts of his body. The warmer areas are where the skin lies over a layer of brown fat. This increased skin temperature reflects the heat being produced in the brown fat. The rich blood supply of brown adipose tissue helps to distribute the heat that is generated by metabolism of brown fat to other parts of the body.

The newborn responds to cooling with an *increase in metabolic rate*. The baby's thyroid gland is stimulated to hyperactivity when he is exposed to cold and his general metabolism increases considerably. There will be a delay of a few hours, and perhaps 12 to 24 hours, before the metabolic rate rises significantly, but thereafter, it will respond to cooling or warming of the body. Although a baby's general metabolism will decrease as he is warmed, the impact of the increase in metabolic rate that took place as a result of cooling at birth will continue for a week or more. The metabolism of a baby who was cooled at birth is higher than that of a baby who did not lose much body heat and it remains elevated throughout the first week to 10 days of life.

Effects of Chilling on a Newborn

As babies who are cooled increase their metabolism, they must increase their oxygen consumption and their use of glucose and brown fat. These babies have a tendency to develop a metabolic acidosis and are in danger of being unable adequately to produce pulmonary surfactant.

As the baby increases his heat production, his oxygen consumption rises sharply. In a thermal environment in which the baby does not lose body heat and thus does not need to increase his metabolism for heat production, his oxygen consumption for his basic body needs is from 4 to 6 cc of oxygen per kilogram per minute. This is at a body temperature of 97.5 to 99°F (36.4 to 37.2°C). With a relatively small reduction in a baby's skin temperature he begins to increase his oxygen consumption, and as he cools to a considerable degree his oxygen need increases accordingly. When the skin temperature drops to between 94 and 95°F (34.4 and 35°C), his basal oxygen need is twice as high. This means a doubling of oxygen need with a drop of body temperature of 3°F (1.7°C). At a body temperature of 92°F (33.3°C) the baby needs three times as much oxygen to meet his basic needs (to remain alive) as he needs at a normal body temperature. Such a great increase in oxygen need may mean that supplemental oxygen may be necessary to maintain body temperature or if the baby cannot breathe well, he may not be able to obtain enough oxygen to sustain life.

MECHANISMS OF HEAT LOSS	PREVENTION OF HEAT LOSS
Evaporation — of moisture on body	Quickly dry off amniotic fluid
Convection — to surrounding air	Protect against cool drafts
Conduction — by direct transfer to cool material	Use warmed blankets to cover Place on warmed surface for care
Radiation — through the air to cooler objects in the room An incubator permits radiation of body heat to the environment outside of the incubator	Insulate with warm clothes and blankets and/or Provide radiant heat and/or Depend on maternal body heat

MECHANISMS OF HEAT PRODUCTION	EFFECTS OF COOLING AND INCREASED HEAT PRODUCTION
Increase in muscular activity and shivering	Increase in oxygen consumption Increase in glucose consumption Possible metabolic acidosis due to lactic acid from anaerobic metabolism
Increase in metabolic rate	Increased oxygen and glucose consumption and possible metabolic acidosis — as above General metabolic rate remains elevated for 7 to 10 days, even after warming
Metabolism of brown fat	Release of fatty acids which contribute to metabolic acidosis Possible inhibition of surfactant production because of a reduction in amount of glucose and available oxygen, and presence of acidosis

MECHANISMS OF HEAT CONSERVATION	PROTECTION OF THE SMALL BABY HANDICAPPED IN HEAT CONSERVATION
Subcutaneous fat	Poorly developed in premature and SGA infants The babies need extra protection against heat loss
Flexed position to decrease surface	Premature infants have less tone than full-term and may not be able to assume a flexed position The relatively large surface of a baby's head and damp hair may require extra protection to reduce heat loss
Peripheral vasoconstriction	Present in prematures as well as full-term

Figure 17-3. Mechanisms of heat loss, heat production, and heat conservation; the effects of these processes on the newborn; and actions that the nurse can take to reduce the serious consequences of chilling. Premature, small-for-gestational age, and sick babies are likely to be seriously handicapped by the effects of chilling because of low glycogen reserves, low reserves for increasing ventilation, and possibly preexisting acidosis. These infants have special needs for protection against heat loss.

Need for calories is high when heat production is high. As the baby is increasing his oxygen consumption, he is equally increasing his use of glucose. This means that when a baby's oxygen consumption is doubled or tripled, his utilization of glucose is likewise doubled or tripled. Although the normal full-term baby may have a reasonably large amount of glucose available to him (stored as glycogen), the small baby has only a small amount accessible in his body for increased metabolism.

With increased metabolism during cold stress a baby can quickly exhaust the glycogen store of his body and become hypoglycemic. A small baby may use all of his glycogen in 4 to 6 hours, and his blood sugar will fall to a very low level. Under such conditions the baby may sustain brain damage, since brain cells are in need of glucose as well as oxygen for adequate development and function.

A baby who is cooled and in need of increasing his metabolism is likely to develop a metabolic acidosis quickly. This is particularly true if his metabolic needs are higher than the amount of oxygen available to carry metabolism to completion. When more oxygen is required than can be supplied to the body, products of incomplete metabolism will accumulate.

Cooling quickly stimulates shivering and brown fat metabolism. Glucose is the source of energy for the shivering and sometimes the glucose metabolism cannot be carried to completion due to an inadequate supply of oxygen. This incomplete (anaerobic) metabolism leads to an accumulation of lactic acid. When brown fat is metabolized, fatty acids are released into the blood. The combined effect of fatty acids from the fat metabolism and lactic acid from the incomplete glucose metabolism is a lowering of blood pH, resulting in acidosis. The pH may even drop as low as 7.0 in the presence of considerable cooling and respiratory distress. A severe acidosis may interfere with essential body functions to a degree that is incompatible with life.

A baby who is cool may not be able to produce surfactant well. Pulmonary surfactant must be continually replaced. Its activity lasts only about 12 hours without replacement and, if production is halted, a baby can lose the surfactant which he had at birth within 12 hours or even in a shorter time. As a result of the loss he can progress to severe respiratory distress. The baby needs glucose and good oxygenation and a good circulation to produce surfactant well. Cooling may greatly reduce the amount of glucose and available oxygen, produce acidosis, and result in a decrease in circulation through the lungs. All of these factors, especially when combined, inhibit production of surfactant. A small baby is in greater danger than a large one of losing his ability to produce surfactant, since the small baby is handicapped by a low reserve of glycogen and a low reserve for increasing his ventilation.

A small baby or one who has respiratory distress is at a considerable disadvantage when he is cooled. A baby who does not have good lung function or who has required resuscitation may not be able to meet the body's doubled or trebled oxygen need for the increased metabolism necessary for heat production. This baby may already have an acidosis from his respiratory difficulty and he is likely to have a superimposed cause for becoming more acidotic.

Ways of Preventing Heat Loss

Delivery Room Care

Chilling of the baby after birth can be considerably reduced when immediate attention is given to minimizing his heat loss while he is in the delivery room. Proper care in the delivery room includes quickly drying the baby's body to reduce heat loss through evaporation of amniotic fluid, replacement of wet blankets with dry ones, and immediate care after birth in an incubator or under a radiant heater. This care is described on page 355.

When a newborn is moved from the delivery room to the nursery, he must be kept well covered with warm blankets. A full-term, healthy baby can be moved out of the delivery room with his mother and observed by both parents without undue cooling, if he is well covered. A corner of a blanket around the baby's head will reduce heat loss from the relatively large surface of his head and possibly from damp hair. When the mother holds her baby in skin-to-skin contact, her body is a source of considerable warmth, particularly when a blanket covers both mother and baby. When inspection of the baby by his parents is done careful attention must be given to ascertaining that the room is warm in order to prevent chilling while the baby is uncovered or that a radiant heat source is provided. A premature baby will probably need to be taken directly to the nursery. Transportation in a warmed incubator will protect him in transit.

Immediate Nursery Care

In the nursery the baby is placed into a warmed bassinet (or incubator) to provide warmth and help him to quickly regain a normal body temperature. Birth weight can be obtained by weighing the baby in a blanket and subtracting the weight of the blanket from the total weight. The baby's initial bath should be postponed until his respirations are stabilized and his body temperature has returned to around 98°F (36.7°C), which is likely to be 3 to 4 hours later. Physical examinations, laboratory procedures, x-rays, and other procedures that may be necessary in the first hours after birth and that require that the baby be exposed or undressed should be done under a heat lamp.

Incubator Care

A premature or low-birth-weight baby, or a full-term baby who has been delivered with difficulty, is placed into an incubator in the nursery as quickly as possible after birth. The incubator is used for control of air temperature, humidity, and oxygen if necessary, and for close observation of the baby, since he does not need covers and clothing in an incubator. When a premature birth is anticipated, the incubator should be warmed well in advance.

Maintenance of a constant air temperature in the incubator and in the nursery does not assure a constant thermal environment for the baby. Other factors, such as the humidity of the air, the temperature of the walls and windows of the nursery, and the amount of covers over the baby, will influence his environmental conditions. Therefore, even an incubator temperature of 93 to 95°F (34 to 35°C) does not ensure that the baby will maintain a basal metabolic rate. An incubator helps to decrease heat loss from a baby, but it does not provide heat; the baby must produce his own body heat, unless he is provided with warmth from a source of radiant heat. See page 716 for additional ways in which to protect the preterm baby in an incubator against heat loss.

When one finds that a baby can maintain a constant normal body temperature in an incubator maintained at a constant temperature, the assumption cannot be made that his thermal environment is satisfactory. The baby may be able to raise his metabolism sufficiently to produce adequate heat to maintain his body temperature even while he is radiating heat to his environment, but the cost to him of such heat production is likely to be great.

Radiant Heat

A source of radiant heat, can be used to supply warmth to a baby. Placed above the bassinet or the roof of the incubator, the lamp will radiate heat to the baby. A radiant heater should be used when the baby is first placed in the bassinet or incubator, and at any time that a baby cannot maintain a normal body temperature well, or when outside conditions indicate that the baby needs warmth. Such radiant heat helps to deliver warmth to the baby, reduces his metabolic rate, and serves to return his body temperature to normal more rapidly than with incubator or clothing protection alone.

The baby's metabolic rate increases or decreases rapidly with cooling or warming. Even while the baby's body temperature is still low, his metabolic rate and thus his oxygen need decreases when he is placed into a heat-gaining environment. A gradual rise in body temperature to normal will then take place without undue expenditure of energy.

When it becomes necessary to obtain blood samples and to begin intravenous fluids on the baby, he needs protection from covers, where possible, and heat from lamps. When treatments are necessary it may be advisable to use an open-ended radiant warmer infant care table (page 717).

Need for radiant heat to the baby is lessened if the baby has clothes on, if the incubator temperature is high, at 95°F (35°C) or above, and as he gets older.

Regulation of Incubator Temperature

A baby's surroundings should be such that he can maintain his body temperature between 97.5 and 98°F (36.4 and 36.7°C) axillary, or 98 and 98.6°F (36.7 and 37°C) rectally, without stress. The incubator should be placed against an inside wall of the nursery, since the temperature of that wall does not become as cool or fluctuate as much as an outer wall, and heat loss by radiation is likely less. Even with little exposure to cold surfaces outside of the incubator, the temperature of the baby's incubator may need to be as high as 96 to 97°F (35.6 to 36.1°C) if his weight is under 3 lb (1360 gm) and 94 to 96°F (34.4 to 35.6° C) if he is somewhat larger. With clothes or blankets on the baby, or a heat lamp over the incubator, a somewhat lower incubator temperature may soon be satisfactory. Clothes, however, interfere with good visibility and are ordinarily not used while a baby in an incubator is in need of close observation. A transparent plastic shell heat shield will help to conserve heat (page 717).

A highly desirable method of regulating the warmth of an incubator is through maintenance of the baby's skin temperature at or near a normal body temperature. Many incubators are equipped with a skin thermistor probe, which may be taped to the exposed skin of either of the sides of the baby's abdomen. This probe monitors the skin temperature, and through a control mechanism, regulates the heater in the incubator to increase or reduce heat output in accordance with a predetermined setting for the desired skin temperature.

The temperature of the baby's skin appears to have considerable influence on his metabolic rate. Relatively small changes in skin temperature influence oxygen need. Oxygen consumption is relatively low when the abdominal skin temperature is maintained between 97.5 and 98°F (36.4 and 37.6°C). To maintain such a skin temperature, the control mechanism of the heater of the incubator, to which the skin thermistor is attached, may be set at 97.6°F (36.4°C). A small piece of gauze or cotton should be used to cover the skin probe to insulate it against air currents in the incubator and against direct radiant heat.

When a skin thermistor is not used, it is necessary to monitor the baby's body temperature frequently to determine his need for, and his response to, warmth. Every effort must be made to maintain a warm and stable environment through careful control of the incubator temperature and the surrounding area.

Under any circumstances, with or without control of the incubator temperature according to a desired skin temperature, it is important to monitor the baby's body temperature and his environment frequently and to be concerned that his surroundings are such that he does not lose body heat to the environment. When the baby does not need to expend extra energy to keep warm, his use of oxygen and calories for heat production can be kept at a minimum. He will then not develop the metabolic acidosis and the deficiency of surfactant production that can accompany increased metabolism and an inadequate supply of oxygen and glucose.

When a baby is placed into a heat-gaining environment it is important to guard against too much warming as well as too little. A baby does not tolerate overheating, since his metabolism then also rises. He is likely to become restless and begin to perspire when his body temperature rises to 99.5°F (37.5°C). Overheating is more likely to occur with a full-term baby, who is placed into a heated bassinet for quick regain of normal body temperature, than with a premature in an incubator. A full-term baby, who is likely to be dressed or wrapped in blankets, may become too warm after an hour or two in a warmed bassinet. His body temperature must be monitored every 30 minutes so that the heat in his bassinet can be reduced when he is warm. After the body temperature of a full-term baby returns to normal, external heat is ordinarily not necessary.

Humidity

A high relative humidity reduces evaporative heat loss from the body and may be desirable for a short time, while the baby's temperature is being stabilized and for treatment of thick secretions in the respiratory tract, such as meconium. Use of a nebulizer on the incubator to maintain a high humidity for a prolonged period is inadvisable. It increases the risk of bacterial colonization of the baby's skin and umbilical cord and may result in serious infection associated with waterborne bacteria such as *Flavobacterium* and organisms in the *Pseudomonas* group.

Observations of Body Temperature

After birth, when a baby may have lost heat and he is placed into a heat-gaining environment to help him recover from the loss, the baby's temperature should be taken every 30 minutes. This is continued until his body temperature is stable and until a proper balance between the amount of warmth from the incubator or clothing and from the radiant heat has been determined. After body temperature stability has been attained less frequent checks are required, but monitoring the premature at least every 4 hours for a few days is important. Later a temperature check every 12 hours is adequate unless observation of the baby's behavior indicates the advisability of more frequent monitoring. For the full-term baby a daily temperature check is sufficient after the baby's body temperature has stabilized, unless the baby is exposed during manipulative procedures or there are clinical indications for more frequent checking.

Once a baby's body temperature is stabilized, there should be very little difference between skin and body temperature, taken either by axilla or by rectum. Any one of these readings should be around 98°F (36.7°C), plus or minus approximately 0.5°F. A skin reading can be obtained from a skin thermistor probe, if one is used, but since factors other than loss or gain of body heat may affect a baby's temperature, it is important also to monitor the baby's body temperature. This must be done to determine if the body temperature exceeds the limits of normal. A higher than normal temperature may indicate that the baby has an infection and a low temperature in a warm environment may indicate that the baby is unable to raise his temperature to normal because of a pathologic condition.

Body temperature may be taken by rectum or by axilla. When a temperature must be taken often, frequent insertion of a thermometer into the rectum may be injurious to the rectal mucosa. Axillary temperature readings are dependable, are as satisfactory as rectal readings, and are preferable to frequent taking of a rectal temperature. It is therefore recommended that the baby's axillary temperature be taken after an initial rectal temperature to assure anal patency. The American Academy of Pediatrics, Committee on Fetus and Newborn states that "the taking of temperatures rectally is not recommended."[4] An axillary temperature may be taken by holding the bulb of the thermometer high in the baby's axilla for 3 minutes while pressing the baby's arm gently but firmly against his body.[5] An axillary reading is not considerably lower than a rectal reading, as often assumed; axillary and rectal temperatures taken at the same time are very similar. The axillary temperature reading may be a few tenths of a degree lower than the rectal reading, but sometimes it is even higher than the rectal temperature, especially if

[4] American Academy of Pediatrics, Committee on Fetus and Newborn, *Standards and Recommendations for Hospital Care of Newborn Infants*, 5th ed. Evanston, Ill., 1971, p. 89.

[5] Jane T. Torrance, Temperature readings of premature infants, *Nurs. Res.* 17:312–320 (July–Aug.) 1968.

chilling has stimulated metabolism of brown fat. Both body temperature and incubator temperature should be recorded at each check.

WEIGHT

The mean, or average, birth weight of full-term Caucasian babies is 3400 gm (7 lb, 8 oz). There are, however, wide variations in birth weights of normal full-term infants. Approximately one half of all full-term babies weigh between 2950 gm (6 lb, 8 oz) and 3515 gm (7 lb, 12 oz). A full term baby weighing 2500 gm (5 lb, 8 oz) or less at birth is considered a low-birth-weight baby. A weight of 4080 gm (9 lb) or over at full-term gestation is considered excessive in size. Excessive size may cause dystocia, increasing risk of injury to mother and baby during delivery. Both low-birth-weight babies and those of excessive size are considered high-risk babies and require special observation and care in the nursery.

After 38 weeks gestation male infants are larger than female infants, weighing an average of 200 gm (7 oz) more. This difference, although significant, is not differentiated on the intra-uterine growth chart illustrated in Figure 18-2 (page 475). The normal full-term weights of babies of non-Caucasian races (Negro, Oriental, Indian) are usually somewhat smaller than those quoted above.

An unexplained maternal factor regulates the genetic growth potential of a fetus. Given a normal healthy mother and fetus, the size of the baby will be within approximately a 20 percentile range of the mother's own birth weight. Barring disease processes which are likely to alter fetal growth, all babies born to a mother will be close to the percentile of her own birth weight, if the gestational age and the birth weight of each individual is considered in establishing the comparison. (See Fig. 18-2, page 475, for charting of birth weight against gestational age.) The hereditary influence of the father on size has an effect on the growth period after birth.

Physiologic Weight Loss

All infants lose weight during the first few days of life. The weight loss ranges between 5 and 10 percent of the birth weight. This decrease in body weight is caused by a loss of excess fluid from the body tissues and a relatively low food and fluid intake, which means the baby uses his own body stores during his early days. The weight normally becomes stationary on the third or fourth day of life and then begins to increase (Fig. 17-4). Birth weight is usually regained in 10 to 14 days; some infants are back to their original weight at the end of one week of life. On some days the weight may

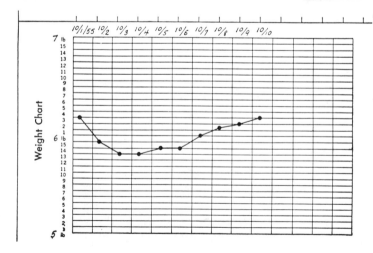

Figure 17-4. Weight chart of an infant weighing 6 lb 3 oz at birth, showing the physiologic weight loss on the first three days, a stationary weight on the fourth day, and a steady gain back to birth weight by the tenth day.

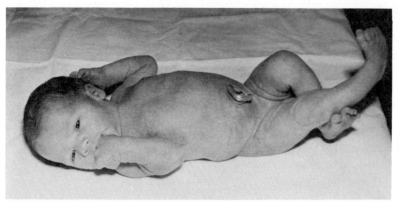

Figure 17-5. A newborn infant 2 days old. His head is large, his eyes are crossed, and lanugo hair is present on his forehead and in front of his ears. The abdomen is prominent and very relaxed and the pelvis is small. The neck, arms, and legs are relatively short. The baby's arms are flexed at his elbows with his hands near his face. The baby's fist is clenched, and he is making attempts to suck his hand. The umbilical cord is clamped and drying. The legs are abducted, flexed, and bowed so that the soles of the feet nearly face each other. The skin on the feet is dry and wrinkled. The baby appears alert and has good muscle tone.

remain stationary, but the general trend is upward, with an average gain of approximately 30 gm (1 oz) per day during the first three months of life.

LENGTH

The average length of the full-term infant girl is 50 cm (19.7 in.) and of the full-term boy, 52 cm (20.5 in.). At full-term lengths range from 45.2 to 50.6 cm (17.8 to 19.9 in.) in girls and from 45.4 to 55 cm (17.9 to 21.7 in.) in boys.[6]

Length is difficult to obtain because the baby normally lies tensely and with his legs flexed; to be measured accurately he must be placed flat on his back and extended as much as possible. It is helpful to mark with a pencil or safety pins the places to which the top of the baby's head and his heels reach. When the baby is moved, the distance between the marks is measured.

[6] U.S. Dept. of Health, Education, and Welfare, National Center for Health Statistics, *NCHS Growth Charts, 1976.* Monthly Vital Statistics Report, Vol. 25, No. 3, Supplement, June 22, 1976.

The greatest increase in a baby's length occurs during the first three months of his life.

SKELETON

The young infant's body has a large amount of cartilage, the bones are soft because of the small amount of mineral deposit, and the joints are very elastic, especially during the first week of life. The great mobility of the joints, which makes the body quite pliable, offers mechanical advantages during delivery, and the flexibility of the skelton allows the bones to bend rather than break if pressure is applied.

The head of the infant is much larger than an adult's in comparison to the rest of the body size, accounting for one fourth of the body length in the infant as compared with one eighth of the adult's body length.

Compared with the head, the thorax and pelvis of the newborn infant are small. The abdomen is prominent due to weak muscles and rather large abdominal organs. The neck, arms, and legs are relatively short. The legs are abducted and flexed and so markedly bowed that the soles of the feet may nearly face each other (Fig. 17-5). The midpoint of the infant is at the umbilicus, compared with the symphysis pubis in the adult, and the sitting height of the infant is almost 70 percent of his total body length.

HEAD

The baby's cranium is large and the face relatively small compared with the adult head, the ratio of face to cranium being 1:8 in the infant and only 1:2 or 1:2.5 in the adult. The jaws are small, and the poorly developed mandible appears to recede; these bones develop further under the influence of mastication. The lower jaw grows more rapidly than the rest of the face.

Molding

The bones of the cranium are loosely held together by membranes at the suture lines, which allow for considerable molding of the head during labor and delivery, especially in prolonged, difficult labor. Molding may make the head very elongated at birth, but the distortion recedes rapidly and is much improved in 24 to 48 hours. The head assumes its normal shape in about one week (Fig. 17-6A, B).

The head of the infant born by cesarean section or by a breech extraction may not become molded during birth and is often characterized by roundness compared with the usual elongation following delivery of a vertex presentation through the birth canal. Following breech presentation the head may be somewhat flattened at the top or at one side because of pressure on it from the fundus of the uterus, especially during labor.

Asymmetry of the face, caused by fetal posture and pressure *in utero*, may be present at birth, but usually diminishes quite rapidly. A relatively common irregularity is a deviation of the mandible from the midline; this results when the baby's chin is pressed against his shoulder and the mandible is pushed to one side.

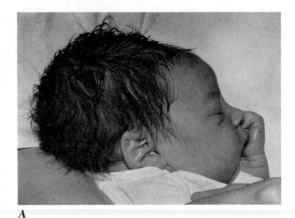

A

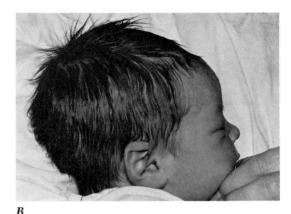

B

Figure 17-6. *A.* Elongation of the head immediately after birth due to molding during labor and delivery. *B.* The same baby 24 hours later when the elongation has receded considerably and the head has assumed a more rounded shape.

The position that the baby assumes during the early weeks of life affects the shape of his head. If he maintains the same position constantly or takes a certain position frequently, temporary deformities may develop since his bones are soft and are not able to resist pressure. If he lies on the back of his head too much, it becomes flattened, and if he is on one side more than the other, his face may become asymmetric. His position must be watched because he likes to turn his head toward the side, seems to prefer one side more than the other, and prefers to turn toward a light if it is not too bright. Changing his position frequently is beneficial. When the infant is too young to change his own position, it is a good plan to alternate the side on which he is placed after each time he is picked up or fed. When he lies on his side, he has a tendency to roll slightly backward; the prone position is therefore best, and it usually appears to be very comfortable. It is wise to recommend to the parents that they use a crib or a bassinet with a firm flat mattress for the baby's sleeping at home.

Caput Succedaneum

A diffuse swelling, known as caput succedaneum, may be present at birth in the soft tissues of the scalp overlying the presenting part of the head. This swelling is due to edema produced by a difference in pressure on the tissues which are pressed directly against the cervix and those which lie over the dilated canal. Circulation is arrested in that part of the scalp which presents over the dilated cervical os. This edema is completely absorbed in one to two days, and the caput rapidly diminishes in size.

Cephalhematoma

Sometimes a swelling, known as a cephalhematoma, appears on the baby's head soon after birth (Fig. 17-7). This swelling is a subperiosteal extravasation of blood due to rupture of a blood vessel and subsequent bleeding beneath the periosteum of one of the cranial bones, usually one of the parietal bones. It is most likely due to trauma of labor and delivery, this trauma probably caused either by friction of the skull against the mother's pelvic bones or by obstetric forceps. A cephalhematoma may occur following either spontaneous or instrumental delivery. The hematoma does not cross suture lines and is therefore limited to the surface of the cranial bone over which it began, but a hematoma may develop over more than one bone. The swelling varies in size, depending on the amount of bleeding; there may be an increase in size during the first few days of life. A superimposed

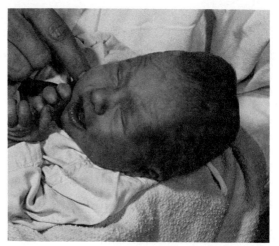

Figure 17-7. A cephalhematoma over the right parietal bone.

caput succedaneum may obscure the swelling of the hematoma until the former has receded. Unlike the caput, a cephalhematoma does not recede quickly and may require weeks for complete absorption. As the hematoma organizes, a hard border may be felt around a soft central area.

A cephalhematoma will disappear spontaneously without treatment, but the area should be protected from further trauma. The hematoma may produce significant amounts of bilirubin as the blood breaks down and is absorbed. Since the hematoma will cause parents considerable concern, they need an explanation of its cause and its expected resolution.

Measurements

The average circumference of the full-term baby's head at birth is 34.2 cm, with usual variations ranging between 32.1 and 36.1 cm in girls and 32.1 and 36.4 cm in boys. The head circumference is approximately 2 cm greater than the chest measurement at birth and remains larger for a few months. A difference greater than 2 cm may be found between the size of the head and the size of the chest in a preterm infant.

The size of the head increases considerably

during infancy because of rapid brain growth; measurements taken at intervals may be valuable in making a diagnosis of failure of brain growth or of a hydrocephalus. The relationship between the head and chest measurements is important, since a disturbance in proper proportion may mean an abnormal development of the head or the chest or may indicate chest or cardiac disease, unless the unusual proportion results from malnutrition or a familial characteristic.

Fontanels

In the examination of the newborn infant, the fontanels are palpated for size and tension. The anterior fontanel, a diamond-shaped area located at the juncture of the two parietal and two frontal bones, is approximately 2 to 3 cm wide and 3 to 4 cm long. The posterior fontanel, which is triangular in shape and located between the occipital and the parietal bones, is much smaller, and on palpation may be found closed, nearly closed, or wide open. The sagittal suture, located between the parietal bones, can easily be palpated; it may vary in size from wide open to almost closed (see Fig. 10-11, page 241, for illustration of fontanels and sutures). Much variation will be found in the size of the fontanels. Owing to an overlapping of skull bones during birth, the size of the fontanels and also the circumference of the head will be smaller shortly after birth than a few days later. When the fontanels are palpated for size, their tension is also noted. An increase in tension may indicate increased intracranial pressure or a hydrocephalus, while a decrease in tension may be found in the presence of dehydration or shock.

THORAX

The thorax is almost cylindrical, with the anteroposterior and lateral diameters the same size. The xiphoid process is often prominent. The average circumference of the chest at birth is 32 cm (12.6 in.), approximately 2 cm less than the circumference of the head. If the chest circumference is less than 30 cm (11.8 in.), the baby is probably low birth weight. In the infant, the ribs are placed horizontally, at right angles to the vertebral column and almost at right angles at the sternum. They are soft, the attached muscles are weak, and little respiratory movement is carried out by the thoracic cage. Most of the respiratory movements are, therefore, accomplished by the diaphragm and the abdominal muscles. When the baby sits up, the ribs begin to slope, they become harder, and the muscles become stronger.

Thymus

The thymus is normally large in the newborn and continues to grow so rapidly that it triples its birth weight by five years of age. Thereafter little change in size takes place for about 10 years, when it finally decreases in size. The thymus is generally not considered a cause of respiratory distress as sometimes previously supposed.

GASTROINTESTINAL TRACT

Inspection of the mouth of the newborn infant reveals it to be shallow, with a flat, hard palate due to the absence of alveolar ridges. Glistening white raised areas, caused by an accumulation of epithelial cells, may be seen on the surface of the hard palate, and sometimes cysts are present on the gums. Neither of these is of significance. The tongue is quite large. The frenum of the tongue is rather short and tight, a condition that does not affect nursing ability because it does not interfere with the use of the tongue in sucking. The newborn infant does not have the ability to move food from his lips to his pharynx and must therefore receive his food on the back of his tongue to be able to swallow it. The salivary glands are immature, and the flow of saliva is minimal until the age of three months, at which time these glands become mature and the amount of saliva increases. The upper lip may be swollen for a short time after nursing, and sometimes a blister, known as the *labial tubercle,* appears in its center immediately following nursing.

Sucking, the means by which the infant gets his food, is assisted by the presence of a series of corrugations in the anterior aspect of the mouth which aid in grasping the nipple, and by strong sucking muscles. Deposits of fatty tissue called *sucking pads* are present in each cheek to prevent indrawing of the cheeks during nursing and to make sucking effective. This mass of fatty tissue, so important in obtaining food, remains even in cases of malnutrition when fat is lost from all other parts of the body; it disappears only when sucking is no longer an essential means of obtaining food.

The capacity of the infant's stomach is difficult to measure; it has the ability to stretch very easily, and it can readily empty its contents into the duodenum. Since its physiologic capacity is greater than its anatomic capacity, it is possible for the newborn infant to take more fluid at a feeding time than the normal capacity of the stomach would indicate it could hold.

The intestinal tract in the infant is longer proportionately than in the adult. It has a large number of secretory glands and a large surface for absorption of food, but is poorly equipped with elastic tissue; the development of musculature is not complete, and nervous control is inadequate. Although the intestinal tract does not function *in utero* in the capacity of digesting and absorbing food, it has some opportunity to use its rather weak muscles. The fetus swallows large amounts of amniotic fluid as early as the fourth month of its intrauterine life (page 102), and a fecal material termed meconium begins to form. This may be expelled *in utero* under hypoxic conditions.

The gastrointestinal tract functions in a much more limited capacity in the fetus than either the circulatory or urinary system and has been active up to the time of birth only to the extent that swallowing and intestinal movements have taken place; nevertheless it is able to assume its functions quite easily. The infant digests and ab-

sorbs a tremendous amount of food in proportion to body weight as compared with an adult. He is quite capable of doing so even before full-term gestation, as is evident in the premature infant. Except for pancreatic amylase, which is deficient for several months, and lipase, which is deficient to a lesser degree, the digestive enzymes seem to be present fairly early in fetal life in an amount adequate to digest simple foods very well, but not complex starches. Hydrochloric acid is produced by the stomach immediately after birth. Absorption of proteins and carbohydrates is very good; the ability to absorb fat is rather poor.

The Stools

The character of the stools of the newborn changes each day during the first week of life. The first stools are meconium, the fecal material that begins to appear in the intestine by the end of the fourth month of fetal life. *Meconium* is a sticky, black, odorless material consisting of lanugo and vernix caseosa swallowed in the amniotic fluid, desquamated cells, digestive secretions, mucus, and bile pigments. The gastrointestinal tract, and therefore also the meconium, is sterile at birth, unless an infection has begun in the uterine cavity owing to ruptured fetal membranes or prolonged labor. Soon after birth it contains ingested bacteria.

Often the first material expelled from the bowel, immediately before meconium, is a thick, grayish-white mucus, called a *mucus plug.* Sometimes the material that is passed prior to the first meconium is a small cylindrical mass, 2 to 5 cm in length, grayish-white in color, and of firm, leathery consistency. This firm material is called a *meconium plug.* It is thick meconium that does not contain bile pigments. A meconium plug may be passed with difficulty and may delay the first stool.

Meconium may be excreted *in utero* under abnormal conditions; or during the birth process, especially in breech delivery, owing to the mechanical result of pressure; or at any time within the first 24 hours after birth. Some meconium is usually passed during the first 8 to 24 hours of life; if none is passed within 24 hours concern for obstruction arises.

The intestinal content changes from meconium to transitional stools and then to milk stools. During the first two to six days the color of the stool changes from black to greenish black, to greenish brown, brownish yellow, greenish yellow, and finally to the yellow color of milk stools. The *transitional stools*, which appear sometime between the second and fourth days, are rather loose, contain some mucus, and are greenish brown or greenish yellow in color. They consist partly of meconium and partly of milk stools.

After the first four to five days the character of the stools depends on the type of feeding. The breast-fed infant usually has yellow, semiformed, curdy stools, which later change to a golden yellow, with a pasty consistency and a characteristically sour odor. Formula feedings cause the stools to be drier, more formed, of a paler yellow or brownish yellow color, and of a rather foul odor. The normal healthy infant may have greenish yellow stools, and curds may be present in those of either the breast-fed or the artificially fed baby. In small amounts, mucus in the stool is not significant, especially in the breast-fed infant.

A minute amount of blood, which follows bowel irritation caused by ingested food or bacteria, may be present in the stools during the first few days and is not significant if the baby does not show any other signs of bleeding. Frank blood, either fresh or old, is abnormal and requires investigation. Blood may be found in the stools if the baby has nursed from a bleeding nipple.

The number of stools per day varies a great deal, tending to be more frequent in the breast-fed than in the artificially fed baby. There may be only one stool daily, but more frequently stools are passed from four to eight times a day in the early days of life. The baby may possibly have a small stool after each feeding. Later the stools become more infrequent. Constipation does not occur in the breast-fed infant and

rarely with artificial feedings. The ingestion of large amounts of milk during the first week or two of life may produce loose stools, but diarrhea of an infectious nature must always be considered a possibility when the stools are loose.

The baby's stools are observed for frequency, color, and consistency. The nurse must consider the day of life and the amount and kind of feeding the baby is taking in judging the normalcy of the color and consistency of the stools. Greenish yellow, curdy stools containing a small amount of mucus are normal in the young infant, and the stools may be loose during the first week or two of life if the baby is ingesting a large quantity of milk. Diarrhea must be considered if the stools are watery. The mother is told of the number and kind of stools she may expect her baby to have and is advised to report watery stools to the physician.

Regurgitation and Vomiting

Regurgitation, or spitting-up, during or soon after a feeding is quite common in the newborn infant, for he has neither the valvular arrangement at the lower end of his esophagus of the adult nor the nervous control that develops later. Some of the feeding may, therefore, escape from the stomach during the first 20 to 30 minutes after a feeding; with the very active baby this may even continue at intervals for a period of 30 to 60 minutes.

Regurgitation can often be reduced by bubbling the baby adequately during and after feedings, by avoiding overfeeding, by handling him gently after feedings, and by positioning. He may be placed on his right side with the head end of the mattress elevated to a 20- to 30-degree angle for a short time after feedings or placed on his abdomen. In these positions the feeding is not pushed up easily and a bubble in the stomach may rise better.

Vomiting may occur during the first two to three days of life; this may be caused by maternal discharges that the baby may have swallowed during passage through the birth canal. The frequency of his vomiting should decrease rapidly; its cause requires investigation if it continues.

A baby may also vomit a feeding if the air he swallowed during a feeding was not eructated immediately after the feeding. When the air leaves the stomach after the baby is placed in his crib, some of the formula may be expelled with the air. Air and food vomited together make the volume appear to be many times the actual amount.

Liver and Spleen

The liver is relatively large, occupying about two fifths of the abdominal cavity, and its lower edge is usually palpable, sometimes 2 to 3 cm below the right costal margin. The liver has served as an important organ in blood formation in fetal life, and it may retain this function to some extent for a few months after birth. Along with its many other functions it is, therefore, one of the extramedullary centers of hematopoiesis, at least to a slight degree, in the newborn infant. Unless the red cell mass at birth was low, enough iron is stored in the liver to carry the baby over the period in which his food, mainly milk, may be iron deficient. This store of iron in the liver is used for hemoglobin formation during the first few months of life; at about the fifth month it is depleted and foods furnishing iron must be added to the diet to prevent anemia, if iron-containing foods have not already been started.

The spleen is also relatively large. Ordinarily, it is not palpable through the abdominal wall, but occasionally its tip can be felt at the costal margin.

GENITOURINARY SYSTEM

Urinary System

The urinary system begins to develop early in fetal life and is ready to function quite adequately at birth. The kidneys have their full number of nephrons at birth, but functional maturation continues postnatally for a variable period of time and is not completed until some time between 6 and 18 months.

Although the kidneys are not essential during fetal life when the placenta is taking care of waste excretion, they assume some function very early. Urine production begins by the end of the first trimester of pregnancy and large amounts of urine are apparently produced by the end of pregnancy. Most of the information about function of the fetal kidney is based on animal studies, but there is reason to believe that assumptions about function of the human kidney can be made from such studies. Amniotic fluid, at least in the latter part of pregnancy, is believed to be largely derived from fetal urine.

Very important adaptation in kidney function must take place quickly in the days after birth. Fluids and electrolytes, previously furnished by the placenta in almost unlimited supply, are much reduced after birth, and the kidney must replace the placenta as the major excretory and regulatory organ. The postnatal kidney must modify its prenatal function of producing large amounts of urine to include conserving fluids and electrolytes.

At the time of birth the kidneys will ordinarily function adequately, but structural and functional development of all components is not yet complete. Maturation continues in the postnatal period in both structure and quality of performance. Development of good renal function is a gradual process, and the adequacy of kidney function continues to increase as the infant grows and develops.

Among some of the differences of the newborn kidney and later maturation are low glomerular filtration rate (GFR), reduced tubular function, and lowered renal plasma flow (RPF). The glomeruli and tubules grow postnatally and the capillary bed increases. GFR, which is only one fourth to one third of that expected for size at birth, gradually increases with age to full function by about 18 months. The newborn can conserve sodium well but has difficulty excreting an increased load of sodium. Renal concentrating ability may be low in the infant. Response to diuresis of water load is inadequate or lacking during the first few days of life. Renal adjustment to various amounts of solutes is fairly good, but when a diet with a high solute load (nitrogen, sodium, potassium, chloride) is fed to a baby and the fluid intake is relatively low, a normal body water and electrolyte balance may be disturbed.

Under favorable circumstances, the needs of the body can be adequately met by the maturing kidney. Stress from disease, drugs, solute or fluid loads, or acidosis will place the newborn into a potentially dangerous position. Fluids and solute loads must be carefully assessed. When parenteral fluids are necessary, the kind and amount must be carefully evaluated. Any necessary drugs are assessed for the kidney's ability for adequate excretion.

Since urine is present in the bladder at birth, the infant frequently voids immediately after he is born, but emptying of the bladder may be delayed for 12 to 24 hours, and sometimes even longer. Many babies have voided within 8 hours, 50 percent have voided by 12 hours, and over 90 percent by 24 hours. There is need for concern if the baby has not voided by 48 hours.

Urinary output may be relatively low, and voidings may be scanty during the first few days of life or until fluid intake has increased, unless the baby is edematous at birth. This edema fluid excreted through the kidneys soon after birth may make the first voidings large and frequent. Ordinarily, however, urinary output is low until fluid intake increases, which will then increase both frequency and volume. The amount of urinary output is greater proportionately in the child than in the adult.

The total amount of urine voided per day is from 30 to 60 ml (1 to 2 oz) during the first two days of life; and the amount then increases up to approximately 200 to 225 ml (7 oz) by the end of one week. The frequency of voiding increases from an average of two to six times per day during the first few days up to 10 to 15 times per day and even up to 20 times a day after the immediate postnatal period. This frequency de-

creases again when the child gains bladder control.

The first urine voided, often shortly after birth, was formed *in utero* and is dilute. After the first voiding, which may be clear and pale, the urine appears cloudy and quite highly colored owing to more concentration and its rather high urate and mucus content. After fluid intake increases, the urine again becomes a pale yellow color. It is practically odorless during infancy.

Uric acid excretion in the newborn is high; it may be deposited in crystal form in the kidneys and produce uric acid infarcts. As these uric acid crystals are passed in the urine, they may appear as red (brick-dust) spots on the baby's diaper and are sometimes confused with blood in the urine.

The number of voidings daily is recorded, and note is taken of amounts that appear either scanty or excessively large. Highly colored, concentrated urine, evidence of uric acid crystals, or observation of abnormal conditions such as blood is charted and reported to the physician. Efforts to increase fluid intake may be necessary when voiding is scanty and infrequent and when uric acid crystals are seen on the diaper.

In physical examination of the newborn, the lower pole of both kidneys may be felt under favorable circumstances, when the flanks are palpated. The bladder in a baby is an abdominal organ, because the pelvic cavity in the newborn is too small to contain it.

External Genitalia of the Female Infant

The external genitalia of both sexes show definite sex characteristics by the time the fetus is three months old, and they are quite well developed at birth. However, the labia majora are somewhat underdeveloped and do not lie in close proximity as in the older child, thereby making the labia minora appear relatively large. A hymenal tag is often present. The vagina contains a mucous discharge, which may be slightly bloody during the first week of life.

The vulva should be cleaned by gentle washing with soap and water; special care must be taken to separate the labia to remove secretion that may collect between the labia minora and majora. At birth there is a heavy layer of vernix caseosa between the labia, which may be washed away over a period of several days. It is impossible to remove all of this vernix at one time without vigorous effort, and it is therefore better to remove a little each day by gently washing between the labia at bath time and whenever the buttocks are cleaned following a stool. This vernix should, however, be completely washed away by the time the baby is discharged from the hospital.

Genitalia of the Male Infant

Although the external genitalia are well developed, the size of the scrotum and penis varies considerably. The scrotum may be edematous and may contain some fluid at birth, but this condition is usually not a true hydrocele and disappears in a few days. The testes have, in most instances, descended into the scrotum by the ninth month of intrauterine life, but occasionally one or both have remained in the inguinal canal or less frequently in the abdomen. Ordinarily, they descend in the next few weeks or months. The prepuce of the penis is usually adherent to the glans and does not separate until after several months of postnatal development.

Care of the genitalia of the male infant consists of cleaning the glans of the penis. *Smegma*, a cheeselike material, collects under the foreskin and, with bacteria added, produces irritation. The time at which retraction of the foreskin is begun varies. Often a circumcision is performed early, and the glans is cleaned each day thereafter. If the baby is not circumcised, some physicians advise retraction of the foreskin beginning a few days after birth; others recommend postponing complete retraction of the foreskin for several months, since an adherent foreskin at birth may separate with further development and is then much easier to retract.

Until the physician has circumcised the baby or has retracted the foreskin for the first time, the nurse may retract it a short distance daily, only as far as this can easily be done, remove the smegma from the exposed part of the glans with water or oil, and then pull the skin back to its original position. Adherence of the skin to the glans will usually prevent the nurse from being able to retract the foreskin completely for the first time during the early days of life. If the physician recommends early complete retraction, he may dilate the prepuce and draw it over the glans. After this first retraction the nurse may be instructed to continue the procedure daily and to use oil to clean the glans of smegma. After retraction the foreskin must be pulled back into its normal position, over the glans, within a few seconds, because its tightness will reduce circulation in the penis, cause edema, and soon make it impossible to draw it forward. A *paraphimosis* would then develop.

Circumcision

A circumcision, surgical removal of the foreskin of the penis, is frequently performed on the newborn baby. Circumcision is said to be done to make cleaning of the glans easier, to help prevent disturbances such as inflammation of the prepuce and the glans, and to lower the incidence of penile carcinoma and repeated infection. Others say that routine circumcision of newborns is not indicated and that the advantages claimed for circumcision are equally present in persons who practice good personal hygiene. A phimosis, a severe degree of narrowing of the foreskin, may necessitate circumcision.

The Committee on Fetus and Newborn of the American Academy of Pediatrics stated in 1971 that there are no valid medical indications for circumcision in the neonatal period. The present Committee has undertaken a review of the data to support arguments "pro" and "con" circumcision of the newborn, and finds no basis for changing this statement.

Nevertheless, traditional, cultural, and religious factors play a part in the decision made by parents, pediatrician, obstetrician, or family practitioner on behalf of a son. It is the responsibility of the physician to provide parents with factual and informative medical options regarding circumcision. The final decision is theirs and should be based on true informed consent.[7]

Circumcision when done is usually performed before the baby is discharged from the hospital if his condition is good, which means that for the normal full-term baby the operation is often done on the second or third day of life. This is at a time when physiologic hypoprothrombinemia would ordinarily be present, but it is usually not a problem because vitamin K_1 is often administered at birth to prevent a transitory deficiency in blood coagulation in the early days of life. A bleeding and coagulation time is sometimes indicated before the operation.

Sometimes a circumcision is performed immediately after birth, before the baby leaves the delivery room, if his condition is good. For most, this is inadvisable so early in life for at least two reasons. The baby is separated from his mother at a critical time of infant–maternal bonding, and the baby is subjected to loss of body heat to the cool environment of the delivery room unless special precautions are taken to provide warmth.

Jewish parents may wish to observe the religious rite of circumcision. Prayers are recited during the circumcision, and it may be performed by a rabbi who is called a *mohel*. Separate facilities are arranged for a ritual circumcision.

A circumcision is usually carried out on the obstetric unit. It is a sterile procedure; the physician uses sterile gloves, instruments, draping towels, and skin preparation solutions. The nurse restrains the baby for the operation on a Y board, which holds the legs firmly separate, or she can restrain him very satisfactorily by grasping his legs and holding them firmly apart.

The baby should not be fed for an hour or more before operation because he may regurgitate his feeding during the operation. The procedure is frequently performed without anesthesia. (Anesthesia, if used, is administered locally.) Early operation is apparently not very painful, but the baby will cry, often because of the restraint as well as from discomfort of the operation. The nurse can sometimes comfort the baby during the procedure; a sterile nipple used as a pacifier may be quite effective.

The baby will usually stop crying as soon as he is removed from the restraints, but the nurse may continue comforting him by holding him for a short time. Perhaps the mother would provide the greatest source of comfort to the baby after his circumcision. There is no contraindication to feeding the baby after his circumcision if he appears hungry. The mother may appreciate the opportunity to give him his feeding, since she will have been anxious over her baby's operation.

After circumcision the nurse must watch the area for postoperative bleeding. If bleeding occurs, the nurse applies pressure to the operative site with sterile gauze and notifies the physician. The dressing on the operative area may be removed after the first voiding if it has been applied loosely; if it was applied firmly, it may remain in place for a day or two. The nurse should ascertain the physician's preference for aftercare. A sterile gauze to which sterile petroleum jelly has been applied may be placed over the penis each time the baby's diaper is changed. The mother may be instructed to continue this care at home until the operative area has healed sufficiently to prevent the diaper from adhering to it.

It may be necessary to retract regularly the foreskin that remains following a circumcision, after danger of bleeding is past, in order to prevent adhesions to the glans during the healing process. If adhesions do form, the doctor will separate them later with a sterile probe or small forceps.

[7] Committee on Fetus and Newborn, American Academy of Pediatrics, "Report of the Ad Hoc Task Force on Circumcision," *Pediatrics 56:610*–611 (Oct.) 1975.

Skin

The skin is dark red or pinkish red shortly after birth and changes to a pinker hue in a week or two. Pallor, especially if accompanied by pale lips and pale mucous membranes, is not normal. The hands and feet are often a slightly cyanotic color for an hour or two after birth, during which time the peripheral circulation improves. A persistent blueness of the hands and feet or cyanosis of other parts of the body is suggestive of heart disease, pulmonary pathology, or birth injury. Between the third and fourteenth days varying degrees of jaundice of the skin may be present.

Petechiae, accompanied by bluish discoloration of the skin, may be seen on the face for a day or two after delivery as a result of pressure during birth. Edema and extravasation of blood into the tissues of the buttocks and genitalia are frequently seen following a breech delivery because of pressure changes in the area lying over the cervical opening, as well as bruising of the tissues as the breech is pushed through the birth canal (Fig. 17-8).

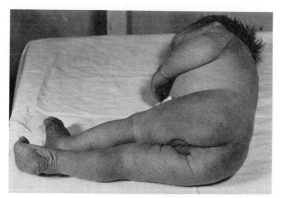

Figure 17-8. Infant delivered by breech extraction—age 18 hours. The legs continue to assume the intrauterine position by remaining in extension, with the toes pointing toward the shoulders. There are edema and extravasation of blood into the tissues of the buttocks and genitalia. This is the result of pressure changes in the area which presented at the cervical opening during labor and bruising of the tissues as the breech was pushed through the birth canal.

Vernix caseosa, a greasy, white, cheeselike material, consisting of an accumulation of secretion from the sebaceous glands and including epithelial cells and lanugo hair, covers the skin at birth. This material may be present as a very thin covering or as a thick layer; it is especially heavy in folds and creases of the skin and between the labia. The vernix caseosa absorbs, rubs off on the clothing, or dries and falls off within the first day, except that present in the creases.

Lanugo hair, the downy covering that develops on the fetus during the fourth month and begins to disappear after the eighth lunar month of intrauterine life, may still be present on certain parts of the body, especially over the shoulders, back, ear lobes, or forehead (Fig. 17-9). Most of the lanugo is lost during the first week of the neonatal period. The covering of the head varies from almost complete baldness to a growth of thick, dark hair extending over the temples; this hair may later be lost and replaced by a new growth. Eyebrows and eyelashes are present, but may be thin and very light in appearance.

An ample distribution of subcutaneous fat gives the full-term baby's skin a soft, elastic texture. The epidermis comes off in flakes during the first week or two of life, and peeling of the skin may be quite generalized. During this time

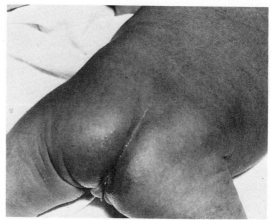

Figure 17-9. A baby's back covered with lanugo hair.

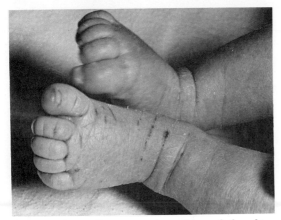

Figure 17-10. Dryness and cracking of the skin, which are often temporarily present in the newborn—this infant is 4 days old.

the skin may be very dry, and fissures at the wrists and ankles are not uncommon (Fig. 17-10). Occasionally desquamation of the hands and feet is seen at birth.

Milia, pinpoint-sized white spots beneath the epidermis, may be seen over the nose and chin during the first one to two weeks. These spots are concretions of sebaceous material that has been retained in the ducts of the sebaceous glands.

The newborn infant's skin is very sensitive. Some babies have benign, self-limited eruptions, called *erythema toxicum* (erythema neonatorum). These eruptions appear as splotchy erythematous blotches, or as firm white papules or hivelike areas on an erythematous base (Fig. 17-11). On some babies they appear and disappear at intervals during the first few days of life, often following slight irritation from clothing or bathing or after a period of crying. Etiology of these eruptions is unknown. There are no apparent related systemic symptoms and treatment is not necessary.

The skin of the newborn is very thin and even minor irritations easily produce rashes and breaks in the skin. *Denuded areas* are seen following even minor, but frequent, irritation of one specific site. The active baby may rub some part of his body, mainly his nose, knees, or toes,

against the crib covers during crying and break the skin enough to cause active bleeding. The skin of the buttocks is likewise irritated easily, and if the baby has frequent stools, the buttocks may become quite raw and sore.

Flat *hemangiomatous areas*, light red in appearance, may be present on the upper eyelids, between the eyebrows, on the upper lip, or at the nape of the neck; these eventually fade and disappear between one and two years of age. *Papillomas* of the skin may be present; they are seen most frequently near or in front of an ear. Babies of Negro or Oriental parents and of parents from Mediterranean countries may have bluish pigmented areas, known as *mongolian spots*, on the back or the buttocks. Babies of dark-skinned races may also have areas of dark pigmentation in certain localized areas, especially over the genitalia and at the base of the nails.

Sweat glands are present over all of the skin, but babies usually do not sweat during the first one to two days of life. Sweating begins on the face at about the third day of life in full-term infants and later over other parts of the body. Sweating will vary markedly with ambient and body temperature, with activity, and with fever. *Sebaceous glands* are active up to and immedi-

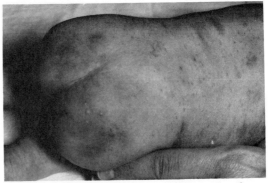

Figure 17-11. Erythema toxicum (erythema neonatorum) on the back of a newborn. Some babies develop these benign eruptions which appear as erythematous blotches or as firm pale-yellow or white papules on an erythematous base. They are likely to appear at intervals after slight irritation from clothing or bathing or after a period of crying.

ately after birth. Shortly thereafter, when maternal androgens are no longer present, they become quiescent and remain so until puberty.

Insensible water loss through the skin can be great in the newborn because the thin skin and relatively large body surface in relation to body mass permit a large loss. Fluid loss through the skin may be very significant in preterm infants and in babies under radiant warmers (page 719).

The baby's fingernails are well developed and may extend well beyond the tips of the fingers. The toenails are also well formed, but may appear embedded at the distal end.

Care of the Skin

Care of the skin of the newborn during the hospital stay has changed from time to time. About 40 years ago the so-called "dry" technique of skin care began to replace the use of soap and water or oil baths, because there was evidence that the less handling the skin received, the less the irritation, and consequently the less the danger of infection. Thereafter, the hazard of staphylococcal infections among infants in newborn nurseries brought about another change. A bath with a liquid detergent containing 3 percent hexachlorophene was often used in an effort to reduce the rate of skin and nasal colonization by staphylococci and possibly reduce the incidence of skin infection.

A number of recent studies have raised questions concerning the toxicity to the central nervous system of 3 percent hexachlorophene preparations when used daily for total body bathing of newborns. According to the *FDA Drug Bulletin*, December, 1971, the FDA and the Committee on Fetus and Newborn of the American Academy of Pediatrics have "jointly concluded that the use of hexachlorophene for total body bathing of infants in hospital nurseries or at home is not recommended." In its place the committee recommends the following procedures:

At present we recommend dry skin care, washing with plain soap and water or tap water alone for skin

care of the newborn infants. It should be emphasized that the most important factor in the transmission of infection from infant to infant is hand contact. This can be minimized by scrupulous hand washing before entering the nursery as well as just before and just after handling each infant. Either an iodophor preparation or 3% hexachlorophene emulsion is recommended.[8]

Following the above recommendations the question of a possible increase in staphylococcal infection was raised. Since then some hospitals have reported cases of staphylococcal infection, manifested mainly by a pustular dermatitis or impetigo. Where bacterial outbreaks have appeared, the FDA has permitted use of hexachlorophene temporarily for once-daily bathing of infants.

The "dry" technique is used between soap and water baths. It may also be used if a soap and water bath is postponed because of a baby's adverse condition or postponed until the baby has regained a normal temperature. Sometimes the "dry" technique is used throughout the baby's hospital stay. In this method of care, water or oil is not used on the baby's skin, with the exception of small areas that need special attention. As soon as possible after birth, blood on the baby's face and scalp is washed away with cotton balls or a soft washcloth dipped into warm water, and the baby is wrapped in a warm blanket. No attempt is made to wash or wipe off the vernix caseosa. To avoid undue chilling, the baby may be wrapped in the warm blanket before the blood is removed from his face and scalp.

The vernix acts as a vanishing cream and rubs into the skin or off onto the clothes within 12 to 24 hours. It remains for a longer time, however, in the creases and folds of skin where a heavy deposit may be found. Instead of being protected, these areas may become irritated if vernix is left indefinitely, and it should therefore be removed in 24 to 48 hours.

[8] U.S. Department of Health, Education, and Welfare, Public Health Service, Food and Drug Administration, *FDA Drug Bulletin*, December, 1971, Rockville, Md.

The dry technique does not eliminate daily morning care. The only omission is use of soap and water or oil. Inspection of the condition of the skin and of the eyes, nose, mouth, ears, umbilicus, and genitalia must be done as thoroughly as any observation made during the more traditional bath. Special care must be taken to inspect the creases behind the ears, around the neck, in the axillae, and in the groin for skin irritation. The skin may become very dry and peel in large flakes after a few days, and dry cracks may appear around the wrists and ankles (Fig. 17-10). This drying is not significant except insofar as it causes the mother concern; the nurse explains that it is a temporary condition of the skin that does no harm and that after a few days the flakiness and cracks will disappear. It is important for the nurse to note and report to the physician moist irritated areas, pustules, or water blisters which may be impetigo and therefore may need special attention.

Even with the dry technique it is necessary to use some water on the baby's skin, but the amount is minimal. The face is washed with clear, warm water and a soft washcloth to remove regurgitated formula or mucus. The vernix that remains in the axillae may be spread as cream to other parts of the body during the first day or two; after that the axillae are wiped with a wet cloth during daily morning care unless the skin in that area is dry. The groin and buttocks are washed with warm water each time the diaper is changed and sometimes bland soap is necessary. Some authorities recommend using petroleum jelly or an ointment for the diaper area, but others are opposed to such use during the hospital stay because they believe a moist skin is more susceptible to infection than one that is kept completely dry. When lubricants are used on the diaper area, they must be used from an individual container for each infant to avoid cross contamination.

After a thorough inspection of the skin, the morning care is completed and the baby is dressed in clean clothes. Fingernails and toenails may need trimming if they extend beyond the ends of the fingers and toes.

If plain soap and water is used for bathing, the first bath is postponed for several hours until the baby has regained his normal body temperature or longer if the baby's condition warrants protection against exposure. It is given as a sponge bath to avoid getting the umbilical cord wet. The baby should be protected against chilling by keeping as much of the body covered as is possible during the bath or by working under a radiant heat lamp.

Infants are very susceptible to skin irritation. They may develop a heat rash, especially in the neck region and in the groin, if they become too warm for even a short period of time. Occasionally pinpoint- or pinhead-sized erythematous papules or vesicular lesions develop. Such irritations are often treated by washing the affected area and keeping it dry and by using less clothing. A baby may develop a chafing, called *intertrigo*, where two moist surfaces rub together, especially in the creases of the neck, in the axillae, and in the groin. These areas are also washed and kept as dry as possible, and cornstarch may be applied. Abrasions may occur on the heels, toes, or knees from kicking or rubbing against the sheets. Further irritation is prevented and healing takes place if the areas are bandaged. Although a baby's skin is very sensitive and frequently shows signs of minor insignificant irritations, the nurse must be alert for evidence of infection, which requires immediate treatment and precautions against spread to other infants.

Frequent diaper changes and careful cleaning of the buttocks of urine and stool are important in prevention of raw buttocks; such care is essential when there is evidence of skin irritation. If the buttocks become sore, an ointment such as petroleum jelly, zinc oxide, or one of several commercial preparations, such as vitamin A and D ointment or methylbenzethonium (Diaparene), may be applied; it helps keep the stool off the raw area and aids in the healing process. Exposure to air helps in healing; during exposure the baby's diaper is placed under him, but is not pinned on. The baby must be protected against chilling while exposed. Treatment may be alternated by exposing the buttocks to the air while the baby is asleep and applying an ointment when he is picked up to be fed.

UMBILICAL CORD

The umbilical cord begins to discolor and shrink soon after birth; within a few days the stump has shriveled and turned black, and a red line of demarcation has begun to appear at the juncture of the umbilical cord with the skin of the abdomen. This skin may extend just to the base of the cord, or it may extend up onto the cord a short distance. By the sixth to tenth day the cord has atrophied to a dry black string; it then sloughs off and leaves a small granulating area, which heals entirely in another week (Fig. 17-12). The amount of granulation tissue is determined by the amount of Wharton's jelly that was present in the umbilical cord. Occasionally there is a delay in separation of the cord into the third week of life, but this is not significant if the cord appears dry and healthy.

The blood vessels at the base of the umbilical cord are sealed off by the formation of thrombi, but final obliteration does not occur until toward the end of the neonatal period when the thrombi organize and the vessels become fibrous cords. Until this anatomic closure has occurred, the blood vessels are portals of entry to pathogenic organisms.

An umbilical hernia may develop, but strapping of the area is not recommended. A strap or abdominal band offers no benefits and may cause skin irritation or infection. The hernia usually disappears during the baby's first year.

Care of the Umbilical Cord

Care of the umbilical cord immediately after birth has been described in Chapter 15. To avoid serious hemorrhage from the cord stump, it must be observed closely during the next 24 hours for evidence of bleeding; inspection may be necessary every one-half to one hour until it appears quite evident that bleeding will proba-

bly not occur. The danger of bleeding is greatest when the cord contains a large amount of Wharton's jelly, which shrinks and leaves a previously tight ligature or tight clamp loose. In some instances bleeding does not occur even when the

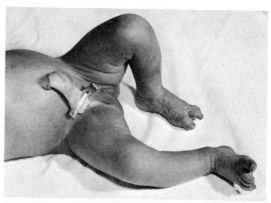

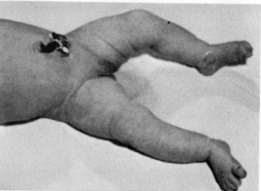

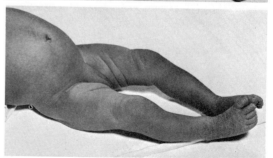

Figure 17-12. Mummification and separation of the umbilical cord. *Top:* Appearance of the umbilical cord six hours after birth. *Center:* Appearance of the umbilical cord four days after birth. *Bottom:* Appearance of the umbilicus one day after the separation of the umbilical cord.

ligature is loose because a blood clot has formed at the end of the cord stump. This clot may become loosened, however, with manipulation or movements of the baby, and bleeding may then occur. The quickest way to stop bleeding from the cord is to apply a sterile hemostatic forceps. This should be placed as far away from the abdominal wall as possible, allowing for adequate room to apply another ligature or clamp should the forceps in some way injure the cord itself and make hemostasis at this point impossible. After bleeding has been controlled with the hemostatic forceps, the nurse or doctor can apply another ligature or clamp, using aseptic technique.

In daily care of the umbilical area, it is important that asepsis be maintained until healing is complete. Until then, pyogenic bacteria can produce an infection that may even extend to the peritoneum, to the liver, or into the blood stream. Careful hand washing before caring for the area is important. Moisture in the area should be kept at a minimum by avoiding putting the baby's diaper on so high that the cord is moist for long periods from a wet diaper. An umbilical cord dressing is currently not used.

Daily care of the umbilical cord often consists of wiping the stump and the area around the umbilicus with an antiseptic. Alcohol, 60 percent, is frequently used. It also acts as a "drying" agent. Some physicians recommend painting the cord with a bacteriostatic such as triple dye. After the cord drops off, further treatment may not be used or the granulating area may be cared for by wiping with an antiseptic until it is completely healed. This may take another few days.

As she cares for the cord, the nurse should note any signs of infection and report these to the physician immediately. There should be no odor or moistness of the cord while it is mummifying. If it is moist, which is indicative of a mild infection, or if there is a moist granulating area at the base of the cord with a slightly mucoid or purulent discharge, the physician orders a culture of the discharge to identify the organism and further treatment, sometimes application of an antibiotic ointment.

The mother should be instructed in the care of the umbilicus before the baby leaves the hospital. If the cord is still on, she is told that it will soon be found loose and that there will probably be a small amount of bloody discharge from the navel for a few days, but that the navel should appear more healed every day. She should be instructed concerning precautions to keep the area clean and advised not to give the baby a tub bath or to allow the navel to get wet until the scab has come off and the area is completely healed. It is advisable to give the mother an opportunity to care for the umbilicus before she leaves the hospital, especially if she has anxiety over care of the umbilical cord.

HORMONE REACTIONS

Breast hypertrophy, uterine bleeding, and vulvar or prostatic hypertrophy may occur in the genital organs of newborn infants. These changes are produced by maternal or placental hormones which have been transmitted through the placenta and are temporarily present.

A number of those changes probably result from a dominant influence of maternal steroids, particularly estrogens, which are at a high level in the mother's blood just before labor. These easily cross the placenta. After birth the tissues of the newborn that were stimulated by the steroids soon regress to their normal state of development, and some of the changes that occur are due to the sudden withdrawal of maternal hormones.

The moist, congested, external genitalia, hymenal tags of tissue, and vaginal discharge, at first watery and later a thick, white mucoid material, are a result of the endocrine substances that affect the genital organs. The maternal hormones present in the fetus and their subsequent withdrawal and exhaustion following birth are considered responsible for the hypertrophied vaginal epithelium, resembling the adult type, which is present at birth, and for the desquamation and mucosal changes with regression to an infantile type of tissue, which takes place in two to three days. Within a week or two after birth, congestion of the genitalia has disappeared, and vaginal discharge decreases.

Bleeding from the vagina, which occurs in some infants during the first neonatal week, is also caused by a temporary imbalance in the endocrine system, which produces hyperemia of the pelvic organs and subsequent bleeding. This pseudomenstruation is considered physiologic, occurring because of the activity of the maternal hormones transmitted to the baby *in utero* and subsequently withdrawn at birth.

Another manifestation of reactions produced by maternal hormones is breast enlargement, with swelling and tenseness; this may occur in babies of either sex during the first week of life (Fig. 17-13). A milky fluid, called witch's milk, may be secreted from the engorged breasts. Engorgement and secretion are much more pronounced in some babies than others. They also disappear in approximately one month.

IMMUNITY

Antibodies to diphtheria and tetanus and antiviral immune bodies against measles, smallpox, mumps, poliomyelitis, and probably some other infectious diseases pass from the mother to the infant through the placenta, provided the mother herself has an immunity to the disease. There is very little or no inherited immunity to whooping cough or herpesvirus. This relative, not absolute, inherited passive immunity lasts for varying periods of time; for some infections the period of resistance may be very short, while for others it may be active for several months. The average half-life for the passively transferred IgG immunoglobulins is between 20 and 30 days. Their concentration in serum drops quite rapidly thereafter and reaches a low level between two and four months of age. This period is referred to as physiologic hypogam-

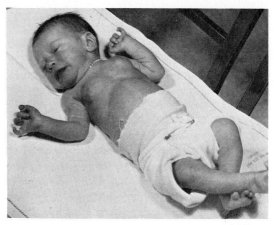

Figure 17-13. Breast engorgement in the newborn infant. Engorgement may occur in an infant of either sex during the first week of life.

maglobulinemia. There is no immunity to many of the organisms to which the neonate is most apt to be exposed; for example, the staphylococcus and cold and flu viruses. This makes good asepsis essential in the care of all newborns.

In addition to providing protection for the newborn, the passively acquired IgG antibodies may interfere with active antibody production while they are present. Immunization with killed vaccines, however, such as diphtheria and pertussis, is usually begun at 2 to 3 months. Live virus immunization, with the exception of polio, is delayed until the end of the first year of life. Exposure to antigens in the environment results in an increase in gamma globulin in the baby's first years of life.

Placental transfer of antibodies is discussed on page 84 and deficiency of antibodies in the newborn is described on page 816.

NERVOUS SYSTEM

The brain of the newborn is in a period of rapid growth at the time of birth. The nerve cells, called neurons, are formed primarily between 10 and 18 weeks gestation. The adult number of neurons is established quite early in the baby's development. After this period of neuronal development, a period of rapid brain growth begins. The brain growth spurt appears to start at about midpregnancy and continues well into the second postnatal year. Further gradual growth of the brain continues until its maturity is reached.

In the weeks and months immediately following birth the brain grows rapidly, and a number of functionally important processes take place. Glial cells, which form a protective and supportive framework for the nerves throughout the brain and spinal cord; dendrites, the short, thick protoplasmic projections of the nerve cell body that receive impulses; and synapses, junctions where two neurons come into functional contact, multiply and grow. Myelination progresses.

John Dobbing states:

The demonstration that the human brain growth spurt is much more postnatal than was formerly thought creates a new opportunity to ensure one important positive . . . , by actively promoting good bodily growth at the time when this most important organ is passing through its own vulnerable period of growth.[9]

The newborn's motor coordination is quite sophisticated. Some of his behaviors are necessary for survival, and some have no apparent immediate usefulness. Many actions show good motor control; others demonstrate immaturity of the central nervous system and poor cerebral influence. Poor nervous system control makes the baby "jumpy"; he startles easily, at times his chin quivers, and frequently he has tremors (quivering movements) of short duration of the arms and legs. Much of the baby's motor behavior seems to be under control of the spinal cord and the medulla.

Although the nervous system is relatively im-

[9] John Dobbing, The later development of the brain and its vulnerability, in *Scientific Foundations of Paediatrics*, edited by John A. Davis and John Dobbing. Heinemann, London, 1974, p. 576.

mature at birth, cortical activity appears to have more influence on behavior than has been suspected in the past. The newborn is able to turn toward sounds, follow objects with his eyes, take food when hungry, cry when hungry or in pain, maintain good postural muscle tone, show spontaneous alertness and activity, and become quiet when comforted.

Certain behavior patterns, including those which regulate intrauterine movements, are present before the baby is born, but it is after birth that behavior becomes more coordinated and comes under the higher levels of control. Development takes place rapidly. Soon certain pathways that control the activity of various muscles are used, nerve fibers make new connections with one another, more complex behavior patterns develop, and the higher cerebral levels begin to function. Gradually, coordinated movements, conditioned reflexes, habits, inhibitions, and discriminations develop.

The brain matures rapidly and in an integrated orderly process. Each added function is incorporated with those already present. As development proceeds, more and more regulation of behavior is taken over by the cerebral cortex. Generalized mass movements are replaced by specific individual responses. Rapid development of consciousness, arousal, and responsiveness to surroundings indicates ongoing brain maturation.

Reflexes

The baby is born with certain reflexes that are significant to note as evidences of normal development. Their presence or absence and the time at which they appear or disappear are indicative of progress. The manner in which they are used gives evidence of the functioning of the nervous system. For example, a weak or absent reflex may indicate the presence of a lesion in the central nervous system. Certain reflexes, which are evidences of immaturity, are normal only in the newborn infant. With normal development of the nervous system, they disappear in the first few months of extrauterine life.

A baby's reflex response may depend upon his behavioral state. While one response may be diminished when tested during light sleep, another may be checked during this state or deep sleep. Sucking may change a response. Some reflexes are present in all states. Some should not be tested when the baby is sleepy; an alert period may be the most desirable time to check reflexes.

Moro Reflex

The Moro reflex is a vestibular reflex that demonstrates an awareness of equilibrium in the newborn infant. It requires certain nerve tracts which are present and can be elicited at birth, unless there has been damage to either the central nervous system or the peripheral nerves.

The Moro reflex is tested when the baby is lying quietly. It is more easily elicited when he is undressed. A sudden stimulus, such as jarring of the table on which the baby lies, sudden jerking of his blanket, or a sudden change in posi-

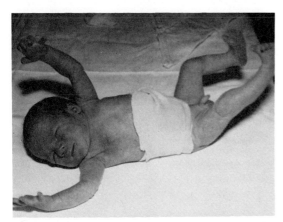

Figure 17-14. The Moro reflex. A sudden stimulus causes the baby to stiffen his body, draw up his legs, and throw his arms up and out. He will next bring his arms forward as in an embrace position and he may begin to cry. The response of the arms and legs is symmetric in the normal infant. The semiflexion of the thumb and index finger of each hand, forming the shape of a C, which normally occurs during the Moro reflex, can be seen on this baby's left hand. (Note the mottling of the skin, which is probably due to circulatory instability and exposure.)

tion elicits the response. The baby stiffens his body, draws up his legs, and throws his arms up and out and then brings them forward as in an embrace position (Fig. 17-14). It may be noted that he also semiflexes the thumb and index finger of each hand, forming the shape of a C and extends the remaining fingers. The baby often begins to cry at the end of his embrace gesture. Movement of the arms is the most prominent feature of this reflex. Their movements should be symmetric. When one arm does not come forward, the possibility of an injury to the arm, the clavicle, or a nerve must be considered.

If the Moro reflex is absent at birth but present on the following day, its previous absence may have been due to edema of the brain; the reflex returns when the edema subsides. If this reflex is present at birth but absent soon thereafter, increasing edema of the brain or slow bleeding due to intracranial hemorrhage is considered as a possible cause of its disappearance. If brain injury has occurred during delivery, the reflex is absent at birth and for the next several days; it will return, however, in three or four days if the damage is not too severe.

The characteristics of the Moro reflex pattern depends upon gestational age. In the immature baby, below 30 weeks gestation, the Moro reflex is not well developed and is barely apparent or easily exhaustible. The second phase of the reflex, the flexion component, becomes stronger as the infant matures; it is not fully developed until after 35 weeks gestation. While checking the Moro reflex it is well to note separately the degree of abduction at shoulders and extension and flexion at elbows, and also the ease with which the reflex is elicited. The Moro reflex normally disappears two to three months after full term.

Tonic Neck Reflex (*The Asymmetrical Reflex*)

The tonic neck reflex is a postural reflex in which the baby assumes a fencing position. When this reflex is present, it will be noted that, as the baby lies on his back and rotates his head to either side, the arm and leg on the side

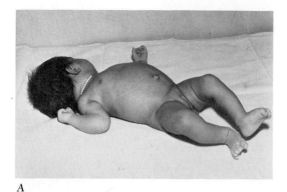

A

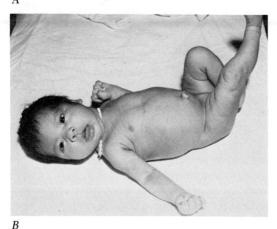

B

Figure 17-15. The tonic neck reflex. *A.* As the baby lies on her back with her head turned to her left side, her left arm and left leg are partly extended and her right arm and right leg are flexed. *B.* As the baby turned her head to the right side, she extended her right arm and right leg and flexed her left arm and left leg.

to which his head faces are partly or completely extended and the opposite arm and leg are flexed (Fig. 17-15). The tonic neck reflex develops in the fetus by 28 weeks, and it disappears in the newborn by the age of two or three months. The reflex is more marked and persists longer in spastic babies.

The Neck Righting Response

If the head of a healthy full-term newborn is turned to one side, his trunk will follow. The receptors of the neck righting reflex are located in the muscles and joints of the neck. It is present at birth and strongest at the age of three months. This reflex is the first of several that develop to help the baby to restore the normal position of his head in space and maintain the normal postural relationship of his head and trunk. Other righting reflexes will develop as the baby gets older to help him to roll over, to get on his hands and knees, and to sit up.

Grasp Reflex

The grasp reflex is present in both the hands and the feet. The baby will grasp an object placed into his hands, hold on tightly for a short time, and then drop it (Fig. 17-16). The grasp of a full-term baby may be strong enough to support his weight and lift him to a standing position. Holding a finger firmly against the sole of the foot just below the toes will elicit a plantar grasp causing all of the toes to turn downward at the same time. Although grasping is a reflex at birth, it later becomes voluntary and purposeful. The reflex is strongest at full term, becomes much weaker by two months, and usually disappears by the age of three months. Sucking movements enhance the grasp reflex.

Traction Response

The traction response can easily be tested at the same time as the grasp reflex. After the baby has grasped the examiner's fingers with both hands, he is gently pulled into a sitting position.

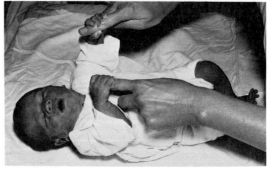

Figure 17-16. The grasp reflex. The baby will grasp an object placed in his hands and hold on tightly for a short time.

The examiner uses his other fingers to assist the baby in his grasp. A vigorous baby will show flexion tone in his arms by flexing his elbows, will show good ability to support his head so that it does not lag completely, and he will hold on to the examiner's finger with a strong grasp.

Withdrawal Reflex

The withdrawal reflex (from unpleasant stimuli) is well developed in every healthy newborn, full-term and premature. It is present from any point of the skin, but is most easily assessed when the sole of the foot is stimulated.

Placing, Standing, Crawling, and Walking Reflexes

To check the placing response the baby is lifted with both of the examiner's hands under the baby's arms and around his chest. He is held so that his insteps touch the protruding edge of a table. If he is alert at the time of this test, he will flex his knees and hips and lift his feet and place them on the table. If his trunk is lowered after this placing movement, his leg extensors become activated, and he makes a response with a standing movement.

The full-term, alert baby will make crawling movements when he is placed on his abdomen and stepping movements when he is held in an upright position, leaning slightly forward, with the soles of his feet touching the surface of a table (Figs. 17-17 and 17-18). These reflexes are present in the premature but are weak, and the baby walks on his toes. The walking reflex becomes much better developed by 36 weeks ges-

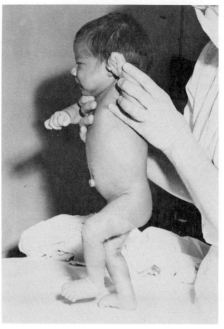

Figure 17-18. Stepping movements. (Note that this baby's umbilical cord has separated and fallen off, but the skin of the abdomen which had extended up on the umbilical cord a short distance appears quite prominent.)

tation. It disappears by three or four weeks of age. The walking reflex must disappear before voluntary walking can take place.

Feeding Reflexes

The newborn has a number of reflexes that are important to obtaining food; these are all very active in the normal full-term infant.

ROOTING REFLEX The rooting reflex, by which the baby searches for food, functions whenever his cheek is touched with a hand, the mother's nipple, or any other object, or when the baby smells milk. The baby immediately moves his head toward the source of stimulation and opens his mouth in anticipation of food. The intensity of this reflex should be noted.

SUCKING, SWALLOWING, AND GAG REFLEXES The sucking, swallowing, and gag

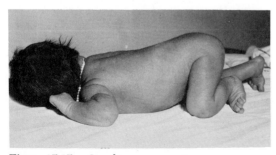

Figure 17-17. Crawling movements.

reflexes, responsible for getting food to the stomach, are all active in the full-term, alert newborn but may be easily exhausted or uncoordinated in the premature baby. The gag reflex, however, is usually present in prematures, even those unable to suck and swallow.

The fetus makes lip movements that simulate sucking from 18 weeks gestation onward, but a true sucking reflex does not seem to appear before 24 weeks. Strong sucking apparently does not occur until the last part of gestation. The sucking reflex is so well developed at full term that the baby may suck his fist or thumb immediately after birth, and sucking movements are stimulated whenever anything touches his lips. An absent or weak sucking reflex indicates immaturity, narcosis, or intracranial injury. Sucking is slow, weak, and present in only short periods, or even absent, in a baby who is depressed by maternal medication.

Fetal swallowing reflexes normally occur *in utero* and have been demonstrated at 12 weeks gestation. It is estimated that the fetus swallows as much as 500 ml of amniotic fluid daily near term, but the frequency of fetal swallowing and other influencing factors are not known. This swallowing apparently strengthens the pharyngeal and esophageal musculature. Adequate strength of swallowing is as important to nursing as good integration of tongue and lip movements in sucking activity. Suck and swallow must be coordinated for adequate feeding movements.

HUNGER AND SATIETY REFLEXES Hunger and satiety reflexes cause the baby to cry when he is hungry and to know when he has had enough to eat.

Protective Reflexes

Many of the baby's actions are protective or defensive in nature. Among others, not described above, are the ability to yawn; hiccup; clear the respiratory tract by coughing and sneezing; blink when the eyes are exposed to bright light; shiver when cold; resist restraint, thus demonstrating a muscle and joint sense;

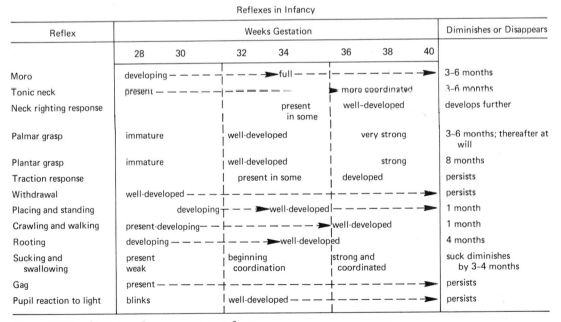

Reflexes in Infancy

Reflex	Weeks Gestation							Diminishes or Disappears
	28	30	32	34	36	38	40	
Moro	developing – – –		– – ➤full – – –		– – – – – –		– – – ➤	3–6 months
Tonic neck	present – – – – – –		– – – – – –		➤ more coordinated			3–6 months
Neck righting response				present in some	well-developed			develops further
Palmar grasp	immature		well-developed		very strong			3–6 months; thereafter at will
Plantar grasp	immature		well-developed		strong			8 months
Traction response			present in some		developed			persists
Withdrawal	well-developed – – –		– – – – – –		– – – – – –		– – ➤	persists
Placing and standing		developing – – ➤well-developed			– – – – – –		– ➤	1 month
Crawling and walking	present-developing – –		– – – – – –		➤well-developed			1 month
Rooting	developing – – –		– – – ➤well-developed					4 months
Sucking and swallowing	present weak		beginning coordination		strong and coordinated			suck diminishes by 3–4 months
Gag	present – – – –		– – + – – – –		– – – – – –		➤	persists
Pupil reaction to light	blinks		well-developed – – –		– – – – – –		➤	persists

Figure 17-19. Certain reflexes present in infancy.

withdraw from painful objects; and cry when disturbed by pain or any other discomfort.

Many more reflexes have been studied and identified, but more important than observing the presence of individual reflexes is observing the baby's ability to coordinate movements and to respond to his environment. The full-term newborn has the ability to organize his motor capabilities quite well, he has good sensory and perceptual capabilities, and he shows good ability to learn.

Vision

A newborn's vision is much more advanced at birth than has previously been supposed—tests show that his visual acuity varies from around 20/150 to 20/290—and it continues to develop rapidly in the immediate postnatal weeks. Retinal development is quite advanced and the baby has a well-developed visual cone system except for seeing color. Myelination of the optic nerve is completed within a few months after birth.

A newborn's eyes are large at birth compared with the rest of the body. The pupils are small, and they react well to light. A premature of 28 weeks gestation will blink at a bright light and by 32 weeks the baby will close his eyes to a bright light. The cornea is clear. The red reflex is present under ophthalmoscopic examination. The eyes move well in response to vestibular stimuli and in following objects.

At birth, the eyes of all babies are blue or slate blue-gray. They become their permanent color at approximately three months of age, but pigmentation of the iris may not be complete for one year. Tears are not usually seen in the eyes of babies for several months, but basic tear production is possible and lacrimation is usually normal.

A full-term baby opens his eyes to see, and he is often able to fixate on near objects, about 7 or 8 inches from his face, as soon as he is born. The baby's stare may be uniocular (with only one eye). He may stop crying and become quiet as he is gazing and observing. If he is sucking he may stop to concentrate on what he sees. The baby seems to have a preference for fixation on certain types of objects—the human face, complex patterns, and distinct black and white contrasts.

When an object on which a newborn's eyes are fixed is moved, he may soon follow it successfully. He can follow an object with his eyes within a few hours after birth, and he may turn his head to follow when he is 2 or 3 days old.

The capacity for visual alertness differs considerably among newborns. A few do not respond early to faces or bright objects or do not follow well. Unless the baby is in an alert state, one cannot be sure of his visual abilities. Some babies, however, who are only partially alert or are drowsy may become alert when they are presented with something to see.

Within the month after birth the baby's periods of visual activity become longer, fixation and following develop considerably more, and the baby is able to use both eyes simultaneously. Visual acuity continues to develop well, and the baby soon becomes very curious and interested in his surroundings.

Hearing

The auditory nerve and the membranous labyrinth are well developed quite early in gestation. The fetus *in utero* has been noted to react to external sound stimuli in the twenty-sixth week of gestation, and a fetus born as a premature, as early as 28 weeks gestation, is able to hear sounds.

The newborn infant can not only hear well, but he appears to be able to make fine discriminations in sounds and he can usually locate the general direction of the sound. Many babies respond to sound such as a voice by alerting and looking for the sound. Some sounds appear to be meaningful and comforting to the baby. Sudden loud noises usually cause the newborn to startle, to blink, or to change his respiratory rate. A baby usually learns quickly to be somewhat unresponsive to irritating noise.

Newborns are able to coordinate vision and

hearing, at least to some extent. Sensitivity to auditory stimuli seems to be quite well correlated to capacity for visual pursuit.

Smell

Development of the olfactory sense is not clear, but there is reason to believe that the sense of smell is quite well developed at birth. Babies appear to be sensitive to stimuli of odors, to grimace with unpleasant odors, and to discriminate between different odors. The baby is believed to search for food when he smells milk.

Taste

The literature on the degree of taste sensitivity is controversial, but it appears that babies show distinct reactions to different taste substances. Taste buds in the fetus have matured by the beginning of the second trimester of gestation, and there appears to be some evidence that the fetal taste system is functional *in utero*.

The newborn appears to be able to differentiate well between pleasant and unpleasant tastes. The baby increases his suck and swallow movements with sweets and grimaces, stops sucking, or rejects unpleasant tastes, such as a salty or sour or bitter taste.

Tactile Senses

Skin, muscular, and vestibular senses are highly developed before birth. Tactile sense begins to function in the fetus before any of the other senses, because much of fetal stimulation is cutaneous.

The area around the fetus's mouth is the first to become sensitive; response to stimulation of the lips and the perioral area has been observed as early as 7.5 weeks menstrual age. More and more skin surfaces then become sensitive to cutaneous stimulation in an orderly sequence of development—the oral area, the genital area, and the palmar and plantar surfaces respond earlier than the intervening areas. Reflex response to cutaneous stimulation is at first limited to the earliest matured portion of the

neuromuscular system, but as more and more regions mature reflex response becomes more refined.

Since the newborn's tactile senses are very well developed at birth, he will respond to contact stimuli, and he will cry from pain, pressure, heat, cold, hunger, and other discomforts. Pain sensitivity appears to develop further after birth and to increase steadily during the first few postnatal days. The baby can also be expected to respond with pleasure and quiet to soothing touches—patting, cuddling, carrying, changing position, and rocking.

The newborn's lips and cheeks are very sensitive to touch from the beginning. The baby will search for food when his cheek is touched, and he will purse his lips and begin to make sucking movements whenever they are touched.

Sleep and Awake States

For many years it was believed that the newborn functioned mainly by reflex activity and unpatterned behavior, because the cerebral cortex was practically inactive at birth. Investigations, which began as recently as 20 years ago, have shown that newborns are capable of a great deal of organized behavior, they can interact well with their environment, and each infant's reaction to the influences of his environment is unique.

The way in which a baby will respond at any given time depends on his state of consciousness at that time.

Six different states of sleep and wakefulness, which range from deep sleep to intense crying, are now generally recognized. The way in which a baby responds to stimuli at a particular time is determined largely by his level on the sleep–awake continuum. Criteria of the six states as described by T. Berry Brazelton are as follows[10]:

[10] T. Berry Brazelton, *Neonatal Behavioral Assessment Scale, Clinics in Developmental Medicine, No. 50.* Spastics International Medical Publications, Heinemann Medical Books, London, and Lippincott, Philadelphia, Pa., 1973, pp. 5–8.

Sleep States

1. Deep sleep with regular breathing, eyes closed, no spontaneous activity except startles or jerky movements at quite regular intervals; external stimuli produce startles with some delay; suppression of startles is rapid, and state changes are less likely than from other states. No eye movements. . . .

2. Light sleep with eyes closed; rapid eye movements can be observed under closed lids; low activity level, with random movements and startles or startle equivalents; movements are likely to be smoother and more monitored than in state 1; responds to internal and external stimuli with startle equivalents, often with a resulting change of state. Respirations are irregular, sucking movements occur off and on. . . .

Awake States

3. Drowsy or semidozing; eyes may be open or closed, eyelids fluttering; activity level variable, with interspersed, mild startles from time to time; reactive to sensory stimuli, but response often delayed; state change after stimulation frequently noted. Movements are usually smooth. . . .

4. Alert, with bright look; seems to focus attention on source of stimulation, such as an object to be sucked, or a visual or auditory stimulus; impinging stimuli may break through, but with some delay in response. Motor activity is at a minimum. . . .

5. Eyes open; considerable motor activity, with thrusting movements of the extremities, and even a few spontaneous startles; reactive to external stimulation with increase in startles or motor activity, but discrete reactions difficult to distinguish because of general high activity level.

6. Crying; characterized by intense crying which is difficult to break through with stimulation. . . .

In addition to the behaviors that are usually described for each of the six states of consciousness, babies have different responses in heart rate, blood flow, muscle tone, and EEG patterns.

Sleep States

In the *deep sleep state*, sometimes called *quiet sleep*, the baby is sound asleep, he does not respond to stimuli unless they are very disturbing, and even if he does arouse for a short time he may return to a deep sleep. This sleep state is quite obviously not the time to try to feed the baby, since he is likely not to awaken for a feeding even with stimulation, and it is not the appropriate time to try to check a baby's ability to respond to various stimuli or to check his reflex capability.

In *light sleep*, which is also called *active sleep* or rapid eye movement (REM) sleep, the baby is more responsive to stimuli, such as hunger or handling, than he is in deep sleep. Sucking movements and smiling have been observed in newborns in REM sleep. The baby may have brief periods of fussing in light sleep.

Caretakers who are not aware of the baby's sucking movements or smiling in light sleep may think the baby is ready to awaken and play. They may attempt to feed him when he is really not ready to eat or to play with him when he is not awake. The baby may remain in light sleep for a while, or go into deep sleep again, or awaken.

The full-term newborn sleeps from 16 to 20 hours a day in the first two weeks of life, for an average of 4 hours at a time. While asleep, periods of active sleep alternate with periods of quiet sleep in a fixed pattern with about equal time of each kind of sleep or perhaps 60 percent active sleep and 40 percent quiet sleep. A sleep cycle, which is a period of active sleep through a period of quiet sleep to the beginning of another period of active sleep, averages about 60 minutes, varying from 30 to 70 minutes. This means that within approximately every hour of sleep a baby is in both an active and a quiet state of sleep. As a baby gets older he spends more time in quiet than in active sleep; this is attributed to increasing maturation of the central nervous system.

Parents can learn to observe behavioral differences in their baby's levels of sleep, to know the baby's behavior when he is ready to go to sleep, to base their care on the baby's cycle, and to note when he begins to sleep fewer hours and to sleep longer periods at night. The total amount of sleep decreases very little in the first few months, but the periods of sleep become more consolidated.

Awake States

In the *drowsy state* the baby semidozes. He opens and closes his eyes, is relatively inactive, and reacts to sensory stimuli with delay. From this state he may awaken fully or he may return to a sleep state. A drowsy state is not a good time to attempt to feed the baby or to interact with him. Feedings are best given in the fully awake states.

In the *alert state*, Brazelton's state 4, the baby pays considerable attention to his environment. This is also called a *quiet awake state*. The baby watches and follows voices and faces. This state is of short duration in the newborn, but becomes longer and more frequent as the baby gets older.

In the normal newborn who is not affected by maternal medication, there is usually a short period of intense alerting behavior immediately after birth, before the baby begins a period of sleep. This is shown in the first period of reactivity in Figure 18-5, page 494.

In Brazelton's state 5, which may also be called an *active awake state*, the baby's eyes are open, but he does not have the distinctly bright, alert look of the quiet awake state. The baby moves about quite a bit in this active awake state, he may have periods of fussiness, he is sensitive to stimuli like hunger and noise, and he may begin to cry.

In the *crying state* the baby is communicating discomfort and his need for attention. Crying is his only means of letting someone know he is uncomfortable. He may be hungry, tired, cold, or have pain. A newborn normally cries lustily whenever he is hungry or uncomfortable. Hunger is the most common cause of crying. A weak, whining, grunting, or poorly maintained cry is not normal.

When a baby is crying he may soothe himself and go to a lower state or he may need help from others to become quiet. A comforting maneuver that a newborn uses to soothe himself is the hand-to-mouth movement. He may quiet himself by sucking on his fingers or fist or sometimes just making sucking movements with his mouth. He may also pay attention to voices or faces and remain quiet for awhile in this way.

A crying baby may also be uncomfortable from a wet diaper, abdominal discomfort, a distressing temperature, or close restraint, or he may be fussy because he needs to be held. Some babies are not disturbed by a wet diaper, while others are quite uncomfortable when they are wet. If a crying baby is not hungry or wet, he may need to be picked up and patted for an air bubble, he may need more or less cover or a change of position, or he may need to be picked up and held and rocked to quiet.

Some babies need much more help than others to quiet and some need different methods of quieting at different times and under different circumstances.

Newborns have a total of 7 to 8 hours of wakefulness in a 24-hour period with each period of wakefulness being from 1 to 2 hours in length.

Posture and Muscle Tone

The young baby prefers the position to which he was confined *in utero*. The newborn may be restless in an unaccustomed position and will often fall asleep easily when he is "folded" into his most comfortable posture, called his *position of comfort*. Observation of the baby for preference of position for his head and extremities will be useful in reconstructing his fetal posture, which in general is one of flexion. Observing the baby's position of comfort will often explain an unusual appearance of certain parts of his body such as facial asymmetry, pressure marks on the chest, and a peculiar position of the legs (Fig. 17-8).

The baby can gradually assume a less "folded-up" position, but he continues to prefer a somewhat flexed posture for a period of time; even in sleep this is not relaxed. He usually sleeps with his hands near his head or chin. If he is on his back when he awake, he takes the tonic neck reflex position. Whenever he moves his arms about, they remain flexed at the elbows and move from the shoulders. This brings his hands near his face, which he frequently scratches, or where he may stick his fingers in his eyes, which fortunately, he usually closes (Fig. 17-20). At the end of the neonatal period this flexion is much less noticeable, but it is not until later in infancy that the arms move at the elbows. The fists are kept clenched for the first eight weeks. Control over muscle movements always begins at the proximal and moves to the distal parts.

The normal full-term newborn should have good muscle tone. The baby maintains his extremities in a flexed position (Fig. 17-21). Any attempt to straighten out an extremity or passively manipulate it will demonstrate his strong flexor tone. Although the baby's head and back will need support when he is picked up, a sensation of good tone should be conveyed when he is handled. Limpness or relaxation, with little or no resistance when an attempt is made to restrain the baby or change his position, is not a normal reaction and may mean that the baby is suffering from shock, narcosis, or intracranial injury, or occasionally from some type of muscle disorder. The premature baby normally has less

tone than the full-term and may lie with his arms and legs in extension.

When the baby is in the prone position, he can pick his head up momentarily and rotate it from side to side, and he often moves a short distance with a crawling motion. When he is

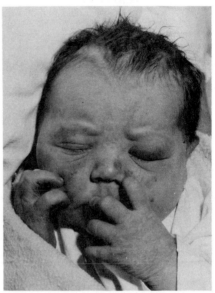

Figure 17-20. Newborn infant—18 hours old. With the arms remaining flexed at the elbows and moving from the shoulders, a baby frequently scratches his face. This baby has edema and redness of his right eyelids, which are probably the result of trauma to the lids during instillation of silver nitrate and/or a chemical conjunctivitis.

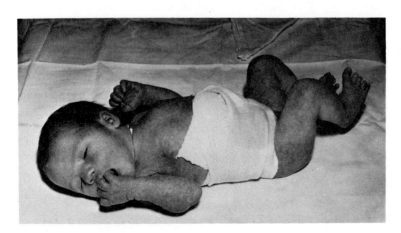

Figure 17-21. Full-term newborn—2 days old. This baby demonstrates good muscle tone. He keeps his extremities in a flexed position. The baby is in a drowsy state with one eye open and one eye closed. Note that he has his hands to his mouth, a maneuver often used by babies to comfort themselves.

held against the shoulder, he will attempt to, and can, hold his head up for a moment, but the neck muscles are not strong enough to maintain this position and his head soon drops back. He is unable to raise his head from the supine position; he can turn his head to either side from this position, but prefers one side more than the other.

A baby's head must be given considerable support when he is picked up because the muscles of his head and neck are not strong enough for him to hold it up. To keep his head from falling back, the person picking him up must place one hand, with fingers spread, under his head and shoulders while the other hand supports the lower part of his body, either by grasping his legs firmly or by placing the hand under the buttocks. To give the baby a feeling of security, he should be held firmly whenever he is picked up or moved.

HUNGER

At varying intervals the baby will show signs of hunger by becoming restless, crying fretfully, moving his head about in search of food, and sucking on his fingers, clothing, or anything he finds near his mouth. The time at which the baby first desires food depends somewhat on his size, the type of labor and delivery, and the amount of analgesia his mother received. He may show signs of hunger immediately after he is born, or he may have little or no desire for food for 24 hours. The baby usually falls asleep immediately after he is fed, but may stay awake and even cry for a short time before he sleeps. After a feeding period he should sleep quietly from one to several hours, only to awaken again when uncomfortable because of hunger or a wet diaper.

SUMMARY

The general appearance of the normal full-term newborn immediately after birth is that of an infant with a large head, short neck, narrow chest, prominent abdomen, and short arms and legs, which are sharply flexed (Fig. 17-5). He assumes his intrauterine position, lying somewhat curled up with his back rounded, his arms bent and lying across his chest, and his legs flexed on his abdomen unless his intrauterine position was a breech presentation, in which case his legs are usually extended with the toes pointing toward the shoulders. His skin is tight because of a thick layer of subcutaneous fat, and it is at least partly covered by vernix caseosa and often with lanugo hair on certain parts of the body. His color is pink or pinkish red except for a slight cyanosis of the hands and feet. His body may be cool, and his temperature may be below normal unless he has been well protected against heat loss. The baby should be crying lustily immediately after birth, and he usually draws up his arms and legs and clenches his fists during periods of crying. His Moro reflex should be complete and his grasp reflect strong. He may begin to suck his thumb or his fist almost immediately after he is born.

The baby's appearance and behavior at the time of birth are affected to some extent by the duration of labor, type of delivery, and amount of analgesia the mother received during labor and delivery. His head may show very little to a considerable amount of molding with overlapping of the cranial bones; a caput succedaneum may be present; and there may be an asymmetry of the face due to pressure from intrauterine position. Edema and ecchymosis of the presenting part are sometimes observed. The baby may be quiet but alert; may cry readily following minor stimulation; may be irritable and easily startled; or may be sleepy and listless.

During the first few days the baby recovers from the stress of birth. The period of transition from intrauterine to extrauterine existence is characterized by some instability of the various systems. This instability shows itself in many ways; tremors and quiverings, gagging, choking, poor sucking, regurgitation, irregular pulse, and hyperactivity during sleep, even awakening every few minutes, may be included in these manifestations.

Within a few days to a week the effects of birth and sudden change of environment have been largely overcome. Molding of the head has receded; cdcma of the presenting part has disappeared; the face has become symmetrical; temperature maintenance has improved; the respiratory, circulatory, and digestive systems are functioning better; and the posture is more relaxed. The normal newborn will have good color and good muscle tone, cry lustily, sleep approximately 20 hours a day, awaken only when hungry or uncomfortable, eat well, and gain weight steadily.

Newborns have been observed to be in different sleep and awake states which range from deep sleep to light sleep, to drowsy, to quiet awake, to active awake, to crying.

At about 28 weeks of gestation, the time when extrauterine life may be possible, a baby begins to show some degree of alertness that apparently is not present earlier. He can be aroused from sleep and will remain alert for a few minutes, and he may occasionally show spontaneous alerting. By 32 weeks a newborn may alert spontaneously, his eyes may remain open for awhile, and roving eye movements appear. By 37 weeks alertness is increased and the baby cries vigorously when awake. By full term the baby has distinct sleep and awake periods and he responds well to stimuli.

When in a quiet awake (alert) state the normal newborn is likely to focus his eyes on faces and objects and to follow them even within a few hours after birth. He will respond to a variety of sounds and is likely to try to locate sounds.

Babies differ a great deal in how they respond to stimuli: how active they are, the amount they fuss and cry, how alert they are, and how easily they are quieted. Babies are capable of responding in an organized way in each state of sleep or awakeness and can control the kind of input they get from their environment. They can close out repeated unwanted stimuli just as easily as they can respond to significant and interesting stimuli.

Most babies move easily from one state of consciousness to another. Some, however, do not move easily and smoothly between states and do not spend much time in some states. They sleep or they cry and spend little time in the drowsy or quiet awake states. Normal babies will differ considerably from one another in their behavior and therefore in the care that they need.

As the baby develops postnatally he will reduce the total amount of time he sleeps, his sleep and wakefulness periods will lengthen, and he will shift from daytime to nighttime sleeping.

BIBLIOGRAPHY

Artal, Raul, and Rosen, Mortimer G., Fetal response to sound, *Contemp. Ob/Gyn* 5:13–16 (May) 1975.

Assali, Nicholas S. (ed.), *Biology of Gestation*, Vol. 2: *The Fetus and Neonate.* Academic Press, New York, 1968.

Avery, Gordon B. (ed.), *Neonatology.* Lippincott, Philadelphia, Pa., 1975.

Avery, M. E., Wang, N. S., and Taeusch, H. W., Jr., The lung of the newborn infant, *Sci. Am.* 228:74–85 (Apr.) 1973.

Behrman, Richard E. (ed.), *Neonatology. Diseases of the Fetus and Infant.* Mosby, St. Louis, Mo., 1973.

Boddy, K., and Dawes, G. S., Fetal breathing, *Br. Med. Bull.* 31:3–7 (Jan.) 1975.

———, and Mantell, C., Observations of fetal breathing movements transmitted through maternal abdominal wall, *Lancet* ii:1219–1220 (Dec. 2) 1972.

Brazelton, T. Berry, *Neonatal Behavior Assessment Scale, Clinics in Developmental Medicine, No. 50.* Spastics International Medical Publications, Heinemann Medical Books, London, and Lippincott, Philadelphia, Pa., 1973.

Brück, Kurt, Heat production and temperature regulation, in *Physiology of the Perinatal Period*, Vol. 1, edited by Uve Stave. Appleton-Century-Crofts, New York, 1970, Chapter 16.

Dahm, Lida Swafford, and James, L. Stanley, Newborn temperature and calculated heat loss in the delivery room, *Pediatrics* 49:504–513 (Apr.) 1972.

Davis, John A., and Dobbing, John (eds.), *Scientific Foundations of Paediatrics*, Heinemann, London, 1974.

Dawes, Geoffrey S., Breathing before birth in animals and man: An essay in developmental medicine, *N. Engl. J. Med.* 290:557–559 (Mar. 7) 1974.

———, *Foetal and Neonatal Physiology.* Year Book Medical Publishers, Chicago, Ill., 1968.

Edelmann, Chester M., and Spitzer, Adrian, The maturing kidney, *J. Pediatr.* 75:509–519 (Sept.) 1969.

Erickson, Marcene, *Assessment and Management of Developmental Changes in Children.* Mosby, St. Louis, Mo., 1976, Chapter 5, "Sleep."

Evans, Hugh E., and Glass, Leonard, *Perinatal Medicine.* Harper and Row, Hagerstown, Md., 1976.

Faber, Myron M., Circumcision revisited, *Birth Family J.* 1:19–21 (Spring) 1974.

Gill, Thomas J. III, Transfer of immunity to the fetus, *Contemp. Ob/Gyn* 1:53–57, (May) 1973.

Gryboski, Joyce D., The swallowing mechanism of the neonate. I. Esophageal and gastric motility, *Pediatrics* 35:445–452 (Mar.) 1965.

Harding, Paul G. R., The metabolism of brown and white adipose tissue in the fetus and newborn, *Clin. Obstet. Gynecol.* 14:685–709 (Sept.) 1971.

Heim, Tibor, Thermogenesis in the newborn infant, *Clin. Obstet. Gynecol.* 14:790–820 (Sept.) 1971.

Hodgman, Joan E., Freedman, Robert J., and Levan, Norma E., Neonatal dermatology, *Pediat. Clin. North Am.* 18:713–756 (Aug.) 1971.

Humphrey, Tryphena, Function of the nervous system during prenatal life, in *Physiology of the Perinatal Period*, Vol. 2, edited by Uve Stave. Appleton-Century-Crofts, New York, 1970, pp. 751–796.

Johnson, S. H., and Grubbs, J. P., The premature infant's reflex behaviors: Effect on maternal–child relationship, *JOGN Nurs.* 4:15–20 (Mar.–Apr.) 1975.

Korner, Anneliese, Visual alertness in neonates: Individual differences and their correlates, *Percep. Motor Skills* 31:499–509 (Oct.) 1970.

Lenard, H. G., Sleep studies in infancy: Facts, concepts, and significance, *Acta Paediatr. Scand.* 59:572–581, 1970.

———, von Bernuth, H., and Prechtl, H. F. R., Reflexes and their relationship to behavioral state in the newborn, *Acta Paediatr. Scand.* 57:177–185, 1968.

Lockman, Lawrence A., Neurologic assessment in the first year of life, *Postgrad. Med.* 50:80–85 (July) 1971.

MacKinnon, J., and Harvey, David, The assessment of organ function in the newborn, *Br. J. Hosp. Med.* 14:395–403 (Oct.) 1975.

Mistretta, C. M., and Bradley, R. M., Taste and swallowing *in utero*, *Br. Med. bull.* 31:80–84 (Jan.) 1975.

Oliver, J. K., Jr., Temperature regulation and heat production in the newborn, *Pediatr. Clin. North Am.* 12:765–779 (Aug.) 1965.

Pang, Leila Mei, and Mellins, Robert B., Neonatal cardiorespiratory physiology, *Anesthesiology* 43:171–196 (Aug.) 1975.

Patient Care, Circumcision: A balanced report on facts, not conjecture; the arguments for and against routine neonatal circumcision; Guidance for parents and recommended surgical techniques (illustrated), 5:56–*86 passim* (July 15) 1971.

Popick, Gregory A., and Smith, David W., Fontanels: Range of normal size, *J. Pediatr.* 80:749–752 (May) 1972.

Prechtl, H. F. R., The behavioral states of the newborn infant. A review, *Brain Res.* 76:185–212, 1974.

Preston, E. Noel, Whither the foreskin? A consideration of routine neonatal circumcision, *JAMA*, 213:1853–1858 (Sept. 14) 1970.

Schulte, F. J., Neonatal brain mechanisms and the development of motor behavior, in *Physiology of the Perinatal Period*, Vol. 2, edited by Uve Stave. Appleton-Century-Crofts, New York, 1970, pp. 797–841.

Silberstein, Richard M., and Dolgin, Joseph, The cephalic reflex: An aspect of the rooting reflex, *Clin. Pediatr.* 6:305–306 (May) 1967.

Silverman, William A., and Parke, Priscilla, The newborn: Keep him warm, *Am. J. Nurs.* 65:81–84 (Oct.) 1965.

Smart, Mollie S., and Smart, Russell C., *Infants, Development and Relationships.* Macmillan, New York, 1973, pp. 74–101.

Solomon, Lawrence M., and Esterly, Nancy B., Neonatal dermatology. I. The newborn skin, *J. Pediatr.* 77:888–894 (Nov.) 1970.

Spitzer, Adrian, Renal Physiology: Impact of recent developments on clinical nephrology, *Pediatr. Clin. North Am.* 18:377–393 (May) 1971.

Stave, Uve (ed.), *Physiology of the Perinatal Period*, Vols. 1 and 2. Appleton-Century-Crofts, New York, 1970.

Stone, L. Joseph, Smith, Henrietta T., and Murphy, Lois B. (eds.), The capabilities of the newborn, in *The Competent Infant*. Basic Books, New York, 1973, Chapter 3.

Walton, David S., The visual system, in *Physiology of the Perinatal Period*, Vol. 2, edited by Uve Stave. Appleton-Century-Crofts, New York, 1970, pp. 875–888.

18

Clinical Management
of the Normal Newborn

Clinical management of the newborn begins with an appraisal immediately after birth of the baby's ability to make a satisfactory adjustment to extrauterine life. Repeated assessments are then carried out in the following hours and days to determine the baby's gestational age, his stage of development, his ongoing adaptation to his environment, his general physical condition, and his behavioral abilities.

Assessment of the newborn's gestational age, physical condition and adaptation, and abilities is essential to providing the baby with appropriate care. Since one general overall plan of care will not be suitable for all newborns, the cumulative observations and assessment of the baby's first hours and days of life are used for planning the baby's medical and nursing care and for assisting the parents in developing their approaches to his care.

ASSESSMENT METHODS

Several tools have been developed as aids to a systematic assessment of the newborn for determining his stage of development and for assessing a number of different abilities. Included are the (1) Apgar score; (2) intrauterine growth charts; (3) scoring systems for clinical assessment of gestational age; (4) physical examination; and (5) Brazelton neonatal behavioral assessment scale. All of these scales of development and observation will be needed to make a complete

evaluation of a newborn's abilities and an appropriate plan of care.

The Apgar Score

The Apgar score, described on page 356, is important as an initial screening tool and is used for assessment of the infant immediately after birth. It reflects the condition of the baby after the stress of labor and delivery, and it provides a quick assessment of those functions that must immediately begin adapting to extrauterine existence and are necessary to sustain life. From this score one can roughly determine the degree of alertness or depression of the infant after birth. In the Apgar assessment the immediate response of the cardiovascular and respiratory systems to extrauterine change are evaluated, and a perfunctory idea of the state of the lower centers of the nervous system can be obtained by observing the muscle tone and reflex irritability of the infant.

The Apgar score is important for early recognition of any problems. The 1-minute score is used to determine what kind of assistance, if any, a baby needs to adapt favorably to his new environment and the 5-minute score gives an indication of the immediate capacity of the baby to respond to the stress of labor and delivery and the likelihood of problems in the early neonatal period. The Apgar score may be repeated in 5 and 10 minutes if indicated.

The Apgar score, done in the early minutes

after delivery, is important as an initial assessment of the baby, but it has limited predictability of later abilities of the baby. Other assessment methods must therefore also be used for a complete evaluation of the baby.

Categorization According to Gestational Age

A baby born at less than 26 weeks gestation is considered immature; one born between 26 and 37 completed weeks of gestation is called preterm or premature; one born between 38 and 42 weeks gestation is considered a term or mature infant; and a baby born after 42 completed weeks of gestation is considered postterm.

An accurate assessment of gestational age is of great importance to the immediate clinical care of the newborn, since the problems, the needs, and the clinical course are very different for each of the group of infants identified above— the preterm, the term, and the postterm infant.

Gestational age may need to be determined by the use of a number of different criteria. Often estimation of the expected date of full-term gestation can be made fairly accurately by calculating from the day of onset of the mother's last menstrual period. The accuracy of this date is enhanced when it compares favorably with a clinical estimation of the duration of pregnancy from such signs as expected progression of the height of the uterine fundus at various stages of pregnancy and the time when the fetal heart is heard for the first time (see Chapter 7). Sometimes fetal maturity studies, carried out prenatally by examination of the amniotic fluid (pages 612–14) and by fetal biparietal diameter measurements (pages 616–17), are used to estimate gestational age, but these tests are better for assessment of maturity and size than of gestation. They do, however, give supportive data.

After birth, the baby is examined for characteristics that can be used as a fairly accurate assessment of gestational age. This assessment is described in detail below, beginning on page 478. Since a detailed assessment of characteristics requires time, a quick examination for a few clinical criteria as shown in Figure 18-4,

combined with information obtained prenatally, will usually suffice to tentatively place the baby into an appropriate gestational age category for beginning care. A more detailed examination later should be used to confirm or revise the original calculation of gestational age.

Categorization According to Intrauterine Growth

For a number of years newborns with a birth weight of 2500 gm (5 lb 8 oz) or less were arbitrarily classified as premature, and those weighing more were designated full term. It later became evident that almost one third of babies weighing under 2500 gm at birth were full term. For some reason these infants had not developed to a normal size and weight for a mature baby. From this it became apparent that birth weight alone cannot be used as a measure of maturity. The birth weight must be correlated with gestational age to be valuable in estimating the meaning of the weight and how it may relate to the baby's condition.

As the concept that a baby might be small because of intrauterine growth retardation was being accepted through studies by Gruenwald[1] and the necessity of relating birth weight to gestational age was becoming apparent, the Colorado intrauterine growth charts were being developed.[2,3] These charts were used as a means of determining the appropriateness of a baby's weight in relation to that baby's gestational age.

Using an accurate measurement of birth weight and an accurate assessment of a baby's gestational age, the two values are placed on the chart shown in Figure 18-1 at the point where

[1] Peter Gruenwald, Chronic fetal distress and placental insufficiency, *Biol. Neonat.* 5:215–265, 1963.

[2] Lula O. Lubchenco, Charlotte Hansman, and Edith Boyd, Intrauterine growth in length and head circumference as estimated from live births at gestational ages from 26 to 42 weeks, *Pediatrics* 37:402–408 (Mar.) 1966.

[3] Frederick C. Battaglia and Lula O. Lubchenco, A practical classification of newborn infants by weight and gestational age, *J. Pediatr.* 71:159–163 (Aug.) 1967.

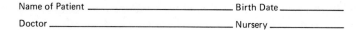

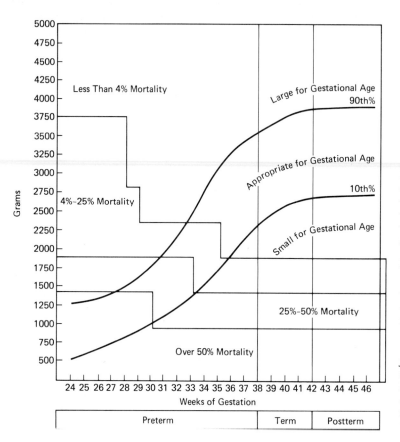

Figure 18-1. Each newborn can be classified by birth weight and gestational age with the use of this chart. It is easy to recognize the baby as large, appropriate, or small for his gestational age and provide him with the appropriate care immediately after birth. This illustration may be used as a wall chart in the nursery to provide for quick recognition of the "at-risk" baby. Neonatal mortality risk is also shown. [*Reproduced from Frederick C. Battaglia and Lula O. Lubchenco, "A Practical Classification of Newborn Infants by Weight and Gestational Age," J. Pediatr. 71:159–163, 1967, p. 161.*]

this baby's weight and weeks of gestation intersect. The weight chart of Figure 18-2 may be used instead of Figure 18-1, but it requires more interpretation by the user.

From the chart in Figure 18-1 the newborn can be categorized according to where the point of intersection of this baby's weight and weeks of gestation is found. The baby is thus categorized as appropriate (in weight) for gestational age (AGA); small for gestational age (SGA); or large for gestational age (LGA). At the same time the baby is identified as preterm, term, or postterm.

When each baby is classified according to weight and weeks of gestation, clinical care can be planned in accordance to his expected needs, since it is possible to anticipate the kind of clinical problems peculiar to the category to which the baby belongs. For example, the needs of the full-term, low-birth-weight baby and those of a premature of the same weight are vastly different. Likewise a LGA, preterm baby has very different immediate clinical problems than a term infant of the same weight. The mortality risk, superimposed on the chart in Figure 18-1 provides one more basis for judging the degree of intensive clinical care that the baby will probably need.

For further evaluation of a newborn's size in relation to his gestational age, his length and head circumference are also measured and compared to percentiles of measurements for babies of similar gestational age. Thus a newborn's weight, length, and head circumference may be plotted on the intrauterine growth chart shown in Figure 18-2. From this chart the baby's relative weight, length, and head circumference may be observed. It is possible, using these data, to determine if all of his measurements are appropriate for gestational age; if only growth in weight is affected; if both weight and length are small; or if all three measurements are small. In

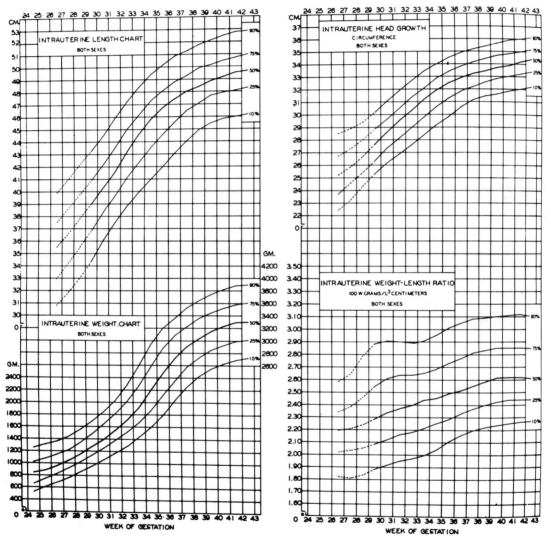

Figure 18-2. Percentiles of intrauterine growth in weight, length, head circumference, and weight–length ratio. This form is usually included as a part of the hospital record of each newborn. [*Reproduced with permission from Lula O. Lubchenco, Charlotte Hansman, and Edith Boyd, "Intrauterine Growth in Length and Head Circumference as Estimated from Live Births at Gestational Ages from 26 to 42 Weeks," Pediatrics 37:403–408 (Mar.) 1966, p. 404.*]

general, mild growth retardation affects only weight and somewhat more severe retardation affects both weight and length. Head size appears to be the last affected and when it is also small, retardation is severe, unless the baby is genetically of small size.

Use of a weight–length ratio helps to further identify the baby who is proportionately of good size or who may have considerable discrepancy between weight and length. The relationship of body weight to body length has been used primarily to detect infants with intrauterine growth retardation, but it may also be used to detect infants who are high-risk because they are too heavy for their length.

The weight–length ratio helps to define the greater retardation in weight than in length and will show the severity of the malnourishment of

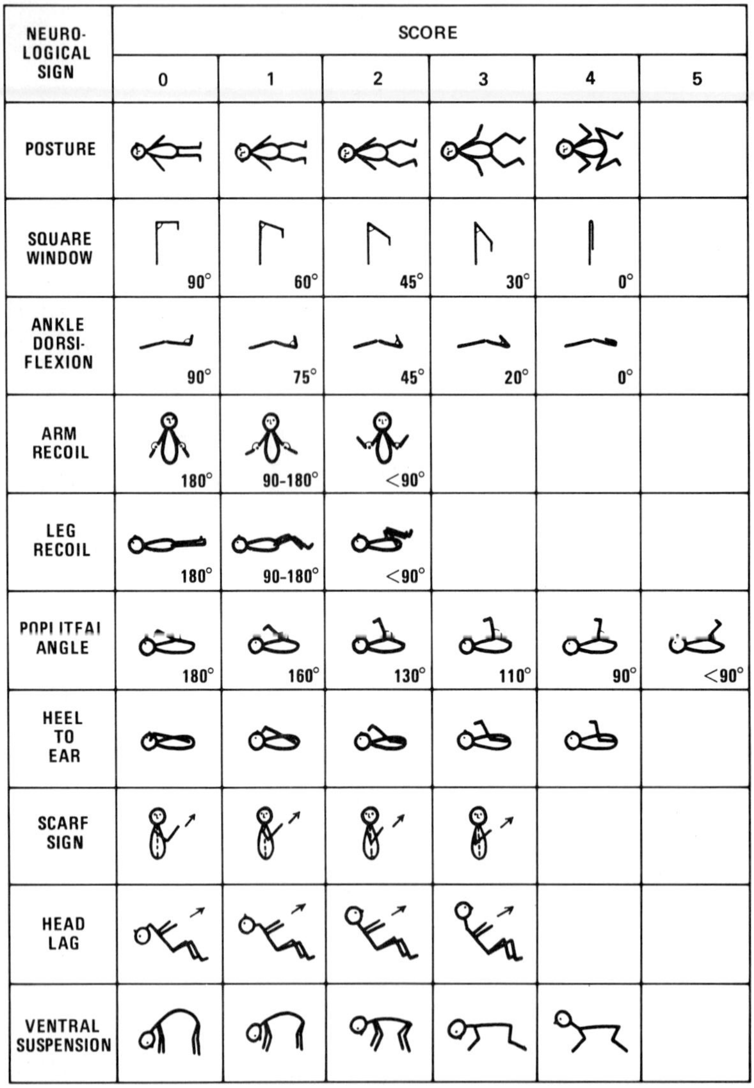

NEURO-LOGICAL SIGN	SCORE					
	0	1	2	3	4	5
POSTURE						
SQUARE WINDOW	90°	60°	45°	30°	0°	
ANKLE DORSI-FLEXION	90°	75°	45°	20°	0°	
ARM RECOIL	180°	90–180°	<90°			
LEG RECOIL	180°	90–180°	<90°			
POPLITEAL ANGLE	180°	160°	130°	110°	90°	<90°
HEEL TO EAR						
SCARF SIGN						
HEAD LAG						
VENTRAL SUSPENSION						

A. Scoring system for neurologic criteria.

Figure 18-3. Clinical assessment of gestational age in the newborn infant. [*Reproduced with permission from Lilly M. S. Dubowitz, Victor Dubowitz, and Cissie Goldberg, "Clinical Assessment of Gestational Age in the Newborn Infant," J. Pediatr. 77:1–10 (July) 1970.*]

the body tissues. It will also show whether a large baby with a weight above the 90th percentile has an excessive weight for size or if the baby's weight is reasonable in relation to the length. Infants who fall below the 3rd percentile for dates are considered malnourished, and those who are above the 97th percentile for dates are overweight.

The weight–length ratio is especially useful when infants are near to or outside extremes of growth on any of the measurements on the intrauterine growth chart, and also when there is a discrepancy between percentile positions of weight, length, and head circumference. The ratio has the advantage of not being influenced by sex or by race.

POSTURE: Observed with infant quiet and in supine position. Score 0: Arms and legs extended; 1: beginning of flexion of hips and knees, arms extended; 2: stronger flexion of legs, arms extended; 3: arms slightly flexed, legs flexed and abducted; 4: full flexion of arms and legs.

SQUARE WINDOW: The hand is flexed on the forearm between the thumb and index finger of the examiner. Enough pressure is applied to get as full a flexion as possible, and the angle between the hypothenar eminence and the ventral aspect of the forearm is measured and graded according to diagram. (Care is taken not to rotate the infant's wrist while doing this maneuver.)

ANKLE DORSIFLEXION: The foot is dorsiflexed onto the anterior aspect of the leg, with the examiner's thumb on the sole of the foot and other fingers behind the leg. Enough pressure is applied to get as full flexion as possible, and the angle between the dorsum of the foot and the anterior aspect of the leg is measured.

ARM RECOIL: With the infant in the supine position the forearms are first flexed for 5 seconds, then fully extended by pulling on the hands, and then released. The sign is fully positive if the arms return briskly to full flexion (Score 2). If the arms return to incomplete flexion or the response is sluggish it is graded as Score 1. If they remain extended or are only followed by random movements the score is 0.

LEG RECOIL: With the infant supine, the hips and knees are fully flexed for 5 seconds, then extended by traction on the feet, and released. A maximal response is one of full flexion of the hips and knees (Score 2). A partial flexion scores 1, and minimal or no movement scores 0.

POPLITEAL ANGLE: With the infant supine and his pelvis flat on the examining couch, the thigh is held in the knee–chest position by the examiner's left index finger and thumb supporting the knee. The leg is then extended by gentle pressure from the examiner's right index finger behind the ankle and the popliteal angle is measured.

HEEL-TO-EAR MANEUVER: With the baby supine, draw the baby's foot as near to the head as it will go without forcing it. Observe the distance between the foot and the head as well as the degree of extension at the knee. Grade according to diagram. Note that the knee is left free and may draw down alongside the abdomen.

SCARF SIGN: With the baby supine, take the infant's hand and try to put it around the neck and as far posteriorly as possible around the opposite shoulder. Assist this maneuver by lifting the elbow across the body. See how far the elbow will go across and grade according to illustrations. Score 0: Elbow reaches opposite axillary line; 1: Elbow between midline and opposite axillary line; 2: Elbow reaches midline; 3: Elbow will not reach midline.

HEAD LAG: With the baby lying supine, grasp the hands (or the arms if a very small infant) and pull him slowly toward the sitting position. Observe the position of the head in relation to the trunk and grade accordingly. In a small infant the head may initially be supported by one hand. Score 0: Complete lag; 1: Partial head control; 2: Able to maintain head in line with body; 3: Brings head anterior to body.

VENTRAL SUSPENSION: The infant is suspended in the prone position, with examiner's hand under the infant's chest (one hand in a small infant, two in a large infant). Observe the degree of extension of the back and the amount of flexion of the arms and legs. Also note the relation of the head to the trunk. Grade according to diagrams.

If score differs on the two sides, take the mean.

B. Some notes on techniques of assessment of neurologic criteria.

Assessment of Gestational Age

Assessment of gestational age is carried out by evaluation of a number of parameters. Such assessment is possible because certain physical characteristics of a baby and neurologic signs change predictably with increasing fetal age. A number of criteria are generally used in assessing age, since trying to base gestational age on the presence or absence of individual criteria is not very reliable.

Since the mid-1960s a number of methods for assessing a newborn's age have been proposed. Some of these evaluations are based on external physical characteristics of the baby, some are based on neurologic examination, and some use both external characteristics and neurologic criteria. A scoring system, developed by Dubo-

EXTERNAL SIGN	SCORE*				
	0	1	2	3	4
Edema	Obvious edema of hands and feet; pitting over tibia	No obvious edema of hands and feet; pitting over tibia	No edema		
Skin texture	Very thin, gelatinous	Thin and smooth	Smooth; medium thickenss; rash or superficial peeling	Slight thickening; superficial cracking and peeling especially of hands and feet	Thick and parchment-like; superficial or deep cracking
Skin color	Dark red	Uniformly pink	Pale pink; variable over body	Pale; only pink over ears, lips, palms, or soles	
Skin opacity (trunk)	Numerous veins and venules clearly seen, especially over abdomen	Veins and tributaries seen	A few large vessels clearly seen over abdomen	A few large vessels seen indistinctly over abdomen	No blood vessels seen
Lanugo (over back)	No lanugo	Abundant; long and thick over whole back	Hair thinning especially over lower back	Small amount of lanugo and bald areas	At least 1/2 of back devoid of lanugo
Plantar creases	No skin creases	Faint red marks over anterior half of sole	Definite red marks over > anterior 1/2; indentations over < anterior 1/3	Indentations over > anterior 1/3	Definite deep indentations over > anterior 1/3
Nipple formation	Nipple barely visible; no areola	Nipple well defined; areola smooth and flat, diameter < 0.75 cm	Areola stippled, edge not raised, diameter < 0.75 cm	Areola stippled, edge raised, diameter > 0.75 cm	
Breast size	No breast tissue palpable	Breast tissue on one or both sides, < 0.5 cm diameter	Breast tissue both sides; one or both 0.5–1.0 cm	Breast tissue both sides; one or both > 1 cm	
Ear form	Pinna flat and shapeless, little or no incurving of edge	Incurving of part of edge of pinna	Partial incurving whole of upper pinna	Well-defined incurving whole of upper pinna	
Ear firmness	Pinna soft, easily folded, no recoil	Pinna soft, easily folded, slow recoil	Cartilage to edge of pinna, but soft in places, ready recoil	Pinna firm, cartilage to edge; instant recoil	
Genitals Male	Neither testis in scrotum	At least one testis high in scrotum	At least one testis right down		
Female (with hips 1/2 abducted)	Labia majora widely separated, labia minora protruding	Labia majora almost cover labia minora	Labia majora completely cover labia minora		

Adapted from Farr and Associates, *Develop. Med. Child Neurol.* 8:507, 1966.
*If score differs on two sides, take the mean.

C. Scoring system for external criteria.

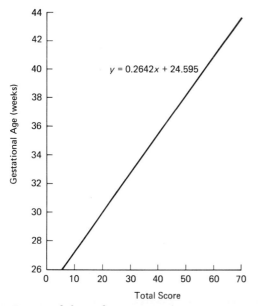

$y = 0.2642x + 24.595$

D. Graph for reading gestational age from total score.

witz, Dubowitz, and Goldberg[4] in 1970, is often used for age assessment. The Dubowitz assessment score, which can easily be learned by nurses, is described below. Since this system is rather detailed, an effort has been made by some persons to select a smaller number of criteria which will be easier to perform and yet give an estimation that is accurate for clinical purposes.[5]

The Dubowitz scoring system uses 10 neurologic and 11 external physical characteristics as criteria for evaluation of gestational age (Fig. 18-3A,B,C,D). The neurologic signs are dependent mainly on development of posture, tone, and primitive reflexes. The external criteria are dependent mainly on stage of development of skin, breasts, ears, and genitalia.

Scoring for gestational age can easily be learned by the nurse and can be done at any time after birth. The score is not influenced by the sleep–awake state of the baby. Each criterion on the scoring system is assessed and given a value from 0 to 4. The score is totaled and the gestational age in weeks is read from the graph in Figure 18-3D.

Scoring can be done by use of the external criteria alone or the neurologic criteria alone. There may be times when it is appropriate, because of the baby's condition or the time involved, to do only one set of criteria at first. When only one set of criteria has been used the score is doubled for purposes of reading the gestational age from the graph in Figure 18-3D. Analysis of the original data showed that the external characteristics, scored collectively, gave a better index than the neurologic criteria, but that the total score, using both groups of criteria, gave better results than either alone. With careful assessment and scoring it should be possible to assess a baby's gestational age quite accurately, with no more than one to two weeks error.

It is obviously not as accurate to assess gestational age from observation of a few developmental characteristics as it is to use a larger number of parameters and a scoring system, and yet a quick appraisal of certain well-defined characteristics has clinical value. It is very useful to determine from a quick appraisal almost immediately after birth if the baby belongs into a term or preterm category of age. To make such a brief, sketchy evaluation of the baby a few physical characteristics that can easily be assessed by quick observation are used. This usually means looking at sole creases, breast growth, ear cartilage development, and progress in development of the external genitalia. These characteristics and their stage of development at several gestational ages are shown in Figure 18-4.

Assessment of Physical Condition

An initial assessment of the baby's physical status, usually done by the nurse, is made immediately after birth, mainly through use of the

[4] Lily M. S. Dubowitz, Victor Dubowitz, and Cissie Goldberg, Clinical assessment of gestational age in the newborn infant, *J. Pediatr.* 77:1–10, 1970.
[5] Demetre Nicolopoulos *et al.*, Estimation of gestational age in the neonate, *Am. J. Dis. Child.* 130:477–480 (May) 1976.

Gestational Age According to Clinical Criteria

Clinical Criteria		36 weeks and less	37 to 38 weeks	39 or more weeks
Sole creases		Anterior transverse crease only	Occasional creases anterior two thirds	Sole covered with creases
Breast nodule diameter		2 mm	4 mm	7 mm or greater
Ear cartilage (pinna)		Little or no cartilage Ear returns slowly from folding	Some cartilage Ear springs back from folding	Stiffened with cartilage Firm erect ear
Scalp hair		Very fine Wooly or fuzzy	Very fine Wooly or fuzzy	Coarse, silky texture Each hair appears as a single strand
Genitalia	Male	Testes in canal, have not yet descended completely into scrotal sac Scrotum small with few rugae	Intermediate	Testes fully descended Scrotum full and pendulous with many rugae
	Female	Labia majora open	Labia majora open	Labia majora closed and cover labia minora and clitoris

Figure 18-4. Gestational age according to several well-defined characteristics and clinical criteria.

Apgar score; auscultation of the chest and heart; a quick appraisal of the condition and appearance of the baby, looking at size, color, muscle tone; and appraisal to rule out gross abnormalities and congenital anomalies. The American Academy of Pediatrics recommends that after the baby's condition has stabilized (usually in 5 to 10 minutes of age) he should be checked for several anomalies not grossly apparent. The Academy suggests the following:[6]

1. The infant's breathing should be observed to see if he can breathe with his mouth closed. (Rule out choanal atresia.)
2. A soft tube should be passed through the mouth a sufficient distance to reach the stomach. (Rule out esophageal atresia.)
3. The gastric contents should be aspirated quantitatively. (More than 15 to 20 ml leads to suspicion of high intestinal obstruction.)

[6] American Academy of Pediatrics, *Standards and Recommendations for Hospital Care of Newborn Infants,* 5th ed. Evanston, Ill., 1971.

4. The patency of the anus should be checked by passing the soft catheter into the rectum if no meconium is seen.
5. The number of umbilical vessels should be counted. Three are normal.

After an initial transitional period, a complete detailed physical examination is done. Frequently such an examination is done by the physician, usually sometime during the first 24 hours. The nurse, however, is the only member of the health care team continuously with the baby and may be the only member available to appraise the baby in the first hours of life. Physical assessment skills have become increasingly important to the nurse, who is assuming increasing responsibility for evaluating the status of infants.

The nurse may do a physical assessment in order to plan appropriate care to assist the baby to make a good adjustment to extrauterine life, to determine any risk factors, and to notify the physician early of any abnormal findings in order to institute necessary medical management early. Nurse and physician physical assessment data may be much the same. As it is pooled and shared, optimum plans can be made for the baby for prevention of difficulty and protection against problems that could arise, for medical management of any problems present, for support of the baby's efforts in his adjustment, and for nurturance of his physical and emotional needs.

History

The obstetric history and the progress of the baby since birth are important sources of information before the actual physical examination is begun. The nurse will want to know the pre-pregnancy, pregnancy, and labor and delivery history, and about the adjustment the baby has made since birth.

Prepregnancy history should include maternal medical complications such as diabetes, hypertension, renal disease, thyroid disease, and how long the disease has existed and how it has been treated, including drugs. A history of any condition that is likely to alter the fetal environment is important. Pregnancy history should also include family history of congenital diseases and history of known drug abuse, child abuse, and psychiatric problems. If the mother has other children, information about the events of their birth and their present health is important. History of abortions or stillbirths should also be included.

Pregnancy history should include expected date of delivery; blood type and Rh factor; serology; history of any bleeding during pregnancy, of any blood pressure elevation; of any infection, and of all drugs or medications taken; weight before pregnancy and weight gain; amount of prenatal care; and data concerning fetal assessment, if such was done. It is also important to know if the pregnancy was planned.

Labor and delivery history should include length of gestation, kind and length of labor and type of delivery, all analgesic and anesthetic agents (how much and when), management of any maternal medical complications, time of rupture of membranes, meconium in amniotic fluid, fetal heart rate and pattern during labor, fetal pH if done, and any maternal fever or bleeding.

The baby's condition at birth, his Apgar score, any resuscitative efforts, gestational age and weight, and his extrauterine adjustment since birth must be included in the history.

Physical Examination

The physical examination must be done in a systematic, orderly manner to avoid overlooking some important observations. Modifications of approach may be necessary depending upon the "state" of the infant, but even modifications can be made in an orderly way. The value of the nurse's physical examination will depend upon her ability to differentiate between normal and abnormal findings and her knowledge of the range of normal for the newborn. A detailed record should be made of the findings of the physical examination in a way that will be useful to others.

The basic methods used in a physical examination of any individual are also used for the newborn. These include inspection, auscultation, palpation, and percussion. The methods should be used in that order, in the hope that the baby will not be disturbed and crying prior to auscultation. General inspection, observing the baby as a whole, and also local inspection, focusing on each anatomic region of the baby, will yield a great deal of information. Auscultation usually means listening with a stethoscope, but sounds such as noisy or grunting respirations and the quality of the baby's cry may also be included. Palpation, feeling by the sense of touch, can be used on every part of the body that is accessible to the examining fingers. Palpation is followed by percussion or tapping where appropriate.

The actual examination of the newborn is reviewed below, pointing out some of the observations that can be made and some of the common findings. No attempt has been made to cover all the possibilities of the examination and all the disorders that can be discovered. Experience gained by examination of many normal newborns will assist the nurse in identifying abnormalities when they arise.

GENERAL INSPECTION An overall inspection will show if the baby assumes the normally expected flexed posture, if he appears to have a normal, firm, strong muscle tone, and if he appears to have symmetrical and easy movement of all of his extremities. He should not appear to be hypotonic or excessively jittery in response to stimuli. The baby's general size in relation to gestational age and the relative size of head, body, and extremities can be evaluated. General inspection should reveal any gross abnormalities. Characteristic facial features may lead to suspicion of Down's syndrome or other genetic disorders.

General inspection also includes looking at skin color for the normally pink or red color, with possibly bluish extremities, or for abnormalities such as ruddiness, pallor, cyanosis, or jaundice. Any abnormalities in respiration may also be observed. Effects of the birth process such as degree of molding of the head and ecchymosis may be observed. Facial expression may show a baby who is comfortable or one in distress. When the baby begins to cry, the quality and pitch of his cry may be evaluated.

HEART AND LUNGS Examination of the heart, lungs, and abdomen are most easily done while the baby is asleep or at least not crying. If the baby begins to cry it may need to be postponed until he quiets.

Observation of the chest is made for the normal breathing pattern of diaphragmatic breathing with the abdomen rising and falling with inspiration and expiration, and for a normal respiratory rate of approximately 40 times per minute. Intercostal or xiphoid retractions, nasal flaring, expiratory grunt or sigh, and tachypnea are abnormal findings. It is also helpful to note if the chest appears high (hyperextended) or low (hypoextended) in the anterior–posterior diameter. Auscultation is made for type of breath sounds, rales, rhonchi, and wheezes. The entire chest, both anterior and posterior, is examined. Sometimes auscultatory sounds are heard better if the baby is crying.

Localization and identification of chest sounds is very difficult in the newborn, and sometimes the sounds are transmitted so well from an unaffected area of the lung to an affected one that the absence of sounds cannot be diagnosed. Auscultation of the newborn chest requires considerable experience.

The heart is examined for rate and rhythm of heartbeat, position of apical impulse, and intensity of heart sounds. Location of apical beat gives information about heart size and location. The apical impulse can normally be seen or palpated at the fifth intercostal space just left of the sternum. A shift in the mediastinum moves the apical impulse away from the affected side of the chest. Therefore a pneumothorax in the right chest moves the mediastinum to the left and the apical impulse farther to the left than normal. When the left chest is affected the apical impulse is close to the midline of the chest or even to the right of midline.

By auscultation of the heart the first and second heart sounds can be clearly heard. They have been described as a rapid lubb-dubb or a toc-tic sound with the second sound being somewhat sharper and having a higher pitch than the first. Murmurs may be heard, but many are transient and disappear by the third day. Heart rate normally fluctuates from 100 to 180 beats per minute. Auscultation of the heart includes listening over the entire precordium, below the left axilla, and posteriorly below the scapula.

The femoral pulses are palpated by applying gentle pressure, perhaps using the middle finger, over the femoral canal. Decreased or absent femoral pulses indicate coarctation of the aorta. The brachial pulses are also palpated for equality with each other and with the femoral pulses.

ABDOMEN The abdomen is inspected for size and contour and for localized bulging. The abdomen is normally cylindrical in shape and there may be slight bulging between the recti muscles. The umbilical cord is inspected for normal drying or for redness and moistness, and it is examined for the presence of two arteries and one vein. Observation of only two vessels raises the suspicion of congenital anomalies elsewhere in the body.

Palpation of the abdomen for softness or tenseness and for masses should be done in a systematic manner, beginning in one of the quadrants and continuing to the others in a clocklike direction. Palpation may first be done lightly and then repeated with deeper pressure.

The edge of the liver of the newborn is normally palpated 1 to 2 cm below the right costal margin. The tip of the spleen can sometimes be felt in the normal newborn in the lateral portion of the left upper quadrant. Examination of the abdomen must include deep palpation for each kidney. With the baby in the supine position a finger is placed at the posterior flank, the costovertebral angle, to provide upward pressure and the other hand presses down toward the finger at the posterior flank. The kidney can be felt as a small oval structure between the hand and finger. Normally the lower pole of each kidney is situated about 1 to 2 cm above the umbilicus. Below this level means enlargement. It is best to palpate the kidneys soon after birth, or at least before 4 to 6 hours have elapsed, since they can be felt much easier when the intestines are not yet filled with air.

If the baby has not passed meconium and if the anus has not been checked for patency it may be done at this time.

HEAD AND NECK The head is inspected for degree of molding, for size, and for soft tissue edema and bruising. The circumference of the head is measured and compared to normal measurements and to measurement of the chest. For measurement of the baby's head circumference the tape should be placed over the most prominent part of the occiput and brought around to just above the eyebrows. Since head circumference is an important measurement of brain size and later measurements are good in-

dicators of brain growth, the head circumference should be measured very carefully and accurately. To check on one's own measurements it is advisable to repeat the measurement a second and a third time.[7] Since measurement of the head may change as molding decreases, it is helpful to remeasure the head a few days later.

The anterior and posterior fontanels are palpated for size and depression or bulging, and then are measured, and the sutures between the cranial bones are palpated for amount of overlapping. For measurement of the anterior fontanel, the anteroposterior and transverse dimensions are measured with the fingers, and the size is recorded. The posterior fontanel may also be measured with a finger. In order to obtain an accurate measurement of the fontanels the width of the examiner's fingers can be measured in centimeters.

Often the baby's chest is measured at the same time that the head is measured. For measurement of chest circumference, the measuring tape is placed at the lower end of the scapulas and brought around anteriorly directly over the nipple line. Three measurements are taken and the average is recorded.[8] Measurement of the abdominal circumference may also be taken at this time, placing the measuring tape around the baby's abdomen at the level of the umbilicus.

The baby's face is assessed for symmetry of the eyes, nose, and ears.

The eyes are checked for size, equality of pupils, reaction of pupils to light, the blink reflex to light, and edema and inflammation of the eyelids. The conjunctivas are checked for hemorrhage and inflamamation and the corneas are examined for a bright and shiny appearance. A hazy dull cornea is abnormal. The eyes are examined for the normal red reflex to check that there is no opacity between the lens and the retina and to rule out cataracts.

[7] Marcene Erickson, *Assessment and Developmental Changes in Children.* Mosby, St. Louis, Mo., 1976, p. 25.
[8] *Ibid.*, p. 35.

Examination of the eyes may be difficult in the newborn because the baby tends to keep his eyes closed. It is usually not helpful to attempt to hold the lids open. The baby is likely to open his eyes when he is rocked from the upright to the horizontal position a few times or by other methods that may alert him.

The ears are inspected for size, shape, position, and anomaly. Low set ears are sometimes associated with anomalies elsewhere. Preauricular tags are relatively common.

Newborns must breathe through the nose, since they cannot ordinarily breathe through the mouth. Patency of the nares or unilateral choanal atresia can be checked by closing first one nostril and then the other, making sure the mouth is closed, and then observing respirations.

The mouth is checked especially for cleft palate. Visualization of the mouth is probably best when the baby is crying. Palpation with a finger is also done since a cleft of the hard palate with intact mucous membrane cannot be visualized. This is also an opportunity to evaluate the strength of the baby's suck.

The neck is inspected for webbing and palpated for presence of lymph nodes and masses.

The clavicles are palpated for crepitus, depressions, bony masses, or ridges to rule out fracture.

GENITALIA   Examination of the male consists of looking for the position of the meatal opening and for any evidence of hypospadius and also inspecting the scrotum for size and symmetry, for hydrocele, and for undescended testicles. The testes should be palpated separately between the thumb and finger of one hand while the thumb and index finger of the other hand are placed together over the inguinal canal.

The female genitalia are examined for size of the labia majora and minora, for amount of protrusion of labia minora from majora, for clitoral size, and for fusion of the labia. Hymenal tags are often normally present, protruding from the vagina. A creamy, mucous vaginal discharge is normally present, and vaginal bleeding is seen occasionally.

SKIN   The skin should be closely observed as each area of the body is examined. Color, consistency, turgor, elasticity, texture, hydration, and areas of desquamation are noted. The examiner is watchful for petechiae, areas of ecchymosis, hemangiomas, eruptions, hemorrhagic manifestations, inflammation, and nevi.

MUSCULOSKELETAL   The spine is inspected and palpated for abnormal curvatures, for masses, tufts of hair over the spine, spina bifida, and pilonidal sinus. The extremities are examined for gross deformities, for extra digits, for webbing, for club feet, and for range of motion.

The baby is examined for congenital dislocation of the hip by placing him supine, flexing his knees, and then abducting both of his hips and knees. Normally both knees can be brought down simultaneously to the examining table. A dislocated hip does not abduct well. Sometimes with dislocation a click can be heard and felt with this maneuver. Asymmetry of the buttock creases and unequal leg length when the baby lies on his abdomen are also present with dislocation.

NEUROLOGIC   Some of the neurologic examination is accomplished throughout the physical examination as the baby is observed for respiratory movements, cardiac action, eye movements, posture and muscle tone, spontaneous activity, spontaneous alertness, the strength of the cry, and the response to stimuli. Fine, rapid tremors are normal, but large coarse tremors are suggestive of pathology.

A few of the baby's reflexes may also be checked to determine neurologic status. These usually include the Moro reflex, grasp, grasp and traction showing ability to bring the head up, standing and walking, and rooting and sucking.

More evidence concerning development of the central nervous system is obtained if a Brazelton neonatal behavior assessment is done. This assessment is described below.

The Neonatal Behavioral Assessment Scale

The Brazelton Neonatal Behavioral Assessment Scale, developed by Dr. T. Berry Brazelton[9] and associates over the past 20 years, is a means of scoring a newborn's interactive behavior. It evaluates the baby's behavior, his responses to his environment, and the ways in which he attempts to control his environment. A number of the items on the scale are psychologic items that permit assessment of some of the baby's capabilities relevant to his developing social relationship with others.

As a result of the work of Brazelton and a number of others it is now known that newborns are really very capable. They can see, hear, attend to various stimuli, shut out stimuli they do not want, and maintain attention quite well when they want to. They can often quiet and console themselves when they are upset. Newborns can communicate their needs very well. They communicate through crying, through smiling, and through paying attention to others. Their motor capability and coordination is quite well developed.

Newborns can explore and learn from the beginning. They can adapt quite easily to most situations presented to them. They are well able to demonstrate individual temperamental characteristics that influence their care. The important thing is for parents and caretakers to understand each individual newborn's capabilities and his particular needs.

The Brazelton behavioral evaluation scale provides for a systematic, organized way of assessing a newborn's varied unique and complex capabilities. By testing the baby's integrated behavior it gives much better evidence of his CNS function than tests of isolated reflexes and

[9] T. Berry Brazelton, *Neonatal Behavioral Assessment Scale. Clinics in Developmental Medicine, No. 50.* Spastics International Medical Publications, Heinemann Medical Books, London, and Lippincott, Philadelphia, Pa., 1973.

neurologic capabilities. The test relies on the higher levels of function of the central nervous system. It tests the newborn's responses to various kinds of stimulation, always taking into account his state of consciousness at the time of each test item. When a baby has been somewhat uncoordinated in a testing, repeated tests will show a curve of either a quick or rather prolonged recovery from an insult. Such evidence may then be a good predictor of future CNS function. Behavioral assessment may also be of special value for observing mother–infant interaction, predicting mother–infant attachment, and helping with a good mother–infant adjustment.

The Brazelton score includes 27 behavioral items, each scored on a nine-point scale, and 20 elicited neurologic responses, scored on a three-point scale. Some of the items are scored according to the baby's reaction to specific stimuli. Others are observed throughout the assessment and scored at the end. Although the main purpose of the examination is behavioral evaluation, neurologic items are included to check the baby's inherent neurologic capacity. Dr. Brazelton also suggests that the examiner make note of how the baby reacts to stress. Does he spit up, thrash around, cry often, hiccough, have much skin color variability, make sucking movements frequently?

The midpoint of the Brazelton scale is the norm for most items. The mean is the expected behavior of a full-term, average-sized baby who had a normal intrauterine environment, a good Apgar score at birth, and did not need special care at birth. The behavior of the third day of life is taken as the expected mean. This is to avoid the discoordinated behavior of the first 48 hours of a number of babies. By the third day the great demands of physiologic adjustment to extrauterine life have decreased and the baby can better attend to other things. Testing can, however, be done earlier than the third day.

Items on the Brazelton scale are repeated as necessary so that the rating can be done on the baby's best rather than his average performance.

Basing the score on the best the baby can do provides a prediction of his capability, given optimum conditions. If the baby has responded poorly to an item the test should be repeated later in the examination to look for a better response. It is always important to consider the baby's state of consciousness when evaluating his reactions to stimuli, since such reactions will vary markedly depending on his state. The optimal state for eliciting each response is printed on the scoring sheet. The six different states of sleep and wakefulness that are generally recognized are described on pages 464–66.

Dr. Brazelton's explanation of the importance of considering state is as follows[10]:

The baby's state of consciousness is perhaps the single most important element in the behavioral examination. His reactions to all stimulation are dependent upon his ongoing state of consciousness and any interpretation of them must be made with this in mind. In addition, his use of a state to maintain control of his reactions to environmental and internal stimuli is an important mechanism and reflects his potential for organization. State sets a dynamic pattern which reflects the full behavioral repertoire of the infant. Specifically this examination tracks the pattern of state change over the course of the examination, its lability and its direction in response to external and internal stimuli. Thus, the variability of state becomes a dimension of assessment, pointing to the initial abilities in the infant for self-organization.

Further assessment of the infant's ability for self-organization are contained in the skills measuring his ability for self-quieting after aversive stimuli. This is contrasted to the infant's need for stimuli from the examiner to help him quiet.

Categories of Behaviors

The items from the Brazelton Neonatal Behavioral Assessment Scale have been arbitrarily organized into certain categories of behavior, which are briefly described below. These categories will give the reader an acquaintance

[10] *Ibid.*, p. 2.

with some of the behavioral items and some of the expected responses. For a complete discussion of all of the test items the reader is referred to the original scale.[11]

Habituation

This rather forbidding term means that an individual reaches a stage where he can block out or stop responding to repeated stimuli. This makes it possible to stop reacting to annoying or irritating stimuli such as noise or bright lights. The normal newborn is well equipped to habituate, making it possible for him to decrease his reactions to repeated disturbing stimuli. Such a response provides time for rest and for reaction to new stimuli.

The Brazelton scale includes items of repeated stimuli of light, sound of a bell and of a rattle, and a pinprick to the heel to assess how soon and how well the baby closes out noxious stimuli or how vulnerable he may be to continued stimulation. This behavior is tested in a sleep state. A normal healthy baby is likely to filter out such stimulation and quit responding to annoying stimulation. His response will change from gross motor movements to no more than an eye blink. He shows that he can reduce his responses and control things himself, without the assistance of others.

Orientation

Several tests are performed to check on the baby's ability to orient or respond to stimuli in the environment. These tests are scored in the quiet awake (alert) state. The baby is assessed for his ability to turn toward the direction of visual and auditory stimuli of an inanimate and an animate nature and also a combination of visual and auditory stimuli.

The above testing assesses the baby's ability to attend to, to focus on, and to respond to stim-

[11] T. Berry Brazelton, *Neonatal Behavioral Assessment Scale. Clinics in Developmental Medicine, No. 50.* Spastics International Medical Publications, Heinemann Medical Books, London, and Lippincott, Philadelphia, Pa., 1973.

uli of a bright object like a red ball, a rattle or a soft bell, the examiner's face, the examiner's voice, and the examiner's voice and face. It can be noted how well he pays attention to the stimuli, how well he concentrates on them, whether or not he follows with his eyes and/or with his head, whether he searches for the source, and how vigorously he alerts and responds. The baby's overall ability to alert, with brightening and widening of the eyes, which is observed throughout the assessment examination, can often be especially observed while testing his orientation ability.

Motor Ability (Maturity)

Several items on the assessment scale, such as general tone, smoothness of movements, pull to a sitting position, and ability to coordinate hand-to-mouth movements, test motor maturity. These items are assessed continually during the examination and scored at the end of the assessment. They are especially observed in an alert state.

The baby's overall general tone and his posture and his passive movements while he is handled are all assessed. This is an overall assessment of the baby's body tone as he reacts to a number of different test items. His motor maturity is also demonstrated by smooth movements of the extremities (in contrast to jerky movements) and by easy range of motion.

A hand-to-mouth reflex is present in all newborns. The baby uses this reflex to control himself and comfort himself. The ease with which the baby does this maneuver and the quickness with which he sucks on his fist show motor maturity and also his ability to quiet himself.

A pull-to-sit maneuver also tests motor maturity. As the baby grasps around the examiner's fingers he is pulled to a sitting position. The shoulder girdle muscles will respond with tone and the baby will attempt to right his head into a position which is in the midline of his trunk and parallel to his body. Since the baby's head is heavy in comparison to the rest of his body, he will ordinarily not be able to right his head for

very long, and it will fall back. When the baby is placed in a seated position he will also attempt to right his head, and it is then likely to fall forward. Most infants will make several attempts to right their heads.

The ease and frequency with which a baby startles is assessed. Tremulousness is also assessed. Tremors may be present off and on, especially after startles and upon awakening. Mild tremors of the chin and extremities can be expected during the first week. Severe tremors may be a sign of prematurity, or metabolic imbalance, or CNS irritation or depression.

Defensive movements, such as baby's attempt to remove a cloth placed over his head also demonstrate motor maturity.

Quieting Ability

Self-quieting ability measures the baby's ability to quiet himself when he is in a fussing state. He may use such actions as hand-to-mouth movement, sucking on his fist or tongue, or attending to a visual or auditory stimulus. Abilities of babies range from those who consistently quiet themselves to those who quiet themselves on occasion, to those unable to quiet themselves. The number of observable activities the baby uses is counted. The ability of the baby to quiet himself shows his capacity for self-organization.

Consolability with intervention is an item closely related to self-quieting. This item, observed after each disturbing maneuver, is assessed by determining how much intervention is necessary to quiet a fussy baby and allow him to move to a lower state. Intervention may begin with simple measures such as the examiner presenting first the face, then the face and voice, then placing a hand on the baby, putting covers over him, and perhaps holding one arm or both of his arms across his abdomen or his chest. Holding the baby's arms may help to quiet him because it interferes with the startle reflex, which is triggered by crying or fussing, and which disturbs the baby. When the simpler measures are not effective, the baby is picked up, rocked and talked to, and, if necessary, offered a pacifier.

Cuddliness

This is an assessment of the baby's response to being held. Some babies do not like to be picked up and held, and others adjust their bodies to that of the adult holding them and settle in comfortably without a struggle and even actively participate. In scoring this item there will be variations in babies from those who actually resist being held most all of the time to those who will eventually settle in to those who settle in well and quickly with their entire body.

Smile is included here with cuddliness because it is one of the behaviors that parents assess along with cuddliness as they interact with their baby. Smiles in the newborn may be mainly reflex grimacing, but they do sometimes appear in response to talking or looking at the baby, and mothers are likely to note them as they interact with their baby.

Changes of State, Activity, Color

Certain items that are continuously assessed are lability of color, rapidity of changes in activity levels, periods of alertness and periods of excitement, number of startles, amount of irritability, and lability of states. Irritability is measured by the number of times the baby gets upset and for what reason.

The number of state changes during the entire examination are counted. Careful record is kept of state and color changes because they are good indicators of stress on the autonomic nervous system, and rapidity of change of states measures the amount of control the baby can maintain with increasing aversive stimulation.

Clinical Use of Neonatal Behavioral Assessment

The Neonatal Behavioral Assessment Scale was developed as a research tool. Any individual who will use it as such needs training to do scoring reliably so that results are useful for investigations and studies. However, this assessment tool can be used as a part of nurses' and physicians' clinical assessment of newborns.

Nurses should be aware of the observations that they can make using this tool or a modification thereof in the ordinary care of each newborn. It will help them assess the baby's responses to his care, assess their own reactions to his responses, anticipate and observe how the baby may or does affect his parents, and use this information to inform parents of their baby's behavior, help them to understand him, and plan for his individual care.

A behavioral assessment tool can be used very profitably with mothers or parents observing, or in discussion with parents, to demonstrate to them their baby's unique abilities. Nurses can, in addition, make a number of ongoing observations of the individual baby's sleep patterns, eating patterns, quieting and/or irritability characteristics, alerting behavior, and so on in their care of the baby while he is in the nursery and give this information to parents. Helping parents to understand and respond to their baby's individual temperament, characteristics, and needs is a very important contribution that can be made by professionals to the baby's future care and development.

Parents can be helped to learn about their baby's sleep and awake states, how quickly he changes states, how much he sleeps and alerts, why the alert state is the best time to feed him and play with him, when he needs to be picked up to be consoled and when this may not be necessary.

Babies differ a great deal from one another in the length of their periods of sleep and wakefulness, in their eating cycle, in how rapidly and how smoothly they move from one state to another, how much they cry, how easily they are soothed. Some babies are neither readily awakened nor easily disturbed by noise or handling, while others are often wakeful and fussy and respond to minimal stimulation. A quiet baby may need periods of stimulation, and an excitable baby may need all sources of stimulation minimized and may need time for quieting. A fussy, crying baby will require a much different kind of care than one who is placid and easily soothed.

Cuddliness is a characteristic that most people like in a baby, and yet there are some babies that resist being held and cuddled. Parents with a baby that does not "settle in well" when held must be helped to understand that their baby's behavior is a part of his individual temperament, that he reacts in that way with other persons, and that his reaction is not a result of their care or a reaction to them personally. They need help to understand that such behavior happens to be the baby's preference.

By use of the behavioral assessment scale or some modification of it parents can learn that their baby is capable of alerting and turning toward their voice, of looking at them and fixating his eyes if they take care to get into his visual field, and of responding positively to gentle touch. The baby must be given time to respond. Parents can learn that the baby shows that he is attending to stimulation by such actions as quieting and settling down if he has been active, or by increasing his activity if he has been quiet, by visual fixation, by listening, by searching for the source of the stimulus. They can also learn how much their baby reacts to stimuli or closes it out.

Parents can learn about their baby's self-quieting efforts and that he should be given time to use them. They may learn that a baby is not necessarily hungry when he attempts to suck his fists.

Parents can learn of the various methods of soothing a crying baby beginning with sight of face, voice, and touch, and moving to picking up and rocking as necessary. They can learn that picking the baby up and rocking him will not spoil him; he may need such help to quiet. Parents can be encouraged to search for a good method for their baby and what seems best for him. Parents' success in soothing their baby has a positive effect upon their feeling of competence.

Among other things that nurses may observe and report to parents or parents may observe and discuss with nurses are:

How clearly does the baby show he is asleep or drowsy or awake?
How does the baby act when he is hungry, or tired, or wet?
How does the baby act when he is satisfied?
How does the baby act when he is dressed and bathed?
When is the baby most likely to be fussy and crying?
How well does the baby quiet himself and in what ways?
How does the baby suck and feed? Does he spit up? Are there any special ways helpful in feeding him?
What are some of the reasons for the baby's crying? How can parents begin to interpret what he is trying to communicate by his cry?

It is apparent that there are many ways in which nurses, physicians, and parents can learn to understand a baby's individuality. An organized assessment form is a very useful way for the nurse to do a systematic observation of a baby's behavior. When the nurse has an understanding of the items usually assessed she will also be alert to the behavior the baby demonstrates as she is giving daily care. All this information should be shared with parents to help them understand their baby's behavior and to interact with him in an effective way.

IMPLEMENTATION OF NURSING CARE

Immediate Care of the Newborn in the Delivery Room

Nursing care of the newborn begins with the baby's birth. In the period immediately after birth the baby must be assisted in establishing and maintaining respirations, and he must immediately be protected against heat loss and provided with warmth. Apgar scoring is done at 1 and 5 minutes, a quick appraisal is made of the baby's overall appearance and behavior, and the entire body is quickly examined for gross anomalies. After respirations have stabilized the baby may also be examined for anomalies not grossly apparent. Suggestions for this examination as made by the American Academy of Pediatrics are described on page 480.

Appropriate identification of the baby and probably prophylactic treatment against gonorrheal ophthalmia are also included in the early care of the newborn. Depending on the mother's and infant's condition, the baby is given to the mother to look at and hold and examine as soon as possible. All the immediate care of the newborn that is given in the delivery room has been described on pages 354–74.

Transitional Care

The greatest hazard in the postnatal period is in the first day of life. The nurse must watch the newborn baby very closely during this period in which he is making drastic adjustments to his environment. Since many neonatal problems begin in the first 6 to 8 hours after birth, the baby's care during this time should be given in a nursery area specially designated as recovery room or transitional care area. There the baby can be closely monitored during this transitional phase and for a longer period of time if necessary. In terms of time the transitional period is usually considered to be the first 6 to 8 hours after birth, but for some babies a longer time is necessary for their conditions to stabilize, with the transitional period extending to an upper limit of 24 hours.

Each baby, regardless of how normal his past history, must be closely observed. Every baby must be assumed to be at risk, at least from choking by mucus, and all must be closely observed. For some babies the risk of postnatal difficulty is particularly great. Conditions that may complicate the postnatal course include intrauterine fetal distress, apnea or hypoxia at birth, prolonged labor, difficult delivery, and complications of the mother during pregnancy, such as antepartum bleeding and diabetes. The nurse caring for newborns should be acquainted with the prenatal, labor, and delivery history of each baby for whose care she is responsible.

Babies in whom difficulty is anticipated may be cared for in an incubator where they are more protected and also more easily observed than they are in a bassinet.

After it becomes apparent that the baby has made a good adjustment to extrauterine life, anywhere from 6 to 24 hours for the normal fullterm baby, he can be cared for in his mother's room or in the central nursery.

Admission to the Nursery

Immediately on admission of a baby to the nursery the nurse will need to have some important information of the pregnancy and the labor and delivery. She will want to know the estimated gestational age according to the mother's history and other assessments that may have been made before delivery; any medical or obstetric complications; the mother's Rh factor and serology; when labor began; when the membrane ruptured; all medications given to the mother during labor (kind and amount); the fetal heart rate and pattern during labor; the Apgar score and any resuscitative efforts. Additional history can probably be obtained later.

The baby's vital signs are checked on admission, and he is measured and weighed. While these procedures are carried out care is taken to avoid exposure and heat loss. The baby should be placed in a preheated bassinet or incubator and he should be provided with an overhead radiant heater. Most of the care can be given under the heat lamp.

The baby's general overall appearance and behavior can also be assessed during admission procedures. It is important to look at relative size of body, head, and extremities; to observe for the normally flexed posture, strong muscle tone, and symmetrical, spontaneous movement of all extremities; to check for a normally pink-red color with perhaps cyanotic hands and feet, forceps marks or bruises, condition of the skin, edema, and a normally strong, vigorous, spontaneous cry.

To obtain the respiratory rate the respirations are counted for one full minute. Since there is little thoracic movement with a newborn's respirations, they are best observed by watching the abdomen rise and fall with inspiration and expiration. The chest should be observed for any retractions. The heart rate is counted for 30 seconds using a stethoscope, listening for the lubb-dubb sounds. Auscultation for heart sounds and breath sounds, may also be made at this time. Each sound should be listened to separately, however. The initial body temperature is taken rectally to check on patency of the anus. Thereafter it is advisable to take the baby's temperature by axilla to avoid injury to the rectal mucosa.

The baby's birth weight is obtained and recorded, and his length is measured by placing him on his back and extending him as much as possible. See page 501 for precautions in taking measurement of weight and page 441 for suggestions for obtaining an accurate length. A measurement of the head circumference is usually taken at this time, and the fontanels may also be palpated and measured. The chest and sometimes the abdomen may be measured immediately after the head has been measured or it may be done later during a complete physical examination.

A gestational age assessment is made, probably using the brief set of criteria in Figure 18-4. Later, and as indicated, a more detailed assessment using the Dubowitz assessment score (pages 478–79) may be used. The measurements and gestational age may be recorded on the intrauterine growth chart shown in Figure 18-2. Using this information it should be possible to differentiate between a preterm baby and a term baby who is SGA and between a normal-sized term baby and a preterm LGA baby. Certain problems can be anticipated by accurate assessment and classification of gestational age.

The baby's identification bracelets are checked to correlate the information on them with the chart records.

As was suggested on page 370, it is desirable to postpone prophylactic treatment of the eyes (which for many years was a traditional delivery room procedure) until admission of the baby to the nursery. If the treatment was not done in the delivery room, it should be carried out as a part of the admission regime. The method of prophylactic eye treatment is described on pages 368–71.

The umbilical cord stump and the surrounding skin is wiped with an antiseptic, usually with alcohol 60 percent; or with a bacteriostatic such as triple dye. The number of umbilical cord vessels can be checked at this time.

A few reflexes may be checked on admission. The Moro reflex and grasp reflex, valuable signs of normal behavior, should be elicited easily. The baby may demonstrate his sucking reflex by attempting to suck on his fist or on anything that comes near his mouth.

Blood on the baby's face and scalp may be washed off with a warm wet cloth or cotton balls. No further bathing is done until the baby has regained a stable normal body temperature or until after the second period of reactivity described below.

Vitamin K, usually ordered as a single dose of 1.0 mg, is given intramuscularly to prevent a transitory deficiency in blood coagulation.

Administration of Intramuscular Medication

The preferred intramuscular injection sites for infants are the muscles of the thigh. The gluteal region, a common site for intramuscular injections, is small and shallow in a baby; this relatively small area increases the possibility of injection in the vicinity of the sciatic nerve.

When the thigh is used for injection, one of two areas is satisfactory. The injection may be made into the large muscle at the upper third of the lateral aspect of the thigh or into the midportion of the anterior aspect of the thigh. For administration into the lateral area the baby is placed on his side, and his leg is held firmly while the injection is made. When the anterior aspect of the thigh is used, the baby is restrained during injection by placing him on his back, extending his leg, and making firm pressure on his knee. Use of the anterior injection site requires precaution against placing the needle toward the inner aspect of the thigh because of important nerves and blood vessels in that area.

Occasionally the baby's arm is used for injection, making the deltoid muscle the site of the injection. Care must be taken that the drug is injected into the muscle, and not into adjacent tissue. The deltoid muscle is used only when the thigh is not accessible or when the baby is receiving many repeated injections.

Before proceeding with a description of care of the newborn over the next several hours after admission to the nursery the early clinical behavior of the baby will be described.

Clinical Behavior in the Transition Period

All infants, mature or immature, well or sick, must go through a period of transition to extrauterine life. This process involves changes in function in all organ systems, a reorganization of functions, and an adjustment of metabolic processes in order to achieve homeostasis. In an observational study of the clinical behavior of newborn infants in the first hours after birth Dr. Murdina Desmond[12] and others found that the normal vigorous newborn went through a characteristic orderly pattern of a series of changes in vital signs and clinical appearance—color, cry, and activity—during the transition phase that consisted of the first 6 to 12 postnatal hours. From their findings they identified a first period of reactivity, a relatively unresponsive interval that usually included sleep, and a second period of reactivity.

Dr. Desmond and others found that an overall predictable sequence of clinical behavior generally appeared after birth regardless of the baby's gestational age or route of delivery. Wide fluctuations, however, were noted in normal infants. The ordinary time sequence of events was considerably altered in babies with low Apgar scores, with maternal medications, with an ab-

[12] Murdina M. Desmond *et al.*, The clinical behavior of the newly born. I. The term baby, *J. Pediatr.* 62:307–325 (Mar.) 1963.

normal intrauterine environment, and with immaturity.

The First Period of Reactivity

The vigorous infant begins this period immediately after birth. The baby responds to the intense sensory stimuli of labor and delivery and the sudden new environment with a predominance of activity of the sympathetic nervous system. As a result the baby becomes intensely active and alert and hypertonic, with outbursts of diffuse purposeless movements, immediately after birth. The heart and respiratory rates become very rapid and transient flaring of the nostrils, retraction of the chest, grunting, and chest rales are likely to appear.

In Desmond's studies, the general trend of the heart rate was a somewhat slow rate at delivery, but immediately thereafter an abrupt rate increase usually took place. The mean peak in heart rate was 180 beats per minute at about 2 or 3 minutes after birth. This tachycardia was brief, deceleration followed, and the rate slowed to 120 to 140 by about 30 minutes after birth.

The respirations were rapid, shallow, and irregular immediately after delivery. The median peak respiratory rate was 82 breaths per minute and this occurred at a median time of one hour after birth. The range of time at which a peak respiratory rate occurred was wide, however. Flaring of the nostrils was common, at least in the first 15 minutes. Transient, brief episodes of grunting and retraction were noted in some babies. Barreling of the chest (an increase in the anteroposterior diameter) was noted to accompany periods of rapid shallow respiration, most commonly between 1 and 2 hours after birth. Barreling disappeared whenever the respiratory pattern changed and recurred with rapid, shallow breathing. Fine rales and rhonchi were heard during the first 15 minutes. Clear thin mucus was present at the mouth in some babies.

The baby's activity immediately after birth was described as one of alerting exploratory behavior. This activity included such actions as movement of the head from side to side, opening and closing of the eyelids, fixation of the gaze for brief periods, sucking, chewing, swallowing, smacking, rooting, grimacing, chewing of the fingers, and protrusion of the tongue. The baby's ability to be alert and explore and to respond to his mother makes this period immediately after birth an important time for maternal–infant bonding. The time is more appropriately used for maternal–infant acquaintance than for other aspects of care, such as prophylactic treatment of the eyes.

The baby's activity also included outbursts of rapid movement of the extremities, increased muscle tone, spontaneous startles, tremors of the extremities and chin, and abrupt onsets and cessations of crying. In some babies intense activity began immediately after birth, while in others there was a brief period of quiet and inactivity at first, although these babies were responsive to stimuli. In general alerting exploratory behavior peaked at one hour. Some babies were constantly active, while most had brief periods of relative inactivity interspersed with periods of active movements. During the periods of relative inactivity the babies usually assumed a characteristic position of increased muscle tone (Figure 17-21, page 467).

The color at birth usually showed some cyanosis, but became pinker with the onset of intense activity. General flushing with crying usually appeared after 15 minutes postnatally.

Bowel sounds were absent at birth but became audible with a stethoscope after about 15 minutes.

A summary of the physical findings of the first period of reactivity is shown in Figure 18-5.

First Period of Rest and Sleep

Following the initial alerting behavior of the first period of reactivity the normal infant becomes quiet and relatively unresponsive to stimuli. He relaxes and is likely to fall asleep. The time of the first sleep of the individual baby and the length of that sleep varies considerably.

The most frequent and characteristic pattern observed in the newborns studied was alerting and exploratory behavior that lasted anywhere

from 30 to 150 minutes and then began to decrease. Intervals of quiet lengthened, and outbursts of activity, spontaneous or in response to mild stimulation, decreased in frequency. Sleep began anywhere from 1 hour to 4½ hours after birth. Often there were spontaneous jerks and twitches and chewing, smacking, and grimacing movements during sleep. Length of sleep varied from a few minutes to 3 to 4 hours.

In some babies the time of alerting behavior was short, less than 30 minutes, and inactivity or sleep began early. Sometimes there were alternating brief periods of activity and inactivity or sleep.

Second Period of Reactivity

A second period of reactivity, which may remain active for a variable period of time, being brief or lasting for several hours, appears when the baby awakens from his first rest or sleep. This hyperactivity sometimes occurs with the third hour, but is more common beginning at the fourth or fifth hour. Responsiveness in this period may be exaggerated and the baby may have brief periods of tachycardia, tachypnea, abrupt changes in tone, color, peristalsis, and mucus. It appears that both sympathetic and parasympathetic responses occur in cycles of short duration during this time.

During the second period of reactivity the heart rate is labile with wide swings in rate varying from bradycardia to tachycardia, depending upon the body's activity. Respirations are variable, decreasing with activity and with crying. There may be very short apneic pauses. Flaring of the nostrils, grunting, and retraction may occur intermittently, especially if the baby has difficulty with mucus.

Mucus appears again during this period. It tends to be thicker than that seen in the period immediately after birth. Presence of mucus is often accompanied by sneezing. The appearance of oral mucus can be a major problem at this time. It may be associated with gagging, swallowing, vomiting, and sometimes choking.

Color changes appeared quickly and frequently during the second period of reactivity. Marked vasomotor responses were evident in the quick changes of deep flushing with crying and rapid decrease in color to a pallor when crying stopped. Circumoral pallor, brief pallor of the body, and brief periods of acrocyanosis with activity or crying were not uncommon.

Meconium is often passed between 2 and 5 hours after birth.

A summary of the physical findings of the second period of reactivity is shown in Figure 18-5.

When the second period of reactivity is finished the normal newborn usually appears to be relatively stable and recovered from the experience of labor and delivery and the influence of any drugs, and he has usually made a good adjustment to extrauterine existence.

The physical findings of normal newborns in the first hours after birth as described above may vary considerably in individual infants, but taken collectively they give a description of the physiologic changes that can be expected in a baby in the transitional period. A number of these events, such as grunting and chest retraction, would be signs of illness if they were present at a different age, or present continuously, or not consistent with other findings at this time. It is nevertheless essential to observe closely any signs that are ordinarily considered evidence of distress to determine if they are only transient or if they persist and lead to difficulty. The baby needs recovery room or transitional nursery care during this time.

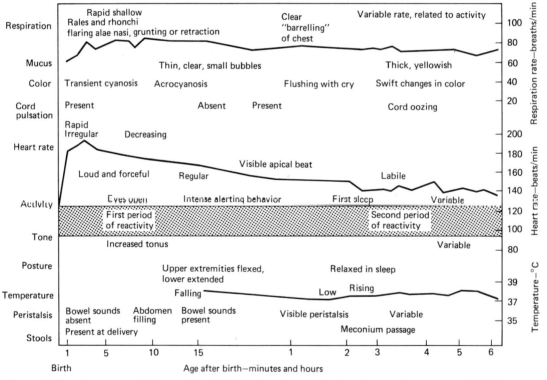

Figure 18-5. A summary of the activity and vital signs during the first hours of extrauterine life (the transitional period) in babies who are not stressed or depressed at birth. [*Reproduced from Helen W. Arnold et al., "Transition to Extra-Uterine Life,"* Am. J. Nurs., 65(10):77–80 (Oct.) 1965. *Copyright October 1965, The American Journal of Nursing Company. Reproduced with permission from the* American Journal of Nursing, Vol. 65, No. 10.]

The period immediately after birth has traditionally been considered a time of crisis for the newborn, but it is important to keep in mind that the baby may also have serious difficulty in the second period of reactivity. There can be problems with choking on mucus, with cyanosis, apnea, grunting, chest retraction, and bradycardia. The persistence of any of these signs of distress must be closely monitored. The nurse must be well informed as to what to expect of the newborn in this important period of transition from intrauterine to extrauterine life and must be aware of the complications that may arise.

It is important to note that, although as a group normal babies of an uncomplicated pregnancy follow the relatively predictable time schedule of transition as described above, an individual baby is unpredictable and variable. This may be related to differences in biologic maturity or in prenatal and birth influences. The nurse must be alert in her observations for those babies who need a much longer than usual time for transition.

The transition period may be complicated and prolonged for babies who begin extrauterine life under adverse conditions. The time sequence of changes in clinical behavior is likely to be considerably altered in babies who have not had an entirely normal prenatal and labor and delivery course. Generally, reactions are slower in babies of low birth weight, in those with low Apgar scores, in those affected by maternal medication, in those born of a complicated pregnancy, and in those with intrinsic disease. The initial tachycardia may be delayed, the period of rapid respiration may be delayed and prolonged, the alerting response may be poor or unsustained, the unresponsive period may be prolonged, and the second period of reactivity may be delayed by a number of hours. These babies may need a day or more of care in the transitional nursery.

An illustration of a baby with a prolonged course of recovery is shown in Figure 18-6. The illustration shows that the baby was vigorous at birth, possibly from the stimulation of labor and delivery and then quickly became depressed from drugs. It also points out that a good Apgar score gives an assessment of the condition of the baby at the beginning of the transition period but does not necessarily predict his subsequent course.

Ongoing Observations and Care in the Transition Period

Admission of the baby to the nursery and the observation made at that time have been described above. Following those assessments the baby needs ongoing observation of his vital signs, of his overall behavior, and for any signs of potential difficulty.

Pulse and respirations should be checked every 15 to 30 minutes in the first hour after birth and then every hour until stable. Finally a check every four hours may be sufficient.

If respiratory distress develops, it is most likely to appear in the early neonatal period. Function of the respiratory system must be closely watched in the transition period so that difficulty can be averted or treated. Observations include respiratory rate and pattern, chest movement, and color of the infant. The respirations may be irregular and occasionally rapid for short periods during the first few hours, but are abnormal if they are sustained at 60 or more times per minute. After a period of adjustment the normal respiratory rate is approximately 40 per minute.

Chest movements must be carefully observed and, if chest retraction persists, it must be described and reported. The respirations should be quiet, with only momentary periods of expiratory grunting. Persistent grunting is not normal and requires investigation for cause. There should be no episodes of cyanosis. Oxygen should be readily available in the transition nursery in case it is needed for respiratory difficulty.

A newborn must be closely observed for accumulation of mucus in his mouth and oropharynx, which may cause gagging and choking. Some babies have difficulty with mucus for several hours after birth. Other babies have mucus

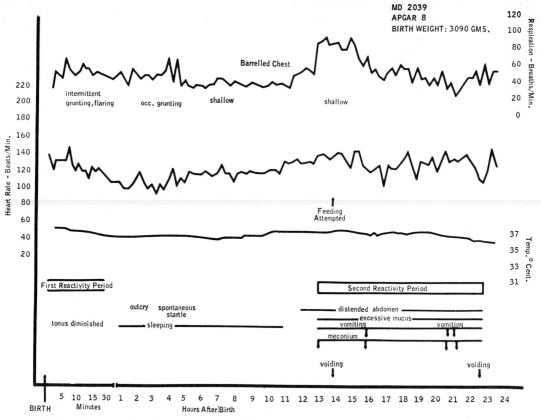

Figure 18-6. Moderate drug depression with vigorous condition at delivery. This 3090-gm infant was born to a 34-year-old multipara after a total labor of 8 hours and a vertex presentation outlet forceps delivery. Medications included promethazine hydrochloride, 25 mg, and secobarbital sodium, 100 mg, intramuscularly 4½ hours, and meperidine, 50 mg (25 mg intramuscularly, 25 mg intravenously), 70 minutes prior to delivery. The infant was vigorous 1 minute after delivery, but tachycardia and rapid respiration did not develop. Tone diminished within 4 minutes after delivery and remained decreased for an 8-hour period. Note shallow respiration, abdominal distention, and relative inactivity. Secondary reactivity was delayed (13 hours) and turbulent. Feeding was attempted at 14 hours, a procedure which may have contributed to problems at this time. After 24 hours the infant appeared to be in good condition. [*Reproduced with permission from Murdina M. Desmond, Arnold J. Rudolph, and Phuangnoi Phitaksphraiwan, "The Transitional Care Nursery: A Mechanism for Preventive Medicine in the Newborn," Pediatr. Clin. North Am. 13(3):651–668, p. 660.*]

immediately after birth, then seem clear, and after several hours have another episode of oral mucus. This may cause choking, gagging, breath-holding, and cyanosis. One cannot assume that a baby who has had a clear period during the early hours of life is in little danger of choking on mucus later in the day when it may appear upon awakening after the first sleep and may be much thicker than earlier. It has been noted that when the baby begins to make swallowing movements it can be anticipated that excessive mucus, and sometimes gagging and vomiting, will soon follow.

Some babies are easily able to clear their mouths and throats of mucus without assistance, but suction must always be immediately available in the nursery. A bulb syringe often clears the mouth sufficiently. Such a syringe should be in the bassinet at all times.

Occasionally a newborn suddenly develops serious respiratory difficulty from obstruction due to accumulation of mucus in the respiratory tract or regurgitation of stomach contents or from a sudden and prolonged period apnea. When such an emergency arises, the nurse must take action quickly to assist the baby and

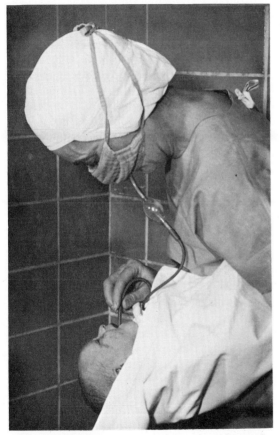

Figure 18-7. Nurse using a plastic or rubber catheter to remove secretions from the baby's mouth and oropharynx. The catheter is placed as far back as possible into the baby's throat and is moved about frequently. Brief suction is made on the mouthpiece of the mucus trap which collects the secretions and thus prevents them from entering the mouth of the operator. The use of postural drainage during this procedure aids in removal of secretions.

also summon medical assistance. Obstructing material must be removed from the mouth and oropharynx, and efforts must be made to reestablish respirations if they have stopped.

Postural drainage can be instituted immediately by holding the baby with head down and neck extended for drainage of secretions by gravity. The nurse should aspirate the baby's mouth and oropharynx. Aspiration may be done with a bulb syringe inserted in the baby's mouth or with suction on a soft catheter introduced into the oropharynx. This catheter, size no. 12 or 14 French, should have one or two holes at the end and be attached to a mechanical suction, or a DeLee mucus trap may be used (Figure 15-9, page 354). Aspiration with a catheter may be more effective in reaching mucus far down in the throat than aspiration with a bulb syringe. The catheter is put into the baby's throat and suction is made on it through the DeLee mucus trap or with a mechanical suction. The position of the catheter should be changed frequently during suctioning. Postural drainage may be used simultaneously with suctioning (Figure 18-7). The baby's head and neck should be slightly hyperextended during suction in either the head-down or the supine position; extension raises the tongue from the posterior pharyngeal wall.

When suctioning mucus, the nurse must keep in mind that vigorous suction in the posterior pharynx can cause vagal stimulation and reflex apnea and bradycardia. Suction must therefore be gentle and brief and done with as little trauma as possible. Very close observation for effects of suction is important, and if the bulb syringe appears to be sufficient, use of more vigorous suction is not advisable.

If the baby is breathing, oxygen administration will improve a hypoxic condition and may improve ventilation. If the baby is receiving oxygen at the time difficulty arises, the oxygen concentration may need to be increased temporarily. If oxygen is not already being given, it may be administered with a mask. If at all possible, the oxygen should be warmed and humidified. Free flowing oxygen to the baby's face, especially if it is not warmed and humidified, should not be used. It causes the baby to respond physiologically as if cold-stressed even though the rest of the body is in a thermoneutral environment. This response comes about because the thermal sensors of the face are more responsive than the skin sensors in other parts of the body.

Sensory stimulation to the baby is sometimes sufficient to initiate respirations during a period of apnea. Flicking the soles of the baby's feet or changing his position may be all that is required, especially sitting him up and rubbing his back gently. If the baby does not breathe following skin stimulation, other measures must be instituted after ascertaining that the airway is not obstructed. If a bag and anesthesia mask and oxygen are readily available, oxygen may be administered by holding the mask over the baby's face and gently applying intermittent pressure to the bag while watching for chest movement. The baby's head should be tilted slightly back and his chin should be held forward during this procedure. Mouth-to-mouth breathing is the method always available to the nurse since equipment is not required. The nurse should be thoroughly familiar with this method, described on pages 364–65.

The body temperature is checked every 30 minutes, especially if a baby is under a radiant heater, until the temperature reaches 98°F (36.7°C). Frequent checks of body temperature are important to ensure that the baby is regaining a normal body temperature quickly. When the baby is placed in a heated bassinet body temperature is used to determine when additional heat is no longer necessary in order to avoid overheating the baby.

The umbilical cord must be closely observed for bleeding and immediately reclamped or retied if necessary.

In addition to watching the baby's color for cyanosis indicating hypoxia, the skin color is observed for pallor indicating low hematocrit or low blood pressure and shock or unusual ruddiness suggestive of polycythemia, and it is checked for jaundice. If the baby's skin appears pale, the color of the mucous membranes should also be noted. The baby's color may indicate that the hematocrit should be checked to determine if it is within a normal range. If presence of jaundice is suspected, it is most easily observed immediately after momentary pressure has been made on the skin. Such pressure, applied to the skin with a finger, causes momentary skin pallor at the pressure area and permits easier visualization of jaundice.

Observation of the baby's activity, cry, and muscle tone is important. Activity can be expected to be alerting, almost hyperresponsive to stimuli, during the periods of reactivity. Quiet and sleep can be expected in the interim between the reactivity periods. The normal cry is lusty and spontaneous at birth and occurs spontaneously at intervals thereafter. Cry and spontaneous activity may be diminished if the baby is depressed from drugs or other conditions of the birth process. Normally the baby maintains a tense posture and moves actively with minimal stimulation. A flaccid, relaxed posture and slow responsiveness to stimuli are abnormal. Twitching, jitteriness, and high-pitched crying are also abnormal.

Babies who are at risk of developing hypoglycemia (low-birth-weight, LGA, complicated pregnancy, labor, and delivery) will require checks for blood glucose values, probably with the use of Dextrostix testing. Hypoglycemia is described in detail on pages 795–800.

The first bowel movement and first voiding, both of which may occur in the delivery room, should especially be noted and recorded as evidences that the intestinal and urinary systems are functioning. Thereafter, a record is continued of each voiding and of each stool.

A detailed gestational age assessment and a physical examination may be done during the transitional period or may preferably be postponed until after the second period of reactivity.

Some time after regaining a normal body temperature the baby may be given his first bath. Included in observations during the bath are the condition of the baby's skin, his body tone, response to touch, and general behavior. The bath may be postponed until after the second period of reactivity. Owing to the hyperactivity of the reactivity periods, sensory input should ordinarily be minimized for the normal baby during these periods. Procedures that are not essential are best postponed until after the reactivity periods are complete and the baby is more stabilized.

The baby is observed for signs of hunger and desire to eat. Unless there is a contraindication to oral feedings, the baby is given his first feeding when he appears to have recovered from the birth and shows a readiness to eat. The appropriate time to offer the baby his first feeding can usually be determined by observation of his reactions during reactivity periods. The baby is more likely to coordinate sucking and swallowing and less likely to have difficulty with gagging and regurgitation when he has become relatively stable. Various aspects of feeding of the newborn are discussed in the next chapter.

Continuing Care After the Transition Period

Included in daily care of the baby are close observation, bathing, feeding, prevention of infection, meeting comfort needs of the baby, facilitating the maternal–infant acquaintance process, and instructing the mother in the care of her baby.

Prevention of Infection

Prevention of infection is an important part of planning for nursery care, and it is also the individual responsibility of everyone concerned with the care of the newborn baby. The first and foremost precaution is thorough hand washing whenever the baby is handled. An antiseptic detergent or a soap or detergent containing hexachlorophene is considered superior to other soap for nursery hand washing.

It is advisable for all persons who will care for newborns to carry out a 2- to 3-minute scrub with iodophor or hexachlorophene at the beginning of each shift. Thereafter the hands should be thoroughly washed with an antiseptic

detergent and running water before and between babies, and before clean nursery equipment is handled. It is especially important that the hands are washed carefully before the baby is fed or the upper part of his body is handled after a diaper has been changed. Jewelry should not be worn by nursing staff. Adequate handwashing facilities should be within easy reach of all bassinets.

Any time that any part of one's face or head (hair, eyes, ears, nose, mouth) is touched with one's hands they are considered contaminated. The hands must be washed again before handling a baby. Persons caring for babies must develop a real awareness of this so that they do not unconsciously touch their face and hair.

To protect the baby from contact with uniforms, all persons wear a gown in the nursery. Nurses and auxiliary personnel wear a short-sleeved gown or scrub dress to permit washing to the elbows. The gown should be changed frequently enough to ensure cleanliness and at least once daily. Cover gowns may be left at each bassinet for staff use while handling an individual infant to prevent cross-contamination between infants. Routine wearing of masks in the nursery is not recommended. Masks become wet from the breath and, if occasionally worn, must be changed at least every one-half hour to be effective. Handling or adjusting of the mask means contamination of the hands and necessitates washing before anything else is handled. When masks are removed, they must immediately be discarded and not worn dangling around the neck.

During her stay in the hospital, the mother is taught the importance of washing her hands before handling her baby and after she has changed his diaper, by explanation of this precaution and reminders when necessary.

A preemployment and annual physical examination of the nursing and auxiliary staff is an essential preventive measure against a newborn's acquisition of infection from nursery personnel.

All personnel must be instructed not to enter the nursery when they develop any signs of an upper respiratory infection, diarrhea or other gastrointestinal upset, skin rashes, or any other infection. Hand washing, gowning, or masking precautions are not adequate in the presence of infection. It is essential that personnel remain away from the nursery until they have fully recovered from any infectious disease. Similar signs of infection in the mother must be especially evaluated as to their seriousness. Depending upon the kind of maternal illness and the prior exposure of the baby, the baby may be separated from his mother and the other babies until the mother recovers, or he may be permitted contact with his mother but isolated from other newborns.

As a safeguard against infection from outside sources the number of persons entering the nursery should be kept to a minimum and people should be screened as to who may or may not enter.

The best possible physical facilities to make nursery care easy will help prevent spread of infection. It is recommended that the bassinets be well spaced, with at least 2 ft between bassinets, and that the aisles be 3 ft in width. Nursery equipment must be simple enough to be easily cleaned. Dry dusting is prohibited in the nursery. Common bathing and dressing tables should not be used. Soiled diapers should be placed in containers with foot-control covers and must not be rinsed in the nursery. All supplies should be autoclaved. Infant clothes and linen are autoclaved or laundered separately with special care.

Infection is more likely to be limited in small nurseries containing no more than 8 to 12 babies than in large units. Contact with a large number of personnel is usually less in small nurseries, and the number of babies exposed if an infection does occur is decreased.

To prevent spread of infection from one infant to another the nurse must observe all babies closely for evidence of infection. Any baby with a fever; frequent and loose stools; discharge from the umbilical area, the eyes, or the vagina; skin lesions; respiratory disease; or any other signs of infection should be isolated from the other babies by incubator or a separate room.

The isolette incubator filters the air coming into it to protect the baby inside. It does not filter the air coming out to protect adjacent infants, but it does serve as protection of other babies by being a physical barrier which may remind caretakers of hand-washing and infection dangers.

When an infant becomes infected parents should not be separated from the baby. They can be taught how to wash and gown when they visit.

Observation and Assessment

It can be anticipated that the normal baby will have made marked adjustments to extrauterine life by the end of the first day, but close observation of behavior and normal functioning of body systems must continue. Included are observation of respiratory function, muscle tone, cry, alertness and responsiveness, color, ability and desire to take food, and bowel and bladder function. For meaningful observations the nurse must be familiar with the normal characteristics of the newborn and be alert to any subtle variations and their meaning.

Many of the observations that were made during the transitional period are continued but may usually be done with less frequency.

The baby's color is observed frequently for pallor, ruddiness, cyanosis, and jaundice. It should be anticipated that the baby's color will normally be pink and neither pale, nor ruddy, nor cyanotic. Jaundice will appear by the second or third day in approximately 50 percent of newborns. If it appears earlier or advances rapidly a serum bilirubin level determination is indicated.

The baby's vital signs—temperature, pulse, and respirations—are checked and recorded once daily unless instability or physical condition requires more frequent assessment.

Stools and voiding are recorded when diapers are changed. The baby's stools are observed for frequency, color, and consistency. In judging normalcy of the stools the nurse must consider the day of life of the baby and the kind and amount of feeding he is taking. Normal changes in character of stools are described on page 445. Urinary output is observed for approximate frequency of voidings, for scanty or excessively large amounts of urine, and for highly concentrated urine.

The baby's weight is usually taken and recorded daily, ordinarily at bath time. In a warm nursery the average newborn may be weighed completely undressed without undue exposure, but small babies, under 2275 gm (5 lb), are protected against temperature changes by weighing them with their clothes on or wrapped in a blanket and the weight of the wrap deducted from the total weight.

While weighing the baby, adequate precautions must be taken to protect him from falling off the scales. An accident can be prevented by placing one end of the scales (the end toward which the baby's head will be placed) near but not against a wall and watching the baby carefully during the weighing instead of concentrating completely on balancing the scales.

The nurse compares the day's weight with the birth weight and with the weight of the previous day and reports to the doctor any great weight loss during the first few days of life as well as a stationary weight or a very slow gain after the first week. The weight is recorded on the baby's hospital record each day and may be charted on a graph (Fig. 17-4, page 440).

The Neonatal Behavioral Assessment Scale described on pages 485–89 is done some time after the transition period, and it may be repeated fully or in part on successive days.

A physical examination may be done after the transition period either for the first time or as a repeat examination. The first physical examination should be done relatively early in the postnatal period, at least within the first 24 hours.

Daily Bath

The baby is ordinarily given a bath each day with either soap and water or according to the "dry technique" described on page 453. The skin is carefully examined at bath time for rashes and irritated areas. Also at this time, as well as

at any other time the baby is handled, the eyes, ears, nose, umbilicus, and genitalia are closely inspected. The daily weight can be taken and recorded at bath time.

The face is washed with clear warm water and a soft washcloth, starting with the eyes and wiping from the inner canthus outward. The mouth area is washed clean of formula and mucus, and the outer ears and the creases behind the ears are washed and inspected for skin irritation. A cotton ball may be used to wash the face, but special care must be taken to moisten it completely to prevent cotton wisps from getting into the baby's eyes and nose, when they would produce irritation. For this reason it is necessary to use a soft towel rather than a cotton ball for drying the face.

In inspecting the eyes, edema of the lids and a purulent discharge from the eyes may be seen within a few hours after birth. This condition is a chemical conjuncitivitis, which may be produced by the silver nitrate used in the eyes shortly after birth (Fig. 17-20). Small areas of subconjunctival hemorrhage, caused by changes in vascular tension during birth, may be present during the first week or two. They apparently do not leave defects.

A baby's eyes do not require daily care other than the removal of accumulated secretions in the corners of the eyes, using a soft washcloth and clean water. They should not be irrigated unless there is a conjunctival discharge. If it is necessary to irrigate the eyes, a physiologic salt solution may be used; the mother is given instructions in its preparation if its use at home becomes necessary.

The newborn is an obligatory nose-breather and needs clear nasal passages, but his nose does not ordinarily need special attention because he sneezes vigorously and frequently to clear his own nasal passages. At birth and during the first hours of life when the baby may have mucus in the nose as well as the oropharynx, the nose is cleared with gentle suction on a catheter or a bulb syringe. If a small amount of mucus accumulates later and is well down in the nostrils, it may be possible to remove this with a twisted piece of cotton that has been moistened with water and the excess solution squeezed out. An applicator should not be used to clear the nose because of the danger of injury.

The ears are washed externally only. It is never advisable to introduce an applicator into the ear canals.

After the face has been cleaned, the creases around the neck are wiped with warm water and they are inspected for irritation. The neck is difficult to clean because of several skin folds, but these can usually be wiped fairly easily if the baby's head is hyperextended but supported in the back so that it does not fall back completely.

The axillae are wiped with a wet washcloth, and if there is still vernix in the axillae in the first day or two it may be spread as cream to other parts of the body.

The umbilical cord is inspected and cared for at bath time as well as several other times daily at diaper changes. Asepsis must be maintained. Careful hand washing before caring for the cord stump is important. The cord stump and the area around the umbilicus is wiped with an antiseptic; alcohol 60 percent is frequently used to promote drying. After the cord drops off the granulated area that is left may be wiped with an antiseptic until it is dry. The umbilical area is always observed for signs of infection, for example, odor or moisture. The baby's diaper should be applied low on the abdomen so that the umbilical cord remains dry.

The groin and buttocks are washed with warm water at bath time and each time the diaper is changed. Use of bland soap is often necessary to wash the buttocks and the crease between the buttocks to clean stool off completely.

The external genitalia in the female are cleaned by gentle washing with soap and water; special care must be taken to separate the labia to remove secretion that may collect between the labia minora and majora. At birth there is a heavy layer of vernix caseosa between the labia, which may be washed away over a period of several days. It is impossible to remove all of this vernix at one time without vigorous effort; it is therefore better to remove a little each day by gently washing between the labia at bath time and whenever the buttocks are cleaned following a stool. This vernix should, however, be completely washed away by the time the baby is discharged from the hospital.

In the male the penis is cleaned of smegma over the exposed part of the glans. Ordinarily the foreskin cannot be retracted in the early days of life and it is pushed back only a very short distance. If the foreskin is retracted it must be pulled back to its normal position within a few seconds to avoid reducing circulation in the penis. If the baby has been circumcised a sterile gauze with sterile petroleum jelly or petroleum jelly alone is placed over the penis each time the diaper is changed until the area has healed. Care of the genitalia and circumcision are described in more detail on pages 449–50.

After the bath the baby is dressed in clean clothes and he is probably ready for a feeding.

Changing and Care of Diapers

A change of the diaper before and after each feeding is sufficient for many babies, but some are uncomfortable from a wet diaper and wake up and cry between feeding times. Others may need more frequent changing because of an irritation of the skin in the diaper area. A diaper needs to be put on the baby snugly, but not so tight as to hamper his movements. It is important for the person applying the diaper to keep a hand between it and the baby while pinning it.

Wet or soiled diapers should be placed in a covered container immediately after removal. If disposable diapers are not used in the hospital, provision is made for rinsing of stool-soiled diapers in a flush sink *outside* the nursery.

Diapers need more attention than any other clothing because a *diaper rash* may develop from what is known as an ammoniacal diaper. A diaper rash consists of a diffuse redness of the buttocks and possibly also blisters and pustules and an irritation of the urethral orifice in the circumcised baby. Bacteria from stool decompose the urea in urine and liberate free ammonia; this causes the ammonia dermatitis. Some commercial antiseptic solutions used for diaper rinses have a marked bactericidal action and are useful in controlling the bacterial growth if directions are carefully followed, but boiling diapers is a safe and satisfactory means of killing the organisms. Three minutes of boiling is sufficient to destroy these bacteria; with a large pan full of diapers, however, it may be necessary to boil them 15 minutes to adequately heat those in the middle of the pan. If ammonia rash is severe, it may be necessary to boil all other clothes that become wet with urine, since ordinary washing does not destroy these bacteria. An ammonia dermatitis is usually not a problem in the hospital; in addition to adequate laundering, many hospitals autoclave all clothes used in the newborn nursery. Commercially laundered diapers are carefully washed to destroy bacteria and to ensure adequate rinsing to remove soap or detergent.

If a baby develops a diaper rash he may need an ointment such as lanolin, A and D ointment, or a commercial antiseptic preparation of powder or ointment applied to the irritated skin. Exposure of the buttocks for "air drying" is also advisable. Long periods of wet diapers and impervious materials such as plastic or rubber as diaper covers should be avoided. These permit bacteria to grow freely in the heat, moisture, and urine held next to the baby with no circulation of air.

Everyone finds many uses for diapers; they often serve as sheets, or towels, or bibs. If diapers have not been boiled, it is unwise to use them for any area of the body other than the buttocks. Another safety reminder: it is never advisable to leave loose diapers or towels or plastic material at the head end of the baby's crib.

Feedings

Feeding of the baby, an important aspect of each day's care, will be described in the following chapter. Breast- and bottle-feeding and preparation of formula will be presented in detail.

Facilitating Mother–Infant Acquaintance

Facilitating maternal and paternal and infant bonding and assisting the parents in learning to know their baby and how to care for him are very important aspects of newborn care. This part of infant care is discussed in detail in Chapter 20.

BIRTH REGISTRATION

Registration of birth is of utmost importance to the baby. The law requires the physician, midwife, nurse, or other attendant at the birth to register, with the local registrar, the name of the child, the date of birth, the place of birth, names of the parents, and any other information that is requested. Proper blanks for registration of birth are obtained from the state department of health. All information must be accurately reported and legibly written. These records are permanently filed with the state bureau of vital statistics. A photographic copy of the birth certificate or some other form of notification of registration is sent to the parents.

A birth certificate is necessary for a number of reasons and must be retained throughout life. The following list of reasons is partial, but demonstrates the importance of this document: to prove place of birth; to prove parentage and legal dependency; to prove age for entrance to school, for right to vote, for right to marry, for social security; to prove right to inheritance of property; to obtain a passport; and for other legal purposes.

The parents should be told of their responsibility for receiving a photographic copy of the birth certificate, or a notice of registration, as absolute proof that their baby's birth has been registered.

DISCHARGE FROM THE HOSPITAL

Although the parents have had adequate instructions and some practice in the care of their baby during the hospital stay, it becomes necessary to adapt this learning to the care of the baby at home. Referral to a public health nursing agency, for one or more follow-up visits by a public health nurse, is valuable for parents who need or wish guidance at home. Such visits provide for assistance with problems that may arise at home and ensure continued nursing supervision for as long as necessary.

If the baby will not remain under the medical supervision of the physician who cared for him in the hospital following his discharge, continuing medical care is planned for by referral to the family physician or to a community agency maintaining a well-baby clinic. In some instances, where financial aid is needed, referral is also made to a family service agency.

BIBLIOGRAPHY

Affonso, Dyanne D., The neonate, in *Childbearing: A Nursing Perspective*, edited by Ann L. Clark and Dyanne D. Affonso. Davis, Philadelphia, Pa., 1976.

Alderman, Mary M. (ed.), Priority care for the newborn, *Patient Care* 8:72–126 passim (July 1) 1974.

Alexander, Mary M., and Brown, Marie Scott, Physical examination. Reflexes in infants, *Am. J. Nurs.* 76:50–55 (July) 1976.

Als, Heidelise, and Brazelton, T. Berry, Comprehensive neonatal assessment, *Birth Family J.* 2:3–9 (Winter) 1974–75.

American Academy of Pediatrics, Committee on Fetus and Newborn, *Standards and Recommendations for Hospital Care of Newborn Infants*, 6th ed. Evanston, Ill., 1977.

American Journal of Diseases of Children. Editorial, Water bugs in the bassinet, 101:273–277, 1961.

Apgar, Virginia, The newborn (Apgar) scoring system: Reflections and advice, *Pediatr. Clin. North Am.* 13:645–650 (Aug.) 1966.

Arnold, Helen W.; Putnam, Nancy J.; Barnard, Betty Lou, Desmond, Murdina M., and Rudolph, Arnold J.; Transition to extrauterine life, *Am. J. Nurs.* 65:77–80 (Oct.) 1965.

Auld, Peter, A. M., Resuscitation of the newborn infant, *Am. J. Nurs.* 74:68–70 (Jan.) 1974.

Avery, Gordon B. (ed.), *Neonatology.* Lippincott, Philadelphia, Pa., 1975.

———, Kraybill, Ernest N.; and Mullick, Umesh C., Examination of the newborn, *GP*, 37:78–94 (Apr.) 1968.

Bancalari, Eduardo, Resuscitation of the newborn, *Postgrad. Med.* 57:89–92 (Mar.) 1975.

Battaglia, Frederick C.; The unique problems of small-for-dates babies; *and* The large-for-gestational age baby—An overlooked problem, *Contemp. Ob/Gyn* 1:35–42 (Mar.) 1973.

———, and Lubchenco, Lula O., A practical classification of newborn infants by weight and gestational age, *J. Pediatr.* 71:159–163 (Aug.) 1967.

Bee, Helen, *The Developing Child.* Harper and Row, New York, 1975.

Behrman, Richard E. A. (ed.), *Neonatology. Diseases of the Fetus and Infant.* Mosby, St. Louis, Mo., 1973.

———, James, L. S., Klaus, M., Nelson, N., and Oliver, T., Treatment of the asphyxiated newborn infant, *J. Pediatr.* 74:981–988 (June) 1969.

Brackbill, Y., Kane, J., Manniello, R. L., and Abramson, D.; Obstetric premedication and infant outcome, *Am. J. Obstet. Gynecol.* 118:377–385 (Feb. 1) 1974.

Brazelton, T. Berry, Does the neonate shape his environment?, *Birth Defects* 10:131–140, 1974.

———, *Neonatal Behavioral Assessment Scale, Clinics in Developmental Medicine, No. 50,* Spastics International Medical Publications, Heinemann Medical Books, London, and Lippincott, Philadelphia, Pa., 1973.

———, Assessment of the infant at risk, *Clin. Obstet. Gynecol.* 16:370–375 (Mar.) 1973.

———, Effect of prenatal drugs on the behavior of the neonate, *Am. J. Psychiatry* 126 II:1161–1166 (Mar.) 1970.

Cahill, Betty, The neonatal nurse specialist—New techniques for the asymptomatic infant, *JOGN Nurs.* 3:34–38 (Jan./Feb.) 1974.

Clark, Ann L., Recognizing discord between mother and child and changing it to harmony, *MCN* 1:100–106 (Mar./Apr.) 1976.

———, and Affonso, Dyanne D., Infant behavior and maternal attachment: Two sides to the coin, *MCN* 1:94–99 (Mar/Apr.) 1976.

Clark, J. Michael; Brown, Zane A., and Jung, August

L., Resuscitation equipment board for nurseries and delivery rooms, *JAMA* 236:2427–2428 (Nov. 22) 1976.

Cook, Larry N., Assessing maturity of the neonate, *Contemp. Ob/Gyn* 1:64–67 (May) 1973.

Desmond, Murdina M., Obstetric medication and infant behavior, *Anesthesiology* 40:111–113 (Feb.) 1974.

———, Rudolph, Arnold, J., and Phitaksphraiwan, Phuangnoi, The transitional care nursery, *Pediatr. Clin. North Am.* 13:651–668 (Aug.) 1966.

———, and Rudolph, Arnold J., Progressive evaluation of the newborn infant, *Postgrad Med.* 37:207–212 (Feb.) 1965.

——— *et al.*, The clinical behavior of the newly born. I. The term baby, *J. Pediatr.* 62:307–325 (Mar.) 1963.

Dubowitz, Lilly, M. S., Dubowitz, Victor, and Goldberg, Cissie, Clinical assessment of gestational age in the newborn infant, *J. Pediatr.* 77:1–10 (July) 1970.

Dubowitz, V., Neurological fragility in the newborn: Influence of medication in labour, *Br. J. Anaesth.* 47:1005–1010 (Sept.) 1975.

Erickson, Marcene, *Assessment and Developmental Changes in Children.* Mosby, St. Louis, Mo., 1976, Chapters 2, 3, and 5.

Evans, James A., Fundamental of infant resuscitation, *Int. Anesthesiol. Clin.* 11:141–161 (Summer) 1973.

Evans, Marian, Adaptation of the infant at birth and intervention techniques for distressed neonate, *J. Nurs. Midwif.* 20:18–28 (Winter) 1975.

Faber, Myron M., Circumcision revisited, *Birth Family J.* 1:19–21 (Spring) 1974.

Farrar, Carrol Ann, A data collection procedure to assess behavioral individuality in the neonate, *JOGN Nurs.* 3:15–20 (May/June) 1974.

Fink, H. William, The newborn at first glance, *Hosp. Topics* 44:99–101 (Mar.) 1966.

Galloway, Karen, Early detection of congenital anomalies, *JOGN Nurs.* 2:37–39 (July/Aug.) 1973.

Grayson, Robert, and Cranch, Gene S., Care of the foreskin, *Am. J. Nurs.* 56:75–76 (Jan.) 1956.

Hervada, Arturo, Nursery evaluation of the newborn, *Am. J. Nurs.* 67:1669–1671 (Aug.) 1967.

Hodgman, Joan, Clinical evaluation of the newborn infant, *Hosp. Pract.* 4:70–86 (May) 1969.

Iles, J. Penny, and McCrary, Marcia, Cuddle bathing can be fun, *MCN* 1:350–354 (Nov./Dec.) 1976.

Johnson, Suzanne Hall, The contemporary neonatal nurse, in *Current Practice in Obstetric and Gynecologic Nursing*, Vol. I, edited by Leota K. McNall and Janet T. Galeener. Mosby, St. Louis, Mo., 1976, Chapter 9, pp. 105–124.

Klaus, Marshall H., and Fanaroff, Avroy A., *Care of the High-Risk Neonate.* Saunders, Philadelphia, Pa., 1973.

Korner, Anneliese, Individual differences at birth, *Birth Defects* 10:51–61, 1974.

Korones, Sheldon B., *High-Risk Newborn Infants: The Basis for Intensive Nursing Care*, 2nd ed. Mosby, St. Louis, Mo., 1976.

Lewis, Michael, and Rosenblum, Leonard A. (eds.), *The Effect of the Infant on Its Caregiver*, Wiley, New York, 1974.

Lipsitt, Lewis P., The study of sensory and learning processes of the newborn, *Clin. Perinatol.* 4:163–186 (Mar.) 1977.

Lockman, Lawrence A., Neurologic assessment in the first year of life, *Postgrad. Med.* 50:80–85 (July) 1971.

Lubchenco, Lula O., Assessment of gestational age and development at birth, *Pediatr. Clin. North Am.* 17:125–145 (Feb.) 1970.

———, Hansman, Charlotte, and Boyd, Edith, Intrauterine growth in length and head circumference as estimated from live births at gestational ages from 26 to 42 weeks, *Pediatrics* 37:403–408 (Mar.) 1966.

McLean, Frances H.; Significance of birthweight for gestational age in identifying infants at risk, *JOGN Nurs.* 3:19–24 (Nov./Dec.) 1974.

Mauer, Daphne, and Mauer, Charles E., Newborn babies see better than you think, *Psychol. Today* 10:85–88 (Oct.) 1976.

Miller, Herbert C., and Hassanein, K., Diagnosis of impaired fetal growth in newborn infants, *Pediatrics* 48:511–522 (Oct.) 1972.

Nicolopoulos, Demetre *et al.*, Estimation of gestational age in the neonate, *Am. J. Dis. Child.* 130:477–480 (May) 1976.

Nitzkin, Joel L. (ed.), Infection control in the newborn nursery, *Hosp. Topics* 53:37–39 (Sept./Oct.) 1975.

Ostwald, Peter F., and Peltzman, Philip, The cry of

the human infant, *Sci. Am.* 230:84–90 (Mar.) 1974.

Patient Care, Circumcision (a series of articles), 5:56–86 passim (July 15) 1971.

Roberts, Joyce E., Suctioning the newborn, *Am. J. Nurs.* 73:63–65 (Jan.) 1973.

Scanlon, John W., How is the baby? The Apgar score revisited, *Clin. Pediatr.* 12:61–67 (Feb.) 1973.

Silverman, William A., and Parke, Priscilla, The newborn: Keep him warm, *Am. J. Nurs.* 65:81–84 (Oct.) 1965.

Smith, Ann Noordenbos, Physical examination of the newborn, in *Maternity Nursing Today,* 2nd ed., edited by Joy P. Clausen, Margaret H. Flook, and Boonie Ford. McGraw-Hill, New York, 1977, Chapter 26, pp. 571–584.

Stone, L. Joseph, Smith, Henrietta, F., and Murphy, Lois B. (eds.); The capabilities of the newborn, in *The Competent Infant.* Basic Books, New York, 1973, Chapter 3.

Usher, Robert, McLean, Frances, and Scott, Kenneth E., Judgment of fetal age. II. Clinical significance of gestational age and an objective method for its assessment, *Pediatr. Clin. North Am.* 13:835–848 (Aug.) 1966.

Van Leeuwen, Gerard, The nurse in prevention and intervention in the neonatal period, *Nurs. Clin. North Am.* 8:509–520 (Sept.) 1973.

Williams, Joann K., and Lancaster, Jean, Thermoregulation of the newborn, *MCN* 1:355–360 (Nov./Dec.) 1976.

19

Feeding the Newborn

The newborn baby may either be breast-fed or artificially fed. Many factors enter into the decision of the method that will be used. Breast feeding is the natural method of feeding the normal newborn and has certain advantages over artificial feeding, but if it is to be a satisfactory experience for both mother and baby, the mother must want to breast-feed her baby. Assuming that the mother's and baby's conditions are satisfactory, breast feeding will usually be successful if the mother has the desire to nurse her baby, and if she gets encouragement during the time the feeding is being established.

Breast feeding is no longer necessary to maintain a baby's good health, or ensure his survival, as it was prior to development of satisfactory artificial feedings, but it has important advantages. Breast milk is the natural and ideal food for the newborn infant. If the mother's diet is adequate, the baby receives from breast milk the nutrients necessary for growth during the early months of life, with the exception of vitamin D and possibly vitamin C. Breast milk is readily digested and assimilated, and feeding difficulties are less frequent and usually less severe than with artificial feedings.

Breast milk is clean, fresh, and readily available at the proper temperature. Breast feeding eliminates the need for preparation of formula and warming of milk before the baby is fed. The milk flow from the breast is well regulated. The baby can suck at the breast until he is satisfied, and there is less tendency to attempt to control

his food intake. Breast feeding helps to meet the baby's and the mother's needs for close relationship if the mother wants to breast-feed her baby; if not, artificial feedings may be more satisfactory for such close relationships.

FACTORS INFLUENCING METHOD OF FEEDING

Psychologic, sociologic, and physical factors enter into whether a mother breast-feeds her baby successfully or unsuccessfully or makes no attempt to breast-feed. Some mothers are very eager to breast-feed their babies; some nurse their babies, but feel that it makes little difference if they must change to artificial feeding; some try to breast-feed even when they prefer to give an artificial feeding; and others are strongly opposed to breast feeding. To some mothers this method of feeding seems repulsive or rather primitive, or they feel that it may be disfiguring or too tiring. Some mothers do not breast-feed because the custom in their community is to give bottle feedings, especially since artificial feedings have become safe and easy. Others believe that they may be criticized by relatives or friends who do not particularly approve of this method of feeding. In some cases the care of the baby by others will be easier if he is fed by bottle. Some women express the belief that their milk may not be good for the baby, or they think they will worry if they do not know exactly how much milk the baby is taking at each feeding.

The husband's interest and encouragement of a woman's desire to nurse her baby are very important to successful breast feeding.

The attitude of the physician and nurse toward breast feeding and the amount of assistance given to the mother in the hospital while breast feeding is being established often determine the mother's success in nursing. The mother may need a great deal of assistance at first, especially if she is insecure, or if her baby does not nurse well initially.

Breast feeding is inadvisable or impossible in some instances because of the mother's or the baby's physical condition. Tuberculosis and certain acute infectious diseases, especially those to which a baby is particularly susceptible, such as whooping cough or staphylococcal infection, are contraindications to breast feeding. Other complications in the mother, such as heart disease, kidney disease, or syphilis, may be contraindications. In come cases of chronic disease and general debility, contraindication to breast feeding is relative and depends on the mother's condition. If breast feeding is started and the mother begins to show evidence of strain, it is discontinued. During acute illness of the mother, breast feeding often must be temporarily discontinued.

Flat or inverted nipples may be impossible for the baby to grasp sufficiently to nurse. Fissured or cracked nipples may necessitate temporary discontinuance of nursing until the nipples heal. If mastitis develops, nursing is temporarily stopped, or it is permanently discontinued.

The return of menstruation is not an indication for weaning, but the baby may have some colic, vomiting, or loose stools on the first day of the menstrual period. Pregnancy is an indication for weaning the baby because of the additional strain on the mother.

The baby's condition may be the factor determining the method of feeding. An immature baby or one with an abnormality, such as cleft lip or palate, may be unable to nurse. Sometimes, in these cases, the breasts are emptied by artificial means until the baby can nurse. The decision may depend on the mother's desire to continue lactation by artificial emptying of the breasts and also on the baby's disability and the period of time required for his recovery.

The prenatal period is the best time to discover the mother's attitude toward nursing her baby and to answer her questions concerning breast and artificial feeding. She will then have information for making decisions and plans.

A mother who is undecided about breast feeding but who does not express adverse feelings can often be encouraged. Mothers often lack information, and they need the sanction of physicians and nurses. They may need help in deciding how to manage feedings when away from home for work or for social activities. Breast feeding is not necessarily restricting, since a bottle feeding can be given when the mother is away. The woman who is planning to return to work can be encouraged to breast-feed during the early weeks of the baby's life.

Any discussion with the mother concerning breast feeding should encourage her to make her own decision. The advantages of breast feeding should not be stressed to such a degree that the mother may develop a feeling of inadequacy or guilt if she decides not to breast-feed or if she cannot do so for a physical reason. If the idea of breast feeding is repugnant to a woman, attempts to persuade her to breast-feed are unwise. Such efforts may lead to mental conflict and may inject or increase feelings of guilt.

A baby's nutritional needs can be met very satisfactorily with artificial feedings and a good mother–child relationship can be established in many ways other than through breast feeding.

NUTRITIONAL REQUIREMENTS

The goal of infant feeding should be a well-nourished baby, fed in a way that is satisfactory to the parents and the baby. To accomplish this the baby may be either breast-fed or artificially fed with a commercially prepared formula, evaporated milk, or cow's milk. The infant's diet should provide an adequate amount of water, calories, and essential nutrients for health and normal growth, and it should be easily digestible. Since the growth and nutritional status of the breast-fed infant is ordinarily excellent, the composition of breast milk is used as a standard for preparation of formulas for babies.

The *requirement* for a nutrient may be defined as the least amount of that nutrient that will promote an optimum state of health. The meaning of the terms "requirement" and "minimal requirement" is the same and the terms are sometimes used interchangeably. The *advisable intake* for a nutrient is generally set at values greater than the estimated requirement because of individual differences of infants and the various conditions that may influence the effect of the nutrient, such as genetic makeup of the baby, environment, activity, storage reserves, and influence of other nutrients.

The *recommended dietary allowances* (RDA), which are revised periodically by the Food and Nutrition Board, National Academy of Sciences, National Research Council differ further from the advisable intake. The RDA recommendations are at least equal to, and generally greater than, the advisable intake. The RDA recommendations are intended to serve as a general guide to provide an adequate nutritional intake for almost every healthy person.

Caloric Needs

Babies require a relatively large intake of food and fluids to cover basal metabolic needs and provide for growth. After an initial postnatal period of a few days, when a relatively small caloric intake appears to satisfy the baby, his caloric needs are high. By several days of age a baby needs 110 to 120 Calories (kilocalories) per kilogram of body weight per day (50 to 55 Calories per pound). Such caloric intake is necessary to provide energy for the baby's relatively high basal metabolic needs as compared with an adult, for his rapid growth, and for his daily increasing activity during the neonatal period. A baby's increasing need for calories is shown by the daily increase in the amount of food that is

necessary to satisfy him during his early days of life. Caloric needs vary greatly for different babies of the same age and size. The active baby, because of increased muscular activity, and the one who cries considerably use more energy than the quiet infant and thus require a higher caloric intake. Needs are based on weight gain, satiety, and general well-being.

There are so many variables involved in caloric needs of infants that it is difficult to state an ideal caloric intake for the newborn. The requirement of 120 kcal/kg-day is a rough rule of thumb of what is sufficient for growth for most babies. Optimal caloric intake should be supplied to the newborn to avoid any malnutrition. Too few calories cause tissue breakdown and divert all food substances into energy. On the other hand, overnutrition may contribute to adult obesity. It is difficult to define excessive intake, but it is well to be aware of the potential. Some babies will not gain weight on 120 kcal/kg-day and need to be fed a higher amount. Others, especially inactive babies, may gain satisfactorily on 90 kcal/kg-day. A weight gain of 15 to 30 gm (½ to 1 oz) per day is considered satisfactory and evidence of good growth.

The distribution of calories in the baby's food is important to well-being. That which seems appropriate for good nutrition for full-term infants and is recommended for full-size infants is as follows: 7 to 16 percent of calories to be derived from protein, 30 to 55 percent from fat, and the remainder from carbohydrate.[1] At least 1 percent of the calories should be supplied by the essential fatty acid, linoleic acid.

Human milk provides approximately 7 percent calories from protein; 55 percent from fat, and 38 percent from carbohydrate. Most commercially prepared formulas fed in the United States supply 9 to 15 percent of the calories from protein, 45 to 50 percent from fat, and the remainder from carbohydrate. An intake of protein of less than 6 percent of the caloric intake is likely to lead to protein deficiency. Extremely

[1] Samuel J. Foman, *Infant Nutrition*, 2nd ed. Saunders, Philadelphia, Pa., 1974, p. 473.

high fat content in the formula may lead to ketosis. Diets supplying less than 30 percent of the calories from fat or more than 65 percent of the calories from carbohydrate are believed to possibly be of low satiety, but little evidence for this is available.[2]

Fluid Needs

Fluid requirement per kilogram of body weight is greater in the infant than in the adult. The baby's increased muscular activity, caloric intake, and basal metabolism demand more water than he will need later in life. An adequate amount of fluid is thus essential to a baby's well-being. Infants have a relatively large percentage of body fluid, but their ability to withstand an inadequate fluid intake is not as efficient as that of an older child or an adult. In addition, infants need more water than older individuals for good excretion of solutes.

The normal newborn's need for fluid intake is between 150 and 200 ml per kilogram (2⅓ and 3 oz per pound) of body weight per 24 hours. Fluid intake may also be expressed in relation to caloric intake and would then be equivalent to 1.5 ml/kcal. That is the statement of the RDA recommendation. Need for fluid is very great in hot weather and may increase to over 200 ml per kilogram of body weight (3 oz per pound) when the temperature is high.

The normal baby will ordinarily easily fulfill his own requirement by taking an adequate amount of breast milk or formula. Offers of water between certain feedings and later intake of orange juice add to the fluid intake of milk. Water must be given frequently if formula intake is inadequate because of poor appetite or poor sucking in the early days of life, if body fluids are lost due to heat, if the baby is under lights or a radiant heater, or if the baby has a fever. It may be necessary to offer water between all feedings when need for fluid is great.

It is important to realize that between 70 and 90 ml of fluid per kilogram (1.2 and 1.5 oz per pound) of body weight is the minimal water requirement for a full-term normal newborn in a 24-hour period to protect him against dehydration. The much higher intake is advised to provide for a generous margin of safety.

When a baby gains poorly or gains excessively the fluid and caloric intake should be calculated to determine the exact intake and to note how it compares with requirements.

Vitamins

When the mother is well nourished the normal newborn can be expected to have adequate vitamin stores at birth. An infant's vitamin requirements are high, however, because of rapid growth, and added vitamins are required, beginning around 10 to 14 days, to provide for good development of rapidly growing bones and tissues. Suggested daily allowances of some of the necessary vitamins are shown in Table 19-1. Recommended intake of vitamins are estimates, which are generally higher than minimum requirements. In addition, intestinal absorption is not constant, and the vitamin content of natural foods may vary considerably. The quantity of the various vitamins present in milk, both human and animal, will vary to some extent with maternal intake.

Vitamin A is present in large amount in human milk, cow's milk, and commercially prepared formulas. Many strained and chopped commercially prepared infant foods and many table foods fed to infants have a good supply of carotene. Vitamin A supplementation for infants is therefore not necessary under usual circumstances. Since vitamin A is stored in the liver, the average intake is more important than the daily intake.

The advisable intake of vitamin A has been tentatively set at 500 IU between birth and one year of age. This is twice the estimated requirement. The same intake is recommended for low-birth-weight babies.

Since vitamin A has been used in excessive amounts and resulted in toxicity, a joint statement on the use and abuse of vitamin A was

[2] *Ibid.*

Table 19-1. Requirements, Advisable Intake, and RDA Recommendations for Selected Nutrients for Infant Diet

Daily Allowance—Birth to Six Months*

Nutrient	Requirement (minimum)	Advisable	RDA Recommendation
Water	70–90 ml per kg	150 ml per kg	1.5 ml per kcal
Calories	90–110 per kg	110–120 per kg	117 per kg
Protein	1.6 mg per 100 kcal	1.9 gm per 100 kcal	2.2 gm per kg
Vitamins			
A	250 IU	500 IU	1400 IU
D	100–200 IU	400 IU	400 IU
C	10 mg	20 mg	35 mg
Fluoride	—	0.5 mg	Fluoridation of water supply where indicated
Iron	6.7 mg	7 mg	10 mg

*Based on data obtained from Domenik Reina, Infant nutrition, *Clin. Perinatal.* 2:373–339, (Sept.) 1975.

RDA recommendations for all nutrients are listed in Food and Nutrition Board, National Academy of Sciences—National Research Council *Recommended Daily Dietary Allowances,* 8th ed., 1974.

issued by the Committees on Drugs and on Nutrition of the American Academy of Pediatrics in 1971. These committees advised against the use of preparations providing more than 6000 IU/dose.[3]

While it is unlikely that a normal infant in the United States who is receiving an adequate diet needs supplemental vitamin A, a deficiency of this vitamin is a common nutritional deficiency in most developing countries of the world. In countries where vitamin A deficiency is prevalent animal fats are rarely eaten and the total dietary fat intake is so low that even if carotenes are present in the diet in moderate amounts they are poorly absorbed.

Vitamin D is essential to the prevention of rickets. It is inadequate in both breast milk and cow's milk, but cow's milk, evaporated milk, and most commercially prepared formulas are well fortified with vitamin D.

A daily intake of 400 IU of vitamin D, which represents at least twice the requirement, is suggested as the advisable daily intake. Since human milk provides only a small amount of vi-

tamin D, breast-fed babies need this supplement.

Use of a supplement is not advisable when dietary sources provide 400 IU daily, as may well be the case for the baby who is eating a large quantity of fortified formula or is taking a liter of fortified milk. In the United States most commercially prepared formulas, evaporated milk, and fresh whole milk are fortified with 400 IU of vitamin D per quart. Except for milk, few foods eaten by infants are fortified with vitamin D; therefore, if a baby's daily intake of vitamin D from milk or formula is below 400 IU some supplementation to raise the baby's daily intake is advisable. However, excessive intakes (above 2000 IU per day) are dangerous and should be avoided.[4] A regular intake of vitamin D is important because it is poorly stored. Sunshine will fulfill some of the need for vitamin D, but ordinarily a baby under one year of age does not receive enough of the vitamin from this source.

Vitamin C is found in human milk in a quantity sufficient for the infant, provided the mother's diet is adequate, but cow's milk is low

[3] American Academy of Pediatrics, Committees on Drugs and on Nutrition, The use and abuse of vitamin A, *Pediatrics* 48:655–656 (Oct.) 1971.

[4] Roslyn B. Alfin-Slater and Derrick B. Jelliffe, Nutritional requirements with special reference to infancy, *Pediatr. Clin. North Am.* 24:6 (Feb.) 1977.

in this vitamin at all times, even when the milk is raw. Heat used to modify cow's milk for infant feeding destroys part of the vitamin C that is present, bringing the total amount even lower and making the addition of ascorbic acid important when artificial feedings are given.

Commercially prepared formulas and fruit juices are fortified with vitamin C. The recommended dietary allowance of vitamin C is 35 mg daily. Two ounces of orange juice will provide the advisable daily intake of vitamin C for a baby; supplementation should be continued until the baby takes this amount of orange juice daily. There are no large body stores of vitamin C, and any excess is excreted in the urine.

Vitamin B complex is present in adequate amounts in human milk, cow's milk, and commercially prepared formulas. Deficiencies are rare in developed countries but may be severe in countries where rice gruel is substituted for milk a few weeks after birth. Toxicity is not a problem because the B-complex vitamins are only minimally stored in the body, and any excess is excreted in the urine.

Vitamin K intake is adequate after the first several days of life for the normal baby taking human milk, cow's milk, or commercially prepared formula. To avoid a vitamin K deficiency in the first few days of life, a baby is given 0.5 or 1.0 mg of vitamin K intramuscularly after birth (see page 432).

Minerals

Most minerals are adequately provided by human milk, cow's milk, commercially prepared formulas, and other foods usually taken by babies. Iron and fluoride are exceptions. The need for iron and for fluoride and the fulfillment of these requirements are described on pages 547–48.

THE FIRST FEEDING

For the normal healthy baby who has good color, good muscle tone, and a lusty cry, evidence of hunger and desire to eat seem to be valid guides for offering the first feeding. Some infants seem to be ready to eat as soon as they are born, and some do not show hunger for several hours. It seems desirable to feed each baby according to his individual needs rather than according to an established routine. A scheduled time for a first feeding at a predetermined number of hours after birth requires some babies to wait long past their initial hunger, while others are offered a feeding when they are not ready to eat. (See also discussion on hypoglycemia on pages 795–800 in relation to first feedings.)

Many factors must be observed and considered in determining the time for offering the first feeding. The baby should be in good condition as determined by vital signs and general behavior. A baby ordinarily shows signs of hunger by a search for food, sucking motions, and crying. When the mother plans to breast-feed, her condition should be assessed to ascertain if she is able and ready to nurse her baby. Type of delivery, analgesia during labor, and need for rest influence her readiness. The mother's desires and plans for feeding her baby are considered. Some mothers want to nurse their babies as soon as possible after birth, either in the delivery room or the recovery room. If mother and baby are in good condition this is a good time to begin breast feeding. The baby is in his first period of reactivity, is alert and active, is likely to suck well at this time, and the feeding will very likely be successful. With an early feeding the baby will get early sucking experience, he will get some food from the colostrum that is present in the breast, the mother's breasts will be stimulated to begin producing milk, and the mother will have the satisfaction of a successful feeding.

If the baby is to be formula-fed the first feeding may be postponed until the second period of reactivity.

Often the first feeding, called a *test feeding* because it helps to assess the baby's ability to swallow fluid, is 10 to 15 ml of sterile water followed by a 5 or 10 percent glucose solution. If the water feeding is regurgitated and aspirated, or if the baby cannot swallow because of an anomaly in the upper gastrointestinal tract, irritation of the respiratory tract is apt to be less from water than from glucose or formula. After it has been ascertained that the baby can take fluid satisfactorily, breast or formula feedings are started.

The baby may be satisfied with a very small amount of food at his first feeding. He often has a need to suck in addition to a need for food and this desire to suck may be satisfied while he is taking his small feeding.

FREQUENCY OF FEEDING

Newborn babies are sometimes fed on a four-hour schedule or possibly a three-hour schedule is used for the babies who are smaller than average. However, a rigid schedule is not satisfactory for newborns because it requires the baby who is alert and hungry before the scheduled feeding time to wait for his feeding and the one who is not hungry to be awakened and urged to take food.

Self-Demand Feedings

A self-regulating (self-demand) feeding schedule permits the baby to eat when he is awake and hungry and to take the amount of feeding that he wishes. This means that the interval between feedings may be from three to six hours and may even vary from every two to every eight hours. The individual baby is likely to vary his schedule from day to day during the first week or two of life.

The normal newborn is a good judge of his need for food. Hunger wakes the baby and he begins to cry. If he is fed when he is hungry, eating is a pleasant experience. The baby also knows when he has had enough to eat. He will stop eating when he is satisfied and he should not be forced to take more food than he is eager to take. Forced feedings are unpleasant, and it is not necessary for a baby to finish the last drop from a bottle.

With a rigid feeding schedule a baby who is hungry early, but must wait until a certain approved time for his feeding, may not eat well. He may have lost his feeling of hunger and he may also be exhausted from crying. When a sleeping baby is awakened to be fed he may not eat well because he is not hungry enough to eat and he is not sufficiently awake. Sometimes the newborn does not wish to eat frequently, or in amounts that seem adequate, during the early days of life; he should not be prodded or patted too firmly in an effort to awaken him and to force him to eat more than he wishes. Even when he appears to be hungry, he may dawdle during the first few days; feedings should be offered with patience and calmness.

With breast feeding it is especially important that the baby is ready to eat when he is taken to the mother for nursing. When he does not have a desire to eat he is not likely to grasp the mother's nipple. The attempt at feeding is unpleasant for the baby, and, in addition, the mother may become concerned over the baby's lack of desire to eat and her ability to feed him.

Most normal newborns eat about six to eight times in a 24-hour period during the first week or two of life, with an occasional day or two of more frequent feedings. During the early days of life there may be considerable irregularity in a baby's need for food, both in the interval between feedings and in the amount of food taken. The baby may wish to have a feeding often on one day and less frequently on another, and sometimes he desires food at frequent intervals during a part of a day and at longer-spaced intervals during the rest of the day.

After three or four days of age many babies have several days on which they want to eat very frequently, sometimes as often as every two hours for at least several times in succession. This frequency will not continue, and the mother who is breast feeding will probably be able to meet his needs by frequent nursing. The nurse, however, must observe the mother to ascertain that she is not becoming too tired and that her nipples do not become sore from frequent nursing. It may be possible to satisfy the baby occasionally with a pacifer, a drink of water, or other attention. Perhaps he does not really need food so often.

A baby establishes a fairly regular schedule after a week or two. As he gets a little older he usually takes from 3 to 4 oz of milk at each feeding and is satisfied for a three- to four-hour period.

BREAST FEEDING

The various aspects of breast feeding will be described below. In addition to a discussion of the factors important in breast milk secretion and the baby's sucking, care of the breasts and nipples during lactation, and the nursing mother's health regime will be presented.

Anatomy and Physiology of Lactation

The secretory portion of each breast consists of 15 to 20 lobes of alveolar glandular tissue; each lobe has its own execretory duct opening into the nipple (Fig. 19-1). Each lobe is further subdivided into smaller lobes, or lobules, containing ducts opening into a larger duct. The lobules in turn are comprised of many acini or alveoli. These tiny sacs, or *alveoli*, lined with a single layer of cells which secrete milk, are the secretory portion of the breast. These secreting cells are surrounded by a capillary network.

Tiny ductules carry milk from the alveoli to

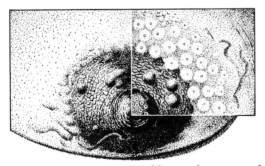

Figure 19-1. Front view of breast showing areola, tubercles of Montgomery, and orifices of milk ducts.

the ducts of the lobules, which in turn open into the larger duct of the lobe; these lead to the nipple and open to its surface (Figs. 6-3, page 114 and 19-3A). The walls of these ductules and ducts contain elastic and muscular tissue. Before it reaches the surface of the nipple, each large duct widens into a *lactiferous sinus*, a minute reservoir for milk (Figs. 6-3 and 19-4A). These sinuses lie just behind and beneath the areolar part of the breast.

The clusters of alveoli or acini, uniting to form lobules with tiny ducts leading into the main duct of each lobule, closely resemble a bunch of grapes. The separate grapes correspond to the alveoli, their small stems to the tiny ducts that lead to a larger one, and the central stem of the grape cluster to the milk duct that opens through the nipple.

The size of the breasts is largely due to the amount of fatty tissue they contain and, therefore, is not indicative of ability to produce milk. Gross anatomy and development of the breasts have been described on pages 14 and 114.

Colostrum Secretion

There is little or no apparent change in the breasts during the first two or three days after the birth of a baby. In this early period, they secrete a small amount of thin, yellowish fluid called *colostrum*. Colostrum contains proteins, fat, sugar, salts, and water, but in different proportions than milk, having less fat and sugar than milk and a greater amount of protein and salts. Colostrum also contains large amounts of vitamins and antibodies. In addition, it contains cells with large masses of fat. These cells are called colostrum corpuscles and are secreting cells that have undergone fatty degeneration. The yellowish color is due to a pigment.

The alveoli, ducts, and ampullae of the breasts are filled with colostrum at the time of delivery, and the alveolar cells continue to secrete colostrum at a slow rate. At the first few nursings the baby receives the colostrum in the breasts in amounts varying from a few milliliters to ½ oz at each feeding.

Lactogenesis

The relatively small amount of colostrum in the breasts is replaced by milk on the second or third day after delivery. A major change in mammary gland function takes place during this time. The breasts begin to secrete a large volume of fluid, which gradually changes in composition from colostrum through a transitional fluid of early milk to mature milk by the end of about one week after delivery. This process, termed *lactogenesis*, is brought about by hormonal influences on the alveolar cells, biochemical changes in these cells, and circulatory changes in the breasts.

With delivery of the placenta and loss of its hormones, the hormonal milieu changes considerably. Estrogens and progesterone in the circulation fall to a low level. These hormones, especially the high level of progesterone, and lack of stimulation are believed to have inhibited milk secretion prior to delivery. As the level of placental hormones falls, secretion of a complex of lactogenic hormones from the anterior pituitary increases considerably. At the same time blood flow to the breasts increases, bringing more hormones and milk precursors to the alveolar cells. The lactogenic complex of hormones, which is made up of prolactin, somatotropin, ACTH, and probably TSH, causes cellular and biochemical mechanisms in the alveolar cells to secrete milk. ACTH and TSH act through the adrenal and the thyroid glands, respectively.

Lactogenesis is further promoted by the baby's sucking and by emptying of the breasts and relief of distention of the alveoli. As the alveoli are emptied they can secrete more milk. Without emptying true milk secretion will not develop. With regular emptying of the breasts milk flows more freely and more abundantly with each nursing. The same complex of hormones that was necessary to start milk secretion is required for continuation of secretion.

The manner in which the breast milk comes in as well as the time of its appearance varies considerably in different women. Sometime be-tween the second and fourth day after delivery, the breasts become heavy, full, and firm. Filling may be rapid, with a distinct change noticeable within a few hours, or it may be much more gradual.

Filling of the breasts is often, but not necessarily, accompanied by congestion or engorgement of the breasts. Engorgement lasts for a day or two and is likely to cause discomfort to varying degrees. Thereafter the congestion disappears, and although the milk supply steadily increases and the breasts are heavy with fullness from milk, they are not uncomfortable. Milk supply may increase rapidly during the first days following its initial secretion, or the increase may be very gradual. It may even be several weeks before the supply is adequate to fulfill the baby's needs completely.

Breast Engorgement

There is considerable variation in the degree of firmness of the breasts as well as in amount of discomfort the mother experiences at the time the milk comes in. Sometimes the breasts produce a large amount of milk without previous engorgement, but usually they become distended and tender to varying degrees and may become markedly uncomfortable. Sometimes the breasts become so full and tense that they are described as being "hard as boards." The distention may pull the skin so tight that it appears shiny. The skin may also be reddened and feel very warm in some areas, and distended veins may be visible. The mother may feel a throbbing in her breasts, with pain whenever they are touched or moved. If the tissues surrounding the nipples become taut, nursing becomes difficult because the baby cannot grasp the nipple and the areolar area adequately.

Engorgement disappears in 24 to 48 hours, and although the milk supply is increasing, the breasts become softer and more comfortable.

Engorgement of the breasts is apparently partly due to an increased vascularity and partly due to an increased accumulation of milk. There may also be secondary lymphatic and venous stasis if the milk cannot be removed. The amount of blood to the breasts increases quite suddenly sometime between the second and fourth postpartum days, and engorgement probably begins with a filling of the breasts with blood. As the breasts then fill with milk, the engorgement increases, especially if they cannot be easily emptied. It may be difficult to withdraw the milk because of occlusion of ducts by the congested tissues surrounding them and/or occlusion from blockage by earlier secretions which are viscous or have become thickened. Retention of milk in the alveoli causes them to become distended and to compress surrounding milk ducts. This compression interferes with the flow of milk. Secondary venous and lymphatic stasis may follow distension of the breasts with the milk that cannot be emptied.

Sometimes during this period of breast engorgement a hard, tender mass is felt in one or both axillae. This mass is glandular breast tissue which also becomes engorged and filled with milk. This congestion decreases in one or two days, and the lump gradually disappears as the milk in it dries up. An ice bag applied to the axilla helps relieve the discomfort.

It was formerly believed that engorgement produced fever, but lactation is not an inflammatory process, and if there is fever at this time some other cause (with rare exceptions) should be suspected.

While engorgement is present, measures are taken to keep the mother comfortable and also to empty her breasts to prevent a decrease in milk secretion. Discomfort is lessened or relieved by support of the heavy breasts, application of ice bags or warm water bottles or packs (whichever feels more comfortable to her), use of analgesic drugs as necessary for pain relief, and sometimes use of oxytocin. Darvon and aspirin constitute the analgesic commonly used. Since the breasts do not remain uncomfortable for a long period, medication is necessary for a short time, and danger to the baby is minimal.

A breast support should be used as soon as the breasts become heavy. It should lift the breasts, suspending their weight from the shoulders, and should not put pressure on any area. Ordinarily the mother wears her brassiere for support, usually the nursing brassiere that she plans to wear throughout the period of lactation. A well-fitting brassiere is often very comfortable (Fig. 19-2).

The pressure created by milk in the breasts can be relieved by emptying them, either by the baby's sucking if he can grasp the nipple or by a breast pump if he cannot nurse well. A warm pack to the breasts, prior to attempts to empty them, may enhance the flow of milk and help bring relief of pressure from milk retention.

The mother needs reassurance that the discomfort of engorgement will subside in a day or two because she may think that the breasts will remain uncomfortable during the entire time that she nurses her baby and become discouraged with nursing. When the breasts become soft and comfortable, the mother may then think

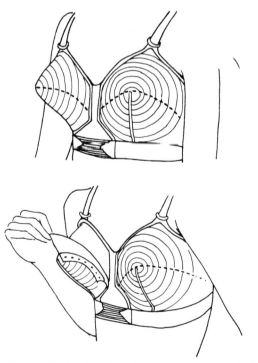

Figure 19-2. Nursing brassiere. Circular-stitched cups give extra support. Cup drops down for nursing.

that her milk supply has decreased unless she is again assured that the breasts are normally comfortable even when they are functioning adequately.

Mechanisms in Lactation

For adequate lactation there must be both secretion of milk in the breasts and expulsion of milk from the breasts.

MILK SECRETION   Secretion of milk begins two or three days after delivery and will continue for months if the breasts are frequently and sufficiently emptied. If little or no milk is withdrawn for a period of time, the milk that accumulates in the alveoli reaches a pressure level that inhibits secretion. If this back-pressure in the alveoli is inadequately relieved over a period of several days, milk secretion decreases; if it is not relieved, milk secretion stops.

Frequent and complete emptying of the breasts stimulates production of milk, and the amount produced depends largely on the amount that is removed.

Milk production can often be increased by nursing both breasts at each feeding time and by increasing the frequency of feedings, if they are not so frequent that the mother becomes tired. Milk production is slow in some mothers, and persistence may be necessary to reach a level adequate to satisfy the baby's needs.

MILK EXPULSION   The expulsion mechanism, also called the *let-down reflex,* must function adequately for proper emptying of the breast. Initiation of the reflex by the baby's sucking on the mother's nipple, or by psychic factors, causes release of oxytocin from the posterior lobe of the pituitary gland. Sensory nerve endings in the breasts, mainly in the skin, are very sensitive to pressure, temperture, pain, and the baby's sucking. Afferent fibers from these nerves travel to and through the spinal cord and to the hypothalamus. Oxytocin is produced in response to impulses along the nerves and released into the circulation from the neurohypophysis (posterior lobe of the pituitary gland). Oxytocin then

reaches the breast tissue through the circulation and causes the tissue surrounding the alveoli of the breasts to contract and propel the milk from the alveoli and the small ducts to the larger ducts opening through the nipple. From these large ducts the milk can then be removed by compression and suction. An active let-down reflex is important to maintenance of milk production. The milk expulsion reflex is easily conditioned and also easily inhibited in response to a number of other stimuli than sucking.

Some mothers experience a prickling or tingling sensation in the breasts before a feeding time. They report that they feel the milk coming in (not referring to the beginning of milk secretion) or that they feel the milk coming down. The mother may notice that milk begins to drip from her breasts at a time when she is anticipating giving a feeding or when she hears the baby cry. During a feeding time she may notice milk dripping from the breast opposite to the one from which the baby is sucking.

Worry, fatigue, pain, emotional conflicts, or other distractions interfere with the let-down reflex, and the baby gets less milk than he could if the reflex were functioning well. Nipple pain and painful uterine contractions sometimes make nursing difficult. To help prevent inhibition of the let-down reflex the mother should be given adequate pain relief if she is uncomfortable, provided with a quiet and undisturbed atmosphere while nursing her baby, and given encouragement that the breast feeding will be satisfactory. Inhibition of the let-down reflex over a period of time may result in breast feeding failure.

Fright, grief, anxiety, or any marked emotional disturbance may result in a decrease, perhaps only temporarily, in a quantity of milk that previously had been satisfactory.

Since emotions influence the secretion of milk in a number of ways, the first essential toward successful breast feeding appears to be a mother's real desire to nurse her baby. A desire to nurse, a state of good nutrition, adequate rest, and a relaxed attitude are important factors in establishing breast feeding and in maintaining the secretion of an adequate supply. The psychic influence on the production of breast milk is so significant that emotional serenity and freedom from worry are especially important. A woman's lack of confidence in her ability to nurse, especially if quantity of milk is slow to increase, may have an adverse effect, and she needs frequent encouragement and reassurance that persistence will bring good results.

Oxytocin is very occasionally administered to a mother during early lactation to initiate milk flow and assists in the ejection of milk when the let-down reflex is inhibited, as in times of stress. Oxytocin may facilitate the flow of milk.

Oxytocin is available for administration as a spray into the nasal cavity, as well as in preparation for injection. It is readily absorbed into the blood from the nasal mucous membrane. It is provided in a plastic squeeze bottle and when used is sprayed into the nostril with a squeeze of the plastic container. A single spray, as a whiff, is made into one or both nostrils two or three minutes before the breast is nursed or pumped. The effectiveness of this treatment is not assured.

The Baby's Sucking

The baby obtains milk by taking the nipple well back in his mouth and closing his lips tightly around the breast tissue, compressing the lactiferous sinuses behind the areolar area to squeeze milk out (Figs. 19-3 and 19-4A), and sucking the milk into his mouth and swallowing it.

For satisfactory nursing a baby must have the nipple well back in his mouth with his tongue pressing the nipple against his palate. When the nipple is far back in the baby's mouth, his gums press on the areolar area of the mother's breast and his lips can close tightly around the breast tissue to permit suction. Eminences across the inner part of the baby's lips are helpful in closing around the nipple. With his mouth firmly around the areolar area of the mother's breast, the baby empties the breast by compression and suction. As he nurses, his jaws move up and down and compress and empty the sinuses.

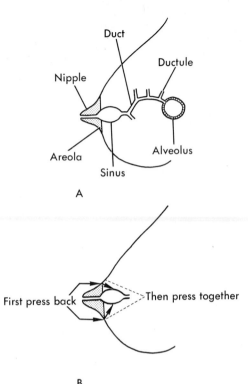

Figure 19-3. *A.* Simplified anatomy of the breast. *B.* Method of areolar expression, showing proper means of compressing sinuses. [*Adapted by permission from George R. Barnes, Jr., Anton N. Lethin, Jr., Edith B. Jackson, and Nilda Shea, "Management of Breast Feeding," JAMA, 151:192–199, 1953, p. 193.*]

Tongue action, which sucks the nipple back and presses it against the palate, and suction will complete removal of milk from the nipple. The milk is then swallowed. This action of compression, suction, and swallowing is continued rhythmically for a short period of time, followed by a few moments of rest, and then resumed. Periods of nursing interspersed with periods of rest are continued until satiety is reached.

A baby does not always take the mother's nipple properly, and although he goes through some of the movements used in nursing, he does not empty the breast satisfactorily. He may close his lips tightly around the nipple only (Fig. 19-4B) and suck vigorously. With this method he obtains very little milk, and the mother's

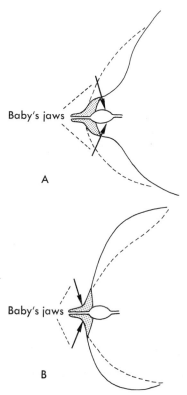

Figure 19-4. Position of baby's jaws in nursing. *A.* Correct position. *B.* Poor position resulting from areolar engorgement. [*Adapted by permission from George R. Barnes, Jr., Anton N. Lethin, Jr., Edith B. Jackson, and Nilda Shea, "Management of Breast Feeding," JAMA, 151:192–199, 1953, p. 194.*]

nipple is apt to be injured by vigorous sucking. He may also attempt to suck with his tongue above the mother's nipple instead of underneath it; this too gives poor results.

If the baby has a good grasp on the nipple, he makes deep sucking movements with the muscles in his cheeks and frequent swallowing movements. When he does not have the nipple in his mouth properly, his jaws move up and down, but suction and swallowing movements are infrequent or absent.

When the baby nurses well, he usually sucks vigorously for a few minutes, stops a few moments to rest, and then sucks again. Some babies rest more frequently than others and

some rest for several minutes at a time. The baby's nursing usually slows as his hunger decreases. He releases the nipple when his hunger and/or his desire to suck is satisfied. Ordinarily the baby does not let go of the nipple during rest periods if he has a good grasp of it. If he releases the nipple frequently, he may not have it in his mouth properly, or he may need to do so to breathe. A baby normally breathes through his nose and can breathe easily during nursing if his nose is not obstructed. He will not have difficulty breathing when his nose is not tight against the breast tissue provided it is not obstructed with secretions.

There are considerable individual differences in the ways in which babies nurse. These differences are described as follows by Dr. George R. Barnes, Jr., and coauthors:[5]

1. "Barracudas": When put to the breast, these babies vigorously and promptly grasp the nipple and suck energetically for from 10 to 20 minutes. There is no dallying. Occasionally this type of baby puts too much vigor into his nursing and hurts the nipple. 2. Excited Ineffectiveness: These babies become so excited and active at the breast that they alternately grasp and lose the breast. They then start screaming. It is often necessary for the nurse or mother to pick up the baby and quiet him first, and then put him back to the breast. After a few days the mother and baby usually become adjusted. 3. Procrastinators: These babies often seem to put off until the fourth or fifth postpartum day what they could just as well have done from the start. They wait till the milk comes in. They show no particular interest or ability in sucking in the first few days. It is important not to prod or force these babies when they seem disinclined. They do well once they start. 4. Gourmets or Mouthers: These babies insist on mouthing the nipple, tasting a little milk and then smacking their lips, before starting to nurse. If the infant is hurried or prodded, he will become furious and start to scream. Otherwise, after a few minutes of mouthing he settles down and nurses very well. 5. Resters: These babies prefer to nurse a few minutes and then rest a few minutes. If

[5] George R. Barnes, Jr., Anton N. Lethin, Jr., Edith B. Jackson, and Nilda Shea, Management of breast feeding, *JAMA* 151:194, (Jan. 17) 1953.

left alone, they often nurse well, although the entire procedure will take much longer. They cannot be hurried.

There are many babies who fall between these groups and others who fall into groups not described because they are less common. The above grouping serves merely to emphasize the fact that each baby nurses differently, and the course of the nursing will depend on the combination of the baby's nursing characteristics, the mother's personality, and the quality of help from the attending nurse. A calm mother with a "barracuda" will be quite a different matter from an anxious mother with an excited ineffective. It is accordingly advantageous to have the same nurse for both mother and baby; a nurse who knows both mother and baby can give more effective help.

Assisting the Mother and Baby

The Early Feedings

For the normal healthy newborn with a healthy mother, breast feeding is usually begun within a few hours after birth. The mother may wish to feed her baby as soon as possible after birth, and the baby is likely to suck well in this first period of reactivity. It is therefore a good time to start and usually proves to be very satisfactory for both mother and baby. When breast feeding is not started within an hour after birth, it is likely to be started in the second period of reactivity.

Once breast feeding is begun, it is continued as the baby has a need for food and for sucking, except that the night feeding may be omitted the first night if the mother so wishes to allow her to obtain additional rest.

During the first few feedings the baby gets only a small amount of colostrum, but early breast feeding, before the mature milk comes in, has several advantages. It appears to have a beneficial effect in early establishment of an adequate milk supply. It may lessen engorgement by keeping the milk ducts open through regular removal of colostrum and breast secretion, which minimizes distention of alveoli from an increased accumulation. If emptying of the breasts is not begun before engorgement appears, emptying them may be difficult.

Early breast feeding accustoms both mother and baby to the nursing process. The mother learns how to handle her baby and to put him to the breast, and the baby learns how to take the mother's nipple. All babies do not nurse well when first put to the breast; practice during the early days usually accustoms the baby to nurse well by the time the breasts secrete a larger amount.

Sucking on the nipples releases oxytocin, which promotes involution of the uterus, beneficial in the early days post partum. The mother is often aware of uterine contractions during nursing and sometimes becomes quite uncomfortable from them. Medication for pain relief may be necessary for comfort, both during and after the nursing period. This discomfort sometimes makes nursing difficult and may inhibit let-down of breast secretion.

Starting the Baby to Nurse

Helping the mother breast-feed her baby is an important nursing skill. The nurse should be available to help the mother the first time she feeds her baby and for as many times thereafter as is determined by the mother's and baby's need for assistance. Some mothers know how to make themselves and their babies comfortable during nursing, how to handle their babies with ease, and how to help their babies grasp the nipple. Others need help in all these methods. Many babies grasp the mother's nipple easily and begin sucking immediately; others need assistance and urging.

In preparing to nurse her baby the mother is advised to wash her hands and to assume a comfortable position. At first it may be easier for her to lie on her side with the head of the bed elevated slightly. Later she may wish to sit up, either in bed or in a chair. It is often easier for the nurse to assist a mother lying on her side than in an upright position (Fig. 19-5). The mother is instructed to turn well over to her side so that the baby does not need to reach up to grasp the nipple. The mother may hold the baby in the

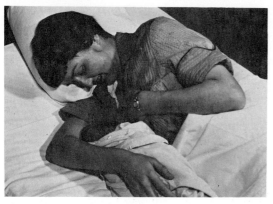

Figure 19-5. Nursing the baby while lying in bed. The nurse has assisted the mother and baby into a comfortable position. A pillow is propped under the mother's head so that she can observe the baby without strain. The mother places her arm around her baby to hold him securely. The baby's head is in a comfortable position, and the mother is turned toward him sufficiently so that he does not have to reach for the nipple. Note that the mother is holding the breast away from the baby's nose with her finger to permit him to breathe without losing a grasp on the nipple. It may be necessary for the nurse to assist the baby to get a good grasp on the mother's nipple and areolar area during his first nursing periods.

curve of her arm, but care must be taken that he is not held in a cramped position. Sometimes the baby is more comfortable if he lies on the bed with the mother's arm securely around him (Fig. 19-5).

After the baby has been placed beside the mother, attempts should not be made to urge him to begin nursing immediately. The baby's rooting reflex is well developed, and he will hunt for the nipple himself if given a few minutes' time. He will either smell the milk and hunt for it or hunt for an object that touches his cheek. Therefore, if the mother's nipple is touched to the baby's cheek he will instinctively turn his head, open his mouth, and grasp it. It may be necessary for the nurse to put her hand on the back of the baby's head to direct him to the nipple, but she should be careful not to place her fingers to his cheeks because he will feel the pressure and turn his head toward the

fingers. The head should not be forced because the baby will fight against this and begin to cry, and he will not grasp the nipple while he is crying. The baby may put his hands to his mouth while he is attempting to grasp the nipple. They may be moved away gently, but he will object to having his hands held down to his sides.

It may be necessary for the nurse to put one hand on the mother's breast and compress the areolar area between thumb and forefinger to make the nipple more prominent or to lightly massage around the nipple to make it stand out prominently. With one hand on the mother's breast to bring the nipple out and the other hand on the back of the baby's head, the nurse can assist the baby to grasp the nipple. She can bring the baby's mouth up to the nipple quickly when he opens it and is ready to grasp, or she can touch the nipple to the baby's cheek and, when his head turns toward it, be ready to put it in his mouth. It is not possible to get the mother's nipple into the baby's mouth by trying to gently pry the mouth open.

Many babies grasp the nipple easily and start sucking immediately, but with others the nurse may have to resort to a number of expedients to persuade the baby to begin nursing. Moistening the nipple by expressing a few drops of colostrum or milk may prompt the baby to take it more eagerly. Allowing the baby to take a few swallows of glucose water from a bottle and then removing it and offering the mother's nipple is sometimes helpful. The nipple in the baby's mouth, which actively stimulates his sucking, and the taste of food seem to increase his interest and effort in sucking on the mother's nipple. He does not have the rubber nipple long enough or obtain sufficient glucose to satisfy and cause him to lose interest.

Occasionally the baby is started at nursing through a nipple shield if he will not, or cannot, grasp the mother's nipple (Fig. 19-6). This glass shield with a large-holed rubber nipple attached is placed over the mother's nipple, and the baby sucks on it. It is ordinarily unsatisfactory for prolonged use because the lacteal sinuses are not compressed during nursing, and the breast can

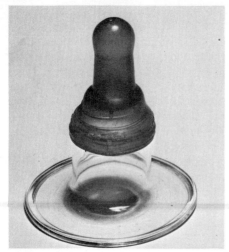

Figure 19-6. A nipple shield which may be used temporarily over the mother's nipple for the baby to suck through if he cannot grasp the mother's nipple. The opening in the nipple has been enlarged to reduce the effort that would be necessary to draw milk through the holes of the nipple. The shield may also be used as a temporary measure if the mother's nipples become very irritated and need protection.

rarely be emptied through it. Nursing through a shield for the first few minutes of a nursing period may help to pull out a flat nipple to make it easier to grasp. Sometimes a nipple shield is used for the entire nursing period for a few times if the baby cannot grasp the mother's nipple or does not suck well, but the shield should be replaced with nursing directly on the nipple as soon as possible. A breast pump may also be used for a few minutes before nursing to draw out a flat nipple.

Flat or even retracted nipples may draw out sufficiently for the baby to grasp when the areolar area is compressed, and they may come out farther when the baby sucks. Sometimes retracted nipples will not pull out, and even the baby who is making vigorous efforts cannot grasp a sufficient amount of the nipple and areolar area for satisfactory nursing. Occasionally when a mother with poorly developed nipples is attempting to nurse, such efforts may have to be discontinued after sufficient attempts demonstrate that the baby is making satisfactory efforts but cannot grasp the nipple adequately. A baby who is attempting to nurse on this type of nipple often grasps the areolar area and through vigorous sucking soon injures the skin.

The nurse must realize that many babies do not nurse well the first week of life and that, if nursing is to be a pleasant experience, the baby must not be forced to take the nipple or urged to nurse longer than he wishes. If the baby becomes upset and begins to cry hard while efforts are made to persuade him to nurse, it is best to pick him up, comfort and quiet him, and then start again. He will not take the mother's nipple while he is crying even though his mouth is wide open and the nipple can easily be placed into it.

It is not advisable to snap the feet of a sleepy baby or make vigorous efforts to prod him, because these usually result in crying and resistance, and they disturb the mother. It is very important to make sure the baby is in an alert state (quiet awake) when feedings are offered. If the baby was picked up for a feeding while in a light sleep state, at the time at which he had a brief fussy period, he may not yet be ready to eat.

When a baby does not nurse after approximately 10 minutes of effort, it is best to stop and try again at the next feeding or whenever the baby seems hungry. It may be necessary to offer a bottle in place of the breast feeding that was refused, but if the baby does not act hungry, he can be put back in his bassinet without feeding. It is permissible to omit a feeding to allow the baby to become hungry, but if he is particularly resistant to breast feeding, starving him will not help solve the problem. In such cases breast feeding is tried at each feeding time, and until the baby takes the breast, a bottle is given after each attempt. Some babies refuse to nurse at the breast for several days and then quite suddenly begin to nurse well.

The mother may become very discouraged when her baby nurses poorly. She needs frequent reassurance that continuing efforts will be successful.

When it is difficult to start a baby on breast feedings, it is especially important to attempt such feedings at a time at which the baby is hungry and fully awake, but not after he is tired from a long period of crying. A self-regulating feeding schedule is more apt to ensure success in the feeding of these infants.

Once the baby begins to suck he will usually continue without difficulty if he has the nipple well back in his mouth. If he takes only one or two sucks and then stops, he undoubtedly is trying to nurse but is not getting a good grasp on the nipple. He needs help to get the areolar area of the breast in his mouth, as he makes further attempts to nurse. The infant's first grasps on the nipple are uncomfortable to the mother. Her discomfort will be lessened if the baby gets the nipple well back in his mouth from the beginning, so that he does not need to make repeated attempts to get a good grasp.

After the baby has sucked for a minute or two and is observed to swallow, the nurse can assume that he will continue to nurse without further assistance. The mother places her arm around the baby to hold him securely and turns toward him sufficiently to make it easy for him to hold onto the nipple. The mother is instructed to keep her breast away from the baby's nose by pressing her forefinger into the breast tissue near the baby's nostrils; this permits him to breathe without releasing his hold on the nipple (Fig. 19-5).

Explanation to the mother that the baby will stop nursing and take a rest every few minutes will relieve her concern when he stops nursing for a few moments and constrain her from prodding. The baby may appear to fall asleep, but will keep the nipple in his mouth and soon begin sucking again. If it seems that he rests for very long periods, he may resume nursing if he is gently patted. His cheek should not be stroked to restart sucking because he may release the nipple to hunt for the object that is touching his cheek. If the baby releases the nip-

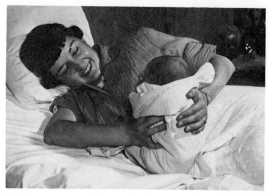

Figure 19-7. Bubbling the baby during a breast feeding in bed. The mother is holding her baby upright after his feeding and patting him gently on the back to raise the air bubble in his stomach.

ple during a rest period, he will usually grasp it again without difficulty unless his hunger or his desire to suck is satisfied. Sometimes the baby is satisfied with 5 to 10 minutes of nursing.

The mother is instructed to hold the baby up after his feeding and pat his back gently to raise the air bubble he has in his stomach (Fig. 19-7). It may be difficult for the mother to do this during the early days of nursing if she cannot move with ease, and she may need assistance from the nurse. When she is sitting up for nursing, and many mothers prefer to do this early, she can usually handle the baby easily (Figs. 19-8 and 19-9). Some mothers like to stop the baby's nursing for an air bubble halfway through a feeding, but this is not necessary with all babies, and if a baby has been difficult to start at the breast it may be wise to wait until the end of the feeding for bubbling.

The baby who breast-feeds reluctantly may need urging for several days, but he usually improves with each feeding and often nurses eagerly after the first time he has nursed well.

The period of engorgement may present difficulty even to the baby who has previously nursed well. The areolar area may become so large and firm that the baby cannot get his mouth around it or cannot compress it. Sometimes the nipple is flattened with engorgement.

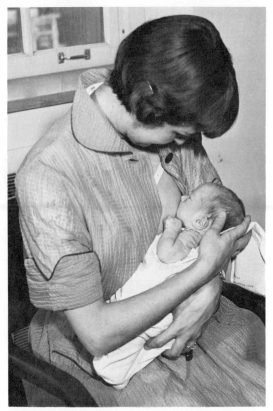

Figure 19-8. Nursing the baby while sitting in a chair. The mother should be in a comfortable chair (preferably a rocking chair) and with her feet touching the floor easily or placed on a stool. The baby is held in her arm in such a position that the upper part of his body is higher than the lower part.

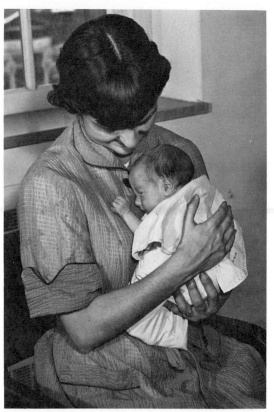

Figure 19-9. Bubbling the baby while sitting in a chair. The mother's body is helping to support her infant in this upright position for bubbling.

The baby may make many attempts to nurse and find it impossible to do so, or he may grasp the nipple only and suck on it alone (Fig. 19-4 B). Either attempt is likely to result in nipple injury.

When engorgement is a hindrance to adequate nursing, the nurse may use the same measures that are used to help a baby nurse on a flat nipple or one that is difficult to grasp. This includes compressing the areolar area between her thumb and forefinger, which may soften it somewhat and may also raise the nipple. Other measures are use of a nipple shield or a breast pump for a few minutes prior to nursing. If the baby is unable to grasp the nipple, the breast may need to be emptied with a breast pump until engorgement subsides. Sometimes the breasts do not soften completely with nursing, but if the baby has sucked well, further efforts are usually not taken. Additional use of the breast pump is often tiring and uncomfortable to the mother.

Length of Nursing Periods

The length of each nursing period is often limited to between one and five minutes at first because the nipples are sensitive, especially in women with a delicate skin, and they may become irritated. It seems desirable, however, to permit the baby to nurse for at least five minutes, and probably longer, at the first feedings. The let-down reflex may be initiated slowly in the early days of nursing. When a nursing period is limited to less than five minutes, the let-down reflex may not have begun to function and the milk ducts may not be emptied during the sucking. Emptying of the breasts is important to stimulation of milk production and emptying may also prevent or reduce later difficulty from engorgement.

Nursing periods are gradually increased to 15 to 20 minutes as tolerated by the mother's nipples. If the nipples become sore after the nursing periods have been increased, it may be necessary to temporarily limit nursing to 5 and 10 minutes to prevent excessive irritation. It is usually possible to resume a longer nursing period in a few days.

After lactation is well established, a nursing period is about 20 minutes in length, but there is considerable variation in the time for any individual baby. The baby determines this by his satisfaction of hunger and his desire to suck. When lactation is well established, most of the milk is emptied from the breast during the first five to six minutes of sucking. When the let-down reflex is active, the milk may flow so rapidly during the first few minutes of nursing that the baby does not need to make much effort to suck, and he may even have difficulty swallowing the milk as rapidly as it is forced out of the breast. Some babies fall asleep after 5 to 10 minutes of vigorous sucking; others continue to nurse for 20 minutes or longer. When a baby continues to nurse for a long period, he may do so because the breasts are not secreting enough milk and he is hungry, or because he nurses so slowly and intermittently that he takes a long time to obtain milk, or because he has a desire to suck for a long time.

A mother may nurse her baby on only one breast at each feeding time or she may nurse him from both breasts each time. Several factors enter into this decision. Sometimes the mother has a definite preference. In the early days of nursing the ease with which the baby takes the mother's nipples and the condition of her nipples are often determining factors. If the baby has difficulty grasping the nipple it seems wise to keep him on one breast for an entire nursing rather than to make the attempt to change him to the opposite side after five minutes of sucking. If the baby grasps the mother's nipple with ease he may easily nurse both sides each time. If the mother's nipples tend to become irritated in the early days of breast feeding, nursing the baby from only one breast at each feeding time permits a longer period of rest for each nipple between nursings.

After the early days of nursing the amount of breast milk produced may be a determining factor in whether one or both breasts are nursed at one time. Emptying of both breasts at each nursing time may stimulate an increasingly greater production of milk, but if the supply of milk is large, the baby may receive a sufficient amount of milk by nursing from only one breast at each feeding. When both breasts are nursed at each feeding time, the mother nurses her baby on one breast 5 to 10 minutes and then changes him to the opposite breast to suck until he is satisfied, but usually not for longer than between 20 to 30 minutes. It is important to alternate the side from which the baby starts his feeding.

Complementary Feedings

The baby may be offered a bottle feeding after breast feedings if the mother's milk supply is inadequate. Water or 5 percent glucose may be used. The baby's need for additional food and fluid is a good guide for complementary feedings. A baby may be satisfied with a breast feeding alone, at least with some feedings. If a baby is still hungry after a breast feeding, an offer of 5 percent glucose from a bottle after the breast feeding often satisfies him during the early days of life. Such a feeding also provides the baby with fluid, which he may need if the amount of breast milk that he obtains is meager.

If the amount of breast milk the mother produces is still small after several days of nursing, a baby may need formula following his breast feeding to satisfy his hunger. There is sometimes a concern that a baby who receives formula from a bottle may develop a preference for bottle feedings. This concern may not be justified for most babies. If the baby is eager to eat he will likely do well at a breast feeding, even if he has previously had a bottle. Also, a baby's satisfaction of hunger at feeding time reduces his frustration and crying, which becomes very upsetting to mother and baby. A baby who is satisfied at a feeding is likely to be hungry again in three to four hours. Giving complementary feedings of formula should thus not interfere with satisfactory nursing periods.

In most hospitals it is customary to weigh the baby before and after each nursing to ascertain how much breast milk the baby receives. To determine this the baby is weighed in exactly the same clothes after nursing as before nursing. The difference in weight indicates the number of ounces of milk taken. A wet diaper or gown may not be changed until after the weight is taken. As soon as the mother is producing an apparently adequate amount of breast milk, weighing should be omitted. Weighing before and after breast feedings should not be continued at home. The baby's demands are the best indications of his needs.

Artificial Methods of Emptying the Breasts

Sometimes the breasts need to be emptied artificially for a few times or even for several days. This may be necessary to relieve the mother of discomfort and to maintain secretion of milk when a baby cannot empty the breasts in the early days of nursing. Sometimes the breasts are artificially emptied to allow fissured nipples to heal with less irritation than they would have with vigorous nursing. Artificial emptying is sometimes used over a prolonged period when the mother of a premature baby wishes to maintain lactation until the baby is strong enough to nurse.

Milk production can be quite satisfactorily maintained for some time by emptying breasts with a breast pump or by manual expression. The breast pump, however, does not have the same stimulation that the baby's sucking has and also may not empty the breasts as completely. A breast pump only applies suction and does not compress the lacteal sinuses as a baby does when nursing. If the breasts must be emptied artificially for a long period, the milk supply may decrease until the baby can again nurse.

An electric breast pump is often used in the hospital for emptying the breasts artificially (Fig. 19-10). By application of intermittent suction with the pump the baby's nursing is imitated, and milk is drawn out of the breast. The amount of force of the suction can be carefully regulated and is indicated on a dial on the machine. The pump should always be started with low suction, which is gradually increased until the milk flows freely. Strong suction at the beginning is painful and may be injurious. The amount of suction is regulated to the needs of the individual mother, but is usually not over 6 to 8 lb of pressure.

It usually takes from 10 to 15 minutes to empty a breast, and it is not necessary to continue with the pumping much longer even if the breast does not become soft. The pump is not as effective as the baby, and in some instances the

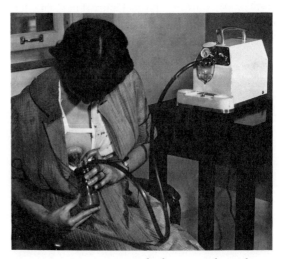

Figure 19-10. Emptying the breasts with an electric breast pump. The mother is taught how to adjust the amount of suction to her needs and tolerance and to apply the intermittent suction that is necessary to draw milk out of the breasts.

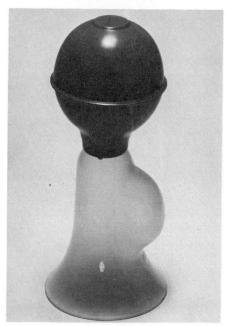

Figure 19-11. Hand breast pump. Suction for drawing milk from the breast is obtained by alternately collapsing and releasing the rubber bulb.

milk cannot be drawn out readily. Nothing more is accomplished in a longer period of time.

A hand pump (Fig. 19-11), working on the same principle as an Asepto syringe, is sometimes used. The suction is obtained by collapsing the rubber bulb, placing the widened end of the syringe over the nipple and the areolar area, and then releasing the bulb. The same process is repeated after each time the bulb has completely expanded. The hand pump is a much slower method than the electric pump and is not satisfactory for prolonged use. It may be used when only a small amount of milk needs to be emptied, as for softening the breast before the baby nurses. Some mothers prefer the hand pump to the electric pump because it causes them less discomfort.

Manual expression may be used to empty the breast. The nurse may do this, but usually the mother is taught. She can best determine how much pressure to use without causing discomfort, and it gives her a method to use at home if

necessary. It takes time to learn to use this technique effectively. On the other hand, mothers often learn to use this method at home as a means of relieving discomfort from a full breast when the baby cannot be nursed immediately or when he cannot grasp the nipple of a full breast.

In preparation for manual expression the hands should be thoroughly washed. The breast is cupped in the hand with the fingers below the breast for support and the thumb above. The forefinger and the thumb should be placed directly opposite each other just behind the areolar area. The thumb and forefinger are next pressed deeply back into the breast tissue (toward chest) and then, without moving the fingers or in any way changing their position on the skin, the thumb and forefinger are brought firmly together well behind the nipple (Fig. 19-12). This motion compresses the milk sinuses (Fig. 19-3 *B*) and milk will drip or flow from the nipple. The pressure is released and the motion of pressure is repeated. The motion of pressing back and then together and then release should be repeated rhythmically at approximately the rate of movement of a nursing baby's jaws. The fingers should not slide forward on the areola during the milking process. It is important to occasionally change the thumb and forefinger to a different position around the areolar area so that all of the sinuses are compressed during the process of manual expression. As manual expression of the breasts is carried out, milk may come only in drops at first, but if the movement of the fingers is correct and if milk is present it will flow in a spurting stream after several repetitions of the movement. It may be wise to express milk from one breast for three to five minutes, then remove milk from the other breast for a similar time, and thereafter repeat the procedure from alternate breasts.

Manual expression may be used for several reasons. Used before nursing, it will soften the areolar area if the area around the nipple is too firm for the baby to grasp. Manual expression of a small amount of milk will relieve a mother's discomfort from a full breast if it is not possible for her to nurse her baby at that particular time.

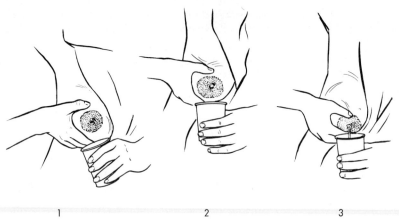

1   2   3

Figure 19-12.   Manual expression of milk. *1.* The hand holds the breast with the fingers supporting it below and the thumb placed directly opposite the first finger. *2.* The thumb and forefinger are pressed deeply back into the breast tissue. *3.* The thumb and forefinger are brought together behind the nipple, without moving them forward or in any way changing their position. When properly done, this movement will express milk from the breast. The milk is collected in a sterile container.

When manual expression is done with ease it can be used to empty the breasts if the baby is unable to nurse for one to several days.

Scrupulous cleanliness must be observed in any procedure used for emptying the breasts. The hands must be washed and the equipment must be sterile. The milk is collected in a sterile receptacle. If it is to be fed to the baby, it is put into a sterile bottle, and if not used immediately, it is covered and refrigerated.

Care of the Breasts and Nipples

The breasts and nipples must be protected from pathogenic organisms. Everyone, including the mother, must carefully wash the hands before touching the breasts. Breast tissue is highly vascular and metabolically active during lactation and is particularly susceptible to infection. The baby's sucking may be very vigorous and is sometimes followed by irritation of the nipples. Some mothers have a particularly sensitive skin, which may easily become abraded or cracked from the sucking. A portal of entry for pathogenic organisms is thus created in addition

to that of the milk ducts leading back into the breast tissue. Sound, uninjured nipples must be kept clean and protected from pathogenic organisms. Those that are abraded or cracked are touched as little as possible, kept clean, and protected against further injury.

Special care, other than cleanliness, is not given to the nipples before and after nursing. Antiseptic solutions should not be used, and boric acid is dangerous since the baby may receive a toxic dose. The usual procedure is to wash the breasts and nipples only once daily, at bath time, using mild soap (sparingly) and water. The skin of the nipples may appear dark because it alters in appearance, and it may become crusty. Attempts should not be made to wash off these crusts. At bath time the breasts should be washed first, and a clean washcloth and towel should be used each day. Niles Newton says [6]:

The standard advice to mothers is to keep their nipples clean. Nipples in our society are well pro-

[6] Niles Newton, *Maternal Emotions.* Hoeber, New York, 1955, p. 45.

tected by clothing from outside soil so that the "dirt" mothers wash off is mostly the natural accumulation of sweat, sebum, and milk.

These nipple secretions are probably very important to the health of the nipple skin by preparing it to withstand vigorous sucking. . . . Sweat with sebum has antibacterial properties. Sebum is an important contributor to the protective covering of the skin, and helps to keep the skin pliable. Sweat may also help to keep the skin pliable and normally acid. The breast milk itself may also contribute to the health of the nipple skin. Newly secreted human milk is very rich in lysozyme—an antibacterial substance.

The result of keeping the nipples "clean" is damaged nipples and excruciating pain in some instances. An experimental study . . . found that mothers washing their nipples with soap solution had more nipple pain on all five days of their hospital stay than the control group who used only water. The pain was both more frequent and more extreme. Nipple pain in turn caused a limitation of sucking and the failure of breast feeding.

Milk frequently leaks from the breasts between nursings, and pads are placed inside the brassiere or binder to absorb it. In the hospital sterile gauze is often used. Disposable breast pads may be used at home, but their cost is often prohibitive and other absorbent material is substituted. Squares of cellucotton may be used.

The nursing mother usually wears a brassiere that gives good support without pressure. Full breasts often give rise to discomfort and even pain because of their weight. A brassiere is often worn at night as well as during the day. A nursing brassiere is not essential if a well-fitted uplift brassiere is worn, but most mothers prefer a nursing brassiere, with its convenient front opening, at first. After a few months a regular uplift brassiere may seem more attractive to some mothers.

Cracked or Fissured Nipples

Nipple pain with the baby's initial grasp on them is common during the early days of nursing. If pain or tenderness persists, its cause is probably not a normal discomfort. The baby's nursing must be observed, since he may have an incorrect grasp on the nipple. This not only causes discomfort at the moment but is likely to result in irritation and fissures. To prevent cracking, the nurse tries to help the baby get an adequate grasp on the nipple.

The nipples should also be examined, under a good light, for irritation. Small cracks or fissures may be visible, but sometimes the first signs of irritation are minute blisters or small petechial spots. Abrasions may become extensive enough to bleed. Even a fissure that is barely visible may be deep enough to bleed, and sometimes the baby swallows blood while nursing. Measures must be taken to prevent further irritation and to encourage healing. Small cracks not only cause the mother much discomfort, but they provide an entrance for bacteria.

To prevent continuing nipple irritation, nursing is either reduced in time or discontinued for a day or two, depending on the extent of the irritation. When it is discontinued, the breast is emptied by one of the artificial methods. If the breast pump is used, it must be applied very gently, since pulling on the nipple with strong suction will open cracks.

A nipple shield is sometimes used temporarily as a protection to tender nipples during nursing (Fig. 19-6). It is not always useful for protection of cracked nipples, because the mother's nipple may be drawn into the shield to a considerable extend as the baby sucks. The nipple is then not rested and may even be traumatized further. The shield is also unsatisfactory if the baby cannot empty the breast quite adequately through it, since breast engorgement adds to discomfort.

An ointment is often applied to tender nipples. It is put on the nipples after each nursing, and squares of sterile wax paper may be used to prevent its absorption into the brassiere. The ointments most frequently used are unmedicated lanolin or vitamin A and D ointment or one of the commercial preparations for treatment of sore nipples, such as Massé nipple cream. The ointment is removed from the nipple with a sterile gauze square before the baby is nursed.

Sometimes the nipples are exposed to the air

for short periods of time after nursing to dry them, which may promote healing. Exposure to dry heat from a lamp, far enough removed to provide only warmth, is also occasionally used. Rubber or plastic shields in a brassiere interfere with good circulation of air and should not be used over irritated nipples. Some mothers do not think it advisable to use moisture-proof protection at any time and will remove the shields from their nursing brassieres from the beginning. Insertion of a small folded cloth in the cups of the brassiere will control leakage. Sleeping without a brassiere at night exposes the nipples to free circulation of air.

The nipples usually heal quite readily when irritation is reduced and treated. Ordinarily they soon become toughened for continued nursing without further difficulty. Occasionally the cracking is severe or recurs. This is most likely to happen when the cause of irritation recurs, such as a baby attempting to nurse from a flat nipple.

Caked Breast

The breasts should normally be comfortable except for some feeling of fullness just before nursing time. If at any time the mother complains of a *sensitive area* in the breast, there is a possibility that a section of the breast, one or two lobules, is not being emptied completely. Usually a hard lump or nodular area, known as a *caked breast,* can be palpated under the sensitive portion. As an abscess may result from a caked breast, particularly if the nipples are sore, the nurse should watch the condition of the breasts closely and notify the physician of a painful area.

Treatment of a caked breast is similar to treatment for engorgement. Good support, application of ice or warmth, and artificial emptying following nursing to try to open stopped milk ducts are used as treatment. If massage is used it should be very gentle since this may bruise the breast tissue, making it more susceptible to infection. It may take several days for a hardened area to soften, but if the mother does not develop a fever, it is ordinarily not serious.

Healthful Regime for the Nursing Mother

Rest

Sufficient rest and relaxation are necessary for adequate lactation. The deleterious effects of fatigue and worry have been described. In the hospital the nurse must be constantly observant of the mother's need for rest. Its importance at home should be emphasized. Encouragement of an understanding person at home and assistance with household work are very desirable if such can be arranged.

The amount of breast milk often increases satisfactorily after the mother leaves the hospital because of the more natural surroundings at home, provided that she rest sufficiently, eats adequately, drinks plenty of fluid, and does not have too many social obligations or family concerns. It may decrease temporarily the first day or two at home, particularly if the mother gets too tired and worried. During these few days the baby may be satisfied with the breast feeding alone if he is nursed frequently or nursed from both breasts. If he is not satisfied or if the breasts do not produce an adequate supply very soon, he will need complementary feedings.

If the mother is tense at nursing time, the baby may not get an adequate amount of milk at an individual feeding. She may find it easier to relax and feel more restful if she lies down while she nurses her baby, but if she had a tendency to fall asleep, it may be better for her to sit in a chair. This is especially true during the night feedings.

It is not necessary for the mother to weigh the baby before and after each breast feeding to know how much milk he is taking. She can determine his satisfaction from his general behavior. If the mother thinks that her baby does not get enough breast milk, a complementary feeding may need to be offered. Many mothers are quite reluctant to give both breast and bottle because they feel it makes too much work and

FEEDING THE NEWBORN 531

that it prolongs the feeding. This method needs careful planning so that the bottle of formula is ready to offer as soon as the baby has finished nursing.

It is advisable to give the baby a bottle in place of a breast feeding occasionally to keep him accustomed to formula and a rubber nipple. Some babies become so accustomed to breast feeding that they refuse a bottle later and present a serious problem if they must be weaned suddenly. Instead of an occasional artificial feeding several times a week, some physicians recommend offering the baby water from a bottle once or twice a day to keep him used to sucking from a rubber nipple. An occasional bottle feeding is important to allow the mother freedom and opportunity for recreation.

Diet

The special need for nutrients and for fluids is described in Chapter 8, "Nutrition," pages 187–89.

Drugs

Information about excretion of many kinds of drugs or combinations of drugs in breast milk is not clear, but it appears that all or nearly all drugs are found in breast milk to some extent. Some drugs apparently cross the plasma–milk barrier in fairly large amounts, while excretion of others into the milk is probably minute. In general, there appears to be somewhat less concern that drugs taken by the nursing mother will affect the infant than there is about drugs that the mother may take during her pregnancy. Since there may be risk to a nursing infant when a mother uses medications, the kind and quantity of drugs must be given serious consideration for each individual mother.

Atropine is contraindicated in nursing mothers; it decreases milk production and may cause intoxication in the baby. Ergot, which is present in many drugs for treatment of migraine headache, crosses into breast milk and may cause vomiting, diarrhea, and weak pulse in the baby.

Bromides, cascara, and senna may cause symptoms in the infant. Oral anticoagulants are easily excreted into breast milk; when such a drug is administered to a nursing mother the baby must be closely observed for bleeding. Since radioactive iodine may be transmitted to a baby through breast milk, it should not be used for diagnosis in the nursing mother.

Alcohol, barbiturates, narcotics, salicylates, caffeine, and nicotine appear in relatively insignificant amounts in breast milk unless large doses are taken by the mother.

Of the kinds of drugs that mothers are likely to use as self-medication it appears that mineral oil and milk of magnesia for prevention of constipation and aspirin for relief of minor discomforts may safely be taken by the nursing mother. Smoking may reduce excretion of breast milk and a small amount of nicotine apparently appears in breast milk. Caffeine may pass into breast milk, but since it apparently does not affect the baby, coffee is not contraindicated for the nursing mother. If alcohol is used, it should be taken in moderation since large amounts can affect the baby.

Oral contraceptives can inhibit lactation. Some of their effect will depend upon how early the drug is started and the dosage prescribed. When begun after the fifth week or later postnatally its effect on lactation may not be noticeable. The risk to the infant, however, is unknown at this time.

It is generally wise to consider that any drug that can pass through the placenta will probably also cross barriers and be excreted in breast milk.

Environmental Contaminants

Fat-soluble chemicals, called chlorinated hydrocarbons, are present in breast milk in variable amounts. These chemicals fall into two categories—agricultural and industrial. Among the agricultural chlorinated hydrocarbon chemicals are DDT and its metabolite DDE, aldrin, dieldrin, benzene hexachloride (BHC) and hexachlorobenzene (HCB). These chemicals concentrate in the fat of organisms, leading to accumulation, they persist in the environment for many years and they have manifested carcinogenicity and other chronic and acute effects in test animals.

Pesticides are usually present in human milk more frequently and in higher levels than in cow's milk, and they may be present in alarming amounts. Data on contamination of infant formula is limited but suggest that the pesticide level is lower than it is in breast milk. The amount of pesticide daily ingested by a nursing baby can equal or exceed the maximum level established for adults by the World Health Organization.[7]

Of the many chlorinated hydrocarbons used for industrial purposes two have been officially reported as found in human milk—polychlorinated biphenyls (PCBs) and polybrominated biphenyls (PBBs). When these chemicals find their way into waterways, fish can concentrate the chemicals in their body to an excessive degree.

When chlorinated hydrocarbons get into the human body they are stored in the body fat. Although much is unknown about mechanisms of storage and mobilization of fat-soluble chemicals, they appear to be mobilized from the body by weight loss and by lactation. The concentration of these chemicals in breast milk appears to be proportional to their concentration in the body fat, which in turn is proportional to level of exposure. As long as there are chemical residues in the fat there will be chemicals excreted in the milk.

A study in Norway on the content of insecticides in human breast milk showed that the concentration of insecticides in human milk decreased from colostrum onward, suggesting that the liberation of insecticides found in body fat is probably greater at the beginning of lactation. These investigators also found considerable fluctuation in the concentration of insecticides in repeated milk samples collected from the same woman a few days apart. In offering an explanation for these fluctuations they state that "it is conceivable that variations in the dietary intake of insecticides can explain, at least partly, the day-to-day fluctuations in insecticide concentration, since mobilization of insecticides from the pool in adipose tissue presumably is more stable."[8]

In order for a mother to make a decision on how to feed her baby she will need to compare the risks and the benefits of breast and bottle feeding, keeping in mind such factors as the nutritional advantages of breast milk, the immunologic qualities of breast milk, and the psychologic benefits, and also remembering that the risks from chemicals are by and large as yet unproven. It is also important to note that use of formula is not a panacea. Formula has its own contaminants such as lead.

Breast milk can be analyzed for level of contaminants if there is reason for concern. If there is a high level of contamination the mother may consider not nursing or nursing only a few days (although the insecticide content has been shown to be highest in colostrum and decreased with increasing duration of lactation), or supplementing breast feeding with bottle feeding to reduce the baby's intake of contaminants.

Contamination of the body with chemicals can be reduced by careful attention to diet, since that is probably the major exposure, unless there is occupational exposure. A major source of PCBs is fish which have lived in fresh water, particularly the bottom-feeding fish such as flounder and sole, the Great Lakes fish such as salmon, and fatty fish such as buffalofish. Ocean fish (cod, haddock, halibut) are usually free of PCB residue.

The pesticides are particularly found in foods of animal origin (meat, dairy products) and in poultry and fish, and especially in the fat of meat. Dairy products of high fat content such as

[7] Stephanie G. Harris and Joseph H. Highland, *Birthright Denied: The Risks and Benefits of Breast-feeding.* Environmental Defense Fund, Washington, D.C., 1977.

[8] Arne F. Bakken and Martin Seip, Insecticides in human breast milk. *Acta Paediatr, Scand.* 65:535–539, 1976.

butter, cream, ice cream should be avoided. Low fat dairy products such as skim milk, yogurt, ice milk are satisfactory.

It is not known how long fat stores retain residue of chemicals nor how long a time of minimal exposure is necessary to reduce the level of contamination of breast milk. A diet low in chemicals may be necessary for several years to bring the chemical residue in breast milk down to a low level. It appears, however, that there are immediate advantages in the breast-feeding mother giving careful attention to reducing dietary exposure, since some of the chemicals in the breast milk may come directly from the diet rather than from fat stores.

Duration of Lactation

The length of time that a mother breast-feeds is determined by many factors. Among these are the mother's desire to continue, her need to return to employment, her general condition, and the amount of breast milk secreted. Some mothers breast-feed for only a few weeks; others may breast-feed for six months or less. Some discontinue nursing within two weeks, before lactation is even well established. Lactation can continue for over a year and in some countries babies are breast-fed for a year or longer.

Normally lactation ceases gradually after 6 to 9 months. The baby nurses less frequently, mammary alveolar cells regress, and less and less milk is formed.

Discontinuance of nursing is usually gradual, progressively substituting bottle or cup feedings and allowing milk production to decrease. If discontinuation of breast feeding must for some reason be abrupt, breast support, application of ice, and analgesics are used as necessary to relieve discomfort from the full breasts.

SUMMARY

It has been said the human milk is for humans and cow's milk is for cows. This is no longer necessarily true, since developments in the preparation of formulas have made it possible to bring the composition of formula close to breast milk composition, and babies thrive well on an appropriate formula. (Unmodified cow's milk is not appropriate for infants.) Breast feeding, however, is advocated for mothers who feel they want to feed their babies in this manner.

Human milk provides the baby with nutrients in the appropriate proportions necessary during the period of rapid growth and high nutritional demand. Certain nutrient interactions may result in some advantages of human milk over formulas. The low protein content of breast milk may favor better absorption of iron, and the fat composition and sodium and phosphorus content may be desirable, although this has not been proven in terms of general health and long-term consequences.

Breast milk is bacteriologically safe and the immune globulins and white cells of colostrum and early breast milk confer substantial immunity to bacteriologic infections, especially enteritis.[9]

The mother who desires to nurse her baby needs a great deal of support and encouragement from her husband, family, friends, and professional staff during the sometimes trying and tiring time when lactation is being established and the baby is learning to nurse well.

Certain practices that will encourage good lactation are:

1. Provide the mother with information on breast feeding in the antepartum period and have her talk with breast-feeding mothers.
2. Avoid fatigue, anxiety, and pain in the puerperium.
3. Provide privacy and a relaxed atmosphere for nursing.
4. Stimulate lactation by starting breast feeding as soon as possible, and do not place a limit on the frequency of feedings or on night feedings.

[9] American Academy of Pediatrics, Committee on Nutrition, Commentary on breast-feeding and infant formulas, including proposed standards for formulas, *Pediatrics* 57:278–285 (Feb.) 1976.

5. Separate mother and baby as little as possible.
6. Organize the days with breast feeding in mind.
7. Avoid anxiety and interference with the letdown reflex by such factors as allowing the mother to get too tired, being unsympathetic or ambivalent about the mother's problems, causing worry about how much milk the baby takes each nursing, and lack of privacy.

ARTIFICIAL FEEDING

The artificially fed baby is ordinarily offered a formula of a mixture of cow's milk, water, and sugar that approximates the composition of breast milk. Most formulas are prepared to have a caloric value of 20 kcal per ounce.

Prior to the early 1960s formulas fed in the hospital were prepared in a special room in the hospital designated a formula room. The ingredients were mixed and terminally heated under rigid conditions that would ensure safety in mixing the proper ingredients and adequate heating and refrigeration to assure bacteriologic safety. Complete sterility could not be assured in each bottle of formula, but the bacterial count of nonpathogenic organisms was low enough to make the formula bacteriologically safe, providing it was quickly refrigerated.

In the early 1960s commercial formula services begun preparing ready-to-feed formulas that the hospital could purchase. At first these formulas were provided in bulk, and the formula was transferred to individual feeding bottles. Later the formula was supplied in individual disposable feeding bottles. More and more hospitals changed to commercially prepared formulas which are safer to use. There is less chance of error in mixing ingredients, the formula is sterile, and refrigeration is not necessary.

Many different formula mixtures, in several different dilutions (caloric strength) and in several different-sized bottles are now available.

These are ready-to-feed formulas in disposable bottles with disposable nipples. Such commerically prepared formula has been terminally sterilized and remains sterile without refrigeration until the bottle is opened. Although there is a large variety of formulas, the majority of them have very similar ingredients.

Formulas

A satisfactory formula must satisfy a baby's requirements for water, calories, vitamins, and minerals; have an appropriate distribution of calories from protein, fat, and carbohydrates; and be readily digestible. Most commercially prepared formulas are quite similar except for specialized formulas for specific purposes, such as the formula prepared for infants with phenylketonuria. Most infant formulas provide 7 to 16 percent protein, 35 to 55 percent fat, and 35 to 65 percent carbohydrate. Most prepared formulas provide 20 kcal/oz.

The American Academy of Pediatrics, Committee on Nutrition published proposed standards for infant formulas in 1967, and similar standards for infant formulas were published by the Food and Drug Administration in 1971.

Recent developments relating to infant formula have prompted the Committee on Nutrition to review formula standards. Some of these developments are production of formulas using vegetable rather than milk protein as a base and more knowledge about the interaction of one nutrient with another (protein with iron, vitamin E with unsaturated fats). As a result of this review the American Academy of Pediatrics, Committee on Nutrition has published a "Commentary on Breast-Feeding and Infant Formula, Including Proposed Standards of Formulas."[10] In this commentary the Academy proposes recommendations toward increasing the practice of breast feeding and makes specific recommendations for standards of infant formulas as to calories, protein, fat, vitamins, and

[10] *Ibid.*

minerals which apply to both milk-based and milk-substitute infant formulas.[11]

The basic constituent of artificial feedings is whole cow's milk or a commercially prepared modification of cow's milk, such as a combination of nonfat milk with demineralized whey or low-solute products. Products are available with a whey content similar to that of breast milk and with a content similar to cow's milk.

Both human and cow's milk provides approximately 20 kcal/oz. This means that the baby who is eating well and having a satisfactory caloric intake will have an adequate fluid intake. However, with the higher protein content of cow's milk compared to human milk the water reserve is larger in breast milk than in cow's milk. In prepared formulas the solute load is between that of breast milk and cow's milk but is usually brought closer toward that of breast milk. (See Table 19-2 for a comparison of human and cow's milk.)

The protein content of human milk is 1 to 1.5 gm percent, which provides approximately 8 percent of the calories. Cow's milk contains 3.3 gm percent protein and provides 16 percent of the calories in cow's milk. The higher protein content in cow's milk comes from its much higher casein content. Human milk has less casein but more whey protein.

The American Academy of Pediatrics recommends a minimum of 1.8 gm protein per 100 kcal and a maximum of 4.5 gm.[12] The level of protein in human milk is about 1.6 gm of protein per 100 kcal. Most commercial formulas in the United States use 2.3 gm protein per 100 kcal. There appears to be no evidence that protein levels above 1.8 gm/100 kcal are an advantage. Increased protein intake increases solute load.[13]

The protein in a formula may be derived from a single source or a mixture of protein sources. A variety of proteins has been successfully used.

In addition to milk-based formulas, there are also formulas that have vegetable proteins as their major protein source, such as soy protein formulas. The American Academy of Pediatrics, Committee on Nutrition says[14]:

The Committee believes the development of milk-substitute formulas for infants is important to child health. The supply of milk protein is marginal and its costs are increasing. Cheaper and more available substitutes that are nutritionally safe are welcome as a means of assisting in the prevention of malnutrition. However, there is risk of fostering other forms of malnutrition if the new products do not provide all nutrients needed by the infant. The nutritional problems to be resolved in making formulas from vegetable proteins are more complicated because milk used as a base for formulas contains nutrients that are not provided by vegetable proteins.

Lactose is the sugar present in both human and cow's milk in a percentage of approximately 7 and 4.5, respectively. In commercially prepared, milk-based formulas carbohydrate in the form of lactose is added to bring the percentage of lactose to that found in human milk. Sometimes other sugars such as sucrose or glucose may be added.

The fat content of both human and cow's milk is variable, but generally averages 3.8 and 3.7, respectively. Fat provides about 50 percent of the calories in human milk and in formulas. The fat content of most formulas is similar. Fat in formula is primarily provided as vegetable and coconut fats. These fats are easily digested and well absorbed, and they contain acceptable amounts of linoleic acid, an essential fatty acid in the diet. Skim milk provides a high protein and carbohydrate intake, but has a very low content of essential fatty acids. Skim milk should therefore not be used as a formula for infant feeding.

Vitamins are added to commercially prepared formulas in an amount that will meet the requirements for the normal healthy baby who is eating well. Iron may be added to any one of

[11] *Ibid.*
[12] *Ibid.*, p. 281.
[13] *Ibid.*, p. 282.

[14] *Ibid.*, p. 279.

Table 19-2. Comparison of Human and Cow's Milk*

	Human Milk	*Cow's Milk*
Water and solid content	Same in both; 87 to 87.5 percent is water	
Calories	Same in both; 20 calories per ounce	
Protein	1 to 1.5 percent; 60 percent of this is lactalbumin, and 40 percent is casein	3.5 percent; 15 percent of this is lactalbumin, and 85 percent is casein
Carbohydrate (in form of lactose)	6.5 to 7.5 percent	4.5 to 5.0 percent
Fat(s)	Variable from time to time, but both have approximately 3.5 percent; differs qualitatively	
	Contains more olein, which is more readily absorbed	Contains more volatile fatty acids, which are irritating to the gastric mucosa
	Digestion of fat easy	Digestion of fat sometimes difficult
Minerals	0.15 to 0.25 percent	0.7 to 0.75 percent; contains more of all minerals with the exception of iron and copper
	Iron content is low in both milks, approximately:	
	1.5 mg/liter	0.5 mg/liter
Vitamins	Varies with maternal intake; vitamin content of cow's milk may also vary with cow's intake	
Vitamin A	Relatively large amount in both milks	
Vitamin B complex	Probably adequate in both milks	
Vitamin C	More is found in human milk	
Thiamine	Higher content in cow's milk	
Riboflavin	Higher content in cow's milk	
Vitamin D	Relatively small amount in both milks	
Vitamin E	Satisfactory level in breast milk	
Digestion	Cow's milk has a higher buffer content and can therefore absorb much more gastric acid than breast milk before it reaches the acidity necessary for digestion. The large amount of casein in cow's milk makes large, tough curds in the stomach as compared with the fine, easily broken-down curds of breast milk.	

*Since cow's milk is the most common substitute for human milk, a comparison of the constituents of each may be valuable in understanding why cow's milk is modified when used in infant formulas. The curd in cow's milk is altered and made smaller and less tough by boiling, pasteurization, homogenization, and by the heat necessary for making evaporated milk. These modification processes change the curd that is produced in the stomach either by altering the casein, or by homogenizing the fat, or by producing both changes, as in the evaporation process. Modification of cow's milk makes it more suitable for infant feeding.

the proprietary formulas; these formulas can thus be obtained with or without iron.

Feeding the Baby

As with breast feeding, it is best to feed the artificially fed baby when he is hungry, according to the baby's self-regulating schedule. The baby is prepared for his feeding by being made dry and comfortable and his bottle is prepared as necessary.

Moderately cold or room temperature formula is usually well tolerated by the baby. The temperature of the formula is relatively unimportant unless it is either too hot or too cold, but a baby's palate is very sensitive to temperature changes, and he usually likes his formula the same temperature each time. Commercially prepared, terminally sterilized formulas, which do not require refrigeration, allow for storage at room temperature. With use of such formula warming is not necessary. When refrigerated formula is used, the bottle of formula is usually placed into a pan of warm water to remove the chill. A lavatory sink *should not be used* for warming formula since the bottle may become contaminated.

The baby is fed either by his mother or the nurse, being held throughout the entire feeding. The person offering the feeding should be pleasant and unhurried and sit in a comfortable chair.

The baby should always be held while he is being fed his bottle. "Propping" a bottle is dangerous because the baby may choke and aspirate milk. There is also the possibility that he may suck considerable air, which causes distention and discomfort, if he takes his feeding lying down. In addition, the baby gets more enjoyment from eating when he is held. He needs the closeness and security that accompany the feeding. The food, which quiets his hunger pains, the feeling of being held, and a pleasant manner during feeding make his eating enjoyable. Although the baby's hunger will cease even when he receives his bottle lying down, he usually gets greater satisfaction if he receives

this feeding in a more comforting manner. Pleasure and satisfaction in eating may help to make adjustments to other situations easier.

The baby should be held in a semireclining position while he eats so that the air he swallows is kept at the top of the stomach contents. To prevent swallowing of even more air than the baby ordinarily swallows while sucking, the bottle must be tilted enough to keep the nipple filled with milk at all times.

The baby may begin sucking as soon as the bottle is offered, or he may feel the nipple with his lips and take it and let go of it several times before he sucks well. Sometimes the baby raises his tongue when he takes the nipple. Although he may make sucking motions when his tongue is above the nipple, the sucking is ineffective, and the nipple must be gently manipulated or removed and replaced until it is above his tongue.

The baby will usually suck well after he has a satisfactory start on his feeding, provided he is alert and hungry and the nipple holes are satisfactory. If he is obtaining formula, air bubbles can be seen going up into the bottle regularly. If air does not appear to enter the bottle, the nipple holes must be checked for clogging.

A baby usually takes his feeding in 15 to 20 minutes. Wide variations from this time may result from an unsatisfactory nipple. If the nipple holes are too small, the baby may obtain very little milk even with vigorous sucking; the feeding may become too prolonged or the baby may become too tired to continue until he has obtained a satisfactory amount of formula. Some newborns cannot suck well on a new nipple, which is often stiff, and need a used nipple that has become softened or one that is made of soft rubber. If the nipple holes are too large, the baby may choke as the milk flows fast, and he may obtain his feeding so quickly that his desire to suck is not satisfied.

There are two kinds of openings for nipples; holes may be punctured in the end of the nipple, or a crucial incision (cross-cut) may be made at the end. Holes in the nipple should be large enough to permit milk to drop freely when the formula bottle is inverted, but not allow it to run in a stream. If the holes in a nipple are too small, they may be enlarged by slight burning of the rubber with the point of a fine needle that is heated to a red heat and quickly plunged through the end of the nipple. Several small holes are better than one large hole because there is less chance of complete plugging of the nipple.

The *cross-cut nipple* (crucial incision) has two 4-mm incisions, at right angles in the form of a cross, at the end of the nipple. Such an opening has a valvelike action, which opens as the infant sucks and closes as the pressure from the baby's mouth is released. The opening cannot be tested by inverting the formula bottle to observe the speed of the drops, but must rather be tested before the nipple is sterilized by milking the nipple on an inverted bottle of fluid.

Nipples used in a newborn nursery should not be touched after they have been sterilized. If a nipple becomes plugged while a baby is being fed or if the flow of milk is too rapid, a completely new unit—bottle of formula and nipple—should be used instead of a change of nipple. Additional bottles of formula should be available in the nursery to permit substitution of complete feeding units as frequently as necessary.

Raising an Air Bubble

When the baby's stomach is full, his sucking becomes slow and intermittent and he gradually falls asleep. The nipple may be taken away for a few minutes and then offered again to determine if he stopped sucking because of satisfaction or because of tiredness. Sometimes satiety seems to be reached when a large air buble fills the stomach; the baby sucks with renewed interest after eructation of air.

Air is swallowed with milk during sucking; if the air is not eructed before the baby is placed in his bed, it will come up after he has been put down and bring milk along with it. Although the amount of milk thus vomited appears to be considerably larger than it actually is, due to the air

that comes up with the food, it may in some instances be necessary to feed the baby again.

To raise an air bubble from the baby's stomach (bubble the baby) he is held in an upright position, to allow the air to rise to the top of the stomach; his body is supported against the mother's or nurse's body or shoulder; and he is gently patted on the back. As the bubble comes up there is a definite belching noise. If the air has not come up after a two- to three-minute period, the baby can be held in a different position for five minutes and then held upright again; if a bubble is not raised during a second attempt, he may be put to bed, preferably on his right side or abdomen. It is then wise to attempt to raise an air bubble before the next feeding. A baby may not eructate air after each feeding, although the bottle-fed baby does so in most instances.

Bringing up the air bubble at the end of a feeding may be sufficient, especially with the breast-fed infant, but if a baby is known to swallow considerable air and ordinarily vomit before he finishes a feeding, it may be necessary to stop once or twice during each feeding to attempt to raise the bubble.

Teaching the Mother

When a baby is artificially fed, the mother ordinarily feeds him during the daytime hours so that she can become accustomed to his reactions and way of eating (Fig. 19-13). The night feedings usually are given in the nursery to allow the mother to obtain adequate rest. The mother needs assistance with the baby's feedings so that she can learn how to hold the baby, how to hold the bottle, to determine when he seems satisfied, and to gain experience with bubbling him.

The mother needs explanation that the amount of formula (or breast milk) that the baby wishes may increase each day for a week or more, but that he will not take exactly the same amount from his bottle at each feeding. When he ordinarily takes 4 oz at a time he may stop after only 2 oz at some feedings; the bottle should not be jiggled to urge him to take more.

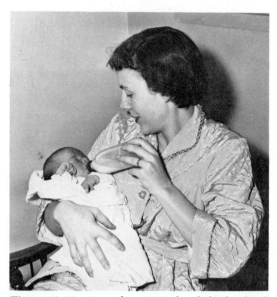

Figure 19-13. A mother giving her baby his bottle feeding. The artificially fed baby should be held for his feeding since it is the only safe way to feed him to prevent choking and aspiration of milk. The baby also needs the closeness and cuddling that accompanies the feeding while he is being held. Mothers enjoy being given the opportunity to bottle-feed their babies in the hospital.

It is also important for the mother to learn that caloric needs and gastric capacity vary greatly in infants of the same size and age and that her baby may not need the same amount that another baby of the same age will take. The question frequently asked, "How much should my baby be eating now?" gives the nurse an opportunity to explain the baby's ability to determine his needs.

Although the mother needs adequate instruction in how to raise the air bubble when she feeds her baby, she also needs reassurance that spitting-up of milk, and some vomiting after a feeding, are normal in the newborn and not always due to inadequate raising of the bubble. She may be told that vomiting decreases as the baby gets older and that it becomes significant only if it continues. Adequate bubbling, gentle handling after a feeding, and making certain that the baby's head is not lower than the rest of his body when he is put to bed all help to decrease regurgitation. Since the amount of food vomited is frequently less than it appears, the mother does not need to be concerned that the baby is not receiving an adequate amount of food unless he does not continue to gain weight. Persistent vomiting, of course, may have a serious underlying cause and may also result in a decrease in body fluids.

The mother needs reassurance that hiccuping is common after a feeding and is not significant. When the baby has hiccups, an attempt can be made once again to raise an air bubble, but further treatment is not necessary to try to stop hiccups; they will soon disappear.

Artificial Feeding at Home

One of the many varieties of prepared formulas, or evaporated milk, or cow's milk may be used for feeding the normal newborn. Foman states that in all except the lowest income group more than 70 percent of infants in the United States receive commercially prepared formulas during the first two months of life. Foman also states that reports from a number of sources suggest that a substantial percentage of the lowest income families in the United States use evaporated milk formula rather than commercially prepared formulas for infant feeding.[15]

Commercially prepared formula is available in powder form, in a liquid concentrate that requires dilution with water before it is fed to the baby, and in ready-to-feed mixture. The ready-to-feed formula may be purchased in 960-ml (32-fl oz) cans from which the formula is poured into feeding bottles, or it is available in 4-oz disposable bottles and nipples. The latter are expensive but convenient for certain purposes, as for use on a trip.

In the early 1950s most commercially prepared formula was in the form of powder. Concentrated liquid formula also became available about that time and within 10 years had largely

---

[15] Samuel J. Foman, *Infant Nutrition*, 2nd ed. Saunders, Philadelphia, Pa., 1974, p. 13.

replaced use of powdered formula. Use of ready-to-feed formula has increased rapidly since 1967.

As to cost, ready-to-feed formula in the 960-ml cans is more expensive than the concentrated liquid which may be purchased in 385-ml (13-fl oz) cans. Ready-to-feed in small individual disposable nursing bottles is most expensive. Fresh fluid milk, as homogenized whole milk or as low-fat (2 percent), costs less than commercially prepared formula, and evaporated milk is the least expensive.

The American Academy of Pediatrics, Committee on Nutrition states that unmodified cow's milk and evaporated milk at usual dilutions do not meet the proposed standards for infant feeding. Growth is satisfactory with cow's milk, but iron deficiency and hyperphosphatemia are common complications, and vitamin C needs to be supplemented. Although not proven, there is some reason to believe that the high salt and saturated fat content of cow's milk may have adverse effects on later health.[16]

After three months of age, fresh cow's milk (whole, 2 percent, or skim) is increasingly used for infant feedings in the United States.

Choosing the Formula

The physician and the mother will consider several factors in determining the kind of formula the baby will be fed at home and its method of preparation. Since the various formulas are quite similar in constituents, most babies can tolerate and thrive on any one of the many kinds available. Cost and ease of preparation can be taken into consideration in choosing a formula unless the baby has special nutritional needs. Sometimes the physician prescribes a specific formula to meet a baby's special needs, as for example, a high-protein or a low-fat content formula or a formula with added iron.

The formula used and the method of preparation may differ for the baby who is fed entirely artificially from that recommended for preparation of an occasional bottle feeding for the breast-fed baby. For the baby who is entirely on artificial feedings, the formula is usually made by dilution of a commercially prepared concentrated formula or by mixing an evaporated milk formula as described below. For the baby who is breast-fed but needs an occasional bottle a commercially prepared formula in powder form, which may be stored without refrigeration after opening, is often used. Occasionally the physician recommends use of undiluted cow's milk for the occasional bottle. It is also possible that the parents will decide to purchase the ready-to-feed prepared formula in single bottle units for the occasional bottle feeding.

Although the frequency and the amount of an infant's feeding are determined by a self-regulatory schedule, the artificially fed baby is usually started on a formula that will fulfill nutritional requirements for his age and size. Thereafter, alterations in formula are made as indicated by the individual baby's response and are determined by growth and satisfaction of hunger.

Commercially Prepared Formulas

A large variety of prepared formulas are available for infant feeding in either liquid or powder form. Many of these preparations have a composition similar to that of breast milk; in some the composition is similar to that of breast milk with the exception of a higher percentage of protein; some have a relatively high-protein and low-fat content; and some have added iron. Vitamins have been added to prepared formulas, making it unnecessary to give the baby additional vitamins while he is eating commercially prepared formula.

Commercially prepared formulas are usually purchased as a concentrated mixture. These require only the addition of water to dilute them to the proper concentration for the infant.

Commercially prepared formulas are also available in ready-to-feed, terminally sterilized, cans or bottles. There are many different milk mixtures available in several size units and in

[16] American Academy of Pediatrics, Committee on Nutrition, *op. cit.*, p. 280.

several different caloric dilutions. These ready-to-feed formulas are generally used in the hospital and are also available for home use. Since they have been terminally sterilized in a closed system, refrigeration and subsequent warming are unnecessary. The ready-to-feed formulas may be prohibitive in cost for prolonged home use but are often desirable for an occasional bottle at any time that preparation of formula is difficult or impractical.

Formula Prepared at Home

Sometimes a formula which is completely home mixed is used for infant feeding instead of a commercially prepared formula. The home-mixed formula is prepared by combining three basic ingredients—evaporated milk (or sometimes whole milk), water, and sugar. The proportions of each ingredient are determined by the infant's caloric and fluid requirements. A formula prepared to approximately 20 calories per ounce usually fulfills the normal newborn's needs. Preparation of such a formula is described below.

MILK The kind of milk used in formula will depend on its safety, its ready availability, its cost, and individual preference. Raw milk should not be used because of its high bacterial count and because of the large, tough curd it produces. Even pasteurized milk should be boiled.

The curd in cow's milk is altered and made smaller and less tough by boiling, pasteurization, homogenization, addition of acid or alkali, and by the heat necessary for making evaporated milk. These modification processes change the curd that is produced in the stomach either by altering the casein, or by homogenizing the fat, or by producing both of these changes, as in the evaporation process. Modification of cow's milk makes it more suitable for infant feeding.

Of the various modifications of cow's milk evaporated milk is the kind most frequently used for artificial feeding during the newborn period. It is readily available, is relatively inex-

pensive, may be stored without refrigeration in the unopened can, and is easy to use in infant formula. The process of evaporation of milk so alters the milk (alteration in casein and decrease in size of fat molecules) that the curd which is produced in the stomach from evaporated milk is smaller and softer than the curd of boiled, whole milk. The curd of evaporated milk is quite similar to that of breast milk. Evaporated-milk formula can also be fed in a higher concentration than whole-milk formula if it becomes necessary to increase a baby's caloric intake above average requirements.

Evaporated milk is decreased in volume to approximately one half of the original volume of whole milk; each fluid ounce of evaporated milk contains 44 calories. It is thus obvious that whole milk cannot be used as a substitute for evaporated milk, nor can evaporated milk be used in place of whole milk, unless the amount of milk and other ingredients is adjusted to a suitable infant formula.

The amount of milk the baby needs varies from 1.5 to 2 oz of whole milk or ¾ to 1 oz of evaporated milk per pound of body weight in a 24-hour period, although this requirement may be less during the first two weeks of life. Protein requirements are fulfilled by 1.5 oz of whole milk, but appetite may not be satisfied by this amount.

WATER Cow's milk is diluted with water, especially in the first few days of life. Since most or all of a newborn infant's fluid intake is formula, the milk is usually diluted up to the amount that will fulfill the total fluid requirement for a 24-hour period. Dilution with water may be continued for several months, although undiluted cow's milk is sometimes fed after a few weeks.

SUGAR Sugar is often used in formula preparation. Sugar furnishes the calories that are needed because of the dilution of the milk. Many sugars are used satisfactorily. Lactose, which is the natural milk sugar, appears to have no advantage over other kinds and may even be less well tolerated. It may cause more flatulence because of its greater degree of fermentation. Cane sugar is easily obtained, is well tolerated by the normal baby, but is sweeter than other sugars. Combinations of maltose and dextrins are sometimes used; they digest and absorb more slowly than some of the other preparations and have a less sweet taste. Corn syrup has been used quite frequently. Many of the sugars contain 120 calories per ounce.

One of several rules may be used to determine the quantity of sugar to add to a formula. One method is to add ½ oz sugar to the day's formula for the first two weeks of life, then 1 oz for four to six months, and then a gradual discontinuance until no sugar is added. Another rule that may be followed is to add $1/10$ oz of sugar per pound of the baby's body weight when whole-milk formula is used and a slightly lesser amount in an evaporated-milk formula. The amount of sugar added to a day's feeding should not exceed 1.5 oz.

To some extent the amount of sugar may be determined by the concentration of the formula and the kind of milk used, and also by the character of the baby's stools. In general, the more concentrated the formula, the less the amount of sugar the baby can tolerate. If the newborn develops loose stools, the amount of sugar in the formula may be reduced. Evaporated-milk formula is sometimes given without the addition of sugar; the concentration of the formula may then be increased fairly early in the newborn period to provide necessary calories.

In preparation of formulas it is important to know the variation in the number of tablespoons of sugar per ounce for the different kinds of sugars. If a tablespoon is used to measure the sugar for a formula, it is necessary to know the number of tablespoons per ounce of the particular kind of sugar that is used.[17]

[17] Cane sugar—2 tbsp per ounce.
Dextri-Maltose—4 tbsp per ounce.
Dexin—6 tbsp per ounce.
Corn syrup—2 tbsp per ounce.

Example of a Formula

Using the above information for formula construction, a 24-hour supply of an evaporated-milk formula that may be considered adequate to meet the needs of a newborn weighing 3600 gm (8 lb) would be calculated as shown on page 543.

This formula may be divided into eight bottles, each containing 3 oz, or six bottles containing 4 oz, depending on the baby's preference for frequency and amount of feeding.

Since this formula furnishes 412 calories, an infant weighing 3600 gm (8 lb) receives 113 calories per kilogram (51.5 calories per pound) in a 24-hour period if he takes all of the formula during that time. This formula also fulfills the baby's fluid needs.

The newborn will not take the total amount of the above formula in a 24-hour period during his first few days of life. He may not take more than 1 to 2 oz at each feeding during his early days. However, his need increases from day to day, sometimes slowly but sometimes rapidly, and he may soon want the full amount of formula. As he grows older he will show dissatisfaction with the proportions of the original formula. Alterations in the formula are then made to satisfy hunger and to meet his growth needs. A more concentrated formula is usually offered. As less water is added to formula, some of the infant's total fluid intake is furnished by orange juice and food high in water content and by drinking water between feedings.

Cow's Milk Feeding

Undiluted cow's milk is ordinarily not used for the newborn's total feedings. It may, however, be used for an occasional bottle by the breast-feeding mother, usually in the form of 2 percent milk.

Undiluted cow's milk has a high solute load, derived from the protein and electrolyte content of the milk. Cow's milk contains approximately three times more protein, four times more cal-

Total fluid requirement approximately 3 oz
    for each pound of body weight   = 24 oz
Total evaporated milk requirement approximately
    1 oz for each pound of body weight   = 8 oz
        (8 oz of evaporated milk × 44 cal per oz)   = 352 cal
Amount of water to be added to the milk to
    make a total of 24 oz of formula   = 16 oz
Sugar   = ½ oz   = 60 cal

        Total   24 oz fluid   412 cal

Therefore the formula prepared may read as follows:

                       Evaporated milk = 8 oz
                       Water   = 16 oz
                       Dextri-Maltose   = 2 tbsp
                               or
                       Corn syrup   = 1 tbsp

(*Note:* Cane sugar is less likely to be prescribed than Dextri-Maltose or corn syrup because it so closely resembles salt in appearance that there is danger of mistakenly using salt instead of cane sugar in the formula. Such an error is likely to result in serious illness of the baby.)

cium, six times more phosphorus, and three times more ash than human milk. In its undiluted state the baby may receive an overload of solutes if he receives his entire milk intake from cow's milk. Interspersed with breast milk or formula, he ordinarily can safely be fed undiluted cow's milk for the occasional feeding when his regular feeding is not available.

Method of Formula Preparation

Preparation of the formula may be a terminal heating method of an entire day's supply of formula or preparation of each bottle as needed. Both methods are described below. Factors that are considered in advising the mother in a method are the kind of formula that will be used, the safety of the water and milk supply, the availability of adequate refrigeration in the home, the mother's ability to utilize the method, and the number of bottles used each day. An occasional bottle may be prepared differently from those for total artificial feeding. Use of safe milk and a pure municipal water supply ordinarily make sterilization of formula unnecessary, at least after the first few weeks.

Terminal Heat Method of Preparation

With the terminal heating method of formula preparation, the entire formula unit, consisting of a bottle filled with the milk mixture, nippled and capped, is exposed to a degree of heat that will destroy bacteria. The day's supply of formula is mixed in a clean container, the required amount for each feeding is poured into clean bottles, nipples and caps are loosely applied to the bottles, and the entire unit is heated at a temperature of 100°C (212°F) for 25 minutes with boiling water and steam in a water bath. It takes approximately 15 minutes' exposure to the boiling water and steam before the formula itself approaches 100°C (212°F). During the total 25 minutes, the formula is therefore at a temperature very close to boiling (98.3 to 99.4°C [209 to 211°F]) for 10 minutes. This amount of heating kills pathogenic bacteria. It does not destroy spore formers, and nonpathogenic heat-resistant bacteria may survive. The bacterial count of the nonpathogenic bacteria is low enough to make the formula bacteriologically safe, but sterility cannot be assured in every bottle. Refrigeration of the formula is thus essential to keep the bacterial count low.

The terminal heating method may be especially useful for preparation of an evaporated milk formula, but is also used to prepare a day's supply of formula from commercially prepared concentrated formula, either liquid or powder form. The concentrated formula is diluted according to directions, poured into clean bottles, subjected to the heating process, and then refrigerated.

Adequate cleaning of bottles and nipples is very important to the safety of terminally heated formula. Cleaning is sometimes difficult because milk solids adhere to the inside of the bottle during heating of the formula. Bottles used daily without thorough cleaning will collect a milk film in which heat-resistant organisms, which can survive terminal heating, may build up and produce a contaminated formula. The bottle, nipple, and bottle cap should be rinsed under cold running water immediately after a feeding and then submerged in cold water to loosen milk solids and coagulated protein. After soaking, the bottles are washed in a warm detergent solution with a brush that reaches the bottom of the bottle so that all particles of formula that adhere to the glass are removed. A detergent is far superior to soap for cleaning formula bottles. Soap combines with milk casein to form a gummy substance that is difficult to remove from the surface of bottles, nipples, and utensils. The bottles are rinsed in hot running water until all detergent is removed, inspected in a good light to be certain that they are clean, and inverted to drain. Nipples and bottle caps should be cleaned in the same manner. A small brush may be used to reach the ball of the nipple or the nipple may be inverted for thorough cleaning. Water should be forced through the nipple holes.

A scum sometimes forms on formula following terminal heating, especially if the formula is cooled too rapidly. This scum may clog nipple holes, necessitating a change of nipple. Careful attention to slow cooling of formula should prevent formation of a film, but it may be desirable to use cross-cut nipples when feeding terminally heated formula, since these usually do not plug.

Terminal heating of a day's supply of formula is a very satisfactory method of formula preparation when conditions for its proper utilization can be met. It seems especially suitable for preparation of formula from evaporated or whole milk, in which three ingredients are mixed. It may be easier to measure and mix milk, water, and sugar in the quantity necessary for a whole day's supply than in small amounts for a single bottle.

Poor cleaning of bottles, permitting a milk film to collect, makes terminal heating unsafe. An adequate number of bottles and adequate refrigeration and space for storage in the refrigerator are necessary to the method. Since the formula must be stored in the refrigerator, warming of each bottle before a feeding to remove the chill may be considered and adds an additional step in use of the method.

Single Bottle Method of Preparation

With the single bottle method only one bottle of formula is made at a time, being prepared just prior to the time it will be fed (see Fig. 19-14). Nursing bottles are filled with an appropriate amount of water, nippled and capped, and terminally heated. A sufficient number of bottles of water for a day's supply are sterilized at one time and stored at room temperature until needed. At feeding time the appropriate amount of concentrated formula is added to one of the previously sterilized bottles of water. Instructions for preparation of a normal dilution formula, which provides 20 calories per ounce, are printed on the can of concentrated formula. The mother can determine from this the amount of water and the amount of concentrated formula, liquid or powder, that must be mixed for a normal concentration of formula.

When the baby gets older, and under desirable circumstances even in the newborn period, sterilization of bottles is not considered essen-

This method enables making one bottle at each feeding by adding Similac Concentrated Liquid or Powdered to bottles and water that have been sterilized previously. Single bottle method is especially useful when a supplement is desired for a breast-fed infant, or for formula preparation when traveling.

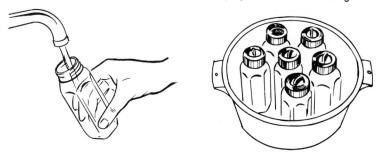

1. To prepare a day's supply of bottles add prescribed amount of tap water to each bottle.

2. Put nipples and caps on bottles loosely. Place bottles on a wire rack or clean cloth in bottom of sterilizer or large covered kettle. Add water to level of water in bottles. Place over heat. After water has come to a boil, cover, and boil for 25 minutes.

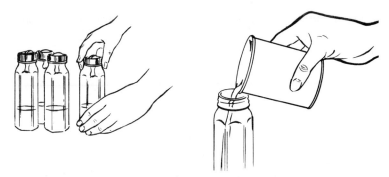

3. When sterilizer is cool to touch, remove bottles, tighten caps and store in any convenient location at room temperature.

At feeding time, wash top of Similac Concentrated Liquid can with hot water and detergent. Rinse and dry. Shake can well and punch two holes in top with clean can opener.

4. Remove cap and nipple from one bottle. Add prescribed ounces of Similac Concentrated Liquid to water in the bottle (equal parts of concentrated liquid and water). Replace cap, shake well to mix, and feed.

If using Similac Powdered, add the prescribed number of level scoops to the water, cap bottle and shake until mixed. One level scoop of powder is used for each 2 oz water.

NOTE: Opened can of Similac Concentrated Liquid should be covered and kept in the refrigerator. Remainder should be used within 24 hours. Opened can of Similac Powdered may be covered with plastic cap and stored in any convenient, cool dry place.

Figure 19-14. The single-bottle method of formula preparation. [*Reproduced with permission from* Preparing Similac Infant Formula for Your Baby. *Ross Laboratories, Columbus, Ohio, pp. 12 and 13.*]

tial. The mother is instructed to carefully wash, rinse, and drain the bottles. The day's supply of water is boiled and stored at room temperature. At feeding time an appropriate amount of boiled water and milk for a single feeding is poured into the clean bottle and fed immediately. When the water supply is safe, it is not essential to boil the water before it is added to the milk.

When milk or liquid formula is used, it is essential to refrigerate the remainder of the milk after the can has been opened. Powdered formula may be stored in the closed container at room temperature.

A few mothers prefer to use the presterilized ready-to-feed formula, which does not require further dilution. It is available in liter containers, as well as in single feeding, glass, disposable nursing bottles. The single bottles, which may be stored at room temperature and require only the application of a nipple, facilitate artificial feeding during travel or when only an occasional bottle is required. When the presterilized, prediluted formula is used from a liter bottle, the amount required for a single feeding is poured into a sterilized nursing bottle, or clean bottle if sterilization is not necessary. The remainder of the formula must be refrigerated after the can is opened. When cow's milk is used, it is handled in the same way.

In the single bottle method it is important to prepare the bottle just prior to the time it will be fed. To prevent proliferation of bacteria, this is especially important when clean instead of sterile bottles are used.

Precautions in Preparation and Use of Formula

1. When a baby does not take all of the formula from his bottle, that which remains in the bottle must always be discarded after the feeding. It is unsafe to use the remaining formula for another feeding, even if the formula is refrigerated.
2. Nursing bottles and nipples should be rinsed immediately after use to prevent milk from drying onto the surfaces. Terminally heated bottles also need to be soaked.
3. Formula prepared in single bottles should be used immediately after preparation.
4. Sterility is not ensured in every bottle prepared by terminal heating and the formula must not be left standing at room temperature. After preparation, the formula should be refrigerated as soon as it has cooled, and when a bottle is removed from the refrigerator it should be fed as soon as the chill has been removed.
5. When evaporated milk or commercially prepared liquid formula concentrate is used, the outside of the can or carton should be washed before it is opened. Refrigeration is important after the can has been opened and the milk should be used or discarded within one day after the container is opened. Use of a powdered formula concentrate is more practical and economical when only an occasional artificial feeding is required.
6. Sometimes a mother who is breast feeding has been told that she may use 2 percent milk for an occasional bottle feeding interspersed with the breast feeding. Some of these mothers stop breast feeding soon after they are home, especially if they become discouraged because of poor lactation. They begin to feed the baby completely artificially. In anticipation of such an event, these mothers should be told that 2 percent milk is not appropriate for a new baby and that they should contact their physician or nurse for formula instructions.
7. Overconcentrated formula imposes a high solute load on an infant which may lead to hyperosmolality and severe illness from dehydration and renal failure. Common offenders in this respect are boiled skim milk and improperly diluted powdered or evaporated milk. It is very important to make sure parents understand the instructions for

formula preparation and also realize that a baby cannot tolerate milk that is more concentrated than the normal dilution.[18]

VITAMIN SUPPLEMENTS

Vitamin deficiency is rare in the United States where vitamin preparations are usually given to breast-fed babies and many of the babies on bottle feedings are given vitamin-fortified formula. In contrast, infants in developing countries may have severe vitamin lack. In these countries the fetuses may not receive adequate vitamins because of a maternal vitamin deficiency, breast feeding may be discontinued early and other vitamin-poor foods are substituted, and vitamin supplementation may be lacking or inadequate.

Vitamins may be given in preparations that contain a single vitamin such as A or C or D, or they may be given in combination in a preparation that combines several vitamins.

A number of vitamin preparations containing vitamins A, C, and D, and also preparations that in addition include vitamin B complex, are available. These multivitamin preparations are usually preferred as supplements, instead of separate administration of several vitamins. Concentrations in water-miscible vehicles are used to avoid danger of aspiration of oil.

Vitamin supplements, especially vitamins C and D and usually A, are prescribed for breast-fed babies and those who do not recieve a formula with added vitamins. Babies who are artificially fed on a proprietary formula, which is prepared with vitamin additions, are not started on vitamin supplements until their feeding is changed to the whole cow's milk. When early feedings do not supply adequate vitamins, administration of supplements is usually begun at approximately one week of age. Some of a baby's vitamin requirements will be met when he is fed vitamin-enriched cereals.

FLUORIDE

Fluoride is a trace element deposited in the mineral of bones and teeth, increasing their hardness. It is considered important in the reduction of dental caries. Many communities have supplemented fluoride intake by adding it to drinking water. Other than fortified drinking water, babies receive very little fluoride from food or drink. Additional fluoride should not be given if the water supply contains an adequate amount because excess fluoride will cause mottling of the teeth. When drinking water is not fluoridated or when the baby is not taking drinking water because of complete breast feeding, the physician may recommend administration of a fluoride. The recommended dose of fluoride is 0.5 mg daily for the infant.

Desirable fluoride supplementation will depend on the fluoride content of the community water supply and upon the amount of that water consumed by the infant. No fluoride supplementation is recommended in communities in which the concentration of drinking water is more than 1 mg per liter.[19]

Preparations of fluoride for infants generally contain 0.1 mg of fluoride per drop. This makes it convenient to adjust the dose as necessary. Parents must be cautioned about the importance of restricting dosage to the prescribed amount.[20]

Combined fluoride–vitamin preparations are widely used, and seem to be better accepted than fluoride preparation alone. The combined fluoride–vitamin supplement, however, makes it impossible to adjust the dose of fluoride without affecting the vitamin dose.

IRON

Iron is an essential nutrient for the body, being an important constituent of a number of enzymes as well as of hemoglobin. The means of

---

[18] Cyril A. L. Abrams *et al.*, Hazards of overconcentrated milk formula, *JAMA* 232:1136–1140 (June 16) 1975.

[19] Foman, *op. cit.*, p. 351.
[20] Foman, *op. cit.*, p. 352.

providing babies with adequate iron intake is given serious consideration because iron deficiency has been found to be a common nutritional inadequacy of infants. The ordinary diet of a baby contributes a relatively small amount of an infant's iron requirement. Either human or cow's milk, which comprises a large portion of a baby's food intake, has a very small iron content. Other foods eaten in limited amounts during the first year, do not ordinarily provide sufficient iron.

Over three fourths of the total iron content in the newborn's body at birth is present in the erythrocytes. There is only a small amount of iron stored in other tissues. The iron from the erythrocytes is retained in the body when the red blood cells break down and it is reclaimed later for hemoglobin synthesis. The amount of iron available from this source will depend upon the initial hemoglobin mass. This amount may be inadequate to meet the baby's needs in later months if this initial hemoglobin level was somewhat low or if he was of low birth weight.

After birth the hemoglobin level falls steadily and the red blood cell count decreases. In the full-term baby recovery of erythrocyte and hemoglobin levels begins at about two months, when hematopoiesis resumes. In the premature baby, the physiologic anemia persists for a longer period of time. The premature has a smaller initial hemoglobin mass and he grows rapidly. His hemoglobin levels may remain depressed four months or longer. As hematopoiesis takes place, iron sources in the body are likely to be depleted, unless preventive measures have been taken. The baby's hemoglobin reading may fall to a level of anemia. Anemia, however, is only one manifestation of iron deficiency. By the time anemia appears, the deficiency is also affecting other tissues and organs.

Infants with low birth weight, full-term babies with a low initial hemoglobin level, and those babies who for some reason have sustained some blood loss are at risk of iron deficiency before one year. These infants may have special iron requirements during the first 18 months of life.

In the past it had commonly been thought that little or no iron was absorbed before three months of life. It is now known that iron will be efficiently absorbed when given to infants early in life and will be utilized in hemoglobin formation. Also, there appears to be no firm evidence that iron additives cause gastrointestinal disturbances in the baby, barring the rare exception. Therefore, the use of iron-fortified food (mainly milk) is considered advisable for prevention of iron deficiency in babies at risk.

The currently recommended intake of iron for normal full-term infants is 0.15 mg/100 kcal. For premature babies and any other infants with special needs the recommended intake is 2.0 mg/kg-day starting at two months or earlier. Formulas may provide anywhere from 0.1 mg to 1.5 mg/100kcal. It is recommended that ordinary formulas should provide 0.15 mg/100 kcal and that iron-fortified formula should provide 1.0 mg/100 kcal. When the formula with the higher level of iron is prescribed for babies at risk of developing anemia it should contain an ample amount of vitamin E and a moderate level of polyunsaturated fatty acids in order to reduce the susceptibility of vitamin E deficiency and hemolytic anemia.

The American Academy of Pediatrics, Committee on Nutrition strongly recommends that when proprietary formula is prescribed iron-supplemented formula be used routinely as the standard rather than as the exception.

It is advisable to meet the iron requirements of the breast-fed baby by including foods that are naturally rich in iron and iron-supplemented foods in the infant's diet. When breast feeding is stopped an iron-fortified formula can be used for the milk that is ordinarily included in the baby's meals during at least the first year of life.

Low-birth-weight babies and those with an initial low iron level may require both iron-enriched milk and medicinal iron or iron-fortified vitamin preparations. Poisoning due to accidental ingestion of medicinal iron is very serious and containers must be kept out of reach of other children.

BIBLIOGRAPHY

Aldrich, C. Anderson, Ancient process in a scientific age, *Am. J. Dis. Child.* 64:714–722 (Oct.) 1942.

Alfin-Slater, Roslyn B., and Jelliffe, Derrick B., Nutritional requirements with special reference to infancy, *Pediatr. Clin. North. Am.* 24:3–16 (Feb.) 1977.

American Academy of Pediatrics, Committee on Nutrition, Nutritional needs of low-birth-weight infants, *Pediatrics* 60:519–530 (Oct.) 1977.

———, Commentary on breast feeding and infant formulas, including proposed standards for formulas, *Pediatrics* 57:278–285 (Feb.) 1976.

———, Fluoride as a nutrient, *Pediatrics* 49:456–460 (Mar.) 1972.

———, Correspondence re iron-fortified formulas, *Pediatrics* 48:152–156; 158–159 (July) 1971.

———, Iron-fortified formulas, *Pediatrics* 47:786 (Apr.) 1971.

———, Iron balance and requirements in infancy, *Pediatrics* 43:134 (Jan.) 1969.

American Academy of Pediatrics, Committees on Drugs and on Nutrition, The use and abuse of vitamin A, *Pediatrics* 48:655–656 (Oct.) 1971.

Anderson, Thomas A., Commercial infant foods: Content and composition, *Pediatr. Clin. North Am.* 24:37–47 (Feb.) 1977.

Applebaum, R. M., The modern management of successful breast feeding, *Pediatr. Clin. North Am.* 17:203–225 (Feb.) 1970.

Avery, Gordon B., and Fletcher, Anne B., Nutrition, in *Neonatology,* edited by Gordon B. Avery. Lippincott, Philadelphia, Pa., 1975.

Barnes, George R., Jr., Lethin, Anton N., Jr., Jackson, Edith B., and Shea, Nilda, Management of breast feeding, *JAMA* 151:192–199 (Jan. 17) 1953.

Bennett, E. J., Fluid balance in the newborn, *Anesthesiology* 43:210–224 (Aug.) 1975.

Brans, Yves W., Neonatal nutrition: An overview, *Postgrad. Med.* 60:113–115 (July) 1976.

Brown, Marie Scott, Controversial questions about breastfeeding, *JOGN Nurs.* 4:45–20 (July–Aug.) 1975.

Countryman, Betty Ann, Breast care in the early puerperium, *JOGN Nurs.* 2:36–40 (Sept./Oct.) 1973.

———, Hospital care of the breast-fed newborn, *Am. J. Nurs.* 71:2365–2367 (Dec.) 1971.

Diamond, Louis K., Letter to the Editor: Iron deficiency and iron-fortified milk, *Pediatrics* 48:666–667 (Oct.) 1971.

Eiger, Marvin S., and Olds, Sally, *The Complete Book of Breast Feeding.* Workman, New York, 1972.

Fitzgerald, Joseph F., Infant feeding: Choosing the right formula, *Postgrad. Med.* 56:47–50 (July) 1974.

Foman, Samuel J., *Infant Nutrition,* 2nd ed. Saunders, Philadelphia, Pa., 1974.

Hambraeus, Leif, Proprietary milk versus human breast milk in infant feeding, *Pediatr. Clin. North Am.* 24:17–36 (Feb.) 1977.

Harris, Stephanie G., and Highland, Joseph H., *Birthright Denied: The Risks and Benefits of Breast-Feeding.* Environmental Defense Fund, Washington, D.C., 1977.

Jackson, Robert L., Long-term consequences of suboptimal nutritional practices in early life, *Pediatr. Clin. North Am.* 24:63–70 (Feb.) 1977.

Jelliffe, D. B., and Jelliffe, E. F. P. (eds.), Symposium: The uniqueness of human milk, *Am. J. Clin. Nutr.* 24:968–1024 (Aug.) 1971.

Jelliffe, E. F. Patrice, Infant feeding practices: Associated iatrogenic and commerciogenic diseases, *Pediatr. Clin. North Am.* 24:49–61 (Feb.) 1977.

Johnson, Nancy Winters, Breastfeeding at one hour of age, *MCN* 1:12–16 (Jan./Feb.) 1976.

Kron, Reuben E., Stein, Marvin, and Goddard, Katharine E., Newborn sucking behavior affected by obstetric sedation, *Pediatrics* 37:1012–1016 (June) 1966.

LaLeche League International, *The Womanly Art of Breast Feeding,* 2nd ed. LaLeche League International, Franklin Park, Ill., 1963.

Lamm, Elizabeth, Delaney, Joanne, and Dwyer, Joanna T., Economy in the feeding of infants, *Pediatr. Clin. North Am.* 24:71–84 (Feb.) 1977.

Lawson, Beverly, Perceptions of degrees of support for the breast feeding mother, *Birth Family J.* 3:67–74 (Summer) 1976.

Mayer, Jean, A new look: Breast or bottle? Liquids or solids? Homemade or store-bought? *Family Health/Today's Health* 8:38–41 (Oct.) 1976.

Morrow, Grant, III, Nutritional management of infants with inborn metabolic errors, *Clin. Perinatol.* 2:361–372 (Sept.) 1975.

Newton, Niles, Psychologic differences between breast and bottle feeding, *Am. J. Clin. Nutr.* 24:993–1004 (Aug.) 1971.

———, Breast feeding, *Psychology Today* 2:34–35; 68–70 (June) 1968.

O'Brien, Thomas E., Excretion of drugs in human milk, *Am J. Hosp. Pharm.* 31:844–854 (Sept.) 1974.

O'Grady, Roberta, Feeding behavior in infants, *Am. J. Nurs.* 71:736–739 (Apr.) 1971.

Reina, Domenick, Infant nutrition, *Clin. Perinatol.* 2:373–391 (Sept.) 1975.

Reynolds, M., Disorders of lactation and the mammary gland, in *Pathophysiology of Gestation,* Vol. I, edited by Nicholas Assali. Academic Press, New York, 1972, Chapter 7.

Rothermel, Paula C., and Faber, Myron M., Drugs in breast milk—A consumer's guide, *Birth Family J.* 2:77–88 (Summer) 1975.

Scahill, Mary C., Helping the mother solve problems with feeding her infant, *JOGN Nurs.* 4:51–54 (Mar./Apr.) 1975.

Schmitt, Madeline H., Superiority of breast-feeding: Fact or fancy? *Am. J. Nurs.* 70:1488–1493 (July) 1970.

Spock, Benjamin, *The Common Sense Book of Baby and Child Care,* Duell, Sloan, and Pearce, New York, 1946, rev. 1957. Also published as *Baby and Child Care,* rev., Pocket Books, New York, 1968.

Steward, Bernice C., and The Association for Childbirth Education, *Best-Fed Babies.* The Association for Childbirth Education, Seattle, Wash., 1960, rev. 1965.

Taubenhaus, Leon J., Bottle propping for infant feeding, *J. Pediatr.* 72:699–672 (May) 1968.

Tyson, John E., Mechanisms of puerperal lactation, *Med. Clinics North Am.* 61:153–163 (Jan.) 1977.

Weil, William B., Jr. Comments on fluid intake, renal solute, and water balance in infancy, *J. Pediatr.* 78:31–32 (Apr.) 1971.

Warshaw, Joseph B., and Wauy, Ricardo, Identification of nutritional deficiency and failure to thrive in the newborn, *Clin. Perinatol.* 2:327–344 (Sept.) 1975.

Wolman, Irving J., Feeding the health normal infant, Clinical Pediatric Handbook II, *Clin. Pediatr.* 11:21–24 (June) 1972.

———, Feeding the healthy normal infant, Clinical Pediatric Handbook II, *Clin. Pediatr.* 11:17–20 (May) 1972.

——— (ed.), The ABC's of artificial infant feeding, Clinical Pediatric Handbook II, *Clin. Pediatr.,* 11:9–12 (Apr.) 1972.

Woodruff, Calvin W., Iron deficiency in infancy and childhood, *Pediatr. Clin. North Am.* 24:85–94 (Feb.) 1977.

World Health Organization Technical Report Series, Nutrition in Pregnancy and Lactation. No. 302, 1965.

Yu, V. Y. H., Effect of body position on gastric emptying in the neonate, *Arch. Dis. Child.* 50:500–504 (July) 1975.

Ziegler, Ekhard E., and Fomon, Samuel J., Fluid intake, renal solute load, and water balance in infancy, *J. Pediatr.* 78:561–568 (Apr.) 1971.

20

Clinical Management of the Postpartum Family

The puerperium[1] is the interval from the end of labor until the return of the maternal physiology to its nonpregnant state approximately six weeks later. This time is also termed the postpartum[2] period.

The puerperium may be thought of as being composed of two distinct periods. During the first two to five days after birth the majority of women in the United States remain in a hospital or maternity home. This may be described as the lying-in period, a rather gracious term which connotes the pace of a less technologic era. During the remaining longer period, the woman gradually resumes her former activities as she and her family work to integrate the new baby into the life of their household.

This is a dynamic and challenging time for the woman and for the family. Remarkable physiologic changes occur very rapidly in the woman's body. Both parents become acquainted with their new infant and learn many new skills and attitudes necessary for infant care. In some sense they become reacquainted with each other after the dramatic experiences of pregnancy and childbirth. Relationships with their other children and with the extended family must be adjusted and renewed. The pattern of day-to-day living changes in response to the sleeping and waking cycles of the infant. It is a time of much joy and fun and family closeness.

[1] From *puer*, child, and *parere*, to bring forth.
[2] From *post*, after, and *partum*, bearing.

But it is also a time of lost sleep, frustration, irritability, and feeling isolated from previous activities, interests, and friends.

This chapter will introduce the basic concepts necessary for the nurse to begin working with families during the purerperium. Emphasis will be on activities which maintain and enhance maternal health and on teaching and anticipatory guidance of parents to facilitate their development as parents and as decision-makers for their own and their child's health.

PHYSICAL ASPECTS OF MATERNAL CARE

Throughout the puerperium, but especially during the first week, the mother's body undergoes a number of rapid changes. Although these are most marked in the pelvic organs and the breasts, the alterations which occurred in all the physiologic systems during gestation are reversed. Changes in the breasts are progressive, if the mother nurses her baby, preparing them for lactation. All other changes are retrogressive. The retrogressive genital changes are termed *involution*.

The alterations producing all of these changes are normal, physiological processes. However, because of the rapidity with which they happen they may be disturbing to the woman unless she understands what is happening to her body. Furthermore, deviations from normal can occur

551

and are most effectively treated if detected early. Consequently, women need information and teaching about the expected physical changes, but they also need systematic physical assessment to monitor the progression of involution.

During the time the mother is in the hospital a physical assessment should be made daily. This provides the ideal setting for teaching and/or reinforcing good health practices. If the mother is discharged very soon after delivery or if she does not deliver in the hospital, arrangements may be made for visitation by a public health nurse. In addition women can learn to observe their own uterine involution and to determine which subjective symptoms ought to be investigated with a health professional. This implies, however, that a significant amount of health education has taken place prior to the birth.

Postpartum Physical Assessment

The purpose of the postpartum physical assessment is to gather data about involutional changes, the mother's awareness of these changes, and her need for nursing care and teaching. An outline is given below. Following the outline is a discussion of the underlying physiology, health teaching, and nursing care pertinent to each area of assessment. The mother should be requested to empty her bladder immediately preceding the physical assessment.

1. *General Observations*
   Throughout the examination the nurse should keenly observe the mother's posture in bed, the ease (or lack of it) with which she moves about, her facial expressions, and her affect. These things are clues to her energy level, her mood, and her general feeling of wellness or illness.
2. *Vital Signs*
   These may be monitored at the time of the physical assessment or at some other time during the day that is routine for the

agency. Late afternoon around 4 o'clock is a common time for daily vital signs since diurnal variations cause most people's temperature to be at its highest for the 24 hours during this period.
3. *Breasts*
   Both breasts are palpated beginning in the axillae and moving toward the nipples, including all four quadrants. The degree of filling and/or engorgement is determined by the consistency of the breasts as well as the presence of milk and the subjective reports of the mother. The nipples are inspected for cracks.
4. *Abdomen*
   Palpation will detect any areas of unusual tenderness as well as the presence of flatulence. Should there be any reason to question intestinal motility (history of general anesthesia, abdominal distention, constipation, etc.) a stethoscope may be used to auscultate bowel sounds.
   A. *Uterus*
      The size of the uterus may be readily determined by palpating it through the soft, stretched muscles of the abdomen. The flat of the hand is placed at the level of the umbilicus and slowly moved downward while gently pressing on the abdomen until the top of the fundus is felt as a firm, globular mass. The height of the fundus is reported in relation to the umbilicus. For example, it is said to be at the level of the umbilicus, two fingerbreadths below the umbilicus, and so on.
   B. *Bladder*
      A full bladder may be palpated and often visually observed because of the flaccid condition of the abdominal muscles. It is particularly important to assess bladder distention during the first 24 to 48 hours post partum, when the urge to void may be dulled.
5. *Perineum*
   A.   Episiotomy
   B.   Hemorrhoids

6. *Lochia*

   Color, odor, and amount of vaginal discharge is noted.

7. *Lower Extremities*

   Both legs should be viewed simultaneously for discrepancies in size and color (see page 562). A check is made for Homan's sign.

Anatomic Changes and Nursing Implications

Care of the mother during the immediate postpartum period, the first few hours after delivery, is described in Chapter 15, Clinical Management During Delivery, pages 378–81. During this immediate postpartum care the vital signs, the contractility of the uterus, and the amount of vaginal bleeding are closely observed. When the fundus remains firm, vaginal bleeding is not excessive, and vital signs are stable, the recovery room care is discontinued. These observations, however, must be continued frequently during the next 12 to 24 hours. In addition, other aspects of physical care assume importance once the first critical postpartum hours are passed.

The Vital Signs

The *temperature* may rise to 38°C (100.4°F) shortly after a long labor, but it should return to normal within 24 hours. For various causes, some unexplained, the temperature may be slightly above normal at times during the first few days of the puerperium, without the patient seeming to be ill. A temperature of 38°C (100.4°F) is the upper limit of normality, and the patient is considered to have a morbid temperature if it reaches that point on any two days after the first 24 hours, providing the temperature is checked at least four times daily. (See Chapter 24, pages 699–704.) The most frequent sites of infection are the uterus, breasts, urinary tract, and respiratory tract. Fever occurring on the same day that the breasts become engorged cannot be attributed to normal breast engorgement. Engorgement does not cause an elevation in temperature except in very rare instances of extreme engorgement when the temperature may be elevated for a few hours. However, if the temperature has been normal for several days or a week and then very suddenly rises to 38.3°C (101°F) or more, a breast infection is often the cause.

The normal *pulse rate* may be slow during the early puerperium, being about 60 to 70 beats a minute or occasionally as low as 50 beats. This is referred to as puerperal bradycardia. It is thought that this is due to the decreased strain on the heart after the birth of the baby and the reduction of the vascular bed with the contraction of the uterus. In 7 to 10 days the rate is usually back to normal. In some cases there may be an increase in the pulse rate, usually following a long, hard labor or a large blood loss at delivery. A tachycardia over 100 beats per minute warrants further investigation and medical consultation, since it may be an early sign of infection, hemorrhage, or pulmonary embolism.

All the vital signs (temperature, pulse, respiration, and blood pressure) are checked three to four times during the first 24 hours after birth. Thereafter, if all are stable, temperature, pulse, and respiration may be monitored daily. The blood pressure is not taken regularly after the first 24 hours unless it has been elevated before, during, or shortly after delivery. In that event it is measured every two to four hours, or more frequently if indicated, until it remains at a normal level for the patient. (See Chapter 22, page 661.)

Breasts

The anatomy and physiology of the lactating breasts, as well as the care of the breasts and nipples of the nursing mother, is discussed in Chapter 19, "Feeding of the Newborn."

For nonnursing mothers breast care is directed at suppressing lactation and giving symptomatic relief to any discomfort which may occur.

The anterior pituitary gland produces and releases the lactogenic hormone prolactin almost immediately after delivery. This stimulates secretion of milk in the breasts. As they fill they become tense and engorged. If the breasts are not emptied, milk secretion is not continued, since the pressure of milk accumulation inhibits further secretion. This process may cause considerable discomfort to the woman until the breasts soften, a process which takes approximately 36–48 hours.

Lactation may be suppressed pharmacologically by the administration of estrogens and/or androgens to inhibit the production of lactogenic hormone. In addition, estrogens are believed to render breast tissue refractory to stimulation by prolactin. Although quite effective in preventing the discomfort of engorgement, these drugs are not without hazard. A 1977 ruling of the Federal Food and Drug Administration requires that women be advised of the risks inherent in taking estrogens for any reason. Because of the relatively large doses required to suppress lactation, some feel the risks of coagulopathy outweigh the advantages of suppressing lactation, particularly since the treatment is not always entirely successful.

If, after discussion with her physician, a woman elects to receive the drug, she will usually be given a single, intramuscular injection of Deladumone, a long-acting combination of testosterone and estradiol. For optimum effect this drug should be administered just prior to the beginning of the second stage of labor. However, because of the many other priorities for care at this time of labor, injection is frequently delayed until after delivery.

Whether or not the mother receives hormones to suppress lactation, some milk will be present in the breasts for varying lengths of time. The mother may observe some slight leaking of milk from the breasts, particularly during a warm shower, when she is cuddling her baby, or when she is sexually aroused. This may continue for several weeks.

If the breasts become uncomfortable from engorgement, symptomatic care is given until resolution occurs in about 24 to 48 hours. Wearing a proper fitting, supportive bra is important for relief from discomfort from the weight of the breasts. Application of ice bags may contribute

to comfort, although some women find application of heat to be more soothing. A mild analgesic such as aspirin or acetaminophen may be given for pain relief as necessary. The breast pump should not be used to remove some of the milk from the breasts, since this will only stimulate further milk production.

Occasionally a mother may decide to breast-feed after Deladumone or other hormones have already been administered. She should be reassured that regular sucking and emptying of the breasts by her infant will be adequate stimulation to milk production, and, that, with a little patience, an adequate milk supply and successful nursing will ensue. Mothers of sick and/or premature newborns have successfully begun breast feeding several weeks after birth. Needless to say such women must be strongly motivated and require support from significant others as well as health professionals.

While performing a postpartum breast examination the nurse should evaluate the mother's knowledge and practice of breast self-examination (BSE) and review this with her as necessary.

The Abdomen

Because of the prolonged distention of the abdominal wall by the pregnant uterus and the possible rupture of the elastic fibers of the skin, the abdomen is soft and flabby. Sometimes the abdominal wall is so stretched that the rectus muscles separate in the midline. In that condition, known as diastasis recti, part of the abdominal wall is formed simply by skin, subcutaneous fat, fascia, and peritoneum. Restoration of the muscle tone requires two to three months and is greatly dependent on the physical constitution of the individual, the number of pregnancies, and the kind and amount of physical exercise.

Many women, especially primiparas, are surprised and disappointed that their flabby abdominal muscles make them look as if they were still pregnant. After the last fatiguing weeks of pregnancy they are anxious to be slim and trim again. An empathetic remark, made at the time of examining the abdomen, will often encourage a woman to ventilate her feelings about how she looks. She can be reassured that this is a temporary situation and that she can speed the return of good muscle tone by doing some postpartum exercises.

The plan for exercising is determined by the type of labor and delivery the mother had and by her energy level and interest. Early exercises are light, require little exertion, and may be begun on the first or second postpartum day. More strenuous exercises are begun later. As at any other time, exercise must be taken with moderation and judgment, started slowly, and increased gradually according to individual tolerance.

Numerous booklets describing exercise regimen are available from pharmaceutical and formula companies as well as other sources. Many communities have organized exercise groups, especially for new mothers, conducted by the YMCA, parent education groups, or other organizations. Several representative exercises are described below.

Deep abdominal breathing: The mother is instructed to breathe deeply four or five times and on each exhalation to contract her abdominal wall. This may be done two or three times daily.

Head raising: This exercise is done while lying flat on the back, without a pillow, and with the arms at the sides. The head is raised from the flat position trying to touch the chin to the chest while at the same time contracting the abdominal muscles. Raising the head is repeated several times; the exercise is done several times daily.

Stretching from head to toe: This exercise is done while lying flat with the arms extended above the head. This tenses both back and abdominal muscles and is useful for postural correction. Similarly, standing tall will improve posture.

Lower back exercise: The mother lies on her back with her knees bent and feet flat on bed or floor. Keeping one knee up, the other leg is slowly lowered to the floor while pressing the lower spine against the bed or floor. The secret to correct performance of this exercise is keeping the spine absolutely flat against the bed or floor.

All of the above exercises may be begun as soon as desired after delivery. In addition to increasing muscle tone they are excellent for relieving backache and tension at the end of the day. As such they may be helpful to the new mother as a means of relaxation for rest and sleep during the first several months post partum.

Kegal exercise: This is an isometric exercise for strengthening the muscles of the pelvic floor. It is advisable for women to develop a habit of doing this exercise during the antepartum period to minimize loss of tone in these muscles during pregnancy. It can be done at any time in any place and will reduce congestion and discomfort in the perineal area, increase the ability to control the muscles at the openings of the urethra, vagina, and rectum, and improve support to the pelvic organs. It consists of gradually tightening the muscles around the vagina and perineum and then just as gradually relaxing them. A good way to practice this in the beginning, in order to know how it is supposed to feel when done correctly, is to stop the flow of urine by contracting the perineal muscles. This exercise should be done many times a day, whenever the woman thinks of it.

Later exercises: Rather strenuous abdominal exercises consist of leg raising and sitting up from a recumbent position. These are illustrated and described in Figures 20-1 and 20-2. In the leg-raising exercise it is recommended that only one leg be raised at one time and then only to about a 45-degree angle. Raising the leg to a 90-degree angle or raising both legs at one time may place too great a strain on the back. Similarly, bringing the body to an erect position in the sitting-up exercise may be too strenuous. Lifting the shoulders and upper back from the

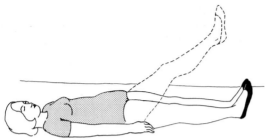

Figure 20-1. Strengthening the abdominal muscles by raising and lowering the legs. While lying on her back, the mother raises her right leg to approximately a 45-degree angle without bending the knee or raising the head and then lets it down slowly. Next the left leg is raised and lowered in the same way. Right and left legs are alternately raised and lowered as the exercise is continued.

A variation of a leg exercise is to bend the right knee and draw the thigh up over the abdomen and then straighten the leg and lower it. Next the left leg is drawn up and lowered in the same way. Right and left legs are alternately raised and lowered.

In either of these exercises each leg is raised and lowered only once or twice at first. Later the number of times is increased.

floor is often as much exertion as is advisable. Complete sit-ups should be done with the knees slightly bent to prevent strain on the muscles of the back and concentrate the effort in the abdominal muscles.

As these exercises require much effort, they must be increased very gradually. Each may be done only once or twice at first and slowly increased to several times twice a day. They should not be carried to the point of fatigue. These exercises are continued for several months. The results will depend on the amount of stretching during pregnancy, the ability of the muscles to regain their tone, and the degree to which the exercises are carried out.

Uterus

Remarkable retrogressive changes take place in the uterus during the puerperium. Immediately after delivery the uterine muscle is contracted so that the walls of the uterus are very thick, its cavity is flattened, and it forms a solid

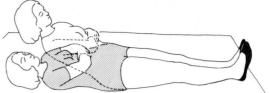

Figure 20-2. Strengthening the abdominal muscles by raising the upper part of the body. This exercise is started while lying on the back, without a pillow, and crossing the arms on the chest. The head and shoulders are raised just enough to clear the floor at first and gradually raised a little farther. Crossing the legs at the ankles may facilitate raising up from the recumbent position.

mass of tissue. The inner surface, where the placenta was attached, is raw and bleeding. After delivery the uterus is about the size of a baby's head and weighs about 1000 gm (2.2 lb). On palpation through the abdominal wall the top of the fundus can be felt at or slightly below the level of the umbilicus.

The uterus remains about the same size for two days and then decreases so rapidly in size that by the tenth day it usually cannot be palpated above the symphysis pubis. Its weight is decreased to about 500 gm (1 lb) at the end of one week. At the end of six to eight weeks the uterus has descended into the pelvic cavity and resumed approximately its original position and size, as well as its former weight of 60 gm (2 oz).

Uterine involution is accomplished by a process of *autolysis* or self-digestion. The muscle cells become much smaller. The protein material in the uterine walls is broken down into simpler components, which are absorbed and cast off, largely through the urine. This greatly increases the nitrogen content of the urine for several days. The change and absorption of uterine tissues are similar to the resolution that takes place in a consolidated lung in pneumonia.

There is evidently a close relation between the functioning of the breasts and of the uterus during the puerperium. Involution usually progresses more rapidly in women who nurse their babies than in those who do not.

The decidua which remained in the uterus

after the placenta and membranes separated becomes differentiated into two layers within two or three days. The outer layer is cast off in the discharge from the uterus, and the inner layer, which contains the bases of the glands and a small amount of connective tissue, remains to regenerate new endometrium. The entire endometrium is regenerated in three weeks with the exception of that over the placental area, which is not completely restored for six to seven weeks. The blood vessels of the placental area become either compressed or thrombosed after delivery of the placenta. It is believed that the large vessels present in the uterus during pregnancy then become obliterated and that new smaller vessels develop.

Progress of uterine involution may be judged by the size and consistency of the uterus and the character, amount, and odor of the lochia. In describing the consistency of the uterus the terms "soft and boggy" or "firm and round" are often used. The size of the uterus is determined by its height and is measured by the number of fingerbreadths the top of the fundus lies above or below the umbilicus. Immediately after delivery the top of the fundus is often several fingerbreadths below the umbilicus. It rises to near the level of the umbilicus within several hours and remains there for a day or two and then descends into the pelvis and decreases in size (Fig. 20-3). The height of the fundus should be measured when the bladder has recently been emptied, because the stretched uterine ligaments permit it to be moved about easily, and a distended bladder may push it up or to one side.

The normal rate of descent of the fundus cannot be stated exactly because of the great variations within normal limits in different individuals, but it is usually not palpable above the symphysis pubis after the tenth day. A daily record of the height of the fundus in the individual patient gives evidence of her rate of progress in involution. The nurse measures and records its height and consistency each day as part of the routine postpartum assessment.

If the uterus is involuting well, the lochia gradually decreases in amount and changes from

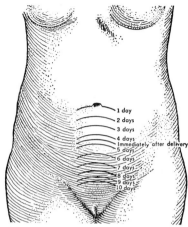

Figure 20-3. Approximate height of the fundus on each of the first 10 days after delivery.

rubra to serosa within a few days and then changes to lochia alba on approximately the tenth day. The amount and color of the lochia are recorded daily.

If the uterus remains soft and large and the mother continues to have a large amount of bright-red lochia, both signs of subinvolution, ergonovine in a 0.2 mg (^{1}/320 gr) dose may be given every four hours for 24 hours or three or four times a day for one or two days. Bright-red vaginal bleeding or expulsion of blood clots may be due to retention of a small piece of placenta or some of the fetal membranes. Involution is usually more rapid when the baby nurses because nursing stimulates uterine contractions.

Afterpains, caused by alternate contraction and relaxation of the uterine muscle, occur in about 75 percent of multiparas. They may be severe and often become worse while the mother is nursing her baby because of stimulation of the uterus. They usually do not last more than 48 hours. The primipara ordinarily does not have afterpains unless her uterus has been distended more than normal. If afterpains persist for much longer than 48 hours or if they are severe in the primipara, the possibility of retention of secundines or blood clots is considered. The pains are aggravated by administration of ergonovine.

Relief of discomfort from afterpains is obtained by pain-relieving drugs. Analgesics commonly given are propoxyphene hydrochloride (Darvon) 32 to 65 mg alone or concurrently with aspirin, or a combination of codeine, 30 to 60 mg (½ to 1 gr), and aspirin, 0.30 to 0.60 gm (5 to 10 gr).

Women often accept afterpains as a discomfort that may be expected after delivery, and they may not inform the nurse of pain. To ensure that the mother is relieved of this discomfort, it is advisable that the nurse tell the multipara that she may have afterpains and that pain medication is available. Breast-feeding mothers may be hesitant to take medications which will be transferred to their infants in the breast milk. They should know that analgesics in the ordinarily prescribed doses are not harmful to the infant. Being tense and in pain, however, may have an adverse effect on the let-down mechanism, thus inhibiting optimum nursing. Pain medication taken 15 to 20 minutes prior to a feeding will often greatly enhance the mother's comfort and enjoyment of her baby.

Cervix, Vagina, Perineum

The cervix, vagina, and perineum, which have become stretched and swollen during delivery, gradually regain their tone during the puerperium. The cervix and lower uterine segment form a flabby, collapsed, hollow tube immediately after delivery and contract slowly. The cervical canal will admit the hand immediately after delivery, two fingers for a few days therafter, and only one finger at the end of a week.

Small lacerations sustained by the cervix during labor heal during the puerperium, but it does not return to its exact predelivery state. The external os, instead of being a smooth round opening, now usually becomes a slightly irregular transverse slit.

Changes in the vagina occur slowly, and it does not return entirely to its original state. It gradually diminishes in size, and the rugae begin to reappear in three weeks. The hymenal ring is replaced by numerous ragged edges of tissue known as *carunculae myrtiformes*. The external genitalia, which have been somewhat distended during pregnancy, become smaller and more flabby. The stretched uterine ligaments become shorter as they recover their tone and regain their former state. Until the ligaments, the pelvic floor, and the abdominal wall are restored to normal tonicity, the uterus is not adequately supported and therefore may be easily displaced. The Kegal exercises described above are important for the rapid restoration of muscle tone of the perineal structures.

Bladder

Immediately after delivery the bladder is edematous and hyperemic. There may be some submucosal extravasation of blood, particularly in the bladder trigone. There is apt to be some swelling and bruising around the urethral meatus as a result of the trauma of delivery. In addition, the bladder has an increased capacity together with a decreased sensitivity to pressure. The renal pelvis and ureters are still dilated as during pregnancy.

Because of the above anatomic variations, there is a tendency for women to have some difficulty voiding during the immediate postpartum period. This tendency is aggravated by the general perineal swelling and tenderness of this period. Women who have had conduction anesthesia have particular difficulty because of the temporary interruption of neural function. Some women, although able to void, cannot completely empty their bladders, leaving residual urine after each voiding. In either case (inability to void or residual urine) the woman is at high risk for urinary tract infection because of the stasis of urine and the traumatized bladder tissues. It is, therefore, of utmost importance that the bladder distention be avoided, by catheterization if all else fails.

Assessment of urinary function is the first step in giving care. Reports of voiding should be elicited from the woman. It is also wise to measure the amount of urine the first several times the woman voids after delivery to determine whether or not a sufficient volume is being eliminated. It is not unusual for 300–500 ml of urine to be eliminated at one time because of the diuresis which occurs during the first couple of days post partum. The abdominal contour should be observed to help determine the presence of a distended bladder. It can be seen as a mass distending the lower abdomen, or it may be palpated above the symphysis pubis. (Figure 14-3, page 305, shows a distended bladder in an undelivered woman.) As the bladder fills it pushes the uterus up higher in the abdomen and/or toward one side. Thus, detecting the fundus away from the midline or higher than normally expected should be reason to strongly suspect a full bladder.

If at all possible, bladder distention should be prevented by urging the mother to attempt to void within two to three hours after delivery. Almost all women are able to be up to the bathroom or at least to a bedside commode by this time. Bedpans should be used only as a last resort, since many women find it difficult or even impossible to urinate in a horizontal position. Since the temporary dulling of sensation in the bladder may prevent the mother from having an urge to void, she may need to be reminded to try urinating at intervals during the first 12 to 24 hours. Before resorting to catheterization the nurse should exhaust all other methods of encouraging voiding such as pouring warm water over the vulva. Sitting in a Sitz bath of warm water is often helpful, especially if the woman is still having difficulty after 24 hours. Applying light pressure or massage just over the symphysis pubis compensates for the lack of abdominal muscle tone and is also useful in preventing residual urine by promoting a more thorough emptying of the bladder.

On the rare occasions when catheterization is necessary, strict asepsis and extreme gentleness are important. Catheterization of a postpartum patient may be difficult. The labia must be gently separated to prevent pulling on the perineal sutures, which causes the mother considerable pain, and yet separated far enough to visualize the meatus, which is frequently difficult to find owing to small lacerations and edema of the tissues of this area. A good light must be directed on the area. The cotton balls used for washing the area around the meatus should be squeezed dry enough to prevent the cleaning solution from running into the vaginal orifice, since this may be a source of contamination to the birth canal. There is danger of carrying lochia into the bladder, since it usually flows freely. A cotton ball placed over the vaginal orifice immediately after cleaning the area around the meatus helps to keep the vaginal secretions from spreading upward.

There is some controversy about whether or not an indwelling catheter should be inserted when a postpartum patient is unable to void or has residual urine. Some practitioners believe this allows the bladder to rest completely and eliminate the possibility of frequent catheterizations. Others believe that there is no more danger of cystitis from frequent catheterizations than from an indwelling catheter and that the muscle may regain its tone more quickly if the bladder fills and is emptied with some regularity. Conclusive research data are lacking to support either position. Any catheterization significantly increases the risk of urinary tract infections. Because of this, prophylactic antibiotics may be prescribed for these women. Fortunately, early ambulation, as well as improved antepartum and intrapartum care, has made this problem less common. Alert nursing care can further reduce the incidence by the skillful use of preventive measures.

For most women urinary function continues normally after delivery. There is a significantly increased urinary output for the first five to seven days due to the elimination of the extra tissue fluids and intravascular volume accumulated during pregnancy. Gradually the renal pelves and ureters regain their tone and by four to six weeks after delivery the urinary tract has resumed its nonpregnant state.

Perineum

The vulva and perineum are bruised and tender for several days following delivery. In addition, most women have perineal sutures used in repair of the episiotomy or occasional lacerations.

Perineal care is given to keep the area clean and dry, to eliminate odor, to promote healing, and to contribute to the woman's comfort. It is the same whether or not there are sutures.

In the past, perineal care was a highly ritualized procedure utilizing a large array of equipment and cleansing solutions and occupying many hours of nursing time. Now, however, it is realized that ordinary washing and careful attention to the usual measures of good hygiene are satisfactory. Because women are out of bed and active quite soon after delivery the nurse's major responsibility is to teach and reinforce the mother's own hygiene practices.

Even if sutures are not present, the perineum should be regarded as an open wound because it is the uterine cavity itself which must be protected from infection. Therefore the principles of hand washing and cleansing from front to back should be strongly emphasized. Washcloths, sponges, or other materials which have come in contact with the anal area should be discarded and never used again around the vaginal and urethral openings. Perineal pads should be applied snug enough to avoid sliding back and forth, possibly transferring organisms from anus to vagina. A clean pad should be used each time the woman goes to the bathroom.

Perineal care should be given by the nurse at least once during the immediate recovery period and at any other time the mother's energy levels or illness indicate the need for such care. The mother is placed on a bedpan and the vulva, perneum, and groin is washed with soap and water, taking particular care to wash from front to back and to avoid any tension on the sutures. Warm water is then poured over the area to thoroughly remove the soap. After drying, a clean perineal pad is usually applied.

Self-care is usually done while showering or while sitting on the toilet. An extra washcloth should be provided the mother specifically for perineal cleansing. A very common and practical piece of equipment is a small plastic squeeze bottle. The mother fills it with warm tap water and uses it to rinse off the perineum after each voiding or defecation. In addition to washing off the lochia, it removes urine which may sting the sutures and the warmth is soothing to the tender episiotomy. The perineum should be blotted dry with toilet tissue, again from front to back.

Perineal sutures cause some mothers considerable discomfort, occasionally for as long as seven or eight days. Others report only mild discomfort for the first few hours.

Ice applied to the perineum immediately after delivery reduces the amount of edema that occurs and thus prevents some of this discomfort. Women who have had a long second stage of labor, required unusual obstetric manipulations, or have extensive episiotomies and/or lacerations are particular candidates for this type of care. A rubber glove partially filled with crushed ice is an ideal size to fit next to the sutures.

After the initial recovery period, heat to the perineum gives some relief of discomfort. Dry heat from a heat lamp may be applied for 20–30 minutes two or three times a day. Perineal care should be given shortly before using the heat lamp to avoid drying lochia on the sutures and skin edges of the episiotomy repair. Sitz baths may be taken several times a day as a means of applying moist heat.

Analgesic ointments or sprays may also provide some relief. The ointments have the additional property of helping to keep the sutures soft and pliable, which prevents a drawing sensation. It is convenient to apply the ointment to a soft tissue which is then placed next to the sutures and held in position by the perineal pad.

If the mother experiences pain while sitting, she may be somewhat relieved by sitting on a large rubber air ring, which is inflated with just enough air to relieve pressure on the perineal area. If the perineum causes the mother much discomfort, analgesic medication may be necessary during the first few days.

Complaints of severe or persistent perineal

pain should prompt immediate investigation, since it may be a symptom of a hematoma or other abnormality (Chapter 24, page 696).

Hemorrhoids, which may have developed (or, if present, become enlarged) during pregnancy, may become more edematous with the straining of the second stage of labor. They are sometimes very painful for a few days post partum, but gradually decrease in size and cause less discomfort as circulation improves.

The mother is kept as comfortable as possible from hemorrhoidal pain by one of several kinds of treatment. Among these are application of either heat or cold, whichever gives most relief, as a heat lamp, warm moist pack, Sitz baths, or ice compresses; witch hazel compresses; analgesic ointment or spray; and rectal suppositories. Witch hazel compresses are analgesic and soothing. Applied for 20 to 30 minutes several times a day they often give considerable pain relief. Small flannel pads saturated with a a solution of witch hazel 50 percent, glycerin 10 percent, and water, commercially available as Tucks, may be used next to the perineal pad. They are placed in contact with the hemorrhoids and are changed as often as they become soiled.

If hemorrhoids were present before pregnancy, they usually subside to previous size during the puerperium. If they were not present before pregnancy, they will probably disappear completely.

Lochia

There is a vaginal discharge after delivery, termed *lochia*. It consists of uterine and vaginal secretions, blood, and the uterine lining that is cast off during the puerperium. During the first few days this discharge is bright red, consisting to a large extent of blood, and is termed *lochia rubra*. As the color gradually fades after two or three days and becomes pinker and more serous, the discharge is called *lochia serosa*. After about the tenth day, if involution is normal, the discharge is whitish or yellowish and is designated *lochia alba*. The normal characteristic odor of lochia is fleshy and resembles menstrual blood. A foul odor is suggestive of infection.

The total amount of the lochial discharge is from 150 to 400 ml. Nursing mothers bleed less totally, but may bleed more during first nursings. Under normal conditions the discharge is profuse at first, gradually diminishing until it entirely disappears by the end of the puerperium. A small amount of blood may be retained during the first day or two and expelled later as clots, without serious significance, and the discharge may be more blood-tinged after the patient becomes active. However, if the lochia is persistently blood-tinged, it may be an indication that the uterus is not involuting well or that a piece of placental tissue has been retained.

A woman should not be alarmed by a sudden gush of blood and clots upon first rising in the morning or after a long nap. While she is recumbent, lochia is apt to pool in the vagina and lower uterine segment for sudden release when she stands up. She can generally expect a slight increase in the amount of lochia when she first goes home from the hospital and increases her activity.

The duration of postpartum bleeding varies with individual women and with whether they are nursing or not. In general, a discharge sufficient to require the use of perineal pads persists for four to six weeks. If desired, tampons may be used after about three weeks or when sufficient perineal healing has occurred to make insertion comfortable.

Blood

A significant leukocytosis is present during and just after labor. A white cell count of 20,000 to 30,000/mm is not uncommon during labor, probably as a result of the physical exertion of this period. The blood count gradually returns to normal during the first postpartum week. During this time the white blood count is not as reliable an indicator of the presence of infection as it is at other times.

During the first postpartum week the increased plasma and red cell volumes gradually accumulated during pregancy are reduced. This results in fluctuations in the laboratory values for hemoglobin, hematocrit, and red cell count. As a general rule of thumb, values which drop much below the level present just before labor are indicative of extraordinary blood loss and anemia.

For at least the first week following delivery, the pregnancy-induced increase in coagulation factors remains present. This places susceptible women at risk to develop thrombophlebitis and suggests the importance of exercising utmost care in preventive treatment (Chapter 24, page 701).

Lower Extremities

Because of the risk of thrombophlebitis (see above), examination of the legs should be a part of the daily physical assessment of all postpartum women. The legs are observed for redness and skin temperature and palpated for tenderness. Edema, which can result from venous occlusion, may be best detected by observing both legs simultaneously, since it is very rare for both legs to be affected. The presence of vascular inflammation will often be indicated by pain in the calf of the leg in response to the application of gentle pressure to dorsiflex the foot. Such an occurrence is known as Homan's sign.

Ambulation is important to prevent postpartum cardiovascular complications. A program of early and progressive activity should be instituted even for women who have had cesarean sections. Indeed, since surgery further increases the risk of thrombophlebitis, ambulation is especially important for these women. Healthy women who have had an uncomplicated pregnancy and vaginal delivery are able and usually wish to be up shortly after delivery.

Additional Aspects of Postpartum Physical Care

Rest and Sleep

Fatigue commonly accompanies the postpartum period. The last weeks of pregnancy are physically as well as emotionally tiring and labor is often exhausting. Added to this is the energy expenditure required to adjust to the new responsibilities of motherhood.

Providing mothers with adequate sleep and intervals of uninterrupted rest and relaxation is a goal which challenges the most skillful of nurses. Physical discomforts, including perineal tenderness, engorgement, and afterpains may prevent rest. Unaccustomed noises in the hospital, a strange bed, or a restless roommate are further difficulties. In addition, hospital schedules, infant needs, physician and nursing visits, telephone calls, family and friends may all interrupt the most carefully planned nap. Yet this rest is essential for the mental as well as the physical health of the mother. Coping with the challenges and joys of a new baby in the family can be almost impossible for a tired mother.

Postpartum women rarely have the energy to assert themselves to demand time for their own needs. Therefore, the nurse has a serious obligation to modify the environment to promote rest and to act as a patient advocate. It is very rare that any hospital personnel must ignore a "Do Not Disturb" sign on a mother's door. Vital signs can be taken a half-hour later; routine chest x-rays can be scheduled at the convenience of the mother rather than the radiology department. Even most medications can be given a half hour earlier or later. As long as the mother remains in the hospital she can take advantage of returning her baby to the nursery for supervision and care while she naps. However, since babies sleep much of their first few days of extrauterine life, most mothers are able to rest with their babies asleep in the crib beside them.

Most hospitals place some restrictions on visitors to the maternity unit in order to protect the mother's time for rest as well as to limit the potential sources of infection. Such restrictions should of course never apply to fathers who need to have free access to their wives and infants. Equally important is the need to provide a visiting time for other children in the family. Multiparas frequently express great loneliness for their older children and the children, particularly preschoolers, should have the opportunity to maintain contact with their mothers and to meet their new sisters and brothers. As long as reasonable precautions are taken to screen visiting children for infectious diseases, there appears to be no increased risk of infection from their presence on the maternity unit.

Since visiting hours are intended for the protection of the patient, it is necessary to modify them whenever individual or family needs are not met by the routine policy. A common example is the single mother who may wish her mother, sister, or boyfriend to have the unlimited visiting hours designated for fathers.

Nutrition and Elimination

An occasional mother will experience nausea or even vomiting immediately after delivery. Most mothers, however, are extremely hungry and thirsty after the physical exertion of labor. Maternity units should be equipped with facilities to provide a light lunch for mothers regardless of the hour of their delivery. Fathers who have done the work of labor support are also usually ready for a snack. Increased appetite and thirst usually persists for the first two or three days post partum.

There is a decided change in weight during delivery and the early puerperium. An initial loss of approximately 5 to 6 kg (11 to 13 lb) occurs with expulsion of the uterine contents. An additional loss of 2 to 2½ kg (4½ to 5½ lb) takes place early in the puerperium. This is due in large part to elimination of the normally increased fluid in the tissues during pregnancy. Even women who were not particularly aware of dependent edema during pregnancy, are amazed to see how skinny their feet and ankles appear several days after delivery. Usually a woman will return to approximately her nonpregnant weight by the end of the sixth to eighth week.

The principles of nutrition for the lactating woman are discussed in Chapter 8.

Concern about the ability to have a bowel movement is relatively common in the puerperium, although it appears to concern physi-

cians more than it does mothers. The sudden loss of intraabdominal pressures, relaxation of abdominal muscles, and the intestinal sluggishness acquired during pregnancy all contribute to the tendency toward constipation. In addition, mothers often fear they will tear their stitches or that a bowel movement will be extremely painful. Most women will not have difficulty if they eat a well-balanced diet with adequate fruits and vegetables and get a reasonable amount of exercise. The urge to defecate should be acted upon promptly. Gentle bearing down serves to relax the anal sphincter and make defecation more comfortable. Stool softeners are often prescribed for several days after delivery.

If a bowel movement does not occur by the third or fourth postpartum day or if the mother is distended and uncomfortable, a suppository or enema may be given. A rectal tube will often relieve distention.

When hemorrhoids are present or a fourth-degree laceration has occurred, suppositories and/or enemas are frequently necessary and the passage of stool may cause severe discomfort. An analgesic given at the time of the suppository or 15 or 20 minutes prior to the enema will usually be helpful, and a Sitz bath immediately after defecating is soothing.

Bathing and Grooming

There is frequently profuse perspiration, especially at night, during the first few days post partum which may add to increased thirst. This gradually subsides and becomes normal by the end of a week. The perspiration sometimes has a strong odor. There may be an appreciable amount of desquamation of the skin.

Opportunity for a sponge bath should be provided as soon as practical after delivery, since the mother will probably feel sticky and sweaty after the work of labor. A few minutes taken to freshen up and brush her hair can make her feel like a new woman.

Mothers may take showers as soon as they feel able after delivery. It is wise for someone to be close by the first time a shower is taken, since even women who have been up and about may become lightheaded or faint in the warm shower.

Tub baths should be delayed for about a week until the cervix has closed as a precaution against infection. Sitz baths, which involve sitting in two to three inches of clean warm to hot water, are exceptions.

Most women feel very feminine during the early postpartum period and enjoy shampooing and arranging their hair, manicuring their nails, and dressing up in pretty nightgowns.

Psychosocial Aspects of the Puerperium

The psychosocial and developmental events which occur as a part of the puerperium are perhaps even more dramatic than the physiologic events. Certainly they have a more lasting effect on the individuals and families involved.

While the puerperium is defined physiologically as the first six weeks after delivery, it is somewhat more accurate to think of the psychosocial and developmental adjustments as occupying the entire three- to four-month period following birth. Some authors have termed this the "fourth trimester." During this time the woman makes gradual adjustments from being pregnant to being nonpregnant and a mother. The baby continues to grow and makes his initial adaptations to family life, behaviorally as well as physically. The entire family responds to new expectations, responsibilities, and routines.

Because of her biologic involvement in childbearing and her subsequent physical interdependence with her infant during lactation, a woman experiences this period in a unique way. The experience is modified for each woman by the number of children she has had, her own childhood and parenting, experiences during pregnancy, the strength of her relationship with her child's father, her own self-concept, and many other things. Yet, there is some common pattern. This pattern should be familiar to nurses so it can be used as a framework for assessment, just as physical and laboratory values are used to assess physiologic homeostasis.

In some respects the change which occurs at delivery is an abrupt one; at one moment there is a pregnant woman and a fetus and at the next moment there is a mother and child. Yet the woman may not feel any more a mother than she did before labor just as a person doesn't suddenly feel married as soon as "I do" is said or suddenly feel educated because a diploma has been granted. Much has gone before to prepare her for this event, and much will follow. Although no longer pregnant, her body is still not what it was before pregnancy. Her uterus still fills much of the abdominal cavity and she still looks pregnant. Her physical state reflects in many ways how she feels. She is in transition; no longer pregnant but not quite feeling herself again and not really feeling like a mother (though she may not know how one feels when "feeling like a mother").

At the moment of birth there is an immediate relief of pain and most women experience a tremendous sense of peace and excitement. Joy is great because both mother and baby have survived the long-awaited and dreaded labor. Usually there is an eagerness to see and touch the baby and a desire to be close to a significant other to share the joy of the moment. During the first hour after delivery women who have had relatively unmedicated labors tend to be quite talkative. They frequently review the recent events of labor. If the opportunity is presented, they will usually inspect and cuddle their infant and may begin breast feeding. They may join the father in making telephone calls to announce the birth to their parents and friends.

Within a few hours after birth the physical exertion of labor as well as the excitement brings on fatigue, and, if she is comfortable and the environment quiet, the woman may sleep soundly for several hours. It has been suggested that failure to obtain this sleep results in a delay of the restorative processes of the puerperium and a sleep hunger which persists for several days.[3]

During the first five to seven days, postpartum women are confronted with various tasks

[3] Reva Rubin, Puerperal change, *Nurs. Outlook* 9:754 (Dec.) 1961.

which they will continue to work out during the whole of the fourth trimester and perhaps, for some women and for some tasks, even beyond. These tasks include:

1. Achieving some closure or resolution of pregnancy, labor, and delivery
2. Replenishing physical and psychic energy
3. Beginning the acquaintance process with her infant
4. Learning infant care skills
5. Reestablishing family life and relationships to include the new infant member

The first few days post partum are characterized by a passivity and dependency not unlike the last trimester of pregnancy. Reva Rubin has very aptly described this time as the "taking-in" phase of the puerperium.[4] Women do indeed take in food, attention, and physical care with obvious enjoyment. They absorb every detail of their infant and their surroundings. It is as if they must fill themselves up after the draining experience of labor before they can give to the very dependent infant. Elements of this need for attention and nurturance continue throughout the puerperium, probably throughout parenthood. The literature on child abuse strongly suggests that mothers without supportive significant others are at risk for maladaptive parenting. The same is very likely true for fathers, although in the United States there are usually more opportunities for men to receive ego support from outside the family, especially during the first year of parenthood.

Gradually the woman moves from a state of predominant dependence to one of predominant independence. The timing of this transition depends on the individual woman as well as her experiences. Women whose pregnancy was medically complicated, whose labor was unusually long, or who had cesarean sections or other operative procedures generally have increased dependency needs over a longer period of time. Multiparas, women whose general health is good, and who view their pregnancies

as positive experiences tend to move more quickly toward independence. On the average this occurs about two to three days post partum and coincides with an increase in physical well-being. By this time the muscular soreness from the work of labor is gone, bladder and bowel function are usually reestablished, engorgement of the breasts is subsiding, fatigue is less overwhelming, and, in general, physical restoration is well underway. After a couple of days acquaintance the baby is beginning to be somewhat familiar, and women begin to plan for going home from the hospital, for resuming their responsibilities. Rubin terms this the "taking-hold" phase.

The observant nurse will easily detect the behavior changes which herald entry into this phase. The mother who has been still dozing when breakfast was served is suddenly showered and dressed with makeup on, waiting for her tray. Lists of tasks to be done and things to be purchased are made out for husbands, mothers, and babysitters. She writes birth announcements and takes a more active role in caring for her infant. Whereas earlier she was comfortable just being instructed, she now is eager to try doing things herself. She has increased confidence in her own opinions of how things should be done. As she begins to plan for the near future she is ready for discussions of public health nurse referrals, household help, other children's response to the baby, contraception, and other pertinent topics.

Nursing care priorities should reflect an awareness of where a woman fits along the continuum of dependency to independency. During the taking-in or dependent phase physical comfort measures should have prominence in the care plan. A back rub, a bed bath, or even a pillow-fluffing can help satisfy needs much deeper than skin care. At this time, too, a woman has an almost compulsive need to talk about her labor and delivery. To anyone who will listen she will give a detailed account of how she knew she was in labor, what her doctor said, how she behaved. She must fit all the pieces together and reconcile them with her ex-

[4]*Ibid.*

pectations for herself. It is most helpful if the nurse who was with her during labor can help her talk out the experience, preferably with the father who was there also. In this way situations which were confusing during the stress of labor can be clarified, questions can be answered, and situations and events verified. Each member of the couple can be reassured of the "goodness" of his or her performance. This is also a valuable means of collecting data about which nursing care measures were helpful or not helpful to the couple, thus enabling the nurse to constantly improve her practice.

During the taking-in phase the mother needs ample opportunity to spend time with her infant. She may use this time to feed, to examine, or simply to watch her baby as he sleeps near her. The nurse can facilitate the acquaintance process by doing a physical examination of the baby in the mother's room, explaining all of the findings, and by pointing out those behaviors and characteristics of the baby which are unique. Although she enjoys her baby, a mother is more inclined at this time to send him to the nursery while she naps or to request a nurse to manage his soiled diapers. Later, as her independence increases, she is more likely to change the diapers herself or at least to ask for help to do so.

The mother's progression toward independence does not mean she no longer needs nursing care, merely that the kind of care is somewhat different. As she assumes responsibility for her own care and that of her infant she needs more guidance and teaching and more positive reinforcement that she is doing things right. She still needs rest, but because of her anxiety about doing everything herself she may have a tendency to overextend herself. Now she needs help to plan for rest periods and to set limits for herself.

The taking-hold phase is often a time of rapid mood swings. As the woman begins to assume more and more of her responsibilities they are occasionally overwhelming and periods of depression are not uncommon. In addition there is a natural let down after the attention in preg-

nancy and the excitement of labor and delivery. The sudden shift in hormone balance, fatigue, physical discomfort, and lack of experience in caring for infants may further add to her feelings of depression. It is often reassuring for the mother to know that virtually all women experience some depression post partum. It is so common, in fact, that it has been termed the "baby blues." Talking about her feelings with her husband, with other women, or with the nurse may be very helpful. It will also be helpful if she receives positive feedback that she is doing well. If the baby goes to sleep when she soothes him, if the nurse praises the way she handles the baby, if her husband says she's a good mother, then her self-esteem will increase and her depression will more likely be mild and transient.

In current maternity practice many women are leaving the hospital before achieving some stability in the taking-hold phase; some may be discharged within a few hours after delivery, and almost all are at home by the fourth or fifth postpartum day. This means that a substantial proportion of women are no longer in contact with the health care system at the time of their greatest readiness to learn about themselves and their infants. Nurses working in traditional postpartum settings must seek ways to resolve this situation. The use of printed instruction sheets and booklets which the mother can keep with her for reference may be useful. Referral to public health nursing services is helpful in areas where this is available. A few hospitals have established outreach services whereby hospital-employed nurses make home visits. Family or pediatric nurse practitioners may establish contact with the woman in the hospital or even prior to delivery and then provide the necessary nursing care from the time of discharge. It can be expected that a variety of patterns of care will emerge in the near future as nurses strive to meet the health needs, as well as the illness needs, of childbearing families.

Yet to be answered in research is the question of the influence of early discharge (24 hours or less after delivery), or even home delivery, on the rate at which a woman moves through the taking-in and taking-hold phases. It may be that this progression will be more rapid if the woman is in familiar surroundings with people she knows and loves. At the present time, however, it seems safe to expect every woman to have some period of increased physical and emotional dependency after giving birth. This has important implications for counseling families, helping them plan for the birth of their infants and for household help and support systems during the first week of the puerperium.

The Growth of Parenting

The process by which an infant becomes attached to his caretaker has been carefully explored and described by Bowlby, Spitz, Ainsworth, and others during the past thirty years. It was not until 1970, however, that systematic efforts were begun to study this process from the maternal perspective.[5] The earlier research made clear that separation from and failure to form an attachment to a primary caregiver resulted in significant disturbances in the child's motor, mental, and affective development. The mother's failure to attach to her infant appears to have equally devastating effects on her offspring.

The mother–child relationship is an interactive one. That is to say, it is two-sided, with each member of the dyad responding to behaviors of the other in such a way that she in turn evokes a response. For example, the mother talks to her infant causing him to turn his head and look at her. The visual contact in turn evokes positive feelings in the mother toward her infant. This relationship begins during gestation as the mother works out the tasks of pregnancy in response to her own bodily changes, her kinesthetic awareness of her fetus, and the role defined for her by the culture in which she lives. If she does not accept her pregnancy as a

positive event, if she does not respond to fetal movement with a growing awareness of the infant as an individual apart from herself, then the attachment process is likely to go awry at an early stage. The survival of the human infant in primitive society required that his mother be sufficiently attached to him to care for him from the moment of birth. Obviously, surrogate mothers and formula feedings no longer make this necessary for the continuation of the species. Nonetheless, most modern mothers are probably positively inclined toward their newborns when they see them for the first time.

Fathers also most likely begin to form an attachment to their infants during gestation as they anticipate parenthood with the mother. This attachment is apt to be stronger the more involved they are in sharing the experiences of pregnancy. Men who watch and feel fetal movement, attend Lamaze classes, and place a high value on children are more likely to be actively involved with their newborns.

Even though a certain attachment to the fetus develops during pregnancy, the emergence of the infant at birth adds an entirely new dimension to the relationship. It is somewhat analogous to being acquainted with someone only through correspondence and then meeting him in person. Now there is an individual that can be seen, touched, and heard, and who can respond in a variety of ways to the surroundings. This individual may be quite unlike the mental image of the letter writer—and of the fetus. Time is required to decide if the reality is as acceptable as the fantasy.

All mothers tend to follow a similar pattern in getting acquainted with their infants. First there is an exploration and identification of the infant. Then, gradually, she claims him irreversibly as her own. This process may occur very quickly or it may require several days to weeks. Figure 20-4 summarizes some of the factors which influence this process.

During the exploration and identification phase the mother can be expected to do certain things with her baby. These behaviors are briefly described below.

[5] Clifford R. Barnett, P. Herbert Leiderman, Rose Grobstein, and Marshall Klaus, Neonatal separation: The maternal side of interactional deprivation, *Pediatrics* 45:197–205 (Feb.) 1970.

FACTORS INFLUENCING MATERNAL-INFANT ATTACHMENT

Personal Characteristics

Relationship with her own parents
Previous experiences with infants
Cultural and/or ethnic background
Age and developmental level

Antepartal Factors

Planned conception
Acceptance of pregnancy as a positive event
Support of family and friends
Health during pregnancy

Intrapartal Factors

Amount of active participation in labor and delivery
Amount of analgesia/anesthesia
Type of delivery (vaginal or cesarean)
Presence of support person(s)

Postpartal Factors

Health and responsivity of infant
Health of mother
Time of initial contact between mother and infant
Opportunity for continued contact and care of infant
Support of significant others
Skill of professionals in providing instruction, consultation, and support

Figure 20-4. Summary of factors influencing maternal–infant attachment.

Touch

The progression of maternal touch has been described by Rubin[6] and verified by numerous other observers. The mother begins touching her infant by stroking his extremities and the outline of his head with her finger tips, then gradually moving toward caressing him with the entire surface of her hand. At the same time she will usually touch and observe him first at arm's length, on her lap, or held slightly away from her body. Finally she will enfold him close to her body with both arms.

Eye-to-Eye Contact

This appears to be an extremely important component of the acquaintance process. Again and again mothers will be observed assuming an *en face* position with their babies. In this position where the two faces are in the same vertical

[6] Reva Rubin, Maternal touch, *Nurs. Outlook* 11:828–831 (Nov.) 1963.

plane each can look into the other's eyes. Mothers interpret their infant's gaze as having many positive intentions and spend much time coaxing their infants to look at them. It is very common on the postpartum unit to hear such comments as "Open your eyes. I know you're in there," "You're really looking me over," "Come on, look at mommy," and to her husband, "She opened both her eyes and looked right at me." (See Figure 20-5.)

As the mother looks at and touches her infant she will begin to attribute to him characteristics that establish him as both unique and a member of the family. That is, she will begin to regard her baby as special and distinctly different from all other babies. Yet she will identify things about him which tie him to his family. Thus she will say the baby looks like her older brother or has her daddy's nose or a temper like Uncle Harry.

If a name was chosen during pregnancy the mother will gradually "try it out" on her baby.

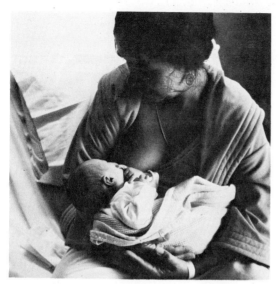

Figure 20-5. Mother nursing her baby in *en face* position.

Sometimes she will decide it doesn't fit and a new name will be chosen. If a name has not been agreed upon prior to birth, sometimes the naming itself can be symbol of claiming the infant as her own.

It should be noted that the attachment process is closely related to the progress of the mother from taking-in to taking-hold. An integral part of what she is taking in is the baby. As the bond with the infant is strengthened and she "feels more like a mother," she begins to assume more responsibility for infant care. She has claimed him as her own and so she begins to take care of him.

Nursing Care to Promote Parent–Infant Attachment

Hospital routines designed primarily for the efficiency and convenience of physicians and nurses have, for many years, done a great disservice to families. Parents have been separated from each other during labor and birth and for much of the lying-in period. Babies were traditionally sequestered away in nurseries to be seen by their mothers only for feeding and by

their fathers only through a window. Changes are occurring, however, and it is hoped that parents will now be able to be together whenever they choose and will have free access to their babies at all times. Consumer input into health care practices has been a valuable force in bringing about the much-needed changes in the care available to childbearing families. Many skilled professionals are now working in a variety of sensitive and imaginative ways to provide both the warmth and security of a family environment and the safety of modern medical technology.

Promotion of healthy parent–infant relationships begins during antepartum care, or even long before. It continues during labor and delivery, when the woman is reassured by the presence of a significant other and a supportive professional. Efforts to enhance the self-esteem of the laboring woman will leave her better prepared to devote the necessary energy to her infant.

Preferably the mother is awake during delivery and both she and the father are participating actively in the birth of their child. In any event, it is important that both parents have the opportunity to see and touch their baby as soon as possible after birth. In animals, there exists a critical or sensitive period for maternal attachment. This is a short period of time, usually less than an hour, immediately following birth, during which the mother animal must have contact with her offspring or she will abandon it. Obviously, adult humans, with their ability to reason, remember, and imagine are not apt to abandon their infants if they do not have contact with them in the first hour of life. Nevertheless there is some evidence that an initial period of separation contributes to maladaptive parenting in individuals who are at risk because of other factors.[7,8]. Equally important is the fact that

[7] M. H. Seashore *et al.*, "The effects of denial of early mother–infant interaction on maternal self-confidence, *J. Pers. Soc. Psychol.* 26:369–378, 1973.

[8] Marshall H. Klaus *et al.*, Maternal attachment: Importance of the first post-partum days, *N. Engl. J. Med.* 268:460–463 (Mar. 2) 1972.

physiologically and psychologically both infant and mother are optimally disposed to begin attachment within the first hour after birth. Therefore, since only extremely rare circumstances necessitate separation, it should be avoided in order to facilitate the development of the parent–infant bond.

Immediately after birth and for about one hour thereafter the infant is in a quiet alert state. (See Chapter 18, page 492.) During this time his eyes are open and he looks around. This is the ideal time for the parents to begin eye-to-eye contact. For this reason, it is recommended that the instillation of silver nitrate drops be postponed until after the parents have spent some time with their infant. While he remains in this first period of reactivity, the infant will often suck well at the breast. This provides him with valuable colostrum and provides his mother with the satisfaction of being a success at her first breast-feeding attempt. In addition, the sucking stimulates oxytocin production in the mother which promotes uterine contraction and minimizes bleeding. Early stimulation of the breast may also prevent, or at least minimize, engorgement.

When the nurse takes the infant to his parents for the first time it is usually wise to spend a few minutes with them inspecting the baby together. The nurse should unwrap the baby and point out the physical characteristics of the newborn which could concern parents who have not had experience with such a young infant. Molding of the head, for example, can look very alarming to the unfamiliar observer. Parents often have questions about the appearance of the genitalia and the umbilical cord. By pointing out forceps marks, caput succedaneum, or fetal electrode marks, as well as the normal variations in the newborn's appearance, parents are reassured that the nurse is aware of these things and judges them to be normal (Fig. 20-6).

After checking over their baby with the nurse most parents appreciate some privacy to be alone with each other and with their baby.

Throughout the hospitalization both parents should have free access to their baby. Hospital

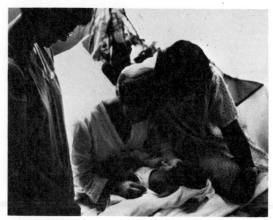

Figure 20-6. Nurse examining baby with parents.

policies should enable the mother to keep her baby with her as much as she wishes and yet be comfortable sending him back to the nursery if she feels the need for a break. It is important to remember that each mother and father will proceed at his or her own pace in developing a relationship with the infant. The nurse should provide support and opportunity for attachment to occur but should not push.

There are a number of ways the nurse can encourage attachment as she cares for the postpartum family. Several suggestions are as follows:

1. Write the baby's first name on the crib identification card and use it when talking to or about him.
2. Serve as a role model for the parents. If they see a nurse cuddling and rocking a baby in the nursery or talking to him or stroking him to quiet him, they will recognize that these are important ways of caring for an infant. The nurse should, however, be cautious not to appear so expert in her handling of the infant that the parent feels she/he can never do as well.
3. Point out the baby's behaviors and help parents to interpret them. For example, some infants prefer to be held up on the shoulder so they can look around, others like to be cradled in the arms. Some infants are able to console themselves quite readily

and are content to look around and "entertain" themselves. Snug swaddling comforts some babies and puts them right to sleep; others fight the confining blankets. Most babies stir and make noises or even cry out briefly in their sleep and then settle themselves again several times before finally waking up all the way for feeding. Learning to wait for the "real" waking up saves the frustration of trying to feed a drowsy baby.

4. Problem-solve with the parents about meeting babies needs. For example, interpreting the meaning of a baby's cry is one of the major concerns of most new parents. Talking together about ways they can distinguish among cries of hunger, discomfort, anger, illness, or just self-expression allows parents to check the validity of their own ideas as well as to obtain suggestions from the nurse.

5. Allow both parents to give as much care to their infant as they wish. Teach skills they are unfamiliar with and provide opportunity for them to practice in a supportive environment. Be sincere in praising them for their progress. The nurse should keep in mind that there is no one best way to do most things. The way the mother does it is likely to be just as good as the standard hospital practice. Incidentally, mothers often need to be reminded of this regarding fathers. Many women discourage men from caring for babies because they "don't do it the way I do."

6. Be accepting of parents' emotions, the negative ones as well as the positive ones. The freedom to let off steam, cry, and feel discouraged without fear of condemnation is important for mental health.

The Father

Many times the father is the most forgotten member of the childbearing family. Unlike the mother and infant, he does not have pressing physical needs which necessitate contact with the traditional system of delivering obstetric care. He is stereotyped as a chain-smoking floor pacer who is quite out of place in a woman's world of birth and babies. Paying the bills has been seen as his chief contribution to the family. More recently he has been given the task of supporting the mother. Fathers are permitted in delivery rooms if the mother is awake and he is prepared to support her; they are encouraged to attend antepartum classes to help the mother. Little attention has been paid to meeting his own needs which arise from the role change to fatherhood.

Interest in the role of the father in the family and in relation to his children has flourished in the past decade, yet much remains to be learned.

Like a woman, a man's adaptation to parenthood depends in large measure on his experiences in his family as he was growing up and on the cutlural expectations or norms for fathers in his society. In the United States at this time the trend appears to be toward an increasing involvement of fathers in pregnancy and in infant care. As more mothers enter the labor force many fathers are assuming a greater share in the day-to-day responsibilities of child rearing. Nevertheless, the nurse should keep in mind that families vary widely in the ways they divide up the tasks of daily living. Assessment of the family interaction is important in determining how each member of the couple is adapting. If the man believes babies are women's work and the mother agrees, all is likely to go well. If the father wants to take a more active role in infant care but the mother is reluctant to give up any of her time with the baby, conflict may occur. Nursing care should be directed at providing the opportunity for both parents to begin parenting with the experts available as consultants. Often communication and role negotiation by the couple can be facilitated by discussing infant care with the nurse. When serious conflicts arise or the nurse feels unable to help, appropriate referrals should be made.

Many men feel isolated from their wives and infants for the first several months post partum. One father described himself as "the fifth wheel in the group." The mother spends much of her time with the infant, and, particularly if she is breast feeding, has a relationship with the infant that may seem to exclude the father. She may be temporarily less interested in issues and activities outside the family and thus be a less interesting conversationalist. Sexual relationships may suffer due to tender episiotomy, fatigue, and night feedings. Mothers should be helped to understand the man's need for her love and support and for some time alone with her without any children.

Sibling Rivalry

Any right-minded preschooler would have to agree with the cartoon concept that a baby isn't nearly so much fun as a puppy. Baby brothers, or even baby sisters, can't do any good tricks. All they do is eat, sleep, cry, and mess their pants. When it comes to playing, they are a total loss. On top of that, they take up enormous amounts of mommy's time that she could otherwise spend much more profitably reading stories or playing ball. On the other hand, few children can resist a baby clinging to their finger. They don't know about grasp reflexes. To them the baby is saying "I like you," because he wants to hold hands. And holding a baby and putting a cheek next to his soft, fuzzy hair is even better than hugging a teddy bear.

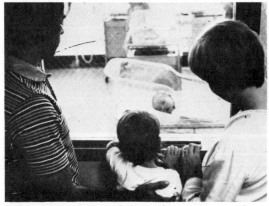

Figure 20-7. Parents helping their two-year-old get acquainted with his new sister.

Children, like their parents, need time to get acquainted with and become attached to the new member of the family. During pregnancy they should share the anticipation and preparation. By helping to put the baby clothes in the drawer and growing accustomed to the empty waiting crib they begin to feel a pleasant expectation. Doll play and talking about what it will be like to have a baby in the house are ways of rehearsing behavior before the actual event happens. After the baby arrives, children enjoy touching, watching, and helping care for him. They also like to look at their own baby pictures to see if there is a resemblance to the new baby and to hear about what they were like when they were babies. Even very young children can be helped to observe the way the baby changes as he grows from day to day. They will soon come to applaud the new accomplishments of their baby in the same way their own accomplishments are applauded by others.

The resentment children feel toward new babies is created by their perceived loss of their valued position in the family. They are outraged at their mother for abandoning them to go to the hospital. When the family is reunited, some children exhibit their anger and frustration by having temper tantrums, regressing in toilet habits, refusing to follow bedtime routines, or any one of a number of disruptive behaviors. It is not uncommon for young children to ignore their mothers upon reunion, refusing to kiss her hello or even sit on her lap, retreating instead to Grandma or the babysitter. For mothers who have spent several days in the hospital very lonesome for their two-year-old, this can be a painful experience.

Helping parents understand normal child behavior and plan ahead for coping with it can do a great deal to minimize the stress for the whole family. It is important for parents to demonstrate to a child that he is still as loved as always and is still very special to them. It is usually necessary, especially with preschool-age children, to plan particular times to do things just with them.

Parents often need help dealing with problem

behaviors during this time. Understanding the reason why a child is having tantrums or refusing to go to bed does not make it any eaiser to live with those behaviors. Neither does it mean parents should indulge the child. They must continue patiently to guide and teach him just as before the baby came. Just as a child must learn that he is no less loved and important because of the baby, he must also learn to share with his brother or sister. While love may be infinite and indivisible, parents' time and energy is not; toys are not; bedrooms are not. Learning to share is a hard but necessary part of growing up.

All children, regardless of age, experience some jealousy or sibling rivalry when a new baby joins the family. This is part of the role realignment that occurs throughout the family system in order to accommodate a new member. Changes are most marked, however, in a first-born when a second child is born and in the "old baby" of the family when a third or subsequent baby is born.

When Something is "Wrong" With the Baby

Whenever any baby is born the parents must resolve their loss of their fantasied, ideal child and form an attachment to the real child. The greater the discrepancy between the reality and the fantasy, the more difficult this task becomes. Anticipatory teaching during pregnancy can do much to help parents appreciate the appearance and behaviors of newborns, so their expectations are reasonably close to the reality of their own infant. In most cases, when a healthy infant is born, disappointments over sex and general appearance are readily overcome. However, when the infant is premature, sick, has an anomaly, or dies, the family suffers severe grief and is in a state of crisis for a period of time.

Different theorists have described various stages which individual families go through in response to a crisis. Initially there is a period of disorganization during which the usual patterns of behavior are inadequate to cope. There is shock and disbelief that such a thing could have happened. Feelings of guilt, anger, and intense

sorrow are common. During this time, a number of physical symptoms occur. There is a constricted, heavy feeling in the throat and chest; sighing and yawning are frequent due to a shortness of breath. There are feelings of exhaustion, emptiness, and unreality. Crying is frequent.

The second stage is one of relative equilibrium. This is a time of information-seeking and resource utilization. Anxiety is somewhat lessened and some problem solving can begin with help. A stage of mobilization or action follows in which the individual or family works out new behavior patterns to resolve the crisis. Finally, there is reorganization. Ideally there will have been growth as a result of mastering the crisis so that the individual or family will emerge stronger and more mature. The stages of the crisis do not follow each other in a discrete sequence. There is considerable overlapping and often a person will move back and forth through several stages during a single day. Thus, information seeking may be accompanied by anger and sorrow and then a period of disbelief or denial may follow.

The progress of families through crises may be modified by whether the event was expected or unexpected. Anticipated crises can be prepared for in advance and the impact can often be softened. Events which originate or are caused by factors external to the family are generally less stressful, presumably because the burden of guilt is lessened. Intact families, characterized by common goals, mutual love and respect, and flexibility of roles, have more resources available to deal with stress and crisis. Similarly, families with strong kinship ties to an extended family generally fare better than isolated nuclear families. In addition, the way the family perceives the situation will influence its response and the ease with which it will be able to accept and cope with the crisis event. Finally, timely intervention by caring professionals can do much to facilitate the development of new coping strategies and the satisfactory resolution of the crisis situation.

The care of parents during a crisis with their

newborn is very similar regardless of the nature of the newborn's problems. However, in order to highlight some of the differences, care is discussed separately for premature and/or sick infants, infants with anomalies, and infants who die. For a more complete discussion of this important topic the reader is referred to the book *Maternal–Infant Bonding* by Marshall Klaus and John Kennel.

Premature or Sick Infants

The birth of a premature infant can always be anticipated, at least for the duration of the mother's labor. In many cases, neonatal illness can also be predicted, as in the case of an Rh-sensitized fetus, an infant of a diabetic mother, or a fetus with intrauterine growth retardation or an abnormal fetal heart rate pattern. Thus parents' concern for their infant precedes birth. Fearing the infant will die, parents may attempt to shield themselves from the pain of loss by remaining aloof from the infant. Anticipatory grief is common and may inhibit attachment to the infant even after the parents realize that their infant is going to get well.

Not only do parents themselves sometimes remain psychologically distant from their newborn, but the medical care system frequently imposes a physical separation of parents and newborn. As specialized, highly skilled, technical care is organized into regional centers it becomes increasingly likely that the newborn will be given optimal care in a center some distance from the parents' home. To the extent that the birth of such infants can be predicted, their mothers should go to the center for delivery. This at least prevents complete separation of the mother and infant for the first several days of life. It is inevitable, however, that parents will have less contact with their premature or sick infant than they would have were the infant full-term and healthy. Thus it is a major responsibility of professionals who work in intensive care nurseries to help parents form realistic expectations of their infant's prognosis and to foster the early development of parent–infant attachment.

Both parents should see their infant as soon as possible even if only for a few seconds. If the mother is awake during delivery and the father is present, then they will, of course, see the infant at birth. Should the mother be anesthetized, the father may see the infant before she recovers from the anesthesia. Even a brief glimpse of the infant helps them to grasp the reality of the situation and often dispels fantasies about the infant's appearance that may be much more frightening than the actual situation. For example, one mother was surprised to see that her 32-week daughter was a complete, if miniature, baby. She had believed that, since she was premature, she was "unfinished" and would be missing some parts of her body.

If it becomes necessary to transfer the infant to a different hospital for care, it is preferable to transfer the mother as well, unless she is nearly ready for discharge. If she is not to be transferred, it is essential that she see and touch her infant before he leaves. The transport team from the intensive care nursery should take a few minutes to give her and the father some information about the nursery. This should be followed up with telephone communication on a regular basis until the mother is able to come to the nursery. The father will frequently accompany the infant to the new hospital.

From the very beginning parents should be encouraged to visit, touch, and care for their infant as much as they are able. Before they go into an intensive care nursery for the first time it is usually wise for the nurse or physician to explain a little of what they will see. The technical apparatus can be overwhelming even if their own infant is not gravely ill. It is usual for parents to be hesitant to touch a very small or sick infant, particularly if he is in an isolette and/or attached to various tubes and machines. Several visits may be required before some parents begin to touch their infant. It is important that this behavior be accepted without pushing the parents. (See Figure 20-8.)

Discussions with the parents about the infant's prognosis should always be optimistic without giving false hope. They should be

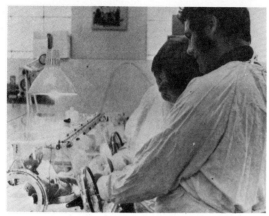

Figure 20-8. These parents are continuing the process of getting to know their premature son by touching him and participating in his tube feedings and other care. They quickly feel he belongs to them and not to the nursery.

helped to realize that, although the infant requires special care for a time, this will not always be the case. As soon as he is well or as soon as he is older he can be treated like any healthy child. Of major help to parents is the identification of one nurse and one physician with whom they can relate during the entire hospitalization. This facilitates the development of a trusting relationship and permits consistency and continuity of care.

When a prolonged hospitalization is required parents are not always able to visit daily. They may live some distance from the hospital, have other children, and so on. Daily telephone communication should be maintained, however. Not only medical progress but also individual behavior and growth and development should be described to the parents. The nurse should remember that in addition to the stress of a sick infant, the parents are coping with all of the other processes of the puerperium, plus family separation, financial stress, and perhaps many other factors. Attention should be paid to their rest and nutrition as well as to their feelings. They should be encouraged to talk and help each other, and appropriate social service referrals should be made whenever indicated.

Prior to discharge, plans should be made for the parents to spend an extended period of time with the baby, becoming familiar with his case. Some hospitals have facilities for parents to live in for as long as necessary to become comfortable with their baby while consultants are readily available. Referral to community agencies are important to provide some assistance during the first several months at home.

Infants with Anomalies

It is paradoxical that, although virtually every pregnant woman worries that something will be wrong with her baby, when an anomaly does occur a common response is "I didn't think it could ever happen to me." The realization that their child is not perfect produces sorrow in all parents. The intensity of their response tends to be influenced by several factors in addition to their own personalities and backgrounds. Among these factors are

1. Whether or not the defect is apparent from looking at the child (e.g., a cleft lip versus an internal, "invisible" anomaly)
2. The extent to which the defect can be corrected, if it can be corrected at all
3. Whether or not there is neurologic involvement; that is, to what extent will the child's growth and development and intelligence be impaired
4. Life expectancy of the child

In general, malformations which require long-term adaptations, especially if they include life-long dependency on the parents, are the most difficult to accept. Defects of the head and face tend to produce stronger reactions than those of other parts of the body.

Early parent–infant contact is important when a baby is born with an anomaly just as it always is with a normal baby. Several studies have shown that parents report feeling better once they have seen their infant. They almost invariably say that the infant looks better than they had imagined. Once the parents feel they are ready to see their baby and then do so, a turning point seems to be reached in their crisis. The longer the contact is delayed the greater the risk for maladaptive parenting. A case report will illustrate some of the tragedies that can occur.

Mrs. R's second daughter was born early in the morning in a small community hospital with a severe bilateral cleft lip and palate. Although it was a normal vaginal delivery, she had general anesthesia. When she awoke and asked about her baby the nurses evaded her questions. She was heavily sedated. Her husband was not permitted to visit and she believed her baby to be dead. In the evening her physician told her of the cleft lip but encouraged her not to see the baby until after surgery. Although she asked to see the baby several times she was not permitted to do so. The baby was concealed behind a screen in the small nursery. One nurse told Mrs. R., "You don't want to see her. She's such an ugly little thing it would only make you cry." Interestingly, the father was permitted to see the baby. Perhaps he was considered "stronger" and better able to "take it."

On the second postpartum day the infant was transferred to a university medical center about six hours drive from the parents' home. On the day of her first lip surgery, ten days later, Mrs. R. first visited her. She was directed to a pediatric ward containing eight infants in identical cribs. She later described her feelings as she entered the ward: "I stopped in the door and just looked around. I suddenly realized that my very own baby was in that room and I couldn't even recognize her because I had no idea what she looked like. I wondered if I could ever be a mother to her."

That child at ten years old is a very pretty little girl due to an unusually fine plastic repair. She is very bright and has no speech difficulties. Her mother refers to her as a tomboy who is "daddy's girl." In sharp contrast to her two sisters, she has always been encouraged to enter into her father's interests and activities. While her sisters take ballet lessons, she plays on the softball team. Although by no means an abused or disadvantaged child, she is obviously regarded as "different" by her mother.

Although the goal of crisis intervention is to help families achieve resolution, for some congenital malformations there can only be partial resolution because the parents are continually reminded of their misfortune by the presence of the child in the home. As the child grows they are constantly faced with new challenges resulting from the malformation. The care of the newborn may be relatively easy compared to the needs of the child for mobility, education, social contacts, sexuality, and so on. These parents have been described by Olshansky as having "chronic sorrow."[9]

Parents Whose Infants Die

The death of a newborn introduces severe conflict. Birth is supposed to be an optimistic, joyful occasion, but now loss and sorrow have occurred. Nurses and physicians who choose perinatal practice are often unaccustomed to dealing with death and feel uncomfortable and inadequate to help. There is a temptation to gloss over the parents grief with such statements as "It was probably for the best" or "You are lucky to have two healthy children at home." Mothers are often transferred from the maternity unit so other babies won't remind them of their loss and so they won't remind the staff.

These and other efforts to "protect" the parents from the impact of their loss are not beneficial, since they discourage the healthy expression of grief. Rather, parents should be helped to face the reality of the infant's death and to support each other in mourning. They need to cry, to express their anger and frustrations, and to talk about the baby and what has happened. Grieving for a dead infant is no different than grieving for the loss of any other loved person.

Parents should be offered an opportunity to see their baby after death, especially if the baby was stillborn or died before the parents could see him. Although this is a painful experience, it promotes healthy resolution of loss by making the death real. Religious and cultural traditions also play an important role in comforting the grieving parents.

Often the death of an infant is the couple's

[9] S. Olshansky, Chronic sorrow: A response to having a mentally defective child, *Soc. Casework* 43:190–193, 1962.

first close experience with death. Even if a parent or other close relative has died, this is very likely to be the first time they have had to make decisions about funerals, burial versus hospital disposal, autopsies, and so on. Therefore, in addition to psychologic support and comforting, they need some very practical information about their options, expenses involved, local laws that pertain, and so on.

Follow-up care of parents whose infant has died is important. Several weeks after the death parents may have many questions that did not occur to them during the disorganized time surrounding the death. This is often an appropriate time to review autopsy findings and to anticipate the need for any genetic counseling. It also permits an evaluation of the parents' progression through the grieving process. Other visits may be scheduled depending on the parents' needs. They should be aware that it is not uncommon for the grieving process to last for six to nine months or even a year. They should be encouraged to ask for help whenever they feel the need. Professionals giving primary health care should be aware of the death and incorporate into the client's care plan a means of facilitating grief work.

PREPARATION FOR DISCHARGE FROM THE HOSPITAL

Planning for going home with the baby is begun well before delivery with the acquisition of a crib and preparation of the room. Nursing care during the antepartum period includes helping parents anticipate their needs for the time immediately after birth. Nevertheless, once the baby is born it is necessary to review these plans and make necessary modifications. The nurse who is responsible for postpartum care should help the parents

1. Evaluate their need for household help and determine how best to meet this need
2. Learn necessary infant care skills
3. Arrange for continued health supervision for both mother and infant

4. Anticipate some of the changes which will occur in their lives during the first three months at home
5. Learn about resources available to new parents in their community

Household Help

The need for household help during the first week or two after delivery is largely a matter of personal preference. A mother who has been ill, had a cesarean section, or is being discharged within a few hours of delivery may have less energy. Many families have a tradition of grandmothers coming to stay and help after a baby is born. Some couples prefer to have this time alone with their baby. It is becoming more acceptable for a father to get leave from his job or take vacation time when his new baby comes home.

If someone will be coming to help, the mother should give some thought to the division of labor. Generally it is best for the mother to care for her baby while the helper takes care of meals, laundry, and cleaning.

When the parents plan to manage without help, it is wise for them to decide what can satisfactorily be left undone and/or what short cuts can be used. For example, they may consider diaper service or disposable diapers for a while to reduce the laundry and make use of convenience foods for some of their meals.

Teaching Infant Care Skills

The more infant care that the parents can perform in the hospital with the nurse available as a consultant, the more they have an opportunity to learn about their baby. In addition to learning how to hold, bathe, and dress their baby, procedures that seem complicated and sometimes cause anxiety, there is much more for parents to learn about the baby's care which is equally, or more, valuable. For example, they must learn to determine the meaning of the baby's cry, signs of hunger and satiety, methods of feeding and bubbling, number and type of stools considered normal; normalcy of regurgitation, sneezing, and hiccuping; methods of turning and positioning; and the value of cuddling and rocking the baby.

Parents need help in learning to care for their baby from a nurse who can put them at ease and give them a feeling of self-assurance. It takes time for an inexperienced parent to develop skills. Encouragement that they are doing well and that they can meet their baby's needs will help them to feel at ease and gain confidence in their ability. To gain skill and confidence the parents need help with the baby's physical care and opportunities to make their own decisions regarding his needs. When they have been helped to find their own answers to questions and have been reassured that their judgment is good, they will be able to meet problems at home more easily.

Parent teaching may be both incidental and planned. Incidental teaching consists of explaining something "on the spot" in response to a specific question or situation. Planned teaching may be more formal. It is scheduled discussion of a particular topic, which may include a demonstration of a skill or a film. Teaching may be done on a one-to-one basis or with a group of parents. Individual teaching has the advantage of addressing the parents' particular needs and concerns in a manner tailored to their level of learning. It may encourage them to raise issues or ask questions which they would hesitate to do in a group. Group teaching is more economical and has the advantage of being able to use the experiences of many people. Parents may learn as much from each other as from the nurse. In addition, they realize that they have fears and questions not unlike those of others.

Readiness to Learn

Regardless of whether teaching is incidental or planned, individual or in a group, the nurse must make an assessment of the parents' readiness to learn. Unless the information has significance for them they will be unlikely to hear and remember what is being taught. It is often necessary to meet other needs of the parents before

they will have the energy to attend to teaching about infant care. When a mother is physically uncomfortable or the couple has urgent concerns about financial affairs, they are likely to be distracted from instruction. Similarly, discussing the baby's bath while the mother is acutely anxious about getting her baby to suck well at breast will not be beneficial.

Level of Learning

The instruction itself should be adjusted to the individual ability of the learner. Care must be taken to use vocabulary that is understandable to the client and to proceed at a pace which allows for thorough comprehension. Repetition may be necessary from time to time. The method of instruction should also be considered. While some parents will learn readily from reading printed directions, others will need a verbal explanation, and still others will need to be shown how. Different topics may require different methods of instruction even for the same parents.

Evaluation

The nurse should be continually evaluating the amount of learning that is taking place. Asking the parents to repeat information back to the nurse is one way of ascertaining their understanding. Providing opportunities for return demonstrations of such manual skills as bathing or diapering is also a valuable means of evaluation.

Although it is by no means exhaustive, the following list contains many of the items of infant care commonly taught to parents.

1. *Feeding.* Holding the bottle so that air does not get into the nipple. Cleaning bottles and making formula. Positioning the baby for breast feeding. Care of sore nipples. How to break the baby's suction on the breast. How to tell if the baby is getting enough to eat (Chapter 19).
2. *Bubbling or burping.* How often and in what position?
3. *Diapers.* Always keep safety pins closed and out of baby's reach. Disposable

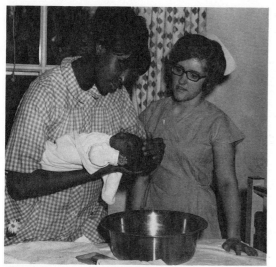

Figure 20-9. The new mother is given an opportunity to give her baby a bath, with the nurse's help and guidance. Holding the baby on her arm and his buttocks securely between her hip and elbow, the mother can support the baby's head with one hand while she washes it with the other.

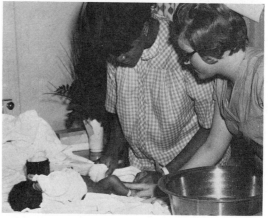

Figure 20-10. Mothers need an opportunity to practice infant care skills with the nurse available as a consultant.

diapers are more expensive but more convenient, especially for trips to grandma's house or pediatric office visits.

4. *Diaper rash.* Frequent change of diapers helps. Bottom should be washed off at each diaper change to remove irritants. Petroleum jelly (Vaseline) or vegetable shortening will protect the skin from moisture of urine. Fair-skinned babies may develop a rash from time to time even with the most conscientious care. Exposing the bottom to air is helpful as are several commercial ointments. Changing laundry soaps may also help sometimes.

5. *Bathing.* Although the bath demonstration is an honored ritual on many postpartum units, mothers will usually not have difficulty bathing their babies if they are taught how to hold them securely and are given an opportunity to practice with supervision. They should practice with equipment similar to that available in their homes, namely, a bar of soap, washcloth, towel, and basin or sink. The plastic bath basins many hospitals use for adult patients make fine baby bathtubs for the first month or two. The kitchen sink is often the ideal place to bathe a baby, since it is a height that avoids bending and usually has a cabinet top next to it to lay the baby on to dry and dress. Until babies can sit alone, it is usually easier to wash them off as they lay on a towel and then lower them into the water for rinsing and playing. A bath need not be given daily but should be an enjoyable time for both parents and baby.

6. *Lotions and powders.* Not essential but enjoyable. Lotions should be mild and nonirritating. Rubbing them in over the baby's body provides pleasurable tactile stimulation. When using powder, care should be taken not to shake it freely over the baby so that he does not inhale the dust. It is best to shake some into the parent's hand and then smooth it onto the baby's skin, taking care to avoid accumulation in folds of skin where it will become moist, cake, and produce irritation. Powder is especially refreshing in warm weather. Cornstarch is an inexpensive alternative for powder.

7. *Umbilical cord.* Falls off in a week to ten days. Alcohol applied at the base of the cord will promote its drying. After the cord drops off the mother may note a few drops of blood on the baby's clothes or bed covers for a day or so. The healing navel can be cleansed with alcohol. A protuberant naval may be indicative of an umbilical hernia. This benign condition will correct itself as the baby grows and the abdominal muscles strengthen.

8. *Pacifiers.* Very useful in meeting the nonnutritive sucking needs of many babies. Can usually be discontinued about four to six months of age as baby gains more interests and has less need for sucking.

9. *Sleeping.* Babies usually sleep through the night by the time they are two or three months old. Parents can help minimize their own loss of sleep by teaching their baby that eating during the night is different from daytime eating. During the night the baby should be allowed to wake up completely before beginning to nurse. He should be fed with a minimum of talking and handling and put immediately back to bed. Most babies will quickly learn to go right back to sleep, particularly if the day feeding is accompanied by cuddling, talking, and playing, and he spends time awake when not eating.

10. *Illness.* Because babies cannot complain of being ill in words, parents are concerned that they will not be able to tell when their baby is sick and should be seen by a physician. The most frequent symptoms of newborn illness are listlessness, loss of appetite, and diarrhea. The parents should know how to take the baby's temperature and should be encouraged to call the nurse or physician if they have any doubts about their baby's health.

11. *Taking baby outside.* It is desirable to take a baby outside from time to time to permit him some exposure to fresh air and sunshine as well as to give parents an oppor-

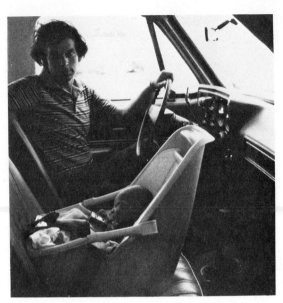

Figure 20-11. Baby snuggled safely in her car seat for the trip home from the hospital.

tunity to go out. Care should be taken that the baby is suitably dressed for the weather. In general he will be comfortable if dressed comparably to the parents. In warm weather protection against sunburn should be assured.

When traveling in a car the baby should be secured in a car seat which is fastened in place by the seat belts. The safest child restraint devices are those which have been crashed tested. Most new models on the market since July 1, 1975, have been crash tested. However, some parents who may receive hand-me-downs or purchase items at garage sales should be cautious. Safety information is available in *Consumer Reports* at the public library as well as from the National Safety Council and some state health agencies.

Continued Health Supervision

Before leaving the hospital the mother should be instructed about making an appointment for a postpartum follow-up visit to her physician. The first medical postpartum checkup after discharge is usually made in approximately six weeks, at about the time the pelvic organs have returned to their normal condition. It includes examination of the breasts and pelvic examination to determine the condition of the perineum, uterus, cervix, and support to the rectum and the bladder. Blood pressure, weight, urinalysis, and sometimes a complete blood count are also included. Attention is also given to the mother's emotional adjustments.

A slight abnormality detected at the six weeks examination can usually be corrected with little difficulty, but if it persists it may result in a more serious problem. If subinvolution, inadequate perineal healing, or uterine displacement is found, treatment can be started. If the cervix is red and eroded, a cauterization may be necessary. All cervical lesions receive careful treatment to prevent predisposition to gynecologic problems later.

The six weeks examination completes the postpartum period, and it is also the beginning of a new period of health supervision. A pelvic examination is usually repeated after six months and one year. Adequate postpartum care over a period of a year may prevent or cure conditions that would otherwise cause trouble in later years.

The first health supervision visit for the infant is generally made at about one month of age. It will include a physical examination and a discussion of infant care and behavior.

If a visiting nurse service is available to the mother, she is referred for a follow-up visit for herself and her baby if she desires. When a referral is not made, the mother is told of the visiting nurse service and how to secure this service should she need assistance.

Anticipation of the First Three Months

It is impossible to predict how life will change for a given family as they mature as parents of a growing infant. Many families have similar experiences, however, and talking about these with new parents often helps them plan ways to help themselves.

Most mothers find the first months with a new baby to be very emotional ones. Mood swings are not unusual. The responsibilities of caring for a new baby occasionally seem overwhelming. Even if it is not her first baby she may become frantic that she can't meet everyone's needs. Mothers should be warned that there will be times when they yearn to be childless again and hate the baby for robbing them of their freedom. Unless a woman realizes the normality of this feeling she may be frightened and will certainly feel guilty and charge herself with being a bad mother. The relationship between the parents can also be strained during this time, particularly if their relationship was not a strong one to begin with.

To help parents begin problem solving so that this time becomes a happy period for maturation as parents and as individuals, the nurse may discuss some of the following things with them.

Organization of Time

The baby will take up quite a bit of time. In addition to the direct care of feeding, bathing, and so on, there will be more laundry and other things. At least for the first month the mother will require extra rest because of easy fatigability. Her husband and other children will also make demands on her time. If her mental health is to be maintained, she will need some time to herself to read a book or sew, work with her plants, or get out of the house for socialization.

Meeting all these needs will require some reordering of priorities. Some things will have to be left undone or done less frequently in order to make time for those things judged most important. A reliable babysitter can be an important asset. Some families can afford help to do housework or may have a willing friend or relative. Fathers are often willing to perform household chores in order to have some time for individual attention from their wives.

Sexuality

This is a frequent area of conflict between couples. Sexual gratification is often postponed during the last weeks of pregnancy. Now when the man desires intercourse the woman may be tired and her perineum may be tender from the episiotomy and/or hemorrhoids. Intercourse may also be painful because of lack of estrogen-induced vaginal lubrication, especially if she is breast feeding.

Women may be confused and embarrassed to find themselves sexually aroused by breast feeding. At the same time sexual stimulation will result in milk leaking from the breast.

If the couple can talk to each other about their feelings and frustrations, they can usually solve their problems satisfactorily. Gentleness, time, and some water-soluble lubricant will resolve the perineal discomfort. Mutual love and a sense of humor will help much of the rest.

Couples should be aware that conception can occur even while the woman is lactating. (See discussion of family planning below.)

Enjoying the Baby

In their zeal to prepare parents realistically for the frustrations of parenthood, professionals often forget to emphasize how enjoyable babies can be. They feel good when you hold them, they are cute to look at, and they grow in marvelous, fascinating ways. They are very tolerant of inexperienced parents, since they have never had parents before just as their parents have never had a baby before. Nurses should strive to increase the new parents' self-confidence to the point where they can relax and have fun with their baby.

Community Resources

Parents should be made aware of the community resources available to them. A directory listing the agencies, any eligibility requirements, and the services they offer would be a valuable service the hospital could provide postpartum patients.

In addition to professional health and counseling agencies, many communities have organized lay groups. Groups of parents with similar interests meet together to help each other. Examples of such groups include the LaLeche League for breast-feeding mothers; and groups for women who have had (or are going to have) cesarean sections, parents of twins, postpartum couples, parents of toddlers, and so on. These mutual support groups are also valuable for parents whose infant is in an intensive care nursery or who has an anomaly. Some groups, like those for parents of children with PKU or spina bifida, are organized on the national level and offer a variety of services to families.

FAMILY PLANNING

It is apropos to discuss the topic of family planning at this time, since it is frequently an area of interest for couples who have just had a baby. New parents should be aware that a woman may become pregnant any time she has unprotected intercourse after delivery, even if she is breast feeding. If they wish to postpone or prevent another pregnancy it is important to give some consideration to the choice of a method of conception control.

The terms "contraception," "birth control," and "family planning" are used interchangeably. Generally speaking, family planning has the broadest connotation; inherent in the phrase is consideration of the physical, social, psychological, economic, and theological factors which affect the family and influence decisions relative to planning for children and utilization of the various contraceptive methods. Contraception, in general usage, refers more specifically to the temporary prevention of pregnancy and gives rise to the terminology of contraceptive methods which are used in order to accomplish this temporary prevention. The term "birth control" has been attributed to Margaret Sanger, a nurse, who in the 1910's began a historical fight for the right of families to limit their size, the right of women to health, and the right of children to the love they may expect through being wanted, planned-for children.

Before any individual or couple uses any method of contraception two decisions must be made: first, a decision to use some form of family planning to prevent or postpone conception, and second, the choice of the method that is most acceptable and workable for the particular individuals concerned. Unless both of these decisions are made freely and with clear understanding of all the implications, the effectiveness of any method will be compromised. Health professionals, therefore, have the obligation to present information about all of the various methods in a manner that can be understood by each client. Attempts to influence the client's decision based on the nurse's or physician's own values are never appropriate.

Among the factors which are likely to influence the decision to use contraception are the following:

Sociocultural: Current trends in family size; effect of the size of the family in which the individuals grew up; stress of a society upon the importance of children; stress any particular society or culture places upon the importance of having a male child to perpetuate the family name; belief of a direct correlation between number of children and proof of virility.

Occupational–economic: The possibility of lengthy separation until the husband's military obligations have been met; economic resources being channeled into the couple's completion of schooling; priority placed on establishing a career; economic ability to provide prospective children with food, clothing, shelter, medical and dental care, and future education.

Religious: All major religious bodies endorse the basic concept of family planning.

Physical: General health of both partners but especially the woman; existence of genetic disorders in the family.

Marital–psychologic: Stability of the couple's relationship; beliefs about the effect of children on marital happiness.

Having arrived at the decision to utilize family planning, still other factors influence the selection of a particular method. In general these

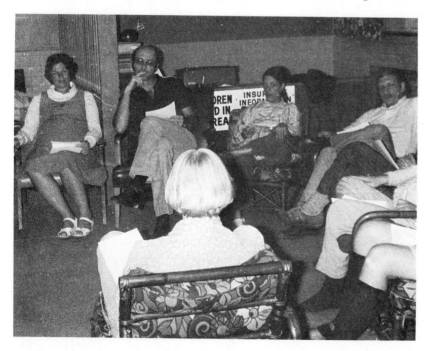

Figure 20-12. Photograph of parents' discussion group.

factors reduce to the acceptability of the method to the individuals involved. Variables which contribute to the acceptability of a method include its cost, its effectiveness, and the ease of using it. Previous experience with a method as well as the extent to which it is used by friends or other members of the family will also have an impact. Women who are hesitant to touch their genitalia will not be likely to choose a method which requires such manipulation for its use. Those who object to "unnatural" drugs or devices will eliminate still other methods from their consideration. The frequency of sexual intercourse may also be a deciding factor. Someone who anticipates infrequent coitus may elect a more episodic means of conception control than those who have an ongoing sexual relationship. In some cases religious affiliation may limit the acceptable ways of avoiding pregnancy. Publicity in the popular press concerning possible side effects and questions of safety may influence many decisions. Furthermore, there are medical contraindications for a number of methods which may preclude their consideration by certain couples. As an example, women with hypertension or a history of thromboembolic disease should not use oral contraceptives.

Because of the multiplicity of the variables involved in decision making it should be clear that "selling" someone a particular method is likely to result in reduced effectiveness in the long run. Even though the professional may feel the client's objections to a method to be irrational, the decision must be made independently by the person who is going to use the method.

Effectiveness of a Contraceptive Method

Failure in a contraceptive method is usually due to either defects in the method itself, human error of the individuals using the method, or a combination of the two. Possible method defects will be noted in the discussion of the specific contraceptive methods. The dominating factor in human error is the strength of a couple's motivation to prevent a pregnancy. Motivation directly affects the degree of regularity with which the contraceptive is used. Without consistent use any method will fail; irregular use of a method constitutes a major reason for contraceptive failure due to human error. Influences of human error, such as the couple's degree of acceptance of the procedure involved may be counterbalanced by their motivation. The other major reason for failure of a contraceptive method due to human error is the improper handling of the technique involved. This may result from an inadequate knowledge of reproductive anatomy and physiology, inaccurate understanding of the method itself and how it works, or an inability to master the skills required by the technique.

While frequently stated in terms of percentages, it is customary to calculate the clinical effectiveness (use effectiveness) of a contraceptive method according to the pregnancy rate per 100 years of exposure. This is done by means of a formula developed in the early 1930s by Raymond Pearl. After having one child, couples not using a contraceptive method average an approximate pregnancy rate of 80 per 100 years of exposure. The effectiveness of a contraceptive method is considered to be high if the pregnancy rate is below 10 per 100 years of exposure; moderate if between 10 and 20; and low if more than 20.

Contraceptive Methods

Since time immemorial people have tried to prevent conception. A wide variety of instruments have been used, ranging from potions, magic, tampons, and penal sheaths of various materials such as handkerchiefs and Saran wrap, to coins, collar buttons, stones, bottle caps, jewelry, carbonated beverages in a bottle released under pressure, or anything else a person thinks will prohibit the spermatozoa from reaching the ovum if it is inserted into the vagina or uterus. This can lead to tragic results such as mutilation or sterility due to infection. It is important to be aware that such dangerous nonmedical and futile attempts are still being made so that efforts may be directed toward finding and guiding such individuals to medical help.

Natural Family Planning

Natural family planning methods, sometimes referred to as *fertility awareness,* are based on the principle that women are fertile only on certain days during the menstrual cycle. These days, which surround the time of ovulation, are known as the *fertile period,* or the *unsafe period,* depending on whether the perspective is one of trying to conceive or trying to avoid conception. Intercourse during this period is quite likely to result in conception, whereas abstinence will prevent conception from occurring.

The obvious problem is determining the day of ovulation and so being able to define accurately the unsafe period. The various natural methods differ in the techniques used to identify this period. At this time all methods leave something to guesswork, although this is currently an active area of research.

The Calendar Rhythm Method

The calendar rhythm method is the simplest of the fertility awareness techniques. The unsafe period is calculated mathematically using the length of previous menstrual cycles as a basis. Before initiating the calendar rhythm method a

SUNDAY	MONDAY	TUESDAY	WEDNESDAY	THURSDAY	FRIDAY	SATURDAY
				1	2 Menstruation begins	3
4	5	6	7	8	9	10
11	12 X	13 X	14 X	15 X	x 16 Estimated date of ovulation	17 X
18 X	19 X	20	21	22	23	24
25	26	27	28	29	30 Menstruation begins	31

Figure 20-13. The rhythm method for a 28-day menstrual cycle. The days marked X are considered "unsafe" days; days on which pregnancy may occur. The estimated day of ovulation is 14 days prior to the next menstrual period. In a 28-day cycle this would be day 14 of the menstrual cycle. Two days should be allowed on either side of day 14 for variations of the time of ovulation from month to month—days 12, 13, 15, and 16 are thus considered unsafe. If ovulation occurred on day 16, day 17 would be unsafe because of ovum survival. If ovulation occurred on day 12, days 10 and 11 would be unsafe because of sperm survival until day 12. In a 28-day menstrual cycle fertilization of an ovum is thus a possibility from day 10 through day 17.

woman should have an accurate record of 6 to 12 consecutive cycles. Based on the fact that ovulation is known to occur 12–16 days prior to the onset of menstruation the fertile phase is calculated to extend from the eighteenth day before the end of the shortest cycle through the eleventh day before the end of the longest cycle. Thus a woman whose previous 12 cycles had varied from 28 to 35 days would have a fertile period extending from day 10 through day 24 of each cycle (see Figure 20-13). Abstinence from intercourse during this entire period would be necessary in order to prevent conception. Unfortunately no woman has assurance that her cycle will remain the same, since it will often be sensitive to change in her routine, strong emotions, physical illness, and other factors.

The Basal Body Temperature

The basal body temperature method utilizes a temperature graph to indicate the time of ovulation and therefore the safe period. The cycles of estrogen and progesterone are responsible for sequential changes in basal body temperature. During the follicular phase (first half of the menstrual cycle) the temperature is approximately one degree lower than during the luteal phase following ovulation. If a woman takes her temperature each morning before rising from bed and graphs it on a chart, the time of ovulation can be noted by observing the rise in basal temperature (Figure 20-14). It must be recognized that temperature variations may also be the result of an illness, sleeplessness, alcohol ingestion, emotional upset, or other factors. Although basal body temperature does not permit prediction of ovulation, the rise in the reading does identify the safe, luteal period after ovulation. Abstinence should be continued until the temperature has remained elevated for three days. This method is often used in conjunction with the calendar rhythm method for a more precise estimation of the time of ovulation.

The Ovulation Method

The ovulation method is also known as the *Billings' method* after John and Lyn Billings,

two Australian physicians who introduced the method into the United States. Dr. John Billings describes this method thoroughly in his book written for the lay person, *Natural Family Planning: The Ovulation Method.* This method depends upon cyclic changes in the consistency of cervical mucus. In response to rising estrogen levels the mucus undergoes distinct changes at the time of ovulation. It increases in amount, making the vagina feel more moist and lubricated, and it becomes slippery and stretches without breaking (Spinnbarkeit). The consistency is not unlike egg white. Following ovulation, progesterone causes the mucus to become thicker and to decrease in amount.

Billings recommends that this method be taught from woman to woman and many communities have organized lay groups for this purpose. After using the method herself for a time a woman is likely to be able to give practical suggestions and support to other women.

When starting to use this method, abstinence is necessary for the entire first cycle while the woman learns to distinguish the types of mucus. She observes the degree of wetness of the labia and vagina and tests the stretchability (Spinnbarkeit) of the mucus by pulling it between two fingers. With practice she will be able to predict ovulation from the characteristics of the mucus. After the first, learning cycle, abstinence is necessary during the fertile phase of each cycle and every other day during the proliferative or follicular phase to enable the woman to detect the fertile mucus.

This method has an advantage over the two previously mentioned methods in that it allows prediction of ovulation and can be used by women with irregular cycles as well as by lactating and premenopausal women.

The Symptothermal Method

The symptothermal method utilizes a combination of all of the above techniques plus other symptoms of ovulation. This method emphasizes the joint responsibility of couples for observing and recording the pertinent symptoms and for interpreting the results. Practicing this method

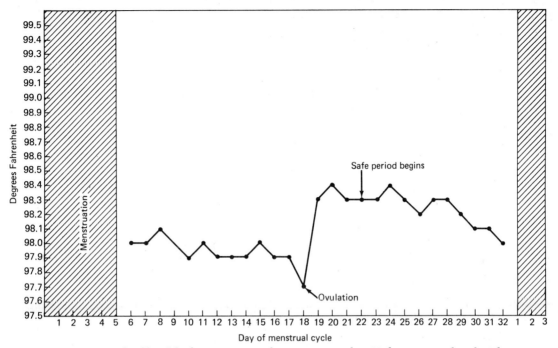

Figure 20-14. A graph of basal body temperature for a woman with a 32-day menstrual cycle. The ovum is considered to be degenerated after 72 hours of sustained temperature increase; thus the safe period begins on day 22 of this cycle.

requires both partners to develop extraordinary sensitivity to the physiology of the woman's body. Taught from couple to couple the instruction includes emphasis on communication and expression of affection by means other than intercourse.

In addition to the day of the cycle, temperature, and mucus, couples using this method observe changes in the dilation and consistency of the cervix and such secondary symptoms as mittleschmerz, abdominal bloating, vulvar swelling, increased libido, and spotting. A complete discussion of this method is contained in *The Art of Natural Family Planning* by John and Sheila Kippley.

All the methods of natural family planning have the advantage of avoiding chemicals and foreign bodies and so may be the only acceptable alternative to total abstinence for some people. To the extent that they heighten the aware-ness of the woman's body and increase communication between partners, they may also enrich the relationships of those who practice natural family planning. Without a strong commitment to both the relationship and the prevention of conception, sexual fulfillment may be sought elsewhere and/or conception control will not be effective.

Mechanical Methods

The mechanical contraceptive methods are those which provide a mechanical barrier between the spermatozoa and ovum or between fertilization and implantation. The mechanical methods most often utilized in the United States are the condom, the diaphragm, and the intrauterine contraceptive devices. Another mechanical method, the cervical cap, is more frequently used in other countries. As the cervical cap is, in some respects, similar in concept to the diaphragm, it will be briefly described at the end of the segment pertaining to the diaphragm.

Condom

The condom is a thin, elastic, and strong sheath of rubber or collagenous material which is unrolled down over the erect male penis. When the male ejaculates, the semen is caught in the condom, thereby preventing its being deposited in the vagina.

Three techniques in using the condom will enhance its efficacy:

1. The condom must be in place before the male penis approaches the female genitalia because of the possibility of spermatozoa being in male urethral coital secretions.
2. When using a plain-ended condom, an overlap allowance of one-fourth to one-half inch should be made for collection of the semen, thereby decreasing the possibility of the condom breaking at the time of ejaculation.
3. As the penis becomes flaccid following ejaculation, it is important that the male withdraw from the vagina immediately following ejaculation while securely holding the edge of the condom so that there is no leakage of semen out the open end of the condom and to prevent the condom from slipping off into the vagina while withdrawing.

If correctly used, the only other reason for possible failure would be due to defects in the condom itself. Defects include weakness of material causing the condom to break from the force of ejaculation, or minute (pinpoint) holes in the condom which would render it ineffective. Condoms made in the United States are under the supervision and quality control of the Food and Drug Administration of the federal government and are unlikely to have imperfections. It is possible to test a condom by overdistending it with water or air and checking for leakage. However, having done this, there is the possibility that such stretching may have weakened the condom for actual use. Although it is possible to

reuse a condom if given proper care, a precaution against breakage during sexual intercourse would be to use a condom only once and throw it away.

There is some discrepancy in the literature as to the effectiveness rate of the condom, with pregnancy rates from 5 to 15 per 100 years of exposure being stated. This discrepancy may be due to variations in the population samples and whether or not the sample included irregular as well as regular users of the condom method of contraception. It might be safe to say that the effectiveness rate of the condom is in the low 90s percentile but probably increases in effectiveness to the mid-90s percentile when correctly used, used in conjunction with a spermicidal preparation such as the contraceptive jellies, creams, or foams, and used consistently with each sexual intercourse.

Condoms, sometimes known as "rubbers," "safes," "sheaths," or "prophylactics," are readily available without prescription and may be purchased dry or lubricated. The cost varies with the make but generally is not exorbitant.

Side effects are limited to possible perineal and vaginal irritation if the condom is not lubricated and there is insufficient female coital secretions or if there is a reaction to the lubricant on the condom. In either situation, contraceptive foam, cream, or jelly, which should be used anyway, is a good substitute. Although the condom is a most widely used method of contraception (either totally, sporadically, or in conjunction with another method such as the spermicidal preparations), many couples do have negative feelings toward it. Some feel the condom dulls sensation, others object to a possible interruption of sexual foreplay to put the condom on, and still others feel that it creates a barrier between them at a time when they desire the feeling of "oneness" which can be attained during sexual intercourse. An additional problem is that the condom has often been associated with prostitutes and disease prevention. Thus, a husband may feel negative and/or a wife feel insulted unless they are reeducated for a change in mental associations and attitudes.

Diaphragm

The dome-shaped diaphragm is made of somewhat thicker rubber than the condom and has a flexible metal spring encased in the rubber rim. This allows the diaphragm to be compressed for ease in insertion and yet retain its shape and provide a snug fit against the vaginal tissues when in place and no longer compressed. The concept is that when the diaphragm is properly positioned with the dome side down, the cervix is covered by the diaphragm, thereby preventing spermatozoa from gaining access to the cervical os.

The dome of the diaphragm is approximately an inch and a half deep at its apex. As each woman is individual in vaginal size and contour, the diameter of a diaphragm may vary from 5½ to 10 cm. In addition, there are three types of diaphragms which differ only in the construction of the metal spring. The type of diaphragm to be used depends upon normal or unusual vaginal size or contour and normal or mild displacements of the uterus or adjacent structures. Due to difficulty or impossibility in fitting, a diaphragm is medically contraindicated for women with severe anteflexion, retroversion, retroflexion, or prolapse of the uterus, or with severe rectocele or cystocele. It is, therefore, essential for the woman to seek medical help for a pelvic examination, evaluation of pelvic structures, determination of the proper size and type of diaphragm, and instructions in using a diaphragm.

The proper position of the diaphragm, which is inserted into the vagina either digitally or with the mechanical inserter, is as follows: posteriorly, the rim of the diaphragm fits behind the cervix into the posterior vaginal fornix; anteriorly, the rim of the diaphragm rests snugly against the soft tissues posterior to the symphysis pubis; and the entire circumference of the diaphragm rests against the vaginal walls. This, then, effectively covers the cervix. It is important that after the woman has inserted the diaphragm she check to make sure it is properly positioned. Proper positioning of a diaphragm is not possible if the diaphragm no longer fits owing to change in size, shape, or position of the pelvis structures. Therefore, a woman should be rechecked for fit and possible change in size or type of diaphragm a few weeks after initial sexual experience, after each childbearing experience, and in the event of any weight gain or loss in excess of 20 lb.

The application of a spermicidal jelly or cream to the diaphragm greatly enhances its effectiveness as a contraceptive method and provides a double protective method. The spermicidal preparation, which is made specifically for use with a diaphragm, is applied to the rim and either the inside or the outside of the diaphragm in such a way as to completely cover the area before insertion. As it takes about six hours for the spermicidal preparation and/or vaginal secretions to immobilize and kill all the spermatozoa, the diaphragm must be left in place for at least six hours following coitus. The woman may then, but not before, douche. One half of the douche is taken before removing the diaphragm and the other half may be taken after its removal if she so desires. If sexual intercourse is repeated within six to eight hours, the diaphragm is left in place and an applicator full of spermicidal preparation inserted.

It is also important that the woman receive instructions on how to remove the diaphragm. Removal is accomplished by the woman inserting her finger into her vagina, bearing down, grasping the upper edge of the diaphragm posterior to the symphysis pubis, and pulling it down and out. She should compress the sides of the diaphragm as it comes out. This was also done for insertion in order to reduce the diameter and makes the insertion and removal procedures more comfortable. Pelvic models are most useful in teaching a woman how to insert and remove a diaphragm. This is followed by practice on herself under supervision after the size and type of her diaphragm are determined.

It is possible for a diaphragm to become dislodged during sexual intercourse. Such a possibility is a potential cause of failure and the inherent limitation of the diaphragm method of contraception. Other major reasons for failure of the diaphragm as a contraceptive method are improper positioning of the diaphragm and inconsistent use. The diaphragm should be periodically checked for wear, pinholes, and brittleness of the rubber. However, if properly cared for through washing, drying, and dusting with cornstarch following removal, a diaphragm should be usable for at least a year, depending on use.

The pregnancy rate for the diaphragm used in conjunction with a spermicidal preparation is approximately 3 per 100 years of exposure for consistent users. The pregnancy rate is much higher without the addition of the spermicidal preparation and in the event of poorly motivated, inconsistent use.

The cost of the diaphragm may be in addition to the medical help received and varies according to size up to approximately $5.00. The diaphragm usually comes in a kit containing the diaphragm, instruction pamphlet, mechanical inserter (optional in use of the method), and a tube of spermicidal jelly or cream. Periodic replenishing of the spermicidal preparation adds somewhat to the cost.

The diaphragm was for some time the "standard" contraceptive method. Of methods previously in common use, it had the lowest pregnancy rate for intelligent, highly motivated women. Some women find the techniques of the method too difficult to learn, since a good understanding of female reproductive anatomy is beneficial. Lack of acceptance of the diaphragm method of contraception is found in women who have a strong aversion to the self-intravaginal manipulation the method demands for insertion, checking position, and removal. Other women object to what they consider the nuisance of inserting the diaphragm, especially on a nightly basis as is frequently recommended for consistent conception protection. Although the diaphragm is usually not felt during sexual intercourse, some couples have the feeling of a barrier between them.

The *cervical cap*, while relatively unknown in the United States, is widely accepted and used in European countries. This discrepancy has been credited to its historical development and differences in cultural background relevant to mastering the technique of the method. The cervical cap is made of either rubber or a clear plastic, Lucite. The latter is known as the firm cervical cap and has the advantage over the rubber of being able to be worn for a number of days before removal.

The rounded, cone-shaped cervical cap fits over the cervix into the vaginal fornices. It stays in place due to a snug, but not tight, adherence to the vaginal fornices and a partial vacuum which is created between the dome of the cap and the cervix. The cervical cap is indicated in women who want a diaphragm-type of method, but, due to anatomic or functional reasons, cannot use a diaphragm. It is contraindicated for women with either an extremely long or short cervix, cervical erosions, nabothian cysts, deep cervical lacerations, or acute or subacute inflammatory conditions of the adnexae.

The pregnancy rate of the cervical cap is 7 to 8 per 100 years of exposure and is generally comparable to the effectiveness of the diaphragm combined with contraceptive jelly or cream method of contraception.

Intrauterine Contraceptive Devices

Intrauterine contraceptive devices, variously abbreviated as IUCD or IUD, are made of a variety of materials, but usually of an inert plastic or stainless steel. Some have the addition of a layer of copper on the surface, usually in the form of a winding of fine copper wire. The qualities of the material used must be such that the device is noninflammatory in the normal uterus, flexible for insertion and removal, and able to retain its "memory" to resume its shape when in position.

IUDs are produced in a variety of shapes. Those most commonly used in the United States at this time are Lippes Loop, Saf-T-Coil, and the Cu-7. The IUDs also vary as to whether or not the device has a cervical appendage. A cervical appendange to the device in the uterus may take the form of "ties," a string, or an extension of the device itself in order to facilitate ease of removal and enable a woman to check periodically to ascertain if the IUD is still in place. (See Fig. 20-15.)

The mechanism of action of the IUD is not known, although several theories have been advanced. One theory holds that the presence of a foreign body increases both uterine and fallopian tube contractions, thus speeding the progress of the ovum through the tube. Even if fertilization should occur, the ovum reaches the uterus prematurely, the endometrium is unready, and implantation cannot occur. A second possibility is that the endometrium forms cytotoxins in response to the foreign body, and these substances either attack the blastocyst directly or somehow interfere with implantation.

Still another theory holds that the IUD stimulates the production of a substance which diminishes the motility and fertility of the sperm. Perhaps some combination of these mechanisms or some as yet undefined mechanism is actually responsible. In any case it seems certain that the larger the surface area of the device the lower the failure rate. Some researchers believe this to be the reason for the success of those devices which utilize a winding of copper wire, although there is some evidence that copper ions exert a contraceptive effect of their own.

Insertion of an IUD is medically contraindicated in the presence of pregnancy or suspected pregnancy; acute or subacute pelvic inflammatory disease; acute cervicitis; myomas

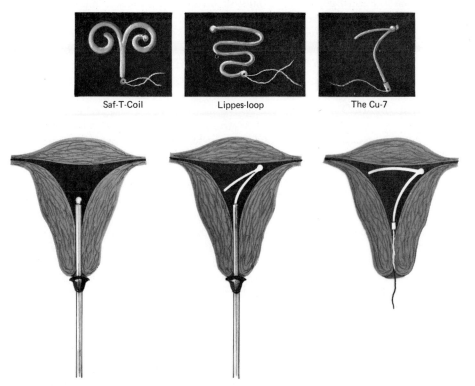

Saf-T-Coil   Lippes-loop   The Cu-7

Figure 20-15. The three IUDs most commonly used in the United States are pictured above. Below is a schematic drawing of the insertion of a Copper 7. The IUD is pulled into the introducer forcing it into a straight line. After preparation of the patient, the uterus is sounded to minimize the risk of perforation. The introducer is then inserted just inside the internal cervical os. The IUD is extruded from the introducer tube into the uterine cavity where it resumes its original shape. The introducer is then withdrawn.

which distort the uterine cavity; suspected uterine carcinoma; unexplained abnormal uterine bleeding or heavy menstrual flow; and in a woman with a history of postpartal endometritis or an infected abortion within the preceding six weeks.

The insertion of an IUD is a medical procedure requiring strict sterile technique. The procedure is preceded by a thorough pelvic examination, in part to determine the position of the uterus. A uterine probe is used to determine the direction and depth of the uterine cavity. The actual procedure for inserting an IUD will vary according to the device being inserted. Generally, a tenaculum or long Allis clamp will be used to grasp the cervix for the purpose of applying traction to straighten the cervico-uterine canal. The woman may feel a short, sharp pain at this time. She may also feel a cramp when the uterine probe passes through the internal cervical os, another cramp when the inserter with the device passes through the internal cervical os, and, depending on the device used, another cramp when the IUD is positioned in the uterus.

Following insertion, women usually experience a varying amount of spotting or bleeding and cramps. Spotting may continue for a few days and some women have a light intermenstrual bleeding during the first menstrual cycle postinsertion. Two or three longer and heavier menstrual periods are not uncommon postinsertion. The menstrual periods may gradually return to what a woman had before insertion or remain slightly more heavy. Cramps usually vary from being light and of brief duration in multiparas to being severe and lasting several days in nulligravidas who may require analgesics. Other side effects include the possibility of syncope, which most often occurs only in nulligravidas immediately postinsertion, and an unresolved question regarding the incidence of pelvic inflammatory disease with the IUDs. A general feeling among authorities at this time is that the incidence of pelvic inflammatory disease is essentially the same as that in the general population without an IUD, but necessary

data are lacking for any definite conclusions. Perforation of the uterus is rare. There is no evidence for believing that the IUDs are carcinogenic, cause ectopic pregnancies, or increase the incidence of prematurity or malformations in the limited number of infants born of women with an IUD *in situ*. It is sometimes necessary for an IUD to be removed and a different size of the same device or a different device used. If this does not effectively alleviate the situation, a different contraceptive method is recommended. The usual reasons for removal are severe, unremitting cramps and heavy bleeding.

Research and statistics compiled in relation to the IUDs generally emphasize pregnancy rates, expulsion rates, removal rates for various reasons, and continuation rates. The pregnancy rate of the IUDs has varied from under 1 to 5 per 100 years of exposure depending on the size and shape of the device. Unrealized expulsion of an IUD, more common in the young nulligravida, contributes to failure of an IUD as a contraceptive method. IUDs are, however, second only to the oral contraceptives ("pills") in effectiveness and have the advantage of not needing daily or monthly thought and supplies.

The cost of IUDs from the manufacturer varies according to the type of device. They usually come to the physician in a set including inserters. Added to this is the cost of a medical visit and a Papanicolaou smear.

Psychologically, again, some women who are adverse to inserting their finger into their vagina may object to checking themselves after each menstrual period if they have a device with a cervical appendage. The couple would need to resolve any moral or religious conflict for themselves. A very favorable psychologic reaction has been that the intrauterine contraceptive device method of conception protection is quite apart from the sexual act itself.

Spermicidal Preparations

The spermicidal preparations are those which contain a spermicidal ingredient which inactivates spermatozoa, combined with an inert base as the vehicle. The nonreactive base constitutes the bulk of such a preparation and also serves as a mechanical block to the cervical os. Most of the spermicidal preparations have an acid pH of 4.5, thereby ensuring a vaginal environment which is hostile to the mildly alkaline spermatozoa-containing semen. This is particularly important in the area of the external cervical os as the cervical secretions are slightly alkaline at the time of ovulation and therefore receptive to the spermatozoa.

These preparations are made, and are so designated, to be used alone, i.e., not in conjunction with a diaphragm. As a group they must exhibit certain common features: high ability to immobilize and kill spermatozoa; widespread vaginal distribution of the contraceptive method with the initial thrust of the penis; and the formation of a surface film which withstands coital activity. The spermicidal preparation is inserted near the cervix. Subsequent distribution over the cervix and throughout the vagina is accomplished through coital movements. Possible contraceptive failure due to inadequate distribution of the spermicidal preparation is inherent in the method.

Patient directions for all the spermicidal preparations, except the sponge and foam method, include the following imperative principles for effective use: reapplication of the method if sexual intercourse does not occur within one hour from the time of insertion; reapplication of the method before each sexual intercourse; reapplication of the method if the woman gets up, or walks around, or goes to the bathroom after insertion but before sexual intercourse; and no douching until at least six hours after sexual intercourse. Douching before six hours have elapsed may dilute or remove the spermidical preparation before complete inactivation of the spermatozoa has occurred, thereby rendering the method ineffective.

The spermicidal preparations generally have higher failure rates than any of the mechanical methods, perhaps due to a less well motivated group of patients as to routine use. On the other hand, women who lack motivation in attaining consistent use of the mechanical methods may be more regular in their use of a spermicidal preparation, thus affording greater conception protection for these women than would other methods. Spermicidal preparations are readily available in drug stores without prescription and are easy to use.

The cost of the spermicidal preparations varies according to type and brand but generally it is not prohibitive.

The major complaint of couples using spermicidal preparations has been one of "messiness." This relates to both the type of product (with the exception of the vaginal foam tablet and the suppository) and postcoital leakage of all the spermicidal preparations to a greater or lesser degree. A reduction in postcoital leakage, owing to a smaller amount by weight, constitutes one of the advantages of the aerosol foam as a spermicidal preparation. At the other end of the spectrum, the sponge and foam method has considerable relative "messiness." The suppository is the least esthetic of all the spermicidal preparations since when adequately dissolved it drains freely over the perineum during coitus as well as postcoitally. If this is annoying to the woman, her sexual pleasure may be diminished. Postcoital drainage can be controlled by placing tissues or a clean towel between the legs against the perineum. This will absorb moisture and make the woman more comfortable. Some couples also have a negative feeling toward a certain amount of "clock watching."

In addition to the foregoing, each spermicidal preparation has features specific to it alone, as mentioned in the following enumeration of the methods.

Jellies and Creams

The jellies and creams are tubed products which come in a kit containing an applicator and instructions. It is important that the instructions be followed so an adequate amount of the preparation is inserted to prevent dilution of the agent by the vaginal secretions. In order to deposit the spermicidal preparation near the cervix, it is recommended that the woman, who is lying down, insert the applicator in a down and backward direction the full length of the vagina and then withdraw it about ½ inch before pushing the plunger.

Aerosol Foam

The aerosol foam is a variation of the cream spermicidal preparation in which the agent has been compressed into a container under pressure with a gas such as Freon. Foam is released when the applicator is pressed against the container and the remainder of the procedure is the same as that for the jellies and creams.

Vaginal Foam Tablets

The vaginal foam tablet is a round, flat, white, 1-gm tablet which contains a spermicide, a bacteriostatic agent, and ingredients which produce a carbon dioxide foam when the tablet is moistened. While lying down, the woman moistens the tablet with a little water or saliva. She waits a moment to see or hear if it fizzes, then immediately inserts it into her vagina, pushing it as far as she can with her finger. If the tablet does not fizz when moistened, it should be discarded and another tablet used. An interval of five minutes must be allowed between insertion and sexual intercourse in order for the foaming action to occur which distributes foam throughout the vagina. Additional foaming action and dissolution of the tablet comes at the time of ejaculation.

A complaint related to the vaginal foam tablet has been an irritative vaginal reaction and a "burning" sensation felt by both husband and wife during the foaming process. Women with an aversion to inserting their finger into their vagina may object to this method.

Although the vaginal foam tablet has generally been considered one of the least effective of the spermicidal methods, it is well accepted by poorly motivated, low socioeconomic, minimally educated groups because of the simplicity of technique involved. As such, it may be more effective for these women than other methods, owing to greater willingness to use it, thereby yielding increased regularity of conception protection.

Suppositories

It is extremely important that products advertised for "feminine hygiene" are not mistaken for the spermicidal suppositories used as a contraceptive method. The cone-shaped contraceptive suppositories contain a spermicidal ingredient incorporated into a cocoa-butter or glycerogelatin base. They have a melting point of slightly below body temperature which makes them a poor choice of method in areas with a combination of hot weather and lack of refrigeration. As the average melting time of the suppository at body heat is around 10 minutes, a suppository should be inserted into the vagina at least 15 minutes before coitus. This waiting period may be objectionable to some couples. The suppository is considered to be one of the least effective of the spermicidal preparations.

Sponge and Foam

The sponge and foam method of contraception involves a small watermoistened sponge to which a spermicidal powder or liquid is applied. The sponge is then gently squeezed to form a foam and inserted into the vagina with as little loss of content as possible throughout the procedure.

There is an almost total reserve foaming power which allows for sexual intercourse to take place any time within six hours after insertion at which time foam is generated by the coital movements. If more than six hours elapse from the time of insertion to the time of sexual intercourse the sponge is removed, additional spermicidal powder or liquid is applied, and reinserted. The sponge must not be removed until at least six hour after sexual intercourse. If later or repeated coitus is desired before this six hours has elapsed, a second, smaller sponge is inserted in front of the first sponge.

The sponge and foam method is one of the least effective of the spermicidal contraceptive methods. However, the method is simple and some women seem to gain confidence that an effective method is being used when they see the foam-filled sponge.

Oral Contraceptives

There are basically two types of oral contraceptive therapy in widespread use: the combination and the sequential. Both types provide a regular cyclic menstruation and are thought to inhibit ovulation.

The combination type of oral contraceptive was the first type to be developed and derives its name from the fact that each pill consists of a combination of synthetic preparation of an estrogen and a progestogen. The main variations among the different formulations of the combined oral contraceptives are the dosages, relative proportion of the estrogenic and progestogenic components, and which estrogenic substance (ethinyl estradiol or mestranol) is used with which of the available progestogens. These variations result in a spectrum of pills with somewhat different minor side effects, which, in addition to the choice of the sequential type, allows for a certain amount of changing of the pill to best accommodate the individual woman's adjustment to the hormonal therapy.

The sequential type of oral contraceptive also derives its name from its formulation and administration. Sequential therapy consists of two different pills to be taken during the menstrual cycle. The first type of pill consists of an estrogenic substance only for three fourths of the pill-taking sequence. The pills taken for the remainder of the pill-taking sequence (usually five days) are a combination of the estrogen with a progestogen. The thinking underlying the development of the sequential oral contraceptive was twofold: (1) that the sequential administration of estrogen and a progestin more closely approximates the physiologic production of hormones by the ovaries, and (2) the later knowledge that estrogen alone could produce the antifertility action. The progestin is added to control the bleeding caused by the administration of estrogen alone and to produce a predictable withdrawal bleeding.

The mechanism of action of the oral contraceptives is not completely understood. It has long been known that suppression of the production of the pituitary gonadotropins (specifically, for contraception, the follicle-stimulating hormone and luteinizing hormone) can be effected by any of the sex hormones: progesterone, estrogen, and androgen. The administration of synthetic steroid preparations effectively inhibits the development of a graafian follicle and the subsequent event of ovulation, without which there is no ovum to be fertilized. However, the antifertility effect of steroids is not dependent on inhibition of ovulation. Other possible methods of action are under investigation and include hypotheses on the effect of hormonal contraception on ovarian responsiveness to gonadotropic stimulation, biogenesis and/or catabolism of ovarian hormones, factors within the fallopian tubes, spermatozoa capacitation, and endometrial changes.

The "menstruation" of a woman on oral contraceptives is actually a pseudomenstruation produced by the administration and then withdrawing of the hormonal substances and more appropriately termed "withdrawal bleeding." The characteristics of the withdrawal bleeding differ between the combination and sequential types of therapy due to the different action each type has upon the endometrium. The combined estrogen-progestin oral contraceptives produce stromal edema, predeciduation, and some degree of glandular involution yielding in a few cycles a thin, hypoplastic-appearing endometrium. This accounts for the characteristic shorter duration and scantier flow noticed by women taking the combination contraceptive pills. In contrast, the sequential type of therapy yields an anovulatory pattern during the estrogen phase and an incomplete progestational endometrium transformation during the combined estrogen–progestin phase. Therefore, neither the predeciduation or thinning out of the endometrium occurs and a woman taking the sequential contraceptive pills will not notice as much change in her "menstruation."

As already mentioned, the minor side effects

a woman may experience while taking the oral contraceptives depend on a combination of her individual biochemical and physiologic response to the formulation of her pills and the properties of the progestin being utilized. For example, the progestin norethindrone in one of the combination type of pills is androgenic in character. In contrast, the progestin norethynodrel in another one of the combination type of pills has estrogenic characteristics. Thus, for example, a woman inclined toward hirsutism might have an exacerbation of these tendencies on the former type of pills and would probably be more satisfied with the use of the latter type. The minor side effects experienced by women on oral contraceptives have often been compared to those of early pregnancy, e.g., nausea, fatigue, breast tenderness. Much of the literature on the minor side effects is based on the extensive research conducted with the first oral contraceptive: a 10-mg pill. Subsequent reduction of dosage has effected a responsive reduction in the incidence and severity of the minor side effects. Intermenstrual ("breakthrough") bleeding is not uncommon and can usually be controlled with dosage or pill prescription changes.

The continuing major issue in the utilization of the oral contraceptive methods is the question of their safety. Of particular concern is the possibility of existing relationships between the hormonal contraceptive formulations and thromboembolic phenomena; endocrine and metabolic effects, especially diabetes and liver function; cervical carcinoma; and heart disease. Oral contraceptives are generally contraindicated for women with a history of thromboembolic disease or hepatic disorders and premenopausal women who have a diagnosis of breast cancer. Diabetics, women with hypertension, and those over age 40 should also use some other form of contraception. The continuing research that is being done on the safety of the oral contraceptives is not minimized by the awareness that final evaluation of them as the most effective of all the contraceptive methods must be carefully weighed. The dangers of childbirth for an individual woman as well as the health and social benefits for families and society which can be accrued through widespread oral contraceptive programs must be considered.

The oral contraceptives are virtually 100 percent effective if taken as directed. A woman on the combination therapy is much less likely to become pregnant if she forgets one or even two pills than is the woman who forgets one pill on the sequential therapy. This probably accounts for the slightly higher pregnancy rates for the sequential in contrast to the combined oral contraceptives.

A woman is more apt to remember to take her pills if she puts them next to or on something which is part of her daily routine, e.g., toothbrush, alarm clock, coffee pot, dining table, etc. The drug companies have also devised innumerable aids for remembering to take the pills in the packaging of their products. These include calendar packs, dial packs, punch packs, etc., which give the day or date of each pill that is to be taken. The original pills were to be taken for 20 days starting on day 5 of the menstrual cycle. The woman would then usually start her withdrawal bleeding two or three days after the twentieth pill and start her pills again on day 5 after her period started. These are still the most common directions for the oral contraceptive pills. However, it has been recommended in working with women for whom such a system of counting might be confusing that the woman take her 20 pills, stop for her "menstruation," and start taking her next package of 20 pills on the same day a week later as the day she stopped taking pills. Some drug companies have incorporated this idea into their packaging of pills with 21 days of pills and seven days without: three weeks on and one week off. The woman then would be starting and stopping her pills on the same day throughout the months. This enables the woman to choose the days of the week on which menstruation will occur. For example, by starting the 21 pills on a Saturday she will not ever have her period on a weekend.

A more recent development is the packaging of 28 days of pills in which the last 7 pills are hormonal placebos. The idea behind the packages of 28 pills is that this enables the woman to get into the habit of taking a pill every day, thereby reducing the chance of her either forgetting her pill or being confused as to whether any particular day is a day during which she should take a pill.

The oral contraceptive pills vary slightly in amount of expense per month, depending on brand and dosage, but for many women cost is not prohibitive.

Psychologically, there has been a diverse reaction to the oral contraceptives. One is fear, owing to the large volume of publicity they have received, much of it based on the thus far unresolved questions of safety and subsequent rumor. The other reaction has been very favorable, based on the ease of using this contraceptive method, its being unrelated to the act of sexual intercourse, and its high effectiveness rate.

Folklore

The following are so-called contraceptive methods of long-standing reputation which because of a basic fallacy in concept and low efficacy might well be labeled as folklore.

Douches

Douching following sexual intercourse as a contraceptive method is one of the most prevalent erroneous ideas. The concept is that if a woman douches immediately following ejaculation she will flush the semen out of the vagina before the spermatozoa can enter the uterus. However, the majority of spermatozoa are contained in the first few drops of the ejaculate and are into the cervical canal within 90 seconds following the usual depositing of the semen at the cervical os. As it is highly unlikely that a woman could douche within this period of time, the entire concept is rendered invalid.

A pregnancy rate in excess of 30 per 100 years of exposure has been stated in various reports for couples using this method, which is better than no contraceptive method at all. However, such low efficacy can scarcely recommend the douche as a very reliable method of contraceptive.

Coitus Interruptus

Coitus interruptus, more commonly known as withdrawal or "being safe," is based on the fact that the male can feel when he is about to ejaculate. The method relies on the male withdrawing his penis from the vagina at this moment and ejaculating outside of it, thereby preventing the spermatozoa from being in a location where they could conceivably reach a mature ovum. Such an action demands split-second timing and idealistic self-control by the male, who may not always be psychologically able to withdraw at the climax of sexual intercourse. In addition, if the male is a fraction of a second too late in withdrawing and the first drop or two of semen is deposited in the vagina or if he ejaculates on the external female genitalia, the method may be rendered invalid.

Coitus interruptus is a method which many couples have used at least occasionally and is recommended in the absence of a more reliable contraceptive method. Although some couples have been satisfied with coitus interruptus as a contraceptive method and have used it successfully, it has been noted for many family planning failures. There has also been some objection to coitus interruptus as limiting full sexual gratification.

Breast Feeding

Following delivery there is a period of six to eight weeks of amenorrhea which may be prolonged to as much as a year by breast feeding. Because they are not menstruating many women may believe that they cannot become pregnant. However, ovulation very frequently occurs prior to the reestablishment of menses. Therefore, although conception is less likely to occur while breast feeding fully, this is not a totally reliable means of contraception.

Female Reserve

Some people believe that a woman may not become pregnant unless she has an orgasm at the time of intercourse. This piece of folklore therefore advises the woman to hold back her orgasm and she will not conceive. This belief is totally untrue.

Sterilization

Surgical sterilization of both men and women is available as a means of permanent contraception. For couples where the wife is in the age range of 30 to 44, sterilization is the most common method of contraception (1970 National Fertility Study). The operations are approximately equally divided between men and women.

Male sterilization is effected by vasectomy, the severing of the vas deferens. This destroys the pathway of the sperm from the testicles to the urethra. Female sterilization involves ligating or severing (or both) the fallopian tubes so that the ovum is unavailable for fertilization. Both procedures are permanent and irreversible, although efforts are being made to develop a procedure that can be reversed.

FRAMEWORK FOR POSTPARTUM NURSING ASSESSMENT

I. Physical Restoration

    A. Breasts
    B. Abdomen
    C. Uterus
    D. Lochia
    E. Bladder
    F. Bowels
    G. Perineum
    H. Lower extremeties
    I. Vital signs
    J. Hemoglobin/hematocrit

II. Psychosocial Adaptation

    A. Maternal dependency/independency

    "How do you feel?"
    "May I help you?"

    B. Resolution of pregnancy, labor, and delivery

    "How did your labor (pregnancy) compare with your expectations?"

    C. Parent–infant attachment

    "Many parents are surprised to find they don't immediately feel a rush of parental affection. How is it with you?"

III. Preparation for Going Home

    A. Need for instruction

    Personal health and nutrition
    Infant care skills
    Family planning
    Exercises
    Adjustment of children to new infant

    B. Anticipatory guidance for first three months

    Family relationship
    Sexuality
    Infant growth and development
    Organization of time
    Available community resources

    C. Referrals for continuity of health care

Figure 20-16. A suggested framework for postpartum nursing assessment. Progress in each of these areas should be reviewed daily and accurately noted in the mother's record.

Future Methods

It is a well-recognized, noncontroversial fact that the ideal contraceptive method, combining the features of 100 percent effectiveness, 100 percent safety, no side effects, ease of use with no interference with sexual intercourse, and acceptability to all religions, has not yet been developed. Intensive research continues both in exploration of possible new methods, and in perfecting already existing methods, based on studies of the cause of side effects, possible relationships with disease (safety), and mechanisms of action.

Of vital importance is the development of a so far elusive method of being able to accurately predict the time of ovulation at least four days prior to the event. Such a development would revolutionize the rhythm method and ease the current religious controversy.

The ongoing research with the intrauterine contraceptive devices yields modifications in existing devices relative to size and material used. New shapes are periodically introduced which, with modifications, are all geared toward ease of insertion and a decrease in expulsion rates, pregnancy rates, and bleeding. Still to be resolved is the question of the role of the transcervical appendage in the development of infection.

Research is occurring in the area of ovulation-inhibiting methods or more broadly, with steroid compounds which act as antifertility agents but not necessarily by means of inhibiting ovulation. One such hormonal contraceptive formulation is the "one-a-month pill" consisting of the combination of a long-acting estrogen and progestogen. Another is the long-acting injectable formulation. This is composed of a long-acting progestogen either alone or in conjunction with a long-acting estrogen. Investigations are being made of injections given every one month, every three months, and every six months. Time-release pellets for intradermal implantation are also under investigation. The main difficulties with these formulations are their irreversibility, amenorrhea, and irregular uterine bleeding. A supplement of a short cycle of an oral estrogen each month decreases the incidence of irregular uterine bleeding and produces a satisfying withdrawal bleeding. The latter is of particular importance for many women who, despite their considering menstruation "the curse" or "sickness," feel it is evidence of their femininity and assurance of their not being pregnant.

Another area of research involves the search for a male contraceptive. Most efforts are directed at finding a suitable combination of progesterone which inhibits spermatogenesis and testosterone which will offset the undesirable side effects such as decreased libido. Unlike female contraception, which interrupts a relatively predictable cycle, male contraceptives must suppress a continuous process of spermatogenesis. So far, no male contraceptive has been approved for general use in any country.

SUMMARY

The puerperium is defined medically as the six weeks immediately following delivery. Psychosocially it extends through the first three to four months after birth.

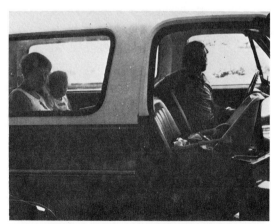

Figure 20-17. Family leaving the hospital for home after the birth of their baby. Notice this mother's way of meeting her two-year-old's needs by sharing the back seat with him while baby sister rides up front with daddy.

Dramatic physiologic changes occur in the woman's body. The nurse must be able to assess the progress of these changes and evaluate their normality.

Equally dramatic psychosocial changes occur in the woman and in her family. The nurse must be aware of the usual pattern of these changes in order to foster parent–infant attachment, role adaptation, and family integration (Fig. 20-16).

Parents require special nursing care when their infants are not full-term and healthy if they are to master this crisis successfully and develop as competent parents.

BIBLIOGRAPHY

Alderson, Margaret, First concerns in the postpartum period, *Patient Care* 9:58–111 passim (Feb. 1) 1975.

Antonucci, Toni (ed.), Attachment: A life-span concept, *Hum. Dev.* 19: entire issue, 1976.

Benfield, D. Gary, Leib, Susan A., Reuter, Jeannette, Grief response of parents after referral of the critically ill newborn to a regional center, *N. Eng. J. Med.* 294:975–978 (29 Apr.) 1976.

Boston Women's Health Collective, *Our Bodies, Our Selves: A Book by and for Women*, 2nd ed. Simon and Schuster, New York, 1976.

Boulette, Teresa Ramirez, Parenting: Special needs of low-income Spanish-surnamed families, *Pediatr. Ann.* 6:613–619 (Sept.) 1977.

Brazelton, T. Berry, *Infants and Mothers: Differences and Development*. Delta Books, New York, 1972.

———, Koslowski, Barbara, and Main, Mary, The origins of reciprocity: The early mother–infant interaction, in *The Effect of The Infant on Its Caregiver*, edited by Michael Lewis and Leonard H. Rosenblum. Wiley, New York, 1974.

Britt, Sylvia Squires, Fertility awareness: Four methods of natural family planning, *JOGN Nurs.* 6:9–18 (Mar.–Apr.) 1977.

Bromwich, Rose M., Focus on maternal behavior in infant intervention. *Am. J. Orthopsychiatry* 46:439–446, 1976.

Brown, Marie Scott, and Hurlock, Joan T., Mothering the mother, *Am. J. Nurs.* 77:438–441 (Mar.) 1977.

Campbell, Sandra J., and Smith, Jean G., Postpartum: Assessment guide, *Am. J. Nurs.* 77:1179, (July) 1977.

Christensen, Ann A., Coping with the crisis of a premature birth—One couple's story, *MCN* 2:33–37 (Jan.–Feb.) 1977.

Clark, Ann L., and Affonso, Dyanne D., *Childbearing: A Nursing Perspective*. Davis, Philadelphia, Pa., 1976.

Clausen, Joy, Efficient postpartum checks, *Nursing 72*, 2:24–25, (Oct.) 1972.

———, Flook, Margaret, and Ford, Boonie, *Maternity Nursing Today*, 2nd ed. McGraw-Hill Book Co., St. Louis, 1977.

Contraceptive Technology, 1974–1975, The Emory University Family Planning Program, Atlanta, Ga., 1974.

Danforth, David N. (ed.), *Obstetrics and Gynecology*, 3rd ed. Harper and Row, New York, 1977.

Donaldson, Nancy, Fourth trimester follow-up, *Am. J. Nurs.* 77:1176–1178, 1977.

Edwards, Margot, The crisis of the fourth trimester, *Birth Family J.* 1:19–22 (Winter) 1973–74.

Greenhill, J. P., and Friedman, Emanuel, *Biological Principles and Modern Practice of Obstetrics*. Saunders, Philadelphia, Pa., 1974.

Gruis, Marcia, Beyond maternity: Postpartum concerns of mothers, *MCN* 2:182–188 (May–June) 1977.

Harrison-Ross, Phyllis, Parenting the black child, *Pediatr. Ann.* 6:605–612 (Sept.) 1977.

Heath, D. H., Competent fathers: Their personalities and marriages, *Hum. Dev.* 19:26–39, 1976.

Hobbs, Daniel F., Jr., and Cole, Sue Peck, Transition to parenthood: A decade replication, *J. Marriage Family* 38:723–732 (Nov.) 1976.

Hubbard, Charles William, *Family Planning Education*, 2nd ed. Mosby, St. Louis, Mo., 1977.

Hurd, Jeanne Marie L., Assessing maternal attachment: First step toward prevention of child abuse, *JOGN Nurs.* 4:25–30 (Jul.–Aug.) 1975.

Johnson, Suzanne Hall, and Grubbs, Judith Pierson, The premature infant's reflex behaviors: Effect on the maternal–child relationship, *JOGN Nurs.* 4:15–20 (May–June) 1975.

Johnston, Maxine, Kayne, Martha, and Mittleider, Kathy, Putting more pep in parenting, *Am. J. Nurs.* 77:994–995 (June) 1977.

Kennedy, Janet C., The high-risk maternal–infant acquaintance process, *Nurs. Clin. North Am.* 8:549–556 (Sept.) 1973.

Kennel, John H. *et al.*, Maternal behavior one year after early and extended post-partum contact, *Dev. Med. Child Neurol.* 16:172–179, 1974.

Kilker, Rosemary, and Wilkerson, Betty, 8-Point postpartum assessment, *Nursing '73*, 3:56 (May) 1973.

Klaus, Marshall H., and Kennell, John H., *Maternal–Infant Bonding*, Mosby, St. Louis, Mo., 1976.

Kowalski, Karen, and Osborn, Mary Ross, Helping mothers of stillborn infants to grieve, *MCN* 2:29–32 (Jan.–Feb.) 1977.

Leonard, Susan Woolf, How first-time fathers feel toward their newborns, *MCN* 1:361–365 (Nov.–Dec.) 1976.

Ludington-Hoe, Susan M., Development of maternicity, *Am. J. Nurs.* 77:1170–1174 (July) 1977.

Lynn, David B., *The Father: His Role in Child Development*, Brooks/Cole Publishing Co., Monterey, Calif., 1974.

McCabe, Susan Nelson, Anticipatory guidance of families with infants in *Family Health Care*, edited by Debra P. Hymovich and Martha U. Barnard. McGraw-Hill, St. Louis, Mo., 1973.

MacFarlane, Aiden, *The Psychology of Childbirth*, Chapters 7 and 8, Harvard University Press, Cambridge, Mass., 1977.

Manisoff, Miriam, *Family Planning, A Teaching Guide for Nurses*, 2nd ed. Planned Parenthood–World Population, New York, 1971.

Mercer, Ramona T., Postpartum: Illness and acquaintance–attachment process, *Am. J. Nurs.* 77:1174–1177 (July) 1977.

Murray, Linda, Searching for safe contraceptives, *Contemp. Ob/Gyn* 9:37–54 passim (May) 1977.

Pritchard, Jack A., and MacDonald, Paul C., *Williams Obstetrics*, 15th ed. Appleton-Century-Crofts, New York, 1976.

Redman, Barbara K., *The Process of Patient Teaching in Nursing*, 2nd ed. Mosby, St. Louis, Mo., 1972.

Rising, Sharon Schindler, The fourth stage of labor: Family integration, *Am. J. Nurs.* 74:870–874 (May) 1974.

Robson, Kenneth S., The role of eye-to-eye contact in maternal-infant attachment, *J. Child Psychol. Psychiatry* 8:13–25, 1967.

———, and Moss, Howard A., Patterns and determinants of maternal attachment, *J. Pediatr.* 77:976–985 (Dec.) 1970.

Rozdilsky, Mary Lou, and Banet, Barbara, *What Now? A Handbook for Couples (Especially Women) Postpartum*. Daisy Publishing Co., Seattle, Wash., 1972.

Schaffer, Rudolph, *Mothering*. Harvard University Press, Cambridge, Mass., 1977.

Schwartz, Jane Linker, and Schwartz, Lawrence H., *Vulnerable Infants, A Psychosocial Dilemma*. McGraw Hill, St. Louis, Mo., 1977.

Sonstegard, Lois J., and Egan, Ellen, Family-centered nursing makes a difference, *MCN* 1:249–255 (Jul.–Aug.) 1976.

Sumner, Georgina, and Fritsch, Joseph, Postnatal parental concerns: The first six weeks of life, *JOGN Nurs.* 6:27–32 (May–June) 1977.

Tudor, Mary J., Family habilitation: A child with a birth defect, in *Family Health Care*, edited by Debra P. Hymovich and Martha U. Barnard. McGraw-Hill, St. Louis, Mo., 1973.

Williams, Janet, Learning needs of new parents, *Am. J. Nurs.* 77:1173 (July) 1977.

Wuerger, Mardelle K., Stepping into parenthood, *Am. J. Nurs.* 76:1283–1285 (Aug.) 1976.

Young, Ruth K., Chronic sorrow: Parents' response to the birth of a child with a defect, *MCN* 2:38–42 (Jan.–Feb.) 1977.

Part Five

The High-Risk Mother and Baby

21

Maternal and Fetal Assessment in High-Risk Pregnancy

In spite of the fact that pregnancy is a physiologic, not a pathologic, phenomenon, approximately 15 percent of pregnancies in the United States are at risk because of maternal and/or fetal factors. Chapter 7 discussed the personal, socioeconomic, and nutritional factors, as well as the medical reasons, why a pregnancy may be at risk. The importance of screening and early detection of women in these categories was emphasized. Watchfulness throughout pregnancy to insure early recognition and treatment of abnormal conditions cannot be too insistently urged.

This chapter will discuss the antepartum care of women whose pregnancies are deemed at risk for any reason. Chapter 22 will discuss obstetric complications, and Chapter 23 will consider complications resulting from preexisting conditions.

GOALS OF HIGH-RISK ANTEPARTUM CARE

The goals for antepartum care of the high-risk pregnant woman are the same as those of all pregnant women. That is, to minimize maternal, fetal, and neonatal mortality and morbidity and to foster the optimum growth and development of both parents and child. The difference, from the nurses' perspective, is one of degree. For the woman whose pregnancy remains uncomplicated little or no intervention is necessary in the traditional sense of illness care. These women and their families usually have sufficient resources to cope productively with childbearing and rely on health care professionals for validation of their well-being, early recognition of any deviations from normal, and instruction and supportive care, the amount depending largely upon the sensitivity of the caregiver. On the other hand, families experiencing a high-risk pregnancy have all the needs of low-risk families—perhaps doubled—plus the need for medical intervention to deal with the pathology. The entire period of the complicated pregnancy becomes very literally a period of intensive care. Indeed, the high-risk obstetric service may be named the Maternal Intensive Care Unit.

How can these goals be achieved? Without offering any easy formula for success, several important factors are discussed here briefly.

1. *Consumer education.*

Health care professionals at all levels should assume responsibility for increasing public awareness about what constitutes quality health care. Consumerism has had some beneficial effects on health care in general as people have insisted on stripping away the medical mystique and becoming partners, if not bosses, in their own health care. Professionals must be responsive to this and enter into dialogue so there can be mutual growth and mutual benefit.

2. *Improved quality of antepartum care for all women.*

Appropriate screening, universally instituted, would detect deviations from normal very early and possibly prevent many high-risk pregnancies. Treatment of clients should meet individual needs. Personnel most qualified to deal with a given problem should be available to the client, and the clients should enter the health care system prior to conception. In this way many genetic, nutritional, and other complications might be averted.

3. *Appropriately trained personnel in adequate numbers.*

This includes perinatologists and neonatologists as well as clinical nurse specialists, midwives, home health aides, and others.

4. *Availability of care.*

Financial barriers to care discriminate against those at highest risk for complicated pregnancy. Low socioeconomic status has the highest degree of correlation with such risk factors as poor nutrition, anemia, toxemia, premature and small-for-gestational age infants, and others. Geographic distribution of qualified personnel is an additional barrier to the availability of care. Because the percentage of women requiring high-risk care is small, a relatively large delivery base (about 15,000 per year) is required to support a perinatal center. Regionalization has been one attempt at making a concentration of skilled personnel and physical resources available within a reasonable distance of all women in the region.

5. *"Team"-directed care.*

Pregnancy offers opportunities for many different professionals to intervene in ways that positively influence the physical and mental health of whole families. This is especially true of the high-risk pregnancy where the needs are varied and may require highly specialized expertise. Such a team approach can be particularly effective when individual members are mature enough to set aside professional territoriality and work in colleagueship for *patient* care rather than medical care or nursing care or nutrition care.

Throughout this text, but especially in the area of high-risk pregnancy, little, if any, effort is made to distinguish between medical management and nursing care. It is believed that the complexity of the services required by families is so great that no one profession can reasonably expect to work alone. In any given situation traditional professional roles may be reversed as in the case of E. C., a very young, frightened, and often hostile girl with chronic renal disease. One of the resident physicians was able to develop a warm, trusting relationship early in her pregnancy. Consequently, it was he who provided the major portion of teaching, supportive care, and general TLC (Tender Loving Care), while the nurse on the team worked with the senior physician to manage laboratory studies and other medical details.

6. *Focus of care.*

Professionals working with childbearing families have as their focus the pregnant woman as an individual who is a member of a family and a community. This is a departure from the traditional medical model which focuses on a pathology and how to cure it.

A FRAMEWORK FOR NURSING ASSESSMENT OF HIGH-RISK PREGNANCY

The dynamics of high-risk pregnancy are the closely interwoven relationships of four overlapping factors: the physiology of gestation, the pathology of the complication, the psychology of pregnancy, and the psychology of illness. It will become clear to the reader that there is much that is unknown about the interaction of these factors. Still, the careful consideration of such interactions can serve as a useful framework for determining the status of a particular woman and, to some extent, that of her family. Such an assessment is useful in establishing priorities of care, determining areas where women and families desire and/or need assistance, and describing outcome criteria which can be utilized to evaluate the effectiveness of the care given.

Physiology of Pregnancy

During gestation striking modifications in physiology occur to meet the demands of the developing fetus. Virtually all the woman's organ systems undergo some change, so that it is accurate to think of pregnancy as an alternate biologic state. Although there are certain commonalities, these changes tend to be individual for each woman and for each pregnancy, so that no two pregnancies are exactly alike even if the same woman is experiencing them. Monitoring the extent and appropriateness of these physiologic changes is an essential part of all antepartum care—high- or low-risk.

Pathology of Complications

Whatever the complication of pregnancy, be it a preexisting chronic illness, an intercurrent acute infection, or an obstetric complication, there will be a specific pathology which affects selected organ systems and alters function. This alteration may be slight or it may be life-threatening. Because of the advances in medical science, many women are becoming pregnant who might not have survived to reproductive age or who might have been infertile in another era. For this reason it is not uncommon to see women with conditions about which the impact on pregnancy (and vice versa) is poorly understood. Conditions such as toxemia or diabetes mellitus have been widely studied and there are many empirical data in the literature to give the practitioner an idea of mortality and morbidity risks, preferred treatment protocols, and so on. Where such data do not exist the practitioner needs a systematic method of determining potential risks to mother and fetus because of the complication. Analysis of the pathology as it affects or interferes with the ordinary physiology and management of pregnancy is one such method. The following three examples will illustrate the problem.

M. J. seeks care at the Maternal Intensive Care Clinic because of pregnancy complicated by mitral valve stenosis secondary to a childhood streptococcal infection. The nurse will recognize that both the increasing cardiac output and the increasing heart rate characteristic of normal pregnancy will likely produce negative effects in this woman. Furthermore, remembering the pattern of these increases, the nurse will be able to foresee that the woman's risks of pulmonary edema, cardiac failure, and other cardiac pathology, will rise in a linear fashion from the third month of pregnancy until approximately the twenty-eighth week, then there will be a plateau-like interval until labor, when the risk is again increased. She will also know that the rapid hemodynamic changes which accompany parturition make the immediate postpartum period the time of greatest risk for congestive heart failure. Applying the old saw that forewarned is forearmed, the nurse can use this knowledge to plan with the woman and other team members for optimum safety at times of highest risk. In this situation the normal physiology of pregnancy adversely affects the preexisting pathology.

R. S. has had intestinal bypass surgery in order to effect weight loss. Although she had weighed in excess of 400 pounds, at the time of her pregnancy she weighed 215 pounds. Because of the loss of several feet of intestines, a significant amount of absorptive surface has been lost. In pregnancy one typically expects a weight gain of approximately 25 pounds because of fetal growth as well as maternal tissue development. In order to insure adequate nutrition to the fetus, careful consideration must be given to high-quality protein foods of high digestibility and in frequent small servings to facilitate maximum absorption. Needless to say, a woman for whom weight loss has been such a priority will need considerable support and instruction about her present need to gain weight.

B. L. has developed severe preeclampsia during the third trimester of her first pregnancy. Preeclampsia is characterized by generalized vasospasm, which interferes with the flow of blood to and from vital organs. Since oxygen and nutrients are carried to the placenta and thus to the fetus by the maternal bloodstream, it can be expected that intrauterine nutrition may suffer as a result of preeclampsia. Indeed, the nurse will understand that it is quite reasonable to expect the delivery of a small-for-gestational-age infant and should alert the neonatal team about this likelihood.

Psychology of Pregnancy

The characteristic emotional and developmental phenomena of pregnancy have been discussed in Chapter 9. It is widely recognized that these phenomena both influence, and are influenced by, the physiologic changes which are occurring simultaneously. At the simplest level, it is the physiology which first makes the woman aware of the fact of her pregnancy. In addition, endocrine changes have been suggested as factors in the mood swings of pregnancy among other things. A passing knowledge of psychosomatics would indicate that the woman's attitude toward pregnancy and motherhood may intensify the nausea, vomiting, fatigue, and other physical irritations of gestation, or, conversely, it may minimize, or even eliminate, them as factors to be considered.

When intervening pathology threatens the life or well-being of the woman herself, or her child, there can be severe obstacles to the orderly progression of attachment and other maternal tasks. The woman's concept of herself as a woman and consequently as a mother may be clouded by an awareness of her "imperfection" in not having what she regards as a "normal pregnancy." Nurses and others in contact with high-risk pregnant women should be particularly sensitive to these feelings, and, whenever possible, intervene to help the woman and her family cope with these difficulties and prepare as well as possible to assume the parenting role. To this end it is usually helpful to spend some time each visit focusing on the "normal" aspects of her pregnancy and the positive findings regarding both herself and her infant. One woman, following a pregnancy cared for in the high-risk obstetric service of a university medical center, said that, although she was convinced she received the best care possible, "no one ever talked to me about having a little baby. I was so excited, but I felt the doctors and nurses only wanted to know about my liver studies."

Psychology of Illness

Society prescribes a specific sick role which allows a person to regress honorably to a position of increased passivity and dependency and to be temporarily excused from meeting some or all of his obligations. Pregnancy, too, is characterized by an increased passivity and dependency, during which the woman is very actively involved in self-reevaluation and in role and relationship adaptation. When these two events coincide, as they often do in a high-risk pregnancy, how do they enhance or inhibit each other?

Pregnancy is regarded as a healthy, usually happy, event. What happens when it is an unhealthy and an anxious time? In spite of ordinary fears for their own well-being and that of their children, most healthy women are hopeful and expect a healthy outcome for themselves and their babies. When the threat to life and health is a very real one because of complications, how can that hope be maintained without giving false hope? These are questions largely without answers which must be considered individually with each client family until some research is available which might give more general direction.

If the complicating condition is one which predates the pregnancy it is useful to have some historical information. The age and developmental stage of the woman at the time of diagnosis, as well as the time elapsed since diagnosis, may give evidence of the degree of acceptance of the diagnosis. As an example, if a young woman becomes a juvenile diabetic during adolescence and the dietary restrictions become a weapon in her struggle for independence from her parents, one would not be surprised to find her in conflict with the nutritionist, whom she places in the role of controlling mother. Similarly, a woman who denies the reality of her diagnosis may place herself and/or her fetus in jeopardy by refusing to accept treatment. One young woman with Gaucher's disease felt well and expressed doubt concerning the accuracy of her diagnosis, although it had been made some five years previously and repeatedly confirmed. She felt if the diagnosis were accurate that she must have a very mild, and, therefore, quite harmless variety. She steadfastly refused genetic counseling and was persuaded by her husband to accept obstetric care at a perinatal center only to please him.

This brief look at the physiology, pathology, and psychology of pregnancy and its accompanying complications points out how closely they influence each other. To examine only some of these factors is to fail to recognize the woman as a whole person. It is only in attempting to assess the interaction of these elements as they relate to an individual that the nurse can form a picture of what it is like for this woman, this fetus, this family, to experience a high-risk pregnancy.

MONITORING MATERNAL WELL-BEING DURING HIGH-RISK PREGNANCY

Because of the unique relationship between mother and fetus, it is somewhat artificial to speak of monitoring maternal and fetal well-being separately. Throughout gestation the woman's nutrition and physical status as well as her emotional status are observed in order to promote her optimum health. The pathology which complicates the pregnancy is followed, using the tests and procedures appropriate to the individual pathology. For example, diabetics will have blood glucose values taken, renal function studies will be routine for those women with kidney disease, and so on. It is important to keep in mind when interpreting the results of these tests that normal values during pregnancy may be significantly different from normal values in the non-pregnant state. (See page 877 for common laboratory values during pregnancy.)

It is not uncommon for periods of hospitalization to be required during the course of a high-risk pregnancy. Sometimes these may be quite extended periods. The diabetic woman may be admitted for diabetic control and teaching. A hypertensive woman or one with renal disease may require complete bed rest and almost continuous monitoring of kidney functions and fetal well-being. Third trimester hemorrhage may dictate hospitalization for other women.

Whatever the reason which precipitates admission to the hospital this is likely to be a very stressful experience for the family. Her very presence in a hospital emphasizes the severity of the risk to mother and infant. In addition, the family is separated and hospitals are universally uncomfortable places to take up residence.

Besides caring for the high-risk pregnancy the team of caregivers must direct their attention in two other directions: facilitating the woman's adaptation to being an inpatient, and assisting the family to modify their lives to accommodate the absence of an important member. The accomplishment of one will help with the other. If the woman knows her children are safely cared for at home by grandma or a neighbor she can rest somewhat easier. If her husband contrives to keep up with his job, manage the household, and still find time to visit her, her contentment will be greater. Conversely, if the family is comfortable in the understanding that both they and the woman are kept clearly informed regarding the plan of care, they will accept the inconveniences easier. If they also see that their wife or daughter or mother is treated with respect and her privacy is valued, a bad situation will be a bit better.

Opportunities for frequent visiting by family members, including children, should be available. If complete bed rest is not necessary, the use of passes to permit an afternoon or day away from the hospital should be considered.

Time passes slowly for these hospitalized women, especially if they feel well. It is a constant challenge to them and to the staff to provide occupation and diversion. Reading, needlework, television, and puzzles become tiresome after a while. It is often helpful if several antepartum women are able to share a room. In such situations they are very helpful to each other and many close friendships develop.

METHODS OF MONITORING FETAL STATUS

The severity of maternal disease is reflected in the growth and development of the fetus. It is difficult, if not impossible, to think of a condition which places the mother at risk without affecting her fetus. Indeed, the fetus is usually the more vulnerable of the two. Thus it is important to attempt to evaluate fetal well-being throughout complicated gestations.

Although at present the therapeutic repertoire for intrauterine intervention remains quite limited, it is often possible to forestall the more calamitous events. This is particularly true during the third trimester. At this time, careful observations of fetal status may permit delivery prior to damage from placental insufficiency. For the fetus whose intrauterine existence is made precarious by chronic hypertension or toxemia, the environment of a modern neonatal intensive care unit may be much more hospitable. On the other hand, determination of fetal lung-maturity may prevent delivery of an infant too immature to adapt successfully to extrauterine life.

Physical Examinations

1. At each antepartum visit the height of the fundus is measured from the symphysis pubis to the upper rim of the fundus. This measurement gives an estimate of the growth of the fetus. Failure of the uterus to grow properly is suggestive of intrauterine growth retardation, while sudden increases in growth may indicate a multiple gestation or polyhydramnios.

2. In addition, the abdomen is palpated to determine uterine contour as well as presentation and position of the fetus. Unusual contours are indicative of anatomic abnormalities of the uterus and often predispose to breech or transverse presentations. Unusual presentation in a normal uterus may suggest an abnormally implanted placenta or fetal anomalies.

3. The woman should be questioned about fetal movement, how it varies over time and how it compares with her other pregnancies. Although fetal movement is quite variable and made even more so by the subjectivity of the reporting, a sudden change in movement bears further investigation. This is especially true if the change is one of decreased movement or of no movement.

4. Auscultation of the fetal heart rate with a standard fetoscope or doptone is an important diagnostic tool for several reasons. The time of initial auscultation with the fetoscope is corroborative evidence of gestational age. Periodic counting establishes the individual baseline for each fetus against which variations can be measured. Bradycardia (less than 100 beats per minute) is associated with congenital heart disease, and tachycardia (more than 180 beats per minute) is suggestive of maternal fever or thyrotoxicosis, or fetal hypoxia, or certain drugs which produce maternal tachycardia.

The presence of a normal fetal heart rate, however, has no predictive value, and the nurse should not be overly reassured by hearing a heartbeat in the face of other ominous signs. Absence of fetal heartbeat should be further evaluated by an ultrasound examination for cardiac pulsation before a diagnosis of intrauterine death is considered.

Amniocentesis

Amniocentesis consists of introducing a needle through the abdominal and uterine walls into the amniotic cavity in order to remove some fluid for examination. After emptying her bladder, the woman is made as comfortable as possible on the examining table. The physician palpates her abdomen for fetal position and to estimate the placental site. It is becoming increasingly common also to employ ultrasonic scanning to pinpoint the placenta and a pool of amniotic fluid removed from fetal vital parts. In this manner the risks of amniocentesis can be reduced to a negligible figure. The abdomen is then prepped with an antiseptic solution, and, using sterile equipment and technique, the physician inserts a long small gauge needle into the

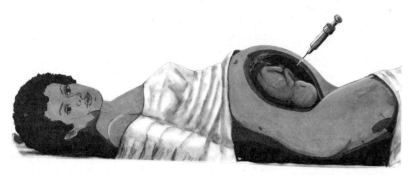

Figure 21-1. Cross section through a pregnant uterus showing the relationship of the amniocentesis needle to the fetus and placenta.

amniotic cavity and withdraws the required amount of fluid, which is sent for the appropriate laboratory analysis (Fig. 21-1).

Prior to the procedure the woman and her family should have a careful explanation of the procedure itself, what information is being sought, and its importance to the fetus. Women have described the pain of the procedure as being comparable to the sensation of having blood withdrawn from the arm. In addition, many describe a pulling sensation as the fluid is being aspirated. The supine position during the procedure is often uncomfortable, particularly as gestation progresses and the uterus grows heavier. Especially during the third trimester, the woman may experience supine hypotension. This, accompanied by her natural anxiety, brings about dizziness, nausea, and occasionally vomiting. She may appear quite pale and feel clammy, although complaining of being too warm. A slight elevation of the head of the examining table or movement to a semilateral position will often prevent this troublesome situation. A cool cloth for her head or throat is often soothing and an emesis basin within easy reach is a wise precaution.

When the amniocentesis is completed the fetal heart tones should be auscultated to be sure there have been no immediate ill effects on the fetus. If the woman has been dizzy or nauseated she will usually feel better if she rests on her side for a few minutes before leaving the examining room.

If blood is aspirated during the procedure it should be analyzed at once to determine whether it is fetal or maternal blood. In the event it is fetal, close monitoring of fetal heart rate for 1 to 2 hours is a wise precaution.

Amniotic fluid may be analyzed for a wide variety of constituents. Only those having the most practical clinical application are discussed here.

Genetic Diagnosis

When amniocentesis is performed for genetic diagnosis, it is generally done as early as is practical, usually about 14–16 weeks gestation. The fluid obtained may be chemically examined, cells floating in the fluid may be examined, or fibroblasts may be cultured from the cells and studied. This latter procedure requires from 3 to 5 weeks to obtain a sufficient amount of material for examination. Genetic disorders characterized by chromosomal abnormalities (trisomies, translocations, and others) and certain metabolic disorders can be diagnosed in this manner.

An additional tool for prenatal diagnosis of genetic defects is the determination of alpha-fetoprotein (AFP), a protein produced by the yolk sac and the fetal liver. This substance reaches its peak at about 14–16 weeks gestation and then declines steadily throughout pregnancy. In the presence of open neural tube defects (anencephaly, spina bifida, meningomyelocele) the amount of AFP in amniotic fluid is increased eight times that of normal.[1]

[1] R. Harris, R. F. Jennison, A. J. Barson, K. M. Laurence, E. Ruoslatti, and M. Seppala, Comparison of amniotic fluid and maternal serum alphafetoprotein levels in early antenatal diagnosis of spina bifida and anencephaly, *Lancet* 1:429–433 (Mar. 16) 1974.

Monitoring of Rh-Sensitized Fetuses

The monitoring of Rh-sensitized fetuses is discussed in Chapter 22, page 649, along with the subject of pregnancy complicated by isoimmune disease.

Maturity Studies

Prematurity is the leading cause of perinatal death. Whenever possible, it is desirable to determine prior to birth whether or not the fetus is capable of surviving in the extrauterine environment. Ideally, then, delivery would be postponed until such maturity is achieved. Unfortunately, the present state of the art does not always permit this. The more commonly used indicators of fetal maturity are discussed below.

LECITHIN/SPHINGOMYELIN RATIO (L/S) A surface-active phospholipid-protein substance known as surfactant normally lines the alveoli of the lungs. Surfactant is produced by the alveolar lining cells of adults and infants and is secreted onto the surface of the alveoli to form a lining film which lowers the surface tension in the alveoli. Surface tension is ordinarily quite high between any two moist surfaces and would therefore be a hindrance to alveolar expansion without the presence of surfactant. For effective respiratory function in the newborn it is essential not only that the potential air spaces are developed but also that surfactant is being produced in sufficient quantities to prevent atelectasis and respiratory distress. (See pp. 785–91.)

Lecithin is the major constituent of alveolar surfactant, and sphingomyelin is one of several related phospholipids which complete its makeup. These substances, produced in the fetal lung, are washed out into amniotic fluid by the respiratory-like movements of the fetal lung and chest and can be measured in amniotic fluid. The ratio of lecithin to sphingomyelin is determined to assess the degree of fetal lung development. The lungs have a developmental sequence that is, in part, independent of gesta-

tional age. The amount of lecithin at a given age varies among individual infants, some producing greater or lesser quantities than the average.

Lecithin is produced beginning at about 20–22 weeks gestation and gradually increases throughout pregnancy, while the amount of sphingomyelin remains essentially the same. Until approximately the thirty-fifth week a less stable form of lecithin is produced, a form more sensitive to acidosis, hypothermia, and other stress. Around thirty-five weeks there is a surge of the major surfactant lecithin, which is very stable and active. This explains in part why premature infants are more susceptible to respiratory distress syndrome.

At the time of the lecithin surge at thirty-five weeks the amount of lecithin rises to more than two times that of sphingomyelin, and thereafter the ratio continues to rise. Thus L/S ratio gives the best prediction for extrauterine survival, since adequate pulmonary function is of critical importance and this ratio is a functional measurement of pulmonary alveolar stability. Although the values may differ from one laboratory to another, according to Gluck, who did the initial work, when the lecithin to sphingomyelin ratio is greater than 2.0 the fetus is considered to have pulmonary maturity and to be unlikely to develop respiratory distress syndrome. Ratios in the 1.0–1.9 range indicate a possibility for the development of respiratory distress, while ratios less than 1 are predictive of severe respiratory distress. If an infant with an immature L/S ratio must be delivered, the neonatal team must be alerted and plans made for immediate respiratory support therapy after birth.

Although research is inconclusive at this time, there is some evidence that several factors may act to enhance or delay surfactant production in addition to the infant's own individual pattern of development. Stress appears to be a factor which promotes earlier pulmonary maturation. Therefore, some conditions such as toxemia, narcotic addiction, intrauterine growth retardation, and premature rupture of the membranes have been associated with an early rise in L/S ratios.[2] Some investigators have suggested that mild diabetes mellitus retards surfactant production, but others have refuted this.

In 1968 Liggins observed that corticosteroid injection of fetal lambs improved the survival ratio when they were prematurely delivered. Since then he has demonstrated similar effects in humans.[3] A national corroborative study is currently under way to determine if this is a safe and useful therapeutic tool. Until the effectiveness of this and other research protocols is established a conservative management approach is usually adopted. Attempts are made to postpone delivery until a mature L/S is obtained, if this can be done safely for both mother and fetus. Repeat amniocentesis is done after a reasonable interval. Depending on the gestational age and the risks inherent in maintaining the pregnancy, this interval may be 3–4 days or it may be 1–2 weeks.

Approximately 5 ml of amniotic fluid is needed for the L/S ratio test, which requires 1–1½ hours to complete. If the test is not to be done for several hours after the fluid is obtained, it must be refrigerated, as the lecithin may deteriorate at room temperature. Bloody or meconium-stained fluid may give false results.

"FOAM" TEST ("Shake" Test, "Bubble" Test). The "foam" test, also called the "shake" test or "bubble" test, is a simple and rapid test for the presence of surfactant in amniotic fluid. Although it is useful as a screening test, it lacks the precision of the L/S ratio and is therefore not as useful for decision making in complex high-risk situations. The test is performed by shaking a 1:2 dilution of 90 percent ethanol and amniotic fluid and observing the foam or bubbles which appear at the surface of the liquid. A complete ring of bubbles which remains for 15 minutes is considered a positive test and is correlated with mature lungs. A negative test is not interpretable and requires a specific L/S determination if immediate information is necessary.

AMNIOTIC FLUID CREATININE The concentration of the metabolic end product creatinine increases progressively in the amniotic fluid as the fetus approaches term. It is assumed that this rise is due to the fetal urine excretion, reflecting increasing muscle mass, as term approaches. Creatinine values of 2 mg per 100 ml of amniotic fluid appear to correlate closely with a pregnancy of 37 weeks duration or more.

However, because this test is only an indirect measure of the vital pulmonary maturity and, for example, could be subject to variation in pregnancies complicated by intrauterine growth retardation, its greatest usefulness is in uncomplicated pregnancies. In situations where confirmation of maturity is desirable before scheduling a cesarean section or elective induction of labor this test appears to be highly satisfactory. A maternal serum creatinine value should be obtained to ensure that the amniotic fluid level is not a reflection of maternal excess.

BILIRUBIN LEVEL IN AMNIOTIC FLUID A marked decrease in the normal amount of bilirubin in the amniotic fluid occurs as the fetus approaches term. The bilirubin virtually disappears in the last month of gestation. Using the optical deviation at 450 nm as an index, a fall in optical density in the last weeks of pregnancy is considered by many to be an assurance of fetal maturity. Exposure of the fluid to light at any time for more than a few seconds may invalidate this test.

CYTOLOGIC STUDIES OF CELLS IN AMNIOTIC FLUID Although the fetus desquamates cells throughout his intrauterine existence, the sebaceous glands become functional and shed cells rather late in gestation. The sebaceous cells are

[2] Louis Gluck and Marie V. Kulovick, Lecithin/sphingomyelin ratios in amniotic fluid in normal and abnormal pregnancy, *Am. J. Obstet. Cynecol.* 115:539–546 (Feb. 15) 1973.

[3] G. C. Liggins and R. N. Howie, A controlled trial of antepartum glucocorticoid treatment for prevention of the respiratory distress syndrome in premature infants, *Pediatrics*, 50:515 (Oct.) 1972.

distinguishable from other shed cells by the presence of lipid globules. The percentage of these fat cells gives an indication of fetal age. The cells are recognized by the use of a Nile blue sulfate stain. In general, a lipid cell count of 20 percent or greater indicates 36 weeks gestation or more. The test may be invalid if the amniotic fluid is contaminated with blood or meconium or if vernix caseosa particles are visible to the naked eye. The test does, however, help to distinguish the premature from the mature infant.

Laboratory Studies of Placental Function

Placental insufficiency is a significant factor in intrauterine growth retardation and in fetal death. Without an adequately functioning placenta, sufficiently supplied by maternal circulation, the fetus cannot obtain enough nutrients and oxygen for health and growth. For this reason measures of placental function are particularly good indicators of fetal well-being.

Estriol Excretion Studies

The measurement of estriol excretion in the maternal urine is particularly well suited to the purpose of estimating both placental function and fetal well-being. As discussed in Chapter 6, this hormone is produced by the joint activity of fetus and placenta and as such requires a certain level of health in both.

Estriol is excreted in the maternal urine in progressively increasing amounts throughout pregnancy. Although values may vary from one laboratory to another, the mean values are usually considered to be as follows: 1 mg per 24 hours at 20 weeks gestation; 8 mg at 28 weeks; 12 mg at 32 weeks; 17 mg at 36 weeks; and 30 mg at term. There is a wide variation in the normal value for any individual in a given 24-hour period. This variation is usually the result of maternal factors such as the completeness of the 24-hour urine collection, amount of fluid intake, kidney dynamics, and the amount of bed rest. It is commonly accepted practice to perform a creatinine measurement on all specimens collected for estriol determination. Because creatinine levels remain fairly constant unless there is an unusual period of strenuous exercise, a creatinine level above 1.0 mg per 24 hours gives reasonable assurance of a complete specimen collection. (In situations where there is significant renal pathology, individual interpretations must be made.)

Because of the normally wide variations in estriol values mentioned above, it is important to keep two things in mind when making clinical interpretations. First, single values of estriol are meaningless by themselves unless they are in the extremely low range incompatible with fetal survival (usually less than 2 mg per 24 hours). Rather, the trend of values over time is more important, with consistently rising values being indicative of fetal well-being regardless of the absolute numbers. Second, in order for a decreasing value to be significant there must be a 50 percent drop from the previous value. This information indicates the necessity for doing serial assays at least three times per week in order to be able to observe developing trends (Fig. 21-2). Daily urine collections are not unusual in situations of grave risk to the fetus.

Urine collections for estriol determination are usually begun about 32 weeks gestation and continued until term. This procedure is often one of the more annoying and stressful aspects of the medical regimen with which the woman is asked to comply. Every effort should be made to give careful instructions about the procedure and its importance and to provide supportive care as needed. Particular emphasis should be placed on the importance of collecting all urine for a 24-hour period. The usual procedure is to begin with the second voiding in the morning and end with the first voiding (inclusive) the following morning. The collection is usually made easier if the woman is provided with a container which fits under her toilet seat as well as a leakproof jar in which to store the urine until it is delivered to the laboratory. Refrigeration is not necessary.

The nurse should be aware that certain drugs may influence estriol values, usually causing

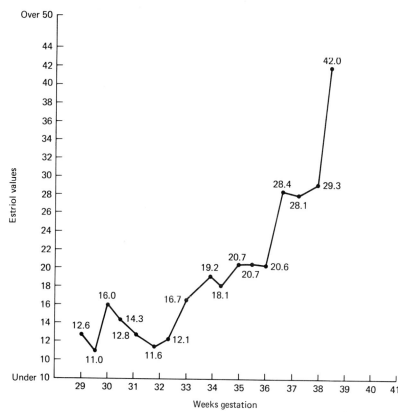

Figure 21-2. Graph of the actual urinary estriol values for a young woman who is a Class A diabetic. Notice that, although individual values may remain unchanged from the previous recording, or may even drop, the overall trend is a rise as gestation progresses.

them to be lowered. Among these drugs are Mandelamine, ampicillin, laxatives containing phenolphthalein, and corticosteroids. Furthermore, in pregnancies complicated by Rh isoimmunization or eclampsia estriol values are not reliable indicators of fetal well-being.

Human Chorionic Somatomammmotropin (HCS)

Human chorionic somatomammotropin, also known as human placental lactogen (HPL), is a hormone produced by the placenta in increasing amounts throughout pregnancy. Like estriol it has the potential of serving as an index of placental function and therefore of fetal well-being. It has the advantage of being a serum study which can be done weekly, thus avoiding the difficulties inherent in 24-hour urine collections. Present methods of assay, however, are expensive and not easily performed in most labora-

tories. With the development of more practical laboratory methodology this test may become a useful adjunct to high-risk pregnancy management. It shows particular promise in the treatment of postdate pregnancies where it has been shown to be useful in predicting which postdate pregnancies involve a dysmature, and therefore at risk, fetus. However, normal values are so variable that interpretation is difficult at present and other tests should be considered together with the HPL.

Electronic Assessment Methods

Ultrasonic Echo Sounding or Sonar

Ultrasonic echo sounding (sonar) utilizes pulsed sound waves of very high frequency, 1–10 million cycles per second. These sound waves are projected as tiny beams of energy

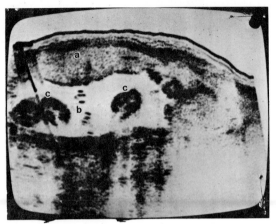

Figure 21-3. Sonogram performed prior to an amniocentesis to localize a safe pool of amniotic fluid removed from fetal vital parts and placenta. Note the marker which shows not only the location but also the depth of penetration required. Structures easily identified are *a*, placenta; *b*, umbilical cord; *c*, cross section through fetal limbs. [*Courtesy of R. O. Friday, M.D., Department of Radiology, Madison General Hospital, Madison, Wisconsin.*]

from a transducer applied directly to the woman's abdomen. They echo, or reflect, from interfaces of tissues of different acoustical density. These echoes are received by the same transducer which transmitted them, converted into electrical impulses, and displayed on an oscilloscope or television screen. In obstetric usage the most common method of display on the oscilloscope is the B-scan; that is, cross-sectional images of the patient are obtained by moving the transducer over the patient. More recent equipment permits this information to be displayed in eight to ten shades of grey (grey scale). A permanent record can be made of the television display by means of photography.[4]

Ultrasound is valuable in many ways in obstetric practice. Pregnancy may be confirmed by visualizing a gestational sac as early as 5 weeks gestation. Likewise, a "blighted ovum" or molar pregnancy may be detected. A pocket of amniotic fluid removed from fetal vital parts can be localized to increase the accuracy and safety of amniocentesis (Fig. 21-3). It is also possible to determine multiple gestations, unusual presentations, and certain congenital anomalies such as anencephaly, hydrocephaly, hydronephrosis, and fetal ascites.

By measuring the biparietal diameter (BPD) of the fetal head and comparing this measurement with a nomogram it is possible to date the gestation. This is presently the most accurate and reliable method of dating pregnancies. By taking serial measurements of the biparietal diameter every two to three weeks and again comparing with the nomogram it is possible to trace fetal growth (Fig. 21-4). In the early stages of intrauterine malnutrition the head will continue to grow at an appropriate rate, but the ultrasound picture will show a discrepancy between the size of the head and the size of the trunk. Body weight and length are affected before head size in intrauterine growth retardation. Later the growth of the head will begin to lag and the ultrasound picture will show a symmetrically small fetus.

One of the most common uses of ultrasound is the localization of the placenta in situations where placenta previa is suspected. In these cases, ultrasound can either confirm or deny placenta previa as the cause of third trimester bleeding and therapeutic intervention can be planned accordingly (Fig. 22-3, page 634).

Ultrasonography as a tool for medical diagnosis is undergoing very rapid exploration and development. As the equipment is refined and personnel gain skill and experience in using it, its capabilities will no doubt expand proportionally. Already fetal movements, including cardiac contraction, can be detected as early as 6–8 weeks gestation, fetal respiratory movements and even detailed fetal anatomy can be visualized. Methods of determining fetal weight are being studied, and fairly accurate estimates are already available from measurements of abdominal and/or thoracic circumference. Perfection of these methods should improve detection of the growth-retarded fetus. If present evi-

[4] Jay P. Sackler and Anthony M. Passalaqua, Diagnostic uses of ultrasound, *Postgrad. Med.* 60:95–101 (Aug.) 1976.

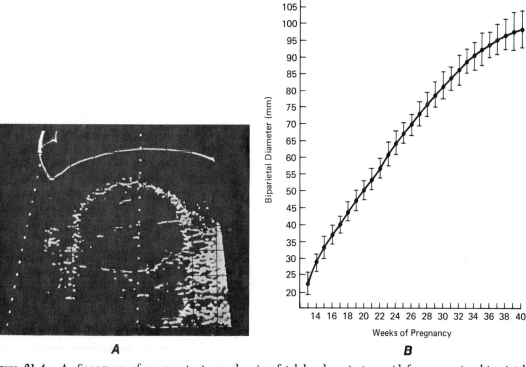

Figure 21-4. **A.** Sonogram of pregnant uterus showing fetal head against a grid for measuring biparietal diameter. This BPD of 79 mm corresponds to a gestational age of approximately 30 weeks on the nomogram shown in **B.** Note the location of the placenta, which is the white area in the lower right-hand corner. [*Courtesy of R. O. Friday, M.D., Department of Radiology, Madison General Hospital, Madison, Wisconsin.*] **B.** Mean fetal biparietal diameter (mm) ± 2 SD for each week of pregnancy from 13 weeks to term (1029 measurements). [*Reproduced with permission from Stuart Campbell and G. G. Neuman, "Growth of the Fetal Biparietal Diameter During Normal Pregnancy," J. Obstet. Gynaecol. Br. Commonw. 78:513–519, 1971.*]

dence concerning its harmlessness to mother and fetus is further substantiated, ultrasound should become an even more important tool in the perinatal care of the future.

When a woman is to have an ultrasonic examination certain explanations are necessary. First, she should be reassured that there are no known ill-effects of the procedure either for herself or her infant. The procedure is a painless one, although the woman may become tired and uncomfortable from the hard examining table. An additional source of discomfort is the fact that the procedure is most successful if the woman has a full bladder. Finally, the woman should expect that a contact medium such as mineral oil

will be applied to her abdomen to facilitate the examination (Fig. 21-5).

Antepartum Fetal Heart Rate Monitoring

Using an external fetal heart rate monitor, the fetal heart rate is recorded in a resting state. The baseline is observed for tachycardia and beat-to-beat variability. Tachycardia over 160 beats per minute or loss of beat-to-beat variability may reflect fetal hypoxia. Such findings are poor prognostic signs. Should a spontaneous Braxton-Hicks contraction occur the heart rate is observed for one of the periodic patterns.

This method of assessing fetal well-being is still in the research phase. It is very time con-

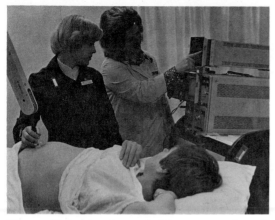

Figure 21-5. As the technician passes the ultrasound transducer over the abdomen a nurse explains to this mother that the upper screen is used to ensure that sound reception is adequate. The lower screen is where the biparietal picture will appear. [*Copyright Sept./Oct., 1976, The American Journal of Nursing Company. Reproduced with permission from Karen G. Galloway, "Placental Evaluation Studies: The Procedures, Their Purposes, and the Nursing Care Involved," MCN, Am. J. Maternal Child Nursing 1(5):300–306 (Sept.–Oct.) 1976, p. 303.*]

suming and would appear to detect only the most seriously compromised fetuses.

Oxytocin Challenge Test (OCT)

The oxytocin challenge test involves the administration of intravenous oxytocin to stimulate uterine contractions while simultaneously monitoring uterine activity and fetal heart rate with an external monitor. It is well known that uterine contractions interfere with uteroplacental blood flow. In pregnancies where there is a diminished fetal–placental reserve the fetus will become hypoxic during a contraction. This hypoxia will be reflected in the monitor tracing as a late deceleration. (For a detailed discussion of fetal heart rate patterns see Chapter 14, pages 316–21.)

If late decelerations occur in response to contractions, and they cannot be corrected by altering the maternal position, the OCT is said to be positive (Fig. 21-6). These fetuses are unlikely to tolerate labor and vaginal delivery and are at very high risk for intrauterine growth retardation, intrauterine asphyxia, and death. In the presence of a positive OCT and a mature L/S ratio labor is induced and a cesarean section performed if warranted by continued late decelerations and fetal acidosis.

The OCT is said to be negative when no untoward changes occur in the fetal heart rate during contractions. The fetus who has a negative OCT is felt to be at no danger from the intrauterine environment for the ensuing week unless there is a change in maternal status. Should there be a change in maternal status, such as the development of toxemia, change in diabetic control, or dropping estriol values, the fetus should be reevaluated. Otherwise the test will be repeated on a weekly basis from about 32–34 weeks gestation until delivery.

OCTs may be interpreted as inconclusive if clear-cut results cannot be obtained. Common causes for these results are insufficient or excessive uterine activity, poor recording of uterine activity because of obesity, edema, or polyhydramanios, and poor recording of fetal heart rate because of excessive fetal activity. Such tests should be repeated within 24 hours.

An OCT may be designated "suspicious" when occasional but inconsistent late decelerations occur. Such tests are usually repeated in 48 to 72 hours.

The woman having an oxytocin challenge test should plan to spend about a half day for this procedure. Although the test itself requires an average of about 90 minutes, it is not uncommon for up to three hours to be utilized. After changing into a gown, the woman assumes a semi-Fowler's position in bed and the external

Figure 21-6. *A.* Fetal monitor tracing of a negative oxytocin challenge test (OCT). Note the regularity of the fetal heart rate at 140 beats per minute in the presence of good quality uterine contractions occurring every 3 minutes. *B.* Fetal monitor tracing of a positive oxytocin challenge test (OCT). Late decelerations occur with each contraction, indicating a likelihood of placental insufficiency.

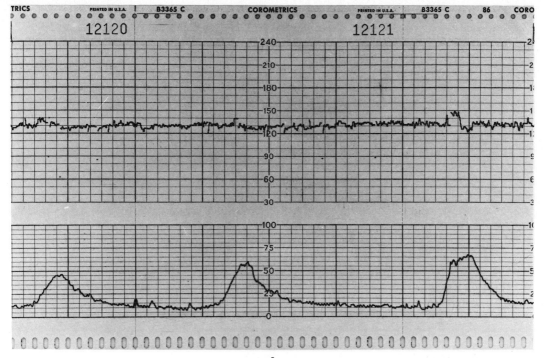

A

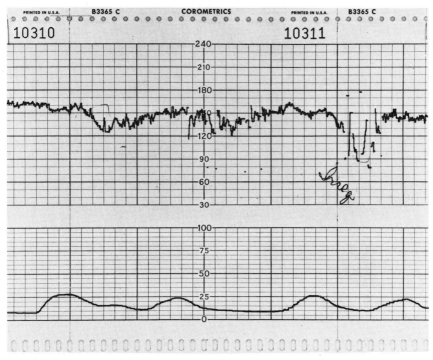

B

microphone or ultrasound transducer is applied to record the fetal heart rate. A tocodynamometer is used to measure uterine activity (Fig. 21-7). After recording 15–30 minutes of baseline fetal heart rate an intravenous infusion of oxytocin is begun by continuous infusion pump. Oxytocin is initially delivered at the rate of 0.5 mU/min with the rate being increased every 15 minutes until contractions of "good" quality occur at the rate of three in ten minutes. The quality of the contractions is subjectively determined by the nurse doing the test. When the monitor tracing has been evaluated the oxytocin is discontinued and the woman observed until contractions have stopped.

The amount of skilled professional time required for this test makes it quite costly as well as inconvenient for the woman and her family. In addition, there is a risk of initiating premature labor. At the present time, however, it gives the most precise assessment of fetal status and its use is indicated whenever there is a risk of placental insufficiency.

The time required for the OCT can be profitably used to develop sound nurse/client relationships, to do informal teaching, and to observe ways the woman and her family cope with the procedure. Many couples have found the oxytocin challenge test to be a useful "dress rehearsal" for labor and have used the opportunity to practice coaching and breathing techniques. They have learned to use the monitor to help them time contractions and breathing patterns. In addition, these periods of intense focusing on

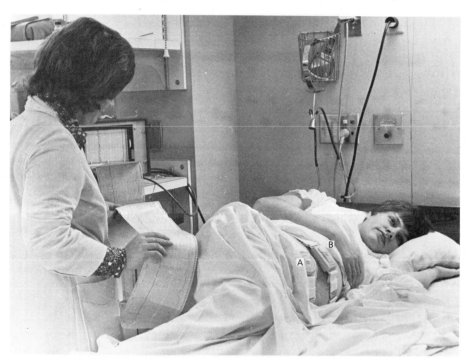

Figure 21-7. This woman is having an oxytocin challenge test (OCT). The ultrasonic transducer (A) and the tocodynamometer (B) are applied to the abdomen to monitor the fetal heart rate and uterine activity, respectively. The nurse is examining the tracing. [*Copyright Sept./Oct., 1976, The American Journal of Nursing Company. Reproduced with permission from Karen G. Galloway, "Placental Evaluation Studies: The Procedures, Their Purposes, and the Nursing Care Involved," MCN, Am. J. Maternal Child Nursing 1(5):300–306 (Sept.–Oct.) 1976, p. 305.*]

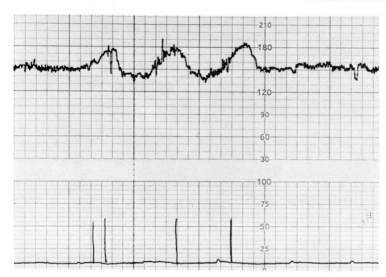

Figure 21-8. Fetal heart rate tracing illustrating a positive fetal activity acceleration determination (FAD). The vertical lines on the uterine activity graph represent fetal movement. Note that the fetal heart rate accelerates from a baseline of approximately 150 beats per minute in response to each period of fetal movement.

the movements and heart rate of their infant may facilitate the attachment process.

Fetal Activity Acceleration Determination (FAD)

Several investigators have noted the presence of transient fetal heart rate accelerations associated with fetal movement. They also observed that these accelerations appeared to be predictive of negative oxytocin challenge tests.[5,6] Performance of this test again requires a period of continuous monitoring of fetal heart rate. The woman is asked to indicate each time fetal movement occurs and the fetal heart rate is observed at the same time. A brief period of fetal heart rate acceleration occurs in association with activity in those situations where there is adequate fetal reserve. If the fetus is inactive, abdominal palpation is used to stimulate activity. Inability to stimulate activity by this method is regarded as a warning sign. The occurrence of 3–4 FHR accelerations with fetal movement is termed a positive FAD (Fig. 21-8). Failure to show accelerations even with external manipulation is termed a negative FAD. If questionable

accelerations occur and/or movements are weak and infrequent the test is termed inadequate.

Since the results of these tests in initial research correlate highly with the results of oxytocin challenge tests, it is being suggested by some authorities that the FAD replace the OCT as a screening test. Only fetuses demonstrating a negative or inadequate FAD would be given an oxytocin challenge test.[7] Like many of the tests used in high-risk obstetrics the value of the fetal activity acceleration determination has yet to be established in widespread use. At this time, however, it appears to be a promising answer to some of the risks and inconveniences of the OCT.[8]

SUMMARY

Approximately 15% of pregnancies in the United States may be classified as high-risk pregnancies. In giving nursing care to the families experiencing these pregnancies it is useful to use a systematic framework. One such frame-

[5] Jay P. Sackler and Anthony M. Passalaqua, *op. cit.*
[6] Barry Schifrin, Rating the fetal stress test, *Contemp. Ob/Gyn* 5:15–17 (June) 1975.

[7] Chang Y. Lee *et al.*, A study of fetal heart rate acceleration patterns, *Obstet. Gynecol.* 43:142–146, 1975.
[8] Chang Y. Lee, P. C. DiLoreto, and Barbara Lagrand, Fetal activity acceleration determination for evaluation of fetal reserve, *Obstet. Gynecol.* 48:19–26 (July) 1976.

work is presented which emphasizes the interaction of four related factors: the physiology of pregnancy, the pathology of the complication, the psychology of pregnancy, and the psychology of illness.

Methods of evaluating maternal and fetal well-being are discussed. Tests of fetal status include those outlined below:

I. Physical Examination
   A. Height of fundus
   B. Uterine palpation
   C. Fetal movement reports
   D. Fetal heart rate auscultation
II. Amniocentesis
   A. Genetic diagnosis
   B. Monitoring Rh sensitization
   C. Maturity studies
      1. L/S ratio
      2. Foam test
      3. Amniotic fluid creatinine
      4. Bilirubin level in amniotic fluid
      5. Cytologic studies
III. Laboratory Studies of Placental Function
   A. Estriol excretion
   B. HCS
IV. Electronic Assessment Methods
   A. Ultrasound
   B. Antepartum FHR monitoring
   C. OCT
   D. FAD

No single method of evaluating fetal status has been proven to be precise enough in itself. Test results must be evaluated along with history, clinical data, wishes of the parents, and available resources. Advances in technology are only as good as the knowledge and wisdom of the practitioners who interpret the results and their courage and skill in acting on their judgments.

BIBLIOGRAPHY

Anderson, Gerald G., Hobbins, John C., and Speroff, Leon, The high-risk patient, in *Medical Complications During Pregnancy*, edited by Gerald N. Burrow and Thomas F. Ferris. Saunders, Philadelphia, Pa., 1975.

Aubry, Richard H., and Pennington, John C., Identification and evaluation of high-risk pregnancy: The perinatal concept, *Clin. Obstet. Gynecol.* 16:3–27 (Mar.) 1973.

Contemporary Ob/Gyn, An updated guide to diagnostic ultrasound, 3:105–109, 114–117 (Mar.) 1974.

Doust, Bruce D., Role of ultrasound in obstetrics and gynecology, *Hosp. Pract.* 9:143–152 (Oct.) 1973.

Freeman, Roger. Clinical dialogue—The oxytocin challenge test, *Contemp. Ob/Gyn* 6:29–40 (Aug.) 1975.

————, and Goebelsmann, U. W. E., Fetal pulmonary maturity and the L/S Ratio, *Contemp. Ob/Gyn* 4:102–108 (Nov.) 1974.

Gallaway, Karen G., Placental evaluation studies: The procedures, their purposes, and the nursing care involved, *MCN, J. Maternal Child Nurs.* 1:300–306 (Sept./Oct.) 1976.

Gluck, Louis, Pulmonary surfactant and neonatal respiratory distress, *Hosp. Pract.* 6:45–56 (Nov.) 1971.

Grant, Kenneth E. *et al.*, Management of high-risk pregnancy, in *Neonatology*, edited by Gordon B. Avery. Lippincott, Philadelphia, Pa., 1975, pp. 51–60.

Greene, John W., Jr., Assessing maternal estriol excretion, *Contemp. Ob/Gyn* 2:61–64 (Sept.) 1973.

Hull, M. G. R., The basis and application of estrogen assays on urine and blood to assess fetoplacental function in late pregnancy, *J. Perinat. Med.* 4:137–162, 1976.

Hunter, John D. W., A look at high-risk pregnancy, *Birth Family J.* 1:10–14 (Fall) 1974.

Kelly, John V., Diagnostic techniques in prepartal fetal evaluation, *Clin. Obstet. Gynecol.* 17:53–74 (Sept.) 1974.

Lee, Chang Y., DiLoreto, P. C., and Logrand, Barbara, Fetal activity acceleration determination for the evaluation of fetal reserve, *Obstet. Gynecol.* 48:19–26 (July) 1976.

Milunsky, Aubrey, and Alpert, Elliot, Part II: Analysis of false positive and false negative alpha-fetoprotein results, *Obstet. Gynecol.* 48:6–12 (July) 1976.

————, and Alpert, Elliot, Prenatal diagnosis of

neural tube defects. I. Problems and pitfalls: Analysis of 2495 cases using the alpha-fetoprotein assay, *Obstet. Gynecol.* 48:1–5 (July) 1976.

Nadler, Henry L., Prenatal diagnosis of inborn defects: A status report, *Hosp. Pract.* 10:44–58 (June) 1975.

———, Indications for amniocentesis in the early prenatal detection of genetic disorders, *Birth Defects* 7:5–9 1971.

Nesbitt, Robert E. L., Jr., The status of perinatal medicine, *Clin. Perinatol.* 1:173–179 (Mar.) 1974.

Ostergard, Donald R., and Kushinsky, Stanley, Urinary estriol as an indicator of fetal well-being, *Obstet. Gynecol.* 38:74–78 (July) 1971.

Picker, Richard H., Robertson, Robert D., Pennington, John C., and Saunders, Douglas M., A safe method of amniocentesis for lecithin/sphingo-myelin determination in late pregnancy using ultra-sound, *Obstet. Gynecol.* 47:722–724 (June) 1976.

Reeder, Leo G., Social factors in maternal care, in *Maternity Nursing*, 13th ed., edited by Sharon R. Reeder, Luigi Mastroianni, Leonide L. Martin, and Elise Fitzpatrick. Philadelphia, Pa., Lippincott, 1976, Chapter 3, pp. 41–52.

Sabbagha, Rudy E., The high-risk pregnancy: The case for serial cephalometry, *Contemp. Ob/Gyn* 8:69–76 (Nov.) 1976.

Sadowsky, E., and Yaffe, H., Daily fetal movement recording and fetal prognosis, *Obstet. Gynecol.* 41:845–850 (June) 1973.

Weiss, Robert R., Macri, James N., and Elligers, Kenneth W., Origin of amniotic fluid alpha-fetoprotein in normal and defective pregnancies, *Obstet. Gynecol.* 47:697–700 (June) 1976.

22

Obstetric Complications

Some pregnancies are high risk because of complications peculiar to pregnancy alone. These complications, which are the subject of this chapter, include:

1. Pernicious vomiting of pregnancy
2. Antepartum hemorrhagic conditions, in particular abortion, placenta previa, and abruptio placentae
3. Premature labor
4. Prolonged pregnancy
5. Isoimmune disease
6. Hypertensive disease of pregnancy; including toxemia
7. Polyhydramnios
8. Fetal death

PERNICIOUS VOMITING OF PREGNANCY

Pernicious vomiting of pregnancy, or *hyperemesis gravidarum*, may develop during the first three months of pregnancy.

Signs and Symptoms

In pernicious vomiting, the nausea and vomiting in the morning may persist for hours; it may occur later in the day, or even at night; or it may be so persistent that the woman will be unable to retain anything taken by mouth. There may be pain in the stomach, hiccups, and gastric pyrosis (heartburn). Thirst becomes severe.

After food is no longer present in the stomach, the emesis is composed of mucus and bile. Considerable weight may be lost during this period.

Whenever vomiting is severe enough to produce nutritional deficiency or dehydration it is considered hyperemesis. If untreated, further deterioration will occur with ketosis, jaundice, fever, and peripheral neuritis. Death may occur from hepatorenal failure.

Etiology

It is the general opinion that all vomiting of pregnancy is of an organic nature fundamentally. Since some degree of "morning sickness" occurs in about one half of all pregnant women, it is believed that all forms of vomiting in pregnancy are due to some factor commonly present in normal gestation. This factor is unidentified, but possible causes that are considered are a toxic element, or a maladjustment of maternal metabolism, or a change in gastric motility. Pernicious vomiting may develop when this factor becomes unusually active or when it is present to an extraordinary degree. Neuroses or psychologic disturbances resulting from all the adjustments that must be made to a pregnancy may, however, exert an important influence and may be superimposed on the underlying organic cause. An interrelation of the toxic or organic and the neurotic factors is generally acknowledged. The extent to which the woman reacts to the underlying cause is somewhat determined by her emotional stability and her mental reaction to the necessary adjustments during pregnancy.

Treatment and Nursing Care

In many instances pernicious vomiting is prevented by management of "morning sickness."

Drug therapy is often useful. A tranquilizer or sedative may be ordered. An antihistamine, antiemetic, and/or anticholinergic drug may give relief of nausea and vomiting if it is not too severe.

Vomiting can often be treated satisfactorily at home, but, if it remains persistent, hospitalization is advised. The goals of therapy are to counter starvation, correct fluid and electrolyte balance, prevent ketosis, and provide help for emotional distress or neurosis. Dehydration and starvation are treated by parenteral fluids, calories, and vitamins, and a gradual resumption of food. The rest, sedatives, and change of environment that can be given in the hospital may be beneficial in resolving emotional conflicts. Tact and understanding and reassurance are important aspects of care.

For the first 24 to 48 hours of hospitalization all food and fluids by mouth, including water and ice chips, are restricted in order to rest the gastrointestinal tract. As patients with pernicious vomiting usually have a bad taste and dry mouth, a refreshing mouthwash is offered frequently.

Carbohydrate, electrolytes, vitamins, and fluid are given parenterally during the first few days. From 2500 to 3000 ml of fluids are given daily.

An accurate record is kept of fluid intake, urinary output, and all emesis.

After this treatment for one to two days, small servings of solid foods—crackers, dry toast and jelly, dry cereal, baked or mashed potato—are given every two hours, or the solid food is alternated with liquid nourishment in small amounts, not more than 100 ml at one time. Hot tea, carbonated fluids, cold fruit juices, and crushed ice are usually easy to retain. Gradually more liquid is allowed so that the mother is taking as much as she desires up to one-half hour before and after the solid food. It is best not to mix the solid and liquid food for a few days. Some parenteral fluids may be necessary during these first few days, depending on the oral intake.

All foods should be served in very small amounts, attractively prepared, and either very hot or very cold. The dishes should be removed from the bedside as soon as the mother has finished eating. Anything that appeals to the mother, or for which she has a particular craving, may be given, although generally fats are restricted and carbohydrates are encouraged during the first few days. The diet is increased slowly to six small meals daily, this being followed by a gradual resumption of a regular diet.

If vomiting should recur after the patient has taken food, the treatment of nothing by mouth and parenteral fluids is repeated, and feedings are then again gradually resumed.

The mother usually recovers quickly with early and persistent treatment. A few continue to vomit to some extent throughout pregnancy. On rare occasions prolonged hospitalization with hyperalimentation may be required in order to maintain nutrition.

The impact of hyperemesis on the fetus is directly proportional to the severity of the disease. If promptly treated and corrected, the fetus should suffer no ill effects. If weight loss and dehydration are prolonged, fetal nutrition may be jeopardized. Maternal ketosis is thought to influence fetal brain development (Chapter 8, page 178).

ANTEPARTUM HEMORRHAGE

Hemorrhage is a life-threatening situation whenever it occurs. If it occurs during pregnancy there are two lives endangered: that of the mother and that of the fetus. As usual in high-risk pregnancies, it is the fetus who is more vulnerable. However, in spite of blood transfusions and modern surgical techniques, obstet-

Table 22-1. Outline of Important Sources of Hemorrhage During Pregnancy

Early to Midpregnancy	Mid- to Late Pregnancy	Intrapartum and Postpartum
Abortion	Placenta previa	Uterine atony
Extrauterine pregnancy	Marginal sinus	Retained placenta
Molar pregnancy	Vasa previa	Lacerations
Tumors of vulva, vagina, or cervix	Abruptio placentae	Uterine inversion

ric hemorrhage remains one of the three leading causes of maternal mortality.

Table 22-1 outlines the major sources of obstetric hemorrhage according to the period of gestation when they are most apt to occur. It should be remembered that there may be considerable overlapping among the groups.

Abortions

Termination of a pregnancy prior to viability (20 to 24 weeks gestation) is known as an abortion. Abortions can be divided into those which are spontaneous and those which are induced. Spontaneous abortions are commonly referred to as "miscarriages" by the lay public. It is important to make this distinction when talking with a client, since the term abortion may evoke negative feelings sometimes associated with induced abortions.

Spontaneous abortions are further classified as follows:

1. *Threatened abortion*—Transcervical bleeding, frequently associated with back and lower abdominal cramping, but no cervical dilatation or expulsion of the products of conception.
2. *Inevitable abortion*—In addition to bleeding there is progressive cervical dilatation and, often, rupture of the membranes with escape of amniotic fluid.
3. *Incomplete abortion*—Expulsion of only part of the products of conception. This may continue spontaneously to completion.
4. *Complete abortion*—As the term suggests, all products of conception are expelled. This

is most likely to occur before the tenth week because the anchoring villi may not be very firmly attached to the decidua at this time. Sometimes the entire decidual lining of the uterus, having the appearance of a triangular sac, may be expelled. More often the vesicular ovum, surrounded only by decidua capsularis, or only the chorionic vesicle, with no decidual lining, is found. The latter usually has a shaggy appearance, or it may be surrounded by a blood clot (Fig. 22-1).

5. *Missed abortion*—The retention of the products of conception in the uterus for eight weeks or more after fetal death.
6. *Habitual abortion*—The occurrence of three or more consecutive spontaneous abortions.

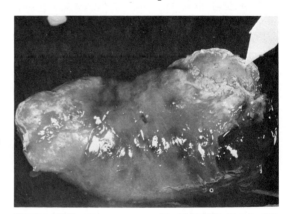

Figure 22-1. Spontaneous complete abortion at 10 weeks of gestation. The arrow points to a part of the amniotic sac that is not surrounded by decidual tissue. This is the mass of tissue that may have the appearance of a blood clot and must be saved for the physician's examination. [*Courtesy of Dr. Madeline J. Thornton.*]

Etiology of Spontaneous Abortions

It is not possible to know how frequently abortions occur. They sometimes happen so early in gestation that the woman was not even aware of her pregnancy, or she may mistake the abortion for delayed menstruation. Estimates about the incidence of abortion suggest that as many as 30 percent of all conceptions terminate in abortion. Three fourths of these occur during the second and third months of gestation.

Well over half of spontaneous abortions are the result of abnormalities of the developing embryo or fetus. In a substantial percentage of pregnancies the fertilizied zygote is intrinsically defective. This may be the result of inadequacies in either the sperm or ovum or due to lethal defects arising from the fertilization of this particular ovum by this particular sperm. Errors in the initial cell divisions also account for some defects. Genetic factors at the chromosome level account for some of these defects as does faulty germ plasm. The latter may result in what is known as a "blighted ovum" or an ovum without an embryo. Abnormality in the development of the placenta is still another cause for abortion.

A number of maternal causes of abortion have been cited. Chronic infections, fibroid tumors, or developmental uterine anomalies may interfere with proper implantation or adequate nourishment of the embryo because of their mechanical effect or because of circulatory disturbances of the decidua.

Acute infections are frequent culprits in abortion. Organisms or toxins may be transferred from the mother to have lethal effects on the embryo/fetus or the fetus may succumb to the effects of very high maternal temperature or anoxia resulting from increased metabolic needs (as in fever) or decreased supply (as in maternal pneumonia).

Endocrine disturbances, especially of the hormones progesterone and thyroid, are also causes of abortion. If there is a true deficiency of progesterone from the corpus luteum, early implantation may not occur. Later, insufficient progesterone may increase uterine sensitivity, contractility, and subsequent expulsion of the pregnancy. Thyroid dysfunction is known to affect both fertility and the ability to carry a pregnancy to viability.

Physical shocks such as falls, blows on the abdomen, jars, jolts, or overexertion are *rarely* the cause of an abortion. They may be precipitating factors when there already exists a marked irritability of the uterine muscle.

Little is understood about the effects of stress, grief, or other psychologic trauma on the incidence of abortion. It can be speculated that extreme anxiety may reduce uterine blood flow, thus placing the fetus at risk for a variety of ill effects, including abortion, premature delivery, and stillbirth. It is to be emphasized that this would indeed be an extreme circumstance.

Exposure of the mother to teratogens, such as drugs or radiation, may be lethal to the embryo/fetus. There is evidence that some industrial chemicals as well as drugs such as alcohol may affect men as well as women, causing germ cell damage. This in turn may result in defective pregnancies, which are either aborted or produce children with anomalies.

A number of groundless beliefs about causes of abortion exist in the tradition of all cultures. Women should be assured, for example, that reaching up or sleeping with the arms over the head will not separate the embryo from the uterine lining. Purgatives apparently have less effect in causing abortion under normal conditions than is generally believed.

The causes of abortions are summarized in Figure 22-2. In simplest form it can be said that pregnancies usually end in abortion either because the products of conception are themselves defective or because the intrauterine environment is hostile.

Prevention

Maintenance of good health and nutrition in both prospective parents is the most important preventive measure. Correction of any disturbance that might interfere with proper implantation or nourishment of the fetus should be accomplished, preferably prior to conception.

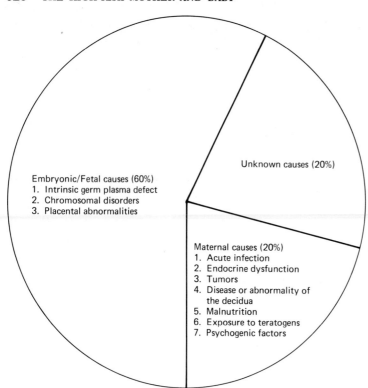

Embryonic/Fetal causes (60%)
1. Intrinsic germ plasma defect
2. Chromosomal disorders
3. Placental abnormalities

Unknown causes (20%)

Maternal causes (20%)
1. Acute infection
2. Endocrine dysfunction
3. Tumors
4. Disease or abnormality of the decidua
5. Malnutrition
6. Exposure to teratogens
7. Psychogenic factors

Figure 22-2. Summary of the more important causes of spontaneous abortion showing the percentages of their occurrence.

Thyroid therapy is used for thyroid dysfunction.

Progesterone has been widely used in an effort to maintain the pregnancy. However, unless there is a true deficiency of this hormone, giving additional progesterone is probably not efficacious. It may in fact be harmful, as progesterone has been implicated in several congenital anomalies.

When abortions are repeated, a careful clinical investigation is recommended to discover possible correctable or preventable conditions. One such investigation is the culturing of the cervix and vagina for the presence of genital mycoplasmas. This organism has been implicated in cases of repeated abortion as well as infertility.[1]

The pregnant woman with a history of spontaneous abortions may be advised to avoid excessive fatigue or physical exertion during the early weeks of pregnancy. Occasionally abstinence from sexual intercourse is suggested. She is usually cautioned to be particularly observant of these precautions at the time menstruation would occur were she not pregnant and at the time she approaches the stage of pregnancy when previous losses occurred.

Symptoms and Treatment

Treatment varies according to the classification of the abortion as threatened, inevitable, incomplete, complete, or missed. The premonitory symptoms, however, are the same for all classifications.

There are vaginal bleeding and pain that is usually intermittent, beginning in the small of the back and finally felt as cramps in the lower part of the abdomen. Since menstruation is suspended during pregnancy, it is a safe precaution to regard any bleeding during this period, with

[1] Hakan Gnarpe and Jan Friberg, Mycoplasma and human reproductive failure, *Am. J. Obstet. Gynecol.* 114:727–731 (Nov. 15) 1972.

or without pain, as a symptom of pending abortion. Because it may be possible in some instances to avert an abortion with treatment, it is advisable for any woman who thinks she is pregnant and who has the slightest bleeding to seek the care of a physician immediately.

In the different classifications of abortion treatment is employed as follows.

THREATENED   It is believed that fetal death has often already occurred when symptoms of abortion appear. Placental hormone production diminishes and the pregnancy cannot be maintained. Bed rest, sedation, and progesterone therapy after symptoms appear do not alter the course of a threatened abortion. The brownish vaginal discharge, which often appears first, is usually followed by true bleeding, uterine cramping, and ultimately expulsion of the products of conception.

Sometimes a small amount of bright-red bleeding, which is physiologic in nature, appears when the fertilized ovum implants. Occasionally, a small amount of bright-red bleeding may be caused by cervical polyps or areas of cervical erosion. About 50 percent of the time bleeding with threatened abortion will cease in a day or two and the pregnancy will continue normally; otherwise it will proceed to termination. Continued bleeding requires a sterile vaginal examination for lesions.

INEVITABLE AND INCOMPLETE   When the bleeding is not profuse in either of these conditions, it may be considered advisable to wait a few hours before interference in the hope that the uterus will expel all of the tissue itself. Blood should be available for transfusion in case bleeding becomes profuse. An oxytocic drug may be given to hasten the process of expulsion of tissue and medication may be needed for pain relief.

The nurse caring for these patients should save all perineal pads for the doctor's inspection. Any tissue or blood clots that are expelled are carefully examined to determine whether or not the abortion has been completed. Since tissue

or clots that are expelled from the uterus sometimes remain in the vagina until the patient changes position, they are often expelled when she sits up to void. The bedpan must, therefore, always be inspected for clots (Fig. 22-1). Catholics believe that every fetus should be baptized, regardless of its immaturity or of the circumstances that have brought about its separation from the mother's body. For instructions for baptism see page 372.

If at any time bleeding becomes profuse, or if the uterus does not soon empty itself completely, operative inteference becomes necessary to remove the retained tissues.

The uterus will usually contract well after it has been emptied and thereby control bleeding. An oxytocic drug will stimulate the uterine muscle to remain contracted. Antibiotics may be administered. If the blood loss has been excessive, blood transfusions are given.

COMPLETE   Treatment and care for a complete abortion consist of observation for bleeding to assure that there is no remaining placental tissue in the uterus.

MISSED   A missed abortion occurs but rarely. In this the embryo or fetus dies and is retained within the uterine cavity, sometimes for many weeks.

A typical history is that the uterus grows quite normally until the third or fourth month, when signs of a threatened abortion may occur. These soon subside, and it is assumed that the pregnancy is progressing normally. Later examination reveals no further uterine enlargement and negative pregnancy tests. Why the uterus does not expel the dead fetus is not known. It is known that a dead fetus can remain in the uterus for months, and even years, without acting as a foreign body or causing symptoms.

Response of the Couple to Loss

The amount of grief experienced by the couple over the loss of the pregnancy is directly proportional to their investment in the pregnancy. Their emotions may range from a sense of relief to profound sorrow. It is typical for the woman to express a feeling of emptiness and, perhaps, of inadequacy. The man's concerns are more apt to center around the woman, since the pregnancy at an early stage is much less real to him than to the woman who has been physically as well as intellectually aware of it.

It is beneficial to both if the couple can share their reactions with each other and be mutually supportive. The nurse should support this relationship by facilitating their talking together, interpreting one to the other if appropriate, and by providing opportunity for them to be together privately.

Facts regarding the etiology of the abortion should be discussed with the couple when and if they are available. History and physical examination of the woman as well as pathology reports on the products of conception may give some insights.

Statements such as "You're young and can have more babies" or "This is nature's way of dealing with defective members" may be theoretically accurate, but they are seldom helpful to grieving parents.

Induced Abortions

Induced abortions may be performed for therapeutic reasons, i.e., because the life of the mother is threatened by the pregnancy or the fetus is known to be defective. With modern advances in obstetric and perinatal care, the medical indications for abortion as a life-saving measure have been almost eliminated. The focus is now changed to the risk of an anomalous child.

Abortions may also be legally induced to terminate an unwanted pregnancy under certain conditions. According to the decision of the United States Supreme Court (Doe v. Bolton and Roe v. Wade) in January, 1973, during the first trimester "the abortion decision and its effectuation must be left to the medical judgment of the pregnant woman's attending physician." After the first trimester, "the State, in promoting its interest in the health of the mother, may, if it chooses, regulate the abortion procedure in ways that are reasonably related to maternal health." After the fetus has reached viability "the State . . . may, if it chooses, regulate, and even proscribe, abortion except where necessary, in appropriate medical judgment, for the preservation of the life or health of the mother."

Methods of inducing abortion are determined in large measure by the stage of gestation. In the first trimester the uterus may be emptied by menstrual extraction, dilatation and curettage (D&C), or dilatation and evacuation (D&E), sometimes referred to as the suction method. After 12 to 14 weeks gestation, the pregnancy is too far advanced for the above methods to be used with safety. Abortion at this time is accomplished either by the intraamniotic instillation of hypertonic saline, the use of prostaglandins, or by hysterotomy.

Menstrual extraction may be performed in an outpatient setting any time up to 14 days following a missed period [42 days from last menstrual period (LMP)]. Without dilating the cervix, a flexible cannula is inserted into the uterus and connected to a vacuum source. The contents of the uterus are then removed by suction.

Dilatation and curettage (D&C) or dilatation and evacuation (D&E) is accomplished by dilating the cervix and removing the products of conception with a ring forceps or a curet or with a vacuum aspirator. Pain relief is provided by an analgesic medication such as meperidine and a block with a local anesthetic of the nerves to the uterus that lie in the paracervical region. The woman is usually discharged from the clinic or hospital on the day of surgery, after assurance that there is no untoward bleeding or pain. She is instructed to report vaginal bleeding greater than a menstrual period and/or persistent abdominal pains. She is also requested to take her temperature daily and to report an elevation over 100°F (37.8°C). She may resume her activities gradually as she feels able. A follow-up visit is usually scheduled for 2 to 4 weeks postoperatively.

Saline or prostaglandin inductions are done in a hospital. Following the instillation of the prescribed solution fetal death occurs, labor begins, and delivery is usually accomplished within 48 hours. For further description of this procedure see page 400.

Hysterotomy is the surgical incision into the uterus through the abdomen. This procedure is frequently accompanied by tubal ligation.

The issue of elective abortion is multidimensional, highly charged with moral, ethical, sociologic, and legal considerations. The woman who chooses this means of ending her pregnancy has often made a very difficult decision. Care from a sympathetic nurse who respects that decision is very comforting. Every effort should be made to make the woman aware of all the options available to her and their realistic outcomes. Following the procedure, information about contraception should be provided as she desires.

Some maternity nurses and physicians, who see their role as bringing life into the world, find it difficult to participate in the care of clients having elective abortions. Staff counseling or rap sessions may help work through these feelings. Anyone is free under the law to refuse to participate in such care for reasons of conscience and may not be penalized for doing so.

Extrauterine Pregnancy

An extrauterine, or ectopic, pregnancy may be defined as a pregnancy that develops outside of the uterus.

Although the fertilized ovum normally travels down the fallopian tube and attaches to the uterine lining, it may become implanted, and begin its development, at any point along the way between the graafian follicle, from which it was expelled, and the uterus, toward which it is moving (Fig. 4-6, page 69). If the fetus develops in the ovary, which is extremely rare, it is termed an ovarian pregnancy. If attachment and development of the ovum occur in the tube, it is termed a tubal pregnancy, this being the most common type of extrauterine pregnancy.

When the ovum attaches itself to the lining of the tube, its history is much the same as when it lodges in the uterus. It erodes into the mucosa, increases in size, and accordingly stretches the surrounding muscle wall. However, the uterine wall is a thick muscular structure and capable of preserving its integrity while being distended. The wall of the tube is very thin and is not designed to meet the strain of a growing mass such as a fetus. As a result, the pregnancy usually terminates within the first three months in one of several ways. A tubal abortion may occur, with the fetus and membranes partly or completely extruded from the fimbriated end of the tube into the peritoneal cavity. The tube may rupture, and the fetus, with or without membranes, may be expelled into the peritoneal cavity or between the folds of the broad ligament. Death and disintegration of the products of conception may take place within the tube.

The point of rupture depends on where the ovum has attached itself. Rupture occurs either because the chorionic villi, which have the power to invade and destroy tissue, have penetrated the wall or because the weakened wall breaks from pressure. Bleeding occurs, varying in amount. A tear that includes a large blood vessel will result in a severe hemorrhage. With abortion through the ampullar end of the tube, bleeding is usually not as profuse or continuous as with rupture of the tube.

The fetus may not be expelled with rupture, or there may be expulsion of the entire products of conception. If the placenta is nearly or completely separated, the fetus dies and may be largely absorbed, or it can be mummified. Rarely, the greater part of the placenta remains attached, and it is possible for the fetus to live and grow and even develop to term. This is called a secondary abdominal pregnancy. The placenta grows out and attaches itself to the other pelvic and abdominal organs.

It is estimated that ectopic pregnancy takes place in approximately 0.3 percent of all pregnancies, with the wall of one of the tubes the most common site of implantation. Tubal pregnancies have a tendency to recur in the same women. Little is definitely known as to their causes but they probably include any condition that interferes mechanically with the downward passage of the fertilized ovum and that favors its lodgment in the tube. This might be true in the case of a diverticulum of the tube or following tubal infection when the lumen would be reduced or distorted as a result of thickening or adhesion of opposing surfaces.

Symptoms

Sometimes the woman does not know she is pregnant, and there may be no symptoms until the tube ruptures. Frequently, however, there is a history of a missed period and slight vaginal bleeding or "spotting." There may also be slight abdominal pain. Early signs and symptoms of pregnancy may be present. The uterus enlarges and decidua develops as in a normal pregnancy. There may be bleeding or menstrual periods may continue, the blood coming from the large vessels in the decidua. If the fetus dies, the decidua will slough off and cause bleeding. Often the first symptom is sudden, excruciating pain in the lower abdomen, which may be on either side or diffuse. The woman suddenly feels faint, becomes very pale, has signs of shock and sometimes coma as a result of hemorrhage into the peritoneal cavity, without appreciable external bleeding. On vaginal examination, the physician finds the changes normally present in the reproductive tract during pregnancy and may palpate an adnexal mass, which is exquisitely tender.

Diagnosis

Diagnosis of an unruptured tubal pregnancy is difficult because the symptoms are often vague. However, for any suspicion of tubal pregnancy several diagnostic procedures are available. A culdocentesis may aid in diagnosis. Intraperitoneal bleeding can often be detected when a needle is inserted through the posterior fornix (Fig. 1-6A, page 9) and blood flows out freely, but failure to obtain blood does not rule out ectopic pregnancy. If the needle puncture of the cul-de-sac is negative, exploration of the area may be made through an incision into the vaginal mucosa and the peritoneum. An affected tube can often be removed through this incision, termed a posterior colpotomy, provided

proper instruments are available for excision of the tube. Adequate precautions must be taken against introduction of infection.

Another exploratory procedure for suspected ectopic pregnancy is a laparoscopy, whereby an instrument for visualization of the pelvic viscera is inserted through a small incision in the lower abdominal wall. If an affected tube is found, a laparotomy is done.

It must be presumed that any woman who is probably pregnant and has sudden abdominal pain and collapse most likely has a ruptured ectopic pregnancy.

Treatment

Usually an operation is immediately performed to excise the affected tube since this condition is very serious. If a diagnosis is made before rupture of the tube occurs, the affected tube is excised as soon as possible to prevent rupture and serious hemorrhage. After rupture, immediate surgery is necessary to remove the affected tube. Blood transfusion to replace the blood loss may be necessary.

The nurse caring for a patient with a suspected ectopic pregnancy should protect her against exertion. She should notify the physician immediately of symptoms of rupture. If rupture has already occurred, she gives the nursing care for shock, as indicated.

For an abdominal pregnancy, surgery is employed upon diagnosis. The placenta usually has to be left in place because hemorrhage cannot be controlled after its removal. If the fetus has died, the vessels supplying the placenta have probably become obliterated and it can be removed more easily.

Hydatidiform Mole and Choriocarcinoma

A hydatidiform mole is a disease of the chorion in which the chorionic villi become cystic and the chorion assumes a grapelike appearance. These cysts may fill the entire uterine cavity. Usually there is no trace of a fetus. This mole is dangerous because its growth may invade the uterine muscle, it may be malignant, or a choriocarcinoma may develop later.

A choriocarcinoma is a very malignant growth which may develop following a normal full-term pregnancy, an abortion, or, more likely, a hydatidiform mole, making follow-up essential.

In the presence of a molar pregnancy, the uterus is typically larger than is expected for gestational age. As the mole separates from its attachment vaginal bleeding occurs. This may occur intermittently or it may be sudden and profuse. Nausea may be unusually severe and signs of toxemia may appear before 24 weeks gestation.

Separation and expulsion of the mole usually takes place in the third or fourth month of pregnancy but may be delayed as long as the sixth month. Complete expulsion of the mole is rare, although fragments are often expelled spontaneously. Since blood loss at the time of expulsion may be severe, the patient must be carefully watched for hemorrhage, and blood should be available for transfusion. A curettage of the uterus is usually performed after expulsion of a mole to remove any fragments of tissue that have remained. With a large mole an abdominal hysterotomy may be necessary for removal.

Chorionic gonadotropin tests may be used as aids in the diagnosis. An increased titer of chorionic gonadotropin is usually present in both molar pregnancy and choriocarcinoma. The urine will give a positive reaction even when greatly diluted. It is best to collect a 24-hour specimen so that an estimate of the total daily output of the hormone can also be made. Ultrasonic scanning of the uterus is useful in diagnosis.

After expulsion of a mole, the woman is advised to avoid pregnancy for at least one year by employing accepted contraceptive measures. Frequent chorionic gonadotropin tests are made with serum or urine. A positive reaction indicates that some living chorionic tissue is left. This may be benign or malignant, but treatment should be reinstituted. This may include surgery or chemotherapy. If the tissue removed is that of a choriocarcinoma the prognosis is more guarded and vigorous treatment is directed toward arresting the malignancy.

Tumors

Small tumors, either benign or malignant, may cause bleeding when associated with pregnancy because of the marked increase in vascularity and pelvic engorgment characteristic of this period. The most common of these tumors are benign cervical polyps. They are readily diagnosed by speculum examination. Malignant tumors of the vagina, cervix, or vulva may be detected upon speculum examination and biopsy.

Placenta Previa

Placenta previa is an obstetric condition characterized by the development of the placenta, either totally or in part, in the lower uterine segment. This condition, which occurs in slightly less than 1 percent of all pregnancies, is subdivided according to the degree to which the placenta encroaches upon the internal cervical os. A complete or total placenta previa occurs when the placenta entirely covers the internal os. In partial placenta previa the os is only partly covered, whereas in a marginal placenta previa (also referred to as a low-lying placenta) only the edge of the placenta reaches the margin of the internal os (Fig. 22-3).

Why the placenta comes to be located in the lower uterine segment rather than in its more usual site in the upper portion of the uterus is not known. It is speculated that endometrial changes associated with such factors as inflammation, age, or closely spaced pregnancies may decrease decidual vascularization and hence nutritional adequacy. For this reason, the placenta grows over a much larger area in an attempt to provide an adequate exchange surface to nourish the fetus. As it spreads out over the endometrial surface it is more likely to impinge upon the cervical os. This theory is somewhat supported by the close correlation between placenta previa and increased parity and maternal age regard-

PLACENTA PREVIA

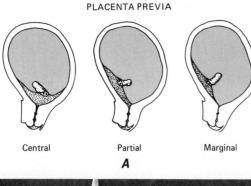

Central   Partial   Marginal

A

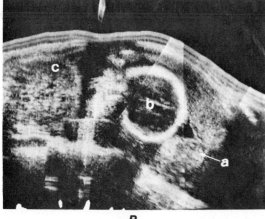

B

Figure 22-3. **A.** Three types of placenta previa are illustrated: complete (placenta totally covers internal cervical os); partial (placenta only partially covers internal cervical os), and marginal, or low-lying (placental edge approaches the rim of the internal os). **B.** Sonogram taken for placental localization. The placenta (*a*) totally covers the internal cervical os (complete previa). The fetal head (*b*) and abdomen (*c*) may also be seen.

less of parity. Placenta previa also occurs more frequently in conditions associated with large placentas such as multiple pregnancy and isoimmune disease of pregnancy.

Symptoms

Painless vaginal bleeding is the classic sign of placenta previa. A review of the physiologic events of pregnancy makes it clear why this bleeding occurs. In the last weeks of pregnancy and during labor the cervix softens, effaces, and begins to dilate. As these changes occur, that part of the placenta in apposition to the internal os is torn from its attachment, causing hemorrhage from the exposed uterine vessels. The same physiology explains why the greater the covering of the cervical os the earlier in gestation hemorrhage is likely to occur. Women with placenta previa may have a history of threatened abortion in the early months of the pregnancy.

Typically, the woman presents at the clinic or hospital in the third trimester with painless, apparently causeless, vaginal bleeding. She often relates awakening in a pool of blood or suddenly seeing blood and clots in the toilet bowl. Assessing the amount of blood loss is difficult as the woman's anxiety tends to exaggerate the amount, particularly if the blood was diluted with water in the toilet. Asking her to compare the amount to a usual menstrual period may provide a somewhat more accurate estimate. It is generally believed that the initial hemorrhage from placenta previa rarely exceeds a few ounces. Bleeding usually stops spontaneously, but may recur periodically without warning until delivery. Each subsequent hemorrhage tends to become progressively more severe.

Placenta previa is commonly associated with malpositions and malpresentations of the fetus, since the placenta occupies part of the space usually occupied by the fetal presenting part. In addition, these women are at increased risk for postpartum hemorrhage, since the lower uterine segment is not capable of contracting and thus does not effectively close the large venous sinuses at the placental site.

Diagnosis

Although unexplained vaginal bleeding in the third trimester is highly suggestive of placenta previa, it is sometimes difficult to verify the diagnosis.

A soft-tissue x-ray may be helpful, but the placenta is not always distinguishable by x-ray. The placenta may be visualized on the film as an area of thickening between the fetal parts and the uterine wall or the bladder. It is not always possible to visualize the placental position, and when the placenta does appear x-ray may not reveal how far down it extends. However, if the placenta is clearly seen in a normal position, the x-ray may help rule out the diagnosis of placenta previa. An additional piece of evidence is the position of the presenting part, especially in a vertex presentation. If the fetal head appears to be displaced from its usual position by a soft tissue mass, or if the presentation is other than vertex, a diagnosis of placenta previa is strengthened.

Sometimes radioisotopes are used to localize the placental position. After the intravenous administration of a radioactive isotope to the mother, the area of greatest radioactive concentration is measured using an external counter or scanning device. The isotope, which is usually technetium, is concentrated in areas of greatest vascularity, hence the ability to localize the placenta. This method is more accurate than x-ray localization and delivers less radiation to mother and fetus, but does require an isotope laboratory and experienced personnel.

Ultrasonography is the safest and most accurate method of diagnosis (Fig. 21-4, page 617). Its use is increasing as the specialized equipment becomes more generally available. (See page 615 for further discussion of ultrasound techniques.)

If fetal maturity has been established by L/S ratio and blood is available for transfusion, a vaginal examination may be done to confirm the diagnosis. Such an examination is done in the cesarean section room under sterile conditions with personnel and equipment in readiness for an immediate operative delivery. The expert practitioner will be able to ascertain not only the presence of placenta previa, but also the extent to which it encroaches upon the cervical os.

Treatment

It is imperative that any woman with bleeding during the third trimester go immediately to a hospital.

Typing and cross-matching for possible trans-

fusion is a first priority and blood should be kept in readiness. The amount of bleeding and the vital signs of both mother and fetus should be monitored. No vaginal or rectal examinations should be done by anyone except under the conditions described above.

Further treatment depends on the extent of the placenta previa, the condition of the mother and fetus, gestational age, and parity.

If the fetus is immature, labor has not begun, and the bleeding is not excessive, a program of observation and support is initiated. The woman remains in or very near the hospital, usually at bed rest. Her hematocrit is monitored to prevent the development of anemia. Each recurrence of bleeding requires a new evaluation of maternal and fetal status, and an appropriate modification of the plan of care.

When the fetus is mature, delivery is the treatment of choice. In the case of a marginal placenta previa or, more rarely, in a partial placenta previa, vaginal delivery may be attempted. This is particularly true if the woman is a multipara and a relatively short labor is anticipated. The membranes are ruptured, allowing the presenting part to drop down. Pressure is thus applied to the placental site, and the blood vessels are at least partially occluded. Continuous electronic fetal heart rate monitoring is indicated to assess the fetal response to labor.

Cesarean section is usually the treatment of choice for placenta previa. When the placenta entirely covers the cervical os, it is difficult to control the bleeding by other means and the infant cannot be born alive by vaginal delivery. Primigravidas and women with the placenta partly over the os are often not easily treated satisfactorily by rupture of the membranes. The cervix and lower uterine segment are very friable because of the vascularity of the placental site. Vaginal manipulation may cause severe lacerations and bleeding. Cesarean section forestalls any possibility of cervical lacerations, and it also decreases the length of time during which the woman may bleed from placenta previa.

As previously stated these women are at increased risk for postpartum hemorrhage and therefore require skilled medical management of the third stage of labor as well as close observation during the immediate several hours post partum. Intravenous oxytocin is usually given as a prophylatic measure post partum.

Abruptio Placentae or Premature Separation of a Normally Implanted Placenta

Sometimes a placenta that is normally placed will separate prematurely, with hemorrhage as the inevitable result. Premature separation of the normally implanted placenta is the term that best describes this condition, but since this wording is rather long, the term *abruptio placentae* is used more frequently.

If blood escapes from the vagina with separation, the hemorrhage is called *external*. If it is retained within the uterine cavity, it is called a *concealed* or *internal* hemorrhage (Fig. 22-4). The latter type is much more severe, but also occurs less frequently.

All degrees of placental separation may take place. The area of separation may be only a few millimeters in diameter, or the entire placenta may become detached. Signs and symptoms vary with the amount of separation.

Antepartum bleeding is sometimes due to a very small amount of marginal detachment of the placenta, but this is not enough to definitely

ABRUPTIO PLACENTAE

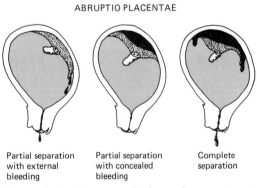

Partial separation with external bleeding   Partial separation with concealed bleeding   Complete separation

Figure 22-4. Degrees of placental separation in abruptio placentae showing both external and concealed hemorrhage.

demonstrate or diagnose. With abruptio placentae, bleeding first occurs into the decidua basalis, forming a hematoma in it and splitting the decidua basalis into two portions—one next to the placenta and one next to the uterine wall. As the hematoma becomes larger, it separates some of the placenta from the uterus. The amount of bleeding may be small and will then not be recognized until delivery of the placenta, when the region of separation can be seen as a depressed area, containing dark, clotted blood. If the bleeding is more profuse, the blood may appear externally by escaping between the membranes and uterine wall. This is external bleeding.

In a concealed hemorrhage the blood remains behind the placenta, or in some instances it may escape into the amniotic fluid by breaking through the membranes. Usually some bleeding will appear externally later, but if the baby's head is tight in the pelvis or if the membranes are tightly adherent, it does not escape readily. In concealed hemorrhage the detachment of the placenta is more likely to be complete, whereas it is generally incomplete when the bleeding is external.

Sometimes with abruptio placentae there is extensive intramuscular hemorrhage, possibly through the entire uterus, which becomes a bluish or purplish color. The muscle may then lose its power to contract. This condition is known as a "Couvelaire uterus."

The cause of abruptio placentae is unknown. Folic acid deficiency has been implicated as an etiologic factor, but investigators have been unable to establish this or to demonstrate that administering folic acid will prevent its occurrence.

Hypertensive disease, especially toxemia, greatly increases the risk of abruptio placentae.

Trauma may precipitate placental separation, although this occurs less frequently than is popularly believed.

Sudden decompression of the uterus, such as may happen when a large hydramnios is emptied too rapidly or a first twin is delivered, can cause the placenta to shear off the uterine wall. Manual manipulation of the uterus during a version may also increase the risk of abruptio placentae.

Symptoms

With external hemorrhage, the chief symptom is an escape of blood from the vagina, frequently accompanied by abdominal pain. The possibility of bleeding due to a placenta previa must be ruled out.

A concealed hemorrhage is an extremely grave complication for both mother and child. The characteristic symptoms are intense cramplike abdominal pain and uterine tenderness and rigidity. In contrast to the flaccid state of the uterus in placenta previa, in the concealed type of hemorrhage from premature separation the uterus is hard in consistency, being described as "boardlike," or 'stony," without alternate contraction and relaxation. It is impossible to palpate the fetus because of the tenseness of the uterine muscle. The fetal heart tones will be absent if a considerable amount of the placenta separates. See Figure 22-5 for signs and symptoms of abruptio placentae as compared to those of placenta previa.

The nurse caring for a mother in the latter weeks of pregnancy, or for a woman in labor, must realize that intense coliclike abdominal pain may be serious. In labor, she should not assume that this type of severe abdominal pain is caused by hard uterine contractions. The abdomen should be palpated to feel the consistency of the uterus and to make certain that the uterine muscle is alternately contracting and re-laxing. With external bleeding the uterus may also remain tense between contractions. There is sometimes a gradual, but marked, enlargement of the uterus with concealed hemorrhage.

Further, the nurse should be alert for signs and symptoms of hypovolemic shock (hypotension; tachycardia; rapid, thready pulse; apprehension). This is a particular risk when hemorrhage is concealed, as blood loss may be marked before a diagnosis is suspected. Another complication associated with premature separation of the placenta is coagulopathy (hypofibrinogenemia and/or thrombocytopenia). Unexpected bleeding from venipuncture sites may be the first sign of this serious condition which is associated with disseminated intravascular coagulopathy.

Treatment

Treatment of abruptio placentae depends on its severity and the extent to which labor has progressed. If contractions have begun and the bleeding is only moderate, labor is ordinarily allowed to proceed normally and unassisted. Rupture of the membranes, so that the uterus can contract around the fetus, may help to control bleeding. Rupture of the membranes also hastens labor and delivery. If labor does not proceed fairly rapidly or if bleeding is profuse, delivery by cesarean section will likely become necessary. Treatment of the accompanying blood loss and shock, if present, is very important and is started before surgery is begun.

In abruptio placentae, as in placenta previa,

PLACENTA PREVIA	ABRUPTIO PLACENTAE
1. Abnormally implanted placenta	1. Normally implanted placenta
2. Vaginal bleeding	2. Bleeding may be concealed
3. Painless	3. Painful
4. Abdomen soft except during contractions	4. Abdomen boardlike and tender
5. Able to palpate fetal outline	5. Cannot palpate fetal outline
6. Coagulation studies within normal limits	6. Hypofibrinogenemia is common

Figure 22-5. Comparison of the signs and symptoms of placenta previa and abruptio placentae. This constitutes the basis for differential diagnosis in a woman who presents with third trimester bleeding.

blood transfusions may be needed. Cross-matching of the patient's blood for a transfusion is done immediately on admission to the hospital so that blood will be available at a moment's notice.

In some cases of abruptio placentae there is a failure of the blood-clotting mechanism due to a decrease in the fibrinogen level and/or platelet level. Frequent tests to assess these factors are made in order that immediate therapy can be instituted should the patient show fibrinogenopenia (less than 250 mg 100 ml of blood) or thrombocytopenia.

If the uterine muscle has lost its ability to contract, owing to dissociation of its fibers by intramuscular hemorrhage (Couvelaire uterus), removal of the uterus may be necessary on very rare occasions to control postpartum hemorrhage.

Complications

Two complications of abruptio placentae warrant further discussion: disseminated intravascular coagulation (DIC) and shock. Although by no means exclusive to abruption, they are commonly enough associated to be reasonably included at this time.

DISSEMINATED INTRAVASCULAR COAGULATION (DIC) Disseminated intravascular coagulation is also referred to as *consumptive coagulopathy.* Either title is sufficiently imposing to indicate the severity of the disease. Normally, the hemostatic mechanism of the body is confined to local areas of vascular damage. Blood does not clot in healthy blood vessels. Some illnesses, however, provoke a generalized activation of the clotting system by stimulating thrombin elaboration and intravascular clotting or by overactivating the fibrinolytic system which prevents stable clotting. A combination of both mechanisms is also seen. The net result for the patient is a hemorrhagic condition. Paradoxically, even when the blood is hypercoagulable in the blood vessels, spontaneous bleeding occurs from the gums, venipuncture sites, and other areas of injury. It is as if all the clotting factors were being used up in tiny intravascular thrombi so that none is left to control bleeding.[2]

Treatment for this disease is directed at eliminating the underlying cause. In obstetric settings this is usually accomplished by delivering the infant and emptying the uterus. Blood products should be available to replace loss due to hemorrhage. Whole blood is the usual choice, as it corrects volume depletion as well as partially replacing blood constituents such as fibrinogen. Occasionally, heparin may be given to stop intravascular clotting and consumption of fibrinogen and platelets and to assist in spontaneous recovery. Heparin does not cross the placenta and therefore may be given prior to delivery without threatening the fetus.

Obstetric conditions which have been associated with DIC, in addition to abruptio placentae, include toxemia, intrauterine death, sepsis, retained placenta, amniotic fluid embolism, and intraamniotic injection of hypertonic saline.

SHOCK Shock results from the body's attempt to protect the vital organs, in particular the brain and heart, from a reduction in effective circulating blood volume. Although there are many causes of shock, the most common is that which results from an acute volume depletion due to hemorrhage.

When blood is lost from the vascular system, venous return is diminished, and consequently cardiac output is reduced. If the loss exceeds approximately 10 percent, or two units of blood, symptoms of shock may be seen. Because pregnant women have a greater circulating blood volume, it is believed that they can tolerate the loss of larger amounts of blood than the non-pregnant woman can. Figure 22-6 illustrates the pathophysiologic events following the sudden loss of large amounts of blood.

Maternal shock due to placental hemorrhage places the fetus in double jeopardy. Not only is

[2] Daniel Deykin, The clinical challenge of disseminated intravascular coagulation, *N. Engl. J. Med.* 283:636–644 (Sept. 17) 1970.

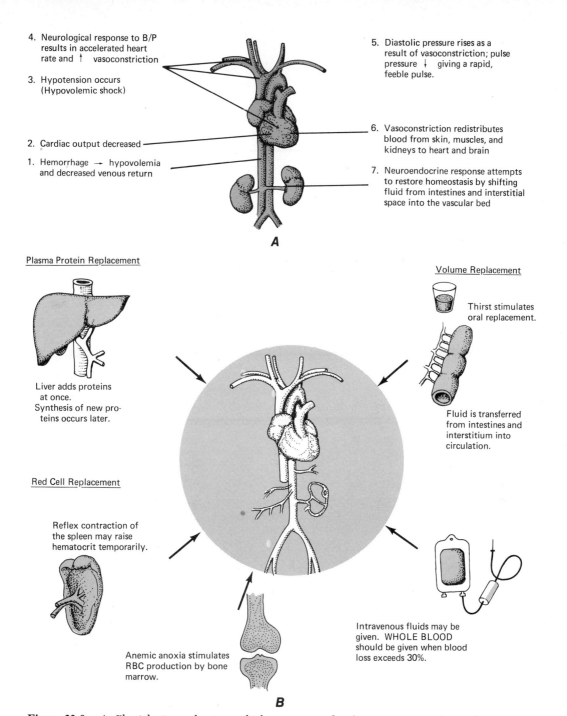

4. Neurological response to B/P results in accelerated heart rate and ↑ vasoconstriction

3. Hypotension occurs (Hypovolemic shock)

2. Cardiac output decreased

1. Hemorrhage → hypovolemia and decreased venous return

5. Diastolic pressure rises as a result of vasoconstriction; pulse pressure ↓ giving a rapid, feeble pulse.

6. Vasoconstriction redistributes blood from skin, muscles, and kidneys to heart and brain

7. Neuroendocrine response attempts to restore homeostasis by shifting fluid from intestines and interstitial space into the vascular bed

A

Plasma Protein Replacement

Liver adds proteins at once.
Synthesis of new proteins occurs later.

Volume Replacement

Thirst stimulates oral replacement.

Fluid is transferred from intestines and interstitium into circulation.

Red Cell Replacement

Reflex contraction of the spleen may raise hematocrit temporarily.

Anemic anoxia stimulates RBC production by bone marrow.

Intravenous fluids may be given. WHOLE BLOOD should be given when blood loss exceeds 30%.

B

Figure 22-6. **A.** Physiologic mechanisms which occur immediately in response to hemorrhage in an attempt to compensate for blood loss and restore homeostasis. **B.** Less immediate mechanisms by which homeostasis may be restored following blood loss. Notice that the ability of the body to compensate is limited, and when hemorrhage is severe, circulatory failure and/or shock may be irreversible unless intravenous replacement of blood is prompt.

639

his source of oxygen diminished by the partial separation of his placenta, but the hypotension and vasoconstriction of the shock mechanisms further reduce fetal oxygenation by reducing maternal blood flow to the placenta.

The nurse must be aware of women who are at risk for hemorrhage and shock and observe them with particular care. Blood pressure is the traditional parameter used in the detection of shock, although it may not be the earliest sign. Blood pressure readings should always be compared with the woman's own baseline, since that which is hypotension for one individual may be a normal reading for another. Tachycardia and a rapid, thready pulse may be the earliest signs of shock, as the heart attempts to compensate for a reduced output by beating faster. Respiration may be rapid and shallow, and the skin, particularly on the extremities, may feel cool and clammy. Often the woman complains of feeling worse or something "being wrong."

Any client suspected of bleeding or shock should have an intravenous infusion running for volume replacement, and transfusion if necessary. It is a good precautionary measure to start I.V.'s in high-risk clients with a needle or intracath of sufficiently large bore to permit blood transfusion. A position of comfort, usually a lateral or semi-Fowler's, and oxygen by mask will improve tissue oxygenation. Constant attendance is necessary to monitor vital signs and reassure the client. Cure is effected by eliminating the cause of bleeding and replacing blood as needed.

The nursing management of women with third trimester bleeding is summarized in Table 22-2.

PREMATURE LABOR

Premature labor is defined as labor occurring prior to 37 weeks gestation. Approximately 8 percent of births in the United States are premature and these account for nearly two thirds of the neonatal deaths.

Evidence appears to be mounting that the signal for labor comes from the fetus, probably because of some genetically imprinted information that tells him nutrition is becoming limited and a change in his environment is necessary for continuing life and well-being. Nevertheless, the exact mechanism which triggers the onset of normal labor remains unknown. For this reason it is not possible to delineate clearly the factors which initiate premature labor. Certain obstetric complications are known to predispose to early labor and delivery. Included among these are

Table 22-2.   Care of the Woman with Third Trimester Hemorrhage

Patient Care Goals	Nursing Interventions
I. Determine extent of blood loss.	1. Obtain history of onset, duration, amount of bleeding, and associated symptoms. 2. Observe perineal pads for amount of bleeding. 3. Monitor vital signs of mother and fetus. (Frequency is determined by severity of clinical symptoms.)
II. Provide volume replacement.	1. Insert intravenous conduit. 2. Request type and cross-match for blood. 3. Administer fluids and blood as prescribed. 4. Monitor intake and output.
III. Minimize chances for further bleeding.	1. *NO* vaginal or rectal exams. 2. Bed rest in position of comfort. 3. Anticipate delivery by cesarean section.
IV. Reduce anxiety.	1. Keep woman and family advised of treatment plan. 2. Share realistic hopes for maternal/fetal/neonatal outcome.

multiple gestations, polydydramnios, hypertension, third trimester bleeding, premature rupture of the membranes, and incompetent cervix. Sometimes it is necessary to interrupt a pregnancy before term because of an unfavorable intrauterine environment or maternal illness. In the majority of circumstances, however, no cause can be determined.

Prevention of Premature Labor

Antepartum care which assists the woman in the maintenance of her own good health is an important factor in preventing premature labor and birth. Good nutrition, although not a prevention for premature labor, does favor the optimum growth and development of the fetus in a healthy mother, and helps prevent a small-for-gestational-age infant.

Little is known that is specifically helpful in preventing premature labor. For some women at special risk bed rest is recommended because it helps to improve uterine blood flow and, therefore, intrauterine nutrition. It may also decrease uterine irritability and the tendency to go into labor, although this is not clearly established.

A few women deliver premature infants because of a condition termed *incompetent cervix.* Termination of pregnancy due to this complication usually occurs in the second trimester, too early for survival of the very immature infant.

Usually after the fourth month of pregnancy, the cervix dilates without the usual painful uterine contractions. The membranes later rupture, labor begins, and an immature fetus is delivered. The etiology of cervical incompetency is not known, but previous trauma to the cervix is a factor in some cases. It usually does not occur in primigravidas. (See Chapter 6, page 112.)

Treatment consists of reinforcing the cervix with a purse-string suture, which is usually placed about the cervix between the fourteenth and eighteenth weeks. Treatment is fairly successful in maintaining pregnancy. When the pregnancy reaches term, the suture may be removed to permit vaginal delivery, or in some cases the suture is left in place and the woman is delivered by cesarean section.

Premature spontaneous rupture of the membranes occurs in 10 to 15 percent of all pregnancies. Not all of these result in premature birth, however. This terminology is somewhat misleading, since the word premature refers not to the duration of the pregnancy but to the fact that the bag of waters ruptures prior to the onset of labor. Obviously this can, and does, occur at term as well as before term.

When membranes rupture, it is essential to determine the gestational age of the fetus. If the pregnancy is at or near term (more than 37 weeks), labor should be induced and a delivery accomplished within 24 hours of the rupture. The risk of infection to both fetus and mother rises quite sharply after 18 to 24 hours of ruptured membranes, and neonates tolerate infection very poorly.

When the fetus is not mature, a more conservative approach is usually taken. Labor is not induced and may even be pharmacologically inhibited. Pregnancy may be allowed to continue until fetal maturity is established, unless symptoms of infection appear (elevated maternal temperature, foul-smelling vaginal discharge). It is even possible that a short period of ruptured membranes may enhance fetal lung maturation. It is suggested that stress stimulates the fetal adrenals to produce corticosteroids, which in turn induce the enzymes which produce surfactant.

Women should be carefully instructed to seek professional evaluation whenever they suspect that the membranes have ruptured, regardless of when in gestation this occurs. Diagnosis of ruptured membranes is discussed in Chapter 12, pages 260–62.

Suppression of Premature Labor

From very early in pregnancy women should be aware of the importance of reporting immediately any contractions which increase in frequency and intensity. Pharmacologic means of stopping premature labor are increasing in effectiveness and availability. These drugs are most useful in early labor. Postponing objective evaluation of the contractions because "it's too early for labor" can result in being too late for most effective use of the drugs.

Women who have been determined to be in premature labor may be candidates for pharmacologic inhibition of labor, provided the fetus is alive but immature, and there are no maternal or fetal indications for terminating the pregnancy. Such indications could include, among other things, bleeding from placenta previa or abruptio placentae, intrauterine infection, erythroblastosis fetalis, severe preeclampsia or placental insufficiency. In addition, cervical dilatation should not be greater than 4 cm, and some authors believe that the membranes should be intact. (See Figure 22-7.)

The drugs most commonly used for suppression of labor include ethyl alcohol and the beta-adrenergic agents, such as isoxsuprine or ritodrine. Alcohol blocks the secretion of oxytocin by the maternal pituitary and also crosses the placenta to block secretion of fetal neurohormones. The beta-adrenergic drugs make myometrial cells less sensitive to oxytocin and prostaglandins. Both drugs are thought to increase uterine blood flow.

```
┌─────────────────────────────────────────────┐
│ Presence of "true" labor                      │
│                                                │
│ Gestational age between 20 and 37 weeks        │
│                                                │
│ Immature fetal pulmonary development            │
│                                                │
│ Cervical dilation less than 5 cm                │
│                                                │
│ No contraindications to continuing pregnancy — For example: │
│                                                │
│         Intrauterine infection                  │
│                                                │
│         Severe vaginal bleeding                 │
│                                                │
│         Severe preeclampsia                     │
│                                                │
│         Placental insufficiency                 │
│                                                │
│         Erythroblastosis fetalis                │
│                                                │
│         Fetal death                             │
└─────────────────────────────────────────────┘
```

Figure 22-7. Criteria for selecting patients for pharmacologic inhibition of premature labor.

Alcohol is administered intravenously as a 10 percent solution in dextrose and water. The goal is to achieve a blood level of 0.12 to 0.16 percent. This is approximately the level that results from three good drinks at a cocktail party (0.10 percent is defined as legal intoxication by most states for driving purposes). Side effects include those of intoxication from oral intake of alcohol and are often quite distressing to the woman and her family. This factor, together with the anxiety precipitated by the threatened loss of their infant, demands a high degree of skill and sensitivity on the part of the nurses and physicians giving care. Labor may be successfully delayed three or more days in up to 66 percent of clients, depending on patient selection. Alcohol is generally unsuccessful if the membranes are ruptured or if the cervical dilatation is greater than 4 cm. When treatment is unsuccessful, attention must be given to the fetus/neonate whose blood alcohol level will approximately equal that of the mother. Personnel expert in neonatal resuscitation should be present at delivery as ventilatory assistance may be necessary due to prematurity and/or respiratory depression resulting from the alcohol.

The beta-adrenergic agents are also administered intravenously in dosages varying according to individual protocols. Adequate hydration of the mother is essential in order to minimize the occurrence of maternal tachycardia and hypotension, the two major side effects of these drugs. The mother should be positioned on her side and her blood pressure monitored every 15 minutes while the drug is being infused. Continuous fetal heart rate monitoring is the safest means of following fetal response. It appears that the beta-adrenergic drugs are more effective than alcohol in stopping labor.

Care of women in premature labor is most appropriately carried out in a perinatal center where personnel have the training, expertise, and equipment to make maximum use of the latest research drugs and techniques. Furthermore, should attempts at arresting labor fail, the infant will be delivered where a neonatal intensive care unit will give him the best chance for

Table 22-3.   Care of the Woman in Premature Labor

Patient Care Goals	Nursing Interventions
I. Maintenance of woman's self-concept as "whole," competent person.	1. Acknowledge normality of feelings of fear and guilt. 2. Provide facts about causes of premature labor. 3. Introduce neonatal team member to family. 4. Share realistic hopes for fetal/neonatal outcome.
II. Maximize fetal oxygenation.	1. Position laboring woman on her side. 2. Prevent hyperventilation by careful coaching, use of rebreathing bag, reducing anxiety. 3. Observe fetal response to labor, using continuous fetal heart rate monitoring. 4. Insure presence of skilled personnel for resuscitation at delivery.
III. Enable woman to conduct labor with minimum analgesia/anesthesia.	1. Reduce anxiety by providing calm, comfortable environment. 2. Remain constantly available to woman and family. 3. Explain all procedures. 4. Keep woman and family informed of progress of labor and condition of fetus. 5. Assist family to support woman as much as they are able. 6. Do not administer analgesics within an hour of anticipated delivery. 7. Monitor fetal as well as maternal response to local and regional anesthesia.

survival. Delivery in the center also avoids the separation of parents and infant, which occurs when only the infant is transported to the intensive care nursery after being born in a community hospital.

Management of Premature Labor

When it is not possible or desirable to arrest premature labor, then the management must be directed at providing an optimal environment for the labor and delivery of a premature infant. The objectives of care for a woman in premature labor include the following (see Table 22-3):

1. To assist the woman through labor in such a way that she is able to maintain ego integration
2. To maximize fetal oxygenation
3. To provide support to enable the woman to conduct her labor with minimal analgesia/anesthesia

The woman in premature labor comes to the laboring experience without the readiness for parturition which characterizes the woman at term. She has not completed the tasks of pregnancy. She is physically and psychologically unready for her baby. The crib and room are not even prepared. In a very real sense, she is a premature mother. In addition, she carries a burden of guilt which may be quite awesome. She fears the loss of her child so, as in all grieving, she asks herself what she did wrong. Her husband, too, will likely feel he should have taken better care of her, not had sexual intercourse, or whatever he imagines may have contributed.

These feelings are a normal part of the grief of parents in premature labor. They should be encouraged to express these feelings and concerns and helped to understand that they are usual and normal feelings. On the other hand, they should be given factual information so they can come to realize at least intellectually, that they did not do something "wrong," that they are not inferior persons.

Fear of losing the child is another real factor. Rubin has described one of the tasks of pregnancy as "securing safe passage for herself and her child."[3] This has certainly not been ac-

[3] Reva Rubin, The maternal tasks of pregnancy, *Maternal–Child Nurs. J.* 4:143–153 (Fall) 1975.

complished as yet by those women in premature labor. A significant manifestation of this fear may be the denial of reality. Some women do not accept labor itself and may put off seeking medical attention, thinking it can't be labor because "it is not time yet." Or, accepting labor, they deny the seriousness of the situation. Much can be done to put this fear into proper perspective and help the parents focus on reality by keeping them well informed of the progress of labor, the fetal status, the plan of care, and the expectations of the professionals caring for them. If it is at all possible during labor, a member of the neonatal team who will be caring for their infant should be introduced to the parents. Depending on the stage of labor and the woman's discomfort, the neonatal nurse or physician can briefly explain what immediate care the infant will be likely to receive, and that the parents will be able to come into the nursery to see, touch, and care for their infant as soon as they wish.

The second objective of care is to maximize fetal oxygenation. The premature is more vulnerable to the stress of labor than is a term fetus. Continuous fetal heart rate monitoring is indicated to constantly assess fetal response to contractions. Blood from fetal scalp samples may be analyzed for blood gases and pH, if indicated by the occurrence of significant fetal heart rate abnormalities.

Women should not labor in a supine position regardless of gestational age because of the risk of the vena caval syndrome. This condition, caused by the compression of the vena cava by the pregnant uterus, results in diminished placental perfusion and, potentially, fetal hypoxia. The left lateral position seems to favor the best placental perfusion, but either side or sitting up is suitable if the woman is comfortable. Women in normal labor often prefer to be out of bed moving about or sitting in a chair.

Maternal hyperventilation should be particularly avoided as it can cause a maternal alkalosis. This in turn may decrease the release of oxygen to the fetus, resulting in fetal hypoxia and acidosis. Hyperventilation may be brought on by

severe anxiety, or it may be the result of improperly performed childbirth breathing techniques. The mother and her coach should be reminded of the importance of the deep, "cleansing breath" at the beginning and end of each contraction and of the necessity to use a normal breathing pattern between contractions. If the mother's fingertips begin to tingle (an early symptom of hyperventilation) it may be helpful for her to breathe in and out into a small paper bag. This will increase the carbon dioxide content of the inspired air.

At the time of delivery the mother should be on her back for the shortest time possible. Some authorities recommend the Sims position for delivery, but this is not usually acceptable in the United States. An episiotomy is generally performed to lessen the risk to the infant of intracranial hemorrhage. For the same reason, outlet forceps may be used to shorten the second stage of labor and reduce the pressure on the fetal head. Someone skilled in neonatal assessment and resuscitation should be in attendance to receive the infant.

The third goal of care is to keep analgesia and anesthesia at a minimum to avoid respiratory depression in the neonate. To do this, expert care and support of the laboring woman is essential. The woman relies on the nurse to help her maintain contact with time and reality and to help her control her own body in order to retain dignity. To meet these expectations appropriately, the nurse must be continuously available to the woman and her family in order to establish and maintain a therapeutic relationship.

Finally, the small premature infant may deliver through an incompletely dilated cervix. For this reason the nurse should be especially sensitive to maternal behavior which signals the approach of second stage of labor.

PROLONGED PREGNANCY

A pregnancy which extends beyond 42-weeks duration is designated *postterm* or *postdate*. The reasons for prolonged gestation are unknown, although perhaps as many as 6 percent of all pregnancies fall into this category.[4]

Effects of postterm pregnancies on the mother are primarily psychosocial in nature. For many weeks she has focused on a time for delivery, only to have that time come and go without a baby being born. In an effort to make appropriate judgments about her care, physicians and nurses cross-examine her in detail about the accuracy of her menstrual dates and other events until she may question what she really knows. If tests or interventions are instituted, her anxiety about her infant and herself will rise markedly. Nursing care should be directed toward helping the woman utilize family and social support systems, providing information and reassurance about fetal assessment, and acting as a sounding board for her fatigue and frustration with "still being pregnant."

Fetal effects due to prolonged gestation are quite variable. Some fetuses will continue to grow, which may lead to dystocia and birth injury because of their large size. Others fail to grow as gestation continues and indeed may even lose weight due to malnutrition. These latter infants, termed *dysmature* or *postmature*, are typically scrawny with long nails; abundant scalp hair; loose, desquamated skin, and a characteristic worried expression on their faces. Dysmaturity is correlated with increased incidence of placental lesions, increased perinatal death, and neonatal morbidity.

With the present methods of fetal/placental assessment, it is not possible to identify which prolonged pregnancies will compromise the fetus until placental insufficiency is fairly advanced. For this reason postterm women should be evaluated for induction of labor. If menstrual dates and other determinants of gestational age are reasonably accurate and the cervix is favorable, an oxytocin induction should be undertaken.

When gestational age is in question or the cervix unfavorable, pregnancy may be continued under very close supervision. Gestational age should be verified and fetal well-being assessed by means of serial estriol determinations and oxytocin challenge tests.

During labor the fetus should be continuously monitored by electronic means as he is at high risk of hypoxia. Particular attention should be paid during the second stage of labor as bearing-down efforts may further compromise placentofetal respiratory reserves. Additional nursing measures include maintaining maternal position for maximal uteroplacental blood flow and providing supportive care to minimize the use of analgesia and anesthesia.

Personnel skilled in resuscitation should be present at delivery. Some authors recommend delaying clamping of the cord to permit an increased blood supply to counteract hypovolemia and dehydration, two threats to the dysmature neonate.[5] Special neonatal care of these infants is discussed in Chapter 25, pages 750–52.

Dysmature babies tend to score lower than term babies on the Brazelton interaction and motor scores and are often described as "difficult" by their mothers.[6] These infant characteristics have the potential for initiating a vicious cycle of parent–infant interaction, which could result in inappropriate infant stimulation, neglect, or even abuse. Nursing care should emphasize helping parents recognize their baby's cues and provide appropriate stimulation to enhance his growth and development. Close follow-up should be assured at least through the first year of life.

ISOIMMUNE DISEASE

Isoimmune disease is primarily a disorder of the fetus and neonate, caused by maternal sen-

[4] Jack A. Pritchard and Paul C. MacDonald, *Williams Obstetrics*, 15th ed. Appleton-Century-Crofts, New York, 1976, p. 797.

[5] Helmuth Vorherr, Placental insufficiency in relation to postterm pregnancy and fetal postmaturity, *Am. J. Obstet. Gynecol.* 123:67–103 (Sep.) 1975.
[6] Tiffany M. Field *et al.*, Developmental effects of prolonged pregnancy and the postmaturity syndrome, *J. Pediatr.* 90:836–839 (May) 1977.

sitization to fetal red cell antigens and subsequent transfer of the resulting antibodies to the fetus. This occurs when the fetus possesses a red blood cell antigen, inherited from the father, that is absent in the mother.

Although the fetal circulatory system is entirely separate from the mother's and the blood of mother and fetus does not mix, it is possible for fetal blood cells to pass through the placenta into the maternal circulation. When these blood cells are incompatible with the mother's blood, she may produce antibodies to them. These antibodies can pass through the placenta into the fetal circulation and destroy fetal red blood cells, sometimes to a severe degree. This condition is known as hemolytic disease of the newborn or erythroblastosis fetalis.

One of 150 births is marked by detectable hemolytic disease of the newborn. The most severe form of the disease is the result of an incompatibility of the Rh, or Rhesus, blood groups. This will be discussed in some detail in the following pages.

An incompatibility may also occur between the ABO blood groups of the mother and fetus. This usually results when there is a type-O mother and a type-A fetus, although it has been known to occur with a type-B fetus. Type-O blood, of course, contains both anti-A and anti-B serum antibodies. This is the most common cause of hemolytic disease, but it is usually mild. It differs from Rh isoimmunization in several important ways: (1) it can occur as readily in a first pregnancy as in a subsequent one; (2) it does not necessarily increase in severity with each subsequent gestation; (3) it does not require intrauterine therapy. Additionally, incompatibility of ABO blood types may protect against Rh immunization. For example, if the fetal red cells are type A, Rh(+) and the mother is type O, Rh(−), the anti-A in the mother's serum will destroy any fetal cells entering maternal circulation before they can stimulate an immune response to the Rh antigen.

About 2 percent of isoimmune disease is caused by other, rare blood groups. Those most often implicated are the Kell, Kidd, Duffy, and MN factors. These antigens, besides being quite rare, are rather weak and do not usually produce severe disease. Sensitization to these antigens is often the result of a previous blood transfusion.

Isoimmune Disease Due to Rh Incompatibility

Isoimmune disease due to Rh incompatibility occurs when Rh antigens enter the blood of an Rh-negative mother and she produces anti-Rh antibodies. These maternal antibodies readily cross the placenta into the fetal circulation. If the fetus is Rh-positive, the antibodies attach to the erythrocytes and cause hemolysis. The antibodies are harmless to the mother herself, since the Rh antigen is absent from her cells, and they are harmless to an Rh-negative fetus.

The hemolytic process may begin early in pregnancy and be so intense as to cause death *in utero* from profound anemia. It may begin later and be mild enough to permit birth of a normal-appearing live-born infant in whom hemolysis continues to a variable, sometimes only mild, degree. To compensate for loss of cells, the hemolytic process is accompanied by an overdevelopment of erythropoietic tissue in bone marrow, liver, and spleen. Anemia and jaundice occur as a result of erythrocyte destruction, and there are many nucleated red blood cells in the circulating blood due to the hyperactivity of blood-forming tissue.

The Rh Factor

The Rh factor, which is a cause of incompatibility between maternal and fetal blood, is really an antigenic system. It was first observed in 1939 by Levine and Stetson.[7] They reported an antibody present in the blood of a woman who had delivered an erythroblastotic, stillborn infant. Her serum agglutinated not only the infant's blood but also her husband's blood.

---

[7] P. Levine and R. E. Stetson, An unusual case of intragroup agglutination, *JAMA* 113:126–127, 1939.

One year later Landsteiner and Weiner published the results of their work with Rhesus monkeys. They had immunized rabbits with Rhesus red blood cells and found that the resulting rabbit serum agglutimated not only Rhesus cells but also the cells of 85 percent of the human population. In other words 85 percent of humans had this antigen on their red cells; 15 percent did not. Those persons possessing the antigen were designated Rh-positive; those lacking the antigen were designated Rh-negative. It was soon discovered that this newly named Rh antigen was the same substance responsible for the fetal death in Levine and Stetson's case report and, indeed, for much of the maternal–fetal blood incompatibilities.

The Rh blood groups vary in their proportions depending on the population under discussion, just as other blood groups do. On the average about 15 percent of the caucasian population is Rh-negative. There are fewer Rh-negative persons in the Negro race (about 8%) and fewer still among Orientals (1–2%).

The Genetics of the Rh Factor

It became evident very soon after Landsteiner and Weiner's discovery that the Rh factor is, in fact, a very complex gene locus. Geneticists are in disagreement about whether there is a single locus with multiple alleles or three very closely linked loci. The clinical relevance is not affected by this technical point, however.

There are five major Rh antigens: C, c, D, E, e. The genetic alternative to D is designated d, although it does not appear to be antigenic. The gene or genes carrying the Rh antigens are, like all genes, located on chromosomes, which are always in pairs—one of which has been derived from the mother and one from the father. An individual then receives one chromosome from his mother carrying a C or c and a D or d and an E or e. He likewise receives one chromosome from his father carrying a C or c and a D or d and an E or e. A single chromosome does not carry both a C and c, a D and d or an E and e; it must be either a large-letter or a small-letter gene. Large letters symbolize the dominant Rh-positive genes, while small letters symbolize the recessive Rh-negative genes.

It can be seen that there are a large number of possible combinations of genes. A person may be CDE/CDE, cde/cde, CDe/cde, cDe/cDE and so on and on. The genotype, or the kind of Rh genes carried by an individual's chromosomes, is determined by laboratory tests using antisera specific to the various antigens.

The D is the most strongly antigenic and as such is responsible for most of the fetal–maternal pathology related to the Rh factor. For this reason, in clinical terminology, Rh-positive means literally D-positive and Rh-negative means D-negative or d. The Rh-positive individual may have two D genes, designated as DD, in which case he is homozygous. Or, he may have one D and one d, designated Dd, and he is then heterozygous. Because the Rh-positive trait is dominant, the presence of only one D makes a person Rh-positive. If both genes are d, the individual is dd, designated Rh-negative.

In addition to the major Rh antigens, a number of variants of C and D are known. Of these only the D appears to be clinically significant. This variant reacts weakly or not at all with anti-D serum and may give a false Rh-negative classification. For this reason, antiserum specific to the D^u should always be used to double-check red cells thought to be D-negative.

Persons who are Rh-negative (i.e., lacking the D antigen) can be stimulated to form antibodies that will destroy Rh-positive (D-positive) red cells. This stimulation occurs when an Rh-negative person is transfused with Rh-positive blood or when red cells of an Rh(+) fetus enter the circulation of an Rh(−) mother. Once antibody formation, or sensitization, has occurred, any further contacts with the antigen will result in a hemolytic reaction. Therefore, if Rh-positive fetal blood cells pass through the placenta into an Rh-negative maternal circulation, antibodies are produced to the fetal red cell antigens. The antibodies then pass back from the mother's blood into fetal circulation, where they hemolyze fetal red cells (see Figure 22-8).

648   THE HIGH-RISK MOTHER AND BABY

Key: ⊕Rh positive ⊖Rh negative ■Rh antibody

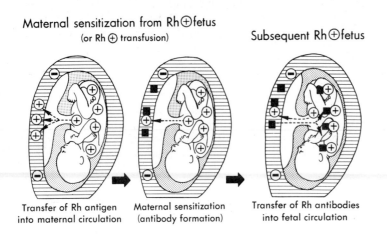

Maternal sensitization from Rh⊕fetus
(or Rh ⊕ transfusion)

Subsequent Rh⊕fetus

Transfer of Rh antigen
into maternal circulation

Maternal sensitization
(antibody formation)

Transfer of Rh antibodies
into fetal circulation

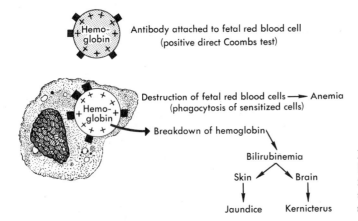

Antibody attached to fetal red blood cell
(positive direct Coombs test)

Destruction of fetal red blood cells ⟶ Anemia
(phagocytosis of sensitized cells)

Breakdown of hemoglobin

Bilirubinemia

Skin   Brain

Jaundice   Kernicterus

Figure 22-8. Erythroblastosis fetalis. [*Adapted by permission from* Erythroblastosis Fetalis, *Ross Clinical Education Aid No. 9. Ross Laboratories, Columbus, Ohio, 1962.*]

How does an Rh-negative woman become pregnant with an Rh-positive fetus? The woman must possess only Rh-negative genes, since that is a recessive trait. Therefore, it is clear that the fetus must have inherited an Rh-positive gene from the father. The mating of an Rh-negative female with an Rh-positive male occurs about 12 times in 100, but not all of the offspring are affected with isoimmune disease. Some of them may themselves be Rh-negative. A review of the genetics will explain how this happens. If the father is homozygous (*DD*), all of his children will be Rh-positive regardless of the mother's blood type. (Remember, *D* or (+) is dominant.) However, if he is heterozygous (*Dd*), a mating with an Rh-negative woman (*dd*) would result (on the average) in half of his children being Rh-positive (*Dd*) and half Rh-negative (*dd*) (see Figure 22-9 for a diagram).

Firstborns of Rh neg.—Rh pos. matings are seldom sensitized. It is believed that the most likely time for fetal cells to escape into maternal circulation is near or at the time of placental separation. This does not allow time for antibody formation to occur and to affect the fetus before birth. First children may be affected if

FATHER   MOTHER

Rh-negative
Homozygous

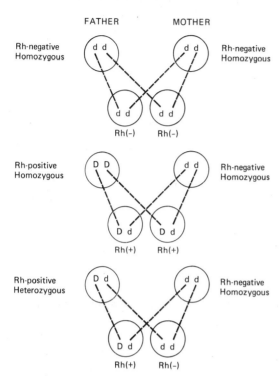

Rh-negative
Homozygous

Rh-positive
Homozygous

Rh-negative
Homozygous

Rh-positive
Heterozygous

Rh-negative
Homozygous

Figure 22-9. Illustration of inheritance of the Rh genes *D* and *d*. The *C* and *c* and *E* and *e* genes are inherited in the same manner.

the mother was previously sensitized by a transfusion or by an abortion which went undiagnosed. Practitioners performing elective abortions are not always knowledgeable or conscientious about the use of RhoGam (see below), and some Rh-negative women are sensitized in this way.

Fetal antigens are not always able to pass through the placenta into the maternal circulation. If they do pass through to the mother they may be rapidly hemolyzed and unable to stimulate antibody formation, as occurs when there is a coexistent ABO incompatibility. Or the mother may not produce any antibodies to them for reasons which are not completely understood.

On the average, about 15 percent of the offspring of Rh-negative females and Rh-positive males will be affected by isoimmume disease if no prophylactic treatment is employed. Once a woman has developed a concentration of antibodies sufficient to cause hemolytic disease in an infant, each subsequent Rh-positive infant is likely to have increasingly severe disease.

Antepartum Diagnosis and Management

Detection and treatment of Rh isoimmunization begins early in pregnancy at the first antepartum visit. At this time the ABO and Rh blood groups should be documented and an antibody screen performed. If the woman is Rh-negative and has no history of a preceding affected infant, it is useful to determine the father's Rh type. If he is negative, the fetus will also be negative and no disease will occur.

If the woman is found to be Rh-positive with no antibodies, a normal pregnancy and delivery is probable, at least with respect to isoimmune factors. However, it is wise to repeat the antibody screen at 28 weeks gestation to rule out the possibility of difficulty from any of the rare blood antigens.

If the mother is Rh-negative and the antibody screen is negative, rescreening is done at 24, 28, and 34 weeks gestation to detect any sensitization that develops during pregnancy. In addition, she will be evaluated to receive RhoGam in the postpartum period (see below).

If the mother is Rh-negative and antibodies are found with an indirect antiglobulin (Coombs) test, titration is made to determine the degree to which they are present. Subsequent monthly titrations will reveal whether the titer rises or remains the same. If the titer remains at or below a *critical* level (usually defined as 1:8) on repeated determinations throughout gestation, the pregnancy will usually be delivered at term with no further treatment.

Detection of an antibody titer above the *critical* level indicates significant sensitization and requires evaluation by means of amniocentesis. Unfortunately the level of the titer does not correlate well with the severity of the fetal disease. A more precise estimate of the degree of fetal illness is obtained by analyzing amniotic fluid samples for bilirubin content. Normally, the amount of bilirubin in amniotic fluid declines steadily throughout gestation until it virtually disappears in the last month. If maternal antibodies are destroying fetal red cells excessive bibirubin will be excreted as an end product of hemolysis by the fetal skin and kidneys. Thus, the more severe the hemolysis the greater the amount of bilirubin in amniotic fluid.

Amniotic fluid is obtained by amniocentesis as described in Chapter 21, page 610. Care must be taken to place the fluid immediately in a light-excluding container, as exposure to light for more than a few seconds will cause deterioration of the bilirubin and may give a falsely low value. The optical density of the fluid is analyzed in a spectrophotometer, which measures the light absorption. Normal amniotic fluid, when plotted on a logarithmic scale, will de-

scribe a straight line from about 350 to 700 nm, but when bilirubin is present a bulge appears in the graph at about 450 nm. The extent of this bulge can be measured and plotted against gestational age to gauge the severity of the hemolytic process.

When the optical density (OD) falls within zone I of the Liley graph (see Figure 22-10), the fetus is only mildly affected if affected at all and may be suspected of being Rh-negative. Zone II indicates a moderate degree of disease. If serial ODs follow the normal downward trend, the pregnancy is usually allowed to continue until 35 to 37 weeks gestation, when labor is induced following confirmation of fetal lung maturity. A reading in zone III is indicative of a severely affected fetus and immediate treatment must be undertaken to avoid permanent disability or death. If the fetus is mature, delivery is effected

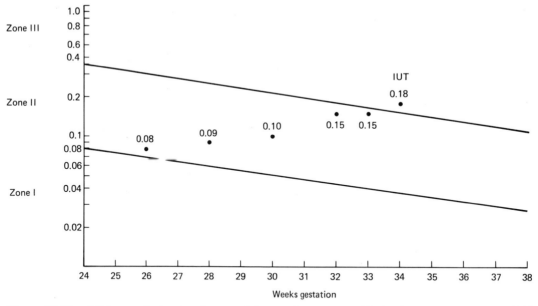

Figure 22-10. A Liley graph showing the optical density for a 29-year-old Rh(−), GIV, PII. Her first child was unaffected; the second was an Rh(−) child; the third pregnancy terminated in a spontaneous abortion at 14 weeks gestation. At the initial antepartum visit at 12 weeks gestation in the present pregnancy the antibody titer was 1:128. Amniocenteses were begun at 26 weeks gestation and continued biweekly and then weekly. At 34 weeks, with an optical density in zone III and a fetal L/S ratio of only 1.8, an intrauterine transfusion was performed. At 36 weeks a 2450-gm male infant with an L/S of 3.6 was delivered vaginally following an oxytocin induction. The infant did well, requiring a single exchange transfusion and phototherapy for hyperbilirubinemia. His parents took him home on the tenth day of life.

at once. When the fetus is not mature, intra-uterine transfusion is undertaken.

Since 1963, intrauterine transfusions have been done on fetuses that would not otherwise be able to survive *in utero* until sufficiently mature to be born. Recently the use of ultrasonography to direct the placement of the transfusing catheter has markedly improved the safety of this procedure. After the insertion of the catheter into the periotoneal cavity of the fetus, a volume of type O, Rh(−) packed red cells commensurate with the fetal weight is infused. These cells, absorbed into fetal circulation, improve fetal anemia and oxygenation. Since these cells are Rh-negative they are not hemolyzed. The transfusions may be repeated at approximately two-week intervals until fetal lung maturity is achieved and delivery can be effected.

Figure 22-11 outlines the steps in diagnosis and management of isoimmunization in pregnancy as described above.

The major threat to the life of the fetus and newborn in hemolytic disease is anemia. Preparations should be made for immediate delivery

room transfusion of the neonate whenever the birth of a severely affected infant is anticipated. Postnatally, hemolysis continues for varying lengths of time and, if untreated, may result in kernicterus, deposition of bilirubin in brain tissue. This irreversible condition may cause profound mental retardation. *In utero* bilirubin is cleared by the placenta and the maternal liver and thus represents no threat to the fetus. For a discussion of the care of neonates with hemolytic disease, refer to Chapter 26.

Prevention of Rh Isoimmunization

Much progress has been made in the prevention of Rh disease with the availability of anti-D immunoglobulin (RhoGam).

The likelihood of maternal infusion with fetal red cells is highest around the time of delivery when placental separation takes place. Normally these fetal antigens would stimulate an active immunity (antibodies) in the mother. However, if a high concentration of anti-D gamma-globulin can be administered, a passive immunity will result. The injected anti-D will destroy the an-

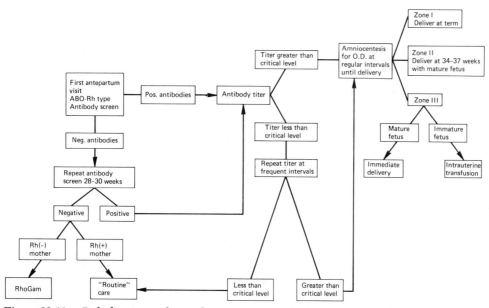

Figure 22-11. Path diagram outlining the management of isoimmunization during pregnancy.

How Rh disease develops...

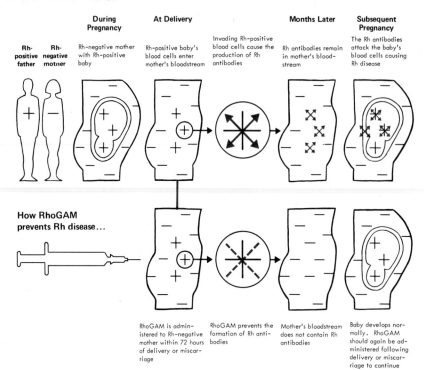

Figure 22-12. How Rh disease develops. How RhoGAM prevents Rh disease. [*Reproduced with permission from Ortho Diagnostics, Raritan, N.J., 1968.*]

tigenic fetal cells before they have the opportunity to stimulate active production of antibodies by the mother (Fig. 22-12)

Since it is not known how long a time period is required for the formation of antibodies, it is recommended that RhoGam be given to the mother within the first 72 hours post partum. A dose of 300 micrograms of the preparation is injected intramuscularly after observing the following precautions:

1. Delivery has occurred within the past 72 hours
2. Mother is D($-$), D^u($-$)
3. Mother is NOT sensitized (negative Coombs test to D or D^u)
4. Infant is D($+$) (or abortus of unknown blood type)
5. Infant is Coombs negative to D or D^u
6. Individual RhoGam dose has been cross-

matched with maternal red cells and is compatible.

Each pregnancy should be followed carefully with antibody screening and RhoGam given after each delivery whether full-term, premature, or abortion.

It should be emphasized that RhoGam cannot reverse or decrease sensitization once it has occurred. In addition, it is only effective against the D antigen, which is the one most commonly responsible for isoimmune disease. Sensitization can occur, however, to other of the Rh antigens or to other blood factors.

HYPERTENSIVE STATES OF PREGNANCY

Hypertension is one of the most serious, and, at the same time, most common complications of pregnancy, occurring in approximately 7 percent of all gestations. It accounts for 15 to 20 percent of maternal mortality, as well as contributing significantly to perinatal morbidity and mortality.

The hypertensive states of pregnancy have been classified by the American College of Obstetricians and Gynecologists into three major categories: (1) toxemias of pregnancy (preeclampsia and eclampsia); (2) chronic hypertension antedating pregnancy; and (3) chronic hypertension with superimposed toxemia. It should be emphasized, however, the differentiation of these disorders is often very difficult. Frequently diagnosis is only possible retrospectively, and then it may be somewhat arbitrary, since the criteria tend to be neither precise nor mutually exclusive.

The proportion of the various categories of hypertensive disease varies somewhat according to the characteristics of a given obstetric population. In general, preeclampsia accounts for between 80 and 90 percent of all hypertension in pregnancy. However, since chronic hypertension is more common in black women than caucasian women, this percentage would be likely to change if the population were largely black. Similarly, both preeclampsia and eclampsia are primarily diseases of primigravidas, so a very young population composed mainly of women in their first pregnancies, such as might be found in some housing developments or university communities, would tend to have a larger proportion of toxemias.

Toxemia

Toxemia is a disease of the last half of gestation characterized by hypertension, edema, and proteinuria. It has been described for as long as written records have been kept. Its occurrence has been attributed to evil spirits, bad humors, and, more recently, to sodium intake and weight gain during pregnancy. Therapy has varied with the theories of etiology and the sophistication of the art and science of medicine. Aligning the woman's body with the magnetic poles of the earth was once a popular treatment as were various herbs and incantations and, perhaps, even "eye of newt; toe of frog."[8]

The cause of toxemia remains unknown today, although much has been learned about the underlying pathology. Research into etiology and physiologic mechanisms is hampered by the lack of suitable laboratory animals, since no species apart from humans is susceptible to this disease.

It is known that functioning trophoblastic tissue is necessary for the occurrence of toxemia, although apparently the presence of the fetus is not necessary, since women with hydatid moles have a markedly increased incidence of the disease. Other predisposing factors include age (very young and very old gravidas), parity (classically a disease of nulliparas), multiple gestations, diabetes mellitus, and chronic hypertension. In addition, the incidence of all toxemia, but especially eclampsia, is significantly higher in less favored socioeconomic circumstances. This has caused speculation that a nutritional basis may exist for the disease. Frequency as well as quality of antepartum care no doubt plays a significant role as well, particularly with regard to eclampsia.

Numerous hypotheses regarding the cause of toxemia have been advanced only to be discarded. One current hypothesis is that of reduced uteroplacental blood flow. A number of investigators have been able to induce hypertension in pregnant dogs or sheep by ligating the uterine arteries and thus producing uterine ischemia. Uterine blood flow is known to be reduced in chronic hypertension and some diabetes mellitus, two of the predisposing factors. Also there is anatomic confirmation that the diameter of the uterine arteries is greater in multigravidas than in primigravidas. It is not decided, however, whether the uterine ischemia is actually the first cause of the toxemia or whether it is the result of some other factor, as yet unknown. Another popular hypothesis suggests that "something" produces an increased vascular sensitivity, accounting for vasospasm which causes uterine ischemia.

[8] William Shakespeare, *MacBeth*, Act III, Scene i.

It is postulated that the ischemic placenta undergoes premature aging and may develop infarcts and other degenerative changes. Catabolic end products from this process are released into the maternal bloodstream, where they bring about a mild disseminated intravascular coagulation. This is aggravated by the hemoconcentration characteristic of the more severe forms of toxemia.

Regardless of where these changes occur in the cause–effect cycle there is agreement that the most basic underlying pathologic change is that of *generalized vasospasm*. If this vasospasm is kept in mind, all of the clinical symptoms of the disease may be explained, as well as the majority of therapeutic interventions.

Symptoms

Toxemia should be thought of as a single disease which exists on a continuum of severity ranging from mild preeclampsia through severe preeclampsia to eclampsia. Patients, however, do not necessarily progress through the disease in this sequence. The woman may present initially with very severe preeclampsia or, less commonly, eclampsia. Mild preeclampsia may progress rapidly to eclampsia or may remain quite stable with only minimum therapy. For this reason an extraordinary degree of vigilance is required in order to control the disease effectively.

The cardinal signs of preeclampsia are three: hypertension, edema, and proteinuria. The presence of hypertension together with either edema or proteinuria or both is diagnostic of this condition.

Hypertension is defined as a blood pressure of 140/90 or a rise in systolic pressure of 30 mmHg or more and a rise in diastolic pressure of 15 mmHg or more over baseline values. The elevation over the individual's own baseline is the more valuable criterion, since many women of reproductive age may have normally low readings, especially in the midtrimester. It is also valuable in detecting preeclampsia when it is superimposed on chronic hypertension. The blood pressure elevation should be noted on two separate occasions taken six hours apart in order to establish a definitive diagnosis. Since this, however, is not a practical procedure in most outpatient settings, treatment is usually begun without meeting this strict criterion.

Blood pressure readings of 160/100 mmHg are indicative of severe preeclampsia. Systolic readings over 200 are usually associated with an underlying chronic hypertension. Patients with systolic pressures over 200 are at significant risk for cerebral vascular accidents and require vigorous medical therapy.

Edema is the least precise of the clinical parameters of preeclampsia though it is often the first one to be detected. Edema of the lower extremities is almost a universal finding in pregnancy because of the mechanical obstruction of veins by the heavy uterus as well as changes in venous pressure. For this reason, edema of the face and hands is given greater significance. A sudden increase in weight (greater than 500 gm or 1 lb per week) without any other explanation is suspicious of developing edema. The woman may complain of a sudden tightness of her rings or of edema present upon rising in the morning. Facial edema may not be apparent to the woman or her family unless the onset is quite sudden. But the nurse who only sees her at weekly intervals may immediately notice a change in her appearance since the last visit.

Proteinuria is indicative of the extent of glomerular damage due to the toxemia and usually appears later than other symptoms. In order to be considered diagnostic, values greater than 1 gm/liter (or 1+ on a standard dip stick) must be detected. Whenever a possibility of preeclampsia exists, care should be taken to obtain a clean voided urine specimen for analysis. Vaginal discharge, characteristic of late pregnancy, readily contaminates the urine specimen and may give a falsely high reading. Twenty-four-hour urine assays are more reliable than a single voiding. Protein values over 500 mg/24 hours are diagnostic of preeclampsia. As preeclampsia becomes severe, urine may be highly concentrated, scant in amount, and contain casts, red and white blood cells, and epithelial cells. Oliguria is a grave prognostic sign.

While mild preeclampsia is characterized by edema and/or proteinuria together with hypertension, as the disease progresses and the vasospasm becomes more severe, other signs and symptoms begin to appear. There is increasing central nervous system irritability as evidenced by headaches, dizziness, visual disturbances, and hyperreflexia. Fundoscopic changes may be seen as a result of the vasospasm and perhaps also because of central nervous system alterations. These changes include retinal edema, arteriolar constriction or spasm, and hemorrhages. Rarely, retinal detachment may occur due to extreme retinal edema. Reattachment is usually spontaneous after delivery and resolution of the disease process. Epigastric pain is a late and ominous symptom. The pain is generally felt to be due to hepatic capsular stretching resulting from edema and/or hemorrhages.

The occurrence of a convulsion or coma, in addition to the symptoms of preeclampsia, is diagnostic of eclampsia. This constitutes one of the gravest complications in obstetrics. Maternal mortality may be as high as 10 percent, while perinatal mortality approaches 25 percent.

All the symptoms enumerated for preeclampsia become more severe with eclampsia. Severe edema distorts the woman's features until she may be unrecognizable. Oliguria or even anuria is noted, and proteinuria varies from a few grams per liter to 30 to 40 gm/liter. Blood pressure averages 180/110 mmHg, although it may be much higher.

Convulsions, both tonic and clonic, occur in eclampsia. At first all muscles go into a state of tonic contraction; then they alternately contract and relax. The convulsions are sometimes preceded by an aura, but often are so entirely unheralded that they occur while the patient is asleep. They ordinarily begin with a twitching of the eyelids or facial muscles. The eyes are wide open and staring, and the pupils are usually dilated. Next the whole body becomes rigid, and then alternate contraction and relaxation of all muscles begin. The twitchings proceed from the muscles about the nose and mouth to those of the neck and arms, and so on, until the entire body is in spasm. The patient's face is usually cyanotic and badly distorted, with the mouth being drawn to one side. She clenches her fists, rolls her head from side to side, and tosses violently about the bed. She is totally unconscious and insensible to light, and during the seizure respirations cease. Her head is frequently bent backward. Her neck forms a continuous curve with her stiffened, arched back. Another distressing feature is the protruding tongue and the frothy saliva, which may be blood stained if the patient bites her tongue. Finally muscular movements become milder, and then the patient lies motionless. After a long, deep breath, respiratory movements are resumed.

Convulsive attacks vary greatly in their intensity and duration. There may be only a few twitches, lasting 10 to 15 seconds, or violent convulsions lasting as long as two minutes. Their number and severity increase with the seriousness of the patient's condition.

The patient lapses into a coma after a convulsion. This also varies in length and profundity, her condition during the intervals being very suggestive of the probable outcome of the disease. Some patients have no recollection of the seizures and may even fail to remember anything that happened within several hours, or even days, before the attack.

During the acute stage the respirations are, as a rule, labored and noisy, and cyanosis may be present. The temperature is often normal or rises to 38.3°C (101°F). It may go as high as 39.4°C (103°F) or 40°C (104°F), in severe cases, and this is a serious prognostic sign.

When eclampsia develops during late pregnancy, labor may begin and the baby be born spontaneously, or the fetus may die, after which the condition begins to improve and the stillborn infant is delivered later.

When eclampsia occurs in labor, contractions usually increase in force and frequency, thus hastening delivery, after which the condition begins to improve. Death or expulsion of the fetus is usually followed by improvement within 12 to 24 hours (coma may continue a few hours or a day) and by ultimate recovery, provided adequate treatment is continued and the condition has not become critical before delivery or death of the baby.

In postpartum eclampsia the convulsions occur soon after delivery—almost always within the first 24 hours.

The most frequent causes of death in eclampsia are congestive heart failure, cerebral vascular accidents, and complications of obstetric operations. Improved antepartum care as well as better methods of treatment for both preeclampsia and eclampsia have led to a significant decrease in maternal and perinatal mortality.

Prevention

Eclampsia is considered to be a preventable disease in almost every circumstance. A woman who assumes responsibility for her own health care, seeks antepartum consultation, and recognizes changes in her body needing evaluation will be diagnosed and treated before eclampsia occurs. Preeclampsia, treated knowledgeably, can almost always be controlled so it does not progress to convulsions. Professionals caring for pregnant women have a serious responsibility not only to recognize and treat early symptoms but also to instruct their clients in what signs and symptoms to report immediately. Every effort should be made to develop a relationship where the woman, though not overly dependent, feels free to call with questions at any time. In this way she is unlikely to delay reporting important symptoms because she doesn't "want to bother you."

Preeclampsia is not preventable at present. Although good antepartum care has markedly reduced the mortality and morbidity due to the more severe forms, there is no evidence that any feature of even the best antepartum care has reduced the overall incidence of preeclampsia.

In the recent past, several measures widely prescribed to prevent preeclampsia have been proven to be of no value and, in fact, potentially harmful. Restriction of dietary salt and caloric intake as well as the use of diuretics have been shown to be detrimental. Severe electrolyte imbalance can result from limited sodium intake, particularly if combined with the use of thiazide diuretics. In fact, there is growing evidence that increased salt intake may be necessary to maintain the positive sodium balance of a normal pregnancy. This is usually accomplished by advising the woman to salt her food to taste, since she will doubtless be increasing her overall food intake.

Weight control is likewise of no value in preventing preeclampsia. As discussed in Chapter 8, inadequate weight gain is associated with an increased incidence of small-for-gestational-age infants.

Diuretics have failed to demonstrate any reduction in the incidence of preeclampsia in double-blind studies. Rather, they have been associated with severe maternal electrolyte imbalance, fetal and neonatal hyponatremia, and neonatal thrombocytopenia. By reducing the effective intravascular volume, diuretics may actually promote vasospasm, thus further reducing uterine blood flow. Furthermore, when given prophylactically throughout pregnancy they may mask the development of early signs of impending toxemia.

Although a cause–effect relationship between nutrition and toxemia has not been proven, there is some reason to believe that a good diet, high in protein, may be helpful. Periods of rest, preferably with the woman lying on her side, may enhance uterine blood flow. Certainly these two precautions are beneficial enough to the woman's general health and well-being that no harm can be done in emphasizing them, even without proof they will prevent toxemia.

Since early detection of the beginning symptoms of preeclampsia is so beneficial, it would presumably be even more beneficial to detect those women who are going to develop preeclampsia before clinical symptoms appear. In 1974, Gant and his associates found that women between 28 and 32 weeks gestation, who later developed toxemia, demonstrated an increased sensitivity to the pressor effects of angiotensin II. In addition, he found that these same women demonstrated a rise in diastolic blood pressure of at least 20 mmHg when turned from a lateral to a supine position. Initial reports indicated that more than 93 percent of the women who showed the rise in diastolic pressure subsequently developed toxemia. Subsequent studies have failed to replicate this high percentage, and the clinical value of this observation is unconfirmed but seems to warrant further investigation.[9]

Gant's blood pressure screening procedure has come to be known as the "rollover test" and is a useful addition to antepartum screening procedures. At a regular office visit between 28 and 32 weeks gestation the woman is positioned in a left lateral recumbent position and her blood pressure taken every 5 minutes until the diastolic reading is identical on two consecutive determinations. Then the woman rolls over to a supine position and her blood pressure is taken immediately and again in five minutes. An increase in diastolic pressure of 20 mmHg or more over her established baseline is termed a positive rollover test.[10] Knowing which women are apt to develop toxemia would help the practitioner focus attention and time on those clients at greatest risk. It does not prevent the disease since no prophylactic therapy is known. Experiments with reduced physical activity or even bed rest are being conducted but no evidence is available at this time.

Treatment

The only cure for toxemia is delivery of the pregnancy. Therefore, if delivery is undesirable because of the immaturity of the fetus, efforts are directed at controlling the symptoms to insure both maternal and fetal safety until delivery can be reasonably undertaken. The extent and

vigor of medical intervention depends on the severity of the disease at any given time. Constant reevaluation and modification of the plan of care is usually necessary.

The most usual situation is for a woman who has been receiving regular antepartum supervision to present in the third trimester at a regular appointment with some generalized edema and a slight elevation in blood pressure. Proteinuria may or may not be present. A diagnosis of mild preeclampsia is made. The woman is advised to maintain bedrest, notify the nurse or physician of any subjective change in status, and return to the office or clinic in 3 to 4 days. A mild sedative (usually sodium phenobarbital) may be prescribed to make bed rest more palatable as well as for its anticonvulsive effects. Bed rest, especially on the left side, facilitates venous return, promotes diuresis, and enhances uterine blood flow. Public health nurse consultation may be sought to monitor blood pressure at home. A case summary will illustrate this care.

M. W., a 19-year-old primigravida, presented in the physician's office at 37-weeks gestation with a blood pressure of 138/90 (previous readings were 100–110/70), 2+ to 3+ edema of feet, legs, and hands, and a trace of protein on the urine dip stick. She had gained 2½ lb since her last visit ten days earlier. The diagnosis of preeclampsia and its implications were carefully discussed with M. W. and she was advised to go on bed rest at home and return to the office in four days. She was encouraged to lie on her left side as much as possible and to get up only to go to the bathroom or to eat. When M. W. returned to the office four days later she still had some dependent edema, but her blood pressure was 112/76, her urine contained no protein, and she had lost 1800 gm (4 lb) from diuresis. This woman was followed closely until 39 weeks gestation when she went into labor spontaneously and delivered a 3150-gm (6 lb 15 oz) girl. Except for continued edema and slight elevation of blood pressure to 130/90 during labor, there were no further clinical manifestations of preeclampsia.

For this woman bed rest was a reasonable request, which she was readily able to carry out. She had previously resigned from her job, had no other chil-

[9] Norman F. Gant *et al.*, A clinical test useful for predicting the development of acute hypertension in pregnancy, *Am. J. Obstet. Gynecol.* 120:1–7 (Sept. 1) 1974.

[10] Ronald A. Chez, and Norman F. Gant, The supine pressor response test, *Contemp. Ob/Gyn* 5:67–69 (May) 1975.

dren, and lived with her husband who was able to rearrange his work commitments to allow time for him to be very nurturant toward his wife.

In contrast, consider the following case.

V. L., a 22-year-old gravida three, para one, lived in a mobile home eight miles from town and nearly three miles from her nearest neighbor. Her husband, a long-distance truck driver, was away from home 11 out of every 14 days. During this time V. L. was alone with her three-year-old daughter. Bed rest in these circumstances would be virtually impossible unless the nurse used tact and resourcefulness to help this family problem-solve. In this case daytime child care and help with grocery shopping were arranged through a local church and a home health aide visited every other day. Later, the husband was able to negotiate with his company for some short-distance drives for several weeks of the pregnancy. At 38 weeks a 2700-gm (6 lb) boy was delivered following induction of labor.

When bed rest at home does not improve the symptoms, or when the presenting symptoms are more severe, hospitalization is necessary. The goals of therapy are to decrease central nervous system irritability, control the blood pressure, promote diuresis, monitor fetal well-being and, ultimately, to deliver the infant.

The newly admitted woman is placed on bed rest, and environmental stimuli are kept to a minimum. Loud talking, bright lights, and unnecessary traffic in and out of her room are to be avoided. Reflexes are checked at frequent intervals for hyperactivity and the presence of clonus is noted. Sodium phenobarbital or some other mild sedative or tranquilizer is usually prescribed. Careful explanation of all procedures as well as the overall plan of care will further alleviate the woman's anxiety.

Renal function is evaluated by means of creatinine clearance tests and 24-hour urine protein determinations. A strict intake and output record is kept to detect any changes in volume of urine. Weight obtained at the same time each day, indicates the extent of diuresis.

An amniocentesis is usually done to deter-mine fetal lung maturity. Twenty-four-hour urinary estriol is measured as an indicator of fetal/placental function, and/or an oxytocin challenge test (OCT) or fetal activity determination (FAD) may be done. If the fetus is near term and has a mature L/S ratio, labor will usually be induced after the maternal symptoms have been controlled for 12 to 24 hours. If preeclampsia is severe, delivery may be necessary before optimal fetal maturity for both maternal and fetal welfare.

The woman who does not respond to bed rest and sedation with lowered blood pressure and diuresis must be treated more aggressively. The usual therapy is magnesium sulfate, administered either intramuscularly or intravenously. This drug is an effective anticonvulsant as it decreases central nervous system irritability by acting directly on the central nervous system as well as at the myoneural junction. A secondary effect is the lowering of blood pressure due to vasodilation. Patients receiving magnesium sulfate by either route should have an intravenous conduit in place, receive nothing by mouth, and have an indwelling catheter in the bladder to permit hourly assessment of urinary output.

When magnesium sulfate is given intramuscularly the initial dose is usually 10 gm (20 ml of a 50 percent solution). It is divided so that 10 ml are given into each buttock; 1 ml of a 1 percent local anesthetic agent is usually added to each 10 ml of magnesium sulfate solution to reduce the discomfort of the injection. If the patient is still hyperactive in 4 to 6 hours and if urinary output is satisfactory, magnesium sulfate may be repeated in a 5 gm dose.

Intramuscular administration of magnesium sulfate should be deep into the gluteal muscle, preferably into the ventrogluteal area. It is advisable to discard the needle used to draw the solution from the ampuls and to attach another sterile dry needle to the syringe for administration of the drug. In this way it is possible to avoid any irritant solution on the outside of the needle. As injection of the medication is made, the needle may be moved about to obtain a wider dispersion of the drug. The area of ad-

Table 22-4. Nursing Management of Inpatients with Toxemia

Patient Care Goals	Nursing Interventions

I. Decrease central nervous system irritability.	1. Modify environment to ensure rest and quiet.
	  a. Eliminate noise, bright lights, other harsh stimuli.
	  b. Minimize number of personnel giving care.
	  c. Initiate painful and/or intrusive procedures after sedation.
	  d. Promote comfort at bed rest.
	2. Explain all plans and procedures simply and briefly.
	3. Administer sedative drugs as prescribed.
	4. Be alert to changing clinical status.
	  a. Assess knee-jerk reflexes.
	  b. Determine subjective symptoms (irritability, headache, blurred vision, epigastric pain).
	  c. Keep emergency support materials readily available (e.g., O_2, suction, airway, $MgSO_4$, sedatives).

II. Control blood pressure.	1. Measure and record B/P (frequency is determined by severity of clinical symptoms). 2. Have B/P taken by the same person using the same cuff whenever possible. 3. Administer antihypertensive drugs as prescribed (usually when diastolic pressure exceeds 110 mmHg).

III. Promote diuresis.	1. Encourage continuous bed rest in left lateral position.
	2. Monitor renal function.
	  a. Dip-stick exam for urine protein.
	  b. Collect 24-hour specimen for protein and creatinine clearance.
	3. Monitor effects of therapy.
	  a. Record accurate intake and output (minimum output: 20ml/hr).
	  b. Weigh daily at same time using same scale.

IV. Monitor fetal well-being.	1. Auscultate and record FHR. 2. Instruct and support during amniocentesis. 3. Collect 24-hour urine specimen for estriol determination. 4. Perform FAD and/or OCT. 5. Reassure parents realistically, based on available data.
V. Deliver the infant.	1. Review parents' knowledge of labor and delivery. 2. Give instructions about induction of labor and electronic fetal heart rate monitoring. 3. Introduce parents to intrapartum nurse prior to onset of labor. 4. Introduce parents to appropriate neonatal staff.

ministration should be massaged and a dry, warm pack applied.

Intravenous administration of this drug is becoming more common. It avoids the painful intramuscular injection, but also has the added safety of a more predictable action, which is more readily controlled. In contrast, medication injected intramuscularly may have quite variable absorption rates and, once injected, cannot be retrieved. A frequent dose schedule for intravenous magnesium sulfate is a "loading" dose of 4 gm followed by the continuous infusion of 1 to 2 gm per hour. Magnesium blood levels are often used to determine the rate of flow.

Regardless of the route of administration, certain clinical criteria must be met prior to the administration of any subsequent doses. These criteria are: (1) respirations greater than 12 per minute; (2) urinary output at least 30 ml per hour; and (3) presence of the knee-jerk reflex.

Magnesium sulfate is eliminated from the body chiefly by the kidneys, and if the urinary output is low, it may be retained in the blood until a high, dangerous concentration is reached. This may depress respirations and cardiac action. The patient must be watched for respiratory depression. It is believed that this depression does not occur until after the knee-jerk reflex disappears.

A further safeguard against magnesium overdose, as well as a means of assuring doses sufficient to prevent convulsions, is the monitoring of maternal magnesium blood levels. Magnesium equilibrates fairly readily across the placenta so the fetal blood level reflects that of the mother, and the neonate may have respiratory depression if born with high magnesium blood levels. Maternal blood levels of 4 to 6 mg per 100 ml are usually sufficient therapeutically and do not cause neonatal depression at birth.

An intravenous calcium preparation, 10 percent calcium gluconate, is an immediate antidote to magnesium sulfate. It should always be available at the patient's bedside in case of respiratory or cardiac arrest. (See Figure 22-13.)

Occasionally magnesium sulfate alone is not sufficient to reduce central nervous system irritability and sodium phenobarbital is given as well. Smaller doses of the barbiturate are necessary when used together with magnesium sulfate. Barbiturate should be avoided in labor, since there is no available antagonist.

An antihypertensive drug is sometimes required to lower blood pressure. When the diastolic pressure cannot be reduced below 110 mmHg with magnesium sulfate alone, a drug such as hydralazine (Apresoline) may be given. This drug has the advantage of dilating peripheral vessels, and thus does not diminish uterine blood flow. Care should be taken to maintain the diastolic pressure no lower than 90 mmHg in order to maintain placental perfusion.

As soon as the maternal condition is stabilized and fetal maturity is established, induction of labor is begun with continuous oxytocin infusion as described in Chapter 16. The magnesium sulfate is continued through labor. In preeclampsia the uterus is highly responsive to oxytocin and vaginal delivery can almost always be achieved. Continuous fetal heart rate monitoring should be employed to assess the fetal response to labor.

In the unfortunate event that the disease progresses to eclampsia immediate efforts are directed toward control of convulsions, stabilization of blood pressure, and maintenance of renal function. Usually 4 to 6 hours are sufficient to control the symptoms and stabilize the patient. Delivery should then be accomplished with dispatch.

The intracranial pressure is frequently raised in patients with eclampsia, and they are therefore very irritable, so that any stimulation may start a convulsion. To this end there are innumerable details to be considered. Every effort is made to keep the patient as quiet and free from stimuli as possible. A quiet, darkened room is important. Every act must be performed as

---

PRECAUTIONS FOR WOMEN RECEIVING MAGNESIUM SULFATE

1. Continuous nursing attendance

2. Intravenous conduit in place

3. Foley catheter connected to drainage

4. $MgSO_4$ given *ONLY* when:

   Respirations > 12 per minute

   Urine output > 20 ml per hour

   Knee jerk reflexes clearly present

5. Calcium gluconate available at bedside

Figure 22-13. Summary of care of women with toxemia of pregnancy who are receiving magnesium sulfate.

quietly as possible. The nurse should walk lightly and guard against kicking or striking the bed. Talking should be in low tones, doors should be opened and closed quietly, and papers should not be rustled or furniture scraped. Since any manipulation may excite a convulsion, the patient should not be disturbed more than is absolutely necessary. Only the care essential for treatment and for observation should be given.

Constant nursing care is necessary, and the patient must never be left alone for even a second. She must be carefully observed for any change in condition and especially for twitchings, cyanosis, and excessive mucus. Someone must be present to prevent the patient from injuring herself during convulsions and to remove mucus from the respiratory passages as it collects.

Restraint during convulsions should be as mild as possible, since resistance increases the patient's excitement while her need is to be quieted, but she must be protected against falling out of bed and against injuring her tongue. During a convulsion there is great danger of the patient's biting her tongue unless something is placed between her teeth at the very onset to prevent their closing on the tongue. A small roll of bandage, a clean cloth tightly rolled, several tongue depressors wrapped with gauze or a piece of thick rubber tubing may be used and must be at the bedside, available for immediate use. Hard wooden mouth gags are not satisfactory because of the danger of bruising or cutting the mucous membranes or even breaking a tooth.

Careful watching and proper positioning are necessary to keep the patient from aspirating excessive pulmonary secretions and vomitus. The comatose patient, or one who is vomiting, is usually turned on her side and the foot of the bed elevated to favor drainage of secretions from the air passages. Suction may be necessary to remove mucus. The pulmonary secretions may be greatly increased. Fluids should never be given orally, for fear of aspiration.

The blood pressure, urinary output, tempera-ture, pulse, and respirations are checked at least every hour and more frequently if clinical conditions warrant. A decrease in the urinary output or a rise in any one of the other signs is considered unfavorable. An indwelling catheter is usually inserted so that the urinary output can be carefully watched. It should be at least 30 ml per hour. The fetal heart tones are checked at regular intervals. Labor frequently begins after eclampsia develops; if not, labor should be induced as soon as the patient's condition is stable. Examinations, however, are kept to a minimum.

Sedatives are administered, sometimes in fairly large doses. The respirations must be closely observed. Magnesium sulfate is used to lower blood pressure and control convulsions.

A 5 to 10 percent dextrose in Ringer's lactate solution may be used to provide fluids, electrolytes, and caloric intake and to overcome acidosis. From 2500 to 3000 ml total fluids are usually given in a 24-hour period. Output must be closely monitored to avoid circulatory overload.

As in the case of preeclampsia induction of labor is by oxytocin infusion. Cesarean section will usually not be done except for obstetric indications or fetal distress.

Regardless of the severity of the antepartum toxemia, the woman remains at risk for convulsions for at least 24 hours post partum. For this reason vigilant care and medical treatment is continued until diuresis occurs and definite improvement in all symptoms is noted.

Prognosis

In general, the prognosis for preeclamptic patients is good when treatment is prompt. If improvement is not evident with bed rest and medical treatment, delivery of the baby is effective. Recovery is usually quite prompt after delivery, with disappearance of all signs of toxemia in 10 to 14 days (Fig. 22-14). In some patients hypertension persists, but it is thought that most such patients have underlying chronic hypertension. There may be a recurrence of toxemia, at least to a mild degree, in subsequent pregnancies.

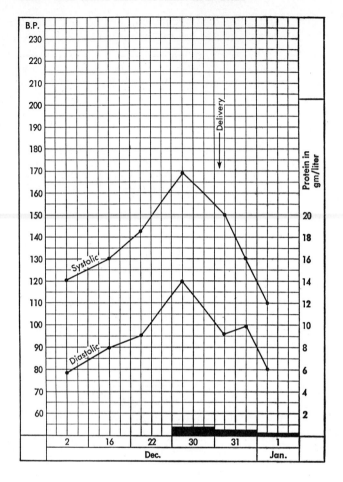

Figure 22-14. Fall in blood pressure and decrease in protein are rapid after delivery of a woman with severe preeclampsia.

The final outcome of eclampsia depends on many factors. The prognosis is more favorable after delivery, especially when the urinary output increases. When signs and symptoms increase, the outlook is unfavorable. The patient may die due to pulmonary edema, cardiac failure, or pneumonia due to aspiration of mucus, blood, and fluid, which may be drawn into the lungs by the deep, stertorous breathing. Exemplary nursing care can virtually prevent this latter complication.

When recovery begins, it is comparatively rapid. In 24 to 48 hours the urinary output may be as high as 4 to 6 liters per day. An increase in the urinary output is the first sign of improvement. Edema disappears in four to five days, and as the woman loses all this fluid, there is a marked difference in her appearance. The patient soon begins to feel well unless she has developed aspiration pneumonia or other infection. The weight decreases rapidly, the blood pressure drops to normal in about two weeks, the protein and casts disappear from the urine in about a week. All symptoms subside in two to four weeks.

In preeclampsia the primary risk to the fetus is intrauterine growth retardation, resulting from poor placental perfusion. In addition, premature delivery may be necessary because of the severity of maternal disease as well as the increasing risks to the fetus of remaining in an environment of malnutrition. Intrauterine death may occur as a result of placental insufficiency, eclamptic convulsions, or abruptio placenta. The neonatal risks are chiefly those of the small-for-gestational-age infant and/or the premature infant. Overall perinatal mortality in toxemia is estimated to be approximately 25 percent, with eclampsia accounting for most of this.

Prior to postpartum discharge from the hospital, the nurse should sit down with the woman (and her family if she desires) and review the course of events, answering any questions she might have. Implications for follow-up health care, contraception, and future pregnancies should also be discussed.

If the woman is not normotensive by four to six weeks postpartum, chronic hypertension is suspected and further medical evaluation is indicated. The use of oral contraceptives is contraindicated in hypertensive women, so alternate forms of contraception should be considered until confirmation of normal blood pressure readings. If the woman is a primigravida, the chances are good that she will not have toxemia in future pregnancies. If, however, there is a predisposing factor, such as diabetes mellitus, which will still be present during subsequent gestations, she should take particular care to alert physicians to her risk at the time of any future antepartum care.

Chronic Hypertensive Disease

Hypertensive disease, also termed essential hypertension or hypertensive vascular disease, is not a true toxemia of pregnancy but is frequently first recognized in pregnancy. It presents some of the symptoms of a toxemia. Although hypertensive disease is not peculiar to pregnancy, it is considered with the toxemias because pregnancy may be an aggravating factor. The patient with essential hypertension often develops a superimposed preeclampsia or acute toxemia. Hypertensive disease in pregnancy is seen most frequently among pregnant women in the older age group, in multigravidas, and in obese women. It appears that the greater incidence of hypertension during pregnancy in

women over 30 years of age is the result of preexisting or latent hypertension, which predisposes to development of blood pressure elevation during pregnancy. When the tendency to develop hypertension in later years exists in any woman, she is more likely to develop an increase in her blood pressure during pregnancy.

Signs and Symptoms

Evidence of this disease is variable. Frequently the only sign of chronic hypertensive disease in pregnancy is hypertension before the twenty-fourth week of gestation. In many of these women a persistently elevated blood pressure and possibly slight changes in the retinal blood vessels are the only evidences of the disease throughout pregnancy. Signs are typically present from the onset of pregnancy, unlike in patients with acute toxemia. These women usually feel well with the possible exception of having headaches. A small percentage of patients have a more advanced disease and show varying degrees of cardiac, renal, and/or retinal damage. Blood pressure readings may vary from slight elevation to levels of 300/160 mmHg and are frequently normal during midtrimester. Marked narrowing and tortuosity of the retinal blood vessels and retinal exudates and hemorrhages may be present if the disease is severe, especially if the kidneys are involved. Proteinuria and edema are ordinarily not present, as in an acute toxemia, unless there is severe renal involvement.

About 25 percent of patients with chronic hypertensive disease in pregnancy develop a superimposed preeclampsia. This is apt to occur earlier than preeclampsia ordinarily appears, and is likely to be a more severe form. This development may be manifested by a sudden exacerbation of previous signs, sudden weight gain, edema, protein in the urine, and retinal hemorrhages and exudates. Fetal growth retardation is frequently seen and is a major risk.

Diagnosis

It may be difficult to differentiate between hypertensive disease and preeclampsia unless it is definitely known that the woman had hypertension before her pregnancy. Examination of the eyegrounds may show hemorrhages and exudates which are not always present in preeclampsia. The response of the blood pressure, weight, urinary output, and protein output while the patient is under treatment of bed rest and dietary control may be of value in diagnosis.

Sometimes chronic hypertensive disease cannot be differentiated from preeclampsia until some time after delivery. The differential diagnosis can usually be made during the puerperium since in preeclampsia the blood pressure usually falls rapidly to normal, the weight decreases rapidly, and the casts and protein disappear from the urine in from two to four weeks. In chronic hypertension, although the blood pressure falls somewhat and protein, if present, decreases as the condition improves, by the end of the puerperium the blood pressure is still elevated and casts and protein may be present in the urine (Fig. 22-15).

Treatment and Nursing Care

Observations of blood pressure, weight gain, and proteinuria are important. Hypertensive disease cannot be prevented through antepartum care, but evidence of disease can be recognized early and proper treatment instituted to minimize its effects and decrease the major risks of preeclampsia and intrauterine growth retardation.

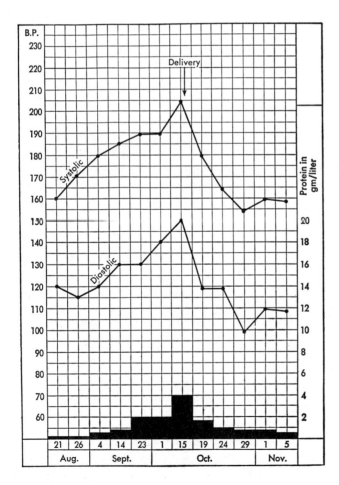

Figure 22-15. Persistence of high blood pressure and protein after delivery of a woman with severe chronic hypertensive renal disease, who additionally had a superimposed preeclampsia during the last month of gestation. Compare this with Figure 22-14 which shows rapid recovery from severe preeclampsia following delivery.

Patients with mild hypertensive disease frequently need only careful evaluation of their cardiovascular status, close observation during pregnancy, and instructions to report untoward symptoms early. Considerable rest and limitation of activity are very important. The more severely ill patient and the one who develops an acute toxemia require hospitalization and intensive treatment.

Careful assessment of fetal growth and evaluation of placental function is important.

Hospital treatment and nursing care are approximately the same as for preeclampsia: rest in bed, a high-protein diet, adequate fluids, and close observation of the patient's general condition.

To discover any change in condition, the weight is checked frequently, sometimes daily, the blood pressure is taken once or more daily, and an accurate record of the fluid intake and output is kept. The urine is examined for protein. Headache, dizziness, and/or visual disturbance should be noted and reported to the physician immediately.

Kidney-function tests and examinations of the cardiovascular system are often made. The results of such findings, the severity of symptoms, and the response to treatment determine subsequent care.

Prognosis

If hypertensive disease is mild and if preeclampsia is not superimposed, the pregnancy usually continues without hazard. Severe hypertension, cardiac or renal involvement, advanced retinal changes, and a superimposed preeclampsia may endanger the mother and may be associated with death of the fetus. Many physicians believe that pregnancy is contraindicated and may recommend that it be terminated in the small number of patients who have a severe form of the disease. If a superimposed acute toxemia develops, there is a high incidence of fetal death *in utero* and an increased incidence of abruptio placentae. When such a condition does not respond to intensive treatment, the physician may recommend early delivery of the baby.

These patients are likely to have a recurrence of an acute toxemia in subsequent pregnancies.

HYDRAMNIOS

Hydramnios (sometimes referred to as polyhydramnios) is the presence of an excessive amount of amniotic fluid. The normal amount of fluid near term is between 500 and 1000 ml, or slightly more. An amount of over 2000 ml is considered excessive. Between 2000 and 3000 ml of amniotic fluid is relatively common; much larger amounts may develop but occur infrequently. Any amount over 3000 ml is considered clinically significant.

The cause of hydramnios is not clear. It is known to occur frequently in association with fetal malformations and in pregnancies complicated by diabetes and severe erythroblastosis. Amniotic fluid may be increased in amount in twin pregnancies and sometimes in the toxemias of pregnancy. The increase to an excessive amount of fluid is usually gradual, but in rare cases it occurs suddenly.

Diagnosis of hydramnios is usually made through clinical observation, since it is difficult to estimate or measure the amount with accuracy. The uterus enlarges more than expected for the period of gestation. Palpation of the fetal small parts, hearing of the fetal heart tones, and ballottement of the fetus may be difficult.

Symptoms caused by hydramnios result from the pressure of the enlarged uterus on adjacent organs and are related to the degree of distention. Pressure against the diaphragm may cause distress. Edema of the lower extremities occurs frequently. Generalized abdominal discomfort may develop. However, maternal discomfort may be only slight, since the increase in fluid is usually very gradual. Labor tends to begin prematurely. The uterine muscle may become atonic due to excessive stretching.

Occasionally, maternal symptoms of shortness of breath are severe as a result of hydramnios. Amniocentesis unfortunately affords only a very short period of relief and in women in the latter weeks of pregnancy may be associated with premature labor. This usually precludes amniocentesis as a useful procedure for relief of hydramnios unless labor and delivery are desired. However, some practitioners have had favorable results in chronic hydramnios with removing 500 to 700 ml of fluid every 3 to 4 days to allow the fetus to reach maturity.

FETAL DEATH

Fetal death late in pregnancy is usually recognized by the mother through the absence of fetal movements. It is a subjective, but a significant sign, and warrants further investigation. The mother may suspect that movement has ceased when the fetus actually is healthy but becomes less active as he nears term. On the other hand, even when fetal movements have ceased, the mother may believe she feels movement and it is difficult for her to accept any other fact. Death of a fetus, or suspected death, causes the mother much concern over carrying the dead fetus and a great deal of worry over what she may or may not have done to cause his death. She needs a great deal of reassurance that she could not have avoided his death and both parents will need much immediate emotional support and, later, guidance in future pregnancies.

Fetal life must be assumed until diagnosis proves that death has occurred. Sometimes this diagnosis is difficult and takes considerable time. Some diagnostic methods will obviously depend upon the period of gestation.

In the early months of pregnancy failure of uterine growth over a period of several weeks is significant. Negative pregnancy tests point to fetal death, but sometimes a pregnancy test may remain positive for several weeks because the placenta may continue to produce chorionic gonadotropic hormone for a few weeks after fetal death.

Later in pregnancy absence of fetal heart tones is strong evidence of fetal death but not infallible. Urinary estriol becomes very low (less than 2 mg per 24 hours) and is a very useful confirmatory test. X-ray shows overlapping of skull bones several days after death. Ultrasound findings include characteristic echoes from the head and thorax, as well as evidence of overlapping skull bones. Amniotic fluid may be analyzed for the presence of creatinine phosphokinase (CPK), which is markedly elevated in fetal death after 48–72 hours. The uterus fails to grow and may even become smaller.

In many women labor will begin spontaneously within a few weeks after fetal death, but induction of labor is usually carried out when the diagnosis is definitely confirmed. Prolonged retention of a dead fetus presents some danger of fibrinogenopenia in the mother, and it is psychologically disturbing to her.

A dead fetus usually shows maceration and peeling of the skin at birth, and the amniotic fluid is small in amount and meconium-stained or reddish in color.

BIBLIOGRAPHY

Aure, Beverly, Intrauterine transfusions: The nurse's role with expectant parents, *Nurs. Clin. North Am.* 7:817–826 (Dec.) 1972.

Avery, Gordon B., *Neonatology: Pathophysiology and Management of the Newborn.* Lippincott, Philadelphia, Pa., 1975.

Burrow, Gerard N., and Ferris, Thomas F., *Medical Complications During Pregnancy.* Saunders, Philadelphia, Pa., 1975.

Chesley, Leon C., What is the long-term prognosis for eclamptic patients, *Contemp. Ob/Gyn* 7:137–143 (June) 1976.

Contemporary Ob/Gyn, Symposium: Therapeutic approaches to premature labor, 8:58–86 (Dec.) 1976.

———, Symposium: Disseminated intravascular coagulation. Part II, 1:69–91 (June) 1973.

———, Symposium: Disseminated intravascular coagulation. Part I, 1:71–106 (May) 1973.

Donald, I., New diagnostic horizons with sonar, *Br. J. Radiol.* 49:306–315 (Apr.) 1976.

Dudrick, Stanley J., Copeland, Edward M. III, and MacFadyen, Bruce V. Jr., Long-term parenteral nutrition: Its current status, *Hosp. Pract.* 10:47–58 (May) 1973.

Fong, Susie W. *et al.*, Intrauterine transfusion: Fetal outcome and complications, *Pediatrics* 45:576 (Apr.) 1970.

Fraser, I. D. *et al.*, Intensive antenatal plasmapheresis in severe rhesus isoimmunization, *Lancet* I:6–8 (Jan. 3) 1976.

Greenhill, J. P., and Friedman, Emanuel A., *Biologial Principles and Modern Practice of Obstetrics*, Saunders, Philadelphia, Pa., 1974.

Johnson, Daniel F., and Kennan, Alfred L., Rh immunoglobulin and its use in preventing erythroblastosis, *Wis. Med. J.* 67:424 (Sept.) 1968.

Lanzkowsky, Philip, Erythroblastosis fetalis, *Pediatr. Ann.* 3:7–34 (Feb.) 1974.

Lindheimer, Marshall D., and Katz, Adrian I., Sodium and diuretics in pregnancy, *Obstet. Gynecol.* 44:434–440 (Sept.) 1974.

Louka, M. H., and Lewis, G. C., Obstetric and gynecologic bleeding, *Hosp. Med.*, 12:44–59 (Aug.) 1976.

McGurn, Wealtha Collins, Mechanisms of shock: Pathophysiology, therapeutic measures, and nursing intervention, in *Advanced Concepts in Clinical Nursing*, edited by Kay C. Kintzel. Lippincott, Philadelphia, Pa., 1971, pp. 181–201.

Pritchard, Jack A., and MacDonald, Paul C., *Williams Obstetrics*, 15th ed. Appleton-Century-Crofts, New York, 1976.

Roberts, John M., and Moy, W. Joseph, Consumptive coagulopathy in severe preeclampsia, *Obstet. Gynecol.* 48:163–166 (Aug.) 1976.

Sabbagha, Rudy E. *et al.*, Sonar biparietal diameter, Parts I and II, *Am. J. Obstet. Gynecol.* 126:479–490 (Oct. 15) 1976.

Tietze, Christopher, and Lewitt, Sarah, Legal Abortion, *Sci. Am.* 236:21–27 (Jan.) 1977.

23

Medical Complications of Childbearing

Both the pregnant woman and her fetus may be at risk because of the existence of a chronic organic disease in the mother or because of an acute illness occurring during gestation. These illnesses are likely to result in a suboptimum intrauterine environment, which places the fetus at a disadvantage for normal growth and development from the very beginning of life. At the same time the normal physiologic adjustments of pregnancy may severely stress maternal organs already impaired by a chronic illness.

Ideally, women who are at risk for complications should be identified prior to pregnancy. Counseling at this time will enable them to make more informed decisions about childbearing as well as provide time to correct remedial conditions and stabilize others so that each woman begins pregnancy in her optimal state of health. Women (and their families) whose pregnancies are concurrent with a chronic disorder should expect that medical supervision will be more intense, office visits will be more frequent, more diagnostic studies will be done, antepartum hospitalization may be necessary, and the cost will be much greater both in dollars and in stress. On the other hand, they can also expect a generally favorable outcome for both mother and infant, provided they are given access to the quality of care that is possible today in perinatal intensive care settings.

INFECTIONS IN PREGNANCY

Since no special privileges of immunity are conferred with conception, pregnant women are susceptible to any infectious agents which can affect the general population. Sexually transmitted organisms as well as others may cause disease in the mother and adversely affect the health of the unborn child. A disturbing characteristic of many of these infections is that, while the maternal disease may be very mild, or perhaps even asymptomatic, severe developmental anomalies and even death may occur in the embryo/fetus. (See Table 23-1.)

The TORCH Complex

The letters in TORCH stand for toxoplasmosis, rubella, cytomegalovirus, herpes virus, and other agents. The "other agents" most commonly refers to group B beta-hemolytic streptococcus as well as syphilis and gonorrhea.

Toxoplasmosis is caused by the protozoa, *Toxoplasma gondii*. It is transmitted through the ingestion of raw or undercooked meat as well as in the feces of cats. Women should be cautioned to cook meat thoroughly, particularly pork, which should never be eaten rare. House cats which do not kill and eat the raw meat of small rodents are probably not a threat. If the woman

Table 23-1. Infections In Pregnancy

Infection	Causative Organism	Mode of Transmission	Maternal Symptoms	Fetal/Neonatal Effects
Toxoplasmosis	*Toxoplasma gondii*	Maternal: Raw meat; cat feces Fetal: Transplacental	Asymptomatic or headache, malaise, low-grade fever	IUGR,* microcephaly, hydrocephaly, chorioretinitis, hepatosplenomegaly; death frequent; if lives, MR* and developmental lag
Rubella	Rubella virus	Maternal: Pharyngeal secretions Fetal: Transplacental	Pharyngeal inflammation, lymphadenopathy, macular rash	Cataracts, hemolytic anemia, congenital heart defects, MR, deafness
Cytomegalic inclusion disease	Cytomegalovirus	Maternal: Most body fluids; sexual intercourse Fetal: Transplacental, contact with infected birth canal	Asymptomatic or, rarely, mild mononucleosis-like symptoms	IUGR, microcephaly, MR, deafness, congenital heart defects
Herpes genitalis	Herpesvirus hominis, type II	Maternal: Sexual intercourse Fetal: Contact with infected birth canal; less often transplacental	Painful vesicles in genital area	Mild: few skin lesions, recovery likely Severe: viremia, CNS involvement, high mortality rate
Streptococcus	Beta-hemolytic streptococcus, group B	Maternal: Ascending genital tract organisms Fetal: Ascending through ruptured membrane; contact with infected birth canal	Amnionitis, puerperal sepsis	Septicemia, meningitis, mortality high
Syphilis	*Treponema pallidum*	Maternal: Sexual intercourse Fetal: Transplacental	Vary with stage of infection; may be asymptomatic, chancre, rash, etc.	Midtrimester abortion; congenital syphilis (septicemia, skin lesions, anemia, jaundice, periostitis)
Gonorrhea	*Neisseria gonorrhoeae*	Maternal: Sexual intercourse Fetal: Contact with infected birth canal	Often asymptomatic, urethritis, cervicitis, pelvic inflammatory disease	Ophthalmia neonatorum
Chicken pox	Varicella virus	Maternal: Airborne viruses Fetal: Transplacental	Characteristic skin lesions, high fever	Congenital varicella, rare but mortality is high
Mumps	Mumps virus (myxovirus group)	Maternal: Airborne viruses Fetal: Transplacental	Parotitis, fever	Spontaneous abortion, premature birth, stillbirth; congenital anomalies

*IUGR, intrauterine growth retardation; MR, mental retardation.

has concerns because of her cat she may have someone else handle the kitty litter and pay particular attention to good hand washing and other hygienic practices.

Toxoplasmosis in the adult is frequently asymptomatic. If symptoms do occur they are mild and nonspecific, consisting of malaise, headache, myalgia, low-grade fever, and occasionally a macular rash. The organism readily crosses the placenta causing congenital infection. The infected infants exhibit a variety of serious conditions, including intrauterine growth retardation, microcephaly, hydrocephaly, chorioretinitis, jaundice, and fever. They rarely live more than a few days. Less severe infections may not be diagnosed until later in infancy when the child may present with mental retardation, seizures, chorioretinitis, or developmental lag.

Because it is generally asymptomatic in the adult, detection during pregnancy is usually possible only through screening. A serologic test for the detection of antibodies may be done. At the present time such screening is not recommended as a routine for all pregnant women. Women at particular risk because of dietary habits or who have special concern arising from their pets may be screened.

Should an active toxoplasmosis occur during pregnancy, treatment may be considered. The drug of choice is pyrimethamine, a folic acid antagonist, which is not without its own risks for the developing fetus. For this reason there must be a definitive diagnosis of infection as well as a careful consideration of the risks of the teratogenic effects of the drug versus the risks of damage to the fetus from the infection.

Rubella, or German measles, is a mild virus infection in children and adults which can produce a severe malformation syndrome in the fetus.

The virus is spread person to person in pharyngeal secretions. Symptoms include pharyngeal inflammation, lymphadenopathy, and a macular rash, which typically begins on the face and spreads to the trunk. It is not un-common for the disease to be subclinical and go unnoticed by those affected.

Transplacental transmission results in infection of the fetus. The severity of its effect depends on the developmental stage of the fetus at the time of infection. The first trimester with its rapid organogenesis is the most sensitive period and infection during this time may result in congenital anomalies in the form of cataracts, hemolytic anemia, congenital heart defects, mental retardation, and deafness. Approximately one fourth of fetuses exposed during the first trimester will be born with this multiple malformation syndrome. Even when the infant does not appear affected, he or she can shed live viruses for many months after birth. Precautions should be observed in the newborn nursery to protect employees who may be pregnant or at risk to become pregnant.

The percentage of women of childbearing age who have no serologic evidence of previous rubella infection has been reduced from 25 percent to 10 percent with the introduction of the vaccine. Since the vaccine consists of attenuated live viruses it should never be given to pregnant women, as the attenuated viruses cross the placenta in the same way as the wild variety and with equally disastrous outcomes. Before children are immunized their mothers should be ascertained either to be already immune themselves or at no risk to become pregnant during the ensuing two months. Pregnant women who have no serologic evidence of past infection should receive the vaccine early in the postpartum period when adequate protection against pregnancy in the next two months has been assured.

Cytomegalovirus (CMV) is a member of the herpesvirus group of which five are known to infect humans. Besides CMV these include the varicella/zoster virus (responsible for chicken pox/shingles), the Epstein-Barr virus, herpes simplex virus type I (cold sores), and herpes simplex virus type II.

Cytomegaloviruses are ubiquitous agents, and it has been estimated that nearly 100 percent of the population are affected in some parts of the world. The incidence tends to be lower in more favored economic environments where sanitation standards are higher. The infection is rarely symptomatic, although a mononucleosis-like syndrome has been described in young adults. Viruses are shed for as long as several years in saliva and urine. It has also been cultured from semen and from cervical smears, indicating that there may be a venereal transmission.

The significance of this virus in pregnancy lies in its ability to cause fetal infection. Although studies are difficult to do because of the typical absence of any symptoms of maternal infection, it is felt that the most critical time is during the second month of gestation. Infants are affected in much the same way as in rubella infection. They are small for gestational age, microcephalic, and mentally and developmentally retarded. Deafness and congenital heart defects have also been observed. When maternal infection occurs in the last trimester infants have been known to become infected during passage through the birth canal. These infants shed viruses but do not exhibit clinical symptoms.

At present there is no way known to prevent infection or to treat the congenital disease. Tragically, most diagnoses are made retrospectively after the birth of an infant with multiple malformations.

Herpes simplex virus, type II, is one of the antigenic types of *herpesvirus hominis.* It generally causes disease below the diaphragm (herpes genitalis), in contrast with type I which produces disease above the diaphragm, most notably the "cold sore," herpes labialis.

Herpes genitalis is a sexually transmitted infection, characterized by exquisitely painful vesicles surrounded by an erythematous area which progress to shallow ulcers, pustules, and crusts with healing occurring spontaneously in about 10 days to 2 weeks. These occur on the cervix, vaginal wall, and vulva and may extend to the buttocks and thighs. The virus may then enter a latent phase and be harbored by the individual indefinitely, giving rise to recurrent infections

when the virus is activated. Numerous modes of therapy have been attempted, but all have been unrewarding. Symptomatic treatment in the form of Sitz baths, wet compresses, lotions, and analgesics can provide some relief from the discomfort.

The maternal infection may be transmitted to the fetus and neonate. The usual mode of transmission is through contact with cervical and vaginal vesicles on the way through the birth canal, although a few cases of transplacental transmission have been documented. The neonates at greatest risk are those whose mothers had an onset of a primary herpes infection shortly before delivery. If the virus is present at birth 40 percent of vaginally delivered neonates will be infected. Since this infection is frequently fatal for the neonate, a cesarean section is generally recommended for the woman with active herpes lesions. Should premature rupture of the membrane occur, cesarean section should be performed prior to four hours elapsed time since rupture in order to prevent ascending infection.

Group B beta-hemolytic streptococcus is currently attracting notice as a factor in both neonatal and puerperal infections. It has been associated with urinary tract infections, septic abortions, stillbirth, and serious neonatal disease. It is estimated that it constitutes part of the normal flora of the genital tract in about 15 percent of the women of childbearing age. The fetus may become infected by organisms ascending through ruptured membranes or from passage through an infected birth canal.

This infection can be devastating in the neonate as it often runs a fulminate course ending in fatal streptococcal meningitis. Because of this many practitioners routinely culture the cervix and vagina of women presenting with premature labor or ruptured membranes. Early identification of group B streptococcus may permit antibiotic therapy in the neonate before the infection is overwhelming.

Efforts to eliminate the organism in the mother by prenatal screening and antibiotic therapy have not proved practical. Success requires treating the woman's sexual partner as well as herself, and even then recolonization is frequent.

Syphilis in a pregnant woman is a serious condition meriting prompt and efficient treatment. Once the leading cause of fetal and neonatal mortality and morbidity, it is now an entirely preventable disease. Yet the incidence of congenital syphilis is increasing as a reflection of increased incidence of parental syphilis as well as a tragic commentary on the inadequacy of antepartum care.

The first, and absolutely indispensable, step toward efficient treatment of syphilis in pregnancy is a diagnostic test. In all but eight states prenatal serologic test is required by law. Even without the force of law omission of such an examination from antepartum care would be indefensible.

The serologic screening test should be done early in gestation in order to permit treatment of the mother prior to the sixteenth week of gestation. The *Treponema pallidum* spirochetes cannot penetrate the early placenta but may begin to do so any time after the fourth month.

Positive serologic tests identified after the sixteenth week should nevertheless prompt treatment for the mother's health as well as for the transplacental treatment of the fetus. All cases of syphilis should be reported to public health officials in order that all contacts can be identified and treated.

Penicillin is used as treatment in all stages of syphilis. It is a safe, effective treatment which quickly eliminates the infectiousness of the disease, prevents later complications, and effectively prevents congenital syphilis. It is easier to administer than the drugs formerly used, rarely has serious toxic effects, and does not require a long period of treatment. Adequate penicillin levels are usually maintained for about two weeks. Even though the mother does not have a negative serology by the time she delivers, a nonsyphilitic baby can be expected if she has shown a favorable response to treatment by monthly quantitative blood tests. Several

months may elapse following treatment before a negative maternal blood test is obtained. A rapid drop in titer is expected after treatment of early syphilis. Even a small drop is considered a favorable response in late or latent syphilis, in which the decline may be quite delayed and very gradual. Retreatment is indicated in cases not showing the normally expected response.

Gonorrhea, once considered conquered by penicillin, is reaching epidemic proportions in the United States. In 1975 there were one million reported cases in this country.[1] The enormous increase in the incidence of this disease is felt to be due to the high percentage of infected individuals who are asymptomatic (70–80 percent) and to increasing antibiotic resistance. There has been a 30-fold increase in the amount of medication needed for cure between 1950 and 1977. In February, 1976, a penicillin-resistant, beta-lactamase-producing gonococcus was isolated.[2]

Diagnosis of gonorrhea is made by culturing the *Neisseria gonorrhoeae* from the endocervical canal. Routine screening cultures are currently recommended at the first antepartum visit, with repeat cultures at 36 weeks gestation for those women at high risk for reinfection.

Although the majority of cases are asymptomatic, the vaginal discharge from an infection may become profuse and purulent. It may cause great discomfort from irritation and itching of the vulva, or even excoriation of the mucous membrane, and sometimes abscesses of the vulvovaginal glands. The chief danger to the mother in an untreated gonorrheal infection is that, after delivery, the organisms may travel from the lower genital tract to the uterine cavity and the fallopian tubes. There they cause inflammation, or possibly a general postpartum infection. Sterility may be one of the results of an untreated gonorrheal infection.

---

[1] *VD Fact Sheet 1975,* U.S. Dept. Health, Education and Welfare, Public Health Service, Center for Disease Control, Venereal Disease Control Division, Atlanta, Ga.

[2] Michael R. Spence, Genital infections in pregnancy, *Med. Clin. North Am.* 61:139–151 (Jan.) 1977.

The greatest danger to the infant is infection of the eyes during passage through the birth canal. This is the reason for the special care given to the eyes of the neonate described on pages 368–71.

The treatment of choice is intramuscular aqueous procaine penicillin G, 4.8 million units. Probenecid, 1 gm, is frequently administered concomitantly to maintain high serum levels by blocking tubular secretion of the penicillin.

Tuberculosis

Although the pregnant woman with tuberculosis must receive special care, routine roentgenograms as a part of antepartum care, to detect early lesions, are currently not often advised. If infection is found, both the infection and the pregnancy need ideal management. It appears that pregnancy does not exert an adverse effect on tuberculosis, but the progress of the disease must be halted. To promote resolution and healing, the mother receives the care she would ordinarily have for a tuberculous infection without a superimposed pregnancy. This treatment remains essentially unchanged during pregnancy. Long-term planning is essential for adequate rest and supervision. Suitable arrangements must be made for the care of the baby since the mother will be unable to care for her baby until her disease is arrested.

To reduce the physical strain of labor, a low forceps delivery is usually considered advisable for shortening the second stage. Excessive sedation and inhalation anesthesia are avoided, insofar as possible, to prevent suppression of the cough reflex. During delivery and the postpartum period good drainage of secretions is maintained to prevent accumulation in the bronchi. The mother is not allowed to nurse her baby because of the danger to the baby from exposure to the disease and also the added strain this would place on her.

With adequate long-continued care the tuberculous patient may usually be carried safely through pregnancy without ill effects.

Tuberculosis is rarely transmitted to the fetus,

and there seems to be no predisposition to the disease. The baby may easily be infected by his mother after birth from droplet contact. Accordingly, he is not allowed to nurse and the mother should not care for the baby in any way. BCG vaccination of the infant may be considered, but this does not decrease the need for preventive measures against infection of the baby.

If a woman becomes pregnant after a tuberculosis infection has responded well to treatment, but while the lesion is still somewhat unstable, she is given all possible safeguards during pregnancy, labor, and the puerperium. Hospitalization during a part of the pregnancy and for a longer than usual period during the puerperium is advisable.

Pregnancy is usually safe without danger of recurrence of tuberculosis when a period of two years has elapsed after the lesions have been well controlled. Safety increases with time since this allows for more effective healing.

Urinary Tract Infections

During pregnancy alterations occur in the collecting systems of the urinary tract which favor the development of infection. These alterations, evident as early as the tenth gestational week, consist primarily of a dilatation and hypokinesis of the kidney pelves and ureters. The result of these anatomic changes is a relatively static column of urine in the upper collecting system which facilitates the ascending migration of organisms to the kidney itself. Therefore bacteriuria is more likely to result in pyelonephritis in the pregnant woman than in the nonpregnant woman. In fact, pregnant women with untreated bacteriuria have a 30 percent incidence of acute pyelonephritis.[3]

Whether or not pregnant women have an increased susceptibility to bacteriuria per se has not been conclusively established. The pathogenesis of bacteriuria and bladder infections is the same regardless of the gravid state. That is,

[3] H. G. Dixon and H. A. Brant, The significance of bacteriuria in pregnancy, *Lancet* i:19–20 (Jan.) 1967.

organisms migrate from the rectum to the urethra and thus to the bladder. This migration may be facilitated by careless perineal wiping and sexual intercourse. Whether the vaginal environment or other factors are more favorable toward this migration of organisms during pregnancy is not known. It is known from epidemiologic studies that 3 to 7 percent of pregnant women have bacteriuria and that this is frequently asymptomatic. If untreated, about one third of these women will develop acute pyelonephritis because of the static column of urine which provides a pathway from the infected bladder to the kidney.

Urinary tract infections, principally pyelonephritis, are associated with an increased incidence of premature labor and thus pose a potential hazard to the fetus. It does not appear that the mother is at increased risk for chronic renal disease because of acute pyelonephritis in pregnancy unless there are abnormalities leading to repeated infections which antedate the pregnancy.

Because bacteriuria is apt to progress to an acute pyelonephritis and because it is so frequently asymptomatic, routine screening for this disorder should be an integral part of antepartum care. There are a number of inexpensive, commercially available, screening cultures that can be done easily by the nurse or physician in the office/clinic setting. Positive findings on such a screening test should be followed by a conventional urine culture in the clinical laboratory. The woman should be carefully instructed and assisted, if necessary, in the collection of a midstream specimen following careful cleansing of the vulva with a nonbacteriostatic soap. If the urine cannot be plated for culture immediately it should be refrigerated to prevent bacterial multiplication prior to plating. Findings of 100,000 bacteria per ml of urine indicate infection and require treatment for the eradication of the bacteriuria.

Antibiotics of choice for bacteriuria are those which achieve high urinary, as opposed to high serum, concentrations. Sulfisoxazole (Gantrisin, Azo-Gantrisin) and nitrofurantoin (Furadantin) are commonly used drugs. In addition, the woman should be instructed in ways to enhance the natural body defenses against infection. She can do this best by increasing her fluid intake and spending several periods each day in the left lateral position to increase blood flow to the kidneys.

Women who have had positive urine cultures should be recultured upon completion of the course of drug therapy. Cultures should be repeated each month for the remainder of gestation and again at six weeks post partum, since recurrence is common. Successful treatment of bacteriuria can decrease the incidence of acute pyelonephritis from 30 percent to less than 5 percent. Failure to eradicate the bacteriuria or persistent recurrence is indication for a complete urologic evaluation after the anatomic changes of pregnancy have been reversed (six weeks post partum).

Should pyelonephritis occur, the woman will typically complain of sudden paroxysms of pain in the region of the kidney in addition to the usual symptoms of a bladder infection (frequent micturition, urgency, burning on urination). The kidneys may be swollen and very tender to palpation and the woman may have a fever and sometimes chills. A catheterized urine specimen will contain bacteria and pus and possibly protein.

Bed rest and increased fluid intake are begun. A urine culture is done to identify the causative agent in order than an organism-specific antibiotic may be prescribed. After the specimen is obtained for culture a broad-spectrum antibiotic is begun, pending results of the culture which takes 24 hours to grow. Prompt treatment is essential to prevent fibrosis of tissue which may result from the inflmmation.

CHRONIC RENAL FAILURE

Women with chronic renal failure for whatever reason typically have impaired fertility. However, should conception occur a successful pregnancy is possible.

The gravest threat to both mother and fetus is uncontrolled hypertension. This accelerates the progress of renal insufficiency and causes intrauterine malnutrition and its attendant risks.

Proteinuria is markedly increased during pregnancy in these women. However, this is most likely a result of increased glomerular filtration rate and not an indication of progression of the underlying disease.[4]

Very careful management throughout gestation by a multidisciplinary team which includes a nephrologist will be essential. In addition to the immediate stresses of the pregnancy, the family will likely need some support and counseling related to child rearing because of the nature of the mother's chronic disease and her lifespan expectations.

THYROID DISEASE

Modifications in thyroid structure and function in pregnancy are discussed on page 124. To summarize, there is an elevated T_4 and T_3 because of an increase in thyroxine binding capacity. However, the free T_4 and T_3 remains unchanged from the nonpregnant state, resulting in normal peripheral thryoid activity (Fig. 23-1). Hyperplasia of the gland is a common physiologic finding during pregnancy.

Hypothyroidism

It is a popular, though undocumented, notion that hypothyroid women have reduced fertility. Whether or not their ability to conceive is affected, they are much less likely to carry the pregnancy successfully to term. There is an increased incidence of all forms of fetal wastage as well as premature labor and the birth of infants who are severely handicapped both physically and mentally.

Thyroid hormone crosses the placenta with some difficulty and probably not in its intact

[4] B. S. Strauch and J. P. Hayslett, Kidney disease and pregnancy, *Br. Med. J.* 4:578–582 (Apr.) 1974.

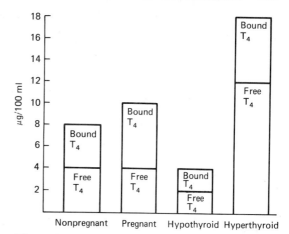

Figure 23-1. Comparison of thyroid hormone levels in nonpregnant and pregnant women with the levels typical of hypo- and hyperthyroidism. Note that the amount of free, and thus active, thyroxine remains unchanged in pregnancy, although the total amount increases due to the action of estrogen which enhances protein-binding capacity.

form but as either an inorganic iodide or some as yet undefined organic iodide. It is evident from the above discussion, however, that passage is essential for normal fetal growth and development, especially prior to the time when the fetus is capable of synthesizing his own thyroxine (approximately 12 weeks gestation). Maternal hypothyroidism therefore requires full thyroid replacement in the form of exogenous hormone.

Hypothyroidism is only rarely diagnosed during pregnancy. A fairly common situation arises, however, when a young woman who is already taking thryoid extract seeks antepartum care. Not infrequently the thryoid extract was prescribed without adequate documentation of hypothroidism because of adolescent complaints of obesity, fatigue, and/or menstrual disorders. Even though the majority of these women will probably be euthyroid, it is wise to continue the therapy until delivery, since normal thyroid function will be depressed for several weeks following the discontinuation of exogenous therapy. Even transient periods of hypothyroidism may threaten the outcome of the pregnancy.

Hyperthyroidism

The incidence of thyrotoxicosis in pregnancy is approximately 0.2 percent or one in every 500 pregnancies.[5] Diagnosis during pregnancy is difficult because many of the symptoms of normal pregnancy are similar to those of hyperthyroidism. (See page 124.)

The appropriate treatment during pregnancy is medical rather than surgical and consists of the administration of antithyroid drug in dosages sufficient to maintain the patient as very slightly hyperthyroid. Since both propylthiouracil (PTU) and methimazole (Tapazole) readily cross the placenta, fetal thyroid is protected by keeping the mother in the slightly hyperthyroid range. This goal is achieved by monitoring the T_4 and the free thyroxine index (FTI) at frequent intervals (every 2–3 weeks) and adjusting the drug dosage to maintain the T_4 at 1.4 times the upper limit of normal for the laboratory and the FTI at or near the upper limits of normal.

The woman should be advised about the importance of taking the prescribed drug regularly in order to maintain relatively stable blood levels. She and her family will usually benefit from a discussion of the personality changes (emotional lability and irritability) which result from the disease process. Understanding that this is a result of the hyperthyroidism, and it will improve with therapy, may lessen the impact. At the same time these are also typical emotional responses to pregnancy, so it is also important to provide the usual counseling about maternal emotions and development.

Infants born to mothers who have received antithyroid therapy should be monitored closely during the newborn period for evidence of hypothyroidism. Neonatal hypothyroidism due to *in utero* exposure to PTU or methimazole is transient, responds favorably to treatment, and has rarely been associated with long-term effects on growth and development.

[5] K. R. Niswander, R. Gordon, and H. W. Berendes, *The Women and Their Pregnancies.* Saunders, Philadelphia, Pa., 1972.

CARDIOVASCULAR DISEASE

Rheumatic heart disease and congenital heart defects are the most common cardiac complications of pregnancy, since these are the heart conditions most likely to affect women of childbearing age. Of these, mitral stenosis is by far the most common lesion. Although the particular pathology may dictate some specific therapy, there are some general principles of management that pertain to all pregnant women with heart disease.

Activity and Rest

Pregnancy places significant demands on the cardiovascular system of healthy women (Chapter 6, pages 126–35). As normal gestation advances there is a progressive decline in cardiac reserve and an increasing tendency toward tachycardia with even mild exertion. This is particularly evident during the third trimester. In a study of women with asymptomatic or only mildly symptomatic heart disease it was found that cardiac output failed to increase during pregnancy to the expected normal levels. The increased incidence of prematurity and low-birth-weight babies in women with heart disease is further evidence that the heart cannot always meet the demands of the growing fetus.[6]

The physiologic alterations which may place increased stress on cardiovascular functioning during pregnancy are summarized in Figure 23-2.

For these reasons, limitations of activity with frequent rest periods seem a wise precaution for the pregnant woman with heart disease. The extent of these limitations will depend primarily on the severity of the cardiac disease. The American Heart Association classifies persons with heart disease into four functional categories, depending on their symptoms in response to activity. Those who are asymptomatic

[6] Kent Ueland, M. J. Novy, and J. Metcalfe, Hemodynamic responses of patients with heart disease to pregnancy and exercise, *Am. J. Obstet. Gynecol.* 113:47–59 (May) 1972.

Physiologic Alterations in Pregnancy Which Stress
Cardiovascular Function

1. 20-25% increase in O_2 requirements

2. 25% increase in cardiac output

3. 50% increase in plasma volume

4. Weight gain due to

    a. Increased maternal and fetal body bulk

    b. Salt and water retention

5. Sudden hemodynamic changes at delivery

    a. Splanchnic vessel engorgment

    b. Sudden decrease in intraabdominal pressure

Figure 23-2. Normal physiologic changes of pregnancy which may place stress on the heart of a woman with cardiovascular disease.

with exertion are termed Class I; those who are symptomatic with strenuous activity are Class II. Class III contains those who are symptomatic with ordinary activities of daily living, and Class IV is reserved for those who are symptomatic with even very mild activity. Clearly the woman who fits into Class I will require fewer restrictions during pregnancy than those in more severe classes.

As early as possible in gestation, the family should sit down with the nurse and attempt to work out a systematic plan for the woman to rest and reduce her workload. Such planning cannot be limited to establishing a schedule of nap times. Discussions of task reassignment may evoke strong feelings of what is "proper" for various family members to do. The woman may feel so guilty about the unfinished tasks that, even though she is lying down for the prescribed time, she does not rest. Providing for the care and safety of small children in the home may necessitate obtaining help from neighbors, extended family members, day care centers, or others.

For some women prolonged hospitalization may be necessary, although the benefits of such

a step should be carefully weighed against the stresses of a disrupted family and the discomforts of being in a hospital. Frequently a well-planned rest and activity schedule at home is more beneficial, particularly if household help and public health nursing are available.

When the woman is not lying down she should wear pressure-graded elastic stockings to prevent pooling of blood in the lower extremities and promote venous return to the heart. These stockings should always be applied before arising from a period of rest in the lateral position.

Fear and worry are additional sources of stress on the heart. Although no one is likely to go through a nine-month period totally free from anxiety—especially not the nine months of a high-risk pregnancy—expert nursing care can reduce this stress. Factual information about the interrelationships of pregnancy and heart disease should be available to the family in a form they can understand. All planning should be done with the woman and her family as active participants. The nurse should strive to enhance the family's ability to support each other as well as providing support herself.

Nutrition and Fluids

The importance of nutrition during pregnancy has been repeatedly emphasized. For the woman with heart disease this is especially important, since she and her fetus are already faced with factors which predispose to intrauterine malnutrition.

Because of her restricted activity there may be a need for fewer calories for the cardiac patient. Avoiding excessive weight gain is quite important because of the increased cardiovascular hazards resulting from obesity. A diet containing 80–100 gm of protein and enough calories to sustain an even progressive weight gain of 15 to 20 pounds is usually recommended. Consultation with a nutritionist is important. If weight gain is low, urine may be checked for ketonuria.

Fluid and sodium restriction are contraindicated during pregnancy. Diuretics are unnecessary unless cardiac disease is severe and the risk of decompensation and pulmonary edema is high. Diuretics other than thiazides are usually selected and careful attention must be paid to electrolyte balance.

Intrapartum Care

Generally a vaginal delivery at term provides the safest intrapartum experience for the woman with heart disease.

Every effort is made to reduce strain and facilitate circulatory activity—a useful goal for any laboring woman. The left lateral position is preferable and constant nursing attendance should be available to provide support. Continuous fetal heart rate monitoring is indicated and the mother's ECG may be monitored as well.

Pain relief is important because of the added cardiac work produced by pain. Analgesics should be used judiciously, keeping in mind the fetal effects of the drug. Conduction anesthesia in the form of epidural or caudal is frequently recommended. Care should be taken that the woman is well hydrated to minimize the danger of cardiovascular side effects from the anesthesia.

Delivery is usually by low forceps extraction to avoid the strain of maternal bearing-down efforts.

Postpartum Care

Dramatic hemodynamic changes occur in the mother at the time of delivery and separation of the placenta. For this reason, the immediate postpartum period probably constitutes the period of greatest risk for the cardiac patient. Careful and frequent monitoring of maternal vital signs in a recovery room setting is crucial during this time. Immediate cardiac consultation should be available should symptoms of congestive heart failure or other complications arise.

Early ambulation should be encouraged to prevent venous. thrombosis. As in the antepar-

tum period, elastic stockings should be worn to prevent pooling in the large dilated veins of the lower extremities.

Both parents should have immediate and continued access to their newborn. The nurse should, however, be sensitive to signs of fatigue in the mother and help her set limits for herself to conserve energy. Decisions about infant feeding should be considered very seriously in the light of the mother's capacity for activity. Breast feeding may place too great a strain on her heart. In addition to the physiologic demands of lactation, the mother would be less able to delegate infant care to the father and others if she were breast feeding.

Discharge planning should include a consideration of the mother's ability to undertake the care of her baby and resume her daily activities and will necessarily involve the family.

DIABETES MELLITUS

Before the availability of commercially prepared insulin in 1921, diabetes and pregnancy rarely occurred together. Few juvenile diabetics lived to reproductive age and those who did were frequently sterile. In the rare instances where pregnancy did occur the maternal and perinatal mortality was enormous. Currently, after more than 50 years experience with insulin, maternal mortality has been virtually eliminated, but perinatal mortality remains as high as 10 to 20 percent. This is well above the 2 to 3 percent perinatal mortality for the general population.

Diabetes is a highly complex disease that affects multiple body systems. There remains much about it that is poorly understood. The physiologic and psychologic interactions with pregnancy are many and, perhaps, even less well understood. Perhaps more than any other high-risk pregnancy this situation calls for the expertise of many highly specialized disciplines working as a team with the client. No single professional has the skill and knowledge to meet all the needs of these families experiencing a di-

---

Classification of Diabetes in Pregnancy

Class A — Pregnant women whose blood sugar is abnormally elevated only during pregnancy. Dietary regulation is adequate for control and no insulin is required. Fetal survival is high.

Class B — Pregnant women whose diabetes is of less than 10 years duration, whose disease began at age 20 or older, and who have no vascular involvement.

Class C — Pregnant women whose diabetes began between age 10 and age 19, whose disease has lasted 10-19 years.

Class D — Pregnant women whose diabetes has lasted 20 years or more, whose disease began before age 10, and who may have vascular involvement and benign retinopathy.

Class E — Pregnant women in whom calcification of the pelvic arteries has been demonstrated on x-ray. (This classification is not employed in current practice.)

Class F — Pregnant women whose diabetes has caused nephropathy (proteinuria, azotemia).

Class R — Pregnant women whose diabetes has caused proliferative retinitis (changes in the retina of the eye causing progressive loss of sight).

Figure 23-3. White's classification of pregnant diabetics according to age at onset, duration, and severity of their disease. [*Priscilla White, Pregnancy and diabetes, Medical aspects,* Med. Clin. North Am. *49:1019 (July) 1965.*]

abetic pregnancy. For these reasons it is strongly recommended that care for pregnant diabetics be concentrated in regional perinatal centers where the necessary human as well as mechanical resources for expert individualized care can be made available.

The experience in one perinatal referral center confirms the value of such a delivery system, at least with respect to perinatal mortality. During the four-year period from 1973 to 1977, 90 diabetic pregnant women were cared for by the Maternal Intensive Care Team at the Wisconsin Perinatal Center in Madison. During this time only two neonatal deaths occurred. One of these deaths was the result of severe erythroblastosis fetalis, while another neonate succumbed to multiple major malformations. No fetal deaths occurred.[7]

Effects of Diabetes on Pregnancy

The potential impact of diabetes on pregnancy is very impressive. This impact, however, can be significantly lowered by maintaining good maternal diabetic control throughout the antepartum and intrapartum periods. The frequency and severity of complications is also influenced by the duration and severity of the diabetes.

Dr. Priscilla White has classified diabetes in pregnancy according to the age at onset and duration of the disease as well as the extent of diabetic complications.[8] These classifications are given in Figure 23-3.

It is possible for a woman to be classified in one category and, at a later time, require reclassification because of progression of her diabetes and/or elapsed time. Generally speaking, the further down the alphabet the woman is classified the greater the risk to her fetus.

The incidence of toxemia is markedly increased in diabetics. Whereas approximately 7 percent of all pregnancies are complicated by toxemia, 25 to 50 percent of diabetic pregnancies are affected, depending on the diet, quality of antepartum care, diabetic control, and diabetic complications. Polyhydramnios affects as

---

[7] Luis B. Curet, Personal communication, April 8, 1977.

[8] Priscilla White, Pregnancy and diabetes, Medical aspects, *Med. Clin. North Am.* 49:1015–1024 (July) 1965.

many as 25 percent of diabetic pregnancies, and vaginal and urinary tract infections are very common.

All forms of fetal wastage are increased in the diabetic, particularly third trimester intrauterine death. The fetus is extremely vulnerable to maternal ketoacidosis as well as to the placental insufficiency which may accompany more severe diabetes.

Infants of diabetic mothers are classically thought of as large for gestational age. Maternal hyperglycemia results in fetal hyperglycemia. This in turn causes increased fetal islet cell stimulation and subsequent high insulin levels. This fetal insulin, needed to metabolize the large glucose loads which cross the placenta from maternal circulation, acts as a growth factor, causing increased deposition of glycogen, fat, and probably protein. Thus, these infants are both longer and heavier than the norm for their gestational age. However, macrosomia is not invariably present in infants of diabetic mothers. Women in White's classifications D through R are more likely to deliver infants who are small for gestational age because of insufficient placental perfusion.

Congenital malformations occur in 5 to 10 percent of diabetic pregnancies. While the precise reasons for this risk is not clear, it is supposed to be a result of some intrauterine environmental factor (e.g., hypo- or hyperglycemia) rather than of a genetic, inherited factor. Evidence for this is found in studies which reveal no increased risk for anomalies when the father rather than the mother, is a diabetic. The most common malformations are congenital heart defects, neurologic defects, small left colon syndrome, and caudal regression syndrome. The latter syndrome, unique to infants of diabetic mothers, is characterized by imperfect development from the waist down and may be associated with cleft lip and palate, congenital heart defects, and upper limb abnormalities.

Complications which may be anticipated in the neonatal period include respiratory distress syndrome, hypoglycemia, hyperbilirubinemia, and hypocalcemia.

Parents often ask about the likelihood of their child having diabetes. The mode of inheritance of diabetes is a matter of some controversy among geneticists. A likely hypothesis is that it is a multifactorial condition. That is, a number of genes are responsible for the trait (polygenic rather than monogenic), and environmental or nongenetic factors contribute to its expression. It is generally believed to be inherited as an autosomal recessive with reduced penetrance, but whether the disease itself, a predisposition to the disease, or still another characteristic is inherited has not been clarified. Congenital diabetes is virtually unknown. The stronger the family history, however, the greater the likelihood of the child manifesting the disease at some time in his life. The older he gets the greater his risks. For example, if only the child's mother is diabetic his chances of having diabetes by age 25 is 8 percent, but the chances of his being diabetic by age 85 increase to 25 percent.[9] Absolute risk values or percentages contain much guesswork. In general, however, infants of diabetic mothers are about 22 times as likely to become diabetic at some time in their lives than are individuals in the general population.[10] It is important to note that good health practices, especially good nutrition and maintenance of optimum body weight, can reduce the risk significantly.

Effects of Pregnancy on Diabetes

A thorough knowledge of the normal alterations in carbohydrate metabolism during pregnancy is essential to the understanding of the effects of gestation on diabetes and, in fact, to the understanding of medical management. The reader is referred to Chapter 6, pages 148–52, for a review of these changes (Figure 23-4).

During the first half of pregnancy the major factor having an impact on carbohydrate metab-

[9] J. M. Darlow, Charles Smith, and L. J. P. Duncan, A statistical and genetical study of diabetes. III. Empiric risks to relatives, *Ann. Hum. Genet.* 37:157–173 (July) 1973.

[10] David Rimoin, Inheritance in diabetes mellitus, *Med. Clin. North Am.* 55:807–818 (July) 1971.

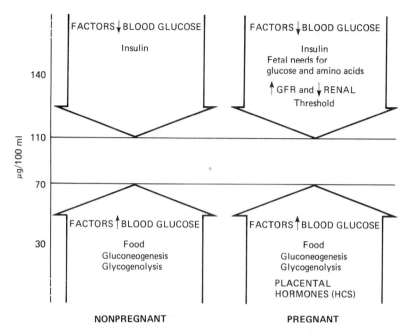

Figure 23-4. Factors which operate to maintain appropriate blood glucose levels in nonpregnant and pregnant women. Although new factors are added during pregnancy, the net result for the healthy woman is normoglycemia.

olism is the fetal need for glucose and amino acids. It is believed that the fetus, like the brain, can utilize only glucose for energy needs. Glucose is transported rapidly across the placenta by facilitated diffusion, effectively lowering maternal blood glucose. The active transport of amino acids to the fetus also reduces the amount of "raw materials" available to the maternal liver for gluconeogenesis. The net result of all this is a tendency toward hypoglycemia. If, in addition, the woman is bothered by decreased appetitie or nausea and vomiting of pregnancy, the blood glucose levels may fall dangerously low. As blood glucose levels fall, fat is broken down into fatty acids to serve as an auxiliary fuel source. These fatty acids cross the placenta to the fetus, where they are potentially hazardous to neurologic development.

In view of the above discussion it is apparent that the diabetic pregnant woman will need to increase her carbohydrate intake during the first half of gestation, and she may also need to decrease her insulin dosage. Care should be taken throughout pregnancy to distinguish between ketoacidosis which results from inadequate insu-

lin dosage and that caused by starvation or inadequate carbohydrate intake. The treatment for the first is more insulin, while the treatment for the second is more carbohydrate.

The increasing supply of placental hormones, principally human chorionic somatomammotropin (HCS), has caused the second half of pregnancy to be characterized as diabetogenic. A woman with a predisposition to diabetes may display glucose intolerance and/or clinical diabetes at this time. Her pancreatic activity is adequate to meet normal needs, but she has no reserve capacity to increase insulin production to compensate for the insulin antagonism of HCS (Fig. 23-5). The insulin-dependent diabetic can accommodate to this challenge of pregnancy only by increasing her dose of exogenous insulin. Very careful control of blood glucose levels are necessary to prevent ketoacidosis, which is a common cause of intrauterine death.

An additional factor operating during pregnancy is the change in renal function characterized by an increased glomerular filtration rate without a commensurate increase in tubular reabsorption. As a result, glucosuria is not well

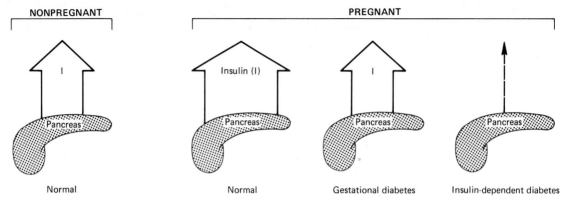

Figure 23-5. Diagrammatic representation of the way in which the pancreas compensates during pregnancy for the insulin antagonist effects of the placental hormones (principally HCS). Notice the pancreas of the gestational diabetic, although producing insulin, does not increase its output of this substance during pregnancy. The pancreas of the insulin-dependent diabetic produces no insulin for all intents and purposes.

correlated with blood glucose. Therefore urine tests cannot serve as determinants of appropriate insulin dosage.

The influence of pregnancy on long-term complications of diabetes has not been conclusively demonstrated. It is known that the better the diabetic control the less likelihood there is for nephropathy, retinopathy, and other complications to occur. Since pregnancy is a period of time when blood glucose levels may be particularly difficult to control it is at least theoretically possible that pregnancy contributes indirectly to the progression of diabetes. Conversely, many women are more rigidly controlled during pregnancy than at any other time because of the fetal intolerance to hyperglycemia as well as to wide fluctuations in blood glucose. Furthermore, women are frequently motivated to become better informed about their disease during this time and thus, perhaps, improve their health practices for future living.

Diabetic Screening

The first step toward improving pregnancy outcome in diabetic pregnancies is an efficient screening program for early diagnosis. As discussed in Chapter 7, a blood glucose determination should be a part of routine antepartum care

for all women. Typically, this is done at about 28 weeks gestation when the placental hormones are beginning to exert their greatest influence. However, early screening in the first trimester is indicated for any woman whose history suggests she may be at particular risk. Factors in the history which prompt earlier screening include family history of diabetes, previous large-for-gestation-age infant (birth weight over 4000 gm), previous unexplained stillbirth, neonatal death or congenital anomalies, recurrent infections (especially monilial vaginitis and urinary tract infections), obesity, and glycosuria.

Prior to the screening blood glucose the woman's dietary pattern should be reviewed. If she is eating less than 200–250 gm of carbohydrate per day she should be instructed in a diet which will provide this intake for three days before the screening test. Failure to do this may result in a false positive test, since the pancreas will be unable to respond appropriately to the sudden, unaccustomed carbohydrate challenge.

When the two-hour postprandial blood test is used for screening, blood glucose values of 140 mg/100 ml or less are considered normal. An ordinary meal containing 100 gm of carbohydrate provides a more physiologic test than the commerically prepared glucose drinks, although the drinks have the advantage of convenience. The motivation of the client as well as her ability to follow directions should be assessed as a means of selecting the appropriate test methods.

Fasting blood glucose or the glucose tolerance test may also be used for screening. The same precautions of three days of high carbohydrate intake should be observed as for the postprandial test. Fasting blood glucose levels of 120 mg/100 ml or less are considered to be within the normal range. In evaluating the glucose tolerance test in pregnancy it is important to remember that the fasting value will be lower than in nonpregnant individuals but that the two- and three-hour values are normally higher. Norms for each individual laboratory should be consulted.

Gestational Diabetes

Gestational diabetes is an abnormal glucose tolerance during pregnancy with a return to normal after delivery. Women who manifest this disorder are variously described as prediabetics, subclinical diabetics, or potential diabetics. They are individuals who do not have the capacity to increase insulin production sufficiently to compensate for the diabetogenic effects of the placental hormones. Maternal and fetal complications are significantly increased. Although dietary control is usually sufficient without exogenous insulin and there is a return to normal glucose tolerance post partum, these women are at increased risk to develop diabetes later in life. This is especially true if they do not maintain a normal body weight.

The impact of a diagnosis of gestational diabetes on the woman and her family is likely to be crisis-provoking. The necessity for adopting a dietary regimen, the added threats to the pregnancy, and the long-term implications of a difficult chronic disease may be, at least temporarily, overwhelming. Careful instruction and frequent contacts with supportive professionals can do much to facilitate the mobilization of the family's coping behaviors.

The gestational diabetic woman requires the same close supervision as the insulin-dependent

diabetic. Evidence of placental insufficiency and possible jeopardy to the fetus must be carefully checked. Even when the diabetes is very mild, the hazard of placental insufficiency increases toward term gestation. Pregnancy should not be permitted to continue postterm.

During the postpartum period the woman should obtain appropriate nutritional consultation for weight control and receive instructions about health maintenance to prevent or detect later development of overt diabetes.

Insulin-Dependent Diabetes

Initial clinical assessment of the insulin-dependent diabetic pregnant woman should include a thorough discussion of her experience with diabetes, her knowledge of the disease, and her own methods of managing her disease. Such discussions can provide valuable information about the individuality of the woman, her coping patterns, and probable needs and responses.

One of the primary goals of diabetic management in the nonpregnant individual is to foster independence in the client so that she can competently adjust her own glucose–insulin balance to meet the needs of daily living and minor illnesses. Some of this independence must necessarily be relinquished during pregnancy because of the necessity for using blood glucose rather than urine tests for the regulation of insulin dosage. It is therefore crucial to a satisfactory working relationship between client and professional that the woman be encouraged to assume as much autonomy in her care as she desires and is capable of achieving. An openness in communication will foster mutual trust which can only benefit the client and her developing fetus.

Antepartum Care

Over and above the usual goals for all antepartum care there are two major objectives for care of the insulin-dependent diabetic. These are (1) to maintain careful diabetic control, and

(2) to evaluate placental function and fetal well-being.

Diabetic control is achieved through the balance of dietary intake and insulin as determined by periodic blood glucose determinations. Diet should be reviewed in consultation with a nutritionist who will assist the woman to define a dietary pattern compatible with her cultural and personal food preferences, life style, and economic status. Caloric intake should be sufficient to permit a weight gain of approximately 25 pounds. This will vary according to activity level and other factors, but in general a diet of 1800 to 2200 calories is satisfactory. The diet should contain 80–100 gm of protein and carbohydrate equivalent to 40 to 45 percent of the calories. In order to avoid the wide fluctuations in blood glucose, the carbohydrate content should be evenly distributed throughout the day. Regularity in both the timing and the content of meals and snacks is very important in order to avoid insulin reactions. The diet may require frequent alterations in response to symptoms of pregnancy such as nausea, heartburn, and pressure of the uterus on the stomach. A bedtime snack is desirable to reduce the risks of the overnight fast.

It is often helpful to both client and nutritionist if the woman keeps a diet diary of all foods and beverages and the time she eats them. Reviewing this diary may assist the nutritionist to diagnose problem areas, and it is also an excellent means of teaching meal planning, calorie counting, and food values.

Insulin dosage is adjusted on the basis of blood glucose levels obtained at frequent intervals throughout gestation. Biweekly or even weekly blood tests are not uncommon. Practitioners differ in their approach to blood glucose collections. Some use a profile of three two-hour postprandial samples on a single day, others use fasting blood samples, and others may use a combination. The therapeutic goal is to maintain the fasting level below 120 mg/100 ml and/or the postprandial level below 150 mg/100 ml. The usual insulin prescription to achieve this goal is a combination of an intermediate or long-acting insulin with regular insulin in the morning and, often, an additional dose of regular and/or intermediate insulin in the late afternoon or evening. It is to be expected that the insulin requirements will gradually increase throughout gestation, especially during the second half. It is usual for the insulin dosage to increase 70 to 100 percent over prepregnancy amounts.[11] It is important to emphasize that urine tests are not reliable indicators for modifying insulin dosage during pregnancy.

As the third trimester begins, evaluation of fetal/placental function becomes paramount. An important cause of intrauterine fetal death is placental dysfunction. Early recognition of signs of impending failure permits life-saving intervention. Maternal insulin requirements provide a crude indication of placental function, since insulin is inactivated by the placental hormones. Failure to require increasing insulin doses or, more ominously, a sudden drop in insulin requirements should cast suspicion on the efficiency of the placenta.

Twenty-four-hour urinary estriol determinations are evaluated two to three times per week, beginning at approximately 32 weeks gestation. Weekly oxytocin challenge tests (OCT) and/or fetal activity acceleration determinations (FAD) are also started at about 32–34 weeks gestation. Any test results indicative of placental insufficiency should suggest the need for prompt assessment of fetal maturity and possible delivery. See Chapter 21, pages 614–21, for a discussion of these tests.

Management of the diabetic pregnancy can almost always be accomplished in an ambulatory setting. Periodic hospitalization, however, may be necessary for the woman who is in poor diabetic control, who has ketonuria, or who demonstrates evidence of placental insufficiency. In addition, a brief period of hospitalization may be the most efficient means of conducting a concentrated program of health education.

[11] Philip Felig, Diabetes mellitus, in *Medical Complications During Pregnancy*, edited by Gerard N. Burrow and Thomas F. Ferris. Saunders, Philadelphia, Pa., 1975.

Intrapartum Care

Historically, it has been good obstetric practice to perform cesarean sections routinely on all diabetic women at 35 to 37 weeks gestation. Since the incidence of intrauterine fetal death was known to be highest during the last three to four weeks of gestation, this practice was a reasonable preventive approach. Cesarean section was preferred over vaginal delivery because, even if the condition of the cervix permitted induction at this early time, the fetus tolerated labor poorly and often succumbed during the intrapartum period.

Currently several factors are changing this practice. The ability to closely monitor placental function and to assess fetal response to labor by continuous fetal heart rate records and scalp capillary blood gases permits both the longer continuation of pregnancy and the potential for safe conduct through labor. In addition, the development of reliable biochemical tests for fetal lung maturity allows the timing of delivery when adequate neonatal pulmonary function is more assured. As long as there is adequacy of placental function, as evidenced by rising urinary estriol values and negative oxytocin challenge tests, many centers are allowing the pregnancy to continue until near term to give the fetus the benefit of intrauterine growth. Near term, personal and obstetric readiness for labor are increased and induction of labor is facilitated.

During labor, or in preparation for cesarean section, maternal blood glucose levels are maintained by the intravenous infusion of glucose or other sugars and regular insulin. There is an attempt in some centers to maintain maternal glycemia under 100 mg/100 ml for several hours prior to delivery. This appears to reduce the risk of neonatal hypoglycemia by providing the fetus an intrauterine period of "withdrawal" from the high glucose loads previously available from the mother.

For the diabetic woman, as for all high-risk pregnant women, laboring is a highly mechanized event. It requires extraordinary skill and sensitivity on the part of the nurse to integrate all of the data from patients and machines and make sound judgments about care. Even greater expertise is needed to permit the laboring woman to maintain her self-esteem and to control her labor and birth in ways that are safe and acceptable to her and to the father. If possible the couple should be attended during labor by physicians and nurses whom they have known through pregnancy. The father or another supportive person should be present throughout labor and delivery. As soon as initial assessment has been made of the infant at birth to insure adequate respirations, the parents should be offered their infant to see, touch, and hold. Unless there are either maternal or neonatal complications the mother may initiate breast feeding during the first one to two hours of life. Emphasis during a high-risk labor must always be on the family—never on the gadgetry.

Postpartum Care

Endocrine and metabolic changes occur precipitously with the termination of pregnancy. The contrainsulin effects are abruptly stopped and insulin requirements are markedly decreased for the first few days post partum. Regular insulin is usually given on a sliding scale, depending on the amount of glycosuria, for two to three days before intermediate or long-acting insulin is prescribed. It typically requires three to six months for the insulin requirements to return to their prepregnant level.

The diabetes may be quite brittle for a time after delivery, and the nurse must observe the patient closely for signs of insulin reaction, hyperglycemia, and acidosis. The tendency toward postpartum infections in increased in the diabetic and even mild infections can severely compromise diabetic control.

The stress of diabetic reregulation, the possibility of an infant who requires special observation and care, as well as the usual anxieties and discomforts of involution may combine to delay comfortable mother–infant contact. Mothers need help to understand and accept themselves if there is not an immediate flood of maternal feeling. Parental attachment can be facilitated by flexible, family-centered policies which permit free access of parents to their infants.

Nutrition consultation should be obtained prior to discharge from the hospital. Emphasis will be on nutritional requirements for lactation, if that is appropriate, and on caloric intake to achieve optimum weight.

Referral to community health agencies, if not initiated antepartally, should be accomplished at the time of discharge. Telephone follow-up within two or three days of going home is quite helpful for all mothers, but especially for those who have had a high-risk pregnancy. For some women the postpartum period is a time of considerable let-down after the intense, almost constant, attention they received during the final weeks of their pregnancy. A period of weaning from the intensive care team members may be necessary.

Observation and special care of the infant of a diabetic mother is discussed on pages 800–802.

GENETIC DISORDERS

There has been a rapid increase in knowledge about the role of heredity in health and disease in the past 20 years. It can be anticipated that dramatic development will continue in this area, giving rise to new challenges in philosophy and ethics, as well as medicine and science.

Since the transmission of genetic disorders requires reproduction by definition, it is relevant and important that perinatal practitioners have some knowledge of basic genetic principles and when to utilize experts as consultants to their clients.

Three categories of genetic disorders suggest a need for action in terms of health teaching, counseling, or direct intervention. In the first category are those genetic disorders that have special implications for the course of the pregnancy itself. The second category consists of dis-

orders which can be predicted to affect the fetus and which may suggest the desirability of prenatal diagnosis. The third, and largest, category contains those diseases of a hereditary nature which are likely to affect the parents and/or their offspring in later life, for example, cardiovascular disease.

The first category of genetic diseases includes such common genetic factors as Rh and ABO blood incompatibilities. Polygenic or multifactorial conditions such as diabetes mellitus, hypertension, and heart disease also belong to this category. Other genetic disorders present in the mother may present so great a risk that the advisability of pregnancy is seriously questioned. Such disorders include Marfan's syndrome, sickle cell anemia, and acute intermittent porphyria. Others require only slight modifications in care. Achrondroplasia, for example, will almost always necessitate a cesarean section because of the abnormal pelvis structure. Otherwise pregnancy progresses normally.

A number of genetic disorders are beginning to be found in pregnancy simply because newer advances in the treatment of these diseases are permitting individuals to reach reproductive age in better states of health. One such example is phenylketonuria. Because of early screening and dietary treatment, many PKU children are now adults having their own children. Women with PKU who wish to bear children should reinstitute a low phenylalanine diet prior to conception and continue it through gestation. If this is not done the fetus will suffer mental retardation from intrauterine exposure to the high maternal phenylalanine levels, even though he himself does not have PKU.

Parents who have a significant risk for having seriously affected offspring, whether or not they themselves are affected, are concerned with the second category of genetic disorders. These include the chromosomal abnormalities such as Down's syndrome and other trisomies and inherited biochemical abnormalities such as Tay-Sachs, galactosemia, and maple syrup urine disease. Both parents and professionals should realize the limitations of amniocentesis for antenatal diagnosis, and it should only be considered when there is a legitimate risk and useful information can be obtained. The most common indications for genetic amniocentesis include maternal age over 35, presence of trisomies or autosomal recessive disorders in previous offspring, translocation in one parent, and X-linked disorders. The procedure for this diagnosis is discussed more fully in Chapter 21.

Category three, diseases which occur later in life, affects virtually everyone. These do not warrant interruption of pregnancy or even alteration in fertility rates. They do, however, provide opportunities for preventive health management and give direction for future screening. For example, families with strong histories of heart disease should be particularly careful to avoid obesity and maintain good patterns of nutrition and physical exercise. Breast cancer in the family should prompt more frequent and perhaps more sophisticated screening procedures for this disease.

Genetic History

Documentation of family history is the most efficient means of gaining information necessary for genetic intervention. A three-generation pedigree which denotes the health status of all first- and second-degree relatives of the fetus should be obtained for all obstetric clients (Table 23-2). Less than half an hour is required and much valuable information can be acquired. It is

Table 23-2. Percentage of Genes Shared in Common with Different Relatives

Degree of Relatedness to Fetus	Percent of Genes Shared in Common	Examples
First-degree relatives	50%	Parents, siblings, own future offspring
Second-degree relatives	25%	Grandparents, aunts, uncles, half-sibs
Third-degree relatives	12½%	First cousins, great-grandparents

best to begin with the couple and ask them first about their own parents, then about all of their siblings, and finally about all their children and stepchildren. Sometimes it is desirable to obtain information about their siblings' children (first cousins to the fetus) in order to get indirect evidence of carrier states in the parents. Once the pedigree has been drawn, it should be determined whether these individuals are alive or dead, their ages, reproductive history, past and present health and/or cause of death. Any affected relatives should be denoted by a full name, including maiden name, and medical validation should be obtained whenever possible. All spontaneous abortions should be included together with any information about them that is available (Fig. 23-6).

Specific questions about inherited disorders may help the couple relate more complete information. For example: Are there any instances of mental retardation or bleeding disorders in your family? The racial and ethnic background may be of importance for some couples.

At the time of the family history the couple should be asked if they have any special concerns. Frequently parents overestimate their risks, and this provides an opportunity to put their fears in reasonable perspective and, usually, to be reassuring.

Genetic Counseling

When family histories or other screening procedures indicate the presence of genetic disorders or when a couple's anxieties about inherited disorders is very high, genetic counseling should be recommended.

The purpose of genetic counseling is to provide information about the risk of occurrence or recurrence of a genetic disorder in a family and about alternatives available so that families can make the best reproductive decisions. Counseling is sought or recommended principally at three times during the family life cycle: prior to conception, during pregnancy, and during the immediate postpartum period. Reasons for obtaining counseling include a positive family his-

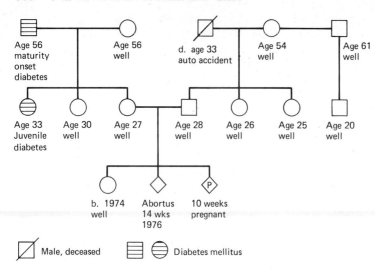

Age 56
maturity
onset
diabetes

Age 56
well

d. age 33
auto accident

Age 54
well

Age 61
well

Age 33
Juvenile
diabetes

Age 30
well

Age 27
well

Age 28
well

Age 26
well

Age 25
well

Age 20
well

b. 1974
well

Abortus
14 wks
1976

10 weeks
pregnant

Male, deceased   Diabetes mellitus

Figure 23-6. Fictitious family pedigree showing first- and second-degree relatives of the fetus. Note the mother's family history of diabetes as well as her previous spontaneous abortion. She should be screened early in gestation for blood glucose levels.

tory for hereditary disorders; consanguinity in the mating; membership in specific population groups (e.g., Ashkenazic Jews because of Tay-Sachs); age of parents; prior exposure to environmental agents such as x-rays or narcotics; habitual abortions; and previous birth of an affected child. Family history is the most common reason in the preconception and prenatal periods, although maternal age is also a very frequent reason during pregnancy. When counseling is sought post partum it is almost invariably because of the birth of an affected child.

The first step in providing counseling is to establish as accurate and precise a diagnosis as possible. The family history provides the first information but is not exhaustive. Chromosomal studies and/or carrier screening tests may be done on the couple. Photographs of affected offspring or other relatives are often helpful. If there has been a previous stillbirth or neonatal death, it is useful to have a photograph as well as a full-body x-ray done at autopsy to accompany the autopsy report. Direct examination of living affected family members may be desirable. Many syndromes share common symptoms. Failure to distinguish between them because the differences are overlooked may substantially alter the estimate of risk.

Once a diagnosis has been established, the

mode of inheritance must be determined. For a great many disorders this is already established and can simply be looked up in one of several reference books designed for this purpose. In other situations the mode of inheritance can be inferred from a detailed family history, and in still others there may be no one certain transmission mechanism.

The determination of the mode of inheritance permits the designation of recurrence risks, which are usually stated as the probability that any particular mating will result in an affected offspring. When Mendelian modes of inheritance apply, risks can be established based on those laws of genetics. In the absence of Mendelian patterns, empirical risks may be determined, based on the frequency of occurrence of the disorder in the population, family history, and other factors.

In addition to the mathematical risk figure it is important to have information concerning the prognosis for affected individuals. Disorders which require long-term, costly treatment may prompt a family to make decisions that are quite different from those it would make when the disorder is fatal at birth or soon after. Physical deformities create different stresses than do mental deficiencies, and so on.

Having assembled all this information the

counselor must then relate it to the family in terms they can understand. Reproductive options that are available to them should be described. Some of these include not having children, adopting children, antepartal diagnosis, early diagnosis, and treatment of neonates (e.g., PKU). Every effort should be made to ascertain the family's comprehension of the information given to them. Follow-up sessions may be necessary, particularly if the initial counseling is done at a time of grief over a newborn or recently diagnosed child. A nondirective approach should be used as much as possible so that the family, not the counselor, truly makes the decisions about their conceiving and bearing children.

Whenever family composition warrants it, genetic implications for unaffected children in the family should be included. Their risks for being carriers of the disorder which affects their sibling has definite implications for their own reproductive futures.

AGE AS A RISK FACTOR IN PREGNANCY

Women in their early twenties have been described as the most biologically fit for reproduction. But is there an optimum age socially or psychologically or developmentally for a person to become a parent? This is a question which awaits discussion and investigation. For the present, it can only be said that women at either extreme of the reproductive life span are at increased risk for both medical and social/psychologic complications of childbearing.

Adolescence

Pregnancy during adolescence received considerable attention in the middle and late 1970s from virtually every facet of society. Birth rates have steadily increased in the under-16 age group while declining in all other age groups. Such pregnancies, generally beginning outside of marriage, place significant stress on the young women involved, their families, and society as a whole.

The girl, not yet a woman, still developmentally occupied with her own physical and psychologic growth, is thrust into a role for which she is ill-prepared. She needs very special nutritional care to insure proper growth for her child, as well as for her own continued physical growth. Because of her physiologic immaturity, nutritional status, and frequent reluctance to seek early antepartum care, she is at increased risk for toxemia, premature labor, low-birth-weight infant, and operative delivery.

All too frequently, teenage pregnancy means the interruption of education, which may substantially alter the girl's future life chances. Premarital conceptions are highly correlated with marital disruptions, as approximately three out of four teenage marriages end in divorce. If the girl does not choose to marry, she must make other very difficult decisions related to her future and that of her child. More and more single women are not relinquishing their infants for adoption but are choosing to raise them alone. This has implications for the support services, financial as well as social, needed to help these mothers.

While services for unwed mothers are rather widely available, little or no attention has been paid to the unwed father. What are his needs for counseling, for education? What are his rights with regard to his unborn child? Social and health agencies and the courts are beginning to address these issues, but there is much yet to be done.

Even more neglected are the parents of these adolescents. Professionals waste little time and no sympathy on these parents who are doubly in crisis. The quality of their parenting is called into question by the out-of-wedlock pregnancy. They hurt for themselves and they hurt for their child, whom they love. In addition, they must deal with the loss of their grandchild if adoption is elected or with adjustment to their new relationship to their daughter as a single parent.

Many references are available which deal more comprehensively with individual aspects of care for the adolescent pregnant girl. The reader is referred to these for assistance in individualizing nursing care for this vulnerable segment of the childbearing population.

The "Elderly" Obstetric Client

Pregnant women age 35 and over are defined as obstetrically elderly. These women are at greater risk statistically for such obstetric complications as placenta previa, abruptio placenta, postpartum hemorrhage, dysfunctional labor, toxemia, and small-for-gestational age infants. Some distinction should be made when evaluating individual women between primigravidas and multigravidas. In many studies parity increases as a function of age, so that it may be the number of pregnancies rather than the age that is responsible for some complications.

Age alone, however, appears responsible for the increased incidence of genetic disorders in neonates whose mothers are over 35. The most striking example of this is the risk of trisomy 21, Down's syndrome, which increases from an overall incidence of one in every 600 to 700 births to one in 100 after the mother reaches age 35 and about one in 50 after age 40.[12] This is believed to be due to aging of the ova which, of course, are developed during embryonic life and remain stored in the ovary until released at a monthly ovulation.

The nurse should also assess the "older" woman's attitude toward her pregnancy, with particular reference to the woman's own developmental stage, as well as that of the family. If this is a first pregnancy, is it timed at this stage of her life because of recent marriage, a period of infertility, or because of priorities given to career development at earlier ages? Each of these, as well as other possible reasons, are apt to affect her perception of herself and her child in different ways. If this is not a first pregnancy, how old are her other children? Mothers of teenagers will likely respond in different ways

[12] H. Eldon Sutton, *An Introduction to Human Genetics.* Holt, Rinehart, and Winston, Chicago, Ill., 1975, pp. 61–63.

than mothers of toddlers. What about the father? Is he pleased and supportive, or does he blame this "mistake" on his wife's failure to take effective contraceptive measures?

There are many other areas important to consider and few of them are unique to any maternal age. The nurse who considers each client as a special individual and includes her as a partner in recognizing and solving her own health problems will have little difficulty in serving childbearing families across the reproductive age span.

BIBLIOGRAPHY

de Alvarez, Russell R., The kidney in pregnancy, *Hosp. Pract.* 8:129–140 (May) 1973.

Bennet, Margaret, *The Peripatetic Diabetic.* Hawthorn Books, New York, 1969.

Bowes, Watson A., Jr.: Detection and treatment of tuberculosis, *Contemp. Ob/Gyn* 6:43–48, 1975.

Burch, G. E., Heart disease and pregnancy, *Am. Heart J.* 93:104, 1977.

Burrow, Gerard N., and Ferris, Thomas F., *Medical Complications During Pregnancy.* Saunders, Philadelphia, Pa., 1975.

Clark, Ann L., Adolescence, in *Childbearing: A Nursing Perspective*, edited by Ann L. Clark and Dyanne D. Affonso. Davis, Philadelphia, Pa., 1976.

Cranley, Mecca S., and Frazier, Sue A., Preventive intensive care of the diabetic mother and her fetus, *Nurs. Clin. North Am.* 8:489–499 (Sept.) 1973.

Contemporary Ob/Gyn, Newest strategy for syphilis control, 8:117–125 (Sept.) 1976.

Dickens, Helen O. *et al.*, One hundred pregnant adolescents: Treatment approaches in a university hospital, in *Vulnerable Infants*, edited by Jane L. Schwartz and Lawrence H. Schwartz. McGraw-Hill, New York, 1977.

Duhring, John L., Diabetes in pregnancy: How to diagnose and treat it. *Contemp. Ob/Gyn* 9:117–124 (Feb.) 1977.

Felig, Philip, Body fuel metabolism and diabetes mellitus in pregnancy, *Med. Clin. North Am.* 61:43–66 (Jan.) 1977.

Frye, Barbara A., and Barham, Barbara, Reaching

out to pregnant adolescents, *Am. J. Nurs.* 75:1502–1503 (Sept.) 1975.

Gabbe, Steven G., Mestman, Jorge H., Hibbard, Lester T., Maternal mortality in diabetes mellitus—An 18-year survey, *Obstet. Gynecol.* 48:549–551 (Nov.) 1976.

Hallal, Janice C., Thyroid disorders, *Am. J. Nurs.* 77:418–432 (Mar.) 1977.

Harger, Edgar O. III, and Smythe, Alexander R. II; "Pregnancy in women over forty, *Obstet. Gynecol.* 49:257–261 (Mar.) 1977.

Hayter, Jean, Fine points in diabetic care, *Am. J. Nurs.* 76:594–595 (Apr.) 1976.

Hubbard, Charles William, *Family Planning Education*, 2nd ed. Mosby, St. Louis, Mo., 1977, pp. 173–212.

Innerfield, Ronald, and Hollander, Charles S., Thyroidal complications of pregnancy, *Med. Clin. North Am.* 61:67–87 (Jan.) 1977.

Kaplan, Alan L., Smith, Julian P., and Tillman, Alvin J. B., Healed acute and chronic nephritis in pregnancy, *Am. J. Obstet. Gynecol.* 83:1519–1525 (1 June) 1962.

Kimball, Chase Patterson, Emotional and psychological aspects of diabetes mellitus, *Med. Clin. North Am.* 55:1007–1019 (July) 1971.

LaBarre, Maurine, Emotional crises of school-age girls during pregnancy and early motherhood, in *Vulnerable Infants*, edited by Jane L. Schwartz and Laurence H. Schwartz. McGraw-Hill, New York, 1977.

Leontic, Emilio A., Respiratory disease in pregnancy, *Med. Clin. North Am.* 61:111–128 (Jan.) 1977.

Lindheimer, Marshall D., and Katz, Adrian I., Managing the patient with renal disease, *Contemp. Ob/Gyn.* 3:49–55 (Jan.) 1974.

Milunsky, Aubrey, Genetic counseling in obstetric practice, *Contemp. Ob/Gyn* 8:105–111 (Sept.) 1976.

———, *The Prevention of Genetic Disease and Mental Retardation.* Saunders, Philadelphia, Pa., 1975.

Nahmias, A. J., Josey, W. E., and Naib, Z. M., Herpes simplex virus infection of the fetus and newborn: Clinical, laboratory and epidemiological aspects, in *Prenatal Infections, International Symposium of Vienna*, edited by Otto Thalhammer. Georg Thieme, Stuttgart, 1971.

Prazar, Greg, and Felice, Marianne, The psychologic and social effects of juvenile diabetes, *Pediatr. Ann.* 4:59–71 (June) 1975.

Pritchard, Jack A., and MacDonald, Paul C., *Williams Obstetrics*, 15th ed. Appleton-Century-Crofts, New York, 1976.

Sever, John L., Cytomegalovirus: Devastation in the nursery, *Contemp. Ob/Gyn* 9:29–34 (Mar.) 1977.

Steinmann, Marion, New gonococcus strain troubles CDC, *Contemp. Ob/Gyn* 9:23–28 (Mar.) 1977.

Ueland, Kent, Pregnancy and cardiovascular disease, *Med. Clin. North Am.* 61:17–41 (Jan.) 1977.

———, and Metcalfe, J., Heart disease in pregnancy, *Clin. Perinatol.* 1:349–367 (Sept.) 1974.

Whalley, Peggy J., and Cunningham, F. Gary, Short-term vs. continuous antimicrobial therapy for asymptomatic bacteriuria in pregnancy, *Obstet. Gynecol.* 49:262–265 (Mar) 1977.

Wolf, Lorraine, The nurse's role in genetic counseling, in *Family Health Care,* edited by Debra P. Hymovich and Martha U. Bernard. McGraw-Hill, New York, 1973.

24

Complications of the Puerperium

The major complications of the puerperium are hemorrhage, puerperal infection, thrombophlebitis, mastitis, and urinary tract infections. Mortality from these conditions has been reduced to almost zero since the general availability of blood and blood products as well as broad-spectrum antibiotics. Nevertheless it is important that the nurse be well aware of the pathology and treatment and which women are at greatest risk. In many, if not most, situations the conditions are avoidable if expert care is given. In those unavoidable situations, early detection and treatment can prevent the more serious illness.

When the postpartum mother is ill there are implications well beyond the physical effects of the complication. Infections may dictate her separation from her infant. Even if there are no medical reasons for separation, her energy levels may be so low that she is unable to extend herself to become acquainted with her newborn. Discharge from the hospital is often delayed, causing increased financial burden as well as extended separation from her home and family. Because of the illness and/or the necessary medications, lactation may be inhibited, thus extending the time required to establish a satisfactory nursing pattern. In some instances it may be necessary to abandon breast feeding altogether. When she returns home, the mother may still require extra help if only because she tires more readily.

In short, the physically debilitating effects of the mother's illness, together with concern and anxiety, use up family energies that would otherwise be directed at reintegrating the family after the addition of a new member. Such far-reaching ramifications clearly demand that first-quality health care be given in order to prevent the occurrence of postpartum complications whenever possible.

POSTPARTUM HEMORRHAGE

Postpartum hemorrhage includes all excessive bleeding which occurs from the time of the infant's birth until the puerperium is ended at six weeks after delivery. Primarily, however, it refers to hemorrhage, which occurs immediately after the separation of the placenta or during the first one to two hours postdelivery.

Healthy women generally lose approximately 300 ml of blood at the time of a normal birth. If an episiotomy is done or a perineal laceration occurs, an additional 100 to 150 ml may be lost. Loss of more than 500 ml of blood is termed a hemorrhage. Blood loss prior to the separation of the placenta should be slight with a short gush coming at the time of separation. Following delivery of the placenta, uterine contraction should be immediate with blood flow decreasing to an amount approximating a heavy menstrual flow during the first two hours post partum and steadily declining thereafter. Any oozing from the vagina is abnormal and warrants immediate investigation.

Excessive bleeding occurring after 24 hours postpartum is called a *late* or delayed postpartum hemorrhage. This is discussed below.

Causes

The most frequent cause of postpartum hemorrhage is *uterine atony*, or impaired tone of the uterine muscle. There are many sinuses or blood spaces between the muscle fibers directly underneath the placenta. As separation of the placenta takes place, the uterine muscle normally contracts, and the sinuses are closed off with eventual thrombus formation. When the muscle fibers fail to contract and the vessels are not constricted, hemorrhage takes place.

Uterine atony is frequently due to exhaustion of the muscle. This exhaustion may follow either a prolonged or a precipitous labor; it may be due to overdistention of the uterus with a multiple pregnancy, a large baby, or hydramnios; or it may be caused by too much massage of the fundus in the third stage of labor. Sluggish muscle, as evidenced by poor contractions during the first and/or second stage of labor, can also be expected to contract poorly after this third stage. The uterine muscle may also fail to contract well when there has been premature separation of the placenta, which allowed bleeding into the muscle, or when fibroid tumors are present. Whenever any of these conditions has been present during labor, the nurse must be particularly careful to check the state of contraction of the uterus during the first few hours after delivery.

Lacerations in the reproductive tract constitute the second major cause of postpartum bleeding. Perineal and low vaginal wall tears usually do not bleed profusely, but those which occur in the cervix or high in the vaginal vault may be so deep and extensive that they open large blood vessels. Cervical or high vaginal wall lacerations are most likely to follow operative deliveries, especially if the cervix is not completely dilated, but they occur occasionally even with spontaneous births. In some deliveries the labia become torn, and if these lacerations extend into the clitoris, they may also cause profuse bleeding.

Pieces of *retained placental tissue* or blood clots, or incomplete separation of the placenta during the third stage, comprise a third cause of blood loss. These keep the muscle from constricting the blood vessels adequately. As long as the entire placenta is attached, there is no danger of hemorrhage, but if partial separation occurs or if even a small piece of the placenta remains adherent, the torn vessels at the point of separation may bleed because the part that is still attached interferes with complete constriction of the sinuses. Incomplete separation of the placenta may be due to poor uterine muscle contractions or defective decidua or early manipulation of the uterus during the third stage of labor.

Symptoms

Bleeding in postpartum hemorrhage may be visible externally immediately, may be entirely internal, or may be present both externally and internally. Ordinarily there is a steady flow of blood from the vagina, and it is very important to recognize that this slow loss may be adding up to an excessive amount. Sometimes the cervix is closed with a clot, and a large amount of blood may be collected in the uterus with only a serous discharge draining from the vagina. When the uterus is palpated through the abdominal wall, it is found to be large and boggy. If pressure is applied, large amounts of blood clots and of fresh blood can often be expressed through the vagina. For this reason it is particularly important to palpate the fundus every 10 to 15 minutes for the first hour after delivery.

Other symptoms are those associated with hemorrhage. However, the pulse and blood pressure may not vary much from normal until a large amount of blood has been lost and then may change quite suddenly. When signs of the effect of blood loss appear, the patient will have a weak, rapid pulse, low blood pressure, rapid shallow respirations, a pale color, cold perspiration, dizziness, faintness, air hunger, restlessness, and anxiety, and progress to a state of profound shock.

Prevention

Prevention of postpartum hemorrhage should begin early in the pregnancy with identification of those women who are at increased risk. A hematocrit should be done early in gestation and repeated at 28 and 36 weeks. (See Chapter 7, page 171.) All pregnant women should take supplemental iron to prevent anemia. If anemia is present aggressive measures should be taken to correct it as soon as possible. Maintenance of good health and nutrition and prevention of infection will likewise reduce the risks for postpartum hemorrhage.

During labor the existence of any factors predisposing to uterine atony should be noted. These include hypotonic dysfunctional labor, prolonged or precipitous labor, overdistention of the uterus (large baby, multiple gestation, hydramnios), great multiparity, and antepartum bleeding. When one or more such factors occur the possibility of postpartum hemorrhage should be anticipated. Venous blood is drawn for typing and cross-matching in readiness for transfusion if needed, and a hematocrit is done. It is usually a wise precaution in such circumstances to have an intravenous conduit in place of sufficient diameter to permit administration of blood should sudden bleeding occur.

No effort should be made to express the placenta until signs of separation appear, but then it should be expressed immediately and inspected carefully to ensure its being intact. Since anesthesia sometimes has a relaxing effect on the uterus, speed in completing any operative procedure and repair of lacerations, thus decreasing the length of anesthesia, may prevent blood loss. Loss of blood from an episiotomy should be kept at a minimum since this loss added to that from the uterus may bring the total amount close to 500 ml.

After labor is completed, the danger of hemorrhage is greatest during that critical hour immediately following. The patient must be watched closely during this period, both to prevent bleeding and to detect bleeding early, making prompt treatment possible. In addition, every newly delivered woman should be taught what her contracted uterus feels like and where she should be able to palpate it. She can then participate in the prevention of postpartum hemorrhage.

Treatment

The primary goal in the management of hemorrhage is self-evident: stop the bleeding by correcting the cause. The second goal is to maintain adequate circulating blood volume to prevent shock and anemia. Prevention of infection is the third goal.

Bleeding which occurs during the third stage of labor is generally due to partial placental separation. Efforts are made to expel the placenta as soon as possible with manual removal being employed if necessary.

When bleeding occurs after the placenta is delivered, uterine atony, which is the most common cause, is considered first. The fundus can very readily be palpated. If it is relaxed, the bleeding most likely is due to failure of the muscle fibers to constrict the blood vessels. If the fundus is firm, the bleeding is probably not from an intrauterine source, and it becomes necessary to look for and repair lacerations.

When the cervix is to be inspected for lacerations, it is necessary to draw it down into view because the entire birth canal is so relaxed and edematous that a speculum or digital examination is unsatisfactory. Retractors are necessary to hold the vaginal walls apart, and a sponge or ovum forceps is used to grasp and expose the cervix. Any sharp instrument will tear the soft cervical tissues. A good light must be provided for this procedure. Most physicians routinely inspect the cervix after operative deliveries. Others believe that small lacerations will heal spontaneously and that the added manipulation is unnecessary. Suturing the bleeding edges controls hemorrhage due to tears of the reproductive tract.

Obviously, when the uterine muscle is atonic, the first step in controlling hemorrhage from this cause is stimulating the muscle to contract. This is done by massage and administration of oxytocic drugs. The fundus should be compressed against the symphysis pubis, or between the hands, and vigorously massaged (Fig. 15-21). Oxytocin medication, 10 oxytocic units (international standard), or ergonovine, 0.2 mg ($1/320$ gr), may be used intramuscularly.

An intravenous drip of oxytocin, 10 units or more in 1000 ml of an appropriate solution, is started if bleeding persists or a tendency to uterine muscle relaxation continues. This may be given more rapidly than the oxytocin drip used for stimulation of labor since its purpose now is to stimulate strong contractions of the uterine muscle. The oxytocin drip may be given over a period of several hours. It is continued until the uterus remains well contracted without massage.

Bimanual compression of the uterus may be employed if abdominal massage and oxytocics are not effective in controlling bleeding. In performing this procedure the physician presses one hand quite deeply into the abdomen and massages the posterior aspect of the uterus while at the same time he inserts the other hand (gloved) into the vagina and massages the anterior aspect of the uterus by rubbing his fingers against the uterine wall. This procedure provides considerably more stimulation to the uterine muscle than can be given with abdominal massage alone, and it also compresses the venous sinuses of the uterus. The uterine muscle may soon contract sufficiently to control bleeding, but if it does not quickly do so, bimanual compression may need to be continued for an indefinite period. In rare instances, when all measures fail to stop bleeding, it becomes necessary to remove the uterus.

Since retention of even a small piece of placental tissue may prevent the uterus from contracting firmly, the treatment of hemorrhage from this cause is immediate removal of the retained fragment. It is to avert this occurrence that the placenta is carefully inspected after its expulsion. If the placenta is not intact, the physician introduces his gloved hand into the uterus and removes the retained portion, making it possible for the muscle to contract properly to close the open blood vessels.

Supportive therapy and replacement of blood are started whenever it appears that blood loss will be above usual. While blood is being obtained for transfusion, intravenous fluids of 5 percent dextrose in Ringer's lactate solution or plasma are given to maintain an adequate blood volume. Since administration of blood is quite obviously the best replacement for blood loss, replacement of blood is begun promptly when bleeding becomes excessive. When much blood has been lost, transfusions may be given several days in succession. Although the blood loss is restored, a patient who has had a postpartum hemorrhage may not recover as quickly as one who has had no complications.

The patient may show signs of shock by the time the bleeding has been controlled and needs the rest, quiet, and supportive therapy that is ordinarily employed for any excessive bleeding. She should be kept warm and comfortable. Elastic stockings or leg wraps enhance venous return and prevent pooling of blood in the lower extremities which may predispose to thrombophlebitis. Vital signs are observed frequently to note the patient's response to blood loss and to its treatment. Contraction of the uterine fundus and amount of vaginal bleeding are checked frequently.

As soon as the immediate danger from the bleeding has been averted, attention is directed toward prevention of infection. A patient who has had considerable blood loss is very susceptible to infection. In addition, the internal manipulations sometimes necessary for control of bleeding increase the opportunities for the introduction of organisms. For these reasons it is not unusual for a broad-spectrum antibiotic to be administered prophylactically.

When bleeding becomes profuse after the termination of the third stage it is usually the nurse, not the physician, who must assume responsibility for emergency treatment. Fortunately, this is a rare emergency, but every nurse involved in perinatal care should be prepared to think and act quickly should the need arise. The first action upon discovery of bleeding is to massage the uterus in order to bring about contraction to control bleeding. The patient *must never be left*. Rather the nurse should summon help in whatever way is possible while continuing to massage the uterus and reassure the patient. Intravenous fluids should be started and venous blood may be drawn for typing and cross-matching depending on the extent of the bleeding.

In anticipation of such emergencies when a physician may not be immediately available it is common to have standing orders for oxytocic drugs which the nurse may administer at her discretion. The usual procedure is to start an intravenous infusion of 20 units of oxytocin in 1000 ml of an appropriate solution.

Above all, the nurse must remember that severe hemorrhage from a relaxed uterus can usually be prevented if the fundus is kept firmly contracted, by massage if necessary, during the first hour or more after delivery.

Delayed Postpartum Hemorrhage

Although the definition of delayed, or late, postpartum hemorrhage indicates that it can occur any time after 24 hours postdelivery, it ordinarily occurs a week or more after delivery. Since the majority of women are at home when it occurs, the possibility of bleeding should be briefly discussed as a part of the patient teaching during the postpartum period.

The usual cause of this late bleeding is the retention of a placental fragment. It may be due also to failure of some of the decidua to go through regressive changes, thus hindering proper uterine involution. Treatment usually consists of the oral administration of ergonovine (0.2 mg four times a day), although it may sometimes be necessary to do a curettage of the uterus to remove the retained fragment. Although bleeding may be excessive, it responds quickly to conservative management.

Placenta Accreta

Placenta accreta is a rare but extremely dangerous complication which occurs in 1 of 2000 deliveries. It is due to the abnormal adherence of part or all of the placenta to the uterine wall. It is associated with abnormalities of the endometrium, apparently resulting from some past trauma, infection, surgery, or endocrine imbalance. As the placenta implants, the chorionic villi invade the myometrium, sometimes penetrating as far as the serosal layer.

If the placenta accreta is partial, then the normally attached portion of the placenta will separate at delivery as usual, but the portion adherent to the myometrium will not detach. Hemorrhage thus occurs because of a partially separated placenta. Complete placenta accreta will not separate, and no bleeding will occur unless manual attempts to remove the placenta tear portions from the uterine wall.

Hemorrhage from placenta accreta can be catastrophic. Abdominal hysterectomy is done as soon as a diagnosis is made to stop the bleeding. Prognosis is good if prompt operative action has been taken and blood loss has been replaced by transfusion.

Hematomas

A hematoma may develop in the connective tissue of the vulva or under the vaginal mucosa from injury to a blood vessel in these tissues. Injury to a blood vessel may occur during delivery (without laceration of the superficial tissues of the vagina or vulva), or the injury may be due to puncture of a vessel during repair of an episiotomy. Bleeding into the tissues may be slow, but continuous. These tissues become very distended, and the patient may experience a great deal of pain. The hematoma may not be visible, especially if the bleeding is under the vaginal mucosa. Intense pain in the perineal area, due to stretching of tissue, may be the only evidence of a hematoma for some hours. Any complaint of such intense pain should prompt the nurse to carefully examine the perineal area and to notify the physician of her findings in addition to reporting the pain.

A vulvar hematoma becomes visible as a swelling develops on one side of the vulva. Later a purplish discoloration of the skin over the swollen area appears. A vaginal hematoma may not be detected until pressure symptoms lead to an examination. A soft mass is then found to protrude into the vagina or rectum. Even with an examination the amount of blood lost is hard to determine since the hematoma may extend upward into the broad ligament. Blood loss into such a hematoma may be excessive.

Treatment consists of incision of the hematoma, removal of blood clots, ligation of the bleeding vessel, blood transfusion to combat the effects of blood loss, and antibiotics for prophylaxis against infection. If the hematoma is small, it can usually be left untreated, slow resorption taking place.

PUERPERAL INFECTION

Puerperal infection results from the entrance of pathogenic bacteria into the female reproductive tract before or during labor or in the puerperium. It is a dreaded complication in the puerperal patient, and has evidently been so considered since the days of Hippocrates. Until the past century this veritable scourge was so utterly baffling that it was regarded as a dispensation of Divine Providence and was therefore accepted with the same philosophic resignation as earthquakes and cyclones.

In dramatic contrast to this unresisting attitude is the present knowledge concerning the cause and prevention of this disease. It is now known to be a wound infection and therefore practically preventable. It is to be ascribed to the carelessness of mankind rather than to the indifference of Providence. This change in attitude was due very largely to the devoted work of three men who were deeply stirred by the tragic frequency with which young women died in so-called "childbed fever." These men were

Ignaz Semmelweis, Oliver Wendell Holmes, better known to Americans as a poet and humorist, and Louis Pasteur, each contributing his own special observations to the sum total of knowledge which was to mean so much to mothers of today. Also, the teachings of Lister concerning antisepsis and the introduction of sterile rubber gloves by Dr. Halsted, of Johns Hopkins Hospital, have had the same life-saving effect on obstetric patients as on all surgical patients.

With the development of antibiotics the treatment of puerperal infection has become more satisfactory. Continued development of new chemotherapeutic agents since their introduction has made therapy ever more specific. Formerly treatment of puerperal infection could be directed merely toward helping the patient build up general resistance to the disease.

In 1843, Oliver Wendell Holmes read a paper before the Boston Society for Medical Improvement, entitled "The Contagiousness of Puerperal Fever." In this paper he presented striking evidence that in many instances something was conveyed by doctor or nurse from an ill person to a maternity patient, with puerperal fever as a result. He was attacked and ridiculed for his theories, and some of the leading obstetricians declared that it was an insult to their intelligence to expect them to believe that an agent invisible to the naked eye could work such havoc.

In 1847, Ignaz Semmelweis, of the Vienna Lying-in Hospital, decided as a result of some of his investigations that puerperal fever was a wound infection, and that septic material was introduced into the birth canal on the examining finger of the doctor or nurse after contact with an infected patient or cadaver. Accordingly, he required that all vaginal examinations be preceded by washing the hands in chloride of lime, after which precaution the mortality from infection dropped from 10 percent to less than 1 percent. In 1861, Semmelweis offered his theories and conclusions in a masterly work on this subject, the title of which may be translated as "The Etiology, Conception, and Prophylaxis of Child-

Bed Fever," but the actual cause of the disease was still unknown.

About 1879 Pasteur demonstrated what is now known as the streptococcus, in certain patients suffering from puerperal fever. René Vallery-Radot wrote:[1]

Pasteur, wrote M. Roux, does not hesitate to declare that that microscopic organism (a microbe shaped like a chain) is the most frequent cause of infection in recently delivered women. One day, in a discussion on puerperal fever at the Academy, one of his most weighty colleagues was eloquently enlarging upon the causes of epidemics in lying-in hospitals; Pasteur interrupted him from his place. "None of those things cause the epidemic; it is the nursing and medical staff who carry the microbe from an infected woman to a healthy one." And as the orator replied that he feared that microbe would never be found, Pasteur went to the blackboard and drew a diagram of the chain-like organism, saying: "There, that is what it is like!" His conviction was so deep that he could not help expressing it forcibly. It would be impossible now to picture the state of surprise and stupefaction into which he would send the students and doctors in hospitals, when, with an assurance and simplicity almost disconcerting in a man who was entering a lying-in ward for the first time, he criticised the appliances, and declared that the linen should be put into a sterilizing stove.

Very slowly the teachings of these earnest men were adopted by the medical profession, with the result that in well-conducted hospitals the precautions that have been described in preceding chapters are rigidly observed.

Adding the use of antibiotics, either prophylactically or as treatment, to these precautions has dramatically reduced the death rate, and today one woman in about 25,000 births dies of puerperal infection, instead of 1 in 10, as in

[1] René Vallery-Radot, *The Life of Pasteur.* Translated from the French by Mrs. R. L. Devonshire. Doubleday, Page & Co., Garden City, N.Y., 1923, p. 291. (Quoted in *Classical Contributions to Obstetrics and Gynecology* by Herbert Thoms, p. 191.)

much earlier days. In the year 1864, 23 percent of the patients at the Maternité, in Paris, died of puerperal infection. Among the deaths associated with childbirth, less than one fifth are now due to sepsis as compared with over one third as late as 1935.

To the nurse there is considerable significance in Pasteur's characterization of the infected mother as an "invaded patient," since the nurse's care of the patient should be enormously influential in preventing this "invasion." In this connection she may well ponder Florence Nightingale's assertion that: "The fear of dirt is the beginning of good nursing." Certainly the obstetric patient cannot be well cared for unless the nurse has this "fear" in her heart.

Puerperal infection, then, in the light of present information, is regarded as a wound infection, the placental area being invaded by pyogenic bacteria which are introduced into the reproductive tract before, during, or after delivery. This is true in cases of abortion as well as in term deliveries. The warm, dark, moist uterine cavity with its rich supply of blood and serum and a reduced amount of oxygen offers the optimum growth conditions required by most bacteria. Infection of the raw and bleeding placental site may occur at any time during labor or the 10 days following, although the danger of infection decreases steadily after the first day post partum. Puerperal infection may be due to many kinds of bacteria, either singly or in various combinations. The streptococci, staphylococci, colon bacilli, gonococci, and gas bacilli are some of the causative agents.

Infection may sometimes develop even though bacteria are not brought in from outside sources. It is then produced by organisms already present in the reproductive tract and is known as *autogenous infection.* Many bacteria are normally harbored in the vagina, living there as saprophytes and ordinarily doing no harm. With vaginal or operative deliveries or in instances where the membranes have been ruptured for a long period of time before delivery, these organisms may ascend or be carried to the uterine cavity, and an infectious process may thus originate. This autogenous infection is more likely to occur when the tissues are bruised by prolonged labor or operative delivery than when birth has been spontaneous.

Diagnosis

A diagnosis of puerperal infection is made when the patient's temperature rises to above 38°C (100.4°F) after the first postpartum day and remains elevated for over 24 hours if no other explanation can be given for the fever. Morbidity has been defined by the Joint Committee on Maternal Welfare as a temperature of 38°C (100.4°F)—if taken at least four times daily—on any two of the first 10 postpartum days, with the exception of the first 24 hours.

Symptoms

The symptoms vary greatly according to the infecting organism and according to the site and extent of the inflammation. The area of involvement may vary from a small lesion, or an infection of the perineal incision, to a generalized infection. If the streptococcus is the causative organism, the local reaction may be slight, but these bacteria sometimes pass into the lymphatic system and bloodstream, causing a septicemia.

In mild types of infection, the patient's course may be entirely normal for the first few days, after which she may complain of chilliness or have a chill. Her temperature will be elevated, ranging between 38°C (100.4°F) and 38.3°C (101°F), and it may remain elevated for a few days, after which it will drop again to normal as the patient recovers.

The severe type of puerperal infection, formerly so dreaded, is characterized by an abrupt rise of temperature, sometimes as early as the second postpartum day, reaching 39.4°C (103°F) or 40°C (104°F). The pulse is usually rapid, and chills are not uncommon. There is likely to be abdominal tenderness. Headache, malaise, deep pelvic pain, and weakness are frequent. The condition of the lochia depends on the infecting organism. In infection by some organisms the lochia may be profuse and have a foul odor.

Areas of Involvement

Infection during the puerperium occurs most often in the uterus and, if mild, is an *endometritis,* or inflammation of the uterine lining. It causes slight chills followed by fever and a rapid pulse. The uterus may be somewhat relaxed and tender. The infection may remain limited to the uterus. More severe infections, however, leave the uterus by way of the lymphatics or veins to involve progressively the parametrial tissues, the peritoneal cavity, and the entire body with the production of a generalized systemic infection.

If the uterine musculature is involved, the infection is known as a *metritis;* when it spreads through the lymphatics or bloodstream to the connective tissues around the uterus, it is termed a *parametritis,* or a *pelvic cellulitis.* Involvement of these tissues may also occur following infected cervical tears. The symptoms vary from only mild chills and fever to severe chills, high temperature, rapid pulse, and general malaise. Another manifestation of infection is a *peritonitis;* the infection spreads from the endometrium to the peritoneum, usually through the lymphatics, but sometimes by the bloodstream or by surface extension through the fallopian tubes. Included among the symptoms are pain and abdominal distention, vomiting, chills, fever, rapid pulse, and restlessness and anxiety. This infection may remain localized in the pelvic peritoneum or may spread to the entire peritoneal cavity, where the rapid absorption of toxins into the blood may have serious effects. Bacteria may gain entrance into the bloodstream through the lymphatics or veins and thus cause a *septicemia.* A *thrombophlebitis* is another form in which the infection manifests itself.

Treatment and Nursing Care

Preventive

Puerperal infection is such a serious complication that the greatest effort should be made to prevent it. The nurse's part in prevention of this complication is an important one. The need for cleanliness in giving patient care and use of aseptic technique when indicated have been stressed throughout this book. To review a few precautions, careful hand washing by all personnel each time a mother is given care is of utmost importance. Anyone with a bacterial respiratory infection or a skin lesion is not allowed to care for obstetric patients. This is also true for any person having recently cared for an infectious patient, especially one having a streptococcal infection.

Deliveries must be conducted with surgical asepsis, but precautions in the delivery room alone are not enough. Infection can be carried to the mother during labor or the early puerperium. Individual bedpans should be provided to prevent organisms that are nonvirulent for one patient from being carried to another in whom they might cause an infection.

Treatment of a vulvitis, vaginitis, or other local infection during pregnancy is a factor in the prevention of puerperal infection.

A woman who has had a long, hard labor, who has injury to the birth canal, or who has anemia due to blood loss is less able to resist infection than one who has had an easy, normal delivery. It is therefore important to keep up the woman's resistance during a long labor with adequate rest and fluids and to prevent blood loss or to replace such loss when necessary. Tears of the reproductive tract and uterine exploration add to the dangers of infection.

Although puerperal infection is easier to treat at the present time than it was in former years, prevention remains a very important factor. The ready availability of antibiotics for prophylaxis is not enough. It is still important to conscientiously employ aseptic technique in every instance. A few patients continue to die of infection in spite of much more effective treatment than formerly was available.

Curative

The treatment of puerperal infection has been revolutionized since the discovery of the antibiotics. When the offending organism is known from lochial or other cultures, the antibiotic specifically effective against it is used.

Curative treatment is also directed toward increasing the mother's resistance to infection. Increased fluid intake is of importance; often from 3000 to 4000 ml or more are provided in 24 hours. If the patient cannot take the necessary amount of fluid by mouth, intake is maintained by parenteral administration of fluid. Easily assimilable food with high-caloric and high-vitamin content is given at frequent intervals. Provision is made for adequate rest and sleep. If there is pain, adequate analgesic medication is given.

The patient is usually placed in a semisitting position, or the head of the bed is elevated to promote free drainage of lochia. Fowler's position may impede upward extension of infection from the pelvis.

The uterine muscle is maintained in a state of contraction, since this tends to prevent extension of bacteria through the uterine walls and also the absorption of toxins. Ergonovine may be given over a period of 24 to 48 hours. This also aids in expulsion of blood clots and/or pieces of membrane if these are present in the uterine cavity.

Blood transfusions are widely employed to aid in increasing the patient's resistance. They help overcome the toxic effects of the disease and the anemia that may develop. Blood transfusions given after blood loss during delivery may be a preventive measure against infection. A patient with a puerperal infection should be promptly and completely isolated, preferably in a room off the obstetric unit. The nurse who cares for this mother must not care for other obstetric patients.

Gonorrheal Infection

In a postpartum infection due to the gonococcus, some patients have moderately elevated temperature, usually not over 38.9°C (102°F), and may develop abdominal tenderness. Others remain afebrile and asymptomatic. If the infection spreads, it is usually by surface extension from an endometritis; if infection is not treated early, it is very likely to produce an inflammation of the tubes, which may result in closure of the fimbriated openings. Accordingly, it may be impossible for ova to enter the tubes subsequently. Unlike other infections, gonorrhea is not conveyed to a patient on instruments or examining fingers, but is previously present in the vulvovaginal glands. The patient is usually not very ill, and the infection is readily arrested and cured by the administration of antibiotics. When a gonorrheal infection is discovered in the antepartum period, it can be cured before delivery.

VENOUS THROMBOSIS

The overall risk for venous thrombosis or thrombophlebitis during pregnancy and the puerperium is more than five times that of non-pregnant women of comparable age and health. The risk is significantly greater during the postpartum period with antepartum occurrence being rather unusual.

There are several reasons why the puerperium is a high-risk period for venous thrombosis. First, there is a change in blood coagulability during pregnancy, which is accentuated postpartum. Increasing levels of coagulation factors are present as gestation progresses, and there is a shortening of partial thromboplastin time. Following delivery there is evidence of a very low-grade activated coagulation related to events occurring in the placenta and uterus in the third trimester and at the time of delivery.

Distensibility of the veins is greatly increased during pregnancy both by humoral and mechanical factors. Thus blood more readily pools in the lower extremities even after the pressure of the enlarged uterus is removed by delivery.

Because of the tendency toward venous stasis the coagulation factors mentioned above may concentrate in the lower limbs, whereas they would be cleared by the liver if blood flow were normal.

Although there is an increased risk for venous thrombosis post partum, it rarely occurs unless there is also present one or more predisposing factors. For this reason, one should be particularly alert for the development of this condition when one or more of the following factors exists:

History of thrombophlebitis or thrombo-
    embolism
Immobilization
Surgery (e.g., cesarean section; tubal ligation)
Toxemia
Hemorrhage, particularly if severe and shock
    has occurred
Puerperal infection
Varicose veins

Thrombosis may occur in either superficial or deep veins. The superficial type, which involves the saphenous vein, is seven times more common than deep vein involvement, which affects the iliofemoral, femoral, and popliteal veins. (Other names for iliofemoral involvement are *phlegmasia alba dolens* and *milk leg.*) Thrombosis of the uterine and pelvic veins is most often associated with puerperal infection.

Early ambulation is considered the best prevention of venous thrombosis. A woman should be assisted out of bed as soon as possible following delivery, even when she has had a cesarean section. If it is necessary for her to remain in bed for a prolonged period she should be instructed in and assisted with active and passive leg exercises. Care should be taken that she does not spend long periods of time with the head of the bed or the knee gatch elevated so that venous return will not be impeded by pressure or position.

Symptoms of thrombophlebitis include leg pain, edema, and increased skin temperature in the affected area. If a superficial vein is involved it may be so inflamed and indurated as to be palpable as a hard cord in the leg. Deep vein involvement causes rerouting of blood to the surface vessels, causing redness and warmth of the entire leg. Since bilateral disease is uncommon, it is useful in examining the woman to compare the circumferences of the legs at ankle, calf, and thigh. Edema will result in a discrepancy in size. Pain on dorsiflexion of the foot (Homan's sign) is considered highly suggestive of thrombophlebitis. Occasionally there may be a rise in systemic temperature during the acute phase of the illness.

Treatment of superficial vein disease is usually only symptomatic. Hot, moist packs are applied to relieve inflammation and reduce discomfort. The foot of the bed is elevated six to eight inches to provide the assistance of gravity to venous return, and pressure gradient elastic stockings are worn. A cradle may be used to keep the bed clothes off the foot and leg if necessary for the woman's comfort. Antiinflammatory drugs and analgesics may be ordered. While on bed rest the head of the bed should not be elevated except for brief periods during meals. The sitting position increases the angle at the hip and inhibits venous return. Occasionally anticoagulant therapy may be initiated as prophylaxis against the involvement becoming deep. This is particularly true if the disease occurs during pregnancy or if there is a history of previous thrombophlebitis and/or pulmonary embolism.

More aggressive therapy, which includes anticoagulation, is indicated when there is deep vein involvement. Heparin is given to achieve rapid anticoagulation, and the patient is then maintained on Coumadin so that her clotting time remains two to three times that of the control. When treatment is initiated prior to delivery the use of Coumadin is contraindicated, as it readily crosses the placenta and may cause hemorrhage in the fetus and neonate. Coumadin is also found in breast milk, and if it is used by nursing mothers, vitamin K supplements should be given to the infants. Most physicians recommend cessation of breast feeding in these circumstances. Anticoagulant therapy is usually continued for a month to six weeks after an episode of deep vein thrombosis.

As soon as the acute symptoms subside the patient should be encouraged in a program of progressive ambulation, since exercise increases circulation.

Pulmonary embolism is the greatest danger from venous thrombosis. The fatality rate is not accurately known because of the difficulties involved in reporting statistics. However, it is a grave medical emergency. Chest pain, even if transient, should arouse suspicion. Other symptoms include tachypnea, tachycardia, and apprehension. Auscultation of breath sounds may reveal rales and a friction rub. Diagnosis is confirmed by ECG, chest x-ray and/or lung scan. Ultrasonography may be used if this equipment is available.

Patients diagnosed to have pulmonary embolism are most appropriately cared for in a medical intensive care unit where optimum expertise is available to meet this serious emergency.

MASTITIS (INFLAMMATION OF THE BREAST)

Mastitis is caused by invasion of breast tissue by pathogenic organisms. They may be brought to the breast by the hands of the mother or her attendants or the infection may be caused by bacteria which are ordinarily present in the lactiferous ducts but do not invade the tissue until it is injured. Fissured nipples allow bacteria to enter by way of the subcutaneous lymphatics. Also, bruising of breast tissue by massage or other manipulation predisposes to infection and allows those bacteria already present in the lactiferous ducts to invade deeper tissues. Stasis of milk in a duct or overdistention of breast tissue does not in itself cause infection, but may injure the tissue and allow bacteria to enter more readily.

Various kinds of organisms may be responsible for breast infections, but the causative agent is most frequently the staphylococcus. If the baby becomes a staphylococcal carrier by acquiring this organism in the nursery, he may easily carry the infection to the mother.

A breast infection may develop at any time during lactation, but is most frequently seen between the first and fourth weeks post partum. The mother who has been feeling well suddenly develops chills and fever. Her temperature rises to 39.4°C (103°F) or 40°C (104°F) very quickly, and her pulse rate increases. One of the lobes of the breast becomes red and painful and feels hard to palpation. Formerly this infectious process progressed until the mother became chronically ill and progressively weaker and frequently developed abscesses, which sometimes had to be incised and drained. Healing was often slow and painful, and destruction of breast tissue sometimes extensive. With present-day treatment the mother almost always recovers quickly.

Treatment and Nursing Care

Preventive

Breast infections can largely be prevented by care of the breasts and nipples during the puerperium. The nurse may help to prevent this complication by cleanliness and gentleness in breast care, prevention of fissured nipples, treatment of fissures if they do occur, proper care of engorged breasts, and prompt reporting to the physician if any signs of infection develop.

Curative

Treatment generally consists of breast support, application of ice bags while the breast is indurated and painful, and administration of penicillin, or a combination of antibiotics. If treatment is instituted early, the infection usually subsides in a day or two. With the use of antibiotics the inflammation almost always resolves without abscess formation.

Controversy exists about whether or not to discontinue breast feeding when mastitis occurs. Some authorities believe that it should be stopped immediately and the breasts allowed to "dry up." The rationale for this approach is that the less stimulation there is to the breasts the more quickly the infection will disappear, and that the mastitis may recur later if nursing is continued. Others prefer to continue lactation to avoid the distention of the breasts that occurs when emptying of the breasts is suddenly stopped. In addition, if lactation is allowed to continue the infant has the benefit of continued breast feeding. Important factors in making this choice are the mother's wishes as well as her own general health and that of her infant. When lactation is to be continued, the nursing is temporarily stopped and the breast is emptied manually or by a pump. The milk is discarded during the time the mother has a fever. Breast feeding can usually be resumed in one to three days.

CYSTITIS AND PYELITIS

The slight lesions which are generally present in the bladder mucosa following delivery favor development of cystitis, especially when catheterization is necessary or when residual urine, which becomes infected easily, is present. There are always stretching and trauma of the base of the bladder during labor and delivery. This causes mucosal edema and hyperemia. There is also a temporary loss of bladder tone, due to pressure and minor injury, that makes the mother less sensitive to bladder fullness and gives her an increased bladder capacity. This may result in overdistention of the bladder, in complete inability to void, or in residual urine, thus predisposing to cystitis. The urethra is also subject to trauma during delivery with the result that voiding may be difficult or impossible. Primiparas and women who have had operative deliveries usually have more difficulty in emptying their bladder than women who previously have borne children or whose labor has terminated spontaneously.

As a preventive measure against cystitis it is important to observe the mother closely for evidence of a full bladder or residual urine. The distended bladder may sometimes be palpated above the symphysis pubis, or the uterine fundus may be felt laterally, having been pushed aside by the full bladder. Some mothers complain of discomfort and constant desire to void, some void small amounts frequently, and others have neither discomfort nor desire to void. With residual urine the mother frequently voids in small amounts, and, in a number of cases, the residual urine may be of sufficient quantity to make the bladder easily palpable. Since the bladder is less sensitive after delivery than under normal conditions, the mother may retain an undue amount of urine without discomfort.

Catheterization is deferred until the mother has been given opportunity to void spontaneously. If it does become necessary to catheterize, the procedure must be done very carefully since the chances of introducing bacteria from the vulva are great. When a mother is unable to void, some physicians recommend that an indwelling catheter be left in the bladder to avoid catheterization every few hours. Others believe that the indwelling catheter is as irritating as frequent catheterization and that the mother will regain tone more quickly if the bladder is allowed to fill. When an indwelling catheter is used, the nurse must use all possible precautions against organisms ascending up the inside of the catheter or alongside it.

Cystitis, then, is due to bladder trauma, stagnant residual urine, and bacteria that have gained entrance to the bladder. Symptoms usually begin several days post partum. These patients often have suprapubic or perineal discomfort, frequent and painful urination, or a feeling of not having emptied the bladder completely. The temperature may rise to 37.8°C (100°F) or even to 38.3°C (101°F). Microscopic examination of a catheterized specimen will show pus cells, bacteria, and often red blood cells.

Treatment consists of making certain that the bladder is emptied completely, forcing fluids, and administering drugs to cure the bacteriuria. A culture of the urine is taken to determine the causative organism, and an antibacterial drug specific for the organism is administered for a few days with excellent results.

Postpartum pyelitis may recur after a previous infection or first appear post partum. The onset of symptoms is usually about the third day post partum, but may occur as late as the twenty-first day. The most frequent complaints are pain in the flank, frequency of urination, dysuria, chills, and fever. Microscopic examination of the urine shows pus cells and bacteria, most commonly the colon bacilli. The symptoms are similar to those occurring in antepartum pyelitis but less severe.

Treatment consists of increased fluid intake, bland diet, rest in bed, and administration of an antibacterial drug. Cultures of the urine are taken every four to eight weeks posttherapy to determine that it has become free of bacteria.

SUBINVOLUTION

When the uterus does not return to its usual size and consistency as rapidly as is normal, the condition is termed subinvolution. The uterus is larger and softer than it should be for the particular postpartum period, and the lochia is more profuse and brighter red in color. This condition may be due to retention of placental fragments or a part of the fetal membranes, or it may be caused by an endometritis. Treatment consists of administration of ergonovine and antibiotics or curettage as dictated by the patient's status.

MENTAL DISTURBANCES

Psychotic complications of pregnancy and the puerperium are relatively uncommon. They most frequently occur in women who have a history of previous psychiatric episodes. It is believed that pregnancy is merely the nonspecific precipitating crisis which triggers their illness.

Neurosis, on the other hand, is a relatively frequent accompaniment to the postpartum period. Some studies have indicated that as many as 25 percent of women experience "nervous symptoms" during the postpartum year. Undoubtedly many of these symptoms are regarded merely as idiosyncratic behavior by the woman and her family and do not appreciably disrupt their living patterns.

Perhaps as many as 4 or 5 percent of women experience a reaction strong enough to require psychiatric intervention. Depression is the most common manifestation of these neuroses, although it may take the form of anxiety states, phobias, obsessions, hypochondriasis, or other symptoms.

It is speculated that neurosis develops either as a reaction to the immediate circumstances of the new infant and family responsibilities, or that childbirth has brought to the surface deep-seated conflicts regarding the woman's own femininity and general self-concept. Symptoms rarely occur before one or two weeks post partum when the mother is home and the full weight of her new responsibilities has been felt. Women who are single and/or separated from their families are more frequently affected, suggesting the enormous importance of supportive significant others.

In situations where there is a solid family structure to initiate the woman into motherhood and give support to her and the new father as well as older siblings, this transition is likely to be easier. Such structures exist in diminishing numbers, however. For most women, the practice of limiting postpartum follow-up to a pelvic examination at six weeks after delivery is a dis-service. In that period of time maladaptive behaviors can be well established.

Nurses who work with childbearing women should be alert for signs that the pregnancy or the infant is not being accepted. In addition efforts should be made to assess the available support systems for each woman and to help her identify persons or agencies to whom she can turn for help. Facilitating good mental health is as important as preventing physical complications of pregnancy and the puerperium.

BIBLIOGRAPHY

Burrow, Gerard N., and Ferris, Thomas F., *Medical Complications of Pregnancy*. Saunders, Philadelphia, Pa., 1975.

Diddle, A. W., Postpartum hemorrhage, *Hosp. Med.* 4:91–104 (Jun.) 1968.

Edwards, Margot, The crisis of fourth trimester, *Birth Family J.* 1:19–22 (Winter) 1973–74.

Greenhill, J. P., and Friedman, Emanuel A., *Biologic Principles and Modern Practice of Obstetrics*. Saunders, Philadelphia, Pa., 1974.

Kaji, Lennart, and Nilsson, Ake, Emotional and psychotic illness following childbirth, in *Modern Perspectives in Psycho-Obstetrics*, edited by John G. Howells. Brunner-Mazel, New York, 1972.

Louka, M. H., and Lewis, G. C., Jr., Obstetric and gynecologic bleeding, *Hosp. Med.* 12:44–59 (Aug.) 1976.

Pritchard, Jack A., and MacDonald, Paul C., *Williams Obstetrics*, 15th ed. Appleton-Century-Crofts, New York, 1976.

Seligman, S. J., Anaerobic therapy in sepsis after cesarean section, *N. Engl. J. Med.* 292:268 (30 Jan.) 1975.

25

High-Risk
Newborn Infants

High-risk newborns are infants who need even more intense care in the first hours after birth than that described for the normal term newborn and who will most likely need intense care for a much longer period of time. Predisposing factors that are likely to place the newborn into a high-risk category are conditions which exist within the infant at birth, such as immaturity and/or abnormal development or disease, and maternal and environmental conditions that have not permitted optimum fetal development or that make adjustment to extrauterine life difficult.

This chapter will deal with identification and care of babies who are born preterm (prematurely), infants of full-term gestation who are underweight, babies who are large for their gestational age, and infants who are born postterm. Certain illnesses and other abnormalities of newborns, which make them high risk, will be described in Chapter 26.

For a number of years birth weight was used as a measure of a newborn's gestational age. Babies weighing 2500 gm (5 lb 8 oz) or less were considered premature and those above a weight of 2500 gm as term infants. A baby with a period of gestation of less than 37 weeks was also classified premature, but the weight classification took priority for statistical purposes and for planning of public health programs. It then became increasingly evident that birth weight was not valuable for identifying gestational age. About one third of babies weighing under 2500 gm at birth are term infants, who for some reason have not grown according to a normal rate. Also some babies who weigh over 2500 gm are prematures as far as aspects of development other than weight are concerned.

In 1961 the Expert Committee on Maternal and Child Health of the World Health Organization, in recognition of the fact that a large number of babies fell within the definition of prematurity who were apparently not premature, recommended that the concept of "prematurity" in the previous definition should give way to the term "low-birth-weight." This meant that the term low birth weight was to be given to all babies, regardless of gestational age, who weighed 2500 gm or less. It also meant that the term "premature" was reserved for babies born at less than 37 weeks gestation (less than 36 completed weeks).

Accurate assessment of gestational age is necessary to distinguish true premature infants from full-term, low-birth-weight babies, and to differentiate full-sized infants born prematurely from full-sized term babies. Methods of gestational age assessment have been described in Chapter 18, pages 476–80.

In order to plan appropriate care for a newborn, it is important to classify each baby by gestational age as being preterm, term, or postterm and also by weight as being appropriate-for-gestational age (AGA), small-for-gestational age (SGA), or large-for-gestational age (LGA). Looking at Figure 25-1, which has been adapted

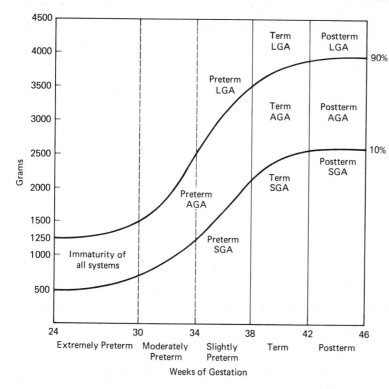

Figure 25-1. Classification of newborns by gestational age and by birth weight according to Figure 18-1, which was reproduced from Frederick C. Battaglia and Lulu O. Lubchenco, "A Practical Classification of Newborn Infants by Weight and Gestational Age," *J. Pediatr.*, 71:159–63 (Aug.) 1967. This illustration identifies the nine groups of infants discussed in the text and also identifies degrees of prematurity of preterm infants. Problems common to the different groups of infants are listed in Table 25-1.

from Figure 18-1, page 474, it is apparent that a baby may be placed into one of nine groups of infants. He may be at term and appropriate for gestational age or he may be at term and large-for-gestational age or small-for-gestational age. If the baby is preterm he will also be classified as appropriate-for-, small-for-, or large-for-gestational age. The same three classifications for size also apply to the postterm baby.

A classification according to gestational age and birth weight, therefore, identifies babies at risk. The increased risk of morbidity and the type of morbidity is suggested by the group into which the infant falls. The neonatal mortality rate for these groups can be seen in Figure 18-1, page 474. It is apparent that a baby may be small because he is preterm and in addition to that be small-for-gestational age. Such a situation would put the baby at risk for both prematurity and poor intrauterine growth. Term and postterm babies may be identified in the same way. Birth weight and gestational age are the

two parameters that can be used very effectively to identify the baby at risk. (See Figure 25-1.)

Term infants with a weight appropriate for gestational age are in the optimum range for both birth weight and gestational age. Given appropriate care, they should have the least number of problems unless they have complications of such a nature as congenital anomalies or infection. The term infant, according to both the mother's dates and the clinical estimates, who has an appropriate intrauterine growth for gestational age, who is born to a mother without complications, and who does not have intrauterine anomaly or disease is considered a *low-risk infant*. Infants who fall into any of the other eight classifications require observation for problems specific to that category (Table 25-1).

Babies who are within the limits of appropriate weight but are close to the tenth percentile or the ninetieth percentile may have some of the problems of babies in the tenth or the ninetieth percentile groups. These babies are in the

Table 25-1.   Common Problems of Several Different Groups of Infants at Risk Because of Variations in Their Gestational Ages and Birth Weights*

Preterm			Term	Postterm	All Ages
Extremely Preterm	*Moderately Preterm*	*Slightly Preterm*	*SGA*	*SGA, AGA, LGA*	*LGA*
Immaturity of all systems	Birth asphyxia Hyaline membrane disease Apneic spells Susceptible to retrolental fibroplasia Susceptible to body heat loss Feeding problems Jaundice Infection Necrotizing enterocolitis Patent ductus arteriosus	Temperature instability Slow to feed Slow to gain Prone to jaundice	Fetal distress Birth asphyxia and aspiration Meconium aspiration Hypoglycemia Cold stress Polycythemia	Postmaturity syndrome Fetal distress Birth asphyxia Meconium aspiration Hypoglycemia Cold stress Polycythemia Persistent fetal circulation	Hypoglycemia Polycythemia Trauma owing to mechanical problems at delivery RDS if preterm

*The importance of determining the proper classification of each baby at birth is apparent from the different problems that should be anticipated. It can be seen that even if a term small-for-gestational-age baby and a preterm baby were of the same birth weight they could have a list of very different management problems.

appropriate weight category, but they border on the risk category.

One fact to be noted is that the division between preterm and term classification has been variously given as 37 weeks gestation and 38 weeks gestation. The World Health Organization definition of prematurity in 1961 stated that a baby born prior to 36 completed weeks of gestation was a premature. This put the division of preterm and term at 37 weeks gestation. The American Academy of Pediatrics, Committee on Fetus and Newborn, in 1967, recommended the use of the words preterm, term, and postterm to indicate length of gestation, wishing to use terms referring to time alone rather than to imply evidence of maturity in classification. When the Colorado classification of newborn infants was devised the words preterm, term, and postterm were used, and the division between preterm and term was placed at 38 weeks. (This

is seen in Figure 18-1.) This classification differed from that of the World Health Organization for prematurity but was acceptable to the American Academy of Pediatrics, Committee on Fetus and Newborn.[1]

Several reasons were given for placing the division between preterm and term at 38 weeks. The distribution of births by gestational age is such that the peak birth rate is at 40 weeks gestation, with 80 percent of deliveries occurring between 38 and 42 weeks. Also there is evidence that seems to indicate that babies born between 37 and 38 weeks are not as healthy as term infants.[2] It is not now known if a different classification by gestational age may be necessary for other racial groups, but the present division seems satisfactory for now.

[1] Lula O. Lubchenco, The high risk infant. *Major Probl. Clin. Pediatr.* 14:2–3, 1976.
[2] *Ibid.*, pp. 2–4.

Infants who are appropriate for gestational age but are preterm or postterm will not have problems because of inappropriate weight, but they will have the special problems of immature babies and of postterm babies.

Small-for-gestational-age babies are at special high risk. They may be preterm, term, or post-term. For some reasons these babies have not developed appropriately *in utero* and they are growth-retarded. If the small-for-gestational-age baby is also preterm, the baby has the problems of both immaturity and inappropriate intra-uterine growth.

When a small baby, under 2500 gm, is born, it is very important to identify the baby correctly, because the problems of the preterm infant are not the same as those of the baby who may be small because he is growth-retarded. As for example, the preterm baby is susceptible to hyaline membrane disease because of immaturity of the lungs, whereas the SGA baby is likely to have mature lungs, especially if he is at term, but is susceptible to lung problems from birth asphyxia and aspiration pneumonia. The preterm baby may have nutritional problems because of immaturity of suck and swallow and of the gastrointestinal tract, while the SGA baby may be mature enough to take food and fluids well but have problems with hypoglycemia because of inadequate nutritional stores laid down *in utero*.

Large-for-gestational-age infants may also be term, preterm, or postterm. Frequently the LGA baby is the infant of a diabetic mother. If the baby is preterm he is predisposed to the problems of immaturity such as respiratory distress, jaundice, and bleeding, as well as the metabolic problems associated with the mother's diabetes. It is very important to the baby's care that he be recognized as a preterm infant so that his large size will not be misleading and that he will receive care appropriate to his immaturity. This kind of baby often looks big enough to be treated as a term baby unless he is identified as preterm through careful gestational age assessment.

Each category of babies has its own specific high-risk problems. Knowing how a newborn is classified helps caretakers to anticipate problems and prepare to treat them. (See Table 25-1.) Good anticipatory care helps to reduce considerably the complications of the postnatal period and also the long-term complications.

The several different classifications of infants that have been briefly described above will now be discussed in greater detail.

THE PRETERM (PREMATURE) BABY

The terms preterm and premature will be used interchangeably in this chapter. The term low-birth-weight is also often used in speaking of a preterm baby, but since a low-birth-weight classification includes both preterm and term babies under 2500 gm, it does not appear to identify the preterm baby specifically.

The preterm baby has a number of special problems because of the immaturity of his body systems, but the magnitude of these problems will depend to a considerable extent upon the degree of the baby's prematurity. Neonatal mortality rises progressively with increasing degree of immaturity.

In addition to identifying an infant as preterm, the degree of maturity must also be established. This can be done quite precisely by determining the baby's estimated weeks of gestation and using gestational age to identify the baby rather than the broad overall preterm categorization. For example, saying that "a baby is of 32 weeks gestation" gives everyone involved in the baby's care an idea of his developmental stage and a basis for beginning to plan his care.

Degrees of Prematurity

Since different degrees of prematurity present different problems, preterm babies have been divided into three groups called extremely premature, moderately premature, and borderline premature.

Both Usher and Lubchenco consider babies born at less than 30 weeks gestation as belonging into a group called *extremely premature* or *preterm*.[3, 4] These babies are at the borderline of viability and require sophisticated management to improve their chances of survival. Babies at these early gestational ages are likely to have a large number of complex interrelated problems. When at all possible babies of less than 30 weeks gestational age should be delivered in a hospital equipped to give intensive care from the moment of birth. These babies need optimum support to give them the best chance possible to survive with good physical and neurologic function and to prevent impairment of function through CNS damage. Within recent years the chances of survival for babies of 28 to 30 weeks gestation has become reasonably good; for babies of 24 to 27 weeks the outlook is improving but is still very poor.

The *moderately premature baby* is defined by Usher as one of 31 to 36 weeks gestation.[5] Lubchenco defines the *moderately preterm infant* as one born between 30 to 34 weeks.[6] These babies have a number of physiologic handicaps and require the same care as the extremely premature baby, but their chances of survival are good. There is definitely an advantage for these babies to be born in a hospital that can provide intensive care from the beginning because optimum care must be intense and early.

The *borderline premature* is defined by Usher as a baby of 37 to 38 weeks gestation.[7] Lubchenco defines the *slightly preterm infant* as one of gestational age from 34 to 38 weeks.[8]

The slightly preterm baby often looks like, and acts like, a full-term baby. These babies have characteristics of both preterm and term infants. One half of these infants weigh over 2500 gm at birth. Although these babies progress reasonably well and neonatal mortality is low, it is important to recognize them as preterm and give them the care they need for their physiologic handicaps. Slightly preterm babies may need close attention to their environmental temperature, they may be slower to feed adequately at breast or bottle, they may be slower to gain weight, and they may be more prone to jaundice than full-term infants. Borderline prematures may not need the care of an intensive care nursery, but they need special observation and care if they are cared for in a low-risk nursery.

Causes and Prevention of Preterm Birth

Adequate antepartum care, started early and continued throughout pregnancy, is an important factor in prevention of preterm births. With good antepartum care, the mother is kept in the best possible health, and abnormal conditions are detected and treated as soon as they arise. This will help bring the mother and baby to the end of pregnancy in the best possible condition.

Premature labor occurs without known cause in a fairly large number of cases. In others, such as multiple pregnancy, premature rupture of the membranes, placenta previa, and hydramnios, preventive measures against the cause are not known. Hospitalization of the mother, however, increases the infant's chance of survival, and with premature labor it may be possible to stop the labor long enough to give additional time for maturation of the baby's lungs. Delay of labor and enhancement of lung maturation are described on pages 612 and 641.

Conditions in which prevention of premature birth may be possible by early diagnosis and adequate treatment include the toxemias of pregnancy, syphilis, chronic diseases such as diabetes and cardiovascular–renal disease, incompetent cervical os, urinary tract infection, acute infectious diseases, and genital tract abnormalities. Syphilis is not the important cause of premature delivery that it was in the past because of earlier prenatal care and more effective treatment of the disease. Some premature births caused by genital tract abnormalities may

[3] Robert H. Usher, The special problems of the premature infant, in *Neonatology*, edited by Gordon B. Avery. Lippincott, Philadelphia, Pa., 1975, pp. 157–188.
[4] Lubchenco, *op. cit.*, p. 143.
[5] Usher, *op. cit.*
[6] Lubchenco, *op. cit.*, p. 145.
[7] Usher, *op. cit.*
[8] Lubchenco, *op. cit.*, p. 146.

be prevented by preconceptional examination and treatment. Certain fetal abnormalities, another factor in premature deliveries, may be prevented by advising the mother to avoid exposure to virus infections and drugs.

Premature induction of labor is sometimes necessary because of maternal complications, but it is performed as late as the mother's health and/or the fetal environment will permit in order to give the infant the longest possible intrauterine existence. In some of these cases pregnancy can be prolonged by hospitalization of the patient, which may improve the disease or slow its progress. However, recognition of the possibility of an adverse intrauterine environment for the fetus must be considered, and premature delivery may be in the best interests of the baby. Assessment of the fetal environment and fetal well-being is described on pages 610–21.

Incidence and Cause of Deaths

The incidence of premature births varies widely, ranging from 4 to 12 percent of the total births in different countries; in the United States the incidence is approximately 8 percent of all live births. Although the mortality rate of infants has decreased during the past 25 years, especially since the establishment of neonatal intensive care units, prematurity is still the leading cause of infant deaths. Most deaths of immature infants occur during the first month of life, with the first day being the most critical period. Approximately two thirds of all infant deaths in the first month of life are related to immaturity. Many deaths are caused by respiratory distress.

The mortality rate of premature infants is inversely proportional to gestational age and birth weight. Babies born prior to 28 weeks gestation have a neonatal mortality rate which may be 50 percent or more. At 31 weeks gestation the mortality rate has decreased to 8 percent, and by 36 weeks gestation it is 2 percent as compared to 0.2 percent at term. Similarly mortality is very high for the baby weighing less than 1000 gm (2 lb 4 oz) but decreases considerably for the

baby weighing 1500 gm (3 lb 5 oz) and even more for the baby weighing 2000 gm (4 lb 7 oz).[9]

Effectiveness of premature care should be gauged by a reduction of sequelae in later life as well as by decreasing neonatal mortality rates. Reduction of sequelae is much more difficult to measure, but recent reports do indicate that about 90 percent of babies who were under 1500 gm (3 lb 5 oz) at birth and survived are mentally and neurologically intact on follow-up examinations.[10]

Characteristics at Birth

Characteristics of the preterm baby will depend upon the baby's weeks of gestation at birth. They will range from a great deal of immaturity to characteristics similar in many respects to the full-term newborn. It can be anticipated when the baby is born preterm that he will have immaturity of all systems—pulmonary, cardiovascular, gastrointestinal, and renal—and that the baby will have problems with temperature control, with metabolic adjustments, and with jaundice. A number of the problems created by the baby's immaturity may be interrelated, and all require that the baby be given specialized care.

Development of the lungs and particularly of adequate production of surfactant is the major factor influencing a preterm baby's survival after birth. Without adequate and ongoing production of surfactant the baby will develop respiratory distress syndrome, a common cause of severe illness and death of the preterm baby.

Since adequate respiratory function is absolutely essential to the baby's survival, the amount of surfactant produced by the fetal lung must be checked prior to a preterm delivery whenever time permits. This should make it possible either to provide intensive care to the mother to prolong her pregnancy and allow fetal

[9] Usher, *op. cit.*

[10] G. Rawlings, A. Stewart, E. Reynolds, *et al.*, Changing prognosis for infants of very low birth weight, *Lancet*, i:516, 1971.

lung maturation, or to facilitate lung maturation through administration of steroids to the mother. When time does not permit enhancement of further lung maturation, preparation must immediately be made for intensive care of the baby after birth.

Although lung maturation is vital to extra-uterine survival, maturation of other systems is also of great importance. Unless the intrauterine environment is hostile, the longer the baby remains *in utero* the greater his chances of survival. In some babies surfactant production in the lungs is adequate relatively early, at 35 weeks or less, but other systems may not mature at the same rapid rate. A mature L/S ratio does not mean a mature baby. If lung maturation is the only consideration prior to delivery, the baby may have a number of problems of other body systems because of their immaturity. It is important, therefore, to consider overall development of the baby whenever that is possible prior to a decision for a preterm delivery.

Externally the preterm baby appears thin and scrawny. The baby's weight is usually under 2500 gm (5 lb 8 oz), the length is often under 47 cm (18½ in.), and the head circumference is frequently under 33 cm. Babies of 24 to 30 weeks gestation usually weigh between 500 and 1500 gm (1 lb 2 oz and 3 lb 5 oz). Moderately preterm infants, of 31 to 36 weeks gestational age, range in weight from 1500 gm for the smallest of these babies to over 2500 gm (5 lb 8 oz) for the largest. Babies between 37 and 38 weeks gestation weigh between 2500 and 3250 gm (5 lb 8 oz and 7 lb 3 oz).

The preterm baby's head is usually round and it is relatively large. Growth of the head is rapid in fetal life compared with growth of the rest of the body, especially in the earlier months, and the head is therefore large in relation to the body when the baby is born. There is a relatively large disproportion between the circumferences of the head and the thorax in the premature baby; that of the head usually being more than 3 cm greater than the chest circumference. The younger the baby, the greater the disproportion between head and chest size.

The preterm baby's neck and extremities are short, and his trunk is broad and long. The eyes are prominent, and the tongue is large. The ears are soft and flabby and hug the scalp. The thoracic cage is less rigid than that of the full-term infant; the abdomen is round and full, and hernias are common. The mammary glands are small, do not become engorged, and do not secrete milk. The genitalia are small.

The thin skin, through which the blood vessels can readily be seen, is delicate, loose, and wrinkled, and has prominent lanugo hair. Increased jaundice is common; it appears earlier, is more severe, and lasts longer than in the full-term infant. Fingernails and toenails are soft but, contrary to popular belief, extend to the ends of the digits. Very little subcutaneous fat is present; this is true even when the infant is born close to the full gestation period, because fat is deposited rapidly in the last month of intrauterine life (Fig. 25-2A, B). Body temperature is subnormal and may be markedly unstable.

There is a greater tendency toward respiratory distress in the preterm baby than in the full-term; this may be manifested by rapid respirations, dyspnea, attacks of cyanosis, and periods of apnea. There is a tendency to snuffles due to mucus in the nose and large adenoids, which fill the nasopharynx.

The cardiovascular system may take hours or days to adjust to extrauterine life. The baby is susceptible to hypovolemia and hypotension. Perfusion of tissues and organs may be poor.

The infant may be inactive, and his cry is often feeble, whiny, and monotonous. Gagging, swallowing, and sucking reflexes are weak or absent. The infant has a lowered tolerance of the alimentary tract with a tendency to vomiting and diarrhea; abdominal distention is more common than in the full-term baby. The stools tend to be infrequent due to hypomotility of the intestinal tract; they are sometimes loose and frequent owing to lowered food tolerance, but may be so infrequent that they dry out and become constipated. The preterm infant loses a larger amount of weight relatively than does the

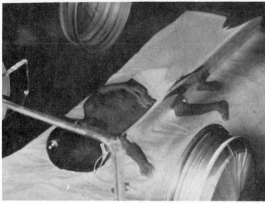

A

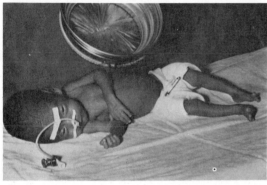

B

Figure 25-2. A. A premature infant, 23 days old, weighing 850 gm (1 lb 12 oz). Note the paucity of subcutaneous fat. (Distortions in the picture are a result of the curving glass of the incubator. It was considered unwise to open the incubator for the purpose of photography.)
    B. The same premature baby 3 weeks later. Note the large head as compared with the rest of the body. Blood vessels are visible through the thin skin of the abdomen. A polyethylene tube is in place for feedings.

full-term baby, and he does not regain it as quickly as the normal infant.

Impairment of renal function and a poor water and acid-base metabolism may cause edema or dehydration, and acidosis. A heightened capillary fragility increases the tendency to hemorrhage, and defective hematopoiesis causes anemia.

Hepatic immaturity with bilirubinemia, hypoglycemia, coagulation defects, and hypoproteinemia is common in the early days of life. Interruption of pregnancy results in curtailment of placental transmission of minerals and vitamins and immune substances and thus may be the cause of rickets, anemia, and/or infection. Congenital malformations are believed to be more common in the premature baby.

When birth occurs before organs are well developed, it is not surprising that the mortality rate is high, and it is quite apparent that the premature baby requires expert medical and nursing care from the moment of birth.

Medical and Nursing Care

The delivery room and nursery should be ready at all times for emergency care for a newborn, with equipment for resuscitation and conservation of body heat, but when a woman is known to be in premature labor, it is possible to make additional plans and thereby avoid loss of time in instituting prompt treatment.

The pediatrician and the nursery staff should be notified of the impending birth so that they can begin preparations for the baby's care. Preparation should be made to reduce to a minimum the amount of time required to get the baby into an ideal environment. Plans can be made for extra personnel in the delivery room to give special attention to the baby. This infant may need the undivided attention of a physician and a nurse in the delivery room and constant observation after he is moved into the nursery.

If facilities are not adequate to care for the baby where he is born, which may be in a small community hospital, it is important to meet the immediate needs of the baby—establish respiration and apply external heat—and then make arrangements for transfer to an institution where adequate equipment and qualified personnel are available.

Care of the preterm baby will be described under broad headings covering common problems of the various systems, instead of as a progressive day-by-day observation and plan of care. Although the baby has several simultaneous immediate (and also more long-term) needs of the respiratory system, the cardiovascular system, and other systems, as well as thermal requirements, each system will be described in its immediate and also more long-term adjustments before another system is discussed.

Respiratory System

Asphyxia at Birth

Asphyxia at birth is commonly present in preterm infants. The more preterm the baby the greater the chance of asphyxia. The immature respiratory center is the underlying cause of asphyxia, but causes of the premature delivery, such as antepartum bleeding, or complications of the delivery, such as breech presentation, may also contribute to difficulty in onset of breathing.

The principles of resuscitation, described on pages 360–67, apply to the preterm as well as the term baby. It is particularly important to anticipate impending asphyxia and to have personnel skilled in resuscitation present at a premature delivery. Trauma should be avoided by using the simplest measures first in resuscitation. Bag and mask resuscitation is often adequate to establish respirations, but endotracheal intubation may be necessary, especially with the extremely premature baby. Special care to provide adequate warmth during resuscitation is especially important for the preterm baby.

Periodic Breathing

Periodic breathing may be described as a pattern of breathing in which there are periods of apnea of 5 to 10 seconds followed by periods of ventilation of 10 to 15 seconds at a rate of 50 to 60 per minute. The overall respiratory rate is 30 to 40 per minute. With such an irregular respiratory pattern it is necessary to count the respirations for at least one full minute to obtain an overall rate and in some cases it is advisable to count for two minutes and divide by 2. There is no change in heart rate or color during the period of apnea in the periodic breathing, in contrast to the apneic episodes described below.

Periodic breathing occurs in up to 50 percent of preterm infants, depending upon the degree of immaturity. The more immature the baby the more frequent the periodic breathing. After 36 weeks gestation periodic breathing is much less frequent,[11] although it may also be present in full-term infants.

Apnea

Apnea is usually defined as a period of respiratory arrest of more than 20 seconds duration and/or an arrest accompanied by bradycardia and cyanosis. Apneic spells should be distinguished from periodic breathing. Preterm babies are especially prone to apnea. With sustained monitoring, apneic spells can be detected in almost every newborn of less than 37 weeks gestation, particularly those with birth weight of less than 1.25 kg.[12] With a conceptual age of more than 36 weeks the frequency and severity of apneic spells decreases considerably.

Apneic spells do not occur during the first day after birth, but thereafter they are likely to increase during the first postnatal week. In very immature babies the spells of apnea may occur for several weeks. Apneic spells may be accompanied by bradycardia and poor muscle tone, but not necessarily. Bradycardia and flaccidity are more likely when apnea is prolonged, but bradycardia may also occur from the beginning. Bradycardia also occurs without apnea.

Most apneic spells in preterm babies occur because of neuronal immaturity of the central respiratory control mechanisms. Apneic spells may present along with pressing or stretching such as occurs during or after feeding, particularly if the baby aspirated, during bowel movements, with lung disorders, and probably some other activities. Any adverse condition may interfere with the rhythmic breathing of the preterm baby; this includes hypoxia, hypoglycemia,

[11] Schulte, F. J., Apnea, *Clin. Perinatal.* 4:65–76 (Mar.) 1977.
[12] *Ibid.*

hyperbilirubinemia, hypocalcemia, and others. Since adverse conditions can be heralded by apneic spells, they should be ruled out when apnea first appears.

The baby susceptible to apnea must be monitored for respiratory and/or heart rates with monitors which include an apnea alarm, so that apneic spells can be terminated. The time set for the alarm must be individualized for each baby according to how soon functional changes such as cyanosis and hypotonia are noted. This time will vary for different babies. Routine monitoring of all preterm infants under 34 weeks or below 2000 gm for 10–14 days, and until no apneic episodes have occurred for several days, is advisable.

The majority of apneic spells can be successfully terminated by gentle stimulation of the baby by touching, rubbing the foot, gently stroking or patting the trunk, or just moving the baby slightly. To avoid opening the incubator frequently, the baby's mattress can sometimes be gently moved for stimulation from the outside. When resuscitative measures are necessary, use of a bag and mask with the same oxygen concentration the baby is receiving or with room air is ordinarily effective. A bag and mask should always be available in the incubator. For severe, prolonged, and repetitive apneic spells artificial respiration may be considered.

Respiratory Distress Syndrome

Premature babies are especially susceptible to respiratory distress syndrome (hyaline membrane disease). This disease occurs in babies who do not have an adequate amount of surface-active material for good postnatal pulmonary function. Surfactant may be deficient at birth because of extreme immaturity of the alveolar lining cells or because of diminished or impaired ongoing production.

Respiratory distress syndrome is most likely to develop in the extremely premature and moderately premature infants. Its incidence lessens with increasing maturity, but infants of borderline prematurity may develop the disease and should be carefully observed for signs of respiratory distress during the first 12 hours of life.

The signs and symptoms of hyaline membrane disease and its treatment are described along with other respiratory problems on pages 785–91.

Use of Oxygen

Administration of oxygen is often necessary to preterm infants because of their respiratory problems, but it requires precise control to avoid giving too much oxygen and to prevent the serious consequences of hyperoxia. Preterm infants, especially the more immature ones, are very susceptible to retinal arteriolar vasoconstriction and eye damage, resulting in partial or complete blindness (retrolental fibroplasia), if the Po_2 rises above 80 mmHg. Use of oxygen and precautions in its administration are described on pages 767–72.

Thermal Regulation

Preterm babies are very susceptible to heat loss and to the effects of cooling. A baby has a large area from which to lose heat, since he has a large surface area in relation to body mass. This is even more pronounced in the preterm baby. Also, the thermal insulation of a baby is low because of a relatively small amount of subcutaneous fat. A preterm baby has a very scant amount of subcutaneous fat and readily conducts heat from his warm inner body to his skin. The preterm baby, with his rather poor muscle tone, is also apt to assume a more flaccid and stretched-out posture than a full-term baby and thus expose much of his body surface to the environment. A preterm baby therefore becomes cooled even more quickly than a full-term infant of normal weight.

Heat production by shivering and muscular activity is difficult for the preterm baby because of his smaller muscles. These babies also have only a very small supply of glycogen, since much of this is stored during the last six weeks of intrauterine life. They may therefore suffer from lack of sufficient available glucose when need for heat production is high. Also lung function is often poor, reducing available oxygen. With a small glycogen store and deficient oxygen supply, acidosis can develop early. The potential consequences of insufficient warmth are increased morbidity and mortality.

Ways of preventing heat loss immediately after birth have been described on pages 355–56. The ways in which a baby loses body heat, the means by which he produces body heat, the effects of chilling, and the ways of preventing heat loss during daily care have also been described in detail on pages 432–40. The following discussion will highlight some of the important aspects of protection against heat loss in the preterm infant.

Since preterm babies, and also other low-birth-weight babies, must be protected against heat loss, they are cared for in an incubator until they have gained some weight and gained stability. The incubator makes it possible to regulate the environmental temperature more easily and to take care of most of the baby's needs without removing him from that environment. It also makes it possible to maintain a desired oxygen concentration, to automatically control circulation of air, and to regulate humidity as desired. The incubator serves as an isolation unit. It filters the air coming into it, protecting the baby from the nursery environment and isolating him from others in the nursery. Several types of incubators are available, one of which is shown in Figure 25-3.

It is important to note that an incubator alone does not protect the baby from radiant heat loss from his body. A warm incubator provides a warm air temperature, but does not protect against variations in the environment outside the incubator. The baby radiates heat from his body to the inside surface of the Plexiglas cover of the incubator. The temperature of the Plexiglas cover is affected not only by the incubator air temperature but also by the room temperature. Thus the temperature of the inside surface of the Plexiglas may be very different from the temperature set on the incubator thermostat, and the radiant heat exchange between the baby

and the Plexiglas may be considerably affected by the room temperature. A baby can be protected from such radiant heat loss in several ways—by some control of the temperature outside of the incubator, by a radiant heater over the roof of the incubator, by a heat shield, and by clothing.

Care can be taken that the temperature outside the incubator is not unduly cold. Incubators can be placed against inside rather than outside walls of the nursery and away from cold windows or air-conditioning vents. Likewise, it is important to watch that the incubator does not become overheated from sunlight through a window. Babies of full-term have a sweating response, but babies below 36 weeks gestation

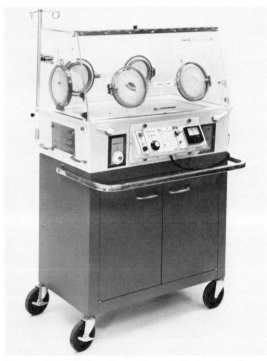

Figure 25-3. Ohio Servo-Care Isolation Incubator. The incubator is equipped with controls for regulation of environmental temperature, oxygen concentration, and relative humidity. The environmental temperature control may be used manually or with the skin thermistor, as described on page 438. [*Photograph courtesy of Ohio Medical Products (Division of Airco, Inc.), 3030 Airco Drive, Madison, Wisconsin 53707.*]

generally show a limited response and below 30 weeks gestation no sweating response. This means that overheating of the small preterm baby is even more serious than it is in a full-term infant.

A radiant heater placed over the roof of the incubator will provide the baby with heat, keeping him from dissipating his own. A radiant heater is used when the baby is first placed in the incubator, at any time when outside conditions indicate that the baby needs warmth, and when it appears that the baby cannot easily maintain his own body temperature.

A heat shield, a transparent plastic shell, which is made of Plexiglas, can be placed inside the incubator, over the baby, to conserve body heat. This second cover (the first cover is the incubator top or hood) is warmed by the incubator air, which is subject to the incubator's thermostat control, and is not influenced by the room temperature in the same way as the incubator hood or cover. The baby then radiates only to the warm inner plastic wall of the heat shield and not to the incubator walls.

Resistance to loss of body heat is considerably increased when the baby is cared for clothed rather than naked. Babies have often been cared for in incubators without clothes on because it is easier to observe their color, breathing, and activities. It has been found, however, that the range within which a baby can be expected to maintain a normal body temperature without seriously increasing either heat production or evaporative water loss is very narrow for naked babies, and this range does not readily increase as the baby becomes older.[13] A clothed baby does not dissipate heat as easily as a nude one and thus has a wider range of a neutral thermal environment. This provides a larger latitude of safe environmental temperatures, and the consequences of any change in incubator temperature are not as great. When continuous observation of the baby is not required, it is advisable to

put clothes on the baby or at least partially clothe him. Protection of the relatively large surface of a baby's head will reduce loss of body heat somewhat. Note the cap on the baby's head in Figure 25-9.

Often the small baby's incubator temperature is regulated by servo-controlled equipment, whereby the heating device is regulated according to the baby's abdominal skin temperature (page 438). Use of the servo-control device may mask the onset of a febrile state and also the baby's inability to maintain his temperature. It is very important to compare the baby's temperature and the incubator temperature frequently when evaluating the baby.

An alternative to the convection type of incubator is the open-ended radiant warmer infant care table shown in Figure 15-10, page 356. These warmers have been widely used for control of body temperature during resuscitation and other immediate care in the delivery room. Recently these radiant warmers are more commonly being used in the nursery for care of sick babies. The servo-controlled radiant warmer provides adequate thermal control, and it has the definite advantage of being open and providing easy accessibility to the infant. The unit is easy to maintain and easy to clean. Since the open warmer uses room air, it does not need a humidity reservoir, as an incubator sometimes does, which can easily become contaminated. There is some likelihood, however, of cross-contamination, and it is easier to forget hand washing while working with a baby on the radiant warmer table.

Studies have shown that there is an increase in insensible water loss in the baby being cared for on the radiant warmer.[14, 15] This could be a potential problem for a sick infant.

The American Academy of Pediatrics reports

---

[13] J. W. Scopes, Thermoregulation in the newborn, in *Neonatology*, edited by Gordon B. Avery. Philadelphia, Pa., 1975, pp. 99–109.

[14] Kamio Yashiro, Forrest H. Adams, G. C. Emmanouildes, and M. E. Michey, Preliminary studies on the thermal environment of low-birth-weight infants, *J. Pediatr.* 82:991–994 (June) 1973.

[15] Paul R. William and William Oh, Effects of radiant warmers on insensible water loss in newborn infants, *Am. J. Dis. Child.* 128:511–514 (Oct.) 1974.

that radiant heaters have in some cases posed a problem of neonatal hyperthermia. The Academy states that serious overheating can result from mechanical failure of the controls, from dislodgement of the sensor probe attached to the baby's abdomen for monitoring skin temperature and regulation of the heater accordingly, or from manual operation without careful monitoring. Radiant heaters must be used with caution and the adequacy of safety mechanisms should be carefully evaluated.[16]

Radiant warmers have been used mostly for the care of very sick infants. When the baby is improving he is usually moved to a convection-type incubator.

A preterm baby's temperature is checked on admission to the nursery and every 30 minutes until a proper balance between a normal body temperature and the warmth from the incubator has been established. Later the temperature is checked about every four hours. Frequency of checking must be determined by the baby's condition and temperature stability. When the baby is older and the temperature is well stabilized, a reading of twice daily may be adequate. Both body temperature and incubator temperature are recorded after each check. This must also be done when the skin thermistor is used.

As the baby gets older and his temperature becomes stable he is gradually changed to a normal nursery environment. His temperature, color, activity, and weight should be carefully observed during the change. The weight grid shown in Figure 25-4 may give some evidence of the baby's need for additional warmth. If he does not follow the steady upward trend in weight gain indicated on the weight grid, a cause must be sought. Sometimes the baby is using so much of his caloric intake for heat production that he does not gain weight.

The baby may need extra clothing or need to be wrapped in an extra blanket for additional warmth after he is discharged to his home,

which is perhaps not as warm as the nursery, but by that time he should be adjusted fairly well to living in a normal environment.

Meeting Fluid and Electrolyte Needs

Fluid and electrolyte needs of any infant, especially when the baby is sick and unable to meet his own needs by ordinary oral intake, is an important aspect of clinical care of the newborn. The preterm baby, who is often limited in the amount of fluid he can take orally, likely to have additional fluid losses, and often ill, is ordinarily in need of parenteral fluid therapy in the first days of life.

The total body water (TBW) is ordinarily divided into two major compartments: intracellular water (ICW) and extracellular water (ECW). Water constitutes a large portion of the body composition. With increasing gestational age the TBW gradually decreases from 94 percent at the third month of fetal life, to 80 percent at 32 weeks gestation, to 78 percent at full-term gestation. At the same time a characteristic change takes place in the proportion of ECW and ICW. The ECW decreases from 60 percent of body weight at the fifth month of fetal life to about 45 percent at term. The ICW increases from 25 percent in the fifth month of fetal life to approximately 33 percent at full-term. Then during the immediate postnatal period the ECW decreases rapidly from the 45 percent at birth to 39 percent at one week of age. This rapid change is the result of several physiologic changes, including an improvement in renal function.[17]

The electrolyte composition of the body fluid of an infant will depend upon the baby's gestational age. Per unit of body weight the preterm baby will have a larger extracellular ion content than the term baby simply because of more ECW. Conversely, the ICW electrolyte content of the preterm baby is lower because of the

[16]American Academy of Pediatrics, Hyperthermia from malfunctioning radiant heaters, *Pediatrics* 59, Part 2, *Neonatology Suppl.* 1041 (June) 1977.

[17]William Oh, Fluid and electrolyte management, in *Neonatology,* edited by Gordon B. Avery. Lippincott, Philadelphia, Pa., 1975, pp. 471–486.

smaller ICW content. These facts must be kept in mind when electrolyte losses and replacement are considered in parenteral fluid therapy.

In determining fluid loss and replacement it is important to consider factors that affect fluid loss. A considerable amount of solute-free fluid is lost from the body through the skin and the lungs as insensible water loss (IWL). Many factors influence IWL in the infant. Immaturity is a large factor. Low-birth-weight babies may have excess fluid losses because of increased water content in the skin, a thinner epidermis, and an increased skin permeability. The large body surface ratio of the preterm baby in relation to body mass, the lesser amount of subcutaneous tissue, and the large exposed body surface because of the relaxed posture all increase IWL. Inefficient vasomotor control of peripheral vessels may also permit loss. Loss of body fluids will be greater in single-walled incubators than when a heat shield is used. Ambient temperature above the neutral thermal zone, radiant warmers, and bilirubin therapy lights increase water loss. Respiratory distress probably increases loss, but high ambient relative humidity will decrease loss. Activity of the baby, as, for example, with labored breathing, and expenditure of energy in other ways will increase fluid loss.

In calculating maintenance fluid for babies, the above-described insensible water loss must be taken into account. This is especially important when the baby's total fluid intake is by parenteral route instead of being somewhat influenced by a baby's desired intake. A prediction of the water required to replace IWL from the many factors involved cannot be precise, but a range in volume required has been established in some conditions.

Renal function in relation to fluid and electrolyte balance and endocrine control are both somewhat limited, especially when given a large challenge. A baby makes a slow diuretic response to a water load during the first three days of life. After about five days the baby can achieve maximum dilution, but the ability to excrete a water load is still slow. This is even more accentuated in the preterm infant. The urine of preterm infants does not reach the concentration of that of older children upon water deprivation. The low-birth-weight baby has been shown to lose relatively large amounts of sodium. Renal water requirement cannot be exactly estimated, but it will depend upon the amount of solute excreted from the body. The amount of solute potentially to be excreted in the urine depends on the protein and electrolyte intake. Enough water to permit a urine flow of 50 to 100 ml per kg per day will not unduly stress renal concentration or dilution capacity, with a reasonable range of solute excretion.[18]

A baby's hydration status may be estimated by several parameters. Body weight should be assessed at least daily, and if the baby is ill or requiring frequent changes in therapy a record of weight may be necessary every 12 hours. Losses in excess of 10 percent of birth weight in the first three or four postnatal days are excessive.

In assessment of hydration status tissue turgor should also be noted. This is only a rough estimate because of wide variations in the amount of subcutaneous fat in different babies, but a gross degree of dehydration would be detectable. With considerable dehydration the abdominal skin becomes very loose. Edema, as an early sign of overhydration, is easily detected from tissue turgor, at least in the low-birth-weight baby. If dehydration becomes severe the baby may show a sunken fontanel, oliguria, and hypotension.

For fluid and electrolyte therapy it is necessary to estimate the amount of fluids and electrolytes lost and then to calculate fluid and electrolyte needs for daily physiologic maintenance, for replacement of past losses, and for replacement of any current abnormal losses if these are present. Careful monitoring must be done during fluid therapy and adjustments made on the results.

Calculation of fluid deficit for replacement is

[18] R. Neil Roy, and John C. Sinclair, Hydration of the low-birth-weight baby, *Clin. Perinatol.* 2:393–417 (Sept.) 1975.

made on changes in body weight if these are available. The difference in weight is considered the fluid deficit. Otherwise the percentage of fluid loss will need to be estimated from clinical signs of dehydration.

Estimates of electrolyte losses are made from measurement of serum electrolytes. Using serum sodium value as a criterion, dehydration can be classified as isotonic or isonatremic, when the serum sodium value is within the normal range of 136–143 mEq/liter, or it may be hypotonic or hyponatremic dehydration when the serum sodium value is below 130 mEq/liter, or it may be hypertonic or hypernatremic dehydration when the serum sodium value is above 150 mEq/liter. A careful clinical history of fever, diarrhea, vomiting, solute load of formula, and other ways in which fluids and electrolytes become unbalanced is also useful in estimating what kind of dehydration is present.

Calculation of Fluid and Electrolyte Needs[19]

Calculation of fluids and electrolytes for maintenance is done on the basis of insensible water loss and urinary loss. IWL and urinary loss depend upon energy expenditure, and theoretically fluid estimates for maintenance should be calculated on the basis of energy expended. In the newborn the relationships between energy expenditure and body weight are such that body weight can satisfactorily be used in calculations of fluid requirements. The IWL in the newborn has been established at an average of 30 to 35 ml per kg of body weight per 24 hours under normal, standard conditions. This fluid requirement definitely needs to be estimated upward when IWL is increased because of immaturity, high ambient temperature, radiant warmer, and other circumstances that cause excess loss of body fluids.

Water loss in the urine depends on the amount of solutes to be excreted by the kidneys. If 10 percent glucose is used for parenteral fluid and if maintenance electrolytes are added to the

[19] William Oh, *op. cit.*

parenteral fluid, it is estimated that 45 ml of water per kg of body weight per 24 hours would provide for excretion of the solute load by the kidneys without posing a problem to the kidneys in regard to their concentrating ability.

The above calculations are the basis for the recommended amount of 75 to 80 ml of fluid per kg of body weight per 24 hours for *maintenance fluid* in the newborn during the first three days of life. The recommendation of 30 to 35 ml/kg-24 hours for IWL and 45 ml/kg-24 hours for urinary water loss add up to 75 to 80 ml/kg-24 hours.

If the baby has an increased IWL because of one or several of the conditions mentioned above, fluid requirements are increased. Also when a baby is receiving oral formula feedings the solute load to the kidneys is considerably increased, and the fluid requirement is likewise proportionately increased. This accounts for the higher fluid requirement for maintenance in babies as soon as these additional factors become operative. Fluid requirements are often up to 120 to 150 ml or even as high as 200 ml per kg of body weight per 24 hours.

Electrolyte requirements for maintenance mainly involve the sodium (Na^+), potassium (K^+), and chloride (Cl^-) elements that are lost in the urine and the stool. Based on balance study data this amount is between 2 and 3 mEq per kg of body weight per 24 hours for each of the elements.

If there are concurrent fluid losses due to vomiting or diarrhea or other body fluids, the fluid is collected and measured, or estimated if necessary, and replaced in parenteral fluid. The solutes in the fluid that is lost must also be estimated and replaced.

Intravenous fluids are usually necessary in the first days of life of the preterm baby, especially in the very immature baby or one who develops respiratory distress. The baby is ordinarily not able to take an adequate amount of fluid orally in the first days of life to meet his needs nor can he meet his caloric needs. Caloric needs exist immediately after birth and nutritional stores are deficient. Glycogen stores are very low in small babies and the need for glucose is urgent. Since fasting and thirsting have adverse effects quickly in a small baby, water and calories should be provided very early. Intravenous fluids are begun within a few hours after birth.

Fluid administration on the first day is usually given in an amount that will provide the maintenance requirements for IWL and renal loss—75 to 80 ml/kg-24 hours. If the baby is below 1500 gm weight, the fluid for maintenance is higher, probably 100 to 120 ml/kg-24 hours. The fluid administered in subsequent days is usually increased in amount varying from 120 to 160 ml/kg-24 hours for large preterm babies to 150 to 200 ml/kg-24 hours for the extremely preterm. Fluid administration on subsequent days is guided by intake and output record, body weight, urine specific gravity, and serum electrolytes as described below. It does not appear that an attempt must be made to prevent entirely the normal physiologic weight loss of the first few days, but ignoring the loss would likely lead to dehydration.

Ten percent glucose is usually used for fluid administration at first. This will provide for some of the baby's glucose and caloric needs. Sodium is usually not added to the intravenous fluid until 12 or 24 hours of life, especially if sodium bicarbonate has been used or is anticipated to be needed for treatment of metabolic acidosis. Sodium chloride is added starting on the second day of age at a dose of 2 to 3 mEq/kg-24 hours. Potassium supplementation at 2 mEq/kg-24 hours is added as soon as the baby has voided unless serum K^+ is elevated.[20] KCl is not given to a baby before he has voided. If 10 percent glucose causes hyperglycemia, it will be necessary to give a lesser concentration.

The volume of parenteral fluids to be given should always be calculated as to the amount needed by the baby in a 24-hour period. It should be administered at a constant rate over the period of 24 hours so as not to stress the baby with fluctuating amounts which may result in erratic blood glucose levels and dehydration.

A constant infusion pump with a volumetric chamber is used in giving the fluids. Fluid needs are always reevaluated every 24 hours on the basis of previous monitoring results. If at some time loss of fluid occurs at an inconsistent rate, a reevaluation of need in 12 hours may be necessary.

The most common infusion site in infants is one of the superficial scalp veins. One of the peripheral veins of the dorsal aspect of either the hand or the foot or a vein in the antecubital fossa may also be used. It is difficult to immobilize the infusion needle in any site other than the scalp, and infiltration is more common. If the baby has an umbilical artery catheter in place for frequent monitoring of blood gases, the infusion may be given through the umbilical artery catheter, but usually only as long as another reason exists for use of an umbilical artery catheter.

Monitoring of the adequacy of parenteral fluid therapy must be done while parenteral fluids are being given. Monitoring includes a record of intake and output, body weight changes, urine specific gravity, serum electrolytes, blood urea nitrogen, and clinical assessment of hydration.

If the amount of fluid administered is inadequate, the urine volume will be reduced, the urinary specific gravity will be increased, and soon there will be a significant weight loss, and thereafter clinical signs of dehydration. If an excessive amount of fluid is being given, the urinary output will be large, and the specific gravity of the urine will be low. Soon fluid retention will lead to edema and weight gain. If overhydration is rapid, pulmonary edema and congestive heart failure can occur.

A good fluid balance is indicated by a stationary weight or an appropriate gain, a urinary specific gravity between 1.008 and 1.012, and no clinical evidence of edema. Weight is taken daily and sometimes twice daily. All urinary output is measured and recorded by weighing the diapers before and after they are applied. A normal range of volume of urine is between 35 and 40 ml/kg-24 hours in the first days and then increasing to between 50 and 100 ml. Urinary specific gravity is checked every 6 to 8 hours. Specific gravity of the urine is an accurate approximation of urinary solute excretion, except when there is significant glycosuria. Then a high specific gravity may reflect the presence of glucose rather than electrolytes. Daily serum electrolyte determinations will give evidence of electrolyte balance. A check of the urine for presence of glucose, and of the blood glucose by Dextrostix, will provide evidence as to how well the baby is tolerating the amount of glucose in the infusion.

Parenteral fluids are continued in the small baby until the baby is able to ingest sufficient food and fluid to meet body needs for maintenance, for replacement of losses, and finally for growth. See pages 779–81 for further discussion of parenteral fluid administration.

Feeding the Preterm Baby

Feeding the preterm baby is made difficult by the lowered tolerance of the alimentary tract; weakness or absence of sucking and swallowing reflexes; relatively high caloric requirement, but a small stomach capacity; poor gag reflexes leading to aspiration; an incompetent esophageal cardiac sphincter; tendency to vomit and to develop abdominal distention; and decreased absorption of some of the essential nutrients. As with other aspects of care, the more immature the infant is, the more difficult the feeding problem.

Meeting the nutritional needs of the low-birth-weight baby very early is important for several reasons. Caloric needs exist immediately after birth. Water is normally lost to the environment by evaporation from the skin and the respiratory passages (IWL), and by excretion in the urine. IWL in the small infant may be very great. Fat and carbohydrate stores are deficient. Glycogen stores are very low in low-birth-weight babies. Antenatal storage of substances such as minerals is low. The baby has a need to grow rapidly at this age, and malnutrition at this early neonatal period may inhibit normal central nervous system development.

Nutritional Requirements

The dietary needs of the preterm baby are those that will meet growth requirements for deposition of new tissue, and maintenance requirements to replace the daily body losses. The adequacy of growth is at present judged according to increments in weight, length, and head circumference. What constitutes optimum nutrition is not clear, but in general an attempt is made to maintain growth within or above the percentiles at birth. It is expected that, with adequate growth, the baby will have an average weight gain of 30 gm each day after the first week or 10 days of life. A weight growth chart that has proven to be very satisfactory is shown in Figure 25-4. It is apparent from this figure that the extremely preterm baby may not begin weight gain as soon after birth as the larger preterm baby.

In planning feedings for the preterm baby careful consideration must be given to gestational age as well as weight because the gastrointestinal capacity, metabolic rates, and fuel and water requirements will differ for different gestational ages. The caloric, water, electrolyte, mineral, and vitamin requirements of the preterm infant will depend on the rate of utilization and expenditure of substances, absorption of substances, excretion of substances, and body stores.

CALORIES   Caloric requirements are usually met if the baby receives 120 kcal/kg (55 kcal/lb) of body weight per day by the end of the first week of postnatal life. This recommended intake should be reached as soon as possible, but it usually takes a week to 10 days to achieve it. If the baby's metabolic rate is increased because of an environmental temperature outside the neutral thermal range, or increased muscular activity, or illness, the caloric requirements for growth increase. Caloric requirements for good growth must be found for the individual baby.

WATER   The actual clinical requirements for water vary considerably, depending upon the

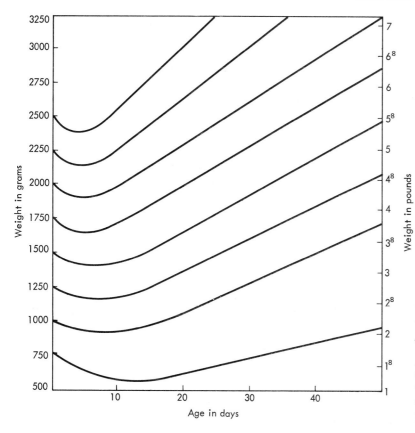

Figure 25-4. Premature weight chart. [*Reproduced with permission from Joseph Dancis, John R. O'Connell, and L. Emmett Holt: "A Grid for Recording the Weight of Premature Infants,"* J. Pediatr., *33:570–572 (Nov.) 1948, p. 571.*]

condition of the baby. Fluid requirements and how such needs are met prior to the time the baby is able to take sufficient oral fluids has been described above.

When the baby is able to fulfill his food requirements orally, he ordinarily obtains a sufficient amount of fluid in his formula.

Babies who receive between 140 and 160 ml of water per kg of body weight per day are usually in positive water balance. Some infants, however, require 180 to 200 ml per kg per day.[21] If the baby takes the necessary caloric intake of 120 kcal per kg per day from a formula that has 24 kcal per 30 ml (1 oz), the daily fluid intake will be 150 ml per kg of body weight per day, which is likely to fulfill the requirement. Some babies may be able to achieve this intake by three or four days after birth. Others, however, do not have the stomach capacity to take such a quantity of fluids orally at first and require intravenous fluids and calories for a number of days.

PROTEIN Protein requirements appear to be greater for preterm infants than the 2 to 2.5 gm/kg-day that is adequate for full-term infants. Currently 3 to 4 gm/kg-day is recommended for the preterm baby.[22] Use of most any one of the commercial formulas will meet this need if the

[21] Marshall H. Klaus, and Avroy A. Fanaroff, *Care of the High-Risk Neonate*. Saunders, Philadelphia, Pa., 1973, p. 79.

[22] Gordon B. Avery, and Anne B. Fletcher, Nutrition, in *Neonatology*, edited by Gordon B. Avery. Lippincott, Philadelphia, Pa., 1975, pp. 839–897, p. 862.

baby can take the recommended amount of fluid and calories.

MINERALS   In addition to daily requirements, the preterm baby needs a diet high in calcium and phosphorus because the perinatal storage of many substances normally occurs during the last trimester of pregnancy. The baby born before full term has a low storage of calcium and phosphorus and a considerable need for these minerals because of rapid growth.

VITAMINS   The premature infant's need for vitamins is high because of low antenatal storage and the demands made by rapid growth. Information concerning vitamin requirements of the premature is not complete, but prophylactic administration is considered important. The baby may not obtain enough vitamins in his milk, and then the daily requirement is given in the form of supplements.

Of particular importance are vitamins A, D, and C. The fat-soluble vitamins, A and D, may not be absorbed well from formula, especially when polyunsaturated vegetable fat has been used in preparation of the formula. Vitamin D is important for the absorption and use of calcium and phosphorus; it is thus very important early and in adequate amounts for preterm babies, who have a tendency to develop rickets.

Most commercially prepared formulas, usually used for feeding preterm infants, contain vitamin supplements, but the supplementation is only adequate when the baby takes about a liter of formula. Since this is quite obviously impossible for the small baby, vitamin supplementation is begun in 5 to 10 days.

Vitamins are given in a water-miscible preparation, which can be mixed with milk or water and given with the feedings. In the small, weak premature there is danger of aspiration if oil is used. Tri-Vi-Sol or Poly-Vi-Sol, 0.5 ml daily, is usually recommended in addition to the vitamins that the baby will receive from the commercial formula.

Vitamin K_1 is important in prothrombin formation and therefore in blood coagulation. It is administered at birth because the prothrombin value decreases in all infants during the first few days of life, thus increasing the blood clotting time. It is particularly valuable in prematures because of their tendency toward hemorrhage. Vitamin K_1 is administered prophylactically in a dose of 0.5 to 1.0 mg, by intramuscular injection, soon after the baby is born. One dose is usually adequate, except in special circumstances such as evidence of hemorrhage or suspicion of intracranial injury. Vitamin K_1 is administered with caution since excessive dosage may be harmful.

Vitamin E, a fat-soluble vitamin, among other properties, plays a role in hematopoiesis. An increase in the life span of red blood cells and in reticulocyte formation is correlated with the level of serum vitamin E. A deficiency in vitamin E increases red blood cell hemolysis, and a hemolytic anemia, characteristically seen in preterm babies at 6 to 10 weeks of age, has been associated with this deficiency.

Vitamin E absorption is poor in a preterm baby of less than 32 weeks gestation, and its absorption has been shown to be decreased in prematures who are also receiving iron supplementation. The iron interferes with intestinal absorption of vitamin E.

Currently, the recommendation is to give vitamin E, 25 IU daily, beginning at 34 weeks conceptual age and to continue this for at least six weeks, and to delay giving supplemental iron until the third month in infants less than 36 weeks gestation. These recommendations may change if vitamin E by injection proves effective.[23]

IRON   In anticipation of a late occurring iron deficiency anemia, the preterm baby is given iron supplementation when the baby has attained vitamin E sufficiency, at about three months of age. Iron supplementation is given at 2 mg/kg-day beginning at two months or earlier during the first year either as medicinal iron in the form of Fer-in-Sol or through supplemented

[23]*Ibid.*, p. 864.

formulas and other iron-supplemented commercially prepared baby foods.

Feeding Schedule

Feedings in preterm babies, especially the very immature, used to be withheld for 48 hours or even much longer to give the baby an opportunity to come to tolerate feedings somewhat better. With this the threat of hypoglycemia was great, the baby was starved, and lost body fluids were not replaced. How early to begin feeding the baby is no longer the serious decision it used to be because the baby is now given intravenous feedings until oral intake is adequate. Early oral feedings will, however, help the baby to begin to gain weight early.

Intravenous fluids are usually begun within the first hours after birth. Early intravenous fluids provide the baby with fluid and some calories and reduce the incidence of hypoglycemia, dehydration, and hyperbilirubinemia. An infusion of 10 percent glucose in water is usually used at first. Sodium bicarbonate may need to be added if acidosis is present. If the baby will not be able to tolerate oral feedings early other nutritional supplements will be added. See pages 733 and 779.

The first oral feeding should be withheld until the baby has made a reasonable adaptation to extrauterine life. He should be breathing normally, have good color and muscle tone, and should be warm. The first feeding is usually a very small amount of sterile water—only 1 to 2 ml for the very small baby and possibly up to 4 to 5 ml for the baby weighing 2000 gm (4 lb, 7 oz). As in full-term babies, sterile water is less injurious than glucose or milk if it is aspirated. Aspiration under any circumstances is serious, however, because of the lung irritation from the other gastric contents, including HCl. The first feeding may be given as early as three to six hours after birth, or it may be postponed for a day or even for several days. After the first water feeding, milk feedings are slowly begun.

The preterm baby's stomach capacity is very small at first. Overfeeding may lead to regurgitation or vomiting, abdominal distention, and respiratory embarrassment. Feedings are therefore given in small amounts and at frequent intervals.

The volume of the first feeding is very small, and it is kept low until the baby's tolerance can be determined. A general plan for early feedings may be somewhat as follows.[24]

For the baby weighing less than 1000 gm (2 lb 3 oz)—first feeding of 1 to 2 ml; subsequent feedings, between 12 and 72 hours, feed formula every hour, and increase 1 ml every other feeding to a maximum of 5 ml; continue a gradual increase until finally reaching a feeding of formula every 2 hours in a quantity of 10 to 15 ml.

For the baby weighing 1000 to 1500 gm (2 lb 3 oz to 3 lb 5 oz)—first feeding of 3 to 4 ml; subsequent feedings, between 12 and 72 hours, feed formula every 2 hours, and increase 1 ml every other feeding to a maximum of 10 ml; continue a gradual increase until finally reaching a feeding of formula every 2 to 3 hours in a quantity of 20 to 28 ml.

For the baby weighing 1500 to 2000 gm (3 lb 5 oz to 4 lb 7 oz)—first feeding of 4 to 5 ml; subsequent feedings, between 12 and 72 hours, feed formula every 2 to 3 hours, and increase 2 ml every other feeding to a maximum of 15 ml; continue a gradual increase until finally reaching a feeding of formula of 28 to 37 ml every 3 hours.

For the baby weighing over 2000 gm (4 lb 7 oz)—first feeding in an amount of 10 ml, subsequent feedings between 12 and 72 hours, feed formula every 3 hours, and increase 5 ml every other feeding to a maximum of 20 ml; continue a gradual increase until finally reaching a formula feeding of 37 to 50 ml every 3 to 4 hours.

With any of these feedings it is very important to go back one step, returning to the next lowest volume, any time that the baby indicates that he is not tolerating the feeding. It may be necessary to remain at the lower volume for a few feedings and then again attempt to increase the amount.

Early feedings are always exploratory, and adjustments are made according to the baby's

[24]*Ibid.*, p. 863.

demonstration of ability to tolerate volume. Increases in volume of feeding will depend on the baby's ability to tolerate the amount offered. The nurse must observe the baby very closely during feedings for evidence of sufficiency. The small baby cannot indicate when he has had enough through refusal of food. Signs of distress such as difficulty in breathing, attacks of cyanosis, regurgitation or vomiting, and abdominal distention must also be closely observed and reported. "Spitting up" of feedings in unacceptable and may be harmful in a small baby in whom danger of aspiration is great. When this happens the volume of formula must be reduced. The nurse must use her judgment in discontinuing a feeding before the entire amount is given or in omitting a feeding entirely if the baby has any signs of distress. Subsequent feedings are rescheduled after the physician has evaluated the infant's condition.

Intravenous fluids are given to fulfill fluid requirements of 150 to 200 ml/kg of body weight until the baby is taking an adequate amount of fluid orally. For a small baby this may be for a considerable period of time. The final feeding schedule for the baby should provide an intake of 150 ml/kg of body weight of a formula with a caloric density of 24 or possibly 27 kcal/30 ml (1 oz).[25]

The feeding interval for a preterm baby is usually every two or three hours and for the very small baby even every hour. The interval is determined by the amount of food that the baby is able to take at one time in relation to his total needs for the 24-hour period; the interval is usually shorter for the small baby than for the larger infant and is lengthened as the baby matures. For example, a baby below 1350 gm (3 lb) may be started on a two-hour schedule and changed to a three-hour schedule when he weighs more than 1350 gm (3 lb).

Kind of Food

Commercially prepared formulas are generally used to feed preterm infants beginning with a formula with a concentration of 20 kcal/30 ml (1 oz) and later increasing to a formula that has 24 or 27 kcal/30 ml (1 oz). The formulas with a 24 and 27 kcal/30 ml (1 oz) concentration are generally made up for low-birth-weight babies and will ordinarily fit well into an acceptable caloric distribution for these infants. Some of these formulas will have a higher protein concentration than others and therefore a higher solute load and ash content, but they appear to be within the renal concentration ability of the preterm baby. Some of the formulas have a lactalbumin to casein ratio similar to breast milk (60:40) and, because of added demineralized whey, have a lower solute content. Calcium and phosphorus ratios are also closer to the 2:1 ratio present in breast milk.

When the preterm baby is able to tolerate oral feedings well, it is possible to provide him with both adequate calories and adequate fluid through the use of formulas that provide 24 kcal/30 ml.

While formulas that closely resemble breast milk are called humanized milk they do not supply some of the factors found in breast milk that may be very important to the preterm baby. The immune globulins and the macrophages of colostrum and early breast milk either make or confer a certain amount of immunity to viral and bacterial infections. Either these immune substances or some special factor in human milk such as a low osmolality may protect the baby from developing necrotizing enterocolitis, a serious complication of the small preterm baby. (See page 740.) It may be that the protein quantity and quality, fat quantity and quality, immune substances, and low osmolality make human milk particularly suitable for the preterm baby.[26]

Although commercially prepared "humanized" formulas are commonly used to feed preterm infants, some physicians prefer to feed breast milk, at least to selected infants and for the early feedings, for the factors named above

[25] *Ibid.*

[26] Lewis A. Barness, Nutrition for the low birth weight infant, *Clin. Perinatol.* 2:345–352, 1975.

and for its easy digestibility and ready tolerance. If breast milk is available, it may be used for the early feedings. Formula may then be used for later feedings because of the adjustments that can be made in its protein content, in other nutrients, and in calories, up to 24 or 27 kcal/30 ml (1 oz).

To supply breast milk for early feedings, and for psychologic reasons if the mother wishes to nurse her baby, her lactation may be established and maintained by artificial emptying of the breasts until the baby is able to nurse at the breast.

Methods of Feeding

Preterm babies are fed by intermittent gavage feeding, indwelling nasogastric tube, indwelling nasojejunal tube, intravenous, medicine dropper, or bottle, depending on their size and vitality, ability to suck, and tendency to respiratory distress. The safe way to feed a small premature is to start with an indwelling tube feeding or intermittent gavage, and when it is ascertained that the baby can suck well, make a change to medicine dropper or bottle feeding. A small baby may need tube feedings for a long period of time, this method being continued until he shows signs of sucking ability.

A fetus at the age of 24 weeks can swallow amniotic fluid quite well, and a preterm baby who has reached the age of 30 weeks can both suck and swallow. However, a preterm baby between 30 and 35 weeks frequently cannot fully integrate his swallowing mechanism with his sucking, and he may aspirate his feeding. (Actually such difficulty may arise with the full-term newborn.) Also, between 30 and 35 weeks gestational age the baby has an increased tendency to vomit, and his mechanism for preventing gastric reflux remains immature. Anatomic capacity of the stomach is small, and emptying time of the stomach is slow.

Coordination between sucking and swallowing, and closing and opening of the epiglottis, develops at about 32 to 34 weeks gestation. Prior to 32 weeks gestation a baby should be fed by nasogastric or orogastric tube, at least in the beginning.

Between 32 and 36 weeks gestational age, when offered a nipple, the baby may appear to suck well, but be unable to swallow well, or consistently, or in coordination with his respiration. The nurse must be watchful for such difficulty and proceed with feedings with caution.

The gag reflex of an infant is not complete prior to 32 weeks gestation. Even if sucking is normal the gag reflex may still be immature. This is another reason for tube feeding prior to 32 weeks.

Immature babies have an immature suck pattern for a period of time. After the first day or two of a transient immature suck pattern, mature babies have frequent prolonged periods of sucking bursts, with 10 to 20 sucks in each burst, and they often swallow during a sucking burst. The immature baby has instead short sucking bursts of 3 to 5 sucks, and he swallows preceding or following the sucking bursts.[27] Development of sucking depends upon birth weight and degree of maturity, but an immature suck pattern may persist for some time. With such sucking the baby does not take large amounts of food in a short period of time. It is believed that this may be a developmental protective mechanism which prevents overloading of an esophagus not yet ready to transmit a large bolus. Suck and swallow improve with practice. Sucking is slowed by a stiff nipple, and sucking is not as effective with water or glucose as it is with milk.

In preparation for feeding and to avoid undue exposure, the baby at first is left in the incubator for his feedings, but the upper part of his body is raised and supported in a semiupright position while he is fed. This position is maintained by elevating the head of the incubator mattress, if it is adjustable, to approximately a 30-degree angle or by support to the baby's head and shoulders with the nurse's hand. When the baby is able to maintain his tempera-

[27]Joyce Gryboski, Gastrointestinal problems in the infant, *Major Probl. Clin. Pediatr.* 13:17–23, 1975.

ture, he is wrapped in an extra blanket and held during his feedings.

INTERMITTENT GAVAGE FEEDING A gavage feeding is given through a catheter passed through the mouth, into the esophagus, to just above the cardiac end of the stomach. Formula is poured through a glass barrel of a syringe attached to the catheter.

The size of the catheter is somewhat determined by the size of the infant. For the very small baby a no. 8 French catheter is best, while for the baby weighing approximately 1500 gm (3⅓ lb) a no. 10 catheter is more satisfactory. The distance to which the catheter should be passed is also determined by the size of the infant; each baby should, therefore, have an individually measured catheter. The distance from the bridge of the baby's nose to the tip of the ensiform cartilage of the sternum is measured, and the catheter is marked at this point with a narrow strip of adhesive tape (Fig. 25-5). Two more marks may be made 2 and 4 cm above the first one for further guidance in passing the catheter, or catheters may be used that already have suitable marks on them for guides.

To prepare for the feeding, the catheter, previously measured, the sterile syringe, and warmed breast milk or formula are conveniently arranged. The baby is prepared for his feeding by changing his diaper so that he will be comfortable, and, to avoid handling after feeding, his temperature is taken if it is due to be checked. If the baby has gastric distention, he may be supported in a sitting position for a moment, and an attempt may be made to raise an air bubble. He is then placed on his back on a flat surface with his head in a straight line and on a level with his body, and the catheter is passed through the mouth into the esophagus until the first mark is even with the baby's lips (Fig. 25-5). The catheter is usually passed without difficulty because it is almost impossible for it to enter the larynx, and there is little or no gagging or retching, owing to weakness or absence of reflexes. If the catheter does not enter the esophagus, it will turn on itself and come

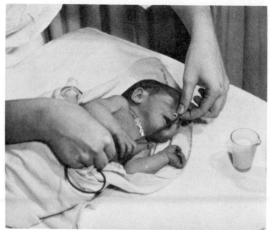

A

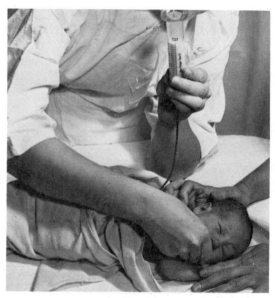

B

Figure 25-5. A. Measuring the distance from the bridge of the nose to the tip of the ensiform cartilage, to determine the exact length of gavage tube to be inserted. The tube is marked at this time.

B. The tube, with the mark at the infant's lips, is held between the nurse's thumb and forefinger while her other fingers are in firm contact with the infant's chin. This assures the nurse that the tube will remain in the same position in the esophagus throughout the feeding. If the infant is active, it is advisable for a second person to hold his hands and head.

out of the mouth. A lubricant should not be used on the catheter because oil may drop into the pharynx.

Occasionally, bradycardia appears with passage of the feeding tube, often immediately on introduction of the tube, owing to a vagal response. If a baby shows a sensitivity to passage of a tube, an indwelling catheter may present less problems.

When the catheter is passed to the first mark,

Oral Catheter Insertion Procedure

1. Restrain infant in dorsal recumbent position with head hyperextended.

2. Select catheter of proper size (premature infants #8, term infants #8-10); check for patency, smoothness of tip.

3. Estimate distance from mouth to stomach by marking on catheter the distance from the bridge of the nose to the xiphoid process.

4. Moisten end of catheter in a medicine glass of sterile water.

5. Insert catheter. Open mouth with one hand and with the other hand gently push catheter over the tongue, down the esophagus and into the stomach.

6. If a whistling sound is heard, or if coughing, aphonia or cyanosis occurs during insertion, the tubing probably has entered the trachea and should be removed immediately and reinserted.

7. Check for correct placement of catheter.

 - Invert free end of catheter into medicine glass of sterile water. If initial flow of air bubbles ceases, the catheter is in the stomach; if they are present with each respiration, the catheter is in the trachea. If no bubbles are observed, tubing may be plugged with mucus and should be removed and another catheter inserted.

 - Aspirate for gastric contents using gentle suction to prevent trauma to the tissues.

 - Place a stethoscope over the left upper quadrant of the abdomen. Quickly inject 1 to 2 cc of air into the catheter and listen for sound of air entering stomach.

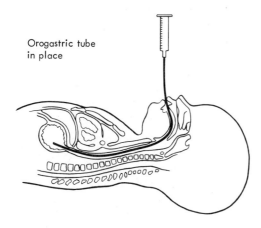

Orogastric tube in place

Figure 25-6. Intermittent infant gavage feeding; orogastric tube in place. [*Reproduced with permission from Ross Inservice Aid No. 6, Ross Laboratories, Columbus, Ohio, 1963.*]

it is just above the cardiac opening of the stomach and is in the best position for the feeding. At this distance it does not stimulate the reflex at the cardiac opening and does not irritate the gastric mucosa. If gastric distention is present which could not be relieved by bubbling the baby before the catheter was passed, it becomes necessary to insert the catheter to the second or third mark so that it enters the stomach and allows the gas to escape. As soon as the stomach is entered, the gas can be heard coming through the tube. When indicated, the stomach contents may be aspirated at this time and then returned to the stomach. The catheter may be left in the stomach for the feeding or may be pulled out to the first mark on the tube so that its eye again rests in the esophagus (Fig. 25-6).

After the catheter has been inserted, the nurse waits a few moments to assure herself that it is not causing the baby distress. Then an accurately measured amount of the feeding is poured into the glass barrel of the syringe, which has been attached to the catheter, and the barrel is elevated to a level at which the formula will flow freely, but not rapidly. The time required for all of the feeding to be given is ordinarily the same as that required for a similar amount by bottle. The tube must be held in place throughout the feeding to ensure that it is not pulled out of its position in the esophagus, which would permit milk to spill into the mouth or pharynx (Fig. 25-5B).

Proper withdrawal of the catheter is important. The tube must be pinched firmly, or bent upon itself, preferably in two places, to prevent milk from dripping into the pharynx, and it is then withdrawn slowly and gently. The baby usually gasps as the tube is withdrawn, especially if it is done quickly, and he may aspirate food that is present in the pharynx.

The baby may be held in a sitting position or picked up immediately after the feeding and held up for a moment to raise air that may be present in the stomach, but the nurse must be careful not to flex his body in a manner that puts pressure on his stomach. It is not customary to bubble all premature babies after gavage, be-cause they get very little air into the stomach with a tube feeding, and bubbling necessitates extra handling, but if the baby has been sucking on the tube or if he has a tendency to regurgitate, it may become necessary to pick him up. Elevating the head of the mattress for approximately 30 minutes following feeding allows for the escape of an air bubble. The baby is gently positioned after feedings, preferably on the right side or the abdomen, since the stomach empties more rapidly in the prone or right lateral positions. For a change in position the baby may be placed on his left side midway between feedings.

INDWELLING NASOGASTRIC TUBE FEEDING An indwelling nasogastric tube feeding is a gavage feeding in which a tube is passed through the nostril into the stomach and left in place from one feeding to another (Fig. 25-7). This method is often preferable to introducing a tube into the esophagus for each feeding, since the very small baby can be fed frequently without the trauma and fatigue that may accompany frequent insertion of a gastric tube. With this method nurses are relieved of the responsibility of inserting a tube each time a feeding is done. Complications that may be encountered with an indwelling tube are a purulent rhinitis due to irritation from the tube and possibly some irritation of the esophagus or gastric mucosa.

A sterile polyvinyl tube, no. 5 French, 38 cm (15 in.) long, is used in most instances. The gastric end of the tube is closed and smooth, with openings along the side near its end; thus, the problem of irritation from the tip is not great. The proximal end of the tube attaches to a syringe; it may also be fitted with a stopper to use in closing the tube between feedings. Before the tube is inserted, it is measured and marked with a small piece of adhesive tape at the approximate distance at which it will enter the stomach. Measurement for the adhesive marker is the distance from the xiphoid process to the tip of the ear lobe and from there to the nostril.

A knowledgeable nurse may insert the tube, passing it through the nostril as far as the

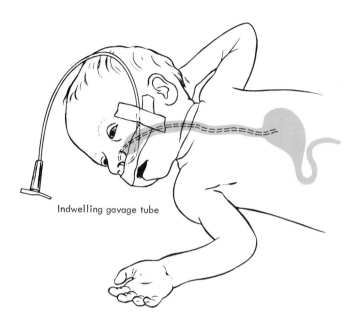

Indwelling gavage tube

Figure 25-7. Indwelling gavage tube. [*Reproduced with permission from Ross Clinical Aid No. 5, Ross Laboratories, Columbus, Ohio, 1960.*]

marker. To make certain that the catheter has not entered the trachea, a stethoscope may be placed over the region of the stomach while a small amount of air is injected into the tube with a syringe; this air can be heard to bubble in the stomach. If the tube enters the trachea, the baby is apt to show signs of respiratory distress. The tube is secured to the baby's face with adhesive tape; it is necessary to secure it quite firmly since the baby may hook his fingers around the tube and pull it out. If the skin of the face shows signs of irritation from the adhesive tape, it may be protected with a prior application of tincture of benzoin.

The baby is positioned on his right side before each feeding is begun, and the head of the mattress, if it is adjustable, is elevated to approximately a 30-degree angle. The nurse then injects 1 cc of air into the tube and at the same time listens with a stethoscope for air entering the stomach, usually recognized by a growling sound. This gives assurance that the tube is still in the stomach. Next the air and any remaining food and fluids are aspirated to determine stomach emptying. This food and fluid is returned to the stomach and its amount deducted from the total feeding to be given to avoid overfeeding

the baby. The feeding is then poured into a syringe barrel and allowed to flow into the stomach slowly by gravity, at about the rate the formula would be taken from a bottle. The infant must be watched carefully for signs of distress and the feeding discontinued if these become evident.

After the total prescribed or tolerated feeding has been introduced, 1 to 2 ml of sterile water are injected to clear the tube of milk. Then a stopper is placed into the end of the tube until the next feeding. The tube should be opened for a few minutes before each feeding is given to allow for escape of air that may be present in the stomach. This may be done by removing the stopper before preparation for the feeding is made.

The nasogastric tube is changed every three to five days, with the new tube being introduced into the opposite nostril. The baby may be given a rest without a tube for two to three hours if it is removed immediately after one feeding and reinserted just before the next.

Nasogastric feedings may also be given by a constant rather than an intermittent method through the use of a slow continuous gravity drip of the formula into the stomach or the use of an infusion pump. Residual gastric contents will need to be checked by aspiration, perhaps even every hour at first and then gradually lengthening the time interval to 2 to 3 hours and finally to 3 to 6 times daily. The formula supply and the syringe will need to be changed frequently, every 4 to 6 hours, so that it will not become contaminated with growing bacteria.

NASOJEJUNAL (TRANSPYLORIC) FEEDING With nasojejunal (NJ) feedings the baby is fed through a silicone or polyvinyl tube which has been passed through the nostril until its tip reaches the distal duodenum or the jejunum. The tube is passed through the baby's nostril into the stomach allowing for adequate length of tubing to pass through the pylorus into the duodenum. This may take a period of time. Placing the baby on the right side may facilitate passage of the tube. Fluid is aspirated through the tube and checked for pH frequently. When the pH of this fluid is found to be somewhere between 5 to 7, abdominal x-rays are taken to check on the position of the catheter tip. In most instances the tube will pass into the distal duodenum or the jejunum with time.

When the NJ tube is in the proper position, feedings are begun, usually with 5 percent glucose at first and then formula in gradually increasing amounts until the baby is receiving adequate daily fluid and caloric requirements in this manner. The feeding may be given in 10 to 15 ml amounts every 2 hours by slow drip, or a continuous infusion pump may be used. Care must be taken not to overload the jejunum with fluid at any one time. Initially the tube may be aspirated every hour to confirm placement and adequacy of gastrointestinal motility. A nasogastric tube may be placed to check on gastric residual and for regurgitation of food through the pylorus. The tubes are washed with 1 to 2 ml of water after a feeding is finished. As with continuous nasogastric feeding, when the continuous method of feeding is used, a fresh formula and fresh syringe must be used every four to six hours.

Nasojejunal feedings have their greatest ad-

vantage in use for babies who have gastric limitations that do not permit an adequate quantity of feedings. They minimize the risk of regurgitation and aspiration because there is ordinarily no gastric pooling. NJ feedings have been used for very sick infants, babies on respirators, preterm babies with apnea requiring ventilation, and other small preterm infants. The NJ tube may be left in place for several weeks if necessary.

Reports about transpyloric feedings have been both favorable and cautionary. Weight gain of the babies fed by this method has been good. Complications have been encountered with use of NJ tubes. Duodenal perforation has been reported. It has been suggested that this is the result of the use of polyvinyl catheters, which harden after they have been in place for a short time. Silicone catheters, which remain soft, are thought to have a definite advantage. It has also been suggested that a relationship may exist between NJ feedings and necrotizing enterocolitis and that there may be possible problems with changing intestinal flora. Rhea *et al.* advise that problems can be decreased by avoiding the use of overly hyperosmolar formula and by the use of open-ended silicone rubber tubing instead of polyvinyl chloride or polyethylene tubes.[28]

Recent studies that have compared nasojejunal feedings with intermittent or continuous nasogastric feedings in small babies have shown that larger volumes of fluid and more calories can be supplied with the transpyloric feedings, resulting in a more rapid return to birth weight. No significant complications were reported.[29, 30] It was concluded from these studies that the nasojejunal method of feeding low-birth-weight infants was safe and effective and was most advantageous in the first two weeks of life. This

[28] James W. Rhea *et al.*, Nasojejunal (transpyloric) feeding; A commentary, *J. Pediatr.* 86:451–452 (March) 1975.
[29] Micheline Van Caillie and Geraldine K. Powell, Nasoduodenal versus nasogastric feeding in the very low birth weight infant, *Pediatrics* 56:1065–1072 (Dec.) 1975.
[30] David H. Wells, and Richard E. Zachman, Nasojejunal feedings in low-birth-weight infants, *J. Pediatr.* 87:276–279 (Aug.) 1975.

method is likely to be used when other methods of oral feedings prove somewhat unsatisfactory.

Intravenous Supplementation of Oral Feedings

When a baby tolerates oral feedings but is not able to take a sufficient amount of nutrients in this manner, the feedings are likely to be supplemented with intravenous infusion. This involves giving an infusion of a supplementary nutrient mixture while at the same time feeding the baby by one of the gavage methods or by nipple.

Glucose, 10 percent, has long been used for supplementation of oral feedings and appears to be adequate when the baby will be able to take food relatively early. More recently glucose and amino acid mixtures or mixtures of glucose, amino acids, and lipid have been used when caloric intake via the gastrointestinal tract is unsatisfactory for a number of days.

One of the superficial scalp veins is commonly used for intravenous infusion in the newborn. A peripheral vein on the dorsal aspect of either the hand or the foot or an antecubital vein may be used. Infusion may also be done by umbilical artery catheter if there are also indications for frequent monitoring of arterial blood gases, but as soon as that indication is past another route is used for infusion because of the risks of umbilical artery catheterization, which include infection, phlebitis, and thrombosis.

Peripheral intravenous infusions require close observation for infiltration, which will quickly cause necrosis of tissue because of the hypertonicity of the solution used for intravenous feeding. Observation for thrombophlebitis and for infection is also important. Maintenance of the intravenous infusion over a period of time may become difficult.

Hyperglycemia may become a problem with intravenous glucose administration, especially in the very small baby who has a poor carbohydrate tolerance. Severe hyperglycemia could lead to cerebral dehydration and excess water loss because of osmotic diuresis. Glucose infusions for very small babies are therefore calculated in terms of milligram per kilogram per minute, or gram per kilogram per hour. Carbohydrate tolerance in these small babies appears to be no more than 6 gm/kg-day in the first day, rising to 10 to 12 gm/kg-day by the end of the first week. Blood and urine glucose determinations must be done two or three times daily until glucose tolerance limits are established. The glucose load will need to be determined accordingly.

Azotemia may develop if the intravenous solution provides excessive nitrogen intake. Careful check of each voiding for volume, specific gravity, glucose, and protein is valuable in monitoring of the baby. A daily weight record is important.

An advantage of intravenous supplementation is that these babies can be fed small volumes orally until their stomachs can accept an adequate amount of food. The danger of aspiration is thus decreased. Weight gain of babies receiving a mixture of nutrients intravenously has been reported to be good.

DROPPER FEEDING   A specially prepared medicine dropper is occasionally used to feed the premature. To prevent injury to the mouth, a ¾-in. piece of rubber tubing is firmly attached to the end of a dropper so that it extends ¼ in. beyond the glass tip.

The baby is supported in a semiupright position in the incubator or held as for a bottle feeding; the method will depend on the importance of continuous incubator care. The milk for the feeding is put into a medicine glass and the dropper is filled intermittently. The tip of the dropper is placed well back on the infant's tongue each time. As the milk is released, it should be directed toward the side of the mouth, and pressure should be exerted on the back of the tongue with the dropper tip to stimulate swallowing. If used too early, this method is dangerous because it may deliver fluid to the back of the baby's mouth that he is unable to swallow. The mouth must be inspected after each dropperful of milk is given to make certain that the milk has been swallowed. Bubbling during and after feeding is important. The head of the mattress is elevated for approximately 30 minutes following each feeding.

The medicine-dropper technique is frequently unsatisfactory; by the time it can be employed safely the quantity of feeding may be so large that it is a slow and tiring method.

BOTTLE FEEDING A small, soft nipple is used for bottle feedings. The nipple holes should be of such size that the milk drops slowly when the bottle is inverted, or a nipple with a crucial incision (cross-cut) may be used.

The baby should be held in the nurse's arm during feeding if he is permitted to be out of the incubator or supported in a semiupright position if he must be fed in the incubator. The bottle must never be propped. The baby will usually open his mouth when the nipple is touched to his lips. If his tongue is elevated against the roof of his mouth, the nipple may be pressed against his cheek and gently manipulated until he brings his tongue down so that the nipple can be placed above it. The baby may then "mouth" the nipple for awhile before he starts sucking. The nurse should stop the flow of milk frequently to coordinate with the baby's attempts to swallow. The baby should be allowed to rest at intervals during feeding, and sufficient time must be taken to bubble him both during and after the feeding. Elevation of the head of the mattress for approximately 30 minutes after feedings may prevent regurgitation of milk, and positioning on the right side is advisable.

During the first bottle feedings the infant may tire before the total feeding is taken. It is not wise to finish the feeding by gavage at this time because the baby may regurgitate as the tube is inserted. The feeding is halted when fatigue is observed, and the next feeding is given by gavage. The total duration of a bottle feeding should not be more than 20 to 30 minutes. Substitution of a bottle for an occasional gavage feeding is resumed after several feedings because the baby's strength improves daily, and his ability to suck well will be strengthened by practice.

With all feedings the baby may need to be bubbled midway in the feeding and again at the end of the feeding. Bubbling may not be necessary when the very weak baby who does not suck is fed by tube, but should always be done at the end of a feeding as soon as he begins to suck on the tube, at which time he will swallow air. The baby who may not be removed from the incubator for feedings is bubbled by being held in a sitting position, supported with the nurse's hands.

To prevent regurgitation, and possibly aspiration, of milk following a feeding the nurse must handle the baby very gently. It is advisable to place the baby on the right side or the abdomen after feedings, since the stomach empties more rapidly in the prone and right lateral positions than in the supine and left lateral positions.[31] This would be especially important for babies who have delayed gastric emptying time or who have difficulty in tolerating the volume of feeding that they require. A rolled towel tucked firmly behind the baby's back will provide support for the lateral position.

If the baby is placed on his right side after each feeding, he should be turned to the left side midway between feeding times to ensure adequate change of position. If the head end of the mattress has been raised, it is advisable to allow it to remain elevated at approximately a 30-degree angle for 30 minutes after feedings, as a further safeguard against regurgitation.

Further Suggestions

The baby must be carefully watched for regurgitation during the first one-half hour or so after each feeding, and the breathing pattern must be closely observed after feedings. Periodic breathing, or apnea, are likely to occur in small babies in about 15 minutes after feedings.

When formula is fed by continuous gravity drip or by infusion pump, great care must be taken to assure that fresh formula and a completely new unit is replaced frequently. As with milk, when formula becomes warm and ex-

[31] Victor H. Yu, Effect of body position on gastric emptying in the neonate, *Arch. Dis. Child.* 50:500–504, 1975.

posed, it will quickly begin to grow bacteria, and it is likely to cause gastrointestinal problems.

A small baby who must be fed by tube should be offered a pacifier or a nipple to suck on as soon as he will and can make the effort. This may be offered during feedings and also between feedings. This will provide the baby with the pleasure and satisfaction of sucking, and it will strengthen his sucking ability.

Feeding should be an enjoyable experience. Even the tube-fed baby can be given some attention that may be satisfying during his feeding if he is talked to, patted, given an opportunity to suck, and rocked if that is permissible.

Parents should be given the opportunity to become involved in their baby's feedings as soon as the baby's condition permits and the parents feel able.

Protection Against Exertion

The preterm baby needs rest and protection from exertion during the first hours after birth and probably longer if he is stressed by illness. Certain procedures must be done early, such as placing monitor leads and temperature probe and starting intravenous fluids, but if there is any care that can be postponed rest will be very helpful to the baby. The baby needs much of his energy to adjust and adapt to his changed environment.

The baby's energy can also be conserved by helping him to maintain his respirations, his body temperature, and his fluid and electrolyte needs without stress. This care has been described, but as an example the reader is reminded of the great deal of energy a baby must use to maintain his body temperature if he becomes chilled.

In ongoing daily care the nurse should organize and plan the baby's care in a way that will reduce undue handling and stimulation and provide for periods of rest. The baby must be protected against becoming tired from too much activity at any one time. Careful observation of the baby's tolerance, and spacing of nursing care

and procedures, can provide for appropriate periods of rest and activity. Care must also be taken that the baby is protected against unnecessary lights and noise and other stimulation that may waste energy.

The Baby's Parents

The preterm baby's parents will be gravely concerned over their small baby. If parents saw their baby briefly at birth, he most likely appeared very tiny and fragile. If, unfortunately, they did not see the baby before he was rushed to the nursery, it is hard to know how they imagine that he looks. When parents see the baby in the nursery, often at first from a distance, he is in an incubator, usually surrounded by physicians and nurses, and often by machines and equipment.

Parents need physician and nurse support to help them understand their baby's illness, all the mechanical equipment, and the care he is receiving, and they need a realistic explanation of his prognosis. Parents have a need to talk with their baby's caretakers frequently, and the caretakers should ask how they can help the parents. Parents should be invited and encouraged to go into the nursery to see their baby as soon as possible. They should be encouraged to see, touch, visit, and finally to care for their baby. They need a great deal of ongoing support, explanation of what is happening, and encouragement to have physical contact with their baby frequently. The parents need to be involved in the baby's care as soon as they feel able, and they should quickly be regarded as a part of the care team rather than visitors.

The first visit to a nursery intensive care unit can be overwhelming and parents need preparation for it. Often their baby has at the least an intravenous infusion running, wires attached for monitoring, an oxygen hood or some other means for administration of oxygen, a radiant warmer or a heat shield, and possibly a feeding tube in place. Other machines and tubes may be attached to the baby. (See Figure 25-8.) In addition to the previous preparation, the person

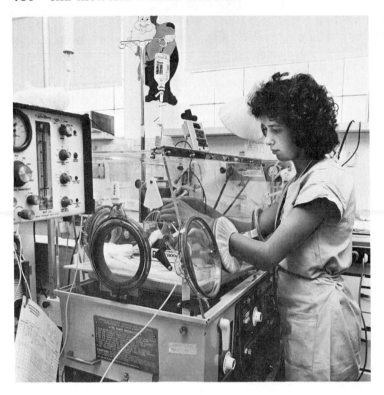

Figure 25-8. The baby in this incubator is receiving a number of treatments. A respirator can be seen to the left of the incubator. The baby is receiving an intravenous infusion and also feedings through an indwelling nasogastric feeding tube by a slow continuous method using an infusion pump. The formula is in the small flask hanging behind and above the respirator. The nurse is checking for gastric residual of formula. Oxygen is being given with an oxygen hood. An oxygen monitor is on the top of the incubator and the cardiac and respiratory monitor can be seen on the shelf against the wall. The lamp above the incubator can be used for radiant heat when necessary. It is apparent why parents may be overwhelmed by their baby's treatments and the technical apparatus, and why they need help in knowing how to visit and touch their baby.

caring for the baby can give parents further explanation at this time and answer their questions.

Parents should be encouraged to touch, talk to, and comfort their baby, but for some, this may take a number of visits, especially if the baby is quite ill. Eventually they are encouraged to participate in much of their baby's care, including feeding, changing of diapers, and other care they feel able to carry out. In order to develop strong parent–child attachments the parents need the same opportunities for touch, eye-to-eye contact, and caretaking that are important with normal newborns. There may be some delay because of the baby's condition, but delay should be no longer than absolutely necessary. The nurse must help the parents to develop an acquaintance with their baby as early as possible.

The importance of early parent contact with their baby and the ways in which the nurse can promote parent–infant attachment is discussed in more detail for all newborns in general on pages 567–73 and for premature and sick infants on pages 573–75.

If the mother had planned to nurse her baby, her breasts may be pumped to stimulate and maintain her milk supply so that she will be able to nurse her baby when he becomes strong enough. Ordinarily, arrangements can be made for the mother to pump her breasts at home, and plans may be made for her to bring the milk to the hospital for the baby's use. Later, of course, she can begin to nurse the baby. The mother who is supplying breast milk for her baby feels good about the valuable contribution she is making to her baby's care.

If at all possible, arrangement should be made for siblings to visit and see the baby through the nursery window to become acquainted, to ask questions, and to feel that they are getting to know the baby. If family visiting is infrequent when a baby must remain in the hospital for a long time after the mother goes home, it is possible for the family to regroup (without the baby), and then it becomes difficult to find a place for the baby. When the mother is discharged from the hospital, frequent visiting, if distance permits, and telephone calls help to keep in close contact.

As time goes on parents need more and more direct contact with their baby if it is at all possible for them to spend such time at the hospital. They need to come to know their baby well, and the mother needs to develop confidence in her ability to care for her baby. As the baby improves the mother should be able to give more and more of his care. Often arrangements can be made for her to spend a day, or several, at the hospital giving complete care to her baby before his discharge.

Sensory Stimulation

Incubator care has in the past isolated the preterm baby from the frequent human contact and the tactile, visual, auditory, and kinesthetic stimulation that the full-term newborn ordinarily receives. It was previously felt that the small baby needed to be isolated from his environment to prevent infection, and that these babies were fragile and needed protection against being handled. Before modern incubators, small babies were wrapped in blankets, placed into an incubator with a glass window on only one side, and handled only once every three hours for diapering, temperature check, and feedings for which the baby was not removed from the incubator. With modern incubators the baby is less wrapped up, and is in an incubator that at least has Plexiglas all around. This makes the baby somewhat less isolated from human stimulation, but an incubator environment is still very monotonous. The incubator separates the baby from much of the sensory stimulation that exists in the environment of the normal newborn, and if the baby is only diapered and fed as necessary the amount of stimulation he receives will be very insufficient.

It is still true that the severely premature baby and the sick baby need to be protected against handling other than that which is absolutely necessary for essential care. All of the energy of these babies must be used for efforts at survival. However, when these babies show improvement and stability in their condition they will profit from being given sensory stimulation.

Research within recent years has shown that newborns are much more capable of organized responses than had previously been assumed. It has also been observed that the preterm baby's ability to see, hear, smell, and respond to touch is quite good. Preterm babies have been observed to gaze at the faces of the nurses who feed them, to respond to handling, and to quiet when someone talks to them.

Early stimulation of the preterm baby may come when parents visit if they are ready to touch, stroke, pat, and talk to the baby. Often parents will assume the *en face* position to look at the baby and thus visually stimulate him. A nursery mobile suspended from the roof of the baby's incubator at a focal plane about eight to nine inches from the baby's eyes will provide visual stimulation, and parents can be encouraged to bring other bright toys. (See Figure 25-9.)

Preterm babies can be removed from the incubator for feedings and extra stimulation as soon as they can maintain their body temperature while out of the incubator during a feeding. At feeding time they can be rocked, patted, talked to, and held in the position in which they can look at their caretaker's face. Holding the baby up for burping also gives him an opportunity to look around. Cuddling and burping can be a part of a gavage feeding as well as a breast or bottle feeding. This feeding and play is ideally done by the parents as frequently as they can be available, but is done by nurses when parents are not there. At times when parents are not available nurses can offer sensory stimuli by talking to the baby, patting him, and managing to be in his visual field during care that involves diapering, temperature taking, feeding, and other care. Nurses should hold the baby for

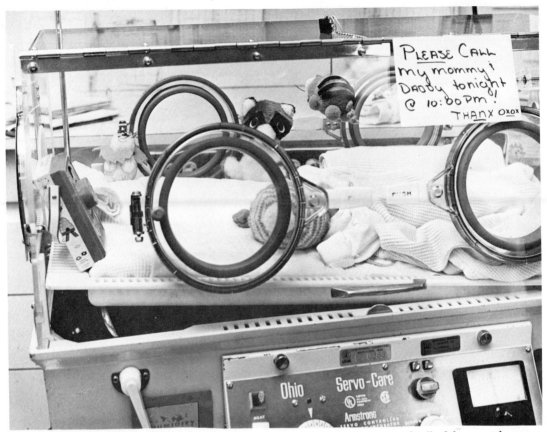

Figure 25-9. The baby in this incubator is progressing well. She no longer needs all of the special apparatus for her care that is shown in Figure 25-8. She is in the incubator because she still needs protection against heat loss. Note that this baby is clothed and covered with a blanket and that she is wearing a stocking cap to reduce heat loss from the rather large surface of her head. This baby is being visited frequently by her parents, and they have brought several toys for her interest and stimulation.

his feedings as soon as that is permissible, and cuddle him and talk to him as they would during feeding of the normal newborns. Nurses and parents may also try to get the baby to follow their head movements with his eyes and to respond to their voices.

Nurses are in a unique position to devise ways that will stimulate these small babies to respond. Nurses also have the information and the knowledge they need to decide when and how much stimulation should be given to each baby, making sure that there is a good balance between rest and activity.

When the preterm baby has matured enough to be moved to a regular bassinet, nurses need to continue to talk to, pick up, and play with these babies around feeding time. Parents should be urged to visit often. Early and frequent parent participation will strengthen the bond between parents and baby.

Sensory stimulation should, of course, continue after the baby leaves the hospital. When parents have been involved in care that encourages sensory stimulation of their baby, they are likely to continue to do so at home and the nurses can help them to understand the importance of this to their baby's continuing development.

Special Problems

Babies who are born preterm are likely to have special problems in their adjustment to extrauterine life because of their physiologic handicaps at birth. The degree of immaturity is very likely to determine the number and the severity of the complications that arise. Some of the problems of the preterm baby, especially those of the respiratory system, of thermal regulation, and of feeding have been described above. A few other problems will be discussed in the following pages. The susceptibility of the preterm baby to hypoglycemia, hyperbilirubinemia, and infection will be described only briefly because these complications are discussed in more detail in Chapter 26. Since patent ductus arteriosus and necrotizing enterocolitis are complications specific to the preterm baby they will be described in this chapter.

Hypoglycemia

Preterm babies may become hypoglycemic, but not necessarily symptomatic. Hypoglycemia may occur in the hours or days after birth presumably as a result of low liver glycogen stores because of their early birth and because of increased metabolic demands after birth. Chilling, asphyxia, and respiratory distress will use glycogen stores quickly. Blood glucose should be checked every four hours until stable.

If intravenous glucose is started in the first hours in the preterm baby, as is recommended for fluid and caloric needs, the blood glucose level is likely to remain above a hypoglycemic level. In the preterm infant a blood sugar level below 30 mg/100 ml whole blood must be viewed with suspicion and a reading below 20 mg/100 ml whole blood (below 25 in plasma or serum) must be considered hypoglycemia and treated. If the preterm baby has not grown well *in utero*, being below the fiftieth percentile in weight, the likelihood of developing hypoglycemia may be greater.

Hyperglycemia

The extremely preterm baby may have a low carbohydrate tolerance and spill sugar into the urine when he receives above his tolerance in intravenous fluids. See page 733 for further discussion of carbohydrate tolerance.

Hyperbilirubinemia

The preterm baby is very likely to develop hyperbilirubinemia and is very vulnerable to the danger of free bilirubin. The preterm baby probably has less ability to conjugate bilirubin than the term baby does. He has less total serum protein and serum albumin for binding bilirubin than the term baby and is likely to have conditions such as acidosis, which may interfere with the binding of bilirubin. Also, since oral feedings are delayed or slow in preterm infants, there is likely to be a delay in evacuation of bilirubin-containing meconium. The preterm baby is in greater danger of developing kernicterus at lower levels of free bilirubin than the term infant. Treatment for jaundice must therefore begin early. See pages 802–809 for further discussion on hyperbilirubinemia.

Infection

The preterm baby must be carefully protected against infection. Immaturity of the baby's organs and a deficiency in resistance to disease give him a high susceptibility. Infection precautions, important in any nursery, discussed in Chapter 18, must be strictly observed.

The preterm baby is very susceptible to upper respiratory tract infections, septicemia, and meningitis. Every precaution should be taken to prevent infection from adults or through aspiration of food. Immaturity of the lungs, presence of asphyxia, and low resistance all contribute to the baby's susceptibility to infections.

The potential for an intrauterine infection, especially pneumonia, is greater in the preterm than in the term baby, because preterm births are more likely to be preceded by a prolonged period of ruptured membranes. When the fetal membranes rupture before labor in the term pregnancy the mother either goes into labor quite promptly or labor is induced. With premature rupture of the membranes in a preterm pregnancy, the pregnancy is allowed to continue to permit further maturation of the fetus. With the membranes prematurely ruptured there is danger of intrauterine infection and exposure of the fetus. See page 641 for management of rupture of membrances in a preterm pregnancy.

Clinical signs of infection are very difficult to evaluate in any newborn, and especially in the preterm baby. Any signs suggestive of infection will need to be investigated by laboratory means as described on page 817.

Necrotizing Enterocolitis

Neonatal necrotizing enterocolitis (NEC) is a very serious disease in the newborn that is characterized by ischemic necrosis of the gastrointestinal tract which frequently leads to perforation. The disease is seen primarily in preterm infants, especially in those who have undergone fetal distress and neonatal hypoxia and shock. Onset is usually in the first week of life but may be delayed into the second or third week. The right colon, cecum, and terminal ileum are most often involved, although the entire colon and small bowel may show lesions. Occasionally only small segments of the ileum are affected, but often large segments of bowel or even the entire bowel are involved.

With necrotizing entercolitis the involved area of the bowel is dilated and the serosal surface is hemorrhagic. Segments of intestine may become agglutinated. The mucosal surface has ulcerations and necrosis and is covered by a pseudomembranous formation of agglutinated inflammatory cells and necrotic epithelium. There is hemorrhage in the submucosa. An ileus develops with the disease. This leads to stasis of intestinal contents and proliferation of bacteria. Many times the bowel perforates; this may be in one place or in multiple places. Perforation of the thin friable bowel is the most common and

the most serious development. Peritonitis and generalized sepsis follow.

The cause of NEC is not certain, but two factors considered most strongly as an initial cause are ischemia of the intestines and the action of enteric bacteria. A period of fetal or neonatal hypoxia and/or systemic shock will bring about a reflexive response in which there is a redistribution of blood, which results in blood being shunted away from the peripheral, renal, and mesenteric vascular beds in order to supply and protect the brain and the heart from hypoxia. The resultant ischemia in the mesenteric vascular bed may then decrease the metabolism in the intestinal mucosa and damage intestinal cells to the point where they may decrease or stop their normal secretion of protective mucus. This exposes the intestinal mucosa to enzymatic autodigestion and allows bacterial invasion. Then, subsequent to the ischemia of the bowel, brought about by the hypotension and hypoxia, there is bacterial invasion of the bowel.

When normal circulation is restored after an episode of ischemia, repair and regeneration of the bowel can take place. However, enteric bacteria and feedings may complicate the changes brought about by the ischemia of the bowel. Along with an adynamic ileus and stasis there may be an overgrowth of bacteria. The gas-forming bacteria, which predominate, may invade the damaged areas of the bowel mucosa and produce gas blebs or small bubbly cysts in the bowel wall (pneumatosis). A third component—the availability of metabolic substrate (the feedings)—adds to the development and progress of the disease by providing good growth material for the bacteria.

The clinical picture of NEC includes the signs and symptoms that could ordinarily be expected to be associated with feeding and bowel problems. The baby may feed poorly and be lethargic. He is likely to have gastric retention because of prolonged gastric emptying. Abdominal distention, especially if associated with rigidity, should be of concern at once. Increase in abdominal distention can be observed by measurement of the abdomen every 4 to 6 hours. Ileus is likely to be present. Bowel sounds or their absence should be checked. A red or shiny abdominal skin may indicate peritonitis. Since the bowel is very friable, abdominal palpation should only be done with utmost care. If emesis occurs it may be bile-stained. Stools become diarrheal and may be blood-streaked. A guaiac test should be done on the stools.

The baby with NEC may develop other signs of illness such as apneic episodes, thermal instability, jaundice, lethargy, and sometimes a shocklike condition.

X-ray of the abdomen of a baby with NEC shows intestinal distention with dilated loops of bowel and pneumatosis (air in the bowel wall). There may also be a pneumoperitoneum (free air in the peritoneum). Sometimes gas is seen in the portal vein, which is a very ominous sign.

The prognosis of necrotizing enterocolitis is very serious. When treatment is successful it often depends on early recognition. Infants at risk require careful observation for signs that are ordinarily relatively nonspecific. As soon as any signs of NEC are detected all enteric feedings are stopped and nasogastric suctioning is started. Intravenous fluid and electrolyte therapy is started, acid–base balance is carefully monitored and maintained, and the circulation is supported with blood and plasma as indicated. Dextran may be given for its effect in countering platelet adherence. Antibiotics, parenterally and topically, are begun, wide spectrum at first, and possibly changed to others when results of blood, urine, and stool cultures are known. Abdominal x-rays are taken every 4 to 6 hours to watch for pneumoperitoneum, obstruction, or peritoneal fluid. A physical evaluation of the abdomen for evidence of perforation is done frequently.

When the baby's condition improves feedings are begun cautiously after 7 to 10 days of nasogastric suction and antibiotics. Feedings are not given earlier than one week.

Surgery may become necessary. Indications for surgery include pneumoperitoneum, actual or impending perforation, peritonitis, and intestinal obstruction. All nonviable or acutely inflamed bowel is removed at surgery, and usually an ileostomy or a colostomy is done. Sometimes a large amount of bowel needs to be removed and malabsorption and short bowel syndrome become a problem. Long-term total intravenous alimentation (page 779) is sometimes necessary for these babies.

Nursing observation of babies with NEC is very important both in recognizing early signs, which have been described above, and after a diagnosis is made in observing changes in the baby's condition. In addition the baby needs supportive care to decrease stress and to promote comfort.

The baby's abdominal area must be protected from trauma. The baby is best cared for without diapers, which put some pressure on the lower abdomen and also involve some pressure on the abdomen during diaper changes. Diapers may also obstruct good observation of the abdomen for any changes in condition. Since the baby is likely to have diarrhea, frequent cleaning of the buttocks and the adjacent area and ointment to the skin are important.

The abdominal area must also be protected from trauma by very careful handling of the baby, preferably not picking him up except when absolutely necessary. The baby needs comforting in other ways than by holding him.

The abdomen must be carefully watched for signs of perforation of the bowel and for peritonitis, for reddening or shininess of the skin, and for increasing distention. Perforation of the bowel may be accompanied by signs of shock.

Vital signs of the baby must be closely observed. Blood pressure change may signal a problem. Apnea or other respiratory problems may suddenly appear. Since a baby on a respirator may not show these changes, he must be carefully observed for other signs. The body temperature may become unstable, and it may drop when shock develops. The temperature must be taken axillary, since taking rectal temperature is contraindicated. Other signs of shock such as change in pulse, change in color to pale or dusky, and limpness may appear.

As with any serious illness of an infant the parents will need support from the nurse. They need an explanation of the baby's condition, the reasons for treatment, and if surgery is done, an explanation of the anticipated postoperative course. They will need help with understanding how the ileostomy or colostomy functions, and assistance in learning to care for it unless an anastomosis is done before the baby goes home.

The role of breast milk in prevention of NEC has been, and is continuing to be, explored. Babies ordinarily do not develop this disease until they have been fed. There is some evidence that formula feedings permit overgrowth of enteric bacteria and that breast milk may provide protection.

A concept of the pathogenesis of acute necrotizing enterocolitis as presented by Dr. Thomas V. Santulli is that after an attack of hypoxia and decreased gut perfusion and mucosal autodigestion has taken place that enteric bacteria will grow well with formula feeding but be controlled by breast milk. With the immature enteric maturity of the preterm baby plus formula feeding an overgrowth of enteric bacteria can take place and the bowel wall can be invaded. With breast milk feeding the baby receives a passive immunity that maintains a normal enteric flora and permits the bowel to repair and recover from the mucosal autodigestion brought about by the insult of the hypoxia.[32]

Gestational age appears to determine a baby's enteric immunity. The full-term baby has relatively good immunity, but the preterm baby is deficient in transplacental IgG, has delayed secretion of IgA, and does not have very good phagocytic action. It is speculated by Dr. Santulli that breast milk may prevent NEC in the preterm baby by providing passive enteric immunity to the baby until its own enteric immunity is established. Dr. Santulli states[33]:

Breast milk contains large amounts of SIgA, smaller amounts of IgG, active lymphocytes and macrophages, specific antibodies against many types of microorganisms (especially against the most important bacterial pathogen of the neonate, *E. coli*), a growth enhancer of gram-positive lactobacilli, an antistaphylococcal agent, complement components, lysozyme, lactoperoxidase, and lactoferrin.

It may well turn out, as it usually does, that nature's evolved wisdom furnishes the better product.

Breast milk used for the purpose of possibly preventing NEC must be fresh mother's milk. Obtaining fresh milk and keeping it uncontaminated may present some special problems. Banked breast milk is not helpful for this purpose because most of the immunologic value of breast milk is lost when it is autoclaved or frozen.

Patent Ductus Arteriosus

The ductus arteriosus, the large blood vessel that connects the pulmonary artery with the descending aorta during fetal life, ordinarily closes by constriction within hours in the normal infant. With the onset of respiration at birth the pulmonary vascular resistance is suddenly lowered and there is a large increase in pulmonary blood flow. Also, with clamping of the umbilical cord, and removal of the low-resistance placental circuit from the circulation, the systemic resistance increases. With the relative fall in the pulmonary vascular resistance and the rise in systemic vascular resistance, each of these resistances become nearly equal very soon after birth, with the pulmonary possibly being a little lower. This permits a small amount of blood flow from the systemic to the pulmonary circulatory system—a transitory left to right shunt. Normally this shunt is not large and with good

[32] Thomas V. Santulli, Acute necrotizing enterocolitis: recognition and management, *Hosp. Pract.* 9:129–135 (Nov.) 1974.

[33] *Ibid.*

oxygenation the ductus arteriosus soon constricts well. The ductus does, however, have the capacity to reopen during the first postnatal days if the Pao$_2$ drops below normal for any reason.

In preterm babies, and especially in those with respiratory distress syndrome, delayed closure or persistence of the ductus arteriosus is common. Persistence of a patent ductus arteriosus may occur in 40 to 50 percent of infants with a birth weight under 1500 gm (3 lb 5 oz). Delay in closure is probably mainly due to (1) immaturity, there being insufficient development of the musculature, and (2) the hypoxemia associated with respiratory distress, which causes the ductus arteriosus to remain patent or to reopen in the early days after birth. Multiple other factors may have some influence.

When the ductus arteriosus is patent, shunting of blood can be from right to left, or from left to right, or bidirectional, depending upon whether the resistance is least in the pulmonary or in the systemic circulation. Persistent patency may lead to severe cardiorespiratory distress.

The more preterm a baby is the less muscular are the pulmonary arterioles. This means that there is a greater difference between systemic and pulmonary resistance in the preterm than in the full-term infant and shunting from systemic to pulmonary circulation is likely to take place. Also, the hypoxia, common in preterm infants, is likely to delay closure of the ductus arteriosus. With these conditions a left-to-right shunt develops. (A small right-to-left or bidirectional shunt may occur in the first hour after birth.) When spontaneous closure of the ductus does not soon occur, but the shunting remains small, it may not cause any serious circulatory problems. If the shunting becomes significantly large, the left ventricle will become overloaded and congestive heart failure may develop.

Pulmonary vascular resistance continues a normal maturational decrease in the next several days and weeks after birth. As the pulmonary resistance decreases there is an increase in blood flow into the pulmonary circulation if the ductus arteriosus is patent. This increase in blood flow through the lungs results in increased pulmonary venous return to the left side of the heart. As the volume of blood returning from the lungs increases, distention of the left ventricle increases and its stroke volume increases. If this process continues the load on the left ventricle becomes increasingly greater. The ventricle may be able to maintain the increased stroke volume; if so, there will be no symptoms. If the heart becomes overextended signs of cardiac failure appear.

When a patent ductus arteriosus is associated with respiratory distress the baby may have respiratory problems because of the increased pulmonary blood flow in addition to those already present because of the status of the lung.

Diagnosis of a patent ductus arteriosus should be made prior to frank evidence of congestive failure. This permits early treatment. With left to right shunting through the ductus an audible murmur develops, the basal heart rate gradually increases, the pulses become bounding so that the dorsalis pedis and palmar pulses may become perceptible, there is a wide pulse pressure, the apical cardiac impulse becomes hyperactive, pulmonary congestion develops, and peripheral edema becomes evident. Congestive pulmonary stress becomes manifest by tachypnea and chest retraction. Apneic spells may develop and increase in severity. Mild cyanosis may develop; it is ordinarily easily relieved by a small increase in ambient oxygen concentration, since the shunt is left to right and not right to left. Echocardiography helps to diagnose the extent of the shunting.

Treatment is likely to consist of administration of diuretics for removal of excess fluid, fluid intake restriction, oxygen as needed, maintenance of a normal blood pH, mintenance of adequate hemoglobin to insure adequate oxygenation, and digitalization as indicated.

When medical management is successful in maintaining the baby, spontaneous closure of the ductus may occur in several weeks. Sometimes surgical closure may be necessary to prevent heart failure. Since surgery in a small preterm infant is accompanied by considerable risk, there has been a search for a means of effecting pharmacologic closure of the ductus. Administration of indomethacin to inhibit prostaglandin synthesis has been reported as successful.[34] Prostaglandin has a relaxing effect on the ductus. With a prostaglandin inhibitor it is hoped that the ductus will close. Study is being continued for any adverse reactions to indomethacin.

Discharge from the Hospital

The preterm baby is usually ready for discharge from the hospital when he is able to maintain his temperature in an average environment, when he is able to eat well from a bottle or the breast and is gaining weight well, and when the mother demonstrates ability and confidence in providing care. Often this time coincides with the time the baby reaches a body weight of about 2250 gm (roughly 5 lb) and a gestational age of 36 to 37 weeks.

Conditions in the home may influence the time of discharge. The public health nurse is important in the transition from home to hospital. Arrangements are often made with a public health nursing agency to visit the home prior to the baby's discharge to help the parents prepare for the baby, and also for visits after he is home to give them further assistance with his care.

A social worker should be a member of the health care team that provides the baby's care. The social worker assists the family with adjustments that must be made in the hospital and in the home, and also with financial arrangements to cover the very high hospital and medical bills.

Physical and mental development of the preterm baby should in general be expected to coincide with that of a full-term baby only when the baby reaches the date when he would have been full-term. Since development is not likely to progress faster extrauterine than intrauterine,

future evaluation of progress should be made from the expected full-term date rather than the date of the baby's birth.

THE SMALL-FOR-GESTATIONAL-AGE BABY

The small-for-gestational-age (SGA) baby is usually defined as one whose birth weight is below the tenth percentile for a given gestational age. SGA has also been defined as a birth weight of more than two standard deviations below the mean for any given week of gestation. This coresponds to approximately the third percentile on the intrauterine growth curves. Defining small-for-gestational age in terms of low birth weight means that gestational age must be relatively closely assessed and that both birth weight and gestational age must be plotted on an intrauterine growth chart. With this definition a SGA baby may be preterm, term, or postterm. The unifying characteristic is a disproportionately small birth weight for gestational age.

Many small-for-gestational-age babies are full-term babies whose birth weight falls below the tenth percentile on the intrauterine growth chart shown in Figure 25-1. This usually means that the term baby who is SGA weighs 2500 gm or less at birth. When weight was being used as a definition of prematurity the SGA term infant was identified as a premature. Now that gestational age assessment is being used to identify the preterm baby, the full-term baby of low birth weight is separated from the preterm and placed into a separate classification designated as term SGA. The full-term SGA baby can be thought of as a baby who is mature but undergrown.

Many descriptive words or phrases have been used for babies who are growth-retarded—small-for-gestational age, small-for-dates, intrauterine growth retardation (IUGR), dysmature, chronic fetal distress, fetal malnutrition syndrome, pseudopremature. All of these terms make some reference to factors of the fetal environment that do not permit the baby to reach

[34] Abraham Rudolph and Michael A. Heymann, Medical treatment of the ductus arteriosus, *Hosp. Pract.* 12:57–65 (Feb.) 1977.

his growth potential as soon as should be expected. Of all the terms that have been used SGA and IUGR will be used in the rest of this chapter.

The SGA baby may be small in weight only, or small in weight and length, or he may be below the tenth percentile in weight, length, and head circumference. The clinical picture of the baby is related to the duration, the intensity, and the time of onset of the growth-retarding influence. With undernutrition weight is affected first, then there is a decrease in growth, indicated by a shortness in body length, and finally if growth retardation is severe the head circumference is affected. Sometimes, however, a baby is hereditarily of small size in all measurements.

When weight alone is diminished and length and head circumference are normal, it is felt that the factor that caused the fetus the distress that reduced its weight occurred only a few days or weeks prior to birth. When distress is of a longer standing, chronic nature, growth in body weight has been curtailed for weeks or months before birth, growth in length has also been retarded, and in extreme cases growth in head circumference was slowed.

Causes of Fetal Growth Retardation

Normal intrauterine growth for body weight, for length, and for growth of other organs is linear between 28 and 37 to 38 weeks of gestation. From 37 to 38 weeks growth of the fetus and placenta begins to fall off somewhat and no longer follows the straight line upward. When for some reason the fetus cannot follow this normal pattern then growth falls off at some earlier time.

Fetal growth may be retarded either because the fetus is unable to grow normally in the presence of an adequate nutritional "supply line," or because a normal fetus does not receive adequate nutrition from the supply line.

Retardation of growth because of factors inherent in the fetus are caused by such problems as chromosomal aberrations (Down's and other trisomy syndromes), congenital anomalies, infections (rubella, toxoplasmosis, etc.), and perhaps other factors that cause subnormal development. A developmental abnormality in the fetus is likely to prevent normal growth of tissues and organs.

The supply line can be thought of as having a maternal and a placental component. Placental causes may be of a pathologic nature such as infarcts, or premature placental separation, or possibly some physiologic limitations, as, for example, being unable to supply adequately all fetuses of a multiple pregnancy. By and large, however, fetal and placental causes account for only a small proportion of fetal growth retardation. Maternal causes are therefore primarily the reason for fetal deprivation. In some cases the mechanism of fetal deprivation may not be known, and in other instances a primary abnormality of maternal circulation may be complicated by secondary pathologic changes in the placenta, but in general the search for cause of fetal deprivation should be made among maternal factors.[35]

Maternal undernutrition and diminished uterine blood flow are two maternal factors commonly considered. Studies done on animals have shown that dietary restrictions in mothers caused reduction in birth weight of offspring. Whether or not maternal malnutrition in human pregnancy has an appreciable effect is not clear. The role of chronic nutrition, prior to conception, in causing IUGR is not well understood either. It is generally believed that the fetus will receive adequate nutrients from the mother if the mother has the necessary reserves. If continuing deprivation of some nutrient depletes maternal reserves the fetus will be unable to get that nutrient. The effect on the fetus will depend upon how essential the particular deficient nutrient is to fetal growth.

Reduction of uteroplacental blood flow is

[35] Peter Gruenwald, Introduction—The supply line of the fetus; Definitions relating to fetal growth, in *The Placenta and Its Maternal Supply Line*, edited by P. Gruenwald. University Park Press, Baltimore, Md., 1975, pp. 1–17.

thought to be a cause of IUGR, because maternal diseases that may cause a reduced placental blood flow are associated with IUGR. These include preeclampsia, chronic hypertensive vascular disease, and advanced diabetes. These conditions can result in significant lowering of fetal weight, and also in fetal mortality and neonatal morbidity. Among other maternal causes of IUGR are smoking, small stature, low maternal age, grand multiparity, inadequate prenatal care, and low socioeconomic class. In many instances the cause of small-for-gestational age cannot be identified.

Incidence and Significance of IUGR

Studies in the United States and Great Britain show that about one third of the babies with birth weight of less than 2500 gm are not preterm but rather term SGA infants. The incidence of SGA births varies from 1.5 to 2 percent of all births.[36]

SGA is second only to preterm as a cause of perinatal mortality. The overall neonatal mortality for IUGR infants is 3.4 percent. This is less than the mortality rate for appropriately grown preterm but more than for appropriately grown term babies. An additional problem with SGA infants is a considerable increase in intrauterine fetal death. Death from intrapartum asphyxia in SGA babies is 10 times higher than for appropriately grown infants. Fourteen percent of all stillbirths and 6 percent of all neonatal deaths occur in babies whose birth weight is less than the third percentile for gestational age.[37]

Clinical Characteristics

The general appearance of the SGA baby varies from normal, at least at first glance, to one of general emaciation, which is more uncommon. The length and the head, chest, and abdominal circumferences are often less affected

by fetal deprivation than the weight. Measurements other than weight may be normal or somewhat lower than normal for an appropriate-sized baby of similar gestational age. The skull sutures may be wide secondary to failure of bone growth. The weight/length ratio is lower than normal. The length is likely to be 50 percent or more greater than the weight in SGA babies, indicating some degree of growth in length in excess of growth in weight. The weight–length ratio is useful for giving some indication of the duration of the malnutrition. Subcutaneous fat deposits and muscle mass may be quite low for maturity. The skin may be thin, loose, and with folds, and may be peeling, dry, and cracked. The umbilical cord may be thin.

Parameters of maturity—sole creases, hair texture, and ear cartilage are similar to those of normal babies of the same gestational age. Breast size may be normal, or it may be considerably smaller due to diminished growth of tissue.

Neurologic maturity is ordinarily not affected and the examination is usually appropriate for actual gestational age. SGA babies are more advanced in motor ability, reflexes, alertness, and ability to take food than preterm infants of similar weight.

Chronic oxygen deprivation *in utero* in IUGR is likely to result in a higher hemoglobin concentration, high hematocrit, and higher erythrocyte count in these babies than in their gestational peers.

The SGA baby has poor glucose control and may have both hyperglycemia and hypoglycemia. Thermoregulation is more limited than in appropriately grown term infants, but better than in premature infants of the same weight.

When growth retardation is severe the SGA baby may have the appearance of the postmature baby described on page 749. SGA and postmaturity syndrome may just be a continuation of the same problem.

Neonatal morbidity and mortality are increased in babies with IUGR. Morbidity is likely to result from perinatal asphyxia, hypoglycemia, hyperbilirubinemia, and polycythemia.

[36] Marilyn L. Renfield, The small-for-date baby, in *Neonatology*, edited by Gordon B. Avery. Lippincott, Philadelphia, Pa., 1975, p. 190.
[37] *Ibid.*

Obstetric Management

Obstetric management of the SGA fetus will depend on suspicion of fetal growth retardation. This may be based on findings that the fundal height is not growing according to what should be expected for the period of gestation, that the uterus remains small, and that the mother is not gaining weight appropriately. On such suspicion it is important to recheck the estimate of gestational age, based on menstrual history and laboratory tests.

Rate of growth of the fetal head may be determined by serial biparietal diameter measurements. When the biparietal diameter grows less than optimal the birth weight is also often low.

When the mother is known to have conditions that are likely to cause a reduced uteroplacental blood flow, such as chronic hypertensive vascular disease or diabetes, evaluations of placental function and fetal well-being are made during pregnancy. These include serial biparietal diameter measurements, estriol determinations, and weekly or semiweekly oxytocin challenge tests or fetal activity determinations. These evaluations are described in Chapter 21.

Having the evaluations of fetal well-being and fetal maturity the physicians must make the decision if it is safe for the pregnancy to continue or if early delivery is advisable. The risks of a hostile, intrauterine environment must be balanced against the problems of early delivery. To avoid the risk of a premature baby who also has IUGR, maturity of the fetus should be attained before delivery whenever possible.

Intrapartum care must be carefully managed whenever IUGR is suspected. Continuous monitoring of the fetus during labor is very important. A fetus with IUGR does not tolerate labor well because the uterine contractions restrict uteroplacental blood flow sufficiently to augment any fetal hypoxia which may already be present. Fetal distress may develop early as shown by late decelerations and loss of beat-to-beat variability. Cesarean section delivery may be indicated to avoid further stress of labor.

With the great risk of birth asphyxia and aspiration in the SGA baby, it is important that the pediatrician or someone equally capable is present at delivery to carry out resuscitation and to give all other care for the baby immediately after birth.

Neonatal Care

Certain problems in the neonatal period can be anticipated in the SGA baby and preparation should be made to manage them immediately.

Birth Asphyxia.

The incidence of fetal distress and birth asphyxia is quite high in the SGA baby. This may produce a difficult resuscitation problem, and plans must be made to manage any breathing difficulty promptly. The baby needs to be dried quickly and kept warm from the beginning. If breathing does not begin quite promptly, it will be necessary to suction the airway, stimulate the baby to cry, and use bag and mask for ventilation, and intubation if necessary. Aspiration of meconium at birth may also present a problem. Meconium aspiration and its management are described on pages 750–51.

Hypoglycemia

Hypoglycemia occurs in almost two thirds of infants whose birth weights are below the tenth percentile.[38] The baby who has suffered from poor nutrition *in utero* will have a decrease in subcutaneous fat deposits and a lack of liver glycogen stores. He will be short on energy reserves of glycogen and fat and very susceptible to hypoglycemia.

The SGA baby needs early feedings, at one to two hours of life, and frequent feedings to provide him with energy. An intravenous infusion of 10 percent glucose at 100 ml/kg-day for the first 12 to 24 hours of life may more easily provide the baby with energy and fluids in the first day than oral feedings.[39] Oral feedings may then

[38] Frederick C. Battaglia, The unique problems of small-for-dates babies, *Contemp. Ob/Gyn* 1:35–39 (March) 1973.
[39] *Ibid.*

be given as the baby can tolerate them. Dextrostix for blood glucose values must be done frequently, every one-half to one hour at first to watch for hypoglycemia. Hypoglycemia is described in more detail on page 795.

Full-term small-for-gestational-age babies usually can take food well soon after birth and they very early take a higher caloric intake in relation to weight than a preterm baby of the same size. Most SGA babies quickly gain back their weight deficit after feedings are begun.

Cold Stress

Lack of subcutaneous fat decreases the thermal insulation and increases the risk of cold stress in SGA babies. If the SGA baby becomes cooled in the delivery room, he quickly uses up his available stores of glycogen. It is therefore very important to protect the baby against heat loss from the moment of birth.

Polycythemia

Polycythemia and *secondary hyperviscosity* develop in SGA babies. This is thought to develop because of the chronic intrauterine hypoxia, which is believed to stimulate the baby's erythropoietin synthesis, which is then followed by an increased synthesis of red blood cells. Polycythemia then can result in blood hyperviscosity and sluggish circulation.

Diagnosis is made by checking the baby's hematocrit. With a hematocrit greater than 65 percent a partial exchange transfusion with fresh, frozen plasma may be indicated to bring the hematocrit down to the 50–55 percent range, and thereby improve the circulation and relieve any symptoms of hyperviscosity.

THE POSTTERM INFANT

The postterm infant is a baby who is 42 weeks or more gestational age at birth. Postterm pregnancy occurs in 10 to 12 percent of pregnancies and of these approximately 5 percent extend beyond 43 weeks of gestation. The baby of a postterm pregnancy is considered to be at risk because somewhere between 20 and 40 percent

of these babies develop a postmaturity syndrome, which puts them at risk.[40] Certain other postterm babies become large infants.

Placental Insufficiency

Placental maturation and function reach a peak near term, and thereafter fetal growth rate is reduced, with cessation of growth occurring at 42 weeks. Diminished placental function during the last month of gestation is not necessarily a pathologic condition but may be critical when any abnormal maternal, placental, or fetal condition exists.[41] Insufficient placental function for good exchange of oxygen and nutrients appears to develop in some pregnancies and when there is also a decrease in uteroplacental circulation it may lead to chronic fetal hypoxia and growth retardation, or to intrauterine asphyxia. Placental insufficiency seems to be fairly likely to occur in prolonged pregnancy when both the normal aging changes in placental function and failure to keep up with fetal growth could have an effect.

Fetal postmaturity may be observed from the thirty-eighth week of gestation on and the chances of the syndrome increases as pregnancy advances beyond term, reaching a maximum at 44 to 46 weeks gestation. With prolonged gestation the likelihood of placental insufficiency increases rapidly. The incidence of postmaturity syndrome is about 3 percent at term and increases to 20 to 40 percent postterm.

The perinatal mortality rate increases two to five times from 42 to 44 weeks gestation and is even much greater after 44 weeks.[42] Intrauterine deaths account for a large number of the perinatal deaths; some of these occur prior to labor, but a fairly large number occur during labor. Respiratory distress due to aspiration of

[40] H. Vorherr, Placental insufficiency and postmaturity, in *Human Placentation*, edited by I. A. Brosens, G. Dixon, and W. B. Robertson. Proceedings of an International Symposium, 29–30 July 1974, Excerpta Medica, Amsterdam, 1975, pp. 109–122.
[41] *Ibid.*
[42] *Ibid.*

meconium-stained amniotic fluid is the most common cause of postnatal morbidity and mortality.

Clinical Characteristics

The postterm baby may be large or small or appropriate in size. When there has been no placental insufficiency in postterm pregnancy the baby is healthy, of normal or large size, well nourished, alert, and active. Some of these babies are large, 4000 gm (8 lb 13 oz) or over. Sixty to eighty percent of postterm infants are in good condition.

When there is placental insufficiency with postterm pregnancy, the fetus is likely to have the clinical signs of the *postmaturity syndrome* or *Clifford's syndrome,* described by Dr. Clifford in 1954. This syndrome is a variation of intrauterine growth retardation described above for the SGA baby. Placental insufficiency, leading to the postmaturity syndrome, may be considered an imbalance between the respiratory and nutritive demands of the fetus and the capacity of the placenta to meet these demands. When the imbalance is acute and extensive fetal death may occur. When the condition is somewhat more chronic the fetus is likely to show signs of wasting.

The baby with signs of postmaturity is often of appropriate length and head circumference but has a malnourished appearance. The baby has failed to grow and has become dehydrated. He is long and thin, looks as though he has lost weight recently, and looks old and "worried." He is open-eyed and alert and looks older than the average newborn. The baby has dry, cracked, wrinkled, and parchment-like skin, with no vernix caseosa. Subcutaneous fat is lacking. With advancement of placental insufficiency meconium is expelled *in utero* due to fetal distress. The fetus's skin, nails, and umbilical cord then become meconium-stained and take on a brownish-green or yellowish discoloration. The baby gives the picture of weight loss *in utero* after a period of appropriate development. The fetus probably does lose weight, since he may

have to meet his needs from his stores of energy, such as subcutaneous fat.

It is important to note that postterm and postmature are not synonymous, although the two conditions are often associated. A postterm baby may be healthy and not develop the postmaturity syndrome. On the other hand, the postmaturity syndrome may develop in fetuses before they become postterm, even before they reach term gestation.

Clinical Management of Postterm Pregnancy

Since 20 to 40 percent of postterm pregnancies are in danger of placental insufficiency and postmaturity, careful evaluation of placental function is carried out when a pregnancy becomes postterm. This is especially important to consider because in some postterm pregnancies placental insufficiency may not be symptomatic in the fetus, but fetal distress may exist nevertheless. Through early recognition of placental insufficiency, delivery can be planned to avoid serious distress in the fetus. Observation of the prolonged pregnancy is the same as for any high-risk pregnancy.

Clinical evaluation of a potentially postterm pregnancy should begin in the first trimester and be continued at subsequent prenatal examinations. A careful history of the last menstrual period, any bleeding, and possibly postpill amenorrhea will be very useful in establishing a fairly accurate evaluation of the length of gestation. Information about the number of weeks of gestation becomes very important when a pregnancy is believed to be past term. Accurate recordings of fundal height at each prenatal visit, the date of onset of fetal movements, and when the fetal heart is first heard are valuable in confirming expected date of delivery. Observation of increases in fundal height and of serial biparietal diameter measurements will assess fetal growth.

Later, failure of fetal growth, as determined by biparietal measurements and poor growth in fundal height and loss of or poor maternal weight gain, suggest the possibility of postmaturity syndrome.

When the pregnancy becomes postdate, observations of placental function and fetal well-being are carried out to determine if the pregnancy should be terminated or if it can safely continue. These tests include measurements of urinary estriol excretion, fetal biparietal measurements, weekly or semiweekly oxytocin challenge tests and/or fetal activity acceleration determinations. These tests are described in Chapter 21.

Failure to obtain amniotic fluid at amniocentesis suggests postmaturity. Amniotic fluid volume decreases rapidly from the thirty-eighth week on, but with postmaturity the volume is greatly reduced, down to 250 ml or even much less. A very small amount of amniotic fluid is usually a sign of insufficient placental function.

When labor is induced or if it begins spontaneously, continuous fetal heart rate monitoring must be done. These fetuses tolerate labor poorly because the temporary restriction of uteroplacental blood flow during uterine contractions augments the fetal hypoxia. Scalp blood sampling may also be indicated during labor. Intrapartum care is crucial, since fetal distress occurs frequently during this time.

Delivery by cesarean section may be indicated. Placental function studies prior to labor may show that the fetus cannot tolerate labor, or conditions for induction of labor may be unfavorable. When labor does take place the fetal heart rate pattern, usually of late decelerations and loss of beat-to-beat variability, may show that the fetus will be unable to tolerate additional uterine contractions and that labor should be terminated by cesarean section.

It is very important to have someone skilled in resuscitation present at delivery. The postterm baby, and especially the baby with postmaturity syndrome, is very susceptible to birth asphyxia and to aspiration.

Neonatal Care

Since the postmaturity syndrome is likely to be a severe aspect of the problems described for the small-for-gestational-age infant, the postmature baby has many of the same complications as the SGA baby. In some aspects the problems may be more severe. Complications should be anticipated so that management can be planned in advance.

Birth Asphyxia

The incidence of fetal distress and birth asphyxia is high in the postmature baby. Monitoring of a postterm pregnancy for placental insufficiency and monitoring of the fetus in labor have been described. During labor of a postterm pregnancy, advance plans must be made for the pediatrician to be present at the birth to assist the baby to establish adequate respirations.

Meconium Aspiration

A baby with the postmaturity syndrome has usually expelled meconium *in utero*. The amount of amniotic fluid in postmaturity is often scant, and with meconium added, produces a thick meconium-stained fluid often described as "pea soup" fluid or "pea soup" meconium. The presence of meconium, along with birth asphyxia, leads to considerable danger of aspiration of debris into the lungs. Aspirated meconium will obstruct air passages and is also very irritating to the lungs. It therefore presents a significant problem to the baby. Babies who aspirate meconium develop respiratory distress, some require long-term care, and some die from the complications.

The mechanism of meconium aspiration is as follows. Intrauterine hypoxia causes the fetus to expel meconium. Hypoxia and acidosis may also cause the baby to gasp *in utero*. With a gasp, either *in utero* or at delivery, the baby aspirates amniotic fluid with meconium in it. A baby with intrauternine distress is more likely to aspirate than the one who is well oxygenated. With aspiration, the air passages and alveoli may become obstructed or a pneumonitis may develop. Bacteria grow well in the meconium-stained fluid, and infection in the lungs can readily develop. If obstruction takes place, the baby may develop atelectasis and further hypoxia, or he may develop emphysema, which may lead to pneumothorax. With pneumothorax additional problems and complications appear. (See Figure 25-10.)

Several investigators have found that the number of symptomatic infants from meconium aspiration can be greatly reduced and that both morbidity and mortality are likely to be considerably decreased if tracheal suction is done immediately after birth.[43]

The meconium-stained amniotic fluid should be removed as quickly as possible from the airways so that it will not be drawn into the lungs. It is suggested that when meconium-stained amniotic fluid is detected, the oral and nasal pharynx should be suctioned as soon as the baby's head is born, using a DeLee suction tube (Fig. 15-9, page 354). Then when the baby is completely born the mouth, pharynx, and nose should again be immediately suctioned. The larynx should be inspected with a laryngoscope and the trachea suctioned if there is evidence of meconium below the cords (Fig. 15-12, page 364). Intubation may be necessary. If a large amount of meconium is present, suctioning may need to be repeated.

Suctioning of the airways should be done as quickly as possible, but will be helpful in clearing the air passages even if the baby has taken a first breath before the procedure was begun. Oxygen is usually given and the baby must be closely monitored for bradycardia during and after suctioning. The baby is usually depressed at birth because of the previous asphyxia, and respirations may be irregular and gasping. Positive pressure ventilation should be avoided until the airways have been well cleared to prevent pushing meconium down into the smaller airways.

After the baby is stabilized, suction of the stomach is also carried out to remove meconium that the baby may have swallowed. This will reduce the chance of aspiration later.

[43] Richard D. Zachman, Postmaturity, *Perinatal News*, Madison General Hospital, Wisconsin Perinatal Center, Southcentral Region, April 1977, pp. 2–7.

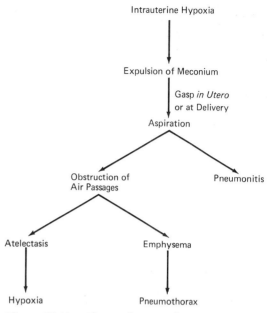

Figure 25-10. The mechanism of meconium aspiration and its consequences.

The baby who has been asphyxiated and/or meconium-stained at birth needs close observation in the nursery, as described on pages 783–85. If aspiration of meconium did occur, it is likely to be followed by respiratory distress, which is described on page 792.

Hypoglycemia

As with the SGA baby, the postmature baby does not have good fat deposits or adequate liver glycogen stores. The baby will lack energy reserves and will be very susceptible to hypoglycemia. Dextrostix checks for blood sugar values must be done at one-half to one hour intervals. Feedings should be early and frequent, beginning at one to two hours of age. Intravenous glucose may need to be given if the baby does not tolerate ample oral feedings.

Cold Stress

With poor stores of subcutaneous fat the baby is subject to quick loss of body heat and the consequences of chilling. He must be well protected against heat loss from the beginning, starting with protection during resuscitation.

Polycythemia

The postmature baby develops polycythemia and secondary hyperviscosity, probably as a result of intrauterine hypoxia. The hematocrit should be checked, and, if greater than 65 percent, the baby may need a partial exchange transfusion with fresh frozen plasma. (See page 814.)

Persistent Fetal Circulation or Persistent Pulmonary Hypertension of the Newborn

An increase in pulmonary vascular resistance in the newborn can cause persistence of blood flow through the foramen ovale and the ductus arteriosus and result in considerable right to left shunting of blood.

In normal infants the pulmonary vascular resistance decreases quite suddenly with onset of respirations and then continues a further decrease in the next several days and weeks after birth. Sometimes this change does not take place normally. The pulmonary vascular resistance then remains abnormally high, and blood does not flow through the lungs easily. Shunting of blood takes place through the ductus arteriosus and foramen ovale which are still patent and do not offer strong resistance. The blood that bypasses the lungs does not become oxygenated. The hypoxia leads to anaerobic metabolism and acidosis. Hypoxia and acidosis tend to increase pulmonary vascular resistance and will permit opening of the ductus arteriosus.

A number of different factors may slow the normal pulmonary and circulatory changes after birth. Delay has been seen in babies with perinatal asphyxia, intrauterine stress, hypoglycemia, and polycythemia with hyperviscosity. Sometimes there appears to be no underlying cause. Several conditions that develop in the postmature baby may cause increased pulmonary vascular resistance. Among these are asphyxia leading to acidosis, polycythemia, and aspiration which may lead to vasospasm.

The clinical signs of this syndrome consist of tachypnea and intermittent or persistent severe cyanosis soon after birth. Chest retractions and grunting are usually absent. A heart murmur may be heard. The PaO_2 is low. Diagnosis is difficult and is done to some extent by exclusion of other pulmonary and cardiac diseases.

Treatment is difficult. Any underlying identifiable cause, such as polycythemia, must be treated. The inspired oxygen concentration is increased to try to reduce the hypoxia. Acidosis should be corrected. If there is no improvement, assisted ventilation may be necessary. There are drugs, such as tolazoline, which are known to be pulmonary vascular dilators, but these are still experimental. Tolazoline tends to dilate all blood vessels. The baby receiving the drugs needs frequent and careful blood pressure checks.

SUMMARY

Placental insufficiency may be a complication of postterm pregnancies. This may lead to a postmaturity syndrome in the baby. Infants with this syndrome often suffer from hypoxia in late pregnancy and during labor, and they may become seriously ill in the early postnatal period. Mortality and morbidity can be lowered by careful observation of postterm pregnancies for signs of fetal distress, by delivery of these babies with the least stress possible, and through assisting the newborn in his adjustment to extrauterine life.

LARGE-FOR-GESTATIONAL-AGE INFANT

Large-for-gestational-age infants are babies whose birth weight is above the ninetieth percentile. They may be preterm, term, or postterm. A term baby weighing over 4000 gm (roughly 9 lb) is above the ninetieth percentile on the Colorado growth chart and is therefore considered LGA. Toward the other end of the weight scale a baby may weigh only 2500 gm but be considered LGA if his gestational age is 33 weeks or less. Such a baby would be immature but overgrown. Again this points out that each baby must have a careful gestational age assessment. It is very important to recognize a LGA preterm infant so that the large size does not mislead his caretakers and he receives care appropriate to his immaturity. Identification and care of the postterm baby who is small for gestational age was described above. It is important to point out here that some postterm babies are large for gestational age.

A number of factors may contribute to accelerated growth *in utero*. The LGA baby may be a normal baby born of large parents. Maternal parity has some influence on weight. The second and third babies are larger than the first; thereafter there is no predictable increase in size. Male babies are characteristically larger than females, and when there is growth acceleration for some reason this could make considerable difference. Race may make a difference. Certain tribes of American Indians, such as the Crow and Northern Cheyenne Indians, have unusually large babies. The specific influence of genetic factors and racial factors or both on intrauterine growth has not been determined.[44]

In addition to the biologic factors that influence growth acceleration, there are some disease conditions that bring about excessive intrauterine growth. The most common of these conditions is maternal diabetes. Babies with Beckwith's syndrome, a condition characterized by gigantism, large tongue, omphalocele, and large viscera, and babies with erythroblastosis fetalis and with transposition of the aorta are usually of excessive size.

Infants of large size usually show an increase in other body proportions as well. The body length and the head circumference are at the upper percentile levels. An exception to a proportional increase is the infant of a diabetic mother who has an increase in total body fat. These babies have an increase of body weight for their height. Along with a large baby there is also a large placenta.

Large-for-gestational-age babies tend to have problems with hypoglycemia and polycythemia and with trauma because of their size.

The fetus of the diabetic mother is exposed to higher than normal blood glucose levels, even in the well-controlled mother. The fetus responds to the higher glucose level with increased insulin production. The insulin facilitates entry of glucose into tissue cells and makes possible the utilization of glucose by muscle and adipose tissue. Insulin inhibits the breakdown of fat to free fatty acids, and it promotes protein synthesis. Insulin is therefore involved in the functions necessary for growth. At birth then the baby has high levels of circulating glucose and insulin, but with severing of the umbilical cord the baby loses the constant supply of glucose from the mother and hypoglycemia soon develops.

The development of hypoglycemia in other neonatal conditions associated with LGA is not as clear, but hyperinsulinemia is known to be associated with erythroblastosis and Beckwith's syndrome, and hypoglycemia is common in LGA babies born of mothers who are not known to be diabetic. It is thought that some mothers who have LGA babies for no known reason may eventually become diabetic. The incidence of hypoglycemia is increased for preterm LGA babies as well as for term and postterm infants.

Polycythemia and hyperviscosity of the blood shows an increased incidence in LGA babies. Infants of diabetic mothers have also been reported to have hypercoagulability of the blood.

Mechanical problems may arise during delivery of LGA babies. Cephalopelvic disproportion may prolong labor and may lead to birth trauma with delivery of the head or to cesarean section delivery. Delivery of the shoulders may be difficult when a baby is large and peripheral nerve injury of the cervical or brachial plexus may occur at delivery.

Management of the large-for-gestational-age baby includes observation for and treatment of the above-named problems. Sometimes birth of a LGA baby can be anticipated from obstetric history and examination. If the mother has previously delivered a large baby another large baby can be anticipated. Careful check for pres-

[44]Lubchenco, *op. cit.*, p. 167.

ence of diabetes in the mother is then also made during pregnancy. Serial measurements of fundal height may give a clue to expect a large baby, and ultrasonic measurement of the fetal head can confirm an anticipated large baby.

Postnatally the LGA baby must be carefully observed for vital signs and behavior, and screening for hypoglycemia and polycythemia must be done to identify the babies who need treatment. This is necessary for all LGA babies, since a significant number of those born of nondiabetic mothers will become hypoglycemic.

Early feedings may counteract the tendency to hypoglycemia. If for some reason the baby cannot take food orally intravenous glucose administration will be necessary. Hypoglycemia and care of the baby of a diabetic mother are described on pages 795–802.

SUMMARY

Care of babies who are at risk for a number of perinatal problems because of their gestational age or their weight at birth or because of both gestational age and birth weight have been described. High-risk conditions range from preterm to postterm births and from small-for-gestational-age to large-for-gestational-age babies. The major difficulties of preterm infants are respiratory distress, thermal regulation, and feeding problems. Small-for-gestational-age babies and postterm babies have problems with fetal distress, birth asphyxia, hypoglycemia, and polycythemia. Large-for-gestational-age babies are also subject to hypoglycemia and polycythemia.

Certain abnormalities and diseases of the newborn that present as high-risk conditions are described in the next chapter.

BIBLIOGRAPHY

Als, Heidelise, Tronick, Edward, Adamson, Lauren, and Brazelton, T. Berry, The behavior of the full-term but underweight newborn infant, *Dev. Med. Child Neurol.* 18:590–602 (Oct.) 1976.

American Academy of Pediatrics, Hyperthermia from malfunctioning radiant heaters, *Pediatrics, Part 2 Suppl.* 59:1041 (June) 1977.

American Academy of Pediatrics, Committee on Fetus and Newborn, Nomenclature for duration of gestation, birth weight, and intra-uterine growth, *Pediatrics* 39:935–939 (June) 1967.

American Academy of Pediatrics, Committee on Nutrition, Nutritional needs of low-birth-weight infants, *Pediatrics* 60:519–530 (Oct.) 1977.

Andrews, Billy F. (ed.), Symposium on the small-for-date baby, *Pediatr. Clin. North Am.* 17:1–202 (Feb.) 1970.

Avery, Gordon B. (ed.); *Neonatology.* Lippincott, Philadelphia, Pa., 1975.

———, and Fletcher, Anne B., Nutrition, in *Neonatology*, edited by Gordon B. Avery. Lippincott, Philadelphia, Pa., 1975, pp. 839–897.

Babson, S. Gorham, Feeding the low-birth-weight infant, *J. Pediatr.* 79:691–701 (Oct.) 1971.

Barnard, Martha Underwood, Supportive nursing care for the mother and newborn who are separated from each other, *MCN,* 1:107–110 (March/April) 1976.

Barness, Lewis A., Nutrition for the low birth weight infant, *Clin. Perinatol.* 2:345–352 (Sept.) 1975.

Battaglia, Frederick C., The unique problems of small-for-date babies, *and* The large-for-gestational age baby—An overlooked problem, *Contemp. Ob/Gyn* 1:35–42 (March) 1973.

———, and Lubchenco, Lula O., A practical classification of newborn infants by weight and gestational age, *J. Pediatr.* 71:159–163 (Aug.) 1967.

Bliss, V. Jane, Nursing care for infants with neonatal necrotizing enterocolitis, *MCN* 1:37–40 (Jan.–Feb.) 1976.

Brans, Yves W., and Cassady, George, Intrauterine growth and maturation in relation to fetal deprivation, in *The Placenta and Its Maternal Supply Line*, edited by P. Gruenwald. University Park Press, Baltimore, Md., 1975, pp. 307–334.

Brown, Bryant J., Gabert, Harvey, A., and Stenchever, Morton A., Respiratory distress syndrome, surfactant biochemistry, and acceleration of fetal lung maturity: A review, *Obstet. Gynecol. Surv.* 30:71–90 (Feb.) 1975.

Brown, Josephine, and Hepler, Ruth, Stimulation—A corollary to physical care, *Am. J. Nurs.* 76:578–581 (April) 1976.

Carson, Bonita S. *et al.*, Combined obstetric and pediatric approach to prevent meconium aspiration syndrome, *Am. J. Obstet. Gynecol.* 126:712–715 (Nov. 15) 1976.

Christensen, Ann Z., Coping with the crisis of a premature birth—One couple's story, *MCN* 2:33–37 (Jan./Feb.) 1977.

Clifford, Stewart H., Postmaturity—With placental dysfunction: Clinical syndrome and pathologic findings, *J. Pediatr.* 44:1–13 (Jan.) 1954.

Conway, Alice, and Williams, Tamara, Parenteral alimentation, *Am. J. Nurs.* 76:574–777 (April) 1976.

Cook, Larry N., Assessing maturity of the neonate, *Contemp. Ob/Gyn* 1:64–67 (May) 1973.

Cornblath, Marvin, Diagnosing and treating neonatal hypoglycemia, *Contemp. Ob/Gyn* 8:95–99, 1976.

Cranley, Mecca S., When a high-risk infant is born, *Am. J. Nurs.* 75:1696–1699 (Oct.) 1975.

Crosse, V. Mary, and Hill, Eileen Elise, *The Preterm Baby,* 8th ed. Churchill-Livingstone, Edinburgh, 1975.

Depp, Richard, The puzzle of postmaturity, *Contemp. Ob/Gyn* 3:109–113 (June) 1974.

Desmond, Murdina M., Rudolph, Arnold J., and Phitaksphariwan, Phuangnoi, The transitional care nursery, *Pediatr. Clin. North Am.* 13:651–668 (Aug.) 1966.

Dubowitz, Lily, M. S., Dubowitz, Victor, and Goldberg, Cissie, Clinical assessment of gestational age in the newborn infant, *J. Pediatr.* 77:1–10 (July) 1970.

Dweck, Harry S. *et al.*, Early development of the tiny premature infant, *Am. J. Dis. Child.* 126:28–34 (July) 1973.

Fanaroff, Avroy A., Kennell, John H., and Klaus, Marshall H., Follow-up of low birth weight infants—The predictive value of maternal visiting patterns, *Pediatrics* 49:287–290 (Feb.) 1972.

Fitzhardinge, P. M., and Ramsey, M., The improving outlook for the small prematurely born infant, *Dev. Med. Child Neurol.* 15:447–459, 1973.

Fogarty, Sarah, The nurse and the high-risk infant, *Nurs. Clin. North Am.* 8:533–547 (Sept.) 1973.

Gluck, Louis, and Kulovich, Marie V., Fetal lung development. Current concepts, *Pediatr. Clin. North Am.* 20:367–379 (May) 1973.

Gersony, Welton M., Persistence of the fetal circulation: A commentary, *J. Pediatr.* 82:1103–1106 (June) 1973.

Goldenberg, Robert L., and Nelson, Kathleen, Iatrogenic respiratory distress syndrome, *Am. J. Obstet. Gynecol.* 123:617–620 (Nov. 15) 1975.

Gregory, George A., Aspiration syndrome in infants, *Int. Anesthesiol. Clin.* 15:97–105, 1977.

Gross, Gary P. *et al.*, Hyperviscosity in the neonate, *J. Pediatr.* 82:1004–1012 (June) 1973.

Gruenwald, Peter (ed.), *The Placenta and Its Maternal Supply Line.* University Park Press, Baltimore, Md., 1975.

———, Growth of the human infant, *Am. J. Obstet. Gynecol.* 94:1112–1132, 1966.

———, Chronic fetal distress and placental insufficiency, *Biol. Neonat.* 5:215–265, 1963.

Gryboski, Joyce, Gastointestinal problems in the infant, *Major Probl. Clin. Pediatr.* 13:12–23; 283–297, 1975.

———, Suck and swallow in the premature infant, *Pediatrics* 43:96–102 (Jan.) 1969.

———, The swallowing mechanism of the neonate. I. Esophageal and gastric motility, *Pediatrics* 35:445–452 (March) 1965.

Heird, William C., and Dirscoll, John M., Newer methods for feeding low-birth-weight infants, *Clin. Perinatol.* 2:309–325 (Sept.) 1975.

Hey, E. N., "The care of babies in incubators, in *Recent Advances in Paediatrics,* edited by D. Hull and D. Gardner. Churchill, London, 1971, p. 171.

James, L. Stanley, and Lanman, Jonathan T. (eds.), History of oxygen therapy and retrolental fibroplasia. *Pediatrics, Part II* [*Suppl.*] 57:591–642 (April) 1976.

Johnson, S. H., and Grubbs, J. P., The premature infant's reflex behaviors: Effect on maternal–child relationship, *JOGN Nurs.* 4:15–20 (May/June) 1975.

Katz, Viola, Auditory stimulation and developmental behavior of the premature infant, *Nurs. Res.* 20:195–201 (May/June) 1971.

Kennedy, Janet C., The high-risk maternal–infant acquaintance process, *Nurs. Clin. North Am.* 8:549–556 (Sept.) 1973.

Klaus, Marshall H., and Fanaroff, Avroy A., *Care of the High-Risk Neonate.* Saunders, Philadelphia, Pa., 1973.

Korner, Anneliese, Early stimulation and maternal care as related to infant capabilities and individual differences, *Early Child Dev. Care,* 2:307–327, 1973.

Korones, Sheldon B., *High-Risk Newborn Infants. The Basis for Intensive Nursing Care,* 2nd ed. Mosby, St. Louis, Mo., 1976.

Kretchmer, Norman, Ecology of the newborn infant, *Birth Defects* 10:19–27, 1974.

Landwirth, Julius, Continuous nasogastric infusion feedings of infants of low birth weight, *Clin. Pediatr.* 13:603–608 (July) 1974.

Lubchenco, Lula O., The high-risk infant, *Major Prob. Clin. Pediatr.* Vol. 14, 1976.

———, Assessment of gestational age and development at birth, *Pediatr. Clin. North Am.* 17:125–145 (Feb.) 1970.

———, Hansman, Charlotte, and Boyd, Edith, Intrauterine growth in length and head circumference as estimated from live births at gestational ages from 26 to 42 weeks, *Pediatrics* 37:403–408 (March) 1966.

McLean, Frances H., Significance of birthweight for gestational age in identifying infants at risk, *JOGN Nurs.* 3:19–24 (Nov./Dec.) 1974.

Michaelis, Richard *et al.,* Activity states in premature and full-term infants, *Dev. Psychobiol.* 6:209–215, 1973.

Miller, Frank C., The significance of meconium during labor, *Contemp. Ob/Gyn* 6:17–19 (Nov.) 1975.

Oh, William, Fluid and electrolyte management, in *Neonatology,* edited by Gordon B. Avery. Lippincott, Philadelphia, Pa., 1975, pp. 471–486.

Pagliara, Anthony S. *et al.,* Hypoglycemia in infancy and childhood. Part I, *J. Pediatr.* 82:365–379 (March) 1973.

Powell, Louisa F., The effect of extra stimulation and maternal involvement on the development of low birth weight infants and on maternal behavior. *Child. Dev.* 45:106–113 (March) 1974.

Rawlings, Grace, Stewart, Ann, Reynolds, E. O. R., and Strang, L. B., Changing prognosis for infants of very low birth weight, *Lancet,* 1:516–519 (March 13) 1971.

Renfield, Marilyn L., Small-for-date baby, in *Neonatology,* edited by Gordon B. Avery. Lippincott, Philadelphia, Pa., 1975, p. 190.

Rhea, James W. *et al.,* Nasojejunal (transpyloric) feeding: A commentary, *J. Pediatr.* 86:451–452 (March) 1975.

Roberts, Joyce E., Suctioning the newborn, *Am. J. Nurs.* 73:63–65 (Jan.) 1973.

Robinson, R., The pre-term baby, *Br. Med. J.* 4:416, 1971.

Rothfeder, Barbara, and Tiedeman, Mary, Feeding the low-birth-weight neonate, *Nurs. 77* 7:58–59 (Oct.) 1977.

Roy, R. Neil, and Sinclair, John C., Hydration of the low-birth-weight infant. *Clin. Perinatol.* 2:393–417 (Sept.), 1975.

Rudolph, Abraham, Cardiac failure in children: A hemodynamic view, *Hosp. Pract.* 5:44–55 (July) 1970.

———, Heymann, Michael A., Medical treatment of the ductus arteriosus, *Hosp. Pract.* 12:57–65 (Feb.) 1977.

Santulli, Thomas V., Acute necrotizing enterocolitis: Recognition and management, *Hosp. Pract.,* 9:129–135 (Nov.) 1974.

——— *et al.,* Acute necrotizing enterocolitis in infancy: A review of 64 cases, *Pediatrics* 55:376–387 (March) 1975.

Sarasohn, Charles, Care of the very small premature infant, *Pediatr. Clin. North Am.* 24:619–632 (Aug.) 1977.

Scarr-Salapatek, Sandra, and Williams, Margaret L., A stimulation program for low birth weight infants, *Am. J. Pub. Health* 62:662–667 (May) 1972.

Schaffer, Alexander J., and Avery, Mary Ellen, *Diseases of the Newborn,* 4th ed. Saunders, Philadelphia, Pa., 1977.

Schifrin, Barry S., Iatrogenic fetal distress, *Int. Anesthesiol. Clin.* 11:119–140 (Summer) 1973.

Schulte, F. J., Apnea, *Clin. Perinatol.* 4:65–76 (March) 1977.

Scopes, J. W., Thermoregulation in the newborn, in *Neonatology,* edited by Gordon B. Avery. Lippincott, Philadelphia, Pa., 1975, pp. 99–109.

Segall, Mary E., Cardiac responsivity to auditory stimulation in premature infants, *Nurs. Res.* 21:15–19 (Jan.–Feb.) 1972.

Shaw, J. C. L., Parenteral nutrition in the management of sick low birthweight infants, *Pediatr. Clin. North Am.* 20:333–358 (May) 1973.

Sinclair, John C., Driscoll, John M., Heird, William C., and Winters, Robert W., Supportive management of the sick neonate, *Pediatr. Clin. North Am.* 17:863–893 (Nov.) 1970.

Silverman, William A., The lesson of retrolental fibroplasia, *Sci. Am.* 236:100–107 (June) 1977.

Stern, Leo, The use and misuse of oxygen in the newborn infant, *Petiatr. Clin. North Am.* 20:447–464 (May) 1973.

Ting, Pauline, and Brady, June P., Tracheal suction in meconium aspiration, *Am. J. Obstet. Gynecol.* 122:767–771 (July 15) 1975.

Torrance, Jane T., Temperature readings of premature infants, *Nurs. Res.* 17:312–320, 1968.

Usher, Robert H., The special problems of the premature infant, in *Neonatology,* edited by Gordon B. Avery. Lippincott, Philadelphia, Pa., 1975, pp. 157–188.

———, McLean, Frances, and Scott, Kenneth E., Judgement of fetal age. II. Clinical significance of gestational age and an objective method for its assessment, *Pediatr. Clin. North Am.* 13:835–848 (Aug.) 1966.

Valman, H. B., Heath, C. D., and Brown, R. J. K., Continuous intragastric milk feedings in infants of low birth weight, *Br. Med. J.* 3:547–550 (Sept. 2) 1972.

Van Caillse, Micheline, and Powell, Geraldine K., Nasoduodenal versus nasogastric feeding in the very low birthweight infant, *Pediatrics* 56:1065–1072 (Dec.) 1975.

Vorherr, Helmuth, Placental insufficiency and post-maturity, in *Human Placentation,* edited by I. A. Brosens, G. Dixon, and W. B. Robertson. Excerpta Medica, Amsterdam, 1975.

———, Placental insufficiency in relation to postterm pregnancy and fetal postmaturity, *Am. J. Obstet. Gynecol.* 123:67–103 (Sept. 1) 1975.

Warrick, Louise H., Family-centered care in the premature nursery, *Am. J. Nurs.* 71:2134–2138 (Nov.) 1971.

Wells, David H., and Zachman, Richard D., Nasojejunal feedings in low-birth-weight infants, *J. Pediatr.* 87:276–279 (Aug.) 1975.

Williams, Paul R., and Oh, William, Effects of radiant warmers on insensible water loss in newborn infants, *Am. J. Dis. Child.* 128:511–514 (Oct.) 1974.

Yashiro, Kamio, Adams, Forrest H., Emmanouildes, George C., and Michey, M. Ray, Preliminary studies on the thermal environment of low-birth-weight infants, *J. Pediatr.* 82:991–994 (June) 1973.

Yu, Victor H., Effect of body position on gastric emptying in the neonate, *Arch. Dis. Child.* 50:500–504, 1975.

Zachman, Richard D., Postmaturity, *Perinatal News.* Madison General Hospital, Wisconsin Perinatal Center, Southcentral Region, April, 1977.

26

Abnormalities and Diseases of the Newborn— Medical Aspects and Nursing Care

The nurse who cares for the newborn infant must have knowledge of those abnormalities and diseases that are peculiar to the newborn period or that originate before or at the time of birth. Because of her close contact with the newborn infant, she is in a position to make valuable observations of the functioning of the various body systems, of deviations from normal behavior, and of appearance of early signs and symptoms of disease. She should be able to recognize early manifestations of abnormalities or disease and understand their signficance. An early report to the physician of any deviation from normal makes early treatment possible. Early treatment often has a profound effect on future development and may be essential for survival.

RESPIRATORY DISTRESS

Respiratory distress may be present at birth, or it may appear after normal respirations have been established. Some babies have difficulty immediately, they are apneic at birth or become apneic after having taken a few gasps; others breathe well at birth, but respirations become inadequate later; and some have apnea at birth and also subsequent distress. Respiratory failure may be due to failure of the central nervous system, resulting in apnea or hypopnea; or it may be caused by difficulty in the respiratory system

itself; or both the central nervous system and the respiratory system may be involved.

Hypoxia may occur before birth. It may develop at any time during the baby's in utero existence, either before labor or at any stage during labor or delivery. Conditions resulting in inadequate oxygenation in the fetus are apt to cause respiratory distress after birth, either immediate or delayed difficulty. Hypoxia is a great hazard to the fetus and the newborn baby. Inadequate exchange of gases affects every tissue in the body and produces changes to a certain, and sometimes irreparable, degree depending on the severity and the duration of asphyxia and the susceptibility of the various tissues. Asphyxia is one of the two most common causes of neonatal death. Sometimes the baby who survives asphyxia has permanent cerebral damage.

Causes of Respiratory Distress

There are many reasons a baby may not breathe at birth or may have difficulty later. Often respiratory distress is caused by a condition that began before birth. It may be of maternal, placental, or fetal origin.

Among complications operative before birth and also often after delivery are (1) illness of the mother due to toxemia, diabetes, or cardiorespiratory disease, (2) antepartum bleeding, (3) erythroblastosis fetalis, (4) interference with umbilical cord circulation, (5) depression of the baby's respiratory center from maternal analgesia or anesthesia, (6) prolonged labor, (7) severe and prolonged contractions, and (8) trauma at birth with resultant cerebral hemorrhage.

Conditions of the baby after birth that may cause respiratory distress are (1) immaturity of the lungs or a deficiency in their function; (2) obstruction of the air passages from aspiration of meconium in the amniotic fluid or aspiration of mucus and blood from the birth canal; (3) congenital defects; and (4) diseases of the infant such as infection and hemolytic disease. It may also be associated with conditions outside of the respiratory system such as intracranial hemorrhage, and congenital anomalies, and metabolic imbalance such as hypoglycemia.

Prevention

Prevention of respiratory distress begins with prenatal care. Advice to the mother in hygienic measures to observe during pregnancy; evaluation of the mother's pelvis for possible dystocia in order to plan management of delivery; early recognition and treatment of complications of pregnancy; and optimum control of preexisting diseases such as diabetes will help to avoid or minimize conditions that may cause fetal hypoxia.

Care given the mother during labor and delivery is very important in prevention of fetal hypoxia or in prevention of conditions that may cause distress after birth. The mother's vital signs must be observed for changes that result from conditions that will also affect the baby. Observation and careful management of bleeding from the uterus, of prolonged labor, and of abnormal uterine contractions are essential in prevention of fetal distress. The administration of analgesic drugs to the mother must be carefully controlled to avoid depression of the baby, a significant cause of newborn respiratory difficulty.

Signs of fetal distress during labor, or during the prenatal period, should alert all responsible for the baby's care to the possible need for resuscitation after delivery and to the necessity of close observation in the immediate neonatal period for later respiratory difficulty. Careful and frequent observation of the rate and rhythm of the fetal heart throughout labor, constant observation during the second stage of labor and during delivery, is the best way to recognize an impending fetal asphyxia. Meconium-stained amniotic fluid signifies that distress has or is occurring. The appearance of golden-yellow amniotic fluid when the membranes rupture and yellow staining of the baby's skin at birth, or staining of the vernix caseosa, are signs of fetal distress during the prenatal period, sometimes days or weeks prior to birth, and of a predisposition to respiratory difficulty after birth.

Oxygen, administered to the mother when the fetus shows signs of distress during labor, may improve the baby's condition by increasing the oxygen saturation of the fetal blood and may prevent severe respiratory depression at birth. Administration of oxygen to the mother may be very beneficial when the fetus is deprived of an adequate oxygen supply due to placental separation, or pressure on the umbilical cord during contractions. If the cause of intrauterine asphyxia during labor cannot be corrected and if labor has progressed to such a stage that conditions are favorable for an operative procedure, the baby may be delivered immediately to prevent further danger from the effects of intrauterine asphyxia. When immediate delivery is not possible a cesarean section may be indicated.

Since trauma at birth may cause respiratory difficulty, every effort is made to avoid injury to the baby during delivery. This applies to a rapid delivery as well as to a difficult one. When delivery is imminent in the absence of the physician, the nurse should not attempt to retard delivery, except for taking measures to control the delivery process and thus prevent rapid expulsion of the baby.

All equipment necessary for resuscitation must be in readiness and in good condition at all times so that any baby with respiratory distress, even when difficulty is unexpected, can be given aid immediately.

When a pregnancy is complicated, assessment of fetal well-being is made at regular intervals to determine if the intrauterine environment continues to be safe and if the fetus will be able to tolerate labor. Findings may show that delivery by cesarean section prior to labor is indicated to avoid distress from hypoxia. Assessment of fetal well-being and fetal maturity is described in Chapter 21.

Signs and Symptoms of Respiratory Distress[1]

All babies should be closely observed during the first hours of life, but, for some, concern over possible respiratory insufficiency is particularly great. Those included are babies born prematurely, babies whose mothers had complications during pregnancy, particularly antepartum bleeding or diabetes, and those who aspirated meconium-stained amniotic fluid or who required resuscitation at birth. Babies in whom the risk of respiratory insufficiency is increased should be under intense observation to detect significant changes early.

The baby should be closely observed for character of respirations, respiratory rate, pulse rate, blood pressure, skin color, and temperature. The frequency of recording of vital signs is determined by the baby's condition. A record is made on admission and every one-half hour at first. The interval may be lengthened to one, two, three, and finally four hours, as indicated by a satisfactory status. The baby's activity, cry, sucking ability, and all other behavior should also be noted and recorded.

A baby who requires close observation is often placed in an incubator where care similar to that given a premature baby can be provided. An incubator facilitates regulation of heat, oxygen, and humidity and also makes observations easier.

Tachypnea

Increase in respiratory rate is a common and easily observable sign of respiratory difficulty in

[1] George Polgar, Practical pulmonary physiology, *Pediatr. Clin. North Am.* 20:303–322 (May) 1973.

newborns. Tachypnea is a very important warning sign of impending trouble. Any increase in elastic recoil of the lungs (i.e., stiffening of the lung as in atelectasis) or increase in resistance of the airways or interstitial lung disease is likely to result in an increase in the respiratory rate. The increased rate does not mean increased effective ventilation but only that more work is being done to try to ventilate the lung.

To observe a trend toward tachypnea, respirations should be counted every 15 minutes during the first hour, every one to two hours for the next 48 hours or longer, depending on the baby's condition, and every four hours until the baby is no longer in danger, or until treatment for distress is no longer necessary. Respirations should be counted for at least one full minute while the baby is quiet.

Rapid respirations are not normal except for a short time in the first and second reactivity periods after birth (see pages 492 and 493). If a rapid rate, usually over 60 breaths per minute, does not show a significant increase after the first hour, and decreases to normal within a few hours the trend is normal. When respiratory rate shows a significant increase over the average rate during the first hour, the trend is abnormal and signifies respiratory distress. The respiratory rate then usually rises to 60 or above and may be as rapid as 80 breaths per minute or even much higher.

Apneic Spells

Periodic breathing is common in premature babies. Most prematures breathe more irregularly than full-term infants. Some prematures have distinct periods of apnea of 5 to 10 seconds duration, alternating with periods of ventilation of 10 to 20 seconds. The respirations of the premature are usually fast during the ventilatory periods, but the average rate per minute may be somewhat low because of the periods of apnea.

Apneic spells, which are periods of nonbreathing that last longer than the ones in periodic breathing (longer than 20 seconds), are not normal and should be considered a sign of respiratory difficulty. Apneic spells are likely to occur in prematures who have some cardiorespiratory or central nervous system stress. The apneic spells are often due to central nervous system immaturity and the stress of disease.

Periodic breathing and apneic spells are described in more detail on pages 714–15.

Chest Retraction

Chest retraction is a valuable sign of abnormality of respiration. It is a sign of increased respiratory work. When expansion of the lung meets increased resistance because of stiffening, atelectasis, or edema, or because of an obstruction of the upper airways, a greater than normal respiratory effort is made.

With an increase in respiratory effort there is an increase in negative pressure in the chest. Since the newborn's chest is very pliable, the increased negative pressure tends to pull the softest parts of the baby's chest inward with inspirations. Pulling inward of these soft parts means retraction of the intercostal spaces, the suprasternal and infrasternal areas, the sternum itself, and the region of the rib cage that corresponds to insertion of the diaphragm.

Chest retraction may range from mild to marked sinking of the intercostal spaces and/or xiphoid retraction with each inspiration. When retraction is severe, the baby may have seesaw breathing, a type of respiration in which the abdomen rises and the chest sinks on inspiration, and the abdomen falls and the chest expands on expiration. Sometimes the lower chest remains continuously retracted when respiration is difficult. Occasionally there is marked expansion of the upper chest, severe retraction at the lower costal margin, and little movement of the abdomen.

Retraction of the chest wall decreases the range of expansion of the lung. With severe difficulty the lung can inflate very little with inspiration, and the chest actually flattens rather than expands. Instead of chest expansion the abdomen expands. In such seesaw type of breathing expansion of the diaphragm permits ventilation of the lower parts of the lung.

A clear description of the baby's chest movements and how and where the chest retracts should be carefully recorded. Retraction of the thorax is proportional to the negative pressure inside the chest. There is quite good correlation between the degree of retraction and the severity of the respiratory difficulty.

Increasing retraction of the chest creates a vicious cycle. The increasing respiratory effort and increasing amount of negative pressure require increased expenditure of energy and thus more oxygen consumption. The increasing degree of retraction, however, decreases effective ventilation of the lung and thus decreases gas exchange. With the increased need for energy for ventilation and increased use of oxygen, the amount of oxygen available for other body functions can become inadequate. Exhaustion from breathing can lead to death. Assisted ventilation may thus be indicated in babies with severe retraction.

Sometimes the chest has a barrel-shaped appearance with distress. The chest is well expanded, with little retraction, but is stiff and does not move easily. Stiff chest movements and hyperexpansion may indicate that the baby's lungs still contain considerable lung fluid, a condition often called "wet lung."

Chin Tug

When a baby's respirations are labored, a tug on the chin may be seen with inspirations. With moderate distress the chin descends, but the lips remain closed. When distress is severe, lips part and the mouth opens as the chin descends during inspirations.

Flaring of the Nostrils

Flaring of the nostrils with inspiration is a reflex response to respiratory distress whereby the baby attempts to widen the nasal passages. Although flaring of the nostrils does not aid breathing, it is a sign of respiratory distress. Often inspiratory flaring of the nostrils alternates with an expiratory grunt.

Expiratory Grunt

An expiratory grunt is abnormal and is evidence of severe distress, especially when it is audible with the naked ear. The grunt is a reflex used by the baby as a protective mechanism to prolong end expiration and improve oxygenation of his lungs. Often an expiratory grunt or moan is the first sign of respiratory distress noticed by the nursery staff. Its appearance should immediately alert the nurse to watch for other evidence of respiratory difficulty, and it should be reported to the physician promptly.

To improve oxygenation the baby approximates the vocal cords and builds up some expiratory resistance behind the partially occluded glottis. The effect of this back pressure, which builds up all the way to the alveoli, and the relatively larger expiratory resistance, is believed to permit the areas of the lungs that are not well aerated to obtain a little more air for gas exchange over a slightly longer period of time. In a sense grunting is a modified Valsalva maneuver, in which the intrapleural pressure during expiration is increased by closure of the glottis and contraction of the abdominal muscles.

A grunting or moaning sound with expiration is made when air is expired past the approximated vocal cords. The respiratory grunt may be short or may be prolonged throughout the entire exhalation. It is sometimes accompanied by a whining or a moaning sound. The respiratory grunt may be audible only when a stethoscope is held near the baby's mouth but often is loud enough to be heard with the naked ear. The sound may be so loud that it is heard throughout the nursery. It sometimes is most apparent when the baby is disturbed by care or treatments.

Prolonged Expiration

Prolonged expiration, which may be difficult to observe because of the baby's rapid respirations, may occur in the presence of lower airway difficulty. With respiratory problems, the expiratory phase of respiration is likely to be prolonged in relation to the inspiratory phase, since air will flow in easier than it will flow out. Bronchi tend to become wider in inspiration. If a relatively higher pressure necessary to expire air through higher resistances can be maintained for a short period, there will be more time for back pressure to enlarge the alveolar spaces that are connected to the more obstructed airways and more chance for air to go into these spaces and for gas exchange to take place. The effect of the prolonged expiration is similar to that of the expiratory grunt.

Cough and Sneeze

Cough is rare in the newborn. It does not seem to be a very well-developed reflex in the baby and may not be present even when there is a large amount of secretion in the respiratory tract or when there has been aspiration.

A baby has a good gag reflex and sneeze reflex and uses both to protect the respiratory system. The sneeze is very common in the newborn. It does not necessarily indicate that the baby has a problem of infection or disease. The sneeze is necessary for clearing of the baby's nostrils. A baby is an obligatory nose-breather who can breathe through the mouth only with great difficulty because of a relatively large tongue and a high larynx which brings the epiglottis very close to the uvula. With nose breathing so important for air passage, sneezing is an important means of keeping the nostrils patent.

Labored Respiration

To summarize some of the signs of labored respiration described above, chest retraction is the most obvious sign of increased work of inspiration. Accompanying this may be descent of the chin, flaring of the nostrils, and rhythmic movement of other parts of the body, such as head bobbing, with respiration. Sometimes there is also a visible rise of the abdominal muscles and other accessory muscles of respiration as expiration is somewhat forced and prolonged. In addition to these signs, the baby may be restless or may be listless and unresponsive.

Color

Generalized cyanosis may or may not be present with respiratory difficulty. When cyanosis is present, the nurse should note the degree of cyanosis, if it is generalized or localized, and if it increases with activity and with crying. Cyanosis of the hands and feet and circumoral cyanosis may be present in the normal baby for an hour or two after birth, but within a few minutes after birth the rest of the body should be pink. A pale or grayish color is a sign of serious disturbance and may be indicative of shock or circulatory collapse.

Cyanosis is not an objective sign of the amount of pulmonary insufficiency. Color of the skin or mucous membranes does not indicate the level of arterial PO_2. By the time frank cyanosis is seen the hypoxemia is already quite far advanced. Cyanosis is not observable until the Pao_2 is down to 42 mmHg or less. To determine how well oxygenation is taking place oxygen tension of the arterial blood must be measured directly whenever facilities are available.

Activity and Muscle Tone

The baby's activity, cry, sucking ability, and all other behavior should be closely observed and recorded. A baby with respiratory insufficiency may be unusually quiet and less active than a healthy baby or the baby may be restless. Usually the baby does not keep his extremities well flexed and thus appears quite limp. His cry may be of a whining or a moaning character, signifying a grunting respiration.

If the baby has been sucking to take food, he is likely to show some difficulty with sucking. Normally a baby does not need to stop sucking to breathe, but the baby with respiratory difficulty may need to stop frequently as if to catch his breath.

Shock

A baby with respiratory difficulty may show signs of shock. He may have systemic hypotension and poor peripheral circulation as evidenced by poor capillary filling when the skin is pressed and then released. The baby may have poor muscle tone and may have difficulty maintaining a normal body temperature. The trend of the blood pressure, pulse rate, respiratory rate, and body temperature must be closely observed and recorded frequently. The heart and respiratory rates of sick babies are usually monitored with the aid of electronic monitors if they are available, but the nurse must also listen to the heart for abnormal sounds and watch the respirations for evidence of abnormal chest movement.

Blood Gas and Acid–Base Disturbance[2]

Blood Gases

A baby with respiratory disease will quickly have a disturbance in arterial blood gases. Poor ventilation is likely to result in a decrease in the partial pressure of oxygen in arterial blood and an increase in the tension of carbon dioxide. With general hypoventilation the arterial PO_2 decreases by approximately the same amount that the arterial PCO_2 increases. This is likely to be the situation when respiration is depressed because of central nervous system depression as may occur at birth.

A more common respiratory problem is one in which there is uneven distribution of ventilation. In contrast to perfusion in the lung, there is a relative hypoventilation of some of the alveoli. When the ventilation–perfusion ratio is uneven, the oxygen tension may be affected more and earlier than the carbon dioxide tension. The carbon dioxide, which diffuses more readily, can be eliminated through the well-ventilated areas of the lung, but oxygen cannot be picked up as easily. The arterial PO_2 will then drop more quickly than the PCO_2 rises. In this situation there is usually a problem with hypoxia but not with excess carbon dioxide in the blood, at least not in the early stages of the disease. In

[2] Sheldon B. Korones, *High-Risk Newborn Infants*, 2nd ed. Mosby, St. Louis, Mo., 1976.

pulmonary disease of the newborn hypoxia is much more common than hypercapnia.

In some cases of uneven ventilation–perfusion ratios blood flow is decreased or bypasses alveoli that are ventilated. This results in an increased retention of carbon dioxide and an increase in arterial P_{CO_2} An elevated arterial P_{CO_2} is called hypercapnia or hypercarbia.

Sometimes, in response to stimuli or in an attempt to correct for lack of oxygen, hyperventilation occurs. With hyperventilation carbon dioxide is blown off in excess and the arterial P_{CO_2} decreases. In this circumstance, oxygen tension level may be normal or continue abnormally low, and the P_{CO_2} will also be low. This situation is almost always iatrogenic with bag and mask ventilation or use of respirator.

Blood samples for measurements of both arterial P_{O_2} and P_{CO_2} are very important laboratory tests that are used to determine the status of respiratory distress and the necessary treatment.[3] The P_{O_2} measurement is necessary to determine the extent of hypoxia, which cannot be judged by the baby's color. The presence of cyanosis will indicate hypoxia but not the degree. Often the baby has already had some of the ill effects of hypoxia by the time cyanosis appears or else the baby's color may not change much even when hypoxia is relatively severe. The P_{CO_2} measurement is used to determine how well ventilation is taking place and also to measure how much carbon dioxide is collecting in the blood.

Poor alveolar ventilation, with resultant hypoxia, leads to abnormal biochemical and physiologic changes in the body. Tissue hypoxia results in anaerobic metabolism, which leads to metabolic acidosis. When adequate oxygen is not available, glucose is incompletely metabolized to lactic acid instead of to carbon dioxide and water. The lactic acid accumulates in

[3] Pa_{O_2} and Pa_{CO_2} refer to partial pressure of oxygen and carbon dioxide in arterial blood. The subscript "a" will usually not be used in this chapter because the measurements of these gases are customarily taken from arterial blood and the symbols "P_{O_2}" and "P_{CO_2}" are understood to mean partial pressure of oxygen and of carbon dioxide in arterial blood.

the body, lowers the pH, and brings about a metabolic acidosis. Anaerobic glycolysis also depletes glycogen stores quickly because more glycogen is required for glucose production when oxygen is not available. Anaerobic metabolism is not very efficient and uses up a great deal of glycogen to produce energy. The result of all this is often hypoglycemia, especially when stores are small.

Cardiopulmonary Consequences of Altered Blood Gases

Constriction of the pulmonary arterioles and a reopening of the ductus arteriosus are other serious consequences of hypoxia. This situation is greatly accentuated if acidosis is also present. When the pulmonary arterioles constrict and the ductus arteriosus opens, there is pulmonary hypoperfusion with impairment of circulation through the lungs and a reestablishment of shunting of blood through the ductus arteriosus and also the foramen ovale. These changes are similar to some aspects of the fetal circulatory pattern. Blood flowing through the lungs is not well oxygenated, and some of the blood may return to the systemic circulation unoxygenated. Hypoxia worsens and hepatic and renal function may be suppressed.

Correction of Blood Gases

Oxygen is administered for treatment of hypoxia, and ventilation of the lungs is necessary if the baby is not able to move air in and out of the lungs adequately. With reoxygenation of the tissues complete glucose metabolism is restored. Production of lactic acid decreases and pH improves with a lessening of metabolic acidosis. The pulmonary arterioles respond with less constriction, and the ductus arteriosus may close again. Circulation through the lungs improves. When oxygen is administered frequent measurements of P_{O_2} are necessary to regulate the concentration of inspired oxygen. It must be administered in an amount that will return the P_{O_2} to normal but not raise it above normal. Requirements for oxygen may change very rapidly as ventilation and circulation through the lungs change. Every effort is made to maintain the P_{O_2} between 50 and 80 mmHg. Use of oxygen is further described on pages 767–72.

The P_{CO_2} measurements are used to determine the amount of ventilation that is taking place. Since P_{CO_2} rises with hypoventilation and decreases with hyperventilation, it is the carbon dioxide tension of the blood, not the partial pressure of oxygen, that gives the correct indication of hypo- or hyperventilation. Carbon dioxide tension is an important measure in determining when ventilation needs assistance. Also when assisted ventilation is being used, the proper level of alveolar ventilation (as determined by the pressure, volume, and rate settings) is regulated on the basis of arterial P_{CO_2} measurements.

Acid–Base Balance

Carbonic acid is one of the products of normal tissue metabolism. It is categorized as a volatile acid because it is constantly converted to carbon dioxide in the blood and eliminated in its gaseous state through the lungs. The respiratory system thus directly controls blood levels of carbonic acid. The concentration of carbonic acid in the blood is determined by the amount of carbon dioxide present (by the P_{CO_2}), and the amount of carbon dioxide in the blood is dependent on the ventilatory ability of the lungs.

Ordinarily the respiratory center of the medulla responds quickly to the need to eliminate carbon dioxide from the body or to conserve it and directs the respiratory rate and depth accordingly. With respiratory disease, however, the lungs may not be able to eliminate carbon dioxide adequately. This retention of P_{CO_2} and its carbonic acid counterpart then results in an acidosis. Measurement of P_{CO_2} is very important therefore in helping to determine how much the retention of carbon dioxide is contributing to an acidosis. Similarly, if hyperventilation is contributing to excessive loss of carbon dioxide the P_{CO_2} level will show that.

An acid–base equilibrium is normally maintained in the body and is necessary to normal function. Normal metabolism produces acids which must be neutralized and excreted from the body. These acids are volatile (carbonic acid, described above) and nonvolatile (or fixed) acids, principally lactic, sulfuric and phosphoric acids. The nonvolatile acids are buffered in the blood and excreted through the kidneys. A buffer is a substance which combines chemically with excess acid or base to modify changes in the body acid–base balance. Normally, when nonvolatile acids, such as lactic acid, are added to the blood, their effect is minimized through the buffering activity of the bicarbonate/carbonic acid system. In this reaction lactic acid is buffered by sodium bicarbonate and converted to sodium lactate and carbonic acid. The sodium lactate is excreted by the kidneys and the carbonic acid by the lungs, as described above. Thus the respiratory center regulates the concentration of volatile acid, and the kidneys control the blood content of nonvolatile acid. The kidneys respond more slowly than the lungs but tend to carry compensatory mechanisms closer to completion.

Any serious illness in a newborn is likely to lead to an acid–base imbalance. Disturbance in acid-base equilibrium is described by a measurement of the acidity of the blood, known as the pH. Abnormalities may result in a lowered pH (acidosis) or an increased pH (alkalosis). The normal pH ranges from 7.35 to 7.45. For normal metabolic processes to take place the acid–base balance must be kept within these very narrow limits. A pH below 7.25 clinically represents considerable acidosis. Although the range between normal and abnormal values is small in numbers, there is a tremendous difference in the acidity of the fluid when there is a small change in the numerical value of the pH.

Acidosis and alkalosis may be of respiratory or metabolic cause or a combination of both. Respiratory acidosis occurs when ventilation is inadequate and pulmonary gas exchange is decreased. Carbon dioxide is then retained in the blood, which means an increased P_{CO_2}. Respiratory alkalosis occurs with excessive elimination of carbon dioxide during hyperventilation. The P_{CO_2} is then low. In newborns the cause of respiratory alkalosis is most frequently mechanical ventilation that is given above physiologic needs.

Metabolic (nonrespiratory) acidosis occurs when there is an increase in nonvolatile acids in the body because of overproduction of acids, or impaired renal excretion of acids, or excessive loss of the base which serves to buffer the acids in the body. In newborns this condition is most likely to occur when hypoxia leads to anaerobic metabolism and an overproduction of lactic acid.

Metabolic (nonrespiratory) alkalosis means an increased concentration of base (bicarbonate). In the newborn this condition is most frequently caused by administration of an abnormally large dose of sodium bicarbonate, usually used to correct acidosis. On occasion, repeated vomiting is a cause.

Sometimes acid–base disturbances are present even when the pH is normal or nearly so. In such instances the body tries to compensate for the abnormality through adjustment in lung or renal function. A normal ratio between the acid and base is partially or fully restored. The pH may then be normal or nearly so, but the values for the acid and base are abnormally high or abnormally low. This is called a compensated acidosis or alkalosis. The original source of the acid–base disturbance may still exist in this condition and the correction of the pH may only be temporary.

The presence of acidosis or alkalosis is determined from pH measurement of the blood. The pH measures the hydrogen ion concentration after any buffer activity has taken place. The pH by itself does not indicate whether an abnormality in the pH is of respiratory or of metabolic origin. To determine its source it is also necessary to measure the Pco_2 and the plasma bicarbonate of the blood. The plasma bicarbonate measures the total bicarbonate concentration, of which the normal values are between 20 and 25 mEq/liter. An example of using Pco_2 and plasma bicarbonate values to determine the cause of acidosis is as follows: a high Pco_2 and normal plasma bicarbonate in the presence of a low pH would mean an uncompensated respiratory acidosis, whereas a normal Pco_2 and low plasma bicar-

bonate with a low pH would mean an uncompensated metabolic acidosis.

Base excess (BE) or deficit is a value that is also important in management of the baby with acid–base imbalance. The base excess is a value that is calculated rather than measured directly. It may be expressed as a positive or negative value, with the negative value also referred to as base deficit. The base excess indicates in mEq/liter the amount of blood buffer base that remains after hydrogen ion is buffered. Normal values of base excess in newborns ranges from +4 to −4 mEq/liter.

Base excess can be calculated from a nomogram when hemoglobin and two of the following parameters are known—the blood pH, CO_2, plasma bicarbonate, or total carbon dioxide content of plasma. In the baby the pH and Pco_2 measurements are usually the ones that are used to calculate base excess.

Blood Gas Measurements

It is apparent from what has been described above that serial measurements of blood gases and of blood pH are very important in care of a sick newborn. These values are likely to change rapidly and frequently when the baby is sick or is receiving treatment such as mechanical ventilation or corrective therapy for metabolic acidosis.

Arterial blood samples are usually taken for Pao_2, $Paco_2$, and pH. The blood may be obtained from one of several sites. In very sick babies, who need frequent checks, a catheter may be inserted into the umbilical artery and left in place. Otherwise, blood samples may be collected from puncture of the temporal, brachial, or radial arteries. With good circulation, blood samples from a warmed heel or finger are acceptable for Pco_2 and pH. The heel or finger should be warmed with a warm, moist pack before the needle stick for obtaining the blood is made. The warmth dilates the capillaries and arterioles so that blood flows freely during collection. The blood sample is then considered to be arterialized capillary blood. When venous stasis is present, as it may be in sick infants, capillary blood samples may vary considerably from arterial blood and the results may be less reliable. If there is a right-to-left shunt through the ductus, a blood sample from the right radial artery, which is preductal and independent of the degree of shunt through the ductus, reflects more closely the oxygen content going to the brain and the eyes than a sample obtained from an umbilical artery.

Capillary blood samples are not reliable for Po_2 determinations. They do not correlate with arterial Po_2 levels. When a premature baby is receiving oxygen, which must be carefully monitored to avoid hyperoxia, blood samples for Po_2 must certainly be obtained from an artery.

Blood samples for blood gases and pH may be taken every 4 hours or somewhat more or less frequently, depending upon the stability of the baby's condition. They are also taken within 15 to 30 minutes after every change in ambient oxygen and after every setting change when assisted ventilation is used.

Differential Diagnosis of Respiratory Distress

Respiratory distress in the first days of life may be caused by many conditions. Among these are hyaline membrane disease, aspiration, pneumonia, asphyxia, central nervous system depression, metabolic disturbances, tracheoesophageal fistula, cardiac problems, and many others. It is important to differentiate between pulmonary, cardiac, CNS, and metabolic causes.

Differential diagnosis can be very difficult, but often a complete history of past events and close observation of signs in the baby will give clues to a likely cause. For example, respiratory distress in a premature infant suggests hyaline membrane disease; in a postmature baby or one who is stained with meconium-stained amniotic fluid suggests aspiration; a history of premature rupture of the membranes and/or prolonged labor may mean pneumonia; excessive maternal analgesia and/or anesthesia may mean central nervous system depression in the infant; choking after feedings and history of hydramnios requires search for tracheoesophageal fistula;

and a baby's inability to breathe with the mouth closed suggests choanal atresia.[4]

A most useful and absolutely essential diagnostic aid is a chest x-ray, which will at least show or rule out such serious problems as a pneumothorax and a diaphragmatic hernia. When diagnosis is difficult a number of laboratory procedures, an electrocardiogram, a lumbar puncture to look for central nervous system problems, and perhaps other tests, may be indicated.

A few of the common causes of respiratory distress will be described after a discussion of intervention and care.

Intervention and Care

Treatment of respiratory distress consists of a number of supportive measures and protection of the baby against further stress. It includes adequate oxygenation, assisted ventilation when indicated, correction of acid–base imbalance, adequate caloric and fluid intake, protection against heat loss, and provision for rest.

For some causes of respiratory distress there will be specific therapy, as, for example, the administration of antibiotics when a baby has pneumonia and aspiration of air from the chest when a pneumothorax is present. In addition, however, a number of the supportive measures described below are important in the treatment of respiratory distress from any cause.

Use of Oxygen

The most important consideration in treatment of infants with respiratory distress is to improve their oxygenation. This is necessary for adequate tissue oxygenation and normal cardiac output and renal perfusion. Without good oxygenation the fetal circulatory pattern will persist, lactic acid will be produced with its resultant acidosis, poor renal function will develop, and shock is likely to develop.

[4] Mary Ellen Avery and Barry D. Fletcher, *The Lung and Its Disorders in the Newborn Infant*, 3rd ed. Saunders, Philadelphia, Pa., 1974, pp. 309–311.

Oxygen can be both very beneficial and very hazardous to newborns, especially prematures, and it must be administered with great care. The desirable amount of inspired oxygen is that which will provide adequate tissue oxygenation without undue risk of damage to certain tissues from an excessive amount.

The oxygen tension or partial pressure is measured in millimeters of mercury. The partial pressure can be thought of as a driving force that determines the degree to which oxygen will move from plasma to tissues.[5] In normal adults the arterial PO_2 (PaO_2) is in the 90 to 100 mm range. Current information indicates that an arterial oxygen tension between 50 and 80 mmHg is satisfactory in the newborn.[6] It should not exceed 100 mmHg in the baby.

With hypoxia anaerobic metabolism takes place, lactic acid is produced, and acidosis develops. The ductus arteriosus and the lung arterioles are sensitive to arterial PO_2 and to blood pH levels. With hypoxia and acidosis the ductus arteriosus opens, and the lung arterioles constrict, raising pulmonary vascular resistance and reducing pulmonary blood flow. This induces further hypoxemia by adversely affecting the ventilation and perfusion in the lung. This leads to a reduction in surfactant synthesis. A vicious cycle is set up of hypoxia which leads to further pulmonary insufficiency, which leads to more severe hypoxia.

Clinical cyanosis is not ordinarily a useful guide for need for oxygen in the infant as it is in the adult. In the newborn the PO_2 will be below 50 mmHg and perhaps even much lower when cyanosis appears. The arterial partial pressure of oxygen will give a much closer idea of the amount of oxygenation of tissues.

Oxygen administration is used clinically when hypoxemia exists in order to improve or maintain oxygenation until the condition causing the hypoxemia is remedied. It is used therefore in

asphyxia and resuscitation, in cardiopulmonary disorders, and in conditions where cerebral tissues are affected by such conditions as meningitis or intracranial hemorrhage.

Increase in oxygen concentration of inspired air (FIO_2) is used in respiratory distress syndrome where shunting in both ventilation and perfusion takes place and in pneumonia, where oxygen cannot diffuse well. The dose of oxygen is expressed as its fraction of inspired air (FIO_2).

Oxygen will act as a vasodilator when hypoxia has caused vasoconstriction. This generally happens at high concentrations of ambient oxygen resulting in a sudden jump in arterial PO_2. If oxygen is then again lowered rapidly and in large decrements, there may be a disproportionate fall in arterial PO_2 and vasoconstriction may follow. A gradual reduction in inspired oxygen concentration will minimize or avoid this flip-flop effect.

A patent ductus arteriosus, relatively common in prematures and also in respiratory distress syndrome, is more likely to close with high oxygen breathing. Closure is not likely to be permanent from this effect, however. It is important to add that, although hypoxemia should be corrected to enhance closure of the ductus, oxygen is not given to attempt closure in the absence of hypoxemia.

Since tissue hypoxia results in anaerobic metabolism and metabolic acidosis, the administration of oxygen will improve metabolism and help correct such acidosis.

Oxygen is administered in concentrations between 21 and 100 percent, depending on the amount needed to keep the baby's PO_2 normal. (Room air contains 20.9 percent oxygen.) Very high inspired oxygen concentration may be necessary in some conditions to maintain adequate arterial oxygenation. Arbitrary limits such as 40 percent (formerly considered safe) cannot be set. Oxygen must be ordered and administered in percentage (concentration) rather than by liters per minute. Flow rates (liters per minute) to oxygen gauges give an indication of how much oxygen flow is required for various environmental oxygen concentrations, but they are

[5] Leo Stern, The use and misuse of oxygen in the newborn infant, *Pediatr. Clin. North Am.* 20:447 (May) 1973.

[6] W. A. Hodson and D. A. Belenky, Management of respiratory problems, in *Neonatology*, edited by Gordon Avery. Lippincott, 1975, p. 271.

not acceptable for guides to oxygen administration.

Several types of oxygen analyzers are available to monitor the percentage of oxygen. One kind requires manual sampling of the ambient oxygen concentration, which must be done at least every two hours. Another kind monitors the inspired oxygen continuously. High and low limits may be preset with an alarm system. Some equipment and respirators may have devices for regulating oxygen concentration but they should not be totally relied upon.

Frequent measurements of arterial blood samples are necessary to determine the appropriate amount of inspired oxygen to be administered and to be able to decrease its concentration as soon as possible. Blood samples may be taken every 4, 8, or 12 hours depending on the severity of the baby's illness, the concentration of the inspired oxygen, and the ease or difficulty of obtaining blood. Blood for PO_2 values is obtained from an umbilical artery catheter or from the radial, brachial, or temporal artery.

Mixtures of oxygen and air may be administered by several methods. When the ambient concentration does not need to be high it may be allowed to flow into the baby's incubator. The incubator, however, is ineffective for high concentration because the portholes need to be opened frequently for infant care. An oxygen hood around the baby's head permits better control of the oxygen concentration and allows a considerable amount of the care of the baby without disturbing the hood. A removable lid on the hood allows positioning and suctioning of the baby without loss of inspired oxygen concentration. Oxygen is heavier than air and is not lost easily. When an oxygen hood is used gas flow through the hood should be at least 2 liters/min to prevent accumulation of carbon dioxide.[7]

Oxygen may also be given by mask, and when mechanical assistance to ventilation is necessary it may be given by mask, by nasal prongs, or sometimes by endotracheal tube.

[7] *Ibid.*, p. 272.

By whatever method oxygen is given it must be humidified and warmed. The gas mixture is bubbled through water which may be warmed by a heating coil. Prolonged use of oxygen by mask is contraindicated. It is very likely to chill the baby even if the oxygen is warmed because the flow of oxygen from the mask over the baby's face results in considerable heat loss by convection. The oxygen hood has somewhat the same effect. A cap on the baby's head helps to protect it. Warming the oxygen is very important. Humidity and warmth are also extremely important with nasal prongs or endotracheal tube administration because the oxygen is then introduced directly over mucosal tissue. Dry air would increase evaporative fluid loss from the mucosa and augment evaporative heat loss. The mucosa also dries easily with dry air and secretions become thick and tenacious.

Hyperoxia

Oxygen has a toxic effect when administered in excess. It is known to adversely affect two organs, and it may have a detrimental effect on other tissues. The retina of the eye may be damaged when the arterial PO_2 rises too high, and the lungs are injured when the concentration of inspired oxygen is high and the period of administration is long.

Bronchopulmonary Dysplasia

The effect of oxygen on the lung appears to be a direct effect of irritation of the lung tissue by the oxygen. A condition called bronchopulmonary dysplasia develops. Changes in lung tissue result in collapse of alveoli, atelectasis, and thickening of alveolar and lung vascular structures. These toxic changes make the lungs less permeable to oxygen and further increase its need. These lung changes clearly show the need for careful assessment of an appropriate, not excessive, amount of oxygen administration to newborns through careful monitoring of arterial oxygen tension. It is important to note, however, that in spite of continuing risk of prolonged oxygen administration, its use may be essential to sustain the baby until he can survive without it.

The danger of high ambient oxgyen, especially above 60 percent, is increased when used with endotracheal tube and IPPV (intermittent positive pressure ventilation). The exact relationship of these three factors in causation is not known.

Retrolental Fibroplasia

Retrolental fibroplasia, a retinopathy of prematurity, was discovered in 1942 as an acquired disease of premature infants. The disease is not present at birth; it results from too great exposure to oxygen. A high arterial concentration of oxygen (Po_2) causes changes in the immature retina of the premature and in the vitreous, and retinal detachment may follow. A retrolental (behind the lens) membrane forms as scar tissue develops (fibroplasia). The opaque tissue or grayish membrane behind the lens results in partial or complete blindness. Before prevention of this disease was known, it was a common cause of blindness in children.

By 1955 the cause of retrolental fibroplasia had been determined, and it is now a less common condition. Its frequency has been reduced by careful use of oxygen for hypoxia only, for the shortest time possible, and at the lowest concentration possible.

In rare cases retrolental fibroplasia occurs when oxygen has not been used or has been used only very briefly.

There appears to be considerable variability in arterial Po_2 at which the earliest phase of vasoconstriction of the retinal vessels occurs. Vascular spasm appears at less than 100 mmHg in some infants. Degree of immaturity and perhaps other factors may contribute to this. The very early phase of vasoconstriction appears to be reversible. Watching for this early period by ophthalmoscopic examination may afford a means of early assessment of potentially toxic reactions in the retina to oxygen, and also another means of monitoring and controlling oxygen

levels during the need for its administration.[8]

While prematures who are receiving continuous oxygen and are being carefully monitored appear to be quite safe against the effects of too much oxygen, small prematures who are resuscitated frequently from apneic episodes with a bag and mask connected to a direct oxygen line may be in danger of receiving too much oxygen. Some of these babies have a fairly normal cardiopulmonary function, do not have large right-to-left shunts of blood, and are ordinarily receiving little or no oxygen, but they have episodes of apnea. During resuscitation with bag and mask and oxygen they are exposed to very high oxygen concentrations which produce high levels of arterial Po_2. It is therefore highly recommended that a self-inflatable bag and mask be kept in the incubator and used with the incubator air for relief of apneic episodes in these babies so that their inspired oxygen concentration is not changed during the resuscitation procedure.[9]

Other Organs

There is increasing concern that vasospasm similar to that of the retinal vessels may occur during hyperoxia in other blood vessels of cerebral origin and thereby reduce the blood flow to other areas of the central nervous system. Certain adverse effects of excessive oxygen have been shown experimentally and suspected clinically, among which are changes in the renal tubules and an increased rate of destruction of red blood cells.

SUMMARY

The desirable amount of inspired oxygen is that which maintains the baby's blood oxygen tension within safe effective limits. If an infant is breathing well and is of good color, he does not need oxygen therapy, regardless of how small he is. If he has respiratory distress, oxygen must be

[8] Leo Stern, op. cit., p. 457.
[9] Leo Stern, op. cit., p. 458.

given in sufficient amount to maintain a normal arterial oxygen tension (50 to 80 mmHg). The Po_2 should not exceed 100 mmHg. Attempting to maintain the inspired oxygen concentration at 40 percent or less to avoid damage is not appropriate; 40 percent may be too much for some babies and too little for others. It is sometimes necessary to raise the inspired oxygen concentration to 60 or 80 percent and even higher to maintain an adequate arterial oxygen tension.

Optimum and reasonably safe use of oxygen requires accurate and careful monitoring of both the amount of oxygen in the blood and the concentration of oxygen in the inspired air. The concentration of inspired oxygen must be measured with an oxygen analyzer at least every two hours. The performance of the oxygen analyzer must be checked daily by calibration with room air and 100 percent oxygen. When possible, constant oxygen analyzers should be used.

A frequent adjustment in the concentration of inspired oxygen is made according to the baby's condition as determined by his arterial oxygen tension. The condition of infants requiring oxygen may improve rapidly. Under these circumstances, the inspired oxygen concentration should be promptly lowered, at least by 10 percent decrements at frequent intervals guided by blood gas measurements.

Correction of acidosis will decrease pulmonary vascular resistance and promote closure of the ductus arteriosus. This diminishes right-to-left shunts and is followed by improved oxygen uptake. As a result, the blood Po_2 level is likely to rise far above normal during oxygen therapy as soon as the blood pH is corrected, unless the inspired oxygen concentration is decreased to levels appropriate to the infant's changing needs. Thus, frequent monitoring of inspired oxygen need must accompany correction of an acid pH.

It is essential to chart both the inspired oxygen concentration, as measured by an oxygen analyzer, and the baby's color every time an adjustment in inspired oxygen concentration is made. The baby's muscle tone, which is a good indicator of the blood pH, should also be noted. When changes are not frequent, charting is important at least every two hours.

The nurse should assume responsibility for rapidly increasing the inspired oxygen concentration if a baby's condition warrants it. This may happen if the baby has aspirated or becomes cyanotic for some other reason.

When the baby is a dusky color his blood oxygen concentration is too low. His arterial Po_2 is below 50 mmHg and perhaps even much lower. Since the ductus arteriosus and the lung arterioles are sensitive to blood Po_2 and pH levels, the ductus arteriosus may open and the lung arterioles may constrict if the Po_2 is less than 40 mmHg. Shunting of blood will then follow. Therefore, when an infant is dusky, oxygen administration is probably best approached from the top. The oxygen flow should be turned high enough to rapidly flood the incubator, quickly achieving a high environmental concentration of oxygen for the baby. A high inspired oxygen concentration is important at the beginning to raise the arterial Po_2 to a level where the pulmonary resistance will decrease and the ductus arteriosus will close. Small gradual increases of oxygen may not increase the blood Po_2 level enough to stop shunting of blood and an irreversible cycle of hypoxemia and shunting may result.

When facilities for blood gas determinations are available these must be done promptly to determine the appropriate inspired oxygen percentage for continuing administration. In a clinical setting without facilities for measuring blood gas, monitoring of oxygen need will have to be done by color, at least temporarily. As soon as the baby's color is pink, the concentration of inspired oxygen should be lowered in decrements of 10 percent every 30 minutes until the baby's color shows signs of becoming dusky. At this point the concentration of inspired oxygen is increased by 5–10 percent, which usually is the appropriate amount to maintain good oxygenation and still not cause hyperoxia.

If the baby becomes dusky after the concentration of inspired oxygen is decreased, raising the concentration slightly may result in return of a pink color. If color does not improve, it is necessary to increase the amount of inspired oxygen to a high level once again and then resume the gradual decrease as before. When it appears that the infant's color will remain good (one to two hours) the concentration of inspired oxygen is decreased further and then discontinued.

When supplemental oxygen is necessary for an immature infant, he should be cared for in a hospital in which inspired oxygen concentration can be regulated on the basis of blood gas measurements. Arrangements should be made for transfer of the baby to an intensive care facility as soon as possible.

Noninvasive continuous monitoring of arterial Po_2 by transcutaneous Po_2 ($tcPo_2$) measurements can be done, but at present the method is not generally available and it may need further testing and development before it can be used reliably for monitoring of arterial oxygen tension. With this method, blood Po_2 is measured transcutaneously on skin arterialized by means of a heated Po_2 electrode. Oxygen diffuses through the relatively thin skin of the baby from the outer capillary layer to an electrode fixed on the skin. Since the capillary Po_2 is lower than the Po_2 in newborns, the arterial Po_2 will need to be determined from the relationship that can be established between Po_2 and $tcPo_2$ if the reading of the $tcPo_2$ is accurate and reliable. If transcutaneous monitoring of arterial Po_2 is developed to the place where it can be used generally, it can eliminate some of the complications of arterial catheters, now commonly used when frequent Po_2 measurements are necessary.

Assisted Ventilation

A baby may need assistance with ventilation in order to adequately move air in and out of the lungs, and/or to keep the alveoli from completely collapsing at the end of expiration.

The baby must move enough air in and out of the lungs to provide adequate oxygen to the tissues and to blow off enough carbon dioxide to avoid a buildup of this gas in the body. Assistance with moving air in an out of the lungs may be necessary (1) if breathing is not adequate in depth or frequency because of respiratory center depression, which may happen when maternal drugs cross the placenta; (2) if the baby becomes tired with breathing, as may happen with the increased work of breathing with hyaline membrane disease; and (3) if partial airway obstruction presents a problem, as may happen with aspiration of meconium. In any of these circumstances the baby is given ventilatory assistance until he has recovered from the underlying problem.

A baby sometimes needs assistance with breathing when the alveoli tend to collapse at the end of each breath owing to an insufficient amount of surfactant. In this circumstance the baby may have the ability to move air in and out of the lungs normally, but each breath is a great effort. In normal breathing some air is retained in the alveoli at the end of expiration, and the next breath can be taken with ease. With a deficiency in amount of surfactant the alveoli collapse at the end of expiration, and each breath requires as much, or almost as much, effort as the first breath. This is the situation in hyaline membrane disease. In this kind of respiratory difficulty areas of atelectasis develop, and there is also little reserve air left in the lungs between breaths. Also blood that flows through the atelectatic areas of the lungs does not become adequately oxygenated, and it returns to the left side of the heart with an inadequate supply of oxygen. This is termed right-to-left shunting of blood through the lungs. Assistance with the kind of breathing difficulty that permits collapse of alveoli involves some method that will help the baby to keep the alveoli open at the end of expiration.

If, along with respiratory difficulty because of collpased alveoli, the baby also has trouble moving air in and out of the lungs because he is tired or has depressed respiration, he will need assistance with both problems at the same time. For assistance with ventilation a baby may therefore need a respirator that will provide (1) intermittent positive pressure ventilation (IPPV) to assist the baby to move air in and out of the lungs, or (2) a system that provides continuous distending airway pressure or continuous positive airway pressure (CPAP), which will counteract the tendency of the alveoli to collapse, or (3) a respirator that provides for the IPPV and also has a mechanism that will provide background CPAP or positive end expiratory pressure (PEEP) to help keep the alveoli open at end expiration. Several methods of ventilation are described below.

Bag and Mask

A bag and mask, with which air can be forced into the lungs when the bag is squeezed, is the simplest method of ventilation. The bag is attached to a face mask held firmly over the baby's face. The bag may be self-inflatable or flow inflated. The self-inflatable bag returns to its original position after it is squeezed. It fills with the surrounding air, which means that it can be used anywhere. The flow-inflated bag is filled by being connected to a source of compressed air or oxygen.

The self-inflating bag has the advantage of not requiring a source of compressed air or oxygen, but it has several disadvantages. It is not possible to accurately regulate the oxygen concentration with this bag, most self-inflating bags do not deliver oxygen above 40–50 percent without an adaptor and may not deliver any air flow without being compressed, and they cannot be used to apply continuous positive airway pressure. The flow-inflated bag and mask setup should be capable of delivering any concentration of oxygen desired and can be used for continuous positive airway pressure and for intermittent positive pressure if desired. The bag should have a preset blow-off valve or a pressure gauge attached in order to enable the person using it to determine the amount of pressure delivered. The operator must, however, rely on clinical assessment rather than a blow-off valve for safety.

Bag breathing may be used for a number of reasons. It can be used for resuscitation in the delivery room for inflation of the lungs and delivery of oxygen to the baby (Fig. 15-11G, p. 363), and it can be used at the bedside for infants who have spells of apnea. For babies in danger of respiratory difficulty a bag must always be available at the bedside in case of emergency. A bag and mask may be used in the nursery to support ventilation and to provide oxygen for the baby who is having some difficulty maintaining ongoing ventilation. In this respect it may be used either to provide intermittent positive pressure ventilation for the baby who needs support with his breaths and/or to provide continuous positive airway pressure to help in keeping the alveoli from collapsing.

When intermittent positive pressure ventilation (IPPV) is used, the mask is held firmly against the baby's face and the bag is squeezed in time with the baby's inspirations. When continuous positive airway pressure (CPAP) is used (with the flow-inflated bag), more gas is permitted to flow into the bag than is permitted to escape; pressure builds up in the system and is transmitted to the baby's airway and alveoli as the mask is held firmly against the baby's face. As the baby breathes spontaneously against this continuous positive pressure, the pressure helps to keep the alveoli from complete collapse at the end of each expiration. Continuous positive airway pressure and intermittent positive pressure ventilation can be used at the same time for the baby who needs that much ventilatory support. Since PO_2 rises significantly with ventilation, it is frequently necessary to ventilate with less oxygen concentration than has been used when the baby has been breathing spontaneously. Frequent blood gas measurements are very important.

When a bag and mask is used to help a baby move air in and out of his lungs, certain checks must be made for proper use of the bag. To avoid inadequate ventilation, the baby should be closely observed (1) for chest movement, especially of the apices, and each inspiration, (2) for improving pink color of the lips, and (3) for breath sounds with each inspiration. The ventilatory rate should be 30 to 50 times per minute, and the depth of ventilation should not be above that normally expected of the newborn. Any long-term ventilation requires checking of blood gases and nasogastric tube for decompression of stomach.

The bag and mask is most useful for short-term use and during transfer of a baby to an intensive care unit. For prolonged assisted ventilation, a more permanent arrangement is necessary. Machines or equipment that provide continuous distending airway pressure or intermittent positive pressure ventilation or both are then used. Continuous positive airway pressure can be set up with tubing, bag, and other equipment not requiring a machine.

Respirators

Continuous distending airway pressure, also called continuous transpulmonary pressure, is used quite extensively for treatment of respiratory distress syndrome, a common neonatal respiratory problem, which is described below. Continuous distending airway pressure counteracts the tendency in this complication of the alveoli to collapse with each expiration and thus is helpful in improving oxygenation. The effects of continuous distending airway pressure are accomplished by continuous positive airway pressure (CPAP), or continuous negative pressure (CNP), or positive end expiratory pressure (PEEP).

With CPAP, a gas pressure greater than atmosphere is applied to the airway continuously during spontaneous breathing. With the CNP a pressure less than atmospheric is applied around the thorax during spontaneous breathing. With PEEP positive airway pressure is applied during the expiratory phase of breathing that is assisted mechanically. CPAP was introduced in 1971 to augment treatment of RDS.[10] Prior to that time artificial airway pressure had been used, but there were many difficulties in adapting it to small babies, and it was only used late in the

[10] G. A. Gregory, *et al.*, Treatment of the idiopathic respiratory distress syndrome with continuous positive airway pressure, *N. Engl. J. Med.* 284:1333–1340 (June 17) 1971.

disease. A year after introduction of CPAP, continuous negative pressure (CNP) was shown to be beneficial.

Continuous distending airway pressure achieves for the baby some of the beneficial effects that the baby achieves for himself when he grunts with expiration. With a grunt the end expiration is prolonged. This maintains the lung at a slightly larger volume for a longer period of time so that gas exchange can take place. This, plus rapid breathing, may prevent complete collapse of alveoli before the baby can take his next breath. The functional residual capacity of the lung thus remains more normal.

When constant distending pressure or end expiratory pressure is applied to the airway during respiration, the alveoli are kept from collapsing completely at end expiration. This improves gas exchange. As the terminal bronchioles and alveoli are kept open, functional residual capacity, that amount of air still remaining in the lungs at the end of the breath, is increased. This allows for continued diffusion of oxygen between breaths. Right-to-left shunting of blood past atelectatic areas also decreases. Blood pumped through the lungs reaches more aerated areas and can pick up oxygen much better. Arterial P_{O_2} increases significantly with continuous distending airway pressure. The exact mechanism by which the arterial P_{O_2} increases is not completely clear, since there is a significant increase in oxygenation even without a very significant change in total ventilation.

Continuous distending airway pressure is also likely to reduce the baby's work of breathing. When the alveoli do not collapse completely at the end expiration they will reopen more easily with the next inspiration. The large amount of effort and energy the baby has been using to take each breath can be reduced. Signs of respiratory distress (retraction) improve.

With CPAP, a baby who is breathing spontaneously is attached to a system that applies a constant distending pressure to the airway. The pressure may be applied to the upper airway by means of a head hood, a face mask, or nasal prongs, or if it becomes necessary to apply pressure to the lower airway, it is done by endotracheal tube. With CPAP, gas is brought into and held in a relatively closed system in a larger amount than is permitted to escape. The gas source should be able to supply any selected mixture of air and oxygen with warmth and humidification. Exhaust tubing and a means of regulating the amount of gas escaping helps to regulate the amount of pressure in the system. A pressure relief valve, a pop-off, inserted into the system, is used to prevent extremely high pressures from accidentally occurring.

If CNP is used, it is administered with a sealed negative pressure tank surrounding the baby's thorax, with the head and oropharynx outside the tank at atmosphere pressure. The negative pressure that is applied around the baby's thorax causes air to be aspirated in through the nose and mouth. The amount of negative pressure applied will determine the amount of positive airway pressure. This technique does not require a means of connecting the system to the baby's airway, but air leaks at all portals of the body chamber may be a problem. Among other problems are a relative inaccessibility of the baby and difficulty in maintaining pressure during care of the baby in the compartment.

Continuous distending pressure is used most effectively in treatment of respiratory distress syndrome (hyaline membrane disease). Indications for its use vary somewhat, but there is fairly general agreement that a Po_2 below 50 mmHg is unsatisfactory. CPAP may be instituted when it has become necessary to raise the concentration of oxygen the baby is breathing to 60 percent to try to maintain the Po_2 at 50 mm. Sixty percent oxygen is an arbitrary choice, since it is not know what percentage of oxygen is toxic to the baby and because of right-to-left shunting higher concentrations of oxygen may not change Po_2 very much.[11] High and prolonged concentration is, however, thought to be more toxic to the lung than the lower percentages.

The amount of carbon dioxide retention is also a factor in determining when ventilatory assistance should be given. A Pco_2 of greater than 70 mmHg warrants ventilatory support in the form of intermittent positive pressure ventilation. When the Pco_2 is elevated but less than 70 mmHg, other factors such as severity of distress, rate of rise of Pco_2, oxygen requirements, and presence of apneic spells are taken into consideration in a decision to provide assisted ventilation.[12]

Episodes of prolonged apnea that are accompanied by severe bradycardia or that do not respond to tactile stimulation require support of ventilation regardless of the blood gas values.[13]

All methods of continuous distending pressure have advantages and disadvantages; a number of these have been enumerated by Affonso and Harris.[14] It appears, however, that CPAP with nasal prongs is a widely used system.

CPAP must be carefully regulated for appropriate humidity and temperature and pressure of the gas. The air/oxygen mixture is passed through a humidifier, and must be carefully observed for appropriate moisture. If the mixture is too dry, the baby's mucous membranes may become dry and thick; tenacious mucus may develop and block the airways. Suctioning of the airways may be necessary every two hours. Excessive humidification causes large droplets of fluid to form in the circuit, and these may get into the airway and cause distress.

The air/oxygen mixture is warmed so that it will not cause the baby to become chilled. Overheating, however, would cause hyperthermia.

The amount of CPAP pressure applied is critical and must be carefully observed. The goal is to apply just enough pressure to help open alveoli and keep them open, but not to overdistend any alveoli that are already considerably

---

[11] W. A. Hodson and D. A. Belenky, *op. cit.*, p. 278.

[12] W. A. Hodson and D. A. Belenky, *op. cit.*, p. 279.
[13] W. A. Hodson and D. A. Belenky, *op. cit.*, p. 279.
[14] Dyanne Affonso and Thomas Harris, CPAP: Continuous positive airway pressure, *Am. J. Nurs.* 76:570–573 (Apr.) 1976.

distended. Improvement in the baby's color and blood oxygen tension can be expected when the pressure level is appropriate. There should be little rise in arterial Pco_2. Blood gases must be monitored frequently, and the CPAP pressure must be checked periodically.

In thinking of levels of pressure in relation to ventilation, the following information may be a guide:

<3 cm H_2O = approximately the same pressure as is normally applied by the glottis.

6–8 cm H_2O = may prevent further atelectasis.

6–10 cm H_2O = general therapeutic range for keeping the alveoli from collapsing completely and preventing atelectasis.

>12–14 cm H_2O = not safe. Probably cannot be achieved with nasal prongs or with face mask.

The baby on CPAP must be observed constantly, since a change in condition may occur quickly. Observation includes looking for cyanosis or ruddiness, checking the heart rate, especially for bradycardia, observing the respiratory rate and pattern, and the baby's tone and activity.

The oxygen concentration in the air/oxygen mixture and the CPAP pressure are adjusted according to blood gas results. They are lowered as soon as the baby begins to improve, so that the baby will not be exposed to oxygen or to extra pressure over any unnecessary period of time.

CPAP sometimes leads to complications of pulmonary air leak or rupture of an alveolus, and reduction in venous return to the heart when airway pressure is too great. Alveoli may become overdistended, decreasing compliance, and eventually the high inspiratory pressure may cause an air leak into interstitial spaces. Air may reach the mediastinal area and cause a pneumomediastinum, or it may break through the pleura and result in a pneumothorax, with collapse of a portion of a lung. Difficulty with air leaks and its consequences may be suspected when the baby's condition suddenly worsens. He quickly develops tachypnea, cyanosis, decreased chest movement on one side, poor air or no air exchange on one side of the chest, displacement of heart sounds, and a general overall appearance of distress. Equipment must be available to remove air from the chest and establish chest drainage.

Some of the CPAP pressure is transmitted through the lungs to the mediastinum. As the lung compliance improves, more of the airway pressure reaches the mediastinum, where it may put pressure on the large vessels returning blood to the heart. This may obstruct venous blood return to the heart and lead to a decrease in cardiac output. The CPAP pressure should be reduced as soon as pressure on large vessels appears to be present.

It sometimes happens that CPAP alone is not sufficient respiratory support, and the baby needs additional mechanical ventilation. A significant rise in CO_2 retention (Pco_2 of 55 to 60 mmHg) often indicates need for more assistance in ventilation; a rise to 70 mmHg is a definite indication.

A respirator provides intermittent positive pressure ventilation (IPPV) to assist the baby to move air in and out of the lungs and may also have a built-in mechanism to provide the baby with positive end expiratory pressure (PEEP) or background CPAP. Such an arrangement makes it possible to assist the baby with adequately moving air in and out of the lungs and also with preventing complete collapse of the alveoli at the end of each expiration.

Respirators are now fairly versatile. This makes it possible to use a machine for IPPV alone or with PEEP or to use CPAP alone or with intermittent ventilation.

Assisted ventilation with the machines described above is a specialized procedure that requires expertise in care and management of the baby and laboratory and x-ray facilities available at all hours. This type of care is given in neonatal care centers. A referral system should be available so that babies who develop respiratory distress can be safely transferred from community hospitals to specialized facilities. When respiratory distress can be anticipated, transfer of mother and baby to an intensive care center can sometimes be arranged prior to the baby's birth.

Correction of Acid–Base Imbalance

Any serious illness in a newborn is likely to lead to an acid-base imbalance. A baby with respiratory distress is in danger of developing hypoxia, hypercapnia, and acidosis. Oxygen is used to correct the hypoxia, and assisted ventilation may be necessary to correct hypercapnia. Acidosis, if it is of metabolic origin, is usually corrected by administration of sodium bicarbonate.

Since blood pH alone does not indicate whether an acidosis is of respiratory or metabolic origin, it is important to obtain a Pco_2 before therapy is started. Accumulation of carbon dioxide in the blood raises the Pco_2 and results in a rapid fall in blood pH, leading to a respiratory acidosis. If the acidosis is almost entirely of respiratory origin, as determined by an elevated Pco_2, therapy with sodium bicarbonate will not correct the acidosis and is then inappropriate treatment. In fact, administration of sodium bicarbonate is contraindicated with severe respiratory acidosis. Sodium bicarbonate gives off carbon dioxide, which these babies cannot blow off with their respirations, and their respiratory acidosis worsens. Mechanical ventilation is the only effective treatment for high Pco_2. Such ventilation is usually given when the Pco_2 is 60 mmHg or over.

If the blood pH is low and Pco_2 is normal or nearly so, the acidosis is of metabolic origin. A combination of respiratory and metabolic acidosis is a common situation.

When acidosis cannot be prevented it must be corrected quite promptly. Intravenous sodium bicarbonate is used to correct a metabolic acidosis. The milliequivalent dose and the volume and route of administration of this base are determined on the basis of the degree of metabolic acidosis and the urgency for correcting the acidosis. Usually the base deficit is determined, and the dosage of sodium bicarbonate is calculated accordingly.

The base deficit can be calculated from a nomogram when the hemoglobin concentration, the blood pH, and the Pco_2 are known. With an acidosis this value will be a negative base excess or base deficit. The dosage of sodium bicarbonate to be given is then computed from a formula which states: mEq of sodium bicarbonate to be given = base deficit $(mEq/1liter) \times 0.3 \times$ body weight in kilograms. The factor of 0.3 in this formula represents the approximate portion of the body weight that is made up of extracellular fluid.[15] It should be noted that there is some disagreement on the true bicarbonate space, the values ranging from 0.3 to 0.6 of body weight. Usually the 0.3 figure is used for calculation. When the dosage of sodium bicarbonate as calculated from this formula has been given, further laboratory studies will determine if a repeat dose is necessary or if sodium bicarbonate should be added to the intravenous drip.

Sodium bicarbonate in the above concentration is available in ampuls of a 7.5 percent solution containing 0.88 mEq/ml. For ease of calculation for clinical use the concentration of sodium bicarbonate in this solution may be considered to be 1.0 mEq/ml.[16] Sodium bicarbonate in the above concentration is hypertonic and may damage blood vessels if used undiluted and will also draw fluid into the vascular system. It must therefore be mixed with at least an equal amount of water for injection, NSS, 5 percent lactated Ringers, or 10 percent glucose water. Some of the dosage may be injected over a period of several minutes and the remainder added to intravenous fluids or all may be added to an intravenous fluid drip. Sometimes when asphyxia at birth is severe sodium bicarbonate is administered as a part of the resuscitation procedure (see page 366). This may be done by clinically estimating the degree of acidosis without waiting for blood pH and Pco_2 values.

Dosage and timing of administration of sodium bicarbonate may need to be modified

[15] Sheldon B. Korones, *op. cit.*, p. 118.
[16] Sheldon B. Korones, *op. cit.*, pp. 117–118.

frequently on the basis of further acid–base measurements. Overcorrection can become a problem. Since carbon dioxide will be released from the sodium bicarbonate that is administered, and this also has to be eliminated through the lungs, ventilation must be good when sodium bicarbonate is given. If ventilation is poor, the carbon dioxide tension of the blood may rise, and respiratory acidosis will develop. Hypernatremia may also become a problem. If more correction is necessary after 15 mEq/kg-24 hr of sodium bicarbonate has been given, *tris* (hydroxymethyl)aminomethane (Tham) may be used. Tham is a base useful in treatment of metabolic acidosis because of its alkalizing effect.

Treatment of Hypovolemia

Babies with respiratory distress, especially hyaline membrane disease, often have a low systemic blood pressure. Systemic hypotension will increase the right-to-left shunting of blood through the ductus arteriosis, especially when the pulmonary artery pressure is high. Babies with hypotension cannot be properly oxygenated and may develop shock.

When hypotension is present it is dealt with by administration of albumin or plasma or small transfusions. Plasma and/or blood is usually given in any amount that equals 10–20 ml/kg of body weight. If hypotension was caused by blood loss the baby may need up to 20 ml/kg for volume replacement.

Blood sampling for laboratory data, especially when done frequently, slowly reduces blood plasma and cell volume. A careful record must be kept of the amount of blood removed. Usually a small blood transfusion is given periodically to replace the blood that was removed for sampling.

Protection Against Heat Loss

An ambient temperature that is high enough to maintain the baby's body temperature at approximately 98°F (36.7°C) axillary or 98.6°F (37°C) rectal is crucial to the welfare of a baby with respiratory distress. If the baby must attempt to maintain a normal body temperature in an environment in which he loses body heat, the amount of oxygen he needs to meet his increased metabolism for heat production is greatly increased. A baby with respiratory difficulties may not be able to meet the body's basal oxygen needs under such conditions. Even when the baby does increase his metabolic rate considerably, he may not be able to maintain his body temperature at a normal level while he is in a heat-losing environment. When oxygen needs cannot be met the baby may need to change to anaerobic metabolism, which may then result in a buildup of lactic acid and metabolic acidosis.

To control the temperature environment, the baby may be placed in an incubator or on a neonatal intensive care unit (Fig. 15-10, page 356). On the open bed of the neonatal intensive care unit the baby is kept warm by a radiant heater. To maintain the body temperature between 98 and 98.6°F (36.7 and 37°C) (when the baby is in an incubator), the temperature in the incubator may need to be raised to 95°F (35°C) or above. It may be advisable to use a heat lamp over the roof of the incubator for radiant heat to the baby and, when possible, to use a skin thermistor for regulation of incubator temperature. A radiant heat lamp is also used to reduce heat loss during any procedure that increases exposure. When the baby is on an intensive care table the skin thermistor is set to keep the skin temperature at 97.6°F (36.4°C) and care is taken to avoid drafts.

Nutrition

Adequate nutrition and good basic hydration are important for support in any disease. Intravenous fluids are therefore started very early in the disease to meet the baby's fluid requirements, to provide some caloric intake, and to ensure an adequate blood sugar level, which is often low in babies with respiratory distress.

Good basic hydration will vary, but in general, 140 to 160 ml per kg per 24 hours will maintain good water balance. For the first few days of fluid administration the average total fluid requirement is somewhat less (page 720). Excess water loss through the skin, especially when the baby is being cared for on an open bed heated by radiant lamps or through the kidneys because of diuresis, may require a much higher fluid intake. A small baby with a large body surface and a small amount of subcutaneous tissue is in danger of evaporative water loss just as much as he is in danger of heat loss.

To recognize water loss the baby's skin turgor should be noted, the urinary output is measured by weighing the diapers or pads used for the baby has a substantial amount of respiratory body weight is checked every 8 to 12 hours. Laboratory studies of urine specific gravity and serum electrolytes also aid in determining fluid need.

Ten percent glucose will prevent hypoglycemia and provide some calories, although not a sufficient amount to meet basal body needs. If the baby has a substantial amount of respiratory distress, and especially if he is a premature, his nutritional needs in the early days of life are often met by intravenous alimentation. Finally, when recovery is proceeding well, formula feedings by tube are begun with caution.

Glucose is offered as the first oral feeding and then a gradual change is made to milk feedings. Intravenous glucose is continued until the baby is able to take enough milk orally to meet his fluid and nutritional needs. See page 720 for further discussion of water requirements of infants, and pages 721 and 733 for intravenous supplementation of oral feedings.

Parenteral Alimentation

Total parenteral nutrition is possible for babies who will be unable to take food over a prolonged period of time. This method of feeding infants has been proven useful for babies with gastrointestinal anomalies that require extensive surgery and for babies with chronic diarrhea and malabsorption syndromes. It has in-

creased survival of such critically ill babies significantly. Total parenteral alimentation has also been used to provide nutrition for low-birth-weight babies whose immaturity makes adequate oral feedings difficult or impossible. Its use for low-birth-weight babies is advised only for selected infants who do not tolerate feedings by other methods.

With total intravenous alimentation the baby is given a constant infusion of a chemically complex mixture that meets the protein, caloric, water, electrolyte, and vitamin needs of the infant for weight gain and positive nitrogen balance. The mixture is made up specifically for the individual baby each day and consists of protein hydrolysate or a mixture of pure crystalline amino acids to provide for amino acid needs, glucose to provide for calories, and minerals, vitamins, and appropriate electrolytes. Complete intravenous nutrition should include fat, a normal part of any diet, in order to avoid essential fatty acid deficiencies. Fat preparations have been widely used in Europe and Japan but have not been approved for use in this country until recently. Administration of fat emulsions requires special precautions to preserve stability. Fat emulsions cannot be mixed with the other solutions and are best given separately and peripherally.

The infusate is administered through an indwelling silastic catheter inserted into the superior vena cava via either the external or internal jugular vein. The fluid is of high osmolality, which requires it to be given slowly into a large central vein where it can be quickly diluted to avoid damage to the blood vessel. The current availability of fat emulsion should make it possible to give a solution of lower osmolality since the fat will provide some of the calories. A constant infusion pump is used to maintain a constant rate of infusion. In general, this method of administering nutrition is used when it is anticipated that parenteral nutrition will be required for at least three weeks.

Initially the infusion fluid is started with low concentrations of glucose and protein. It is gradually increased to full caloric maintenance, which may not be attained before 7 to 10 days in low-birth-weight babies.

Very careful monitoring of the infant is necessary during intravenous alimentation. All intake and output is recorded. The urine is examined for volume, specific gravity, protein, and glucose at each voiding. Dextrostix for blood glucose is done at least every four hours. Blood glucose, electrolytes, BUN, serum proteins, hematocrit, and a number of other blood studies are done once, twice, or three times weekly. The baby's growth rate must be carefully monitored.

Complications of parenteral alimentation generally include sepsis, catheter-related problems, and metabolic problems. The infusion mixture promotes growth of certain organisms and fungi and must be mixed under strictly aseptic conditions. The indwelling catheter is placed in the operating room and is aseptically dressed and cared for thereafter. Strict adherence to placement and maintenance of the catheter reduces complications of malposition, dislodgement, and thrombosis.

Metabolic complications relate to the content of the parenteral solution. Hyperglycemia may occur due to glucose intolerance. Acidosis may develop. Electrolyte imbalance may occur if the required amounts are misjudged, especially when babies have concomitant abnormal fluid losses. The blood urea nitrogen may become seriously elevated from excessive protein content, which must then be lowered.

Refeeding of the baby is begun with great caution and proceeds slowly with small amounts of food. Parenteral alimentation is discontinued very gradually, decreasing both the concentration and the amount of fluids as the baby increases his oral intake.

Total Intravenous Alimentation by Peripheral Vein

Providing adequate nutrition by peripheral vein is very difficult because an adequate infusion mixture is of necessity of high osmolality, making local sclerosing of tissues common, and use of a less hypertonic solution makes it dif-ficult to meet the baby's nutrient needs without exceeding the baby's fluid tolerance. This method has, however, more recently been used with success.

Infusion is made into one of the peripheral veins on the dorsal aspect of either the hand or the foot, or into one of the superficial veins of the scalp. Placing the needle and maintaining it in place often presents a problem.

The nutrient mixture for infusion into peripheral veins is similar to that used for infusion via a central vein, with the exception that the glucose concentration rarely exceeds 10 percent. Glucose is used in a concentration as high as 20 percent for central vein nutrition, since the glucose content in that solution is gradually increased to 25 to 30 gm/kg-day according to infant tolerance. Recently Intralipid has been included in some of the infusions. Intralipid will provide calories without appreciably adding to the overall osmolality. Intravenous lipid cannot be mixed with glucose and amino acids, since the fat emulsion will break down. It is therefore given by "piggy-back" through a Y-connector so that it joins the glucose and amino acid mixture at the entry into the vein. When initiating use of fat emulsion it must be given slowly to observe for adverse reactions. Intralipid makes it possible to meet caloric needs with hyperalimentation of lower concentrations of glucose and protein, supplemented with Intralipid. This means that total alimentation by peripheral vein is possible.

Septic and metabolic complications appear to be lessened with use of a peripheral vein than with a central vein. Phlebitis and local complications from fluid extravasations and tissue sloughs may be a problem, and maintenance of infusion sites for an extended period of time becomes difficult. Infiltration of fluid will result in severe tissue slough if not discovered early.

Stimulation of Sucking During Parenteral Alimentation

The baby who is on prolonged parenteral alimentation does not have the normal experiences of suck and swallow, hunger and relief of hunger by food, nor the taste and touch of food in his mouth. He will not receive the normal suck stimulation important to his normal development unless a special effort is made to simulate feedings. The baby needs to be offered a pacifier and talked to, rocked, cuddled, and played with as he would be at a normal feeding time, or if he cannot be removed from the incubator, he can be given as much of this care as possible while in the incubator. Scheduled times at three- or four-hour intervals for feeding simulation will assure an appropriate amount of stimulation.

When the baby who has been on prolonged parenteral alimentation is permitted to begin feedings he may take one or more weeks to learn to develop a good suck–swallow pattern and to accept food and fluids from a nipple. If he resists taking fluids from a nipple he is given feedings by dropper in very small amounts while he has a pacifier in his mouth. When he has learned to swallow fluid in this way he can be offered a nipple. With the nurse's assistance and patience and effort the baby learns to take a small amount of food orally. Slowly the quantity can be increased. For an excellent discussion on nurses' techniques with feeding infants who have been on parenteral alimentation, as well as other aspects of care, the reader is referred to the article, "Parenteral Alimentation," by Alice Conway and Tamara Williams in the *American Journal of Nursing*.[17]

Position Changes

The baby with respiratory difficulty must have his position changed frequently to prevent pooling of secretions and thus hypostatic pneumonia, to maintain good ventilation, and to promote drainage of lung segments. The baby's position should be changed at least every hour, alternating between sides, prone, and supine positions.

The baby's own breathing ability may be improved when he is placed on his back with the bed elevated at the head at about a 30-degree angle. Since the cartilage in a baby's trachea is soft, and a head-forward position may compress the trachea, the baby's head should be slightly extended with a small towel under his neck and shoulders. Frequent checks are necessary to ensure that the small roll under the baby's shoulders does not slip under his head, causing it to flex. In this back position the diaphragmatic excursion may be better, the angle of the upper airway is reduced, and the upper air lobes may drain spontaneously.[18] This position must not, however, be used for more than one hour at a time.

Suction of Mucus

Removal of mucus and secretions from the respiratory tract is necessary for good ventilation. Suction with a catheter or a bulb syringe may be oropharyngeal, or through the nose, or through an endotracheal tube if one is in place. Keeping the baby's head straight or tipped back slightly during suctioning aids in getting suction to the respiratory tract.

In suctioning, the mouth must always be aspirated first. Putting a catheter in the nose is likely to stimulate the baby to inspire, and any secretions that are accumulated in the mouth and throat are likely to be aspirated. If a catheter is used for suction of the nostrils it must be passed without force, using gentle rotation of the catheter between the thumb and forefinger to advance it. The catheter must be placed quickly without suction and then immediately withdrawn as intermittent suction is applied. Continuous suction is harmful to nasal and oral mucosa and may contribute to collapse of alveoli and developing atelectasis.

A newborn coughs infrequently, but secretions or stimulation with a suction catheter may stimulate a cough. Since the baby is likely to be unable to handle the mucus produced by the cough, the pharyngeal area should be suctioned

---

[17] Alice Conway and Tamara Williams, Parenteral alimentation, *Am. J. Nurs.* 76:574–577 (Apr.) 1976.

[18] Deon Dunn and Amber T. Lewis, Some important aspects of neonatal nursing related to pulmonary disease and family involvement, *Pediatr. Clin. North Am.* 20:487, 1973.

immediately after a cough to avoid aspiration of the mucus back into the lungs.

Suctioning of an endotracheal tube should be intermittent and brief—5 to 10 seconds. Obstruction of an airway for a longer period of time is likely to produce bronchial spasm and hypoxia, vagal stimulation, and bradycardia and arrhythmia.

Bagging with slightly higher inspired oxygen percentage (5 to 10 percent higher than that being administered) before, during, and after suctioning may be indicated. Bagging with increased oxygen concentration helps to prevent a sudden dangerous drop in arterial oxygen tension during suctioning, and it decreases the likelihood of an adverse cardiac response.

Postural Drainage

For a baby with respiratory difficulty, postural drainage, positioning that uses gravity to drain bronchi, may be implemented if symptoms indicate. It is especially useful in cases of prolonged endotracheal intubation and respirator care.

Gravity and pressure are the two main ways in which drainage of bronchial secretions can be facilitated so that gas exchange may be improved. For postural drainage the baby is placed into several different positions, at different times, so that gravity can move secretions from small bronchi to larger bronchi and to the trachea. Knowledge of the anatomy of the bronchi is essential to appropriate positioning.

Percussion with small plastic cups, followed by vibration, are forms of pressure that may be used to facilitate outward movement of bronchial secretions. These are special procedures in the newborn who presents special problems because of his very small tracheobronchial tree and his rapid respirations, especially when sick.

Persons caring for these babies must understand the principles of pulmonary therapy and must be able to carry it out quickly and efficiently to avoid undue fatigue in the infant. Bronchial drainage is fatiguing and stressful. Careful timing of the therapy and close monitoring of vital signs for the effects of treatment is essential. The nurse caring for the baby on an ongoing basis is likely to be the best person to do pulmonary therapy, knowing when and how much treatment the baby can tolerate and how he responds to stress.[19]

Rest

Whereas the development of the normal infant is enhanced by stimulation, the sick baby will not benefit and may well deteriorate from any stimulation in addition to the stress that already accompanies all the procedures that are necessary in his treatment. The sick baby is usually exposed to a number of intrusive procedures and a great deal of noise from the mechanical equipment around him. This causes excessive stimulation and loss of rest and sleep.

In an article written for the Neonatology Supplement of *Pediatrics* J. F. Lucey states[20]:

Picture yourself. . . . You're startled and frightened by loud, strange noises (beepers, voices, roaring respirators, telephones, radios, incubator noise). . . .

You are sleep deprived. Everytime you doze off, somebody gets worried about you. They think you're in a coma. You have to be very careful to breathe *very* regularly. You're not allowed the multiple long pauses (15 seconds or more) of a sleeping, dreaming adult. If you do pause, a bell goes off, waking you up, and somebody slaps your feet or pulls your hair to see if you will or can cry. If you're exhausted or unresponsive, you're in trouble. If you have any jerky movements, you're suspected of having a convulsion.

Every few hours somebody cuts your foot or sticks a needle into your scalp or one of your arteries. Your arms and legs are taped down to boards. Electrodes are attached to your chest. You're immobilized. . . .

We all care "intensely" but in our zeal to care we may have become too enthusiastic and lost sight of the possible therapeutic value of rest, sleep, and quiet. . . .

[19] *Ibid.*, p. 493.
[20] J. F. Lucey, Commentary. Is intensive care becoming too intensive, *Pediatrics* 59, Part 2, Neonatology Suppl.: 1064–1065 (June) 1977.

What should be done? Isn't all this "intensive care" very necessary? I believe it is, but I think we can minimize the stresses it places on babies by some simple changes in the techniques we use.

Since the introduction of continuous transcutaneous oxygen tension monitoring, it has become apparent that the stress caused by such simple procedures as feeding, crying, suctioning, blood sampling, noise, physical examinations, lumbar punctures, and chest physiotherapy may cause repeated episodes of hypoxemia and hypertension. . . . We then find ourselves caught in a vicious circle as these iatrogenic episodes of hypoxemia result in more apnea, requiring more stressful handling and diagnostic studies.

We have much to learn from studies utilizing the new techniques for continuous monitoring of heart rate, blood pressure, and arterial oxygen tension. One of the simplest and most effective things these studies may accomplish may be to remind us of the values of gentle handling and rest, which seem to have been forgotten.

Intensive care surely will require that a number and a variety of procedures will need to be carried out and done so frequently, but these must be balanced insofar as possible with the baby's need for rest. The nurse plays an important role in planning care that provides for quiet periods which permit the baby the sleep that is also necessary for recovery.

As soon as the baby has recovered from his illness reasonably well and is ready and can tolerate stimulation he should be held, talked to, and played with, perhaps especially along with feedings. The parents can play an important role in holding the baby, feeding him, and playing with him at this time.

Disorders of Respiration

A number of causes of respiratory distress have been enumerated on page 758. A few of these conditions will be described in further detail. Since respiratory distress from any cause has many similar signs and symptoms and also requires similar care and intervention, that which has already been discussed will in general be applicable to the conditions described below.

ASPHYXIA AT BIRTH

A normal baby establishes respirations within one minute after birth, often taking his first breath within seconds after delivery. The chemical changes resulting from the brief period of asphyxia during delivery stimulate the respiratory center, but if respirations do not begin almost immediately, the asphyxia increases, and it may then depress the respiratory center rather than stimulate it. If the condition is not quickly reversed, serious damage to tissues or death of the infant may occur.

Failure to breathe at birth, or failure to establish adequate respirations, is usually due to three principal causes: intrauterine hypoxia, drugs, and central nervous system trauma. Infection of the fetus may also be a cause of distress. Many of the conditions enumerated under causes of respiratory distress on page 758, and also less common complications, lead to apnea or hypoxia through depression of the respiratory center. Sometimes the cause of distress originates in the respiratory tract as obstruction of the air passages. More than one condition that will cause apnea or hypoxia may exist at a time, but intrauterine asphyxia is a common cause.

The clinical condition of all babies should be evaluated immediately after birth in order to institute resuscitative measures quickly if indicated.

The time of onset of sustained respirations with resuscitative measures depends on the duration and severity of previous asphyxia, the amount of depression from drugs administered to the mother, or the amount of trauma. An Apgar score below 4 indicates danger to the baby, and the longer the score remains low, the greater the danger. After resuscitation, scoring is repeated during the next 5 to 10 minutes for subsequent evaluation of the baby. The baby is also examined for appraisal of his general condition.

Exposure of the baby should be reduced to a minimum during resuscitative procedures and the hours following. The baby should be kept warm as much as possible while procedures are being carried out and he should be placed into a heated incubator or bassinet as quickly as possible. The baby must be warmed to a skin temperature of 98°F as quickly as possible to reduce his metabolism and oxygen needs to their lowest level.

Subsequent care in the nursery depends on how rapidly and how well the baby establishes good pulmonary function, the cause of the respiratory difficulty, and the findings of the baby's general examination. The baby should be under intensive observation for further signs of respiratory distress, and for the effects of perinatal hypoxia and/or ischemia on other organs.

Numerous organ systems may be affected by an episode of intrauterine asphyxia and this makes management of these babies potentially very complex. It is very important to evaluate the effects of asphyxia on the brain, since the brain is one of the vital organs that may be adversely affected by hypoxia and ischemia. The hypoxia occurs in association with the birth asphyxia. The ischemia, the diminished perfusion of the brain, is usually associated with the systemic hypotension that occurs with bradycardia, either prior to or after birth.

Some of the observations and care of babies following birth asphyxia are as follows:

1. *Respiratory:* The baby with apnea at birth may have normal vital signs, remain alert, and cry spontaneously at intervals as soon as respirations are established, or he may continue for some time to show evidence of severe respiratory distress. Distress is characterized by rapid and labored respirations with chest retraction and cyanosis.

   When the baby has been narcotized as a result of deep maternal analgesia and anesthesia, he may not only have had difficulty in initiating breathing, but may continue to respond sluggishly even after he has cried. Skin stimulation and change of position at frequent intervals are necessary until the effects of the drug have worn off.

   Oxygen administration is continued if the baby continues with respiratory distress after respirations have been established.

   Even when the baby does not require further therapy for respiratory distress, he needs warmth and protection from exposure. Unessential care, such as a bath, can be postponed for many hours. The baby is usually kept in an incubator until he can maintain his own body temperature without stress.

2. *Vital signs* must be checked at least every hour. A check of heart and respiratory rate may be indicated every ½ hour.

   Blood pressure check and maintenance at normal is an important aspect of care. The blood pressure should be taken at birth and every hour for the next 12 hours. The blood pressure should be maintained at normal range with use of fresh frozen plasma or plasma expander such as albumin given at 10 ml/kg.[21]

3. The *hematocrit* should be obtained soon after birth and repeated in 12 or 24 hours if indicated. If the mother had antepartum bleeding, the baby may have a low hematocrit. A hematocrit of 10–12 or lower requires administration of blood. Anemia may not be apparent, however, until after the first day. A hematocrit of 65 or greater is considered polycythemia and usually means that treatment by partial exchange transfusion is indicated.

4. The *blood sugar* should be checked as soon as possible after resuscitation and as frequently as indicated to assure that it remains within a normal range. The blood sugar value should be kept at 45 mg/100 ml or above. An asphyxiated baby, especially if the baby is small, is likely to become hypoglycemic very early. The baby quickly uses glycogen and stores may be meager.

   The brain must have glucose for its energy. A finding from animal data suggests that, even when the systemic blood sugar is normal or above normal in the asphyxiated patient, brain sugar may be less than nor-

[21] A. W. Brann, Jr. and Francine D. Dykes, The effects of intrauterine asphyxia on the full-term neonate, *Clin. Perinatol.* 4:149–161 (Mar.) 1977.

mal. For this reason, blood sugar should be maintained above 45 mg/100 ml. Intravenous glucose solution is started early.[22]

5. *Fluids and acid–base balance:* Intravenous fluids of sodium bicarbonate and glucose may be given, at least during the first few hours after birth, and especially if the asphyxia has been severe. The baby who has been asphyxiated is not able to restore a normal acid–base balance as quickly as the baby who has breathed normally since birth, and he also quickly depletes his glycogen reserve. Sodium bicarbonate and glucose will promote recovery from the biochemical disturbances by restoring a normal acid–base balance and by replacing necessary glucose. The water will help to maintain a normal fluid balance.

6. *Renal function* should be assessed by careful measurement of urinary output, because a decrease in renal blood flow sometimes occurs during intrauterine asphyxia. Need for administration of fluids and electrolytes may also be determined by this assessment of renal function.

7. Observations for *cerebral effects* of asphyxia should include quality and variation in muscle tone, type of cry, presence and quality of sucking reflex, and clinical evidence of seizure activity. Any evidence of seizure activity must be promptly evaluated and treated (see page 837).

A great deal of consideration is now being given to determining if, and how much, brain swelling, along with resultant altered blood flow, occurs in the full-term asphyxiated infant, and how such swelling can be delineated and effectively reduced.

Prognosis

Prognosis following birth asphyxia depends on the degree of asphyxia and the length of time it existed. Delayed respirations may cause permanent damage to brain tissue. Postnatal complica-

tions in babies who had asphyxia at birth are greater than in those who had no respiratory difficulty.

The newborn infant at birth may possibly be able to tolerate anoxia and ischemia to a greater degree than an older individual, but this is not certain. The longer the period of insult, the greater the chances of damage to the central nervous system. Some babies apparently tolerate safely several minutes of apnea, while others have irreparable damage in a very short time. The length of time that anoxia and/or ischemia can be tolerated after birth is likely to be influenced by the amount of insult the baby suffered *in utero.*

Although the possibility of injury to brain cells during asphyxia is present, all asphyxiated babies do not later have manifestations of damage. If injury occurs, it may vary from a very mild degree that is quite inconspicuous to a severe defect in either motor control or intellectual ability, and may manifest itself in a variety of ways such as convulsions, mental deficiency, behavior problems, and cerebral palsy.

IDIOPATHIC RESPIRATORY DISTRESS SYNDROME OR HYALINE MEMBRANE DISEASE

Idiopathic respiratory distress syndrome (IRDS or RDS) and hyaline membrane disease (HMD) are terms often used synonymously. This is the most important cause of newborn respiratory distress, occurring mainly in prematures. It is a worldwide disease and an important cause of death in newborn infants. The disease develops in about one sixth of all premature infants, but the more immature the baby the greater the incidence and the severity of the disease. It has carried about a 25 percent mortality rate, but survival is improving with modern treatment.

Respiratory distress syndrome appears in newborn infants who have a deficiency of the normal surfactant lining of the alveoli. The re-

[22] *Ibid.*

sult of this deficiency is poor stability of aeration (see pages 421–23). The alveoli tend to collapse at the end of each expiration, retaining little or no residual air, and the baby has a generalized atelectasis. Atelectasis is the main pathologic alteration of this disease. The collapse of many of the alveoli reduces the amount of lung tissue capable of expansion and tends to marked respiratory distress. The baby needs to apply a large amount of pressure with each breath to try to open collapsed alveoli and when they cannot be opened he ventilates only a small portion of his lungs.

A material called a hyaline membrane, from which this disease derives its name, often forms in the alveoli and the bronchioles after the disease is in progress. The membrane does not appear until after several hours of breathing and is a consequence, rather than a cause, of the disease. The cause of the formation of the hyaline membrane, which is composed of protein high in fibrin and of cellular debris, is not known.

Immature babies and those who have suffered hypoxia before birth are highly susceptible to the neonatal respiratory distress syndrome. The disease appears in babies who have not reached an age where production of pulmonary surfactant is sufficient for adequate lung function and in those in whom production of surface-active lecithin is not sufficiently rapid to maintain alveolar stability. When conditions are unfavorable, either before or after birth, for ongoing rapid synthesis of surface-active lecithin, postnatal demands cannot be met. Surfactant can quickly be depleted, and, unless it is continually replaced there will soon be a deficiency. The problem in respiratory distress syndrome is the inability to meet the demands of postnatal respiratory adjustment by sufficiently rapid synthesis of surface-active pulmonary lecithin, rather than a problem of an absence of surfactant per se.[23]

The inability to produce surfactant rapidly enough may be a result of pulmonary immaturity or factors which inhibit production. Production of surfactant is inhibited by any condition that interferes with good circulation through the lungs, reduces the amount of oxygen and glucose available to the lungs, and produces a low pH of the blood.

Asphyxia at any time, either before or after birth, interferes with good pulmonary circulation and adequate oxygenation and results in a lowering of the blood pH. Asphyxia due to poor oxygenation *in utero*, or difficulty in breathing after birth, or both, can quickly inhibit production of surfactant. Chilling of the baby after birth may result in a reduction in the amount of available oxygen and glucose and in acidosis, and thus also in the baby's ability to produce surfactant.

Maternal diabetes, maternal bleeding due to placental separation, and any condition that causes intrauterine hypoxia carries an increased risk of respiratory distress in the baby. Such conditions, especially when coupled with prematurity, are likely to result in impairment of pulmonary surfactant production. Cesarean section seems to predispose to hyaline membrane disease, especially when it is done for fetal distress or maternal hemorrhage. In some families a familial factor appears to predispose to hyaline membrane disease, with a tendency for more than one baby in the same family to develop the respiratory distress syndrome. Boys are affected more than girls with hyaline membrane disease.

A deficiency in meeting the demands for production of surface-active lecithin seems to be self-limiting and it disappears if supportive measures such as oxygen and correction of acid–base imbalance are provided and if the baby survives the first two or three days of the disease. Beginning about the third day of life, the capacity to form an alveolar surface film appears better for reasons at present not clear. A spontaneous reversal to a normal condition of the lungs then occurs and recovery from the instability of aeration takes place.

[23] Louis Gluck and Marie V. Kulovich, Fetal lung development. Current concepts, *Pediatr. Clin. North Am.* 20:373 (May) 1973.

Progression of the Disease

Early Clinical Signs

Since loss of potential stability of aeration because of deficient pulmonary surfactant is usually present before birth, signs of difficulty will appear at birth or very soon thereafter. The baby may show definite signs of distress as soon as respirations are established, or his respirations and color may appear normal at first and his condition appear to be satisfactory. An asymptomatic period between birth and appearance of signs of distress is, however, apparently very short or nonexistent when the baby is carefully observed and evaluated. Very soon after birth, often within 5, 10, or 15 minutes, a moan or a grunt with respirations may be noticeable and slight chest retraction is visible. As the condition progresses, signs of distress increase.

Respiratory distress is mild in some babies. In these infants signs of respiratory insufficiency gradually decrease after 12 to 24 hours and recovery is rapid.

Later Clinical and Pathologic Signs

In many babies with hyaline membrane disease respiratory distress becomes progressively more serious. Chest retraction becomes severe due to the large amount of effort that is necessary to inflate the lungs with each breath. The hard pull of the respiratory muscles on the soft thoracic cage causes marked indrawing of the intercostal spaces and of the sternum and breathing may become seesaw. Grunting with expiration increases and in severely affected infants expiration may be accompanied by a whimper or a cry. The respiratory rate rises to over 60 per minute within the first hours of life and may soon rise to 80 per minute or above. The work of the respiratory muscles is great and they may not be able to function continuously as the disease progresses. Apneic periods and a decreasing respiratory rate may appear and are poor prognostic signs.

Since atelectasis is likely to increase during the disease, the baby's marked respiratory effort does not increase the adequacy of his lung function. Cyanosis usually becomes apparent fairly early in the disease and is always present in severely affected babies.

The poor alveolar ventilation with hyaline membrane disease leads to abnormal biochemical and physiologic changes. The baby with respiratory distress is not able to correct the derangement in blood gases and the acidosis present at birth in the same manner in which the baby who breathes normally does. Poor lung function results in a decrease in arterial oxygen tension (PO_2), an increase in arterial carbon dioxide tension (PCO_2), and a lowering of the blood pH. A metabolic acidosis develops with the poor alveolar ventilation, may be superimposed on a respiratory acidosis, and causes the pH to fall considerably. As respiratory insufficiency continues or worsens, acidosis, both respiratory and metabolic, increases.

Pulmonary vascular resistance increases with abnormal blood gases and with acidosis. Shunting of blood through the ductus arteriosus and foramen ovale takes place. A persistent patent ductus arteriosus is fairly common. Considerable shunting of blood will contribute to a reduction in the arterial oxygen tension to a dangerously low level, making the baby's chance of survival poor. In addition to some of the blood bypassing the lungs by way of shunts through fetal blood vessels, all of the blood which does flow through the lungs may not be oxygenated. Some blood may be shunted through the atelectatic areas of the lungs and return to the systemic circulation unoxygenated. The progressive hypoxia in hyaline membrane disease may be due to both poor ventilation of the lungs and to this right to left shunting of blood through nonventilated areas of the lungs and through fetal vessels.

Increasing hypoxia and acidosis also lead to peripheral vasoconstriction. With poor peripheral circulation and possibly systemic hypotension the baby has a pale or an ashen-gray color.

Heat production in babies with hyaline membrane disease is low and hypothermia, which is common in prematures, may be pronounced even in a relatively warm environment.

White frothy mucus may be present in the respiratory tract.

Edema may develop with hyaline membrane disease and there may be pitting in the extremities. Its cause is not known.

The baby with respiratory distress syndrome has poor muscle tone and is limp and unresponsive. Jittery movements due to cerebral irritation sometimes appear. The baby typically assumes a position in which his thighs are widely abducted in a frogleg position, his arms are flexed at the elbows, and his hands lie along each side of his head. This position may be related to the baby's immaturity as well as or instead of the respiratory distress.

It is apparent from the preceding description of hyaline membrane disease that it produces pulmonary, circulatory, and metabolic disturbances. A vicious cycle of events is likely with this disease. A deficiency in pulmonary surface-active lecithin leads to atelectasis and poor lung ventilation. This disturbance results in a lowered arterial oxygen tension, elevated carbon dioxide tension, and lowered pH and acidosis. The abnormal concentration of blood gases and the acidosis lead to pulmonary hypoperfusion, which in turn interferes with production of surface-active lecithin (Fig. 26-1).

Babies who progress beyond the mild stage of the disease, in which recovery begins to be evident within 24 hours, will become progressively worse during the first 48 to 72 hours of life. Labored respiration becomes marked and the respiratory rate may continue to rise. If the respiratory and circulatory systems cannot meet the baby's needs, a severe anoxemia, a rising blood carbon dioxide tension, and a falling pH level may continue in spite of therapy. The baby's color becomes an ashen cyanosis and the respiratory rate may drop to 20 to 30 times per minute with long periods of apnea. If the baby succumbs, death usually occurs within 72 hours, mainly caused by respiratory failure.

Some babies survive even when they have had severe distress. When improvement takes place, it may be rapid and dramatic. Within 48 to 72 hours the baby is usually able to produce an adequate amount of pulmonary surfactant. With this the alveoli become well aerated and the atelectasis disappears. The baby breathes easier by the third or fourth day of life and re-

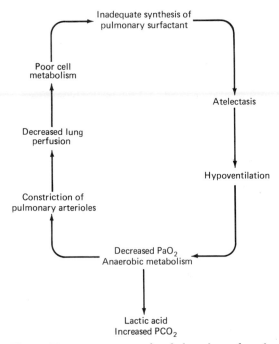

Figure 26-1. A vicious cycle of physiologic disturbances in neonatal respiratory distress syndrome. Inadequate synthesis of pulmonary surfactant leads to atelectasis, a decrease in lung compliance, increased work in breathing, and decreased ventilation. Inadequate ventilation leads to hypoxia, hypercapnia, anaerobic metabolism, and acidosis. As a result of hypoxia and acidosis, the pulmonary arterioles constrict and the ductus arteriosus opens and pulmonary blood flow is decreased. Diminished pulmonary blood flow causes pulmonary ischemia and affects metabolism of the lung. This in turn decreased synthesis and secretion of pulmonary surfactant. The above sequence of events can start at any place in the cycle. For example, antepartum bleeding could lead to hypotension and reduced lung perfusion, asphyxia at birth could lead to hypoxia, hypercapnia, and acidosis, and hypoglycemia in the newborn could lead to poor alveolar cell metabolism. Each of these conditions and also others could start the cycle.

covery proceeds rapidly. Long-term effects are not known. Survival is improving, and more information will become available.

Diagnosis

Hyaline membrane disease cannot be clearly identified by a clinical or laboratory finding, but diagnosis is inferred from clinical signs and symptoms, physical examination, and chest x-ray. A grunt with expiration very soon after birth, often within 15 minutes, chest retraction within the first hour of life, and a respiratory rate of over 60 per minute within a few hours suggest that great effort is necessary to ventilate the lungs. On chest x-ray the lungs show a fine mottling or granular appearance early in the disease and increased opacity later; the x-ray also shows air clearly present in the bronchi and shows hypoexpansion, which suggests atelectasis. A chest x-ray does not give conclusive evidence of the disease, but it aids in diagnosis and is important in ruling out other causes of respiratory distress.

Prevention

Preventive measures against hyaline membrane disease are those which help the baby to be born in optimum condition and which assist him to make the transition to extrauterine life with minimum stress. These include prevention of premature birth, and optimum treatment of complications of pregnancy to protect the baby from intrauterine distress, if possible; protection against causes of asphyxia at birth, and protection against chilling at birth.

Prenatal identification of infants at risk of developing HMD through L/S studies is very important because delivery can sometimes be postponed until the lung matures, or if early delivery is likely or is indicated, glucocorticoids can often be given to accelerate lung maturation. The important finding that accurately predicts increasing fetal lung maturity is an increase in the concentration of lecithin in the amniotic fluid. Amniocentesis and measurement of the ratio of lecithin to sphingomyelin has been de-

scribed on pages 610–13. When the concentration of lecithin is at least two times greater than the sphingomyelin the probability of the baby developing HMD is very small.

Careful evaluation of the lung maturity of a fetus by L/S ratio is a necessary preventive measure prior to elective induction of labor or elective cesarean section. The L/S ratio is usually mature by 36 weeks gestation, but it may be delayed until after 37 weeks. Lung maturation can only be determined by L/S ratio, and with such evaluation inadvertent delivery of a baby with immature lungs can be avoided.

Observation and Treatment

With careful observation of all babies immediately after birth, signs of respiratory difficulty may be detected very early. When the nurse recognizes early signs of respiratory distress and reports these to the physician immediately, the supportive care that the baby needs can be started before respiratory distress reaches a stage of serious physiologic disturbances. As the disease progresses, the nurse's continuous care of the baby often helps to avert serious difficulty if a sudden change in condition takes place, and her ongoing observations and reports to the physician provide him with an overall picture of the baby's progress and need for medical management.

Nursing care and observations of the baby with hyaline membrane disease can be inferred from the preceding description of the characteristics of the disease and its treatment. A brief comment on a number of these aspects of care follows.

Observation of vital signs and signs of respiratory distress must be made and recorded at hourly intervals at least. The baby's body temperature reading must be observed and the incubator temperature adjusted as necessary to raise the body temperature as quickly as possible to approximately 98°F (36.7°C) axillary or 98.6°F (37°C) rectally. Skin temperature, if possible, incubator temperature, and body temperature should be recorded.

The heart rate and respiratory rate must be closely observed. Monitoring machines may be used to monitor heart function and respirations, but these functions must also be closely observed visually and with the stethoscope. The blood pressure must be carefully monitored for variations from normal. A small baby of 1000 to 2000 gm (2 lb 4 oz to 4 lb 7 oz) will normally have a blood pressure of approximately 50/30; one that weighs over 3000 gm (6 lb 10 oz) will have a pressure of around 68/42.

Mucus must be suctioned from the respiratory tract as it appears, and the baby's position must be changed frequently to prevent hypostatic pneumonia.

Apneic spells must be observed, and if breathing does not readily resume, the nurse must stimulate and, if necessary, resuscitate the baby while the physician is called.

Treatment of babies with hyaline membrane disease is supportive. It is directed toward elimination or improvement of each abnormality in the cycle of events described above and includes careful regulation of the thermal environment, oxygen therapy, intravenous fluids to correct acidosis and provide for nutrition, continuous positive airway pressure or assisted mechanical ventilation, and protection from unnecessary exertion. Treatment must be started early in an attempt to avert major pathologic changes or to reverse changes before they become severe.

Treatment for HMD includes all of the therapies described for respiratory distress on pages 767–83. The most important consideration in treatment of infants with hyaline membrane disease is to improve oxygenation. This is essential for normal tissue oxygenation and for normal cardiac output and renal perfusion. Without good oxygenation anaerobic metabolism takes place and metabolic acidosis develops. Also, there will be pulmonary vasoconstriction and right-to-left shunting of blood. With hypoxia and acidosis, pulmonary hypoperfusion and fetal circulatory patterns will shunt considerable blood, which then does not become oxygenated.

The goal of oxygen administration is to maintain the PO_2 between 50 and 80 mmHg. The baby is given enough oxygen to try to correct hypoxia, but great care must be taken to avoid hyperoxia and damage to the eyes and/or the lungs.

Continuous positive airway pressure (CPAP) is a very useful treatment for HMD. Current data suggest that the lung is unable to synthesize surface-active pulmonary surfactant in sufficient quantity when the alveoli collapse with each expiration and need to be reinflated with each inspiration. When such a condition exists, early use of CPAP is believed to conserve surfactant or at least make its production possible by improving oxygenation. Continuous positive airway pressure has effectively reduced the severity of hyaline membrane disease and has markedly reduced the mortality rate.

Continuous positive airway pressure is usually instituted when it has become necessary to raise the concentration of inspired oxygen up to 60 percent or sometimes more in order to keep the PO_2 at 50 mmHg.

The baby with hyaline membrane disease may become very tired from the constant effort to take each breath, and may then need IPPV as well as CPAP. The amount of carbon dioxide retained, as measured by PCO_2, also determines use of ventilatory assistance. A PCO_2 of 70 mmHg usually indicates need for assisted ventilation. Frequent and prolonged spells of apnea also indicate a need for ventilation.

Nutritional support is important for a sick baby for recovery as well as for growth. Intravenous fluids of glucose will be started early for fluid requirements, and if the baby is unable to take oral food for a number of days nutrients of protein and fat may be given intravenously. Careful regulation of intravenous fluids is required and a careful record of intake and output is kept.

The baby with respiratory distress needs protection from all unnecessary handling and exertion. With the baby in an incubator many of the necessary observations can be made without undue handling. Baths should be limited to only those that are absolutely essential, and any unnecessary care should be omitted. The baby needs as much rest as possible.

Use of assisted ventilation and oxygen requires very special care and close observation of blood gases. Special care nurseries have the staff and the facilities to carry out the very sophisticated treatment that is now possible for these sick infants. Such treatment should be provided for these babies, since it has effectively reduced the mortality of hyaline membrane disease in premature infants.

Since the baby with hyaline membrane disease is usually a preterm infant, the care described for preterm infants on pages 715–44 is continued as the baby recovers from respiratory distress. A long period of hospitalization may yet be ahead for the immature infant after recovery from the respiratory problem.

TYPE II RESPIRATORY DISTRESS SYNDROME

Type II respiratory distress syndrome (RDS) bears resemblance to hyaline membrane disease, but has a different history, is more benign in its course, and has a good prognosis. This syndrome has also been called transient tachypnea of the newborn, transient respiratory distress of the newborn, aspiration syndrome, wet-lung disease, and perhaps other names.

Infants with Type II RDS initially may have respiratory symptoms similar to those with hyaline membrane disease, although usually less severe. In the first hours after birth they develop tachypnea, retractions, grunting, and cyanosis. Respiratory rate may be normal or even depressed at first because many of these babies present a picture of oversedation at birth. They may be alert and appear to be in good condition at the moment of birth and have a good Apgar score because of the stimulation of birth and the environment. Then when stimulation decreases, the baby becomes sleepy and may hypoventilate, and have depression of cough,

gag, and swallowing reflexes. Aspiration is a possibility. After a few hours, tachypnea appears and respiratory rate may be as high as 100 per minute or even more.

Grunting respirations begin early. The amount of chest retraction will depend upon the extent of illness and the maturity of the baby, since the chest cage has more stability in the older infant than in the very immature. Flaring of the nostrils is often seen. Cyanosis is usually visible in room air.

A predisposition to this syndrome occurs in infants who are slightly preterm, showing some evidence of immaturity, and with a history of heavy maternal sedation. Sometimes there has been an episode of intrauterine asphyxia, as with maternal bleeding, and sometimes with cesarean section. This history is in contrast to that of HMD, which occurs in more immature babies, who frequently have had a period of perinatal distress.

Whereas babies with HMD have a surfactant deficiency and widespread atelectasis, babies with Type II RDS are likely to have some problem with aspiration and a delayed absorption of lung fluid. (See page 420 for discussion on lung fluid.) Heavy sedation may result in the baby's failure to clear the airway well of mucus. Even when initial suctioning of the airways has been good, depressed gag, swallow, and cough reflexes may permit pooling of secretions in the tracheobronchial tree, especially if the baby is not carefully observed until he becomes reactive. If there has been some birth asphyxia, there may also be a delay in the normal changes in the circulatory pattern, and a delay in the removal of lung fluid by the lymphatics. The chest x-ray shows hyperaeration and overexpansion of the lungs.

Respiratory distress with Type II RDS usually lasts from 24 to 96 hours. Grunting and retraction last 24 to 48 hours and tachypnea lasts somewhat longer. These babies need oxygen during their period of respiratory distress, perhaps even as high as 70 percent for a while, but oxygen need is not as progressive as with HMD.

These babies can easily be hyperoxygenated, and they must be watched very carefully to avoid giving too much. Ventilatory assistance is rarely needed. Hypovolemia is rarely a problem. An acidosis may initially need to be corrected, and intravenous glucose is given for calories and fluids.

Babies who have been sedated require careful observation of their respiratory function, resuscitation as necessary, and continuing observation in the nursery for accumulation of mucus and for ventilatory efforts, at least until through their second period of reactivity. (See pages 492–99 for discussion of periods of reactivity and for observations and care during the transitional period.)

TRANSIENT TACHYPNEA OF THE NEWBORN

With transient tachypnea of the newborn (TTNB), the baby, either full-term or preterm, has an unexplained persistently high respiratory rate, up to 100 or more per minute. Cyanosis is not common, although the baby may need a small increase in percentage of inspired oxygen. Air exchange seems to be good, expiratory grunt is generally not heard, and intercostal retraction is usually minimal. An x-ray can usually be used to distinguish this condition from HMD and Type II RDS. It has been suggested that this transient tachypnea is the result of slow absorption of lung fluid. The lung compliance would be decreased because of the additional fluid and the rapid respirations would then minimize respiratory work. Aspiration of amniotic fluid or mucus has also been considered a cause.

The TTNB syndrome appears to be self-limiting. It resolves in several days. Careful monitoring of respiration and heart rate is necessary, at least at first, to distinguish this syndrome from more serious respiratory distress. Oral feedings may need to be withheld until tachypnea subsides in order to avoid aspiration.

DISTRESS FROM ASPIRATION OF MECONIUM

Aspiration of amniotic fluid containing meconium is apt to be followed by respiratory distress. Meconium may plug small air passages and is irritating to lung tissues. Following aspiration the lungs may have areas of atelectasis due to obstruction and areas of consolidation, and the baby is susceptible to secondary infection of the lungs.

Aspiration of meconium may occur in any condition in which hypoxia causes the fetus to pass some meconium *in utero*. A baby with hypoxia is in danger of aspiration *in utero* or at birth. It may therefore follow any complication of pregnancy or labor that interferes with adequate fetal oxygenation. It may be associated with fetal growth retardation (SGA baby) and with postmaturity—conditions in which intrauterine hypoxia and passage of meconium may occur because of insufficient placental function. A baby with meconium-stained amniotic fluid and meconium-stained skin must be closely observed for signs of distress. The lungs may clear within 24 to 48 hours after aspiration of meconium, but distress may be severe enough to cause a serious illness that requires long-term respiratory assistance, and often it causes death.

The morbidity and mortality from meconium aspiration can be greatly reduced by carrying out tracheal suction before the meconium is pulled into the small air passages. The mechanism of meconium aspiration and prevention of airway obstruction by meconium has been described on page 750 in relation to the postmaturity syndrome.

If a baby does aspirate meconium, he is likely to have tachypnea and labored respirations, which may be gasping. Chest retraction is common. Significant hyperinflation of the chest is usually seen. The chest is enlarged, especially in the anterior–posterior diameter, and there may be a prominent anterior sternal bulge. A chest x-ray shows areas of increased density and areas of overexpansion distributed throughout the lung. The baby may have considerable mucus, which may be meconium-stained. Pneumothorax is a complication of respiratory distress from meconium aspiration. A pneumothorax must be considered whenever there is an abrupt worsening in the baby's condition.

Management of respiratory distress from meconium aspiration will depend upon the clinical course. It will include oxygen, humidification, parenteral fluids, correction of acid–base imbalance, postural drainage and percussion, and perhaps other interventions as described on pages 767–83. Antibiotics may be used if lung infection is suspected.

NEONATAL HEART DISEASE

Many and complex anatomic anomalies involving the heart and/or the great vessels may develop in the fetus. The heart goes through a very complicated developmental process, and a disturbance at any one of the series of changes may result in a congenital malformation.

Some cardiac problems in the newborn are critically serious, complicated cardiac malformations, but others are caused by relatively less serious left-to-right shunts. Among important left-to-right shunt lesions are isolated ventricular septal defect, which is believed to account for between 30 and 40 percent of all congenital heart disease, and atrial septal defect, and patent ductus arteriosus. Serious and sometimes fatal lesions include hypoplastic left ventricle syndrome, coarctation of the aorta, transposition of the great arteries, hypoplastic right ventricle syndrome, and tetralogy of Fallot. Lesions may involve persistent communication between pulmonary and systemic circulation, underdeveloped ventricles or pulmonary artery, stenosis of valves, constriction of vessels such as the aorta, and transposition of vessels. Various combinations of defects may exist.

Some defects are functional and disappear within a few months. Some remain but do not require treatment and do not produce a handicap. Some require surgery to support life, and some are so marked that they are incompatible with life. Congenital heart lesions may be accompanied by anomalies in other parts of the body.

Remarkable advances have been made in recent years in management of babies with heart disease. Diagnostic methods and corrective operative procedures for infants have become much more sophisticated and are now used in the neonatal period. Formerly early treatment was not the case. Centralization of services is necessary for the complex treatment that is now possible for infants with heart disease.

Congenital cardiac anomalies may present no problem until the circulatory adjustments after birth have taken place. Cardiac lesions are not detrimental to the fetus because they do not interfere with the fetal circulatory pattern. With birth and the radical change in the pattern of circulation, a defect in the development of the heart and/or the great vessels is likely to compromise the normal flow pattern and cause cardiac disease. Cardiac problems in the newborn frequently do not appear immediately after birth for several reasons. All of the changes in circulation are not completed immediately after birth and difficulty may not appear until these changes are more complete. Also, compensatory mechanisms may be established and function reasonably well for awhile, until their load becomes too great. The kind of malfunction and its extent will determine how and when signs and symptoms appear.

At birth, when the placental circulation is eliminated and its large low-resistance circuit is removed, the baby's total systemic vascular resistance increases. At the same time expansion of the lungs with air results in a considerable decrease in pulmonary vascular resistance. The result of the increase in systemic vascular resistance, and the decrease in pulmonary vascular resistance is a nearly equal resistance in each system very soon after birth. A small amount of blood may flow from one circulation to another for a short time, but normally, with good oxygenation, the ductus arteriosus closes functionally within 10 to 15 hours. Also pressure changes in the atria close the foramen ovale after birth. Pressure in the left atrium is raised with the marked increase in pulmonary blood flow, and pressure in the right atrium is lowered as aeration of the lungs decreases the pulmonary vascular resistance and as removal of the placental circulation decreases the amount of blood flowing through the inferior vena cava to the right atrium.

The pulmonary circulation is not completely changed immediately after birth, but rather continues to undergo changes during the first six to eight weeks postnatally. In the first several days the pulmonary vascular resistance continues to decrease as the result of further expansion of alveoli. Then, in a normal maturational development, the pulmonary arterioles lose some smooth muscle and dilate still more, bringing about a further decrease in pulmonary arteriole pressure.

With the changes in circulatory resistances that take place at birth and thereafter, problems will arise if there is communication between the systemic and pulmonary circulations, as there is with a ventricular septal defect and a persistent patent ductus arteriosus. At first, when the pulmonary vascular resistance is still relatively high, flow across communication channels may not be great. As pulmonary resistance decreases, however, there is an increase of blood flow into the pulmonary circulation. As a result of such increase there is an increase in the pulmonary venous return to the left atrium and the left ventricle.

The action of the left ventricle will be related to the volume of blood that expands it. As the volume of blood returning from the lungs to the left ventricle increases the ventricle increases its stroke volume. As pulmonary resistance increasingly falls during the first weeks of life, a greater and greater load is placed on the left ventricle as it works against the rising blood volume and as it tries to meet the systemic circulatory needs. As long as the ventricle can maintain its increased stroke volume or has time to develop

hypertrophy, symptoms do not appear, but finally the ventricle becomes overworked and cardiac failure becomes apparent.[24] Any congenital heart lesion in which there is communication between the ventricles or great vessels is likely to show left ventricular failure in time, along with the decrease in pulmonary vascular resistance that occurs with normal maturation during the weeks after birth.

When congenital heart defects are the result of a narrowed opening that cause obstruction to blood flow, heart failure may develop because of the increased systolic pressure that is necessary to effect blood flow across the obstruction. If there is no time for a compensatory hypertrophy to develop, the increased end-systolic volume will dilate the ventricle. An increase in end-diastolic pressure and volume will then occur, and the same problem of overextension and cardiac failure occurs that was described above for shunt lesions. It is because of this that babies with coarctation of the aorta or aortic stenosis develop heart failure almost immediately after birth. A large overload of pressure is applied to the left ventricle before it has had time to develop a compensating hypertrophy. When a lesion is small enough to allow time for adaptive growth, heart failure does not occur until late childhood or adult life.[25]

An elevated left ventricular pressure from either left-sided obstructive lesions or large left-to-right shunts causes an increase in left atrial and pulmonary venous pressure. The pressure may become high enough to cause more exudation of fluid through the pulmonary capillaries than can be removed by lymphatic drainage. Pulmonary edema then develops. Clinical evidence of pulmonary edema appears at lower pressures in infants than in adults.

Pulmonary edema is associated with increased rate and depth of respirations. Increased respiratory effort is the most common sign of heart

---

[24] Abraham M. Rudolph, Cardiac failure in children: A hemodynamic overview, *Hosp. Pract.* 5:44–55 (July) 1970, p. 45.
[25] *Ibid.*, p. 47.

failure in infants, since most cardiac defects that produce heart failure in infancy are associated with left-sided failure. Commonly, there is increased respiratory effort, mild cyanosis, decreased P_{O_2}, and slightly increased P_{CO_2}. When a heart murmur is not detected, it is difficult to differentiate the problem from respiratory disease, at least initially.

The majority of heart defects that produce heart failure in infants are associated with left-sided failure. When left-sided failure persists for sometime, right-sided failure usually develops. Right-sided failure may, however, be primary, as with severe pulmonary stenosis or preductal coarctation of the aorta with patent ductus arteriosus. Right-sided failure does not commonly present with gross edema as in the adult. An early sign is enlargement of the liver. Another early sign of heart failure is increased perspiration, especially around the face and head, particularly noticeable during feedings.

Early recognition of heart disease is important to permit time for transfer of the baby to a specially equipped and staffed cardiac center, and time for cardiac catheterization for diagnosis, and then surgery as indicated. A baby with heart disease in the early days of life may deteriorate rapidly.

For reasons described above, signs and symptoms of heart disease may be absent in the infant, may occur occasionally, or may be constant in a mild or severe form. Signs and symptoms may occur because of a communication between the systemic and pulmonary circulation, or because of an increased load placed on the heart when it is necessary to force blood through narrow passages or stenotic valves.

Cyanosis is a common manifestation of congenital heart disease, but it may be absent or may not appear until later in life. Blueness of the baby's hands and feet is normal for a few hours after birth, but all other parts of his body should be pink. A persistence of cyanosis of the hands and feet after several hours, when oxygenation and circulation should be improved, is considered abnormal. It is suggestive of heart disease, pulmonary pathology, or occasionally

birth injury. Cyanosis without pulmonary disease is usually due to serious cardiac abnormality. Especially in the first week of life, cyanosis may be the only evidence of a cardiac lesion. Cyanosis, which is much more threatening than a murmur, is likely the result of impaired oxygenation because of edema fluid in the alveoli.

A persistent heart murmur is a common sign of a heart abnormality. A precordial murmur in the early neonatal period may be due to delayed closure of one of the fetal openings. It may, therefore, not be significant unless it persists.

Respiratory symptoms commonly precede first detection of a murmur. Rapid, labored respirations, often 60 breaths per minute or more, may precede deterioration to dyspnea and congestive heart failure. Tachypnea requires investigation for respiratory or cardiac cause. When the infant with cardiac disease has predominantly respiratory symptoms he may have congestive heart failure.

Edema may appear early or late.

A baby with cardiac disease may not take his feedings well.

Palpation of the femoral and brachial arteries for pulsation and comparison with each other may help to detect coarctation of the aorta before other signs develop. Pulsations in the femoral arteries are decreased or absent or significantly delayed in coarctation of the aorta because the circulation of the lower part of the body must, to a large extent, be carried on by a collateral circulation. Left brachial pulses may be decreased if the left subclavian arises at or below the coarctation.

While preparing for diagnosis by cardiac catheterization and further treatment, the baby with respiratory problems and edema is treated with administration of oxygen, diuretics, and digitalis.

HYPOGLYCEMIA

The importance of hypoglycemia in the newborn with its serious threat to the baby's welfare has come to be well recognized in recent years and has been found to be more common than previously thought. Hypoglycemia can be the cause of certain early postnatal problems such as a contributing cause of respiratory distress. Much more importantly, it may result in irreparable brain damage. Hypoglycemia is a serious threat to brain cells since the brain can use *only glucose* (not other sugars) for its energy and requires a constant supply. The amount of glucose available to the brain is directly related to the blood glucose concentration. When the blood glucose value is low, there is a real possibility of deprivation of glucose to cerebral tissues, possible permanent impairment of the cells, and residual neurologic defects. The effect upon the brain cells is likely to correlate with the duration of the hypoglycemia.

Since brain damage from hypoglycemia is preventable, the importance of early recognition of a low blood sugar in the newborn and prompt intervention to replace a blood glucose deficiency cannot be overemphasized. Dangerously long periods of hypoglycemia in any infant are unnecessary with current easy diagnostic procedures and knowledge of treatment.

Hypoglycemia may be defined as a significantly low level of *glucose (true sugar)* in whole blood on two reliable repeated examinations that measure the level of *true* blood sugar. Normal blood sugar values in newborns range from 45 to 100 mg/100 ml of blood. A value of 45 mg is considered slightly low and one that reaches a level of 100 mg slightly high. An average between these two values, such as 70 to 80 mg, comes near to an ideal level during the first several days of life. Less than 30 mg of glucose/100 ml of blood is regarded as hypoglycemia. This is considered to be harmful to the baby and may cause symptoms, described below, and will cause chemical brain damage if allowed to persist.

Stated in somewhat more detail, a common definition of neonatal hypoglycemia is as follows: A whole blood sugar level of less than 30 mg/100 ml (less than 35 mg in serum or plasma) in the first 72 hours of life, or of less than 40 mg (less than 45 mg in serum or plasma) after the third

day, in full-term, full-sized infants. In babies of low birth weight the lower figure of normal is 20 mg/100 ml in whole blood or 25 mg in plasma or serum. One low reading is adequate for initiating therapy, but two successive low readings should be used to establish a diagnosis if the baby is asymptomatic.[26]

Dr. Leo Stern states that the levels of blood sugar given above for a definition of hypoglycemia may be dangerously low for some babies. He states that blood glucose levels below 40 mg/100 ml in any infant should be corrected.[27]

During intrauterine life glucose is continuously transferred across the placenta from the maternal to the fetal circulation, supplying a major source of energy to the fetus. At birth, when the baby's energy demands increase, his glucose supply is suddenly cut off. The baby's immediate response to this change is rapid glycogenolysis, using the liver glycogen supply. In addition fat deposits are mobilized for energy.

At birth the blood glucose level in the baby is proportional to that of the mother; venous blood sugar values in the baby are 70 to 80 percent of those of the mother's venous blood sugar level. Variations in values will depend upon maternal expenditures of energy during labor and administration of glucose to the mother during labor. The baby's blood glucose level at birth will depend upon the mother's actual blood glucose level. After birth the baby's blood glucose level falls with a rate varying with the baby's condition and expenditure of energy. In the normal newborn, the blood glucose reaches its lowest level sometime between 1½ and 3 hours of age and then averages around 45 to 50 mg/100 ml of blood. In the normal newborn, without undue postnatal stress, there is a gradual return to higher levels of blood glucose and

[26] Marvin Cornblath, Disorders of carbohydrate metabolism, in *Diseases of the Newborn*, 4th ed., edited by Alexander J. Schaffer and Mary Ellen Avery. Saunders, Philadelphia, Pa., 1977, p. 519.

[27] Leo Stern, Comment on hypoglycemia, in *Care of the High-Risk Neonate*, edited by Marshall H. Klaus and Avroy A. Fanaroff. Saunders, Philadelphia, Pa., 1973, p. 170.

a stability of values by 4 to 6 hours of age. A rise to 60 mg or more/100 ml of blood will occur if the baby has been kept warm; with cooling this value may only average 45 mg. In general, during the first six to twelve hours of life, normal babies who have not been fed will have blood sugar levels between 30 and 125 mg/100 ml of blood with average values of 60 mg/100 ml. After 72 hours most normal infants maintain a blood glucose level of 70 to 75 mg/100 ml of blood. At this age values below 40 mg/100 ml are considered hypoglycemic; values over 125 mg are also abnormal.

Return to normal blood glucose values in a few hours in the *normal* newborn occurs because the baby can make energy and glucose for himself in several ways. He can mobilize glycogen stored in the liver and convert it to glucose and mobilize fatty acids from fat stores and convert them into energy. Stress of low blood sugar increases release of epinephrine from the adrenal gland. The epinephrine mobilizes liver glycogen and inhibits pancreatic release of insulin. With less insulin the blood glucose level tends to remain up.

The level of blood glucose in a fasting newborn is the balance between the amount of liver glycogen that is mobilized and converted to glucose and the amount that is used for energy, vital body functions, and adjustments to extrauterine life. Respiratory distress at birth and chilling quickly use up a supply of glucose. Food and intravenous fluids can augment the body supply of glucose. Food and intravenous fluids can augment the body supply of glucose, but unless both glycogen stores and exogenous supply are adequate the blood glucose level drops to below normal.

When feeding of a baby is started, his blood sugar tends to rise, although fluctuations may remain wide. Early feedings would thus seem to be advantageous to most normal newborn infants.

Hypoglycemia may occur in many conditions. In some babies hypoglycemia is considered idiopathic and may appear in apparently normal healthy newborns. In others, there are predisposing factors, mainly placental dysfunction and neonatal illness.

Hypoglycemia often has its onset with undernourishment *in utero*. Babies of low birth weight, either premature or full-term gestation, are very susceptible to hypoglycemia. Most of the liver glycogen reserve and the fat stores are built up late in pregnancy and normally increase with gestational age. A baby born prematurely does not yet have an adequate glycogen supply or fat store. Placental insufficiency, resulting in intrauterine growth retardation, often means failure of adequate liver glycogen storage and fat deposits, even when the pregnancy continues to full-term, or the store once laid down may be depleted before birth. These babies are usually undernourished and many are under the tenth percentile of birth weight for gestational age. A baby born to a mother with complications such as preeclampsia, renal disease, cardiac disease, chronic infection must be considered susceptible to hypoglycemia. The postterm baby is likely to develop low blood glucose levels. Placental function is apt to decrease after full-term gestation and the baby who remains *in utero* for 42 to 43 weeks or even longer begins to exhaust his stores to satisfy his nutritional needs before he is born. If any of the low-birth-weight babies becomes cooled or has respiratory distress he rapidly uses up his meager stores. A small baby under optimal conditions is low on glucose reserves in 18 to 24 hours. If he became cooled he may be lacking reserves in six to eight hours, and if he was also asphyxiated his reserve is likely to be very low in four hours.

A large baby, over the ninetieth percentile of birth weight for gestational age and the baby born of a diabetic mother are very susceptible to hypoglycemia. The problems of the baby of a diabetic mother are discussed separately on page 800.

Among other conditions that lead to susceptibility to hypoglycemia are a hematocrit of over 65 percent, hypothermia, asphyxia, hypoxia, respiratory distress syndrome, infection, erythroblastosis, and any other condition that results in illness. Any stress condition that increases the metabolic rate requires additional glucose and is likely to deplete a baby's glycogen stores.

Symptoms

Symptoms of hypoglycemia are vague, subtle, and nonspecific to the disorder. It is especially important to be aware of the fact that hypoglycemia in the newborn may be asymptomatic and that diagnosis is made only by blood sugar determination. This makes it important to be alert to a baby's susceptibility and to screen any baby in question.

Among symptoms that may appear in a baby with hypoglycemia are increased respiration; apneic spells; cyanosis; tremors, twitching, and jitteriness, or apathy, limpness, listlessness, poor muscle tone and weak reflexes; unstable temperature regulation; eye rolling; high-pitched cry; and difficulty in feeding. Convulsive seizure may appear late. It is apparent that any of these symptoms may be caused by a number of other conditions.

Diagnosis

Diagnosis of hypoglycemia is made by blood glucose determinations. Since asymptomatic hypoglycemia may be significant, or symptoms may be vague, routine measurement of blood glucose on all low-birth-weight babies, all other high-risk babies, and any apparently normal suspect babies is important. Duplicate screening is important for diagnosis and repeated monitoring must be done until it is certain that the baby's blood sugar level is remaining normal. The nurse has an important responsibility to recognize suspicious symptoms of hypoglycemia and to identify babies with increased risk in order that she may alert all individuals concerned with the baby's care. Such observation and reporting should ensure that rapid assessment and treatment, if indicated, will be fulfilled.

Infants in any risk category require routine screening at least at 1½, 3, and 6 hours after birth. In some nurseries all babies in the nursery are screened between two and four hours of age.

In addition to a laboratory micromethod of testing blood sugar, a reagent test strip (Ames Company Dextrostix) may be used as a screening test. The Dextrostix has an enzyme on the active end of the test strip, which changes color when exposed to glucose. A drop of blood from a finger or heel puncture is put on the active end of the strip, washed off in exactly 60 seconds, and read immediately by comparison to a color chart. The color change of the test strip is proportional to the amount of glucose in the blood. The scale of color ranges from pale gray at 20 to 30 mg/100 ml blood through deepening shades of blue-gray when the amount of sugar in the blood is higher. The color distinguishes between glucose values of 20, 30, 45, 60, and 90 and higher mg/100 ml of blood. The color scheme is accurate, reliable, and dependable, at least at the lower levels of the scale. Laboratory studies may be necessary as follow-up when color changes are doubtful or when confirmation of results is desirable. (See Figure 26-2.)

The Dextrostix enzyme test strip is very useful for occasional or frequent checks since it is readily available and easy to use. It may be used for frequent checks of babies "at-risk," or with suggestive symptoms, or for results of treatment, or for routine screening. Nurses can easily learn to use the Dextrostix. Since timing is of crucial importance in the accuracy of the test, this precaution and all other directions must be carefully observed when the test is done. Some nurses feel more comfortable in using a short, small-gauge hypodermic needle instead of a lancet for the heel stick. The method of heel stick seems immaterial if a large drop of blood, sufficient to cover the entire reagent area, is easily obtained.

Treatment

Prompt administration of glucose will usually establish normal blood glucose levels. The method of administration will depend upon the baby's ability to suck and swallow. The amount and strength of the glucose solution to be given will be gauged by the blood sugar readings.

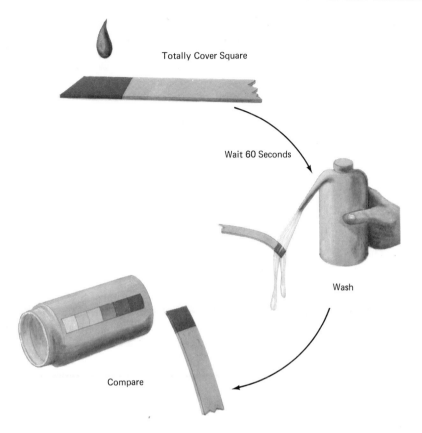

Totally Cover Square

Wait 60 Seconds

Wash

Compare

Figure 26-2. Method of testing blood sugar with a reagent test strip—the Dextrostix. A large drop of blood is put on the reagent end of the test strip, covering it completely. After exactly 60 seconds the blood is washed off with water from a wash bottle and the color of the reagent end of the test strip is compared with a color chart. All directions must be carefully observed. Accurate timing is crucial to the accuracy of the results.

A large baby may be fed a 5 or 10 percent glucose solution orally as soon as his blood glucose value is found to be lower than 45 mg/100 ml of blood. He is usually given the amount of glucose he will take, which may vary from 10 to 30 ml of fluid. His blood sugar level may be monitored in one-half hour after completion of his feeding to determine if he took a sufficient amount of glucose to raise his blood sugar level to normal. Since a hypoglycemic baby may lose his swallowing reflex, the nurse who feeds the baby must proceed with caution. The baby may not be able to take an oral feeding. A gavage feeding may be indicated.

For a small baby the glucose solution may be administered intravenously, usually by peripheral vein. A constant infusion pump will ensure a steady flow of solution as determined to meet the baby's requirement to maintain a good blood sugar level. A hypertonic glucose solution may at first be used. Blood glucose levels are monitored every one to two hours to determine his needs to maintain a normal level.

After a baby's blood glucose level has been raised, subsequent frequent assessments are important until it is determined that the level will remain normal. The cause of the hypoglycemia and presence or absence of complications will determine if normoglycemia will quickly be established or if observation and treatment over a period of several days are necessary. When tolerated, early oral or intravenous glucose feedings are soon followed by full formula feedings with glucose supplementation, if necessary.

In view of the frequency of hypoglycemia in newborns, delayed feedings, a common practice in the past, must seriously be questioned. It would appear that early bottle or breast feedings, if the baby can suck and swallow, or tube feedings or intravenous administration of glucose is important to all babies.

THE BABY OF A DIABETIC MOTHER

The baby born of a diabetic mother is susceptible to certain complications that require intensive care. The baby is usually large-for-gestational age, having received a great deal of glucose because of maternal hyperglycemia. Some babies, however, born of mothers with diabetes are small-for-gestational age because of insufficient placental perfusion. The fetus of a mother with diabetes is very vulnerable to maternal ketoacidosis. Congenital anomalies are more common than in the general population of newborns (see page 680). The possibility of intrauterine death during the last weeks of pregnancy raises concern, and preterm delivery is sometimes necessary. For delivery, labor is often induced and may be rather long and the incidence of cesarean section delivery is increased.

In the past, these babies often were delivered prematurely, a few weeks before term, because of concern over intrauterine death. Currently it is possible to closely monitor placental function and fetal response to the intrauterine environment. This makes it possible to permit pregnancy to continue closer to term in a number of patients. Monitoring during labor may also show that a cesarean section is not necessary as frequently as it was done in the past.

An attempt is made to keep maternal blood glucose levels under 100 mg/100 ml of blood during labor or prior to cesarean section. This gives the fetus an opportunity to adjust to a lower glucose load with a decrease in insulin production and a decrease in hypoglycemic response after birth. It is advisable for the reader to review diabetes mellitus (its effects on mother and fetus and its management) on pages 678–86.

Unusual environmental conditions *in utero*, which lead to the need for marked postnatal adjustment, plus perhaps prematurity and sometimes long labor or cesarean section, result in two major serious difficulties in the newborn—hypoglycemia and respiratory distress. In addition, hypocalcemia and hyperbilirubinemia may present problems in these infants.

The baby of a diabetic mother often grows to excessive size in weight and length. His size is inconsistent with his gestational age. A premature baby may be as large as, or larger than, a full-term. Typically the baby is in the upper percentile on an intrauterine growth chart, unless the mother had some other condition that caused intrauterine growth retardation. The baby's abnormal weight is due to an excess of fat and glycogen in his body tissues. Insulin does not transfer across the placental barrier freely but glucose does. Since glucose passes from the mother's blood to the fetal circulation with ease, the hyperglycemia that is common in the mother keeps the blood glucose in the fetus at an abnormally high level much of the time. This elevated blood sugar level in the fetus exaggerates certain metabolic functions, particularly storage of glycogen and fat and increased insulin production. The excess glucose is converted into glycogen, which is stored in the liver and heart, and into fats, which are stored in fat depots. These large stores result in enlargement of the liver and heart, and in abundant subcutaneous fat. Increased blood sugar from the mother stimulates increased fetal insulin production, which does not cross the placenta to the mother leaving the fetus with hyperinsulinemia.

In addition to excessive size the baby of a diabetic mother may have a puffy cushingoid appearance with round cheeks and short neck; enlarged heart, liver, and spleen; rapid irregular respirations; lethargy at times but an increased Moro reflex and irritability with slight stimulation; and at first a red, tense skin, which later shows jaundice.

James W. Farquhar has described the intrauterine environment and its effects, and the appearance of babies born of diabetic mothers, as follows[28]:

The infants are remarkable not only because, like fetal versions of Shadrach, Meshach and Abednego, they emerge at least alive from within the fiery metabolic furnace of diabetes mellitus, but because they resemble one another so closely that they might well be related. They are plump, sleek, liberally coated with vernix caseosa, full-faced and plethoric. The umbilical cord and the placenta share in the gigantism. During their first 24 or more extrauterine hours they lie on their backs, bloated and flushed, their legs flexed and abducted, their lightly closed hands on each side of the head, the abdomen prominent and their respiration sighing. They convey a distinct impression of having had such a surfeit of both food and fluid pressed upon them by an insistent hostess that they desire only peace so that they may recover from their excesses. And on the second day their resentment of the slightest noise improves the analogy, while their trembling anxiety seems to speak of intrauterine indiscretions of which we know nothing.

If the mother's diabetes can be carefully controlled throughout pregnancy, the baby may not grow to be excessively large for his gestational age, but often times management is very difficult even with excellent medical care and efforts on the part of the mother.

Regardless of size or gestational age the baby is treated as a premature or high-risk baby and cared for in an intensive care unit. He is usually cared for in an incubator for good visibility of his condition and close control of his environment. Observation and treatment for respiratory distress and hypoglycemia are of major immediate concern.

Hypoglycemia

With birth the infant of the diabetic mother suffers from the sudden cut-off of the high glucose supply from his mother and the stimulus

[28] James W. Farquhar, The child of the diabetic woman, *Arch. Dis. Child.* 34:76–77, 1959.

that his pancreas received *in utero* to secrete a large amount of insulin. All newborns have a lowering of blood glucose. The infant of a diabetic, in addition, has a large amount of circulating insulin which will lower his blood glucose level more than normal. As liver glycogen is broken down to elevate the baby's blood glucose level, that elevation of blood glucose in turn causes a further large secretion of insulin, resulting in a still greater hypoglycemia. In many babies the glucose level quickly falls below 30 mg/100 ml of blood, and often goes below 20 mg or even lower during the first few hours, and often even within the first hour. The necessity of immediate blood sugar check after birth and continuing frequent checks is obvious.

In addition to abnormal hypoglycemia the baby of a diabetic mother may be unable to mobilize his excess fat stores. Thus, with hypoglycemia and low serum levels of free fatty acids, the baby has a very small source of energy for certain tissue functions, especially for the glucose-dependent brain and for the heart, which utilizes free fatty acids.

Monitoring and treatment of the infant of a diabetic mother may be somewhat as follows. The blood sugar of the umbilical cord blood may be checked for a baseline. A Dextrostix is done immediately on admission to the nursery and every one-half hour thereafter for three hours. Monitoring following this period may be determined by the baby's response and stability of blood sugar. Laboratory evaluation of blood sugar may also be done once or twice during the first three or four hours and oftener if indicated.

The baby must be given glucose, orally or intravenously, to keep his blood glucose level higher than 40 mg/100 ml of blood, even though elevation of blood glucose may stimulate further insulin production. For the baby who is able to suck and swallow well oral feedings may be started. The baby can usually be fed at one hour of age offering formula of 20 kcal per 30 ml (1 oz) in an amount of 7 ml/kg by gavage or nipple, or the baby may be breast-fed. Possible loss of swallow reflex requires careful evaluation whenever oral feedings are offered. Intravenous administration of 10 percent glucose is started if the baby is unable to take oral feedings, if the Dextrostix falls to 20 mg/100 ml or lower, if the Dextrostix remains below 30 mg on two successive checks, or if the baby becomes symptomatic.

The baby of a diabetic mother is very susceptible to respiratory distress syndrome, regardless of whether he is premature or full-term. The full-term baby's respiratory difficulty is often of metabolic origin. Hyperbilirubinemia is fairly common. Both of these complications are discussed elsewhere in this chapter. Hypocalcemia is a significant complication in babies of diabetic mothers. Many of the signs and symptoms of a low calcium level are nonspecific and similar to those of hypoglycemia. Diagnoses must be made by serum calcium determination. Treatment is administration of calcium gluconate.

NEONATAL HYPOCALCEMIA

Neonatal hypocalcemia may occur early, within the first two days after birth, or "late" when the baby is a week old. A serum calcium level below 7 mg/100 ml blood is usually considered a hypocalcemia.

The "early" hypocalcemia is thought to be caused by perinatal factors and is most likely to occur in preterm infants, babies who have had birth asphyxia, and babies of diabetic mothers. Late hypocalcemia occurs from dietary imbalance of calcium and phosphate.

The cause of hypocalcemia is not completely clear. Several factors are thought to exert an influence. There may be hypofunction of the parathyoid gland, especially in the preterm baby or in perinatal asphyxia or stress. This may lead to a decreased ability to excrete phosphate in the urine. During perinatal asphyxia tissue breakdown adds an additional phosphate load to the circulation. There may also be a maturational delay in responsiveness of the renal tubule to parathormone. This results in hyperphosphatemia with a secondary decrease in serum calcium level. Exchange transfusion with

citrated blood temporarily binds ionized calcium, and rapid correction of acidosis with an alkali decreases the concentration of ionized calcium. It is the ionized calcium that is necessary for use by the cells.

The "late" hypocalcemia sometimes called "seventh-day hypocalcemia" is usually secondary to a high phosphorus load in cow's milk formula. The immature neonatal parathyroid gland is not ready to handle the load. This condition does not occur with breast milk, which contains relatively less calcium and much less phosphate. Presently modified cow's milk formulas have significantly less phosphorus than is present in unmodified cow's milk. Commercially prepared formulas are likely to contain a calcium–phosphorus ratio very similar to breast milk, but a baby who is fed diluted evaporated milk or cow's milk may receive an imbalance of these minerals.

Clinically, the baby with hypocalcemia may show tremulousness, apneic spells, cyanosis, vomiting, and abdominal distension. Carpopedal spasm and convulsions may occur. Symptoms may be confused with those of hypoglycemia, respiratory problems, central nervous system problems, and narcotic withdrawal.

For diagnosis a measurement of serum calcium is made. A value below 7.0 mg/100 ml is considered hypocalcemia. Total calcium levels may drop to 3.0 mg or even lower in severe cases. Roughly about 50 percent of the total calcium is ionized and is available to the cells. The amount of ionized calcium will depend to some extent on the serum protein concentration and on pH.

Hypocalcemia is treated by intravenous administration of calcium gluconate at about 100 mg/kg-day. When symptoms are not dramatic and the baby can take medication orally, treatment may be by oral calcium preparation given in divided doses over 24-hour periods.

HYPERBILIRUBINEMIA

Hyperbilirubinemia in the newborn is an abnormal elevation in serum bilirubin level. It may be caused by an excessive breakdown of red blood cells resulting in accumulation of an unusual amount of indirect bilirubin, or by failure of metabolism of bilirubin to an excretable variety, or a combination of both causes.

Bilirubin is produced when red blood cells break down. Each gram of hemoglobin that is released with red blood cell breakdown gives rise to about 35 mg of bilirubin, which must be conjugated by the liver to be excreted. During fetal life bilirubin is removed from the fetal circulation by the placenta and detoxified and excreted by the mother. After birth the free bilirubin, termed indirect, unconjugated bilirubin, is transported to the baby's liver by serum albumin and there detoxified. Until it is converted, it is insoluble and cannot be excreted. In the liver the indirect bilirubin must be converted by the enzyme glucuronyl transferase to direct bilirubin (bilirubin glucuronide). Direct, conjugated bilirubin is nontoxic, water soluble, and easily excreted into the gastrointestinal tract and the urine. A number of conditions, discussed below, may interfere with adequate excretion of bilirubin. The reader may wish to review a discussion on bilirubin metabolism on pages 429–32.

The concern over hyperbilirubinemia in the newborn is that bilirubin is a toxic substance. Any bilirubin not bound to serum albumin is free to deposit in body tissues—skin, cardiac muscle, kidney, brain. Jaundice of the skin becomes apparent. However, jaundice of the nuclear masses of the brain, termed *kernicterus* (*bilirubin encephalopathy*), is the major concern, since it will leave residual brain damage. Clinical signs of kernicterus are shrill cry, poor sucking, increased lethargy, and later rigidity, spasms, and an opisthotonic position. The amount of unconjugated bilirubin deposited in the brain tissue determines the extent of the neurologic problems.

A nurse's astute observations are important in early discovery and treatment of hyperbilirubinemia. The nurse must observe each baby closely for any evidence of jaundice and report it to the physician promptly. Some babies are known to

be at risk of accumulating excessive bilirubin, but any baby may retain an abnormal amount for any one of a number of reasons. For the baby's color to be judged well, he should be examined in sunlight or white fluorescent light. Yellow-white artificial lights and yellow walls or ceilings give a misleading color. The baby's skin should be blanched by firm pressure with the nurse's thumb or finger over a firm surface such as the baby's forehead or sternum. The color of the underlying skin is observed as soon as the pressure is removed.

Jaundice begins at the face and advances downward on the body, proceeding from face to trunk to extremities and finally to the palms and soles. It is thus advisable to examine the baby undressed. The degree of jaundice and the extent of advancement must then be recorded and reported. Even babies with deeply pigmented skin can be inspected for jaundice of their non-pigmented palms and soles.

Hyperbilirubinemia of physiologic or pathologic jaundice is somewhat difficult to differentiate. In general, however, jaundice is considered abnormal if it appears in the first 24 hours of life, and if the serum bilirubin level rises above 12 mg/100 ml of blood in the full-term baby and 10 mg/100 ml of blood in the premature. A reading up to 12 mg/100 ml of blood has often been considered physiologic but may be pathologic at this level.

A committee on phototherapy in the newborn infant, established by the National Research Council, made the following statements in regard to risks of hyperbilirubinemia and tolerable limits of serum bilirubin levels. Their preliminary report was published in the *Journal of Pediatrics* in January, 1974[29]:

The risks of damage to the central nervous system related to hyperbilirubinemia are increased if jaundice is associated with a history of perinatal asphyxia, respiratory distress, hemolytic disease, acidosis, hy-

[29] Committee on Phototherapy in the Newborn Infant, National Research Council, National Academy of Sciences, Preliminary report of the committee on phototherapy in the newborn infant, *J. Pediatr.* 84:140–141 (Jan.) 1974.

pothermia, low serum albumin concentration, hypoglycemia, or a birth weight of less than 2000 gm. The relation of the serum concentration of bilirubin to that of albumin, for example, the relative saturation of the serum albumin with bilirubin, is probably more important than serum bilirubin concentration alone in determining the ultimate neurologic outcome.

Serum bilirubin concentrations of 20 mg/100 ml or greater are associated with an increased incidence of kernicterus, particularly in infants with erythroblastosis. However, indirect-reacting bilirubin concentrations less than 20 mg/100 ml may also lead to death, neurologic abnormality, and retarded mental and motor development. In low-birth-weight infants, there is an increased risk of impaired neuromuscular development at bilirubin concentrations of 15 mg/100 ml or greater. About 17 percent of premature white infants and 8 percent of premature black infants can be expected to develop bilirubin concentrations greater than 15 mg/100 ml and thus to be at risk. The infants at greatest risk are those weighing less than 1500 gm as well as those with acidosis, hypoxia, hypoglycemia, starvation, hypoalbuminemia, cold stress, sepsis, or hemolysis and those taking drugs that compete with bilirubin for albumin-binding sites. In general, it is accepted practice to try to keep bilirubin concentrations below 15 mg/100 ml in the latter group and below 20 mg/100 ml in all infants, whether full-term or not, even in the absence of the other complicating factors.

In a study on advancement of dermal icterus[30] it was found that generally dermal icterus (1) was not discernible at serum bilirubin levels of less than 4 mg/100 ml, (2) was confined to the face and neck at serum bilirubin between 4 and 8 mg/100 ml, (3) progressed as far as the umbilicus at levels between 5 and 12 mg/100 ml, (4) reached the groin and upper thighs at serum bilirubin levels between 8 and 16 mg/100 ml, and (6) showed on the feet, hands, palms, and soles at serum bilirubin levels of 15 mg/100 ml or higher. Icterus of the hands and feet was present in all infants studied whose serum bi-

[30] Lloyd I. Kramer, Advancement of dermal icterus in the jaundiced newborn, *Am. J. Dis. Child.* 118:454–458 (Sept.) 1969.

lirubin level was greater than 18 mg/100 ml of blood. (See Figure 26-3.)

Low-birth-weight babies tended to become icteric to their palms and soles at lower levels than full-term babies; however, if the hands and feet were not involved the serum bilirubin level did not exceed 18 mg/100 ml of blood. Some infants of low birth weight showed a more rapid progression of skin icterus than full-term babies. Variations in patterns of icterus in some low-birth-weight babies make estimation of bilirubin level by inspection less useful, but progression of jaundice does indicate a rise and a leveling off of serum bilirubin level. Fading of jaundice took place gradually in all skin areas rather than in a progressive pattern.

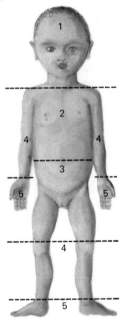

Figure 26-3. Dermal zones of progressive cephalopedal icterus. *1.* Head and neck. *2.* Trunk to umbilicus. *3.* Groin including upper thighs. *4.* Knees and elbows to ankles and wrists. *5.* Feet and hands including palms and soles. See text for further information on progression of jaundice of the skin in a cephalopedal direction. [*Reprinted with permission from Lloyd I. Kramer, "Advancement of Dermal Icterus in the Jaundiced Newborn," Am. J. Dis. Child. 118:454–458 (Sept.) 1969.*]

The author of this report states that estimation of serum bilirubin by advancement of jaundice is not meant to replace laboratory determination of serum bilirubin. It does enable an astute observer to determine the extent of dermal icterus at a given time.

Cause, Course, and Evaluation

There are many causes of hyperbilirubinemia, some somewhat self-limiting and relatively easily treated, others of a serious nature. The accelerated breakdown of red blood cells in the newborn period makes hyperbilirubinemia a common problem. This breakdown results in an accumulation of indirect bilirubin. The enzymes in the liver, which detoxify bilirubin and make it excretable, may be deficient during the first few days of life. When hemolysis is excessive and bilirubin is not excreted it accumulates in the blood and that which is not bound to albumin enters the tissues.

With either abnormal bilirubin production or inadequate liver function the pigment accumulates. Most or all serum bilirubin is bound to albumin. The bound pigment cannot enter the brain but the unbound can do damage. Anything that increases the amount of unbound bilirubin can increase its toxicity. In evaluation of the amount of serum bilirubin it is the bound amount that can be measured. It is not yet possible to measure the unbound bilirubin, which would be most useful. Also, the risk of kernicterus with a specific level of serum bilirubin is not known since many factors besides level determine when it enters the brain cells.

A large group of babies with jaundice of moderate degree have an idiopathic hyperbilirubinemia. The cause and mechanism of this are obscure. The chief problem may be a functional immaturity of the liver. This variety appears after the first 24 hours of life, usually on the second or third day. It should disappear in 7 to 10 days.

Enclosed bleeding, such as a cephalhematoma, considerable bruising from delivery, or central nervous system bleeding may produce significant amounts of bilirubin as this blood breaks down. Hemolytic disease due to Rh and ABO incompatibilities may be a serious cause of jaundice. These problems will be discussed later.

Bacterial infections lead to an increase in destruction of red blood cells. There is an increased incidence of hyperbilirubinemia in prematures and in infants of diabetic mothers. A metabolic disorder that produces hyperbilirubinemia is breast milk jaundice.

When jaundice is apparent bilirubin and hemoglobin determinations are done promptly. These values are useful as base lines for further evaluation. The mother's and baby's blood types are obtained, a direct Coombs' test is done, and the mother is checked for antibodies. A physical examination of the baby is done. The mother and baby are checked for infection. Breast feeding or late start of any feedings may be considered a cause.

Interferences with Bilirubin Metabolism

Most of the bilirubin is transported to the liver bound to albumin. However, the binding to albumin is decreased by acidosis, leaving more bilirubin free to deposit in tissues. Acidosis, and also hypoxia, hypoglycemia, infection, and prematurity are all factors that decrease the resistance of the brain cells to deposition of bilirubin. Thus acidosis not only leaves bilirubin free but also increases the danger of kernicterus.

A low serum albumin level, less than 3 gm/100 ml, is inadequate for ample binding sites and again considerable free bilirubin is available to enter tissues. Bilirubin binding to albumin may also be affected by competition for binding sites by certain chemicals, such as some antibacterial drugs and vitamin K analogues. Also, free fatty acids compete with bilirubin for a binding site on albumin. It becomes apparent that when a considerable amount of bilirubin is unbound kernicterus could occur with low levels of serum bilirubin, even with levels normally considered within physiologic limits.

Certain factors may interfere with detoxification of bilirubin when it does reach the liver. Immaturity of the baby may decrease the amount of bilirubin converted. The enzyme glucuronyl transferase may be inhibited by other factors, two of which are novobiocin and a lipose or an inhibitor substance usually present in breast milk, but in a few women it is present in such large concentration that it inhibits the enzyme from conjugating bilirubin. The inhibition may be of short duration or severe and prolonged. With maturity of the conjugation mechanism the bilirubin level which has been kept elevated by an inhibitor falls in several days to two weeks. When an inhibitor is believed to be the problem the baby is usually fed formula until the jaundice clears and the mother is advised to empty her breasts artifically until she can resume nursing.

Treatment

From the foregoing discussion it is apparent that acidosis, hypoxia, and hypoglycemia must be corrected. Good hydration and early feedings are important. The baby must be carefully examined for infection and treated if indicated. Competitive drugs must be avoided. Serum albumin levels should be checked and albumin administered if it is low and if the serum bilirubin is high.

Early feedings facilitate bilirubin excretion by preventing reabsorption of some of the bilirubin that is present in the gastrointestinal tract at birth. Conjugated bilirubin, which has been excreted into the bowel, cannot be reabsorbed, but it can be converted back to unconjugated bilirubin by the activity of a deconjugating enzyme, B-glucuronidase, present in high concentration in the intestines of the newborn in the early days of life. The unconjugated bilirubin is then reabsorbed by the intestinal mucosa by way of an enterohepatic circulation and is thus recycled through the liver. Since feedings should stimulate gastrointestinal activity and hasten expulsion of meconium, early feedings are considered important in facilitating bilirubin excretion. It is thought that early feedings may

also introduce bacteria into the intestines that will reduce bilirubin to urobilinogen.

Phototherapy

Phototherapy is commonly used for treatment of rising bilirubin levels. The baby is placed under a daylight fluorescent light, unclothed to ensure exposure of as much of his body as possible. The light may be placed over an incubator or a crib, depending on the baby's needs for environment. This supplemental light lowers levels of serum bilirubin due to (1) photooxidation of bilirubin in the tissues, and (2) increased excretion of unconjugated and conjugated bilirubin by the liver.

Dr. Jerold F. Lucey states that the current hypothesis is that the light from the phototherapy penetrates the skin and increases periphral blood flow. This brings more bilirubin to the surface for photodestruction. The breakdown products are rapidly excreted by the liver and kidneys. Also, however, "the major effect of light is to increase, to a significant degree, excretion of *unconjugated bilirubin* by the liver." Since bilirubin cannot ordinarily be excreted by the liver without being conjugated, the light produces some change that cannot be adequately explained that allows the substance to be excreted directly.[31]

Phototherapy has a number of other effects, including vasodilatation of the skin, increased insensible water loss, decreased gastrointestinal transit time, and sometimes skin rashes and bronzing of the skin.

Phototherapy increases considerably insensible water loss. This is believed to be due to increased peripheral blood flow, increased skin temperature, and increased evaporative heat loss. Babies on phototherapy frequently pass loose green stools. The green color is due to excretion of photodegradation products. The looseness is due to increased water content associated with the decreased transit time. Stool water loss is increased. Diarrhea could be masked by this stool pattern.

[31] Jerold F. Lucey, Phototherapy: What it has to offer, *Contemp. Ob/Gyn* 6:51–52 (Nov.) 1975.

A baby under phototherapy may develop a fine skin rash, described as a flea-bite dermatosis. Occasionally, phototherapy causes a transient bronze discoloration of the skin, serum, and urine. The pigment producing the bronze color has not been identified but is not believed to be harmful. A tanning effect (hyperpigmentation) has been noticed in black babies receiving photography.

Phototherapy is a medical treatment that is useful in decreasing serum bilirubin levels, but has some probable hazard in its use. It is therefore carefully considered for use when the bilirubin is rising and other appropriate therapy is not available. The baby is checked prior to therapy for probable etiology of the hyperbilirubinemia, and certain guidelines for treatment are followed. A complete history and physical examination is done, looking for probable cause of increased bilirubin. Laboratory tests include at least total and direct bilirubin levels, hemoglobin or hematocrit, Rh factor and Coombs test, smear for red blood cell morphology, reticulocyte count, serum albumin level, maternal and infant blood types, and antibody screen.

The level of indirect bilirubin is used as a guide for phototherapy. In general it is started when a full-term baby has an indirect bilirubin level above 15 mg/100 ml of blood. For the preterm baby photography is used at lower values—at above 12 mg for the moderate preterm and above 8 mg for the very small preterm. These values may need to be adjusted downward when conditions exist that interfere with bilirubin binding or that decrease the resistance of brain cells to deposition of bilirubin. This includes conditions such as acidosis, hypoxia, hypoglycemia, hypoalbuminemia, and use of other drugs. Phototherapy is not used as a prophylactic treatment and is therefore not started earlier than the values stated, except when the other conditions enumerated are present. Phototherapy may be used as an adjunct to exchange transfusion. More and more information is being gathered on phototherapy, and guidelines may change with a clearer understanding of its effects.

Nursing Observations and Care

The baby receiving phototherapy is completely undressed during treatment to expose as much of his body surface as possible. The baby may be restless at times without clothes on. The nurse may find that one position is more comforting than another to the baby and may also find other ways to quiet the baby. Some position changes must, of course, be considered.

A mask is used to cover the baby's eyes when he is under the light. Commercial masks of adequate thickness or of black felt ovals are available to fit the baby. It is important to be sure that the baby's eyes are closed before the mask is applied. The mask may need to be replaced frequently if the baby is restless. If a bandage is used instead of a mask for shielding the eyes, care must be taken that it is not too tight. Excessive pressure from the bandage may injure the eyes and excoriate the cornea if the baby can open his eyes under the bandage. Mothers often need reassurance that the baby's eyes have been closed under the mask or bandage. The eyes must be examined for discharge and for injury at frequent intervals. (See Figure 26-4.)

For male infants the testes should be shielded

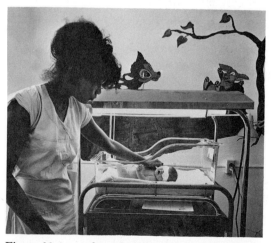

Figure 26-4.   A three-day-old infant receiving phototherapy for nonhemolytic hyperbilirubinemia. Note that the entire body is exposed, but that the eyes are protected by a mask.

from the bilirubin light. This can be done with a diaper.

The baby's vital signs should be observed and recorded every four hours. The temperature especially must be closely observed to be sure it is not elevated.

The baby must be carefully observed for chilling from drafts from air conditioning if he is in an open crib. An incubator must be carefully observed so that the temperature will not become too warm from the light above it. If an incubator with a servo-control is being used, care must be taken that the thermistor is not exposed to direct radiation.

Sensory stimulation is important to the baby. He is taken outside of the light and held for feedings, and his mask is taken off at that time to give him visual stimulation, skin care under the mask area, and inspection of his eyes. Mother–infant contact should be encouraged at feeding time and at other times if they wish. Parents must be kept informed of the baby's progress. Treatment must never be started without first discussing this with the parents.

A careful record of intake and output must be kept. If the baby eats poorly or loses considerable fluid, glucose water is offered between regular formula or breast feedings to compensate for increased insensible water loss.

The bilirubin light must be kept in good condition. The lamps must be adequately shielded, and the bulbs need to be changed after a specified number of hours of use.

Follow-up Care

Direct and indirect-reacting serum bilirubin levels are monitored every 8 to 12 hours during treatment. It is important to know how fast the bilirubin is rising if such is the case and also to know when the trend is downward, since discontinuation of therapy will be determined by results. Since photodecomposition of the bilirubin will occur under lights, the lights must be turned off when the blood is drawn for evaluation. The serum bilirubin is also monitored 12 or 24 hours after therapy is discontinued to observe for possible rebound. The hematocrit should be monitored to detect anemia.

Exchange Transfusion

An exchange transfusion must be considered when the serum bilirubin level rises dangerously. It is difficult to determine the critical level of bilirubin for an individual infant since other relevant factors in the baby's condition are influential in bilirubin entry into the central nervous system. In general, however, an exchange transfusion is considered when the bilirubin level reaches 20 mg/100 ml of blood in the full-term; 16 mg/100 ml in the premature; or rises in excess of 0.5 mg/100 ml of blood per hour. Exchange transfusion is not without risk and is only considered when other treatments have not lowered the serum bilirubin.

Procedure

Fresh blood (*less than five days old*) is obtained. Older blood is undesirable since red cell breakdown releases potassium into the serum, which may cause an electrolyte imbalance, and old blood becomes acidotic. Heparinized blood is preferable because it eliminates the metabolic hazards of the acid-citrate-dextrose anticoagulant. Heparinized blood is especially important in very small babies and in those who are acidotic.

Aseptic technique is absolutely necessary. A disposable exchange transfusion set is desirable. The procedure is carried out on an open-ended radiant warmer infant care table. The baby needs careful regulation of warmth and may need oxygen.

To prepare the baby, his stomach is aspirated to prevent vomiting and aspiration, base-line vital signs are obtained, arrangements are made for continuous heart monitoring during the exchange, and restraint is made. Oxygen and suction equipment should be readily available.

The umbilical vein is the preferred route for an exchange transfusion and can usually be used for the first seven days. Thereafter the extent of thrombosis makes it unavailable, and it is usually necessary to use the femoral vein. A polyethylene or polyvinyl catheter is introduced into the umbilical vein for a distance of 6 to 8 cm until the catheter tip lies in the inferior vena cava. This catheter is attached to a stopcock, and blood is then withdrawn and injected with syringes.

The baby may have an increase in venous pressure and blood volume at birth, and an additional increase in blood volume with transfusion may be dangerous. The venous pressure is therefore checked at the beginning of the transfusion and periodically during the procedure. If the venous pressure exceeds 8 to 10 cm the amount of blood injected may be slightly less than that removed for the first few times or until the venous pressure is normal. Entrance of air into the catheter while checking venous pressure must be guarded against.

The exchange of blood is made by alternately withdrawing and discarding from 10 to 20 ml of the baby's blood and replacing it with an equal amount of donor blood. As a syringeful of donor blood is injected it mixes in the baby's circulation and some of the mixture is then removed with the next withdrawal of blood. A gradual replacement of the infant's blood is thus made. The exchange is proportional to the amount of blood added and removed. The baby's blood with its high bilirubin level is gradually replaced by donor blood. When an exchange is made with a volume of donor blood that is equal to twice the estimated blood volume of the infant (approximately 85 ml/kg body weight), most of the circulating blood at the end of the procedure is donor blood. The maximum volume exchanged is 500 ml of blood. This usually should take about 60 minutes; longer if the baby is very sick.

A small amount of calcium, 5 to 10 ml of a 10 percent calcium gluconate solution, may be administered in divided doses of 0.5 to 1 ml after each 100 ml of blood when citrated blood is used for exchange transfusion. This is given to overcome danger of tetany, which may result from depletion of serum calcium by the large amount of sodium citrate in the donor blood.

When heparinized blood is used, it will affect the coagulation status of the baby for several hours. After use of heparinized blood, protamine sulfate may be given at the end of the transfusion, especially in sick infants in whom metabolism of heparin may be impaired.

Albumin is sometimes given intravenously prior to the transfusion or it is added to the transfusion blood. The albumin is used to attract bilirubin, actually facilitating its movement from the tissues, and thus increasing its removal from the body with the transfusion.

Blood is collected at the beginning and end of the procedure for bilirubin and hemoglobin determination. A blood culture specimen is also collected at the end of the procedure. The umbilical vein catheter is then removed and the umbilical cord is ligated.

Embolism with air or clots, electrolyte imbalance, and infection are known hazards of exchange transfusion but can usually be avoided with care. Cardiac arrest has occurred on occasion, but with careful monitoring and adequate resuscitation this can be avoided.

Careful observation by the nurse of the baby's vital signs and general behavior is essential both before and after transfusion. Incubator care of the baby is desirable to ensure a stable environment, proper concentration of oxygen if required, and easy observation. Vital signs must be monitored frequently, the umbilicus should be checked for bleeding, and the baby's activity and alertness observed. Any change in behavior suggestive of hypoglycemia, kernicterus, sepsis, and cardiac difficulty must be promptly reported. The baby is usually not fed orally for several hours. Further frequent serum bilirubin checks are required. A repeat exchange transfusion may become necessary.

HEMOLYTIC DISEASE OF THE NEWBORN (ERYTHROBLASTOSIS FETALIS)

Hemolytic disease of the newborn is a blood disturbance of late fetal or early neonatal life that may occur when there is a blood-group incompatibility between mother and baby. Incompatibility exists when the fetus possesses a red blood cell antigen, inherited from the father, that is absent in the mother. Fetal blood cells can pass through the placenta into the maternal circulation. When these blood cells are incompatible with the mother's blood, she may produce antibodies to them. These antibodies then pass through the placenta into the fetal circulation and there destroy fetal red blood cells, sometimes to a severe degree.

Hemolytic disease is usually due to incompatibility between an Rh-positive fetus and an Rh-negative mother or between a blood group A or B fetus and its mother. Occasionally hemolytic disease is the result of blood antigens less common than the D antigen of the Rh factor or the A and B antigens of the major blood groups.

Development of maternal sensitization to fetal red cells antigens and transfer of the antibodies to the fetus, resulting in erythroblastosis has been described on pages 645–52.

Signs and Symptoms

The classical signs of hemolytic disease are anemia, jaundice, and edema. In the individual baby any one of these signs may predominate. The disease may be present in a mild or severe form or in any degree between these two extremes.

Clinical manifestations of hemolytic disease and laboratory findings are largely due to hemolysis of red blood cells caused by the antibody-antigen reaction, the resultant end products of hemolysis, and the great increase that takes place in blood production and extramedullary erythropoiesis because of the hemolysis.

Anemia may be present at birth or may develop any time during the newborn period. Severe anemia at birth may cause congestive heart failure. In mild untreated cases anemia may become pronounced in a week or two and the baby's color become quite pale. However,

erythrocytes may be destroyed so rapidly that even where there is only a slight suggestion of anemia at birth, it may become quite evident within 12 hours and profound within a day or two. The erythrocytes may decrease as rapidly as a million cells per microliter per day.

Immature red blood cells, appearing as nucleated cells, are found in the baby's blood in large number. This increased number of nucleated erythrocytes led to the term erythroblastosis fetalis for this disease. Since the presence of many nucleated erythrocytes is only one of several manifestations of this disturbance, the term "hemolytic disease," which better depicts the changes that occur, is considered preferable.

The normal infant has from 200 to 2000 nucleated red blood cells per microliter of blood, whereas the infant with hemolytic disease has from 10,000 to 100,000 and even 500,000 nucleated erythrocytes per microliter of blood during the first 48 hours of life. This means more than 10 and usually from 25 to 200 nucleated red blood cells per 100 white blood cells. Normally the number of nucleated erythrocytes should not exceed 10 per 100 white blood cells at any time during the newborn period. Nucleated red blood cells in the infant with hemolytic disease diminish and disappear within a few days after birth, but this finding does not mean an improvement in condition.

The *reticulocyte count,* which is normally not above 3 percent in the newborn, may be increased, sometimes to a high level. This count is often used as a criterion of severity of illness.

Jaundice is rarely seen at birth, but develops rapidly. It may appear within a few hours, or even within one hour, or sometime during the first day. Jaundice becomes increasingly deep and frequently masks the pallor of the anemia.

Serum bilirubin may be elevated above 3 mg/100 ml of blood at birth and accumulates rapidly thereafter. Levels of 30 to 40 mg/100 ml of blood, or even higher readings, may be reached in a few days if early treatment is not instituted.

The *liver* and *spleen* become *enlarged* due to increased hematopoietic activity. They may be enlarged enough to be palpable at birth or may become palpable during the first week. Cardiac enlargement and murmurs may be present.

The *placenta* may be normal in size, or it may be considerably enlarged, very edematous, and pale in color. The *vernix caseosa* may be normal, or it may have a golden-yellow color, and the amniotic fluid may be greenish-yellow.

Universal edema (hydrops fetalis) may develop. It is usually seen only in stillborn infants or in those who die within a few hours after birth. Fetal cardiac failure due to severe anemia may be a major cause of universal edema. The baby with hydrops fetalis is very waxy in appearance, has a large amount of fluid in all tissues, and has a very low hemoglobin level and red blood cell count.

Course

Hemolytic disease may be so mild that there are no clinical signs of illness, or it may result in such profound changes that death occurs *in utero*. Between these two extremes there are all degrees of illness. Many liveborn babies appear to be in good condition at birth, but rapidly show signs of illness. This course must always be anticipated.

Prognosis

In general, the chances of recovery for liveborn babies are good when treatment is adequate. After the first week prognosis is favorable, and there are no residual symptoms unless kernicterus developed, which may leave the baby with cerebral damage.

The first infant born after maternal sensitization has a fairly good prognosis. When a sensitized mother has once had a child with hemolytic disease, subsequent Rh-positive infants are in danger of developing severe symptoms, and the chances of a stillbirth are greatly increased.

Since fetal death may occur in the last weeks of pregnancy, delivery prior to term, but usually not before the thirty-sixth week, may be considered desirable if amniotic fluid analyses for the amount of bilirubin it contains indicate that the fetus is likely to be in jeopardy and if L/S studies show fetal lung maturity.

Diagnosis

Diagnosis of Rh incompatibility begins in the prenatal period. It is tentatively made before the baby is born with discovery of anti-Rh antibodies in the mother's blood and is confirmed after birth by determining that the baby is Rh positive. See page 649 for antepartum diagnosis and management.

When hemolytic disease is anticipated, the baby is carefully checked at birth for signs of illness. Umbilical cord blood, from the placental end of the cord, is collected for determination of Rh type, blood group, Coombs' test, hemoglobin level, erythrocyte count, nucleated red blood cell count, reticulocyte count, and serum bilirubin. The baby is examined for skin color and general appearance, for color of the vernix caseosa, and for size of liver and spleen. The size and appearance of the placenta are noted.

The umbilical cord blood is immediately tested for Rh type and direct antiglobulin (Coombs') test. The direct Coombs' test is very important in diagnosis since it is positive when there are anti-Rh antibodies in the baby's blood, even in the absence of clinical evidence of disease. The test for Rh type is not always reliable since false negative results may be obtained when anti-Rh antibodies attached to the baby's red blood cells interfere with Rh typing.

The direct Coombs' test reveals the presence of maternal antibodies attached to the red blood cells of an Rh-positive baby (Fig. 22-8, p. 648). Red cells of a baby with hemolytic disease may be coated with anti-Rh antibodies. These antibodies will cause hemolysis of the baby's cells, but may also interfere with the normal agglutinating activity of the typing serum. The baby's cells are thus not agglutinated with anti-Rh serum under ordinary methods of testing and thus appear to be Rh negative. When the baby types Rh negative, it is necessary to exclude the possibility of a false Rh-negative reaction. This false reaction occurs when the maternal antibodies that have been absorbed on the surface of the baby's red blood cells interfere with agglutination tests.

A negative direct Coombs' test excludes the presence of antibodies on the baby's red blood cells; a positive test indicates that antibodies are present on the surface of the cells. The Coombs' test is not specific for anti-Rh antibodies, but in the newborn baby it can be assumed that the antibodies present are most likely antibodies to one of the Rh antigens. The diagnosis of hemolytic disease depends to a large extent on demonstrating by the Coombs' test that the baby's red blood cells are Rh positive and are coated with anti-Rh antibodies unless the incompatibility is caused by the A or B blood group, in which case the Coombs' test is not suitable. If the Coombs' test is negative and the baby's Rh type is negative, the baby can be considered Rh negative and not in need of treatment.

Other significant laboratory findings aiding in diagnosis and giving an indication of the degree of cell destruction are levels of hemoglobin, red blood cells, nucleated red cells, and reticulocytes. The more severe the destruction of cells, the lower the hemoglobin and red blood cells and the higher the number of nucleated red cells and reticulocytes. Other evidence of hemolytic disease, especially if treatment is not instituted immediately, includes early appearance of jaundice and a rapidly rising serum bilirubin level. Jaundice is rarely seen at birth, but serum bilirubin in the umbilical cord blood is often elevated above 3 mg per 100 ml of blood. Since the level of serum bilirubin may rise rapidly, blood examination for bilirubin is repeated every four to eight hours until the possibility of rise to a dangerous level is past.

Treatment

Prompt care immediately after birth is of paramount importance in treatment of hemolytic disease. When the disease is anticipated from past history and from studies made during pregnancy, it is essential to prepare for treatment immediately after the baby's birth. In general the same treatment may be used as for any cause of hyperbilirubinemia, with the exception that the baby's condition may be severe enough to require an exchange transfusion immediately after birth.

An exchange transfusion is used for two problems: (1) to correct anemia rapidly for a baby severely affected with erythroblastosis, and (2) to treat hyperbilirubinemia. In hemolytic disease both of these conditions may be present. Packed cells may be used for partial exchange when severe anemia needs to be treated at birth.

When difficulty is anticipated, Rh-negative, group O blood, which can be used for immediate transfusion if necessary, should be available before delivery. This donor blood can be selected prior to the baby's birth by crossmatching it with the mother's blood, since her blood contains the antibodies present in the fetal blood in similar or greater amounts.

When immediate exchange transfusion is not necessary, ABO-specific, Rh-negative blood which has been typed with the baby's cord blood may be used. This blood should always be compatible with the mother's serum since blood group antibodies have not been actively produced by the baby at birth. If antibodies are present, they are in higher concentration in the mother's serum than in the baby's.

An exchange transfusion not only removes bilirubin, but also many of the baby's Rh-positive blood cells, and Rh antibodies. Bilirubin will, however, continue to accumulate because the baby rapidly forms new cells. These are hemolyzed by the remaining antibodies in his blood.

Accumulation of bilirubin does not cease until the maternal antibodies are depleted, or production of new red blood cells decreases, or the liver is able to convert bilirubin to the conjugated variety which can be excreted. It may be necessary to repeat an exchange blood transfusion in severe, hemolytic disease.

Phototherapy may be used for treatment. It is not a replacement for exchange transfusion but is a valuable adjunct. Phototherapy may reduce the number of necessary exchange transfusions, and it may be effective for mild cases of the disease.

Anemia may occur within one to several weeks when phototherapy has been successful because the baby's Coombs-positive cells continue to be destroyed. Careful follow-up examinations for anemia are made and packed cell transfusions may be indicated.

Hemolytic Disease Due to ABO Incompatibility

Hemolytic disease of the newborn may result from incompatibility between the mother's and baby's major blood groups, the A, B, and O groups. Clinical manifestations of this condition are more common than with Rh incompatibility, but they usually occur in a milder degree. Hemolytic disease due to ABO incompatibility can, however, be as severe as that due to the Rh factor.

Anti-A antibodies are present in the blood of persons who do not have an A factor. Similarly anti-B antibodies are normally found in blood without a B factor. When the mother's blood contains anti-A or anti-B antibodies and the baby's blood contains an A or B antigen, difficulty may arise, since the antibodies may cross the placenta and hemolyze the baby's blood.

Incompatibility exists when the mother is group A and the infant group B, the mother group B and the infant group A, or the mother group O and the infant group A or B or AB. With rare exceptions, however, difficulty is encountered only when the mother is group O and the infant is group A or group B—in actuality, mainly when the mother is group O and the infant group A.

Since antibodies are naturally present in the mother's blood (anti-A and anti-B antibodies in group O blood), prior sensitization is not necessary as with the Rh factor, an antigen to which antibodies are not normally present. A first-born incompatible infant may therefore be as readily affected as a succeeding one. Hemolytic disease may or may not recur in subsequent infants, although the cells of preceding incompatible babies may stimulate formation of additional antibodies in the mother.

Hemolytic disease does not develop in every group A infant born of a group O mother. The reason for this is not definite, but it has been suggested that some maternal antibodies may not cause difficulty or that a protective mechanism functions in the fetus. Some persons apparently have unusual antibodies, termed immune antibodies, as well as the usual ones, designated natural antibodies. These immune antibodies may increase the danger of hemolytic disease.

Jaundice is the main clinical sign of ABO incompatibility, appearing within the first 36 hours of life. The nurse must be alert to its early evidence. Anemia is absent or mild, and the liver and spleen are usually not enlarged. Severe manifestations of illness, although rare, may develop. The direct Coombs' test is negative or weakly positive.

Diagnosis of ABO incompatibility is partly dependent on exclusion of other causes of early jaundice. Laboratory findings of mother and infant aid in diagnosis. The mother is usually blood group O and the infant group A or sometimes group B. The mother's blood is tested for immune anti-A and anti-B antibodies. Finding of a positive indirect Coombs' test with use of adult red cells assists in making a definitive diagnosis. Specific methods of detecting ABO incompatibility are under investigation.

Treatment is directed toward management of hyperbilirubinemia to prevent kernicterus. The serum bilirubin is checked frequently and used as a guide in treatment. Many babies do not require treatment. Exchange transfusion is used as necessary to keep the bilirubin below the danger level of 20 mg/100 ml of blood. Group O blood with a low anti-A and anti-B antibody titer is used.

Progress in Treatment for Rh Incompatibility

Hemolytic disease due to Rh incompatibility is a disease which for many years caused death or disability in the infant. Its cause was unknown until 1940. Since that time rapid advances in knowledge of cause and treatment of the disease have been made, and presently preventive measures are known. It can thus be expected that the disease will not be a serious problem in the future.

A disease that was apparently erythroblastosis was described by Hippocrates 400 years B.C. The 1940s were years of discovery of the Rh factor and its effects, and discovery that replacement of blood could save babies that were born alive. In the 1950s the concept of the value of exchange transfusion was clearly established as a treatment. This was also a time of discovery of bilirubin in the amniotic fluid and the fact that analysis of amniotic fluid proved more valuable in diagnosis of fetal involvement than antibody titer checks of the mother's blood, and that premature delivery could save some babies from serious involvement. During the 1960s discovery was made that intrauterine transfusions could prevent some fetal deaths and permit babies to mature to a further degree than previously without almost certain fetal death. In the late 1960s a method of passive immunization was developed.

With the availability of passive immunization erythroblastosis fetalis should be almost completely eliminated. With immunization the vast majority of women should be protected against sensitization by anti-Rh antibodies.

POLYCYTHEMIA

Polycythemia, an increased red blood cell volume, is likely to cause problems because of hyperviscosity and stasis of blood. Polycythemia in the newborn is usually defined as a venous (or central) hematocrit of 65 percent or greater, or a hemoglobin of 22.0 gm or more per 100 ml. As the hematocrit increases over 65 percent the viscosity of the blood increases markedly for small increases in hematocrit.

A venous sample of blood is preferable to heel-stick blood for making the diagnosis because there is sludging or packing together of blood cells in the distal capillaries when peripheral circulation is sluggish and the hematocrit reading will then be higher.

The hyperviscosity from polycythemia may cause a decrease in blood flow, an increased workload on the heart, an increased blood clotting, and a bleeding tendency. A baby with polycythemia may have signs and symptoms such as plethora (ruddy appearance), cyanosis, respiratory distress, central nervous system abnormalities such as seizures, oliguria, hyperbilirubinemia, and hypoglycemia. The respiratory, cardiac, and central nervous system problems, and the oliguria are likely due to the increased viscosity of the blood. The central nervous system signs and symptoms are important findings in polycythemia because permanent sequelae may recur. The jaundice may be due to greater breakdown of cells and the hypoglycemia due to their greater use of glucose.

Neonatal polycythemia may be due to several factors, but one most commonly mentioned is chronic intrauterine hypoxia. The hypoxia is believed to stimulate a fetus' erythropoietin synthesis, which is then followed by an increase in synthesis of red blood cells. Since SGA and postmature babies are likely to have intrauterine hypoxia, these babies should have their hematocrit or hemoglobin checked at birth.

Once symptoms exist and hyperviscosity is demonstrated a partial exchange transfusion with fresh frozen plasma is considered. It becomes especially important when there is concern over CNS sequelae. The exchange with plasma is done to reduce the red blood cell mass without causing deleterious effects by rapid volume shifts. When the hematocrit is reduced to a range of 50 to 55 percent the blood circulation improves and the symptoms are usually relieved.

INFECTIONS

Infections of the newborn infant may be acquired *in utero*, during passage through the birth canal, and by direct contact with infected personnel and/or environment. Syphilis and some of the virus infections, such as chickenpox, may be transmitted from the mother to the fetus through the placenta. A baby may develop an infection *in utero* when the amniotic fluid is infected. A *Candida (Monilia)* infection (thrush) or gonorrheal ophthalmia may be acquired during passage through the birth canal. Respiratory, gastrointestinal, and skin infections may develop primarily in the birth canal or from postnatal contact.

The newborn is protected against diseases such as measles, smallpox, mumps, and diphtheria for a short time, provided his mother has an immunity. Placental transmission of antibodies and antiviral immune bodies gives him a relative immunity for a variable period of time. For some diseases this period of immunity is very short; for others it lasts several months. The newborn has very little or no acquired protection against whooping cough and chickenpox nor against the common organisms that frequently cause infection. See page 457 for more information on placental transmission.

The remainder of this discussion on infection will center on infections the newborn may acquire *in utero* or in the early postnatal days rather than on the childhood diseases. Sepsis of the newborn is a common cause of morbidity and mortality.

Approximately one fourth of all newborn infections occur within the first 48 hours of life. These often have their onset *in utero*, or are acquired very soon after the baby emerges from a sterile environment. The baby may acquire bacteria before birth, or he may aspirate meconium-stained amniotic fluid or vaginal secretions during birth, or after birth he may aspirate feeding or vomitus, or be contaminated by nursery personnel or environment. Difficult resuscitation at birth predisposes to infection. Exposure to a large variety of microorganisms may be overwhelming to the baby. More than one half of newborn infections occur in the first week of life. A number of the infections that occur after 48 hours imply a nursery-acquired infection. Some infections are secondary to surgical procedures.

Septicemia and meningitis are the serious

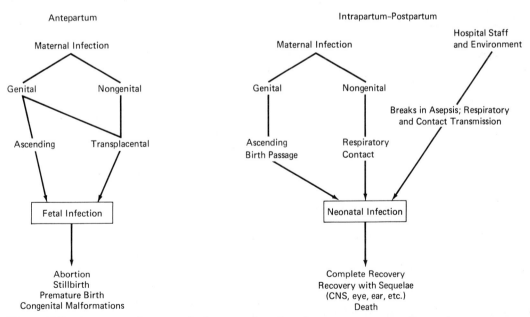

Figure 26-5. Summary of sources of infection and modes of transmission to the fetus and newborn.

consequences of infection in the newborn, making it imperative that diagnosis is made as early as possible. The newborn has a high susceptibility to bacterial invasion of the central nervous system. This susceptibility to meningitis makes early diagnosis and treatment of sepsis in any part of the body mandatory. Any evidence of infection is almost equivalent to anticipation of CNS infection, which often results in death or neurologic damage. Early treatment can reduce the mortality rate considerably. Male infants are twice as susceptible to septicemia and meningitis as females, and as one might suppose the handicaps of a premature make him especially susceptible. The infection rate in prematures is ten times as high as in the full-term baby.

The portal of entry of the organism that infects a newborn is usually not known. *In utero* many infectious agents can cross the placenta and assault the fetus. However, many organisms enter his body from the outside by way of a number of sites, which may include the mouth, nasopharynx, alimentary tract, umbilicus, or the easily traumatized skin. At high risk of infection are babies born to mothers with an infection, or after rupture of the membranes for a 12-hour period, or following a long difficult labor. Under such circumstances bacteria may ascend into the uterine cavity from or through the vagina and contaminate the amniotic fluid. A baby who acquires organisms *in utero* shows signs of infection soon after birth, or at least within the first 36 hours following delivery. Also included in the high-risk category are babies with respiratory distress and those requiring exchange transfusion. The newborn is easily susceptible to pneumonia, especially if he develops atelectasis or if he aspirates food or fluid. Urinary tract infection is more common than in an older child. Skin infections, cellulitis, impetigo, and subcutaneous abscesses are relatively common in the baby. (See Figure 26-5.)

Signs and Symptoms

Typically, a baby with an infection has no specific symptoms. Manifestations are usually vague and those that are present can easily be attributed to many other disturbances. To recognize subtle signs of infection everyone caring for newborns must be knowledgeable about the characteristics of the normal baby and continually alert for subtle signs of illness. A low-grade fever is present in about one half of babies who have an infection, but often the temperature is not elevated, and it may be subnormal. Apathy is common. The baby usually does not suck well and he takes his feedings poorly. Some babies vomit their feedings and some have diarrhea. Periods of cyanosis, irregular respirations, and apnea may be present. Cough is rare even in the presence of pneumonia. Jaundice often appears. The baby may be lethargic at times and hyperirritable at others. He can often be described as just "not acting right" or "not doing well."

The nurse who becomes aware of any suspicious signs must immediately report them to the physician. She should also observe the baby closely for signs of respiratory infection and examine him for redness and discharge at the base of the umbilical cord, for discharge from the eyes, and for vesicles and pustular eruptions on the skin. Although the above observations are important, lack of observable inflammation at the site of infection is not uncommon. The infection may be localized but the site is frequently not apparent. It is likely to give generalized rather than specific reactions and is very likely to spread. Sometimes the infection is generalized, with few, very vague, manifestations of illness.

Deficiencies of Newborns in Resisting Infection

The newborn's ability to resist or overcome infection is very low. His ability to form antibodies is present before birth, but he normally develops in a protective, sterile environment. He has thus ordinarily not been exposed to antigens and has not actively formed his own antibodies. Essentially all of the baby's immunoglobulins at birth are transfers across the placenta of certain types of antibodies from the mother. The level of immunoglobulins rises with gestational age and thus is lower in prematures than in full-term babies. With birth, and stoppage of maternal supply, the level of immunoglobulins falls until the baby later brings it up by his own synthesis. Immunoglobulins have different chemical and physical properties and different names—gamma G, gamma A, and gamma M. The immunoglobulin that almost exclusively passes to the fetus in significant amounts is gamma G.

Gamma M globulin antibody does not cross the placental barrier. Gamma M. globulin antibody is one of the most important antibodies against gram-negative organisms, which are the most frequent invaders of the newborn. This means that the baby does not have gamma M globulin, except rarely, when he may have begun synthesis of the antibody to an intrauterine infection. A postnatal infection stimulates the baby to form antibodies to the foreign antigen, but it takes some time for him to produce significant amounts.

Another important defense mechanism, phagocytosis, seems to be inadequately developed in the newborn: The baby's white blood cells do not engulf and inactivate bacteria as well as adult cells. It appears that the inadequacy of phagocytosis may be the result of a deficiency of some factor in the baby's plasma which aids the white blood cells in the phagocytosis, or the phagocytes may respond sluggishly because they have not had previous practice.

The frequent lack in the newborn of an inflammatory response at the site of a local infection and his inability to wall-off the infection make early diagnosis difficult, and also permits the infection to disseminate rapidly. The baby's lack of gamma M globulin antibodies, his slow response to their production, and his deficiency in effective phagocytosis can quickly result in an overwhelming infection.

Common Causative Agents

The infective organisms of newborns are predominantly gram-negative bacteria. *Escherichia*

coli, usually harmless to adults, is a common cause of infection in newborns. *Klebsiella, Aerobacter, Proteus*, and *Pseudomonas* are also fairly common causes, and sometimes the "water-bugs," such as *Flavobacteria* and *Achromobacter* cause illness in the newborn. Among the gram-positive organisms that may cause newborn infection are streptococci, staphylococci, and pneumococci. In recent years the group B beta-hemolytic streptococcus (not group A), abbreviated frequently as BHS, GBBS, has come to be the most frequent cause of morbidity and mortality of neonatal sepsis. The most serious illness is caused by group B, types I and III.

The chief sources of gram-positive bacteria are the nose, throat, and skin of persons caring for babies. The *E. coli* organism is commonly acquired from the hands of adults. Common sources of other gram-negative organisms are humidifiers, resuscitators, oxygen equipment, incubators, sinks and faucets, and hands of persons handling the baby. *Pseudomonas* is found in many water sources.

The vaginal flora of mothers contains bacteria, among which group B beta-hemolytic streptococci is frequently found. This may cause pneumonia in the baby, especially if prolonged ruptured membranes or long labor permits ample time for intrauterine infection. The group B beta-hemolytic streptococcus is a common inhabitant of the female genital tract. Hospital personnel also have a relatively high colonization rate from throat, vaginal, and anal sources.

Diagnosis

If a mother's membranes have been ruptured for 12 hours or longer or labor has been long and difficult the possibility of infection in the baby should be investigated. A gastric aspirate is collected at birth into a sterile mucus trap. The aspirate is examined for polymorphonuclear cells, not bacteria, since bacteria are likely to be present either with or without infection. The smear of the gastric aspirate is considered positive if one or more polymorphonuclear cells are found per field; not per slide, but per field. If the smear is positive the baby must be closely observed, preferably in an incubator, for abnormal signs and symptoms in order to begin treatment as soon as indicated.

When there is any suspicion that a baby has an infection, cultures and smears are taken of the blood, urine, and cerebrospinal fluid for identification of organisms, their sensitivity to antibiotics, and the extent of their invasion. Cultures are also taken of the throat (pharyngeal wall), the umbilical area, skin lesions, if present, and any other suspicious sites.

The nurse's assistance in effectively obtaining results from specimens is important. Obviously all equipment should be sterile. Chemicals should not come in contact with any of the specimens. All specimens must be taken to the laboratory for immediate examination. Organisms may die in desiccated specimens. Urine that is not taken to the laboratory within one-half hour, or refrigerated, is likely to have an increase in some varieties of organisms and a decrease in other. Blood cultures should not be refrigerated, since bacterial growth is retarded by cold and may cause death of the organism. If a blood culture cannot be taken to the laboratory immediately it should be left at room temperature. It is very important to take spinal fluid to the laboratory immediately after collection. Organisms in spinal fluid are altered or die quickly. Refrigeration is harmful to adequate results.

Other diagnostic studies include a general physical examination, a chest x-ray, and a blood cell count. The white blood cell count is ordinarily elevated with infection, but since it is normally high in the immediate newborn period it is difficult to interpret during the first week. See below for diagnosis of group B beta-hemolytic streptococcal pneumonia.

Treatment

Since infection in the newborn spreads rapidly, therapy is started immediately, before the infecting organism can be identified. Kanamycin and penicillin G, given intramuscularly, are usually chosen for initial therapy. Kanamycin is very effective against almost all of the gram-negative organisms that infect the newborn, with the exception of *Pseudomonas.* Sometimes gentamicin is used instead of kanamycin. Penicillin G (or sometimes ampicillin) is effective against most gram-positive microorganisms, with the exception of resistant staphylococci. When the organism has been identified it may be found that the kanamycin-penicillin treatment should be continued, or that therapy should be changed to an antibiotic specific to the invading organism, as for *Pseudomonas* or penicillin-resistant staphylococcal infection. In the case of epidemic diarrhea caused by enteropathic *E. coli*, neomycin, administered only by the oral route, is used. Treatment with antibiotics is usually continued until spinal fluid and blood cultures have been negative for a week.

Administration of antibiotics to newborns presents some special problems and demands careful consideration. They all have some inherent toxicity to the baby. Metabolism and excretion of antibiotics are different in the newborn than in an older child or an adult, and toxity and dosage must be given special consideration. Kidney immaturity in the baby may reduce excretion of some drugs. Liver immaturity may result in increased amounts of antibiotics in the body and lead to toxicity. The drug may bind to albumin and be in competition with bilirubin. Prophylactic use of antibiotics can be more deleterious than useful. Under some conditions prophylactic use seems important, but the physician will carefully determine the advisability of its use for each individual baby.

In addition to treatment with antibiotics for infection, a number of general supportive measures are important.

1. The baby is usually placed in an incubator for good environmental control. His temperature should be maintained at a 36 to 37°C (97 to 98°F) level. The incubator may make careful observation of vital signs and general reactions easier.
2. Oxygen is given for respiratory distress, and blood gases are checked frequently.

3. Oral feedings may be withheld because of difficulty in feeding and danger of aspiration. Intravenous fluids are used to maintain fluids, calories, and electrolytes.
4. Fresh whole blood or plasma may be given for support in an amount of 10 to 15 ml/kg body weight.

Dr. Pierog and Dr. Nigam have outlined the pathogenesis of neonatal sepsis and the steps in its treatment in *Pediatric Annals.*[32]

Beta-Hemolytic Streptococcal Pneumonia[33]

The baby who develops a beta-hemolytic streptococcal pneumonia becomes seriously ill within a few hours and has a high probability of death within the first day. Tachypnea and grunting appear soon after birth, respiratory distress develops rapidly, and apneic spells may soon develop. Progressive signs of shock quickly appear—poor peripheral circulation, hypotension, and decreased urinary output. Delivery room and nursery personnel should be alert to several early signs suggestive of neonatal infection with beta-hemolytic streptococci. These include a low Apgar score for no known reason, premature rupture of the membranes for 12 hours or longer and the presence of gram-positive cocci in the gastric aspirate, early onset of apnea, and a chest x-ray that is characteristic of respiratory distress syndrome but also shows cardiomegaly.

Treatment of beta-hemolytic streptococcal pneumonia includes antibiotics and supportive measures such as assisted ventilation, intravenous fluids, blood transfusions, and adequate warmth. Penicillin 250,000 U/kg-day or ampicillin 200 mg/kg-day and gentamicin 5.0 mg/kg-day, each divided into two doses are used for antibiotic treatment.

[32] Sophie Pierog and Sarvesh Nigam, Neonatal sepsis, *Pediatr. Ann.* 5:63–79 passim (Feb.) 1976.
[33] Richard D. Zachman (ed.), Neonatal beta-hemolytic streptococcal pneumonia—A serious disease, *Perinatal News,* Madison General Hospital, Wisconsin Perinatal Center, Southcentral Region, Oct. 7, 1977.

Nursery Precautions Against Infection

A number of preventive measures against infection of babies from nursery personnel and environment have been described on pages 499–500. It may be well to reiterate here several important precautions. Thorough hand washing is of utmost importance before clean supplies are handled and before proceeding from one baby to another for care. Personnel with clinical signs of infection should not be in the nursery. Meticulous housekeeping is essential. Routine surveillance of the nursery environment and equipment is important to evaluate the effectiveness of cleaning and maintenance. Since some of the bacteria that cause infection in the newborn thrive in high humidity, routine bacteriologic examination of equipment, such as incubators, suction apparatus, respirators, resucitators, is important in infection control. Use of disposable tubing in suction equipment is strongly recommended. Objective and frequent reevaluation of nursery procedures is strongly advised since some procedures may become traditional without an adequate scientific base.

If a nursery epidemic develops it usually involves staphylococci, *E. coli, Salmonella,* or water bacteria. Skin lesions are often the first sign of a staphylococcal infection, but sometimes there are no manifestations until several days or weeks after the baby is discharged from the hospital. Other members of the family may also then become infected. If the baby is breastfeeding the mother is susceptible to breast infection. Pathogenic strains of *E. coli* are frequently the cause of epidemic diarrhea, a highly contagious newborn infection. Water bacteria present special concern because of the newborn's high susceptibility to infection by gram-negative bacteria.

In case of an infectious epidemic, the infected babies are isolated, ideal procedures in infant care must be strictly enforced, and an attack must be made on the possible source of infection and its spread.

One other measure in infection control is an awareness that every hospital nursery has its own type of bacteria. It is important to know what kind of bacteria these are and their sensitivity to antibiotics.

Thrush

Thrush, or oral moniliasis, is a mild infection of the mucous membranes of the mouth. White, curdlike patches, resembling milk curds, are observed on the tongue, gums, and palate, and inside the cheeks. The patches do not wipe off easily. If they are loosened, there is a raw, bleeding area underneath. The infection usually does not produce systemic symptoms.

A cutaneous infection may accompany oral thrush or may appear alone. It usually begins in the anal region. The infected skin of the perianal region and the buttocks has an appearance very similar to that of excoriated buttocks.

Thrush is caused by the fungus *Candida (Monilia) albicans.* In the newborn the usual source of infection is a vaginal yeast infection in the mother, also caused by *C. albicans.* The infection may spread to other infants in the nursery through careless handling of feeding supplies. Since *C. albicans* is present in stools of infants with infection, or potential infection, careful handling of diapers and hand washing after changing of diapers are important in control of infection spread.

The nurse should inspect a baby's mouth daily. Lesions of thrush are often first seen when the baby is five to seven days old.

Mycostatin (Nystatin) in an aqueous suspension may be used for treatment. It is swabbed over the baby's mouth several times a day. The baby will swallow a small amount of the solution, and this is effective against the fungus in the intestinal tract. Nystatin may also be used prophylactically if the mother has a vaginal yeast infection.

Occasionally thrush is treated by topical application of a mild antiseptic. A 1 percent aqueous solution of methylrosaniline chloride (gentian violet) is applied once or twice daily. Applications are usually made about an hour after a feeding. The mouth is first gently dried of mucus with a sterile cotton applicator. Several days of treatment are sufficient since the lesions heal quickly.

Since gentian violet is a dye that gives the baby's mouth a deep violet color, the mother is told to expect his mouth to be stained if gentian violet is used. The baby usually drools some saliva, which stains clothing. If gentian violet is used on the day of the baby's discharge from the hospital, the mother should be warned to protect the baby's clothing until his saliva is no longer colored.

Infection of the Eyes

An acute conjunctivitis in the newborn is termed *ophthalmia neonatorum.* This term was formerly associated with an eye infection caused by the gonococcus. Gonorrheal ophthalmia is now rare because of prophylactic treatment. Most cases of ophthalmia neonatorum are caused by other organisms.

An infection of the eyes usually manifests itself by the appearance of a conjunctival discharge sometime between the second and fifth days of life. The discharge may be profuse. The eyelids may become red and swollen.

Silver nitrate often causes a chemical irritation of the eyes. In some babies it causes considerable edema and redness of the lids and a profuse purulent discharge. Signs of this irritation are present only in the first day or two after birth. They may appear within four to six hours. The inflammation may be quite severe, but it subsides within a day or two and does not leave harmful effects. Gentle cleaning of the lids or irrigation of the eyes with a warm physiologic saline solution is the usual treatment.

If there is any suspicion that an inflammation of the eyes is infectious in nature, a smear and culture of the pus for identification of the bacteria are indicated. Any discharge from the eyes after the second day of life is caused by bacterial infection. In addition to the gonococcus, many other organisms may cause a conjunctivitis. Among these are viruses, streptococci, staphylococci, and pneumococci, or the infection may be mixed. Treatment is with appropriate antibiotic eye drops or ophthalmic ointment.

A *gonorrheal conjunctivitis* develops following contact with infected vaginal secretions during the baby's passage through the birth canal. It was formerly a common infection of the newborn and one of the leading causes of blindness. At present it is a relatively infrequent infection. A gonorrheal infection in the mother can be cured during pregnancy, and treatment of the eyes at birth is a prophylactic measure against this infection. There is, however, some chance of infection even when prophylactic treatment has been given. Occasionally the medication does not get into the conjunctival sac adequately.

Gonorrheal conjunctivitis usually appears on the second or third day of life. The infection may be unilateral at first, but may soon spread to the other eye. The eyelids become reddened and markedly swollen. The discharge from the eyes is serosanguineous at first, but soon becomes thick and purulent. The conjunctiva is red and swollen. If not treated early, the infection may run a very rapid course and can cause blindness in 48 hours after the first signs appear. Ulceration of the cornea followed by scarring and impaired or loss of vision is a dreaded consequence of the inflammation.

Treatment with penicillin, intramuscularly and by instillation into the conjunctival sac, readily cures a gonorrheal conjunctivitis, but it must be instituted early to prevent corneal ulceration. Treatment is started before results of smear or culture are available because of the urgency. Since conjunctivitis due to other organisms may also be cured by penicillin, the treatment is often effective even when the infection is not caused by the gonococcus.

A baby with gonorrheal conjunctivitis is strictly isolated until the infection has been cured. The eye may be irrigated with a physiologic saline solution while pus is present. Care must be taken to prevent spread of infection to the unaffected eye. Nursery personnel must protect their own eyes from contamination with discharge from the baby's eyes or with irrigating

solution. Persons caring for the baby should never touch their own eyes before they have carefully washed their hands. They may wear glasses while giving care. If the eyes are accidentally contaminated, appropriate treatment is instituted.

Congenital Syphilis

Congenital syphilis is an infection caused by the *Treponema pallidum*, present in the infant at birth. The infection is transmitted from the mother into the fetal blood stream by passage of spirochetes through the placenta sometime between the fifth month of gestation and the end of pregnancy, very occasionally during the fourth month. Mothers who receive antepartum care are tested for syphilis and given adequate treatment. Stillbirth and infant mortality rates due to syphilis have fallen steadily.

Prevention of congenital syphilis depends entirely on preventing transmission of the spirochetes from mother to fetus, through detection of the disease in the mother and effective treatment before or during pregnancy (see page 672).

An infant born of a syphilitic mother, even if she has been treated, is checked to determine if he should receive treatment.

Congenital syphilis may be difficult to detect at birth. Physical signs are usually absent, and the results of a serology test at this time do not prove the presence or absence of the disease. The placenta may show characteristic changes if infection is present. Although in former years babies often had signs of the disease at birth, the possibility of a child's being born with clinical evidence on the skin and mucous membranes is now rare. Signs of the infection are more likely to appear in several weeks, or they may not appear until later in childhood when the manifestations are different than in infancy. The presence of signs at birth usually indicates a severe infection.

The most frequent signs of early congenital syphilis are snuffles and skin eruptions. Snuffles are caused by a swelling of the nasal mucous membrane. This makes breathing and sucking difficult. A profuse nasal discharge, which excoriates the skin with which it comes in contact, soon develops. The mouth and larynx may be infected. The cry may sound hoarse. Skin lesions may consist of eruptions on all or a part of the body; redness, swelling, and peeling of the skin of the palms and soles; and fissures around the mouth, anus, and vulva. The long bones are affected by the disease, and the joints may become swollen and painful. X-rays of the long bones may show bone changes at several weeks of age.

A serologic test is done at birth on a baby born of a syphilitic mother, but the disease cannot be detected by this test in the early months of life. The test becomes accurate sometime between three and six months of age. The test may be negative for a few months even when the baby has the disease because the infant may not yet have developed antibodies. It may be positive for a few months in the absence of disease when there has been a placental transmission of the mother's antibodies. A positive test may, therefore, reflect the mother's rather than the baby's blood condition.

The baby's condition can best be determined by testing the blood in several dilutions once a month or more often over a period of several months. An increasing titer is indicative of the presence of syphilis. A decreasing titer indicates absence of the disease. Subsequent tests are obtained at the age of six months and one year.

Congenital syphilis can be cured with early recognition and treatment. Penicillin is used for treatment in any phase of the disease. The decision to treat depends on the mother's history of disease and her treatment, the presence of symptoms, the serology reports, and the x-ray findings. Early treatment is very important. When the baby has actual lesions, spirochetes are present in the discharge. The baby should be isolated. Persons caring for him should wear a gown and rubber gloves for protection, since the spirochetes may enter through any breaks in the skin. After several days of treatment the contagiousness of the disease is probably past.

The "TORCH" Syndrome

The acronym TORCH is derived from the first letters of four nonbacterial diseases—toxoplasmosis, rubella, cytomegalovirus, and herpes simplex. The newborn ordinarily gets these diseases through placenta transmission from mother to fetus. The TORCH complex has been described on pages 668–73.

THE BABY WITH DRUG ADDICTION

Most babies born to addicted mothers develop signs of acute narcotic withdrawal. At least one half of these babies have moderate to severe symptoms, the rest have mild symptoms and sometimes none. When there are no symptoms the mother may have used only a relatively low dose of the drug. Heroin withdrawal usually begins on the first day, rarely after the third day, but some cases of delayed onset have been reported.

Signs of methadone withdrawal may be delayed for days or weeks after delivery, but moderate or severe symptoms appear in at least 80 percent of these infants. There is actually greater severity with methadone withdrawal than with heroin. This may reflect a higher dose that the mother receives and the pharmacologic characteristics of the drug.

Babies born of mothers with heroin addiction often weigh less than 2500 gm at birth. They may be growth-retarded because of poor maternal nutrition and poor placental circulation, and they may be born prematurely.

Signs of narcotic withdrawal are nonspecific and can be confused with such conditions as hypoglycemia, hypocalcemia, and central nervous system problems. If addiction or a methadone maintenance program is known, withdrawal can be anticipated. If the addiction is not known the diagnosis may be more problematic. Withdrawal from nonnarcotic drugs, such as barbiturates and tranquilizers, may present similar clinical characteristics.

There are many withdrawal signs, but the most common are irritability and a unique kind of coarse flapping tremor. Often there is muscular rigidity. The baby has a hypertonicity and a hyperactive Moro reflex. The baby often has a high-pitched cry, frantically sucks his fists, is not able to rest well, and sleeps poorly. His skin may become irritated from restlessness.

The baby often feeds poorly and inefficiently, not taking much food at one time. He may regurgitate and vomit, which could lead to aspiration, and he has loose stools which may irritate the buttocks.

Marked perspiration is common. The sweating is presumably due to a central neurogenic stimulation of sweat glands.[34]

Respiratory symptoms include tachypnea, sneezing, nasal stuffiness, and a peculiar mottling of the skin.

Convulsions are not common in babies born of heroin-addicted mothers but are more common in methadone and barbiturate withdrawal.

Babies born of mothers using alcohol during pregnancy are abruptly deprived of alcohol at birth and can be expected to exhibit withdrawal symptoms. Initial symptoms appear within the first 24 hours, often within 6 to 12 hours. Withdrawal symptoms generally present as central nervous system manifestations and gastrointestinal symptoms, with irritability and tremors, spontaneous seizures, arching of the back, and abdominal distention commonly present. Alcohol withdrawal and narcotic withdrawal have a number of features in common, but CNS seizure-like activity and tendency to opisthotomos appear to be more frequent with alcohol withdrawal.

Treatment

Therapy should begin with treatment of the mother if possible. She needs care in a facility that is staffed and equipped to follow a high-risk pregnancy and delivery in a hospital staffed and equipped to handle a baby undergoing drug withdrawal.

The baby undergoing drug withdrawal is treated with drugs that will relieve the tremulousness and restlessness and with supportive therapy that will provide him with adequate fluids and calories and keep him relatively comfortable.

A drug commonly used for these babies is paregoric (camphorated tincture of opium) in a dosage of 3 to 5 drops before each feeding and up to 15 to 20 drops for methadone withdrawal.[35] The drug is gradually tapered but may require a number of weeks before it can be stopped. Given to a baby with a mistaken diagnosis it can create an addiction problem. Chlorpromazine and phenobarbital have been used successfully instead of paregoric. Diazepam has also been used successfully, but the intramuscular preparation contains sodium benzoate as a preservative and may present a problem because it interferes with bilirubin binding. Paregoric probably must be used to control methadone withdrawal symptoms, since the other drugs may not give relief.

Water loss is increased in these babies because of their hyperventilation, sweating, and loose stools. Ample fluids must be given and intravenous fluids may be necessary. Body weight must be carefully watched for fluid needs. Calories must be ample because of the baby's hyperactivity and possibly poor intrauterine growth.

Excellent nursing care is very important to these babies. The nurse may be able to soothe the baby and decrease his restlessness by swaddling him and holding him tightly. The nurse must try to decrease all environmental stimuli. Feedings may have to be given in small amounts and at close intervals to maintain required caloric intake. Careful skin care must be given. The baby must be kept warm. It is important to watch for regurgitation and vomiting and to try to position the baby to prevent aspiration.

An important nursing responsibility is to prepare the mother for caring for the baby when he is discharged to his home. This can best be done

---

[34] Leonard Glass, The neonate in withdrawal—Identification, diagnosis, and treatment, *Pediatr. Ann.* 4:25–34 (July) 1975.

[35] *Ibid.*

by involving the mother in the baby's care as early as possible before she is discharged from the hospital. It may be very helpful for a social worker to consult with the mother and for a public health nurse to be involved with home care.

A comprehensive discussion of the problems of the addicted baby and his nursing care has been written by Dr. Loretta Finnegan and Ms. Bonnie Macnew in the *American Journal of Nursing.*[36]

CONGENITAL MALFORMATIONS

An abnormal condition may be present at birth in any part of the body. It may be of a structural or a physiologic nature. A baby may have a single malformation or multiple anomalies. Abnormalities vary from slight to a severe degree. With some the deviation from normal may be so minor that function is normal or only slightly impaired. Others result in disability to varying degrees. Still others are so severe that they are seriously handicapping, unless they can be corrected. Some malformations are incompatible with life.

Congenital malformations are a major problem in infancy. About one-quarter million babies with malformations are born in the United States each year. Congenital malformations are the fourth most frequent cause of deaths in the neonatal period. The extent of developmental abnormalities is not known, since defects of an embryo may be incompatible with intrauterine life and are often a cause of abortion.

Some malformations are genetically determined. Some are caused by adverse environmental conditions that alter development of a normal embryo. Still others may be the result of both genetic and environmental factors. Some abnormalities are the result of an isolated accident in development. Others are of a heredi-

tary nature, occuring either as a sporadic case or as a repeated condition in a family.

Among factors that may cause malformations are maternal rubella, radiation exposure during early pregnancy, maternal age, and chromosomal aberrations. It may be impossible to determine the cause in isolated cases. Specific abnormalities are not related to a specific cause. Several different kinds of abnormalities may arise from one cause, sometimes depending on the time of its action. A specific abnormality can be caused by one of several different factors.

The embryo is most vulnerable to adverse environmental conditions during the early weeks of development, the first 8 to 12 weeks of gestation. It is during this time that organogenesis is taking place. The part of the body that is in a critical stage of development, undergoing rapid differentiation, at the time that an injurious condition exists is in most danger of damage. This part may be arrested in development or become malformed. Thus the kind of abnormality that develops may be determined by the time at which the embryo is exposed to an adverse environment. (See Figure 9-5, page 199.)

Some congenital anomalies cannot be prevented, but increasing knowledge of cause also increases knowledge of precautions that can be taken. Adequate early prenatal care to ensure good health, an adequate diet, and protection insofar as possible against virus diseases, especially rubella, in the early months of pregnancy are valuable in prevention of an adverse environment for the embryo. Avoidance of extensive x-ray treatment during pregnancy is important. All medications taken by the mother should be prescribed by her physician.

Sometimes developmental defects may be suspected before the baby is born. Hydramnios is often associated with a congenital malformation. Dystocia during labor may be due to an anomaly, such as congenital hydrocephalus causing obstructed labor. An x-ray or ultrasound taken late in pregnancy may reveal an abnormality.

Some defects are obvious at birth. Others are not immediately apparent. Some malformations are so obscure that they are not manifested until

---

[36] Loretta Finnegan and Bonnie A. Macnew, Care of the addicted infant, *Am. J. Nurs.* 74:685–693 (April) 1974.

they interfere with normal growth and development. Sudden death in the neonatal period may be due to congenital malformations of the heart, lungs, or brain.

Some babies with malformations cannot make the physiologic adjustments necessary for extrauterine life. Other defects do not seriously interfere with initial function, but make it impossible to meet the demands placed on the body during further development. Some deaths are not preventable because of the extent of malformations. Others may be prevented by immediate treatment. A thorough examination of the newborn infant and close observation of functioning of various systems for characteristic clinical manifestations of internal defects are valuable for early detection and treatment of abnormalities. The nurse can be very helpful in making these observations.

A number of malformations can be corrected surgically. Some of these need early diagnosis and treatment to establish function that will be compatible with life. Other defects may be treated by rehabilitative measures to restore or preserve maximum function.

The birth of a child with an abnormality is accompanied by many emotional and social problems. Parents frequently have a feeling of guilt and self-accusation. They either unconsciously assume or openly express the feeling that they are at fault. They may believe that an anomaly is caused by something they did or omitted to do during the prenatal period. If they cannot think of a cause easily, they may search for one. They will quite naturally be very disappointed, and the baby's disability will sometimes, quite unconsciously, affect their behavior. It will take time for them to accept the reality of the situation.

The intensity of the parent's response to birth of a baby with an anomaly will, of course, be influenced by their personality and background, and in addition other factors will have an effect. Among these are such things as the extent of the defect, the visibility of the defect when looking at the baby, such as a facial abnormality, the amount of neurologic involvement as with cen-

tral nervous system abnormalities, and the possibility of surgical correction of the abnormality.

As always, early parent–infant contact is important. The parents should see the baby as soon as they feel ready. Seeing the baby early is usually helpful to the parents in their adjustment. It gives them the opportunity to know how the baby looks rather than imagining the condition. An imaginary condition may be much more distressful than the real one. Early contact with the baby is very important to good parent–child attachment. As soon as they are ready the parents are encouraged to assist with the care of their baby.

Congenital malformations are grouped into several categories. These include malformations of the skeleton, the central nervous system, the heart and circulatory system, the skin, the urogenital system, the eye, the gastrointestinal tract, and a group of generalized and miscellaneous defects. Certain specific defects are described below.

Central Nervous System

Congenital malformations of the brain and spinal cord vary considerably in location and in extent of involvement.

Anencephalus is a condition in which a considerable portion of the cerebral hemispheres (and the cranium and scalp that lie over them) is lacking. It is not compatible with life.

Hydrocephalus is an accumulation of fluid in the intracranial cavity due to an interference in the flow or absorption of cerebrospinal fluid. It may be caused by a congenital malformation. It is often associated with spina bifida. Evidences of hydrocephalus are an abnormally large head size, tense bulging fontanels, separation of skull sutures, rapid increase in head size, vomiting, and convulsions. It may be necessary to rule out, by lumbar puncture and examination of the spinal fluid, increased pressure due to intracranial hemorrhage. A ventriculoperitoneal shunt is usually performed as initial treatment.

Spina bifida is a development defect in the closure of the bony spinal canal, frequently in the lumbar region. The spinal cord membranes may remain in the canal or may protrude through the defect. Neurologic disability may or may not be present, depending on the extent of the anomaly. A meningocele, in which only the meninges protrude, is not as serious as a myelomeningocele, in which nerve fibers are also present in the sac. Surgical correction may be possible and if done within 24 hours may help to preserve neural function. There is a chance that the protruding sac may break and become infected; meningitis then follows. Infection and dehiscence are complications of surgery.

Circulatory System

Congenital heart disease has been described on pages 793–95.

Gastrointestinal System

Tongue-tie is a condition in which the vertical fold of mucous membrane (frenum) under the tongue, which is normally short and tight in the newborn, extends to the end or nearly to the end of the tongue. It may limit movement of the tongue, which is noticeable when the baby cries, but usually does not interfere with sucking and does not need treatment.

Cleft lip (harelip) and cleft palate are due to failure of the maxillary and palatal processes to close in early fetal life—between the sixth and tenth weeks of gestation. A cleft lip is a fissure in the upper lip to the side of the midline and may vary from a slight notch to a complete separation extending into the nostril. It may be unilateral or bilateral. A cleft palate is a fissure in the midline of the roof of the mouth. This fissure may be small, or there may be complete separation involving both the soft and hard palate. These conditions may occur singly, or the two abnormalities may appear together.

Problems in the newborn nursery are finding the best method of feeding the baby and preventing infection, to which he is very susceptible. The connection existing between the mouth and nose in a baby with a cleft palate permits some of the formula taken into the mouth to come out through the nose. This connection often contributes to respiratory infection. Occasionally a cleft palate alone is not detected immediately after birth. Any feeding difficulty in a baby, especially if regurgitated formula comes through the nose, should be reported to the physician.

Feedings must be skillfully done to have the baby in optimum physical condition for the surgery necessary to correct the defect. Feedings are often given with an Asepto syringe with a rubber tip on the end. A rubber-tipped medicine dropper may be used at first when the feedings are small. Sometimes a soft nipple with large holes, which eliminates hard sucking, is used. Some physicians object to having the baby suck on a nipple at any time, especially when the palate is cleft.

With the Asepto syringe method the rubber tip is placed well back on the baby's tongue. As the formula is squeezed out, it is directed toward the side of the baby's mouth. A feeding is given as rapidly as the baby can take it, but slowly enough to prevent choking. The baby is held in an upright position to facilitate swallowing of milk and to minimize swallowing of air. Frequent bubbling during feedings is necessary since considerable air may be swallowed. Until the baby learns to take feedings well, a suction apparatus should be available in case of aspiration. The mother is taught the feeding technique as soon as the baby is taking feedings well. She is permitted and urged to feed him frequently, in preparation for her care of him at home.

The baby is placed on his side, not abdomen, to prevent rubbing his lip on the bedding. He may need slight restraint of his arms, such as pinning his sleeves to his dress, to prevent irritation of the lip. The lip tends to become dry and may need lubrication with a thin application of an ointment or oil, such as sterile mineral oil.

Since development of the gastrointestinal tract is a very complicated process, malformations can occur anywhere else in the tract. They may be due to arrests in development in early fetal life or to a persistence of fetal structures. These anomalies may cause partial or complete obstruction depending on whether stenosis or atresia is present. The anomalies of the intestinal tract may be single or multiple.

Esophageal anomaly may be present in one of several different forms. Both upper and lower segments of the esophagus may end in blind pouches, or either one or both segments may be connected to the trachea by a fistulous tract. The most common form of esophageal malformation is a *tracheoesophageal fistula,* in which the upper part of the esophagus ends in a blind pouch and the lower segment connects to the trachea.

The baby with esophageal atresia shows signs very early that he has difficulty in swallowing. He usually has an excess amount of mucus flowing from his mouth soon after birth. The nurse in the newborn nursery may be the first to observe this constant, profuse drooling. She should report this observation to the physician immediately. An attempt to pass a catheter into the stomach usually confirms or rules out suspicion of a tracheal anomaly.

If the infant is offered a feeding before a diagnosis is made, further difficulty develops. He may take one or two swallows well and then cough and struggle. Fluid returns through the mouth and nose. Cyanosis and respiratory distress follow. The feeding must be discontinued immediately and suction used to remove the fluid.

Early diagnosis is of paramount importance. It can usually be made by passing a catheter into the esophagus. The catheter meets an obstruction and cannot be passed into the stomach. Some physicians pass a catheter into the stomach of each baby they examine shortly after birth and aspirate his stomach contents. In such instances the diagnosis is made shortly after birth. Hydramnios during pregnancy raises suspicion of a digestive tract obstruction and often leads to early investigation of patency of the eso-

phagus. Radiology may be used to confirm diagnosis.

Respiratory distress followed by pneumonia usually develops early. The baby may aspirate the saliva that fills the upper pouch of the esophagus or aspirate a feeding if it is offered. Digestive secretions from the stomach may pass upward and enter the lungs through the fistulous tract. Although the tendency is to place a baby with excess secretions in a head-down position, any baby with a confirmed or suspected tracheoesophageal fistula should have his elevated to at least a 30-degree angle to minimize upward passage of gastric secretions. Since the infant cannot be fed orally and early develops respiratory distress, surgery is done as early as possible.

The most common abnormality of the stomach is *hypertrophic pyloric stenosis,* resulting from hypertrophy of the musculature of the pylorus—chiefly of the circular muscles. This hypertrophy constricts the lumen of the pyloric opening and thus mechanically interferes with emptying of the stomach. This condition is much more common in male than in female infants.

Pyloric stenosis is not apparent in the immediate new born period. Vomiting usually begins in the second or third week of life, occasionally in the first week. It becomes more frequent and increasingly projectile. The baby vomits during or shortly after a feeding. As a result of vomiting the infant does not obtain an adequate amount of food and fluid. He becomes dehydrated, loses weight, and becomes constipated.

Surgery is almost always necessary to correct pyloric stenosis. The hypertrophied muscles of the pylorus are split, without incision of the mucosa underneath.

Early signs of pyloric stenosis are similar to a *pylorospasm* not associated with hypertrophy of the muscles. Infants with pylorospasm are hyperactive, easily disturbed, and excited. They sleep little, awaken easily, and seem very tense. They vomit frequently during the first few weeks of life. Vomiting occurs suddenly and with considerable force. Slow, careful feeding and bubbling before, during, and after feedings may reduce vomiting.

Intestinal obstruction in a newborn may be complete or partial. It may be located at any level of the small or large intestine. It may be due to stenosis, or atresia, or absence of a portion of the intestine. Evidence appears early, in the first day or two of life. Signs are vomiting, abdominal distention, abnormal meconium, which may be drier or lighter than normal, or absence of stools. Vomiting begins early and becomes more frequent and more severe. The character of the vomitus depends on the level of the obstruction. It may consist of milk and thin fluid only. If the obstruction is below the ampulla of Vater, it contains bile. When the obstruction is as far down as the lower ileum or the colon, fecal material is vomited.

Roentgenograms, even without contrast media, are valuable in diagnosis. There is marked distention of the bowl above the obstruction. Barium is usually not given because of danger of clogging the intestines.

Treatment of intestinal obstruction due to congenital malformations is surgery. Its success will depend on the extent of the anomaly.

Imperforate anus may be caused by a persistent membrane over the anal opening with a normal anus just above the membrane, or there may be complete absence of the anus with the rectal pouch ending some distance above. Direct inspection may reveal the defect. The nurse may discover it when she attempts to take the baby's temperature. A slight depression may be seen where the anal opening should be located. Meconium will not be passed, and the infant may strain, cry, and appear restless. An x-ray will help to determine how much of the rectum or anus is absent.

Surgical correction is necessary. Perineal surgery may establish an opening, but sometimes a colostomy must first be done, followed later by correction of the rectal defect.

Atresia or stenosis of the anus or rectum may be complicated by a fistulous connection with the genitourinary tract.

A *diaphragmatic hernia,* which is a protrusion of the abdominal viscera, to varying degrees, into the thoracic cavity, may be congenital, due to either an absence or a weakness of the diaphragmatic tissue. Symptoms, which include respiratory distress, vomiting, and other evidences of intestinal obstruction, may be present at birth or appear later. Treatment is surgery. It is performed early, before the intestines become distended.

Biliary tract developmental abnormalities, which obstruct the flow of bile into the intestinal tract, cause clay-colored or white stool, bile-stained urine, and early jaundice. The anomaly may or may not be amenable to surgery.

Genitourinary System

Malformations of the genitourinary tract are common, especially in male infants. The development of the genitourinary system is a very complicated process, and any interruption may result in a large variety of abnormalities. Many of these anomalies do not produce symptoms or disturb function. Some cause difficulty sometimes later in life—perhaps at a time of stress on the system. Among the anomalies may be absence, aplasia, or duplication of the kidneys, ureters, or bladder; obstruction of ureters or urethra; and fistulas from the bladder and urethra to the rectum or vagina.

Bilateral renal agenesis, an absence of the kidneys and ureters, causes death within a few hours after birth. It is accompanied by characteristic facial features.

Congenital cystic, or polycystic, kidneys are the most common of kidney malformations. Many cysts, large or small, exist in one or both kidneys. They may not cause symptoms for several years and sometimes not until adult life. This condition will eventually impair kidney function, but it may not be recognized during the neonatal period unless the kidneys are greatly enlarged or irregular.

Exstrophy of the bladder is a partial or complete exposure of the bladder mucosa through an opening in the abdomen. When complete, this defect is due to a failure of union of the abdominal wall, the anterior bladder wall, the symphysis pubis, and the urethra. The opening in the lower abdominal and anterior bladder wall exposes the posterior bladder wall and the ureters on the abdomen.

Ureteral transplants to the bowel and operative removal of the bladder may be necessary; plastic closure may be possible when the exstrophy is not complete. Other anomalies of the genitourinary tract and of the pelvic organs may also be present.

Phimosis is a narrowing of the preputial opening to a degree that makes it impossible to retract the foreskin. Ordinarily it does not interfere with urination, but the opening may be so small that straining is necessary during voiding. The stream of urine is small.

Hypospadias is an anomaly in which the urethra does not extend the entire length of the penis, but rather opens on its lower surface somewhere behind the glans. In severe cases it opens in the perineum. The tip of the penis is bent down. Treatment may not be necessary if the condition is not severe. In other cases a plastic operation may be performed. The urinary flow of these infants should be observed to make certain that the urethral opening is sufficiently large.

A *hydrocele,* an accumulation of fluid in the scrotum, making it a tense, fluctuating, translucent sac, may be congenital. Fluid may be present at birth or may accumulate later. Absorption of the fluid is usually spontaneous. A hydrocele may be accompanied by a hernia.

Undescended testicles make the scrotum appear small. If only one testis is undescended, a difference in size in the two sides of the scrotum is visible. The testes develop in the abdomen and normally descend into the scrotum sometime during the last two months of fetal life. They may, however, remain in the inguinal canal, or even the abdominal cavity, for a longer period of time. Descent is usually spontaneous during the first few weeks of life or at any time up to the age of puberty. An undescended testicle may be associated with hernia.

Musculoskeletal System

Abnormal conditions of the musculoskeletal system may be caused by developmental defects and anomalies of bones and muscles, or they may be the result of an unusual fetal position in utero. Developmental defects may result in the absence of individual muscles, absence of individual bones, supernumerary fingers or toes, union of fingers and toes due to either actual fusion of the bones or webbing of the skin only, and various other deformities.

As the fetus grows, it becomes more and more confined in the uterine cavity. It does not move around as easily as it did earlier in its development, and it may finally maintain a certain posture, at least of some parts of the body. When a certain part is firmly pressed against another bony part, abnormalities, mild or severe, may develop. Unusual positions may result in severe molding of various areas of the body, in asymmetric development, or in a deformity.

Examples of molding due to pressure are abnormal positions of the feet, grooving of the chest due to pressure of the arms against it, and asymmetry of the face from pressure of the chin against the shoulder or the chest. Developmental anomalies or position may cause shortening of muscles and result in contractural defects such as congenital clubfoot or torticollis.

The marked relaxation that characterizes the newborn period diminishes after one week, this being true especially of those muscles and joints which were stretched and strained by fetal position. They become restricted in motion. An example is resistance encountered to leg abduction in the potentially dislocated hip because the muscles splint an unstable hip joint. The joints and muscles that were not strained in utero remain pliant for a longer period of time.

Clubfoot (talipes) is the result of an unequal pull of muscles, producing a deformity in which the foot is turned at an abnormal angle (Fig. 26-6A). Intrauterine position or muscular imbalance is considered a possible cause. The condition is usually bilateral. Diagnosis is sometimes difficult because the foot of the newborn is often normally held in a position similar to a clubfoot.

Since muscular pull may increase the deformity as the muscles mature, corrective measures that change the direction of muscle pull are started early. The method of correction depends on the severity of the condition. One form of treatment consists of passive overcorrection of the position of the foot at frequent intervals during the day. This manipulation may be started before the baby leaves the hospital and is continued at home. The nurses and the mother may be instructed to pull the foot as far as possible in the opposite direction and hold it in that position for a minute each time that the baby is handled (Fig. 26-6B). During manipulation the leg must be well supported under the calf and the knee must be flexed. This protects the lateral ligaments of the knee and the epiphysis of the tibia from strain. The entire foot must be supported to avoid merely bending it in the middle. Bending the foot alone does not correct the shortened heel cord and may result in a rocker foot deformity.

Plaster casts may be applied within a few days after birth. These are changed every one to three weeks to allow for growth of the foot and for further correction. Until the cast is thoroughly dry, care must be taken not to in-dent it with the fingers while handling the baby. It may be necessary to pick the baby up and hold him more than usual after application of the cast until he becomes accustomed to it. After application of a cast the upper leg and the toes must be watched for signs of circulatory impairment. The toes should be warm and a normal pink color—not pale, dark red, or blue. There should be no signs of swelling as indicated by pressure of the edges of the cast against the thigh or the toes. A waterproof material applied to the edge of the cast at the thigh will help to keep it clean of urine and stool.

Congenital dislocation of the hip is a displacement of the head of the femur from the acetabulum. It is much more common in the female than in the male and is more often unilateral than bilateral. Actual dislocation may be present at birth; however, it is usually not actually, but potentially, present. This means that there is in most instances an instability of the joint. This instability is present because the head of the femur is not well anchored into the acetabulum, which is shallow and cartilaginous instead of deep and ossified, and because the joint capsule has poor tone and is stretched. The surrounding muscles, by attempting to splint and protect this soft joint, are actually helping to produce the dislocation.

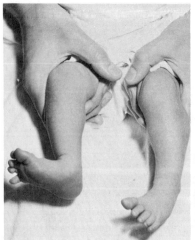 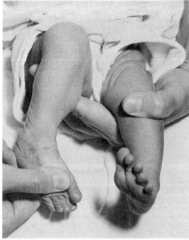

A   **B**

Figure 26-6. A. Talipes calcaneovalgus; right foot moderately resistant. **B.** Pulling the foot downward and inward to overcome the resistance. The nurses were instructed to manipulate the foot in this manner three or four times each time the baby was picked up to be cared for, and the mother was instructed to continue this manipulation at home. If the resistance is not overcome by this treatment, casts will be applied.

The femoral head, which is cartilaginous at birth but begins to have an ossification center at six weeks, remains cartilaginous much longer in these infants, unless treatment is begun early. As the muscles increase in strength and finally as the baby stands, the femoral head is pulled and displaced more and more, the head and the socket are malformed, and the head of the femur is finally completely dislocated.

Early recognition to permit early treatment is important in prevention of an actual dislocation. At the first examination of the baby it may be difficult to recognize a potentially dislocated hip because of the great pliability of the joints of the newborn. By the age of one month and often earlier muscular splinting is evident. The thighs resist abduction. When the normal baby is placed on his back with the knees flexed, his hips and knees can be abducted until they nearly reach the examining table. If a potential dislocation exists, abduction of the affected leg is possible only to one half of this distance. X-ray reveals a persistence of fetal cartilage.

The nurse caring for a baby with a potential dislocation may encounter some difficulty in moving one leg to the side when washing the groin or changing the diaper. Observation of inability to abduct the leg completely is reported to the physician. The baby may also be observed to move this leg less than the unaffected. Other early signs of congenital dislocation of the hip, such as apparent shortening of the affected leg, a higher gluteal and inguinal fold and an additional transverse crease in the thigh, may not be noticeable in the newborn period.

Early treatment of a potential dislocation of the hip is directed toward maintaining the affected leg in complete abduction. The muscle pull then directs the femoral head into the acetabulum, and the pressure thus created stimulates ossification.

A position of abduction may be achieved during the first two months by placing the baby in a prone position whenever he is put to bed and keeping his legs flexed and abducted while he is lying prone. The diaper can be pinned to the sheet to hold the legs in the desired position. Body weight helps to increase the degree of abduction. Another method of keeping the legs flexed and abducted is by the use of a Frejka splint. This consists of a square pillow placed against the infant's diaper and held snugly in place by suspenders or straps. The application of several diapers, in such a manner that there is a very heavy thickness in the center, is another method that may be used to keep the legs widely abducted. Extension of the leg should be avoided when handling the baby.

If treatment is not started early, it may need to be prolonged, and a body cast may be necessary. With early diagnosis and adequate treatment the baby may be able to walk normally at the average age.

The Skin

Nevi may be caused by a hyperplastic development of the blood and lymph vessels or of the epidermis and connective tissue. Nevi made up largely of blood vessels, known as *birthmarks*, are found on various parts of the body. While caring for the baby, the nurse should observe his skin closely for any unusual areas. Birthmarks may be flat or slightly raised. They may range in color from a light red to a darker red or to blue-black. They may or may not have a growth of hair. Birthmarks may be variously described. Some of the most common terms are port wine mark, strawberry mark, and mole. Some lesions regress and disappear. Treatment varies considerably and may not be necessary at all.

The Eye

There are many congenital malformations of the eye. Among them are *congenital cataracts,* which may be caused by a rubella (German measles) infection in the mother in the first three months of pregnancy. This is an important time in the embryonic development of the eye, and the tissue may be particularly susceptible to the effects of the virus. If opacity of the lens is present at birth, it is usually noticeable early as the eyes are observed when the baby opens them in a fairly good light.

Syndromes Caused by Chromosomal Abnormalities

Since 1959, when it was discovered that Down's syndrome (mongolism) was caused by an extra chromosome in the body cells, certain other clinical conditions of previously unknown cause have been found to be associated with the presence of an abnormal number of chromosomes. These syndromes are linked with lack of or acquisition of an additional whole chromosome, or a portion of a chromosome, within the nucleus of a cell, which then continues to reproduce itself.

An irregular number of chromosomes is the result of one of several abnormalities that can occur during cell division, such as nondisjunction during maturation of the sex cells, translocation of a portion of a chromosome, or failure of a chromosome to divide during mitosis as the zygote or early embryo begins development. See pages 59–61 for a description of the mechanism by which alterations in chromosomal distribution may come about.

Some anomalies are linked with abnormalities in the number of sex chromosomes, others with autosomal abnormalities, or possibly a combination of both kinds (Figs. 3-9B and 3-10B, pages 59 and 60). In some of the resulting syndromes the physical anomalies are multiple and severe and mental retardation is common. Among conditions due to an abnormal number of sex chromosomes are rudimentary ovaries and failure to develop full female characteristics, termed Turner's syndrome, and incomplete development of male gonads and other male characteristics, known as Klinefelter's syndrome. Among anomalies linked with an autosome in triplicate are Down's syndrome, D_1 trisomy syndrome, and 18 trisomy syndrome, each resulting in a multiplicity of malformations. Lack of an autosome has not yet been found; this may possibly result in nonviability of the embryo.

Down's syndrome is the name recently suggested for the term *mongolism,* which has long been in use. In this condition mentality is severely retarded, and developmental defects of other tissues are common. Some of the physical characteristics of an individual with Down's syndrome are a small skull, eyes wide set with a lateral upward slope, protruding tongue, short nose with a flat bridge, mobile relaxed joints, poor muscle tone, and often cardiac malformations. Some of the characteristics are not distinct at birth, but become more obvious with age.

Down's syndrome is associated with an extra chromosome, trisomy for no. 21. The extra chromosome is apparently sometimes the result of nondisjunction and occasionally of translocation of no. 21 to another chromosome. There is also a type of Down's syndrome that results from a mosaic pattern, or mixed types, of body cells.

Phenylketonuria

Phenylketonuria (PKU) is a disease of a deficiency of the enzyme phenylalanine hydroxylase, which normally converts phenylalanine to tyrosine. Phenylalanine is an essential amino acid and is necessary for growth, but any excess that is ingested must be degraded, normally by conversion to tyrosine. A baby with phenylketonuria lacks this ability and any phenylalanine not incorporated into body tissues accumulates in the body and eventually spills into the urine.

With phenylketonuria there is progressive mental retardation unless the amount of phenylalanine presented to the tissues is limited to that which is essential. Dietary control must begin early to avoid brain damage. Diagnosis must therefore be made very early.

With PKU the serum phenylalanine level rises rapidly after birth as the baby is fed milk. In most states blood is routinely collected on the day of the baby's discharge from the hospital for examination of an increased amount of phenylalanine. A few drops of heel-stick blood are placed on a filter paper for a Guthrie test. A diagnosis may be made with the test, or a suspicious rise in phenylalanine, which requires recheck, may be found.

An important precaution in the Guthrie test is to make certain that the baby has ingested a significant amount of protein for two or three days prior to the test. If the baby is discharged early, or if there have been feeding problems, or if the baby has vomited, the test may be falsely negative. In cases where feedings have not been sufficient before the baby goes home, the test should be done several days after the baby's discharge. The nurse is usually the person who knows best about the baby's food intake.

BIRTH INJURIES

Trauma during labor or delivery may involve any part of the newborn's body. Some injuries produce only a temporary change, while others cause permanent damage.

Soft-Tissue Injuries

Soft-tissue bruises usually occur in the presenting part of the fetus. Edema of tissues and discolored areas due to an extravasation of blood into tissues may develop in the part of the body that presents at the cervix and vaginal outlet at the time of delivery. This may be the scalp in vertex presentation (caput succedaneum and cephalhematoma), the face in face presentation, and the genitalia, buttocks, and feet in breech presentation (pages 443 and 451).

The face and scalp sometimes have reddened areas or abrasions due to bruising from the obstetric forceps. Occasionally the face has petechial areas for a few days after birth. Subconjunctival hemorrhages may appear following spontaneous as well as instrumental deliveries. They are not considered serious and do not require treatment. Mothers frequently observe this reddened area in the white portion of the baby's eye and inquire about its significance.

Most soft-tissue injuries are not serious. The tissues return to normal in a few days, but should be protected from further trauma during recovery. Breakdown of blood in the tissues may produce hyperbilirubinemia if the bilirubin cannot be excreted rapidly.

Injury to Bones

Injury to bones occurs most frequently to the clavicle and the extremities, rarely to the skull, vertebrae, or ribs. The *clavicle* is the most common site of fractures. It is susceptible to injury when delivery of the shoulders is difficult, but may break during an apparently easy delivery. A fracture is suspected if there is limitation of movement of an arm, if the Moro reflex is unilateral, and if there is spasm of the sternocleidomastoid muscle. However, these signs are not always present. Crepitus may be felt on examination of the clavicle. A roentgenogram will confirm the diagnosis.

Treatment of a fractured clavicle usually consists of immobilization of the arm and shoulder on the affected side. The arm may be placed against the chest wall with the hand lying across the chest and held in place by wrapping a strip of stockinet material around the arm and chest. Complete immobilization is not always done. The infant should be handled carefully to prevent further trauma. When he is picked up, his shoulders should not be pressed toward the middle of the body. The arm on the affected side should not be put through a sleeve daily. When the arm is left out of the sleeve of the shirt or gown, clothing helps to partly immobilize it.

Healing of a clavicle fracture takes place without deformity. A large callus forms within a week and then gradually absorbs. When a fracture is not suspected, it may not be diagnosed until the callus is felt as a hard mass a week or more after birth.

A fracture of one of the extremities may occur if there is difficulty in delivery of an arm or a leg. Spontaneous movement of the involved extremity is limited, and the Moro reflex is not symmetric. These fractures heal rapidly. They heal without deformity when the extremity is immobilized in the corrected position.

Peripheral Nerve Injuries

Injury to peripheral nerves may sometimes occur during birth. The most common involves the *facial nerve*. Temporary paralysis of this nerve is usually due to pressure on it during labor or pressure by a forceps blade during delivery. The affected side of the face is smooth, the eye may remain open, the corner of the mouth droops, and the forehead cannot be wrinkled. This condition is most obvious when the baby cries because the facial muscles on the affected side do not contract, and there is immobility of one side of the mouth. Only the unaffected side of the face moves, and the mouth is drawn to that side. The baby may have some difficulty in sucking during the first few days of life, but this is not always a problem.

Treatment of facial nerve injury is not necessary, but if the eye does not close, it must be protected from injury until it can close. If sucking is difficult for the first few days, it may be necessary to feed the baby with a medicine dropper or a small, soft nipple during this time. Prognosis is good. Improvement begins soon, and recovery is complete in a few weeks. Often this condition is quite transitory, and recovery is complete in a few days.

Brachial palsy is a partial or complete paralysis of certain muscles of the arm due to trauma to nerve fibers of the brachial plexus. The brachial nerves may be injured by pressure, stretching, or actual severance. This injury may occur during delivery from a cephalic presentation when strong traction is exerted on the head during difficult delivery of the shoulders. It may follow breech delivery if traction is made on the brachial plexus as an arm is stripped over the head or if tension is placed on the brachial plexus in making traction.

The site of the injury determines which muscles are affected. The degree of paralysis, therefore, depends on the amount of nerve involvement. The upper arm, the lower arm, or the whole arm may be paralyzed. The Erb-Duchenne (upper arm) paralysis in which the upper part of the plexus (the fifth and sixth cervical nerves) is injured is the most common type. The arm lies limp at the side. It is in a position of extension and is rotated inward. The forearm is in such a position that the palm of the hand faces downward and may even face outward. The baby cannot elevate or abduct the arm. The wrist and hand are normal. The Moro reflex is absent on the affected side. Pain seems to be present at first. The lower arm type of paralysis, which is rare, occurs when the nerves of the lower part of the plexus are injured. The hand and wrist are then paralyzed. The whole arm may be involved, with symptoms of both upper and lower arm type of paralysis. The nurse caring for the newborn should observe any abnormal arm position or diminished arm movements.

Treatment is directed toward restoring function of the involved muscles and preventing contractures of the unaffected ones. Treatment is started as soon after birth as the condition is observed. At first the baby may be placed in a position that keeps his arm abducted and externally rotated and his elbow flexed. The arm is raised to shoulder height, and the elbow is flexed 90 degrees. This position may be maintained in one of several ways. A strip of muslin, tied to the head of the bassinet, may be brought down and tied around the wrist to hold the arm up. With another method the arm may be maintained in the desired position by placing it in a sling made of a folded towel pinned to the mattress. Sometimes the arm is held up by pinning the sleeve of the baby's gown or shirt to the mattress or the top of the crib after the arm has been positioned. Later a splint may be used to hold the arm in the desired position, and massage and exercise may be given. In dressing the baby, the arm should be supported at shoulder level. Clothing should be put on the affected arm first and taken off the affected arm last, and movement of the arm must be gentle.

Prognosis depends on the amount of trauma. If it is slight, caused by edema or hemorrhage around the nerve fibers, the condition soon improves. If the nerves are not lacerated, muscle power usually returns in a few months. Nerve laceration has a more serious prognosis.

Central Nervous System Injury

Injury to the central nervous system is the most serious form of birth injury. *Intracranial hemorrhage*, the most severe form of injury, may be caused by trauma or hypoxia during birth. Rarely, it may be due to a primary hemorrhagic disturbance. The baby's head may be traumatized in a prolonged hard labor, in a difficult delivery, by mechanical injury with obstetric forceps, or in a precipitous labor and delivery.

The shape of the fetal head changes during labor to adapt to the maternal pelvis. Overlapping sutures and soft cranial bones make it possible for the head to accommodate to a pelvic canal of adequate size. Given time, the head can usually make extreme adjustments; when compressed in one direction, it will elongate in another. Excessive molding and overlapping of the cranial bones or sudden molding may, however, cause the meninges or sinuses to tear, resulting in bleeding to a small or large degree. The differences in pressure that cause a caput succedaneum to develop may at times affect the veins of the meninges and the brain in the same area. A short, apparently easy, labor and precipitous delivery are sometimes dangerous because blood vessels may break with sudden changes in pressure during the baby's rapid passage through the birth canal.

Hypoxia and/or ischemia prenatally, during delivery, or following birth is sometimes a cause of brain injury (see page 784). Common causes of hypoxia prenatally are placenta previa, premature separation of the placenta, and complications of pregnancy. Among perinatal causes are hypotension, prolonged, intense uterine contractions, pressure on the umbilical cord, and compression of the head as it passes through the birth canal. Ordinarily the compression is not harmful, but if changes in cerebral circulation are marked and prolonged, reduced circulation and venous congestion may cause hypoxia and predisposition to hemorrhage.

Premature infants are particularly susceptible to intracranial hemorrhage. Their blood vessels are more easily broken than those of the full-term infant, and the tendency to bleed is greater due to a prolonged coagulation defect following birth. Premature rupture of the membranes, breech delivery, and short labor with precipitous delivery—conditions that cause sudden changes in pressure—are more likely to occur in preterm than in full-term delivery.

Trauma to the brain varies in degree from mild to severe. It may be slight, with only edema and no bleeding. When there is bleeding, it may range from a minimal amount due to rupture of a few small vessels to a massive hemorrhage. Large hemorrhages are infrequent and usually fatal. Bleeding may occur from one or more of several sites. It may be subdural, subarachnoid, intraventricular, over the cerebellar area, or into the brain substance itself.

Signs of intracranial injury may be generalized and similar to those produced by several other conditions. Attacks of cyanosis, vomiting, listlessness, and poor sucking may be the only signs of cerebral irritation. These may also be due to other causes, such as respiratory distress and congenital heart disease. Included in signs of cerebral injury are irregular, difficult respirations; a pale, cold, clammy skin; cyanosis at intervals or continuously; an anxious expression, sometimes with the eyes open and staring; restlessness; failure to suck well; forceful vomiting; and a high-pitched cry. Localized muscular twitchings or generalized convulsions may occur several hours after birth. The baby is flaccid at first and in 12 to 24 hours becomes spastic. The fontanels may be tense; the pupils may be of unequal size; Foote's sign, an adderlike, rhythmic protrusion of the tongue, may be present; the neck and spine may become rigid; and the infant may assume an opisthotonic position.

Signs of intracranial injury may be present immediately after birth or may be delayed for several days. With massive hemorrhage there may be few signs, but death may occur soon after birth, or signs may be severe at or shortly after delivery. With slight hemorrhage, due to rupture of small vessels, signs may develop gradually.

The difference in signs of cerebral irritation, cerebral edema, and intracranial hemorrhage is frequently only in degree of severity and length of time they are present. Slight trauma may give rise to mild signs. The baby may be sleepy and listless and suck poorly during the first few days of life. He usually recovers quickly and soon becomes alert, responds more readily, and begins to eat well. Cerebral edema is apt to give the same signs as mild hemorrhage, and it is frequently impossible to determine which is present. With edema the signs usually appear almost immediately after birth and last only three to four days. After this, improvement is rapid and recovery complete.

The Moro embrace reflex is checked on several succeeding days when intracranial injury is suspected. Absence of the reflex immediately after birth with a return in a few days is indicative of cerebral edema. It returns when the edema subsides. With hemorrhage the Moro reflex is often present for 24 to 48 hours after birth, then disappears, and does not return until much later.

To test for increased pressure and for blood, a spinal puncture is done as an aid in diagnosis. It may relieve pressure. Interpretation of findings from a spinal puncture may be difficult. Absence of increased pressure does not exclude intracranial hemorrhage. Presence of blood does not confirm it, since the trauma of puncture may produce blood from injury of a vessel of the spinal canal. A subdural tap may be done.

Treatment is largely directed toward keeping the baby quiet. Rest and a quiet environment may prevent stimulation of bleeding. The baby is handled as infrequently as possible and with utmost gentleness. Care that is not essential, such as bathing, is omitted.

The baby may need additional warmth. He sometimes needs oxygen. He is usually placed in an incubator for temperature control, administration of oxygen if necessary, and easy observation. Following difficult delivery, a baby, regardless of size, may be given premature care

in an incubator until it is ascertained that his condition is good. Instead of lowering the head of the crib following birth, as is sometimes done for drainage of mucus, the crib is positioned on a level or the head is elevated at apprxoximately a 30-degree angle when intracranial injury is suspected. The baby is observed frequently or continuously, depending on his condition, for vital signs and general behavior.

Oral feedings are withheld and intravenous fluids are administered slowly. When feedings are started, they are often given in small amounts until it is ascertained that the baby can tolerate them easily. Feedings are given by a method requiring minimal exertion until it is established that the baby can suck easily. A medicine dropper or a soft nipple may at first be used, and sometimes the first feedings are by gavage.

Vitamin K_1 is usually prescribed for babies after birth. When not used routinely, it is often given prophylactically to a baby delivered with difficulty, or it is used in treatment when symptoms appear. Although hemorrhage is probably not due to a coagulation defect, vitamin K_1 may control the amount of bleeding by minimizing or preventing the transitory defect in blood coagulation which occurs in the early neonatal period.

Sedation may be given, especially if the infant is restless and hyperactive. Phenobarbital, 8 mg (⅛ gr), may be used and may be repeated from two to four times daily, depending on the baby's response to its quieting effect.

Prognosis with intracranial hemorrhage is guarded. Some babies are born dead, and others may die after several days. In those who survive recovery may frequently be complete, or there may be permanent cerebral damage. Sequelae may include convulsions, mental retardation, behavior problems, and spastic paralysis. Cerebral palsy is a common sequela when recovery is not complete. Congenital defects, as well as birth injuries, cause cerebral palsy, but an estimate of how large a factor this may be is impossible. Cerebral palsy may also be caused by other postnatal conditions, such as asphyxia, erythroblastosis, head injury, encephalitis, and other infections, such as whooping cough and measles.

NEONATAL SEIZURES

Seizures in the newborn are often related to significant illness; it is therefore very important to find their cause as early as possible in order to institute early treatment.

Seizures in the newborn differ considerably from those observed in older children. In newborns the seizures are rarely well organized, generalized, tonic–clonic movements. Preterm babies have even less well organized seizures than full-term newborns. It appears that these differences relate to the less well developed neuroanatomic and neurophysiologic systems in the perinatal period.

Signs of Seizures

The most frequent seizure type is characterized as subtle. Its clinical manifestations can easily be overlooked. The major manifestations of this type consist of one or more of the following: repetitive blinking or fluttering of the eyelids; tonic horizontal deviations of the eyes with or without jerking of the eyes; drooling, sucking, or other mouth, cheek, or tongue movements; rowing or swimming movements of the upper limbs or sometimes pedaling movements of the legs. Apnea may appear but is usually accompanied by one of the other manifestations. Less frequently tonic posturing of a limb may be observed. Sometimes a seizure is manifested by clonic movements of a limb which migrate to another body part in no special pattern. As an example, an arm jerking may be accompanied or followed by jerking of a leg. Another type of seizure is a generalized tonic seizure; this is characteristic of the premature. Occasionally a seizure is seen as single or multiple jerks of the limbs.

Jitteriness Versus Seizure

Jitteriness is a movement disorder that should be distinguished from neonatal seizures. It is characteristically a disorder of the neonatal period. It is characterized by movements consisting primarily of tremulousness but occasionally also of clonus. Joseph J. Volpe states that [37]

Distinguishing jitteriness from seizure is readily made if the following four points are remembered. Jitteriness is not accompanied by abnormalities of gaze or extraocular movement, seizures usually are. Jitteriness is exquisitely stimulus-sensitive, seizures are not. The dominant movement in jitteriness is tremor; i.e., the alternating movements are rhythmic, of equal rate and amplitude. The dominant movement in seizure is clonic jerking; i.e., the movements have a fast and slow component. These rhythmic movements of limbs in jitteriness usually can be stopped by flexion of the affected limb. The most consistently defined etiologies of jitteriness are hypoxic–ischemic encephalopathy, hypocalcemia, hypoglycemia, and drug withdrawal.

Causes and Diagnosis

There are many causes of neonatal seizures, but the predominant cause is perinatal asphyxia resulting in hypoxic–ischemic encephalopathy. Other important etiologies are intracranial hemorrhage, intracranial infection, developmental defects, and metabolic disorders such as hypoglycemia and hypocalcemia. Determining the etiology of seizures is critical, since it provides the opportunity to treat specifically. Evaluation of the infant includes careful, detailed history, physical examination, laboratory studies, lumbar puncture, subdural tap, EEG, transillumination of the skull, and other diagnostic procedures that seem indicated from history and physical examination.

Treatment

Continuous or frequent seizures must be treated with urgency because the seizures themselves can result in brain injury. It is therefore

[37] Joseph J. Volpe, Neonatal seizures, *Clin. Perinatol.* 4:50 (Mar.) 1977.

very important to recognize seizures early. Repeated seizures can be accompanied by hypoventilation and/or apnea, and this may result in hypercapnia and hypoxemia. Hypoxemia is a potential cause of brain injury, and it may result in poor circulation and ischemic injury to the brain. Increased intracranial pressure may decrease cerebral blood flow and intracranial pressure can be aggravated by hypercapnia.

For treatment, intravenous glucose administration is started early. It is used to treat hypoglycemia if present and also to maintain blood glucose at high normal or above normal level to assure that the brain cells will receive adequate glucose.

Anticonvulsant drugs are administered if hypoglycemia is not present. Phenobarbital is administered intravenously in a dose of 10 mg/kg over several minutes. A second dose is given in approximately 20 minutes if more anticonvulsant is needed. Occasionally when seizures continue, diphenylhydantoin is also used for anticonvulsant therapy. Phenobarbital is then used for maintenance of anticonvulsant action in a dose of approximately 5 mg/kg-day given in two divided doses every 12 hours.[38]

BIBLIOGRAPHY

Aballi, A. J., Hemorrhagic disease of newborn, *Pediatr. Ann.* 3:35–70 (Feb.) 1974.

Affonso, Dyanne, and Harris, Thomas, CPAP. Continuous positive airway pressure, *Am. J. Nurs.* 76:570–573 (April) 1976.

Altshuler, Anne, Complete transposition of the great arteries, *Am. J. Nurs.* 71:96–98, 1971.

American Academy of Pediatrics, Committee on Nutrition, Special diets for infants with inborn errors of amino acid metabolism, *Pediatrics* 57:783–791 (May) 1976.

Atkinson, Helen C., Care of the child with cleft lip and palate, *Am. J. Nurs.* 67:1889–1892, 1967.

Avery, Gordon B. (ed.), *Neonatology.* Lippincott, Philadelphia, Pa., 1975.

Avery, Mary Ellen, and Fletcher, Barry D., *The Lung and Its Disorders in the Newborn Infant,* 3rd ed. Saunders, Philadelphia, Pa., 1974.

Bacsik, Robert D., Meconium aspiration syndrome, *Pediatr. Clin. North Am.* 24:463–479 (Aug.) 1977.

Barnard, Martha Underwood, Supportive nursing care for the mother and newborn who are separated from each other, *MCN,* 1:107–110 (Mar./Apr.) 1976.

Beard, A. *et al.,* Neonatal hypoglycemia: A discussion, *J. Pediatr.* 79:314, 1971.

Behrman, Richard E. (ed.), *Neonatology.* Mosby, St. Louis, Mo., 1973.

———, The use of acid–base measurements in the cinical evaluation and treatment of the sick neonate, *J. Pediatr.* 74:632–637 (April) 1969.

Brann, A. W., Jr., and Dykes, Francine D., The effects of intrauterine asphyxia on the full-term neonate, *Clin. Perinatol.* 4:149–161 (March) 1977.

Brown, Bryant J., Gabert, Harvey A., and Stenchever, Morton A., Respiratory distress syndrome, surfactant biochemistry, and acceleration of fetal lung maturity: A review, *Obstet. Gynecol. Surv.* 30:71–90 (Feb.) 1975.

Brown, William J., Acquired syphilis, drugs and blood tests, *Am. J. Nurs.* 71:713–715 (April) 1971.

Caldwell, Joseph G., Congenital syphilis: A nonvenereal disease, *Am. J. Nurs.* 71:1768–1772 (Sept.) 1971.

Carroll, Mary Helen, Recognizing narcotic withdrawal in newborns, *JOGN Nurs.* 1:23–24 (May/June) 1972.

Carson, Bonita S. *et al.,* Combined obstetric and pediatric approach to prevent meconium aspiration syndrome, *Am. J. Obstet. Gynecol.* 126:712–715 (Nov. 15) 1976.

Clark, Ann L., and Affonso, Dyanne D., *Childbearing. A Nursing Perspective.* Davis, Philadelphia, Pa., 1976.

Clatworthy, H. W., and Grosfeld, J. L., Danger signals in the newborn, *Hosp. Med.* 9:60–64 (May) 1973.

Committee on Phototherapy in the Newborn Infant, National Research Council, National Academy of Sciences, Preliminary report of the committee on phototherapy in the newborn infant, *J. Pediatr.* 84:135–147 (Jan.) 1974.

[38] *Ibid.,* p. 59.

Conway, Alice, and Williams, Tamara, Parenteral alimentation, *Am. J. Nurs.* 76:574–577 (April) 1976.

Cornblath, Marvin, Disorders of carbohydrate metabolism, in *Diseases of the Newborn*, 4th ed., edited by Alexander J. Schaffer and Mary Ellen Avery. Saunders, Philadelphia, Pa., 1977, pp. 518–528.

———, Diagnosing and treating neonatal hypoglycemia, *Contemp. Ob/Gyn* 8:95–99 (Sept.) 1976.

———, and Schwartz, Robert, *Disorders of carbohydrate metabolism in infancy*, 2nd ed. Volume IV in the series *Major Problems in Clinical Pediatrics*. Saunders, Philadelphia, Pa., 1976, Chapters 1–5.

Cranley, Mecca S., When a high-risk infant is born, *Am. J. Nurs.* 75:1696–1699 (Oct.) 1975.

Cunningham, M. Douglas, and Smith, Franklin R., Stabilization and transport of severely ill infants, *Pediatr. Clin. North Am.* 20:359–366 (May) 1973.

Davis, L., Neonatal respiratory emergencies, *Nurs. Clin. North Am.* 8:441–444 (Sept.) 1973.

Dorand, Rodney D., Neonatal asphyxia, *Pediatr. Clin. North Am.* 24:455–461 (Aug.) 1977.

Dunn, Deon, and Lewis, Amber T., Some important aspects of neonatal nursing related to pulmonary disease and family involvement, *Pediatr. Clin. North Am.* 20:481–498 (May) 1973.

Ehlers, Kathryn, Recognition and management of the high-risk infant with heart disease, *Pediatr. Ann.* 3:41–58 passim (Jan.) 1974.

Eng, G. D., Brachial plexus palsy in newborns, *Pediatrics* 48:18, 1971.

Farrell, Philip M., and Avery, Mary Ellen, Hyaline membrane disease, *Am. Rev. Respir. Dis.* 111:657–688 (May) 1975.

———, and Kotas, Robert V., The prevention of hyaline membrane disease: New concepts and approaches to therapy, *Adv. Pediatr.* 23:213–269, 1976.

Finnegan, Loretta P., and Macnew, Bonnie A., Care of the addicted infant, *Am. J. Nurs.* 74:685–693 (April) 1974.

Fletcher, Anne B., Clinical and biochemical aspects of the infant of the diabetic mother, in *The Neonate*, edited by Donald S. Young and Jocelyn M. Hicks. Wiley, New York, 1976, pp. 285–294.

Fogarty, Sarah, The nurse and the high-risk infant, *Nurs. Clin. North Am.* 8:533–547 (Sept.) 1973.

Fowler, Marsha D., Idiopathic respiratory distress syndrome of the newborn, in *Current Practice in Obstetric and Gynecologic Nursing*, edited by Leota K. McNall and Janet T. Galeener. Mosby, St. Louis, Mo., 1976, pp. 125–145.

Gershon, Anne A., The use of antibiotics for severe neonatal infections, *Pediatr. Ann.* 5:80–88 (Feb.) 1976.

Gersony, Welton M., Persistence of the fetal circulation: A commentary, *J. Pediatr.* 82:1103–1106 (June) 1973.

Gill, Frances M., Thrombocytopenia in the newborn, *Pediatr. Ann.* 3:71–86 (Feb.) 1974.

Gillen, J. E., Behavior of newborns with cardiac distress, *Am. J. Nurs.* 73:254 (Feb.) 1973.

Glass, Leonard, The neonate in withdrawal—Identification, diagnosis, and treatment, *Pediatr. Ann.* 4:25–34 passim (July) 1975.

Gluck, Louis, Editorial. Iatrogenic RDS and amniocentesis, *Hosp. Pract.* 12:11; 17 (March) 1977.

———, and Kulovich, Marie V., Fetal lung development. Current concepts, *Pediatr. Clin. North Am.* 20:367–379 (May) 1973.

Gohari, Parviz, Berkowitz, Richard, and Hobbins, John C., Immediate and long-term risks to IUGR children, *Contemp. Ob/Gyn* 8:79–88 (Sept.) 1976.

Gregory, George A., Aspiration syndrome in infants, *Int. Anesthesiol. Clin.* 15:97–105 (Spring) 1977.

———, et al., Treatment of idiopathic respiratory distress syndrome with continuous positive airway pressure, *N. Engl. J. Med.* 284:1333–1340 (June 17) 1971.

Gross, Gary P. et al., Hyperviscosity in the neonate, *J. Pediatr.* 82:1004–1012 (June) 1973.

Guthrie, Diana W., and Guthrie, Richard A., The infant of the diabetic mother, *Am. J. Nurs.* 74:2008–2009 (Nov.) 1974.

Harris, Michael B., Neonatal host-defense mechanisms, *Pediatr. Ann.* 5:86–95 (June) 1976.

Harrison, V. C., de V. Heese, H., and Klein, M., The significance of grunting in hyaline membrane disease, *Pediatrics* 41:549–559 (March) 1968.

Heird, William C., and Driscoll, John M., Newer methods for feeding low birth weight infants, *Clin. Perinatol.* 2:309–325 (Sept.) 1975.

Hodson, W. A., and Belenky, D. A., Management of respiratory problems, in *Neonatology*, edited by

Gordon Avery. Lippincott, Philadelphia, Pa., 1975, pp. 265–294.

Hsia, David Yi-Yung, A critical evaluation of PKU screening, *Hosp. Pract.* 6:101–104; 109–112 (April) 1971.

Huch, R. *et al.*, Transcutaneous Po₂ monitoring in routine management of infants and children with cardiorespiratory problems, *Pediatrics* 57:681–690 (May) 1976.

———, Lübbers, D. W., and Huch, A., Reliability of transcutaneous monitoring of arterial Po₂ in newborn infants, *Arch. Dis. Child.* 49:213–218 (March) 1974.

Jackson, Pat Ludder, Chronic grief, *Am. J. Nurs.* 74:1288–1291 (July) 1974.

James, L. Stanley, and Lanman, Jonathan T. (eds.), History of oxygen therapy and retrolental fibroplasia. *Pediatrics, Part II [Suppl.]* 57:591–642 (April) 1976.

Johnson, Dale G., Emergency surgical management of life-threatening anomalies in neonates, *Hosp. Med.* 11:69–95 passim (Feb.) 1975.

Jones, M. Douglas, Jr., and Murton, Laurence J., Mechanical ventilation in the newborn with hyaline membrane disease, 6:63–76 (April) 1977.

Kallop, Fritzi, Working with parents through a devastating experience. The birth of a mongoloid child, *JOGN Nurs.* 2:36–41 (May/June) 1973.

Kandall, Stephen R., Control of bacterial infection in the nursery, *Pediatr. Ann.* 5:48–61 passim (Feb.) 1976.

———, Delayed onset of neonatal drug withdrawal symptoms, *Pediatr. Ann.* 4:35–45 (July) 1975.

Kennedy, Janet C., The high-risk maternal–infant acquaintance process, *Nurs. Clin. North Am.* 8:549–556 (Sept.) 1973.

Klaus, Marshall H., and Fanaroff, Avroy A., *Care of the High-Risk Neonate.* Saunders, Philadelphia, Pa., 1973.

Korones, Sheldon B., *High Risk Newborn Infants,* 2nd ed. Mosby, St. Louis, Mo., 1976.

Kramer, Lloyd I., Advancement of dermal icterus in the jaundiced newborn, *Am. J. Dis. Child.* 118:454–458 (Sept.) 1969.

Krauss, Alfred N., Assisted ventilation with bag and mask for neonates, *Pediatr. Ann.* 1:45–52 (Nov.) 1972.

Lanzkowsky, Philip, Iron deficiency anemia, *Pediatr. Ann.* 3:6–31 passim (March) 1974.

———, Erythroblastosis fetalis, *Pediatr. Ann.* 3:7–34 (Feb.) 1974.

Lewak, N., Management of idiopathic hyperbilirubinemia in term infants: Community practices, *Pediatrics* 53:471 (Apr.) 1974.

Lucey, Jerold F., Is intensive care becoming too intensive? *Pediatrics,* Part 2, *Neonatology Suppl.* 59:1064–1065 (June) 1977.

———, Phototherapy: What it has to offer, *Contemp. Ob/Gyn* 6:51–52 (Nov.) 1975.

———, Effects of light on the newly born infant, *J. Perinatal Med.* 4:147–150, 1973.

Lynn, Hugh B., The role of surgery in respiratory emergencies, *Pediatr. Clin. North Am.* 20:323–331 (May) 1973.

Maisels, M. Jeffrey, Bilirubin. On understanding and infuencing its metabolism in the newborn infant, *Pediatr. Clin. North Am.* 19:447–501 (May) 1972.

Mills, Gretchen C., Supporting parental needs after birth of a defective child, in *Current Practice in Pediatric Nursing,* edited by Patricia A. Brandt, Peggy L. Chinn, and Mary Ellen Smith. Mosby, St. Louis, Mo., 1976, pp. 109–129.

Nalepka, Claire D., The oxygen hood for newborns in respiratory distress, *Am. J. Nurs.* 75:2185–2187 (Dec.) 1975.

Passo, Sherrilyn DeJean, Positioning infants with myelomeningocele, *Am. J. Nurs.* 74:1658–1660 (Sept.) 1974.

Penfold, Kathleen McNally, Supporting mother love, *Am. J. Nurs.* 74:464–467 (March) 1974.

Perinatal News, Madison General Hospital, Wisconsin Perinatal Center, Southcentral Region, May 1974, October 1974, and Summer 1976.

Pidgeon, V., The infant with congenital heart disease, *Am. J. Nurs.* 67:290–293 (Feb.) 1967.

Pierog, Sophie, and Nigam, Sarvesh, Neonatal sepsis, *Pediatr. Ann.* 5:63–76 (Feb.) 1976.

Polgar, George, Practical pulmonary physiology, *Pediatr. Clin. North Am.* 20:303–322 (May) 1973.

Ramamurthy, Rajam, and Pildes, Rosita S., Prevention: The key to control of neonatal bacterial infection, *Contemp. Ob/Gyn* 5:59–61 (March) 1975.

Ravitch, M. M., and Rowe, M. I., Surgical emergencies in the neonate, *Am. J. Obstet. Gynecol.* 103:1034–1057 (April 1) 1969.

Renfield, Marilyn, Respiratory distress syndrome, in

The Neonate. Clinical Biochemistry, Physiology, and Pathology, edited by Donald S. Young and Jocelyn M. Hicks. Wiley, New York, 1976, pp. 257–270.

Roberts, Joyce E., Suctioning the newborn, *Am. J. Nurs.* 73:63–65 (Jan.) 1973.

Rooth, Gosta, Transcutaneous oxygen tension measurements in newborn infants, *Pediatrics* 55:232–234 (Feb.) 1975.

Rudolph, Abraham, Cardiac failure in children: A hemodynamic view, *Hosp. Pract.* 5:44–55 (July) 1970.

———, and Heymann, Michael A., Medical treatment of the ductus arteriosus, *Hosp. Pract.* 12:57–65 (Feb.) 1977.

Schaffer, Alexander J., and Avery, Mary Ellen, *Diseases of the Newborn,* 4th ed. Saunders, Philadelphia, Pa., 1977.

Shaw, J. C. L., Parenteral nutrition in the management of sick low birthweight infants, *Pediatr. Clin. North Am.* 20:333–358 (May) 1973.

Sheldon, Roger E., Management of perinatal asphyxia, *Pediatr. Ann.* 6:15–38 passim (April) 1977.

Shin, Yong Ho, and Glass, Leonard, The "torch" syndrome, *Pediatr. Ann.* 5:106–113 (Feb.) 1976.

Shinefield, Henry R., Neonatal septicemia in the premature, *Pediatr. Ann.* 1:12–20 (Nov.) 1972.

Silverman, William A., The lesson of retrolental fibroplasia, *Sci. Am.* 236:100–107 (June) 1977.

Simmons, Michael A., Supportive care in respiratory distress, *Pediatr. Ann.* 6:39–62 passim (April) 1977.

Sinclair, John C., Driscoll, John M., Heird, William C., and Winters, Robert W., Supportive management of the sick neonate, *Pediatr. Clin. North Am.* 17:863–893 (Nov.) 1970.

Smith, David W., and Wilson, Ann C., *The Child with Down's Syndrome.* Saunders, Philadelphia, Pa., 1973.

Solomon, Gail E., Neonatal seizures, *Pediatr. Ann.* 4:35–50 passim (Aug.) 1975.

Solomons, Gerald, Mongolism, *Hosp. Med.* 5:58–69 (Oct.) 1969.

Stern, Leo, The use and misuse of oxygen in the newborn infant, *Pediatr. Clin. North Am.* 20:447–464, (May) 1973.

Thaler, M. Michael, Perinatal bilirubin metabolism, *Adv. Pediatr.* 19:215–235, 1972.

Ting, Pauline, and Brady, June P., Tracheal suction in meconium aspiration, *Am. J. Obstet. Gynecol.* 122:767–771 (July 15) 1975.

Tsang, Reginald, and Steichen, Jean J., Pathogenesis of neonatal hypocalcemia, *Contemp. Ob/Gyn* 5:81–86 (Feb.) 1975.

Volpe, Joseph J., Neonatal seizures, *Clin. Perinatol.* 4:43–63 (March) 1977.

———, Neonatal intracranial hemorrhage: Pathophysiology, neuropathology, and clinical features, *Clin. Perinatol.* 4:77–102 (March) 1977.

Waechter, Eugenia H., Developmental consequences of congenital abnormalities, *Nurs. Forum* 14:108–129, 1975.

———, The birth of an exceptional child, *Nurs. Forum* 9:202–216, 1970.

Wu, Paul Y. K., Phototherapy: Weighing the benefits and risks, *Contemp. Ob/Gyn* 6:53–57 (Nov.) 1975.

Yasunaga, S., Cephalhematoma in the newborn, *Clin. Pediatr.* 13:256–260 (March) 1974.

Young, Donald S., and Hicks, Jocelyn M. (eds.), *The Neonate. Clinical Biochemistry, Physiology, and Pathology.* Wiley, New York, 1976.

Young, Ruth K., Chronic sorrow: Parents' response to the birth of a child with a defect, *MCN,* 2:38–42 (Jan./Feb.) 1977.

Zachman, Richard D. (ed.), Neonatal beta-hemolytic streptococcal pneumonia—A serious disease, *Perinatal News,* Madison General Hospital, Wisconsin Perinatal Center, Southcentral Region, Oct. 7, 1977.

Zanger, N. W. *et al.,* Ophthalmia neonatorum is still with us, *J. Med. Soc. N.J.* 69:674–681 (Aug.) 1972.

Part Six

History and Trends

Trends in Maternal and Infant Care

The state of civilization of any country is said to be reflected in its maternal and infant mortality rates. Since 1915, the number of deaths in the United States has declined, more or less consistently. In 1975, the infant death rate was 1610 infants under one year for each 100,000 live births. In the same year 12.8 maternal deaths occurred for each 100,000 live births. These statistics represented the lowest mortality rates recorded in the United States for these groups. Trends in mortality rates give evidence of great improvement in maternal and infant care over the past 30 to 40 years. They also indicate where more progress is attainable. At the present time the complete maternity care envisioned as early as 1919, when the "Minimum Standards for Public Protection of the Health of Mothers" (Appendix II) were formulated, is not yet available for *all* mothers.

To bring the benefits of complete, high-quality maternity care to each mother, to each family, is the aim of those practicing obstetrics. The combined efforts of many individuals and agencies have contributed to this improvement. Some of these efforts are described in this chapter, others are reviewed in Appendix I, "Historical Developments." Most, if not all, of our new ideas had their beginnings in the activities of the pioneers of the past. Although an arbitrary separation of the past from the present practices and aspirations in maternity care is not possible, certain historical developments have been separated and placed in Appendix I. This will permit the reader of this chapter to give attention to recent developments and progress in the care of mothers and babies, but to have easy access to a history of earlier developments in maternity care by referring to Appendix I.

The nurse plays an important role in the continuing progress in the care of mothers and babies. Her work with each patient is part of a great nationwide effort to improve total maternity care. She will have a better conception of the difficulties to be overcome in securing adequate care for every maternity patient when she is aware of the available community resources for that care and how they came to be what they are today.

Maternal Mortality

Any mother who dies during pregnancy, labor, or the puerperium is registered as a maternal death. The official rate was expressed as the number of maternal deaths per 10,000 live births until 1960. The maternal mortality rate, which was as high as 67.3 deaths per 10,000 live births in 1930, was reduced to 37.6 per 10,000 live births in 1940, to 8.3 in 1950, and in 1967 down to 2.8 deaths per 10,000 live births, or 28.0 per 100,000 live births as now expressed. In 1970 the rate decreased to 21.5 deaths per 100,000 live births. In 1971 and 1972 the rate remained the same at 18.8, but since then there has been a yearly decline. In 1975, 403 women died of maternal causes. As in previous years, this number does not include all deaths of pregnant women but only deaths from complications of pregnancy, childbirth, and the puerperium. The total maternal mortality rate in 1975 was 12.8 per 100,000 live births. The rate for white women was 9.1 and that of women other than white was 29.0. This makes the rate for all other women 3.2 times greater than that for white women.

Figure 27-1 shows a dramatic reduction in the mortality rate from 376.0 per 100,000 live births in 1940 to 83.3 in 1950. This was a period of time during which there was a great increase in hospital deliveries. Since then other develop-

ments and improvements in maternity care have had important influences on the steady reduction in maternal deaths as shown in Figure 27-1 and Table 27-1.

Improved prenatal care has reduced deaths due to toxemias of pregnancy. Development of antibacterial drugs has greatly reduced mortality due to infection. Increased use and availability of blood for transfusion have played a large part in reducing deaths due to hemorrhage and shock. A recent development, that of perinatal centers, which provides intensive care management to high-risk pregnant women in centers that are specially staffed and equipped for ma-

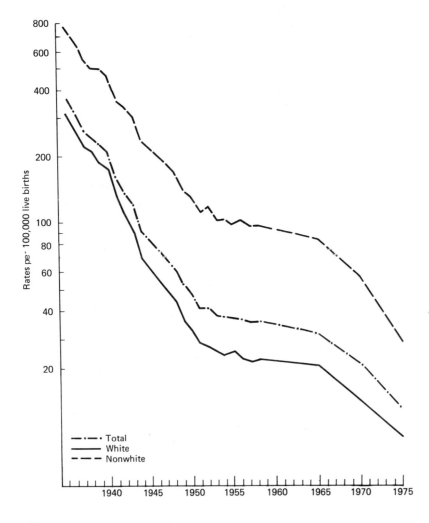

Figure 27-1. Maternal mortality rates by color: United States 1940–1975. [*Source: National Center for Health Statistics:* Infant, Fetal, and Maternal Mortality, *United States— 1963. Public Health Service Publication No. 1000, Series 20, No. 3 and National Center for Health Statistics:* Monthly Vital Statistics Report, *Vol. 25, No. 11, Supplement, Feb. 11, 1977, and U.S. Dept. of Commerce, Bureau of the Census,* Statistical Abstract of the United States, *1976.*]

Table 27-1.   Infant, Maternal, Fetal, and Neonatal Death Rates, by Race: 1940 to 1974

(Deaths per 1,000 live births, except as noted. Prior to 1960, excludes Alaska and Hawaii. See also *Historical Statistics, Colonial Times to 1970,* series B 136–147)

Item	1940	1950	1960	1965	1967	1968	1969	1970*	1971*	1972*	1973*	1974*
Infant deaths**	47.0	29.2	26.0	24.7	22.4	21.8	20.9	20.0	19.1	18.5	17.7	16.7
White	43.2	26.8	22.9	21.5	19.7	19.2	18.4	17.8	17.1	16.4	15.8	14.8
Negro and other	73.8	44.5	43.2	40.3	35.9	34.5	32.9	30.9	28.5	27.7	26.2	24.9
Maternal deaths†	376.0	83.3	37.1	31.6	28.0	24.5	22.2	21.5	18.8	18.8	15.2	14.6
White	319.8	61.1	26.0	21.0	19.5	16.6	15.5	14.4	13.0	14.3	10.7	10.0
Negro and other	773.5	221.6	97.9	83.7	69.5	63.6	55.7	55.9	45.3	38.5	34.6	35.1
Fetal deaths‡	NA	19.2	16.1	16.2	15.6	15.8	14.1	14.2	13.4	12.7	12.2	11.5
White	NA	17.1	14.1	13.9	13.5	13.8	12.4	12.4	11.8	11.2	10.8	10.2
Negro and other	NA	32.5	26.8	27.2	25.8	25.6	22.5	22.6	21.2	19.5	18.6	17.0
Neonatal deaths§	28.8	20.5	18.7	17.7	16.5	16.1	15.6	15.1	14.2	13.6	13.0	12.3
White	27.2	19.4	17.2	16.1	15.0	14.7	14.2	13.8	13.0	12.4	11.8	11.1
Negro and other	39.7	27.5	26.9	25.4	23.8	23.0	22.5	21.4	19.6	19.2	17.9	17.2

NA, not available.

*Excludes deaths of nonresidents of U.S. For 1972, based on a 50-percent sample of deaths.

**Represents deaths of infants under 1 year old, exclusive of fetal deaths.

†Per 100,000 live births from deliveries and complications of pregnancy, childbirth, and the puerperium. For 1960–1965, deaths are classified according to seventh revision of *International Lists of Diseases and Causes of Death;* thereafter, according to eighth revision.

‡Includes only fetal deaths (stillbirths) for which period of gestation was 20 weeks (or 5 months) or was not stated.

§Represents deaths of infants under 28 days old, exclusive of fetal deaths.

Source: U.S. National Center for Health Statistics, *Vital Statistics of the United States,* annual.

ternity care are also contributing to improved care for pregnant women.

In addition to the great decrease in maternal death rate, the morbidity rate has also fallen, and there has been a great improvement in the condition in which the mother returns to her nonpregnant state.

Some results of improved care cannot be measured, since it is impossible to estimate certain results of poor maternity care, as the effects of a period of impairment following complications or the tragic effects of the death of a mother.

The steady and rapid decline in maternal deaths is encouraging, but a fairly large percentage of these deaths are still associated with factors that are considered preventable. That there is much left to be done is indicated by the fact that the decrease in the maternal death rate has been slower for nonwhites than for whites. In 1974 the maternal death rate for nonwhite

mothers was close to three and one half times that for white mothers (Fig. 27-1). There are also regional differences; some areas in the United States have a higher maternal mortality rate than others.

For further improvement, services must be spread to the people who do not yet have excellent care, and the depth of service increased for those who are receiving good care. Every effort must also be made to further reduce morbidity. Adverse influences that certain social, economic, and psychologic conditions have on the welfare of mothers must also be reduced.

Infant Mortality

Infant mortality is expressed in terms of number of deaths in infants under one year of age per 100,000 live births. Prior to 1960 the rate was expressed in number of infant deaths per 1000 live births. Presentation of the rates

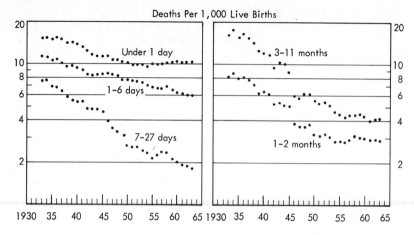

Deaths Per 1,000 Live Births

Under 1 day

1-6 days

7-27 days

3-11 months

1-2 months

Figure 27-2. Infant mortality rates by age: United States, 1933–1964. [*Source: National Center for Health Statistics:* Infant Mortality Trends, United States and Each State, 1930–64. *Public Health Service Publication No. 1000, Series 20, No. 1.*]

per 100,000 live births facilitates comparison of differences in rate from one year to another in categories where frequencies are small, as in age, sex, and color. Like maternal mortality, infant mortality has decreased considerably in the past 40 years (Figs. 27-2 and 27-3).

In 1930 the death rate for infants under one year was 64.6 deaths per 1000 live births; in 1940 it was reduced to 47.0; in 1950 the rate was 29.2 deaths per 1000 live births; and in 1960 there were 26.0 deaths per 1000 live births, or 2604 deaths per 100,000 as now expressed. The death rate of infants under one year of age

reached an all-time low in 1975 according to provisional figures, which places it at 1610 per 100,000 live births or 16.1 per 1000 live births (Fig. 27-3). This means a continuation of the downward trend in infant mortality that began in 1958 and has been even more evident since 1965. It means a decrease in rate in the United States of 38 percent since 1960.

In spite of the lowering trend in infant mortality, much remains to be done. It is considered possible to reduce further the number of infant deaths. Like maternal mortality, infant mortality is higher in the nonwhite than in the white

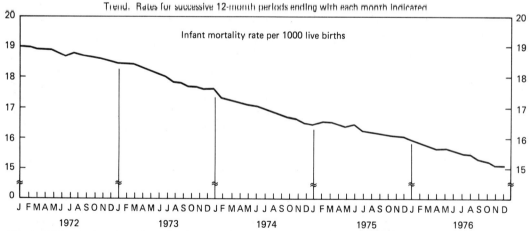

Trend. Rates for successive 12-month periods ending with each month indicated

Infant mortality rate per 1000 live births

J FMAMJ JASONDJ FMAMJ JASONDJ FMAMJ JASONDJ FMAMJ JASONDJ FMAMJ JASOND
1972   1973   1974   1975   1976

Figure 27-3. Infant mortality rate by month: United States, 1972–1976. [*Source: National Center for Health Statistics:* Monthly Vital Statistics Report, *Vol. 25, No. 12, Mar. 8, 1977.*]

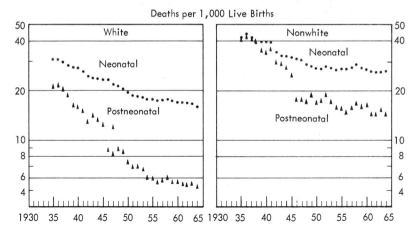

Deaths per 1,000 Live Births

Figure 27-4. Neonatal and postneonatal mortality rates by color: United States, 1930–1964. [*Source: National Center for Health Statistics:* Infant Mortality Trends, United States and Each State, 1930–64. *Public Health Service Publication No. 1000, Series 20, No. 1.*]

group (Figs. 27-4 and 27-5). There are also considerable regional differences. It is apparent from Figure 27-2, showing infant mortality by age, that reduction of mortality rate in infants in the early age groups, the under-one-day group and the under-one-week group, has been slower than for the older infants. In 1975, however, the drop in neonatal mortality in both the white and "all other" population was proportionately larger than in the 2 to 12 month group.

Neonatal Mortality

A neonatal death is one that occurs in the neonatal period, or the first month of life. For statistical purposes this period is limited to the first four weeks after birth. Neonatal mortality is expressed in terms of number of deaths in infants under 28 days of age per 100,000 live births. Neonatal deaths are included in the total infant mortality, but the total mortality rate is subdivided according to various age groups. The neonatal death rate as well as the death rate for separate days of the neonatal period can thus easily be examined.

Since 1921 more than one half of the total infant deaths have occurred in the neonatal period. By 1930 neonatal deaths represented 55 percent of the total infant deaths, and since 1946 neonatal deaths have constituted around 75 per-

cent of the total infant death rate. In 1958 approximately one half of the infant deaths occurred in the first three days of life. The greatest number of neonatal deaths occur in the first day of life. Deaths of babies under one day of age comprised over one third of all infant deaths in 1965. Estimated figures indicate a continuing decrease in neonatal mortality. Provisionally the neonatal mortality rate in 1975 was below 1200 per 100,000 live births, a continuing decrease over previous years (Fig. 27-5).

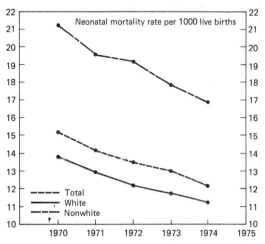

Neonatal mortality rate per 1000 live births

- - - - - Total
———— White
– – – – Nonwhite

Figure 27-5. . Neonatal mortality rates by color: United States, 1970 to 1974. [*Source: National Center for Health Statistics:* Monthly Vital Statistics Report, *Vol. 24, No. 13, June 30, 1976.*]

Although the total neonatal mortality rate for both whites and nonwhites declined in the 1960s, it remained unchanged or increased slightly in some geographic regions and in some age groups. The difference in white and non-white neonatal mortality is wide, provisionally 1170 per 100,000 live births for white and 1580 for all others in 1975. However, the gap between these rates was narrower in 1975 than in any previous year.

Fetal Death Rate

A fetal death is death of a product of conception, irrespective of the period of gestation, prior to its complete expulsion from the mother. State requirements for reporting fetal deaths vary. Some states require registration of all fetal deaths, and others require registration when the fetus has reached a certain gestation period. At present, most states require a report of fetal death when a pregnancy has reached 20 weeks gestation. Tables of fetal death rates therefore often show fetal deaths at 20 or more weeks ges-

tation. Ratios are expressed in number of deaths per 1000 live births (Table 27-1 and Figure 27-6).

Perinatal Mortality

The term "perinatal period" has only recently been widely used, and definitions are not yet standardized. The perinatal period is the time surrounding birth—before, during, and after. A definition widely used for this period is the time from 20 weeks of gestation through 28 days after birth. The term "perinatal mortality" may therefore be applied to deaths of fetuses and infants that occur between the twentieth week of gestational life and the twenty-eighth day of neonatal life, but this range may be otherwise specified in some reported rates.

The perinatal period is very hazardous. At present deaths of viable fetuses and newborn infants make up about 10 per cent of all deaths in the United States. There was a rapid decrease in perinatal deaths during the years of 1935 to 1945, a period of rapid medical and social prog-

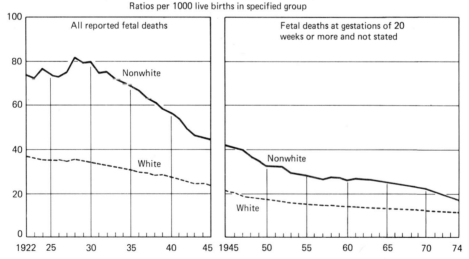

Ratios per 1000 live births in specified group

Figure 27-6. Fetal-death ratios by color: birth-registration states or United States, 1922–1974. [*Source: National Center for Health Statistics:* Infant, Fetal, and Maternal Mortality, United States—1963. *Public Health Service Publication No. 1000, Series 20, No. 3, and U.S. Department of Commerce, Bureau of the Census,* Statistical Abstract of the United States, 1976.]

ress. The decline was slower in the 1950s than in the 1940s. The decrease has been slower in nonwhite than in white groups, but totally it is gradually downward (Figs. 27-5 and 27-6). Continuing reduction can be anticipated as an increasing number of regional perinatal centers are now being established.

The problem of the perinatal period is greater than the mortality rate alone. There is also a high rate of morbidity and of the sequelae that may follow. Morbidity is caused by conditions that existed before birth or occurred during or immediately after birth. The causes of mortality and morbidity are much alike. Reduction in one rate will influence the trend of the other.

Despite reduction in perinatal mortality rate, there is much more to be done to reduce losses. Perinatal casualties—deaths of previable fetuses (as abortions), deaths of viable fetuses and newborn infants, and disability in live infants, as an aftermath of the birth process—are still very high. Dr. Robert E. L. Nesbitt, Jr.[1] has presented seven major factors in prevention of perinatal casualties: These are (1) a multidisciplinary approach to the problem with several health disciplines, including obstetrics, pediatrics, anesthesiology, nursing, hospital administration, and public health, assuming responsibility; (2) wider application of current knowledge of care; (3) raising of living standards of underprivileged groups; (4) preconceptional care to correct defects; (5) continued professional and lay education; (6) avoidance of anoxia and trauma during pregnancy and birth; and (7) continued acquisition of new knowledge. These factors in prevention of problems in the perinatal period are discussed in the original source.

Factors in Improvement in Maternal and Infant Health

The improvement in maternity care over the past two decades can be attributed to several factors. The Children's Bureau laid the founda-

[1] Robert E. L. Nesbitt, Jr., Perinatal casualties, *Children*, 6:123–128 (July–Aug.) 1959.

tion for better care by emphasizing the high maternal and infant mortality rate and the preventability of many of these deaths. Health agencies have made sustained efforts to improve conditions. Advances in medical knowledge have greatly improved the care that can be given. The public has shown more interest. Considerable teaching of the public about maternity care is being done by official and voluntary agencies. Hospitals have increased their facilities for obstetric patients and have improved their care by segregation of the maternity patient from all other patients.

Hospital insurance and an appreciation of the advantages of hospital care induced more mothers to seek this care, which made available to them trained personnel and facilities for emergency treatment. Hospital deliveries in the United States increased in number over the past 35 years, rising from 37 percent in 1935 to 79 percent in 1945 and to 96 percent in 1960. At present the proportion of white births delivered in hospitals is close to 100 percent. A great increase in proportion of hospital deliveries for this group took place during the 1940s. The proportion of hospital births for the nonwhite group is now over 95 percent. A marked increase also occurred in this group since 1940, when the proportion was only 27 percent.

Services that deal with the social and psychological needs of the family are being added to maternal and infant care programs. As a part of complete care, responsibility is now accepted for recognizing the stresses of a complex environment and reducing the effects of these pressures as much as possible.

In spite of these advances in the care of many obstetric patients, much remains to be done for others. In some geographic regions the care of the maternity patient is far from adequate. The mortality rate among nonwhite mothers is still considerably higher than among white mothers (Fig. 27-1 and Table 27-1) and fetal and neonatal deaths among nonwhite infants are notably higher than among white infants (Figs. 27-5 and 27-6).

Providing facilities to make complete maternity care available to every family is a stupendous task. It is a *possible* achievement, since each essential part of the care now known to be necessary has been provided somewhere, at some time, and even now is available to a large number.

Some of the obstacles to be overcome in making available to all mothers the facilities that are now enjoyed by many are ignorance of the need, inaccessibility of some mothers, difficulty in teaching others to influence their day-to-day living, cost, and scarcity of prepared personnel. These are sociologic as well as medical and nursing problems. The first obstacle is being overcome by every instance of good care as well as by present efforts to teach the public the necessity for maternity care and the elements of good care.

To improve the maternity situation further and bring more complete care to all, it is necessary to provide good obstetric care to those of the lower economic groups. A certain proportion of the population is poverty-stricken; they cannot afford adequate food, shelter, and clothing to maintain optimum health. Many of these people delay getting adequate medical care because of the expense involved. Provision of adequate care for these groups is an urgent problem that appears to require community action.

Many studies are being conducted to help identify factors that influence the health of mothers and babies. Studies of perinatal mortality and morbidity are in progress to discover the causes of and means of prevention of fetal and neonatal deaths, of premature births, and of handicapping conditions. The cause of every maternal death is carefully scrutinized.

To improve obstetric and pediatric care, the American Association for Maternal and Infant Health (formerly the American Committee for Maternal Welfare), the American Academy of Pediatrics, and the American College of Obstetrics and Gynecology have developed programs to serve all those concerned with the care of mothers and babies. A mother's charter, equivalent to the Children's Charter formulated in 1930, was adopted by the American Committee for Maternal Welfare in 1941. Very recently a group of concerned citizens formulated "The Pregnant Patient's Bill of Rights," suggested as an addition to the American Hospital Association's "Patient's Bill of Rights" (see Appendix 4).

The American Academy of Pediatrics has a program for developing and improving facilities for the care of the newborn infant. In 1954 it published a manual of *Standards and Recommendations for Hospital Care of Newborn Infants–Full-Term and Premature.* The manual was revised in 1977 and a sixth revision is now published. Since then, other pamphlets providing valuable information for care of newborns have been prepared.

The American College of Obstetricians and Gynecologists published a *Manual of Standards in Obstetric–Gynecologic Practice* in 1959. The purpose of this manual and its revisions is to provide organized groups of recommendations that may be used by obstetric and gynecologic committees and executive committees of hospitals in formulation of local hospital policies according to the available facilities, equipment, and personnel.

It seems realistic to believe that in time the gaps in care will be filled so that adequate care will be available to all mothers and babies. The expected improvement in maternity care in coming years will, however, add to the problems that must be met. Further improvements will require the combined efforts of physicians, nurses, nutritionists, public health personnel in many specialties, social scientists, and all other disciplines concerned with maternal and infant health.

REGIONAL PERINATAL CARE

In the past ten years regional perinatal care centers, which serve large geographic areas have been established for the care of high-risk mothers and newborns.

Regional centers began mainly as neonatal care centers. These centers provided intensive care for high-risk newborns, mainly prematures and babies with major complications, who were transferred to the centers from small community hospitals. In addition to providing intensive care, each center was also committed to updating the education of the health professionals in the region served by the center so that available knowledge and resources could be applied to the care of the infants at the community hospital or the decision could be made to utilize the regional center for the babies' care. The influence of such centers in significantly decreasing neonatal mortality soon became apparent.

When it became more and more apparent that numerous individual, and often small hospitals, could not provide all of the expert care that advances in science made possible, regional centers expanded. More centers were developed and they expanded to include care of high-risk mothers, women who are identified as high-risk by their primary physician and referred to the perinatal center for care. Intensive maternal care at a center includes high-risk ambulatory clinics for antepartum clients who need care by specialists, but do not need hospitalization, as well as hospital care in a facility that is staffed and equipped to provide optimal intrapartum, postpartum, and newborn care.

Perinatal centers serve a designated geographic area. They are staffed with physician and nurse specialists in maternity and newborn care, with nutritionists and social workers, and with all professionals involved in perinatal care. Perinatal centers are places where the advances in the science of high-risk maternal and newborn care can be adequately applied and where staff and equipment can be made available to give expert care to high-risk mothers, fetuses, and newborns. Such professional specialists and the sophisticated equipment necessary for monitoring patients cannot be made available in small hospitals. Perinatal centers are also places where the requirements of health professionals and consumers for optimal maternal and newborn care can be met. An important concept of care in perinatal centers is a team approach to care with the consumer and all the disciplines

that provide perinatal care participating in decision making.

An important responsibility of a perinatal care center is education of the health professionals of the region served by the center. This enhances early recognition of high-risk problems by the professionals providing primary care, assures appropriate care of emergencies, encourages early consultation with experts in the field and transfer to intensive care centers as indicated, and strengthens acceptance of development of regional centers.

Along with establishment of regional perinatal care centers, regional and state perinatal organizations have developed with the major purpose of improving perinatal health care. The membership of each organization reflects a multidisciplinary composition. These organizations have assumed responsibility for education of both health professionals and consumers.

On December 4, 1976 a National Perinatal Association was formed, composed of persons from all disciplines involved in and committed to delivery of high-quality perinatal care. The NPA is to be based on strong regional, state, and area action-oriented groups. One of its important functions will be to assist, strengthen, and facilitate regional, state, and area organizations to accomplish their goals of improving perinatal care.

BIBLIOGRAPHY

Aure, Beverly, and Schneider, Jack M., Transforming a community hospital nursing service into a regional center, *Nurs. Clin. North Am.* 10:275–284 (June) 1975.

Callon, Helen F., Regionalizing perinatal care in Wisconsin, *Nurs. Clin. North Am.* 10:263–274 (June) 1975.

Chase, Helen C., Perinatal mortality. Overview and current trends, *Clin. Perinatol.* 1:3–17 (Mar.) 1974.

Nesbitt, Robert E. L., Jr., The status of perinatal medicine, *Clin. Perinatol.* 1:173–179 (Mar.) 1974.

Pearse, Warren H., The maternity and infant care

programs, *Obstet. Gynecol.* 35:114–119 (Jan.) 1970.

Price, Mary Emily, New perinatal group to tackle national needs, *Contemp. Ob/Gyn* 9:27–28 and 33–34 (Feb.) 1977.

Schneider, Jack M., and Graven, Stanley N., Regionalized OB-GYN care in Wisconsin—Perinatal centers, *Contemp. Ob/Gyn* 3:35–47 (Mar.) 1974.

U.S. Department of Commerce, Bureau of the Census, *Statistical Abstract of the United States,* 1976.

U.S. Department of Health, Education, and Welfare: Public Health Service, Health Resources Administration, *Monthly Vital Statisticals Reports.*

Wegman, Myron E., Annual summary of vital statistics–1976, *Pediatrics,* 58:793–799 (Dec.) 1976.

World Health Organization, Technical Report Series, No. 457, *The Prevention of Perinatal Mortality and Morbidity.* World Health Organization, Geneva, 1970.

———, No. 428, *The Organization and Administration of Maternal and Child Health Services.* World Health Organization, Geneva, 1969.

Appendix 1

Historical Developments*

THE MATERNITY PATIENT IN EARLY TIMES

From the earliest times the birth of a baby has been followed by some form of tribal, racial, or familial ceremony. Among primitive peoples birth, like other mysteries, became the subject of many superstitions, some of which persist to this day. These early ceremonies rarely included any real care of the mother but were feasts or festivals of thanksgiving, sacrifice, or dedication to propitiate the gods or ward off evil spirits.

In primitive society many women delivered themselves, but women have helped each other since the beginning of society. The skillful, or perhaps the more willing ones, became set apart as midwives—women who habitually and for gain assist women in childbirth. The only training of these early midwives was based on experience. When delivery was difficult, priests and medicine men were sometimes called on to help with prayers and incantations.

In early civilizations physicians controlled the practice of midwives and helped with difficult deliveries, although the physician who undertook midwifery was generally scorned. Hippocrates and Soranus did much to improve medicine and midwifery in Greece and Rome. During the Middle Ages in Europe much of this advance was lost. Midwives were of a low type, and executioners and barbers were called in to help with difficult deliveries.

About 1500 the first lying-in wards were

opened where midwives delivered the poor and outcast. In the sixteenth and early seventeenth centuries Ambroise Paré of Paris and the Chamberlens, who migrated from France to England, stimulated medical men again to take an interest in obstetrics. The first school for midwives was established at Paré's instigation at the Hôtel Dieu in Paris.

In the eighteenth century state and national regulation of the education and practice of midwifery began, and the whole maternity situation in Europe greatly improved. Puerperal fever, however, was a veritable pestilence during the seventeenth, eighteenth, and nineteenth centuries. It was so great in hospitals that the public attempted to abolish them. There was no place but hospitals in which poor women could be delivered, and so puerperal fever raged until after 1847 when Semmelweis, in Vienna, demonstrated that washing of hands in chloride of lime solution before examining women in labor would reduce its incidence. The control of this plague, which had interfered greatly with the advance of obstetrics, began. A few years later (1853), after much prolonged opposition from clergy, doctors, and the general public, Dr. James Y. Simpson of Glasgow succeeded in introducing the use of chloroform anesthesia as an aid in obstetrics. Thus the period of modern obstetrics had begun.

MATERNITY CARE ABOUT 1900

In the United States at the beginning of this century the teaching of obstetrics was based on

---

* Historical data in this chapter originally prepared by Anne A. Stevens, R.N.

a thorough understanding of the mechanics of labor and on the acceptance of the teachings of Semmelweis, Holmes, Pasteur, Lister, and Simpson. It included the aseptic technique of normal delivery as well as the technique for various operative procedures and the details of care of certain abnormalities. As in other fields of human activity, the teaching of the leaders was far in advance of the average practice.

Supervision during pregnancy had hardly begun. With rare exceptions, maternity care began when labor began and ended a few days later, seldom more than 14 days.

The institution of modern nursing had improved the general care and comfort of patients in hospitals and in their own homes when they were cared for by privately employed or visiting nurses. There were still many untrained persons giving nursing care. Some of the latter gave excellent care, but many knew little of real nursing and less of asepsis; their work was in no way standardized.

An unknown number of midwives, mostly untrained and unsupervised, were caring for an unknown number of patients. There are no records to tell how many, and estimates varied tremendously because of the great differences in different localities.

In those sparsely populated sections of the country where doctors were scarce, neighbors did what they could to help each other, but many women delivered themselves.

Impoverished mothers used the lying-in wards and hospitals in the cities. Semiprivate and private maternity services were not yet available. Private maternity patients used hospitals only for operative deliveries or in dire emergencies.

In connection with some maternity hospitals, extern services had already been organized whereby doctors and medical students from the hospitals delivered patients in their own homes. The patients were examined as antepartum patients at the hospital clinics and registered for home care. These services were popular among mothers who could not go to the hospital because they would have to leave their home and children with no supervision.

Although there are no records on which to base an exact statement for the whole country, it is undoubtedly true that, except among foreign-born mothers, the family doctor was the *preferred* attendant at delivery.

The attitude of the general public about maternity was the result of false modesty and ignorance. The need for a doctor and perhaps a nurse when the baby came was understood, but the less said about it, the better. Pregnancy was mentioned only in whispers, baby clothes were made in seclusion, and maternity patients concealed their pregnancy as long as possible. Any suggestion of care during pregnancy was frowned upon as an unnecessary and unwarranted interference with nature. Prolonging care or providing any special consideration for the mother after the baby came was regarded as pampering and was seldom indulged in.

When large numbers of patients were cared for, it became apparent to physicians that the deaths incident to maternity were tragically many and often preventable, but maternal mortality rates for any considerable part of the country were not known until after 1915.

THE BEGINNING OF PRENATAL CARE

About the beginning of this century a new understanding of the problems of maternity care developed, and gradually more and more doctors and patients participated in this new program of care.

A new idea often comes to several of those working on the same problem at about the same time, and it is not always possible to know who first promoted it. One of the early leaders was Dr. John William Ballantyne, of the Royal Maternity Hospital in Edinburgh, who cared for and studied a great many abnormalities of pregnancy and labor. In the early years of this century he emphasized the importance of supervising all maternity patients throughout pregnancy instead of giving them no attention before labor unless they became ill. He insisted that much that had been accepted by the maternity patient as sent by God, to be endured with no thought of cure, was preventable by intelligent care. In Paris in 1892, Dr. Pierre Budin initiated consultations for nursing mothers. Later consultations were open for pregnant women also.

In this country, outstanding obstetricians learned to prevent among their private patients several of the complications, abnormalities, and untoward results of pregnancy that so often occurred. These doctors began to urge the patients who registered at their hospital clinics, as well as their private patients, to come earlier in pregnancy and to return for periodic examinations. Their initial examinations included increasing attention to history of previous illnesses. More consideration was given to the patient's general physical condition. The importance of exact pelvic measurements was emphasized. Frequent urinalyses were made. The significance of changes in blood pressure was recognized. Many studies of symptoms of beginning complications and results of treatments were conducted.

Finally, antepartum clinics that were more than mere registrations for care at delivery became an integral part of the maternity services directed by these obstetricians. Later, antepartum clinics became a part of all hospital maternity services, but even in 1918 many hospitals were unwilling to assume responsibility for patients before the seventh month of pregnancy.

Some time before this it had been learned that deaths of babies less than one month old were caused in large measure by the condition of the mother before the infant was born. After this relation between maternity care and neonatal mortality was recognized, the same kind of work begun by a few obstetricians to help save *mothers'* lives was undertaken in connection with baby hygiene work because it was thought it might save *babies'* lives too. This difference in emphasis was the beginning of a great increase in attention given to needs of the pregnant mother for her baby's sake. Unfortunately it was not apparent to any but obstetricians for several years that the real need for the sake of mother and baby was better maternity care during the whole childbearing process, not prenatal care alone.

Prenatal clinics or prenatal nurses were added to the baby health station work of bureaus of child hygiene, settlement houses, church houses, and other agencies concerned with child care. Many private, nonofficial health agencies, whether organized for family work, baby work, or special maternity work, participated in the early development of prenatal care.

The detail of the work in the new clinics was much the same as that being developed by obstetricians in the antepartum clinics of their hospitals. It included a health history, an initial complete physical examination with pelvic measurements, weight, urinalysis, a blood pressure reading, and frequently a Wassermann test. Also, return visits were made at varying intervals for observation and search for signs and symptoms of beginning abnormality, with special care for the patient with these signs or symptoms or any other discomforts. Often a nurse or hospital social worker did some kind of home visiting, at least to patients with apparent social problems. Sometimes the home visiting was done through cooperation between hospitals and visiting nurse societies. Where there was no provision for regular visits, it was not unusual for an interested and enterprising intern to go himself to the home of a patient to persuade her to come to the hospital when her symptoms were ominous and she had failed to return to the clinic as advised. All hospital facilities for consultation and treatment were open to these clinics. Care of patients had the continuity that is possible when it includes the complete service of clinics, delivery rooms, nursing units, outpatient service, and nurseries. These clinics were open only to those patients who were to be delivered in the inpatient or outpatient service of the respective hospital.

In some instances obstetricians examined patients in the unattached clinics. More often young doctors interested in maternity or public health work made the clinic examinations with little or no supervision from an obstetrician. The health station nurses, visiting nurses, or special prenatal nurses did the home visiting. When these patients were ready for delivery or required hospitalization, it was necessary to refer them to another doctor unfamiliar with their problems during pregnancy. The unattached clinics gave supervision to a wide variety of patients—those who could not or did not decide until the last minute where they would be delivered and those who were to be delivered by midwives or by private doctors not offering supervision early in pregnancy.

Development of the unattached prenatal clinics, not connected with hospitals or staffed by doctors and nurses doing the other maternity work in the community, divided the responsibility for medical, and often for nursing, supervision of the patient. This was a disadvantage, since childbearing is a single process from the beginning of pregnancy to the cessation of lactation, and any break in the direction of the mother's care is a distinct loss. However, it was not then a question of continuous or broken care, but a question of separate prenatal care or no prenatal care for all but a few patients.

Various ways in which prenatal work began are illustrated by the following instances. As early as January, 1901, the Instructive District Nursing Association of Boston began an affiliation with the South End Branch of the Boston Lying-in Hospital. In early reports it is recorded that the obstetric nurse received from the hospital the "list of the cases to be visited, of those who have already been confined and of those *who are going to be.*" The nurse visited prenatal patients and taught them to get ready for delivery, to make layettes, and to prepare other necessary articles. "In abnormal or threatening acute cases the nurse takes the temperature and reports all symptoms to the doctor in charge." In 1902, with a second obstetric nurse added to the staff, the first maternity work was done for

private doctors. From then on the work increased.

Visiting nurses going about the districts caring for the sick and the postpartum patients in several cities and towns had probably always given advice to the pregnant women they met. They had not heretofore (according to records obtainable today) taken them under their care as registered patients and attempted to visit them with regularity.

The insistence of the demands for actual physical care of the sick was frequently so urgent as to interfere with the development of this new prenatal nursing service. It was natural to defer visits that seemed to have no urgency compared with the care of those who were ill. Prevention was a new gospel in those days. Besides, each nurse was feeling her way in learning how to do the most for these patients, who were not sick and did not know they needed care. They were interested in clothes for the baby, in planning for care at delivery, and in talking over their fears and questions with a sympathetic listener, but not in the least interested in the nurse's suggestions about taking better care of themselves. This was especially true of those who felt well or were convinced that their discomforts were the lot of all pregnant women and if left alone would take care of themselves.

Although the first prenatal nursing was a minimum of that now known to be effective, the nurses, undoubtedly, discovered abnormalities and were able to secure treatment for patients who otherwise would have had none. Undoubtedly an equally important contribution to the patients was the sympathetic understanding that helped to allay fear and promote a wholesome mental attitude.

In July, 1907, The Association for Improving the Condition of the Poor in New York City—a social work agency that became interested in health work because of the relation between poverty and illness—employed two "teacher-nurses" to visit the pregnant women in families under its care. This work was undertaken in connection with a rest house for mothers that was opened in March, 1907. A report the next year contains this statement: "Teaching mothers before confinement reduces the infant death rate. In 202 cases visited *before* and *after* confinement, there were 9 infant deaths—4.9 percent. In 135 cases visited *after* confinement only, there were 22 infant deaths—17 percent. What would happen to the Infant Death Rate if all mothers were taught and cared for *before* confinement as well as *after*." The Association for Improving the Condition of the Poor also assured extra rest for pregnant women under its care by supplying housekeeping services to those who needed it. This agency continued and increased its health services for expectant mothers.

In 1909 the Women's Municipal League of Boston, under the guidance of Mrs. William Lowell Putnam, supplied to the Boston Lying-in Hospital

. . . a trained-nurse for social service among the hospital's patients. Cases referred to this nurse have been visited during pregnancy, and instructed in the lessons of personal cleanliness and hygiene. Cases requiring medical advice have been referred to the hospital, and some of these cases have been admitted for observation and treatment. Serious complications of labor have thus been prevented.[1]

Beginning in January, 1917, the Metropolitan Life Insurance Company—which offered visiting nurse service to holders of industrial policies—contracted to pay visiting nurse associations for two prenatal visits to maternity patients having these policies. This was a real stimulus to the spread of prenatal nursing. The number of visits increased and also came to include postpartum visits. The example of this insurance company was followed by others. Dr. Louis I. Dublin, of the Metropolitan Life Insurance Company, made many studies of maternity records and is one authority quoted in support of the lifesaving value of prenatal and other maternity care.

[1] From the Annual Report of the Boston Lying-in Hospital for 1909.

In 1917, stimulated by the late Dr. Ralph W. Lobenstine and guided by Mrs. Irene Osgood Andrews and Miss Annie W. Goodrich, the Women's City Club of New York established the first maternity center in this country. Through the center it was planned to secure medical supervision and nursing care for every woman in the district served, from the beginning of pregnancy until her baby was one month old, by coordinating the maternity work of every hospital, private physician, midwife, and nursing agency in the community and by stimulating the development of additional facilities as the need arose. A register was kept of patients cared for and those in need of care. A nurse employed by the center did the home visiting and teaching for these latter patients. Every effort was made to help them arrange for immediate care. A clinic was opened at the center where patients under no other medical care might be examined by an obstetrician and supervised until they could register with a doctor or hospital for care at delivery. Patients to be delivered by midwives were also given medical supervision here.

Classes were developed for the mothers, and a teaching exhibit of baby clothes and mother's supplies was displayed at the center. One of the nurses had office hours every afternoon, and the patients learned to visit the center freely. A special fund provided for a housekeeper service to give mothers needed rest. The patient paid the proportion of the cost she could afford.

"Every woman in the district" was never reached, but the work of the various agencies was coordinated and the amount of service thereby increased. Each nurse gained information from the other nurses as records, routines, and printed "Advice for Mothers" were developed in nursing conferences. Excellent working relations were established with the hospitals, the doctors, and the midwives in the district.

In connection with the opening of the center, the Visiting Nurse Service of Henry Street Settlement established a 24-hour delivery nursing service and gave a month's supervised experience to the students at the Manhattan Maternity

Hospital. This was the first complete maternity nursing service in the city, including prenatal, delivery, and postpartum nursing, that served private physicians as well as the outpatient service of the hospital.

Eventually the Maternity Center of the Women's City Club became a part of the Maternity Center Association—a voluntary organization formed to establish centers throughout Manhattan.

There was little uniformity in prenatal home visiting in the early days. It ranged from a doorstep visit to urge the patient to return to the clinic, to a friendly visit to allay fears and answer questions, to a visit for medical social work, to a real prenatal nursing visit. The latter included a friendly chat and help with situations that disturbed the mother's peace of mind or otherwise interfered with her care. It also included noting the mother's temperature, pulse, respiration, and blood pressure, checking the fetal heart rate, and doing a urinalysis. Advice was given for care of the breasts and relief of discomforts as prescribed by the patient's doctor or by standing orders from the clinic doctor or the medical board. Help was given in arranging for delivery and postpartum care with consideration for the economic situation, housing conditions, and family relationships. Instruction was given in personal and home hygiene, including nutrition, and in preparation for the baby. Plans were made for fitting the baby's care into the home life, to provide for his needs without upsetting everyone else and taxing the mother to the point of overfatigue. Interpretation of the mother's condition and her needs was made to the family, and attention was given to health needs of other members of the family.

By degrees the nursing and clinic procedures became somewhat standardized. Record forms were improved. Routine techniques were printed and distributed. Details, as well as principles, policies, and problems, were discussed at nursing conventions. In time the doorstep or purely advisory visit gave place in all good prenatal work to the more adequate nursing and teaching visit. The content of the visit was adapted to the prevailing medical opinion or modified to suit individual physicians when caring for their patients.

Patients were encouraged by nurses to visit them in their offices when possible for a part of the nursing supervision. These visits did not supplant all home visits, but decreased the number necessary and were an economy in time and money. They were frequently combined with the visit to the physician in the clinic or with attendance at mothers' classes.

In some instances prenatal nurses assumed the responsibility for reaching every expectant mother in the neighborhood, by a door-to-door canvass, because the mother who did not know enough about her need for care to seek it was no less the nurse's responsibility than the one who did. In fact, in the earliest days of prenatal work, the real task was to find the women who did not know that they needed care and to convince them that they did.

Organized prenatal work began in cities and was reasonably well developed there before much was done about it in rural districts; yet this country had many maternity patients living in its vast rural areas. After World War I there was a great stimulation to all public health work. The American Red Cross Public Health Nursing Service, other voluntary agencies interested in health, and state departments of health and education encouraged the development of nursing services in counties and small towns throughout the country. Many of the nurses included some maternity work in their programs.

EXPANSION OF MATERNITY CARE

About the time prenatal work was becoming standardized, the emphasis began to shift from it to "complete maternity care." It was clear that the good accomplished by supervision and intelligent care during pregnancy could be destroyed by poor care at delivery and greatly lessened by insufficient postpartum care. In addition to excellent medical and nursing care, the maternity patient needs sufficient food of the right kind, adequate rest, and attention to social and economic problems—family maladjustments, emotional disturbances, inadequate income, and anything else that interferes with the normal progress of pregnancy, labor, and the puerperium.

As early as 1919 this idea of complete maternity care was formulated in the "Minimum Standards for Public Protection of the Health of Mothers," adopted at the Child Welfare Conferences of national and international authorities called by the federal Children's Bureau (Appendix II). Standards such as these express "what those who were devoting their lives to the study of maternity" considered to be *minimum* requirements. Since these standards were formulated, examinations after the initial six-week postpartum checkup are continued at six-month or yearly intervals. A gradual return to the usual activities and responsibilities, determined by the mother's condition as a whole, is acknowledged as an essential element in good postpartum care. Much closer supervision is advocated for all patients who have, or have had, syphilis, tuberculosis, heart disease, chronic hypertension, diabetes, toxemia, infection, hemorrhage, or any postpartum complication. It is considered important to continue care of the mother during the interpregnancy period and to assure that she is in good health to care for her family and in a healthy condition for another pregnancy.

TEACHING THE COMMUNITY ABOUT MATERNITY CARE

Teaching the community about maternity care is an important part of improving the maternity situation. No less an authority than the late Dr. J. Whitridge Williams is quoted as frequently having said: "When the women of America recognize the value of and need for maternity care they will demand it, and then, and then only, will they get it."

Teaching of maternity care began when individual physicians taught their individual patients about the hygiene of pregnancy. A few physicians at first used printed lists of supplies needed by mother and baby. Later they expanded these to include instructions about the hygiene of pregnancy and the symptoms to be reported immediately to the physician. This individual teaching of the patient by her physician is still being carried out by many. It is very valuable and is continued whenever possible. Classes and pamphlets can serve as supplements, but individual teaching is important in obtaining a good understanding of the patient and her problems and in allaying her fears. It establishes a good patient-doctor relationship. The value of individual teaching cannot be overestimated. However, since the early beginning of prenatal teaching by the physician, much literature has been printed and many classes for mothers and parents are being conducted that supplement the doctor's instructions.

In 1912 *The Prospective Mother*, by Dr. Josiah Morris Slemons, was published. It was one of the earliest books addressed to expectant mothers emphasizing the hygiene of pregnancy. Many books and pamphlets have been written since. In more recent years books for the expectant father and for expectant parents have also been published. Insurance companies added to the prenatal literature by printing instruction sheets for expectant mothers.

In 1913 the federal Children's Bureau published "Prenatal Care," the first of a series of pamphlets for parents. It is significant that the Children's Bureau, created in 1912 and charged with the responsibility for all matters pertaining to the welfare of children, should have begun its series of pamphlets with "Prenatal Care." It thus endorsed the idea that the life of the child begins at conception, not at birth, and that welfare work for children begins with maternity care. This pamphlet has been revised many times since it was first published. A pictorial version of "Prenatal Care" entitled "When Your Baby Is on the Way" was issued in 1961. This is the first visual parent publication by the Bureau.

The first edition of "Infant Care," another Children's Bureau publication, was published in 1914. Since the time that the first edition came out until now, almost 15 million copies have been distributed. This publication has been revised, wholly or in part, many times, and has been translated into eight languages. Many other pamphlets and folders—among them "So You're Expecting a Baby," "Breast Feeding," "Diet and Development Wall Cards," "Your Premature Baby," "Your Child from One to Six," and "Your Child from Six to Twelve"—are distributed each year. During recent years the Bureau has strengthened its efforts in parent education. The list of publications for parents increased, and consultative services were broadened.

The Children's Bureau publications for parents are distributed largely on individual request from parents, often at the suggestion of the physician or the nurse. They are obtained through state health departments, or they may be purchased from the Superintendent of Documents, U.S. Government Printing Office.

Not only the mother but the family and the whole community need to be taught if public attitude toward good maternity care is to be promoted. From the beginning prenatal nurses have taught patients and their families why women need supervision during pregnancy and care afterward and the reasons for each detail of their care.

Mothers' classes and mothercraft clubs were organized by nurses so that prospective mothers might have the benefit of group teaching about their own and their babies' needs. Sometimes expectant fathers were included also. The outlines and briefs for these classes were printed by private agencies and by some departments of health. They were used by nurses all over the country.

About 1916 some of the women's magazines that had long published articles on infant care began to concern themselves with maternity care. They offered, gratuitously or for a small fee, letters and pamphlets of advice on the care of mothers and babies which were prepared by recognized authorities. State and city departments of health and various nursing and health organizations later prepared similar material for free distribution. Magazines have continued providing information. Articles on the care of the individual, as well as articles that inform the public on the needs and programs of maternity care, appear continuously in the popular magazines. Several women's magazines include a regular feature on family or child health by an eminent specialist.

In 1930 the Maternity Center Association of New York City began a campaign to teach every man and woman in the country both the necessity for maternity care and the components of adequate care. The campaign, culminating with an appeal to make Mother's Day, 1931, the beginning of better care for all mothers, was carried through newspapers, magazines, professional and trade journals, club study programs, health-department bulletins, mayors', governors', and health officers' proclamations, sermons, radio broadcasts, and special local meetings. It aimed to direct the attention of everyone to a consideration of the needs of his own community for increased or improved facilities for maternity care. The next year the campaign was repeated in conjunction with the state medical society and with special emphasis on what constitutes good care.

The general public was slow to learn the value of maternity care. However, a decided change in attitude gradually became evident. Pregnancy can be mentioned now, without apologies. The need for maternity care is discussed in the public press as well as in health journals. People are learning that, although childbearing is a natural process, nature alone and unaided by medical science cannot be relied on to keep the mother's body functioning normally under the stresses of certain situations. Many more patients are seeking care and seeking it earlier, but there still are others to be taught.

Mothers' classes increased from 1920 to 1930 and then interest fell off rapidly. Lack of enthusiasm in classes may have been due to a shortage of adequately prepared teachers and a decreasing interest in the material presented. These early mothers' classes placed much emphasis on preparation for home delivery and on early diagnosis and care of complications of pregnancy. Since World War II, however, the number of parents' classes has again increased. They came to be parents' classes, rather than classes for expectant mothers alone. Interest in education for expectant parents increased with interest in "natural childbirth." Many classes now included specific programs in preparation for childbirth.

Classes now aim to give the parents an intelligent understanding of pregnancy and childbearing and provide them with an opportunity to express their feelings and fears. In individual and group discussions many worries over the childbearing process are allayed. This should help to establish good family relations and provide a sound basis for child care. Inclusion of the father in these classes stresses the importance of considering maternity care as a family concern, part of the total endeavor and concern of family life. Through sharing with his wife and with other couples the father learns to cope with the added responsibility that is his. The couple gains in knowledge of facts and is less likely to suffer from superstitions and inaccurate popular beliefs.

The teacher for parents' classes must have a good knowledge of obstetrics, be competent to teach health, be emotionally stable, and have enthusiasm for the subject. Unless these classes are conducted by a well-trained and enthusiastic instructor, they may not be as beneficial as expected.

Education for family living must begin in the home and in the schools. The attitudes necessary to the assumption of the responsibilities of marriage and parenthood are part of the cultural heritage, a most important part. The biologic and psychosociologic facts of human growth and development are included in the basic curriculum of all school systems in direct ratio to the quality of the general instruction.

For further reduction of maternal and infant mortality, education of expectant parents must now move beyond teaching of the basic necessity for early maternity care and the fundamental components of adequate care. It becomes increasingly important to educate toward early detection of high-risk factors in pregnancy and to help parents understand the measures that may be used to decrease such risks. The well-prepared nurse can and should play an important role in parent education leading toward ideal maternity health care and in delivery of quality maternal-child care to these patients.

COMMUNITY HEALTH SERVICES FOR MOTHERS AND CHILDREN

From the very beginning the public health movement stressed maternal and child health. The first White House Conference on Children was called in 1909 by President Theodore Roosevelt. The purpose of this meeting was primarily to discuss the needs of the dependent child, but out of this conference came many recommendations for meeting the problems of mothers and children. One of the most important of these recommendations was for the creation in the federal government of a special bureau for children. As a result the *United States Children's Bureau* was created by Congress in 1912 under the Department of Labor. Since this time the federal government has undertaken to protect the welfare of children. Creation of bureaus of maternal and child health in various state and city health departments quickly followed the establishment of the federal Children's Bureau. In 1946 this federal bureau was transferred from the Department of Labor to the Federal Security Agency, and in 1953, when the former agency became the Department of Health, Education, and Welfare, it was transferred to that department.

In 1969 the HEW Department's Children's Bureau was divided into several separate units. Under the reorganization, maternal and child health programs have been placed into a new organizational unit, called Health Services and

Mental Health Administration. Other programs previously located in the Children's Bureau are administered by other units. The Children's Bureau as such became part of the new Office of Child Development. It was anticipated that the reorganization would strengthen maternal and child health programs.

As a result of recommendations from other White House conferences, which have followed the first at 10-year intervals, there has been much federal and state legislation to promote maternal and child health. At the second conference, standards for the protection of the maternity patient were formulated (see Appendix 2). The Children's Charter, with 19 provisions, was formulated by the third White House conference. The fourth conference made recommendation that the local community should provide care for mothers and children as needed and that the states should set standards of care and give leadership, financial assistance, supervision, and specialized service to the local services, and that the federal government should help states by giving financial support and research and consultation service, and that it should set up standards of care on a national basis. Better training of doctors and nurses and more appropriations for research were recommended.

The Fifth or Mid-Century White House Conference, held in 1950, was called to obtain more facts about the emotional and social development of children and to consider what must be done to give every child an opportunity to develop the mental, emotional, and spiritual qualities necessary for individual happiness. This was the first time that the future parents of this country had an opportunity for active participation. Youth was represented by delegates from its own group at this Mid-Century Conference. The Sixth or Golden Anniversary White House Conference on Children and Youth was held in 1960. Its purpose was to "promote opportunities for children and youth to realize their full potential for a creative life in freedom and dignity."

A real impetus came to rural maternity work in 1921 with the passage by Congress of the Maternity and Infancy Act. This act, administered by the federal Children's Bureau, stimulated the formation of bureaus of child hygiene in state departments of health and made funds available for maternity and infant hygiene work.

The work that developed as a result of the passage of the act has included studies of causes of maternal mortality, neonatal mortality, stillbirths, analyses of mortality rates, and studies of conditions in maternity homes. It provided institutes and practice in well-established clinics so that nurses and physicians might learn the newest methods; also provided were demonstration prenatal clinics and classes and nursing services. Efforts were made to convince localities of the value of these services and inspire their permanent continuance. Included also were instruction and supervision of midwives, campaigns to improve birth registration, traveling child health and prenatal clinics, parental education by group instruction and by the distribution of letters and pamphlets, classes in infant care for girls, and many other related activities.

Federal appropriations ceased in 1929, but the states maintained a program for maternal and child health, and a good cooperative relationship continues between the states and the federal Children's Bureau.

The Social Security Act was passed in 1935. This included, among other programs, annual appropriations for grants to states to improve their health and welfare service to mothers and babies. These grants have been increased several times. The sum of $22,000,000 was originally appropriated. Of this amount $11,000,000 was set aside for maternal and child health services. The rest was to be used for crippled children and child welfare services. All 48 states, the District of Columbia, Alaska, Hawaii, Puerto Rico, and the Virgin Islands received grants. However, each had to give some financial aid. The federal Children's Bureau has the responsibility for the administration of such grants. This money is sent to the state agencies to improve the work of their public health and welfare departments. In recent years an increasing amount of the maternal and child health fund has been spent on professional training. Institutes for nurses have been held, grants have been made to universities for courses in obstetrics and pediatrics, and inservice training programs have been developed. To some extent a shortage of trained personnel has hampered the maternal and child health program.

A special White House Conference on "Better Care for Mothers and Babies" was called in 1938 by the Children's Bureau to consider the particular problems of maternal and infant care. Suggestions made at this conference included appropriation of more money for maternal and child health service and correction of weaknesses in the program. It was recommended that mothers have adequate supervision throughout pregnancy; that delivery care be given by a qualified physician in an approved hospital with facilities for handling complications, or in the home assisted by a specially trained nurse; that postpartum and postnatal medical and nursing supervision be given; and that consultation service be given by obstetricians and pediatricians to the general practitioner.

At the present time a wide range of professional people—including physicians, nurses, social workers, and nutritionists, trained in special branches of their profession—make up the staff of the Children's Bureau. Expert advice can be given to state departments to assist in development of standards of good service. Among its many other responsibilities, the bureau gives advice on adoption policies. There is now a greater interest in improving the care of unmarried mothers and their children. A professional journal, *Children* (formerly *The Child*), is published by the bureau to report on all aspects of its work and all phases of child care. Besides functioning in an advisory capacity to all states, the Children's Bureau also cooperates in an international program for maternal and child care.

It participates in the work of the United Nations International Children's Emergency Fund (UNICEF) and other international agencies.

All states have a bureau or division of maternal and child health in their health departments. Through the local health departments they provide health services for children of all ages and for mothers during and after pregnancy. Services are directed primarily toward a preventive program by promoting health through increasing prenatal clinics, well-child conferences, projects for the care of premature infants, and public health nursing services.

The largest maternity care program ever undertaken in this country was a special wartime project known as the *Emergency Maternity and Infant Care Program* (EMIC), established by an act of Congress in 1943. Under this program the federal government, without state aid and without cost to the family, provided maternity care for wives of enlisted men in the lower pay groups and care of their children during the first year of life. The Children's Bureau was responsible for federal operation of the EMIC program, and state health departments administered it locally. Private physicians and hospitals throughout the country provided necessary care on a fee basis. When Selective Service ended in 1947, the need for this program decreased, and liquidation began July 1, 1947.

The *World Health Organization* has undertaken a program to improve maternity care. The Maternal and Child Health Section was established in 1948. The first World Health Organization Expert Committee on Maternal and Child Health met in Geneva in 1949. A review of child health problems and general surveys of the basic requirements in various countries have been made by maternal and child health advisers. From these it is possible to advise on how best to meet the needs of the countries. The World Health Organization has emphasized the importance of a broad concept of maternity care. It recommends the promotion in young people of a healthy attitude toward parenthood and family life, as well as toward care of mothers during pregnancy, delivery, and the puerperium and care of newborn babies.

"NATURAL CHILDBIRTH"

A discussion of development of maternity care would not be complete without a description of "natural childbirth" and rooming-in, both of which have been instituted in maternity care within the last 50 years. The late Dr. Grantly Dick Read, an English obstetrician, was first to use the term "natural childbirth." In 1933 he published a book by that title in which he described the emotional aspects of pregnancy, labor, and delivery. In 1944, a book written largely for the lay public was published in the United States under the title *Childbirth Without Fear* and in England under the title of *Revelation of Childbirth*.

Dr. Read came to the United States in 1947 under the auspices of the Maternity Center Association to address audiences—professional and general public—on his interpretation of natural childbirth, a method based on the premise that childbirth is a normal physiologic process, but that misunderstanding and fear produce tension and pain. In the practice of natural childbirth, fear is overcome through education of the mother in the physiology of pregnancy and labor. Relaxation during labor is achieved through application of previously learned breathing and relaxation techniques. Support and encouragement during labor by medical and nursing staff are essential. The patient's husband is usually with her during labor, and he has usually attended combined classes for husbands and wives. With natural childbirth the need for analgesia is reduced and many deliveries are spontaneous. The mother has the opportunity to participate in her baby's birth, which is psychologically important to many women.

Following Dr. Read's visit, the late Helen Heardman, an English physiotherapist, who worked with patients being cared for by Dr. Read and other obstetricians, spent several weeks in the United States. She demonstrated the controlled breathing, exercises, and relaxation techniques that prepare women for natural childbirth to doctors, nurses, nurse-midwives, physiotherapists, and patients of the Maternity Center Association and the Grace–New Haven Community Hospital. Mrs. Heardman published a book under the title *A Way to Natural Childbirth*. In this she described exercises to be used during pregnancy, the controlled breathing and relaxation necessary during labor, and postpartum exercises for restoration of relaxed muscles.

The application of the principles of natural childbirth was instituted at the Grace–New Haven Community Hospital in 1948, under the auspices of the Yale University Schools of Medicine and Nursing and the Maternity Center Association, under the direction of Dr. Herbert Thoms. This program worked out very satisfactorily and thereafter was used in part or completely in other hospitals.

Another method of preparation for childbirth has more recently been introduced. This method, known as the Lamaze method of natural childbirth, differs from Dr. Read's principally in the physical preparation of the mother. The Lamaze method is a psychoprophylactic method of preparation through which the mother actively participates in childbirth. It was developed by the late Dr. Fernand Lamaze, a French physician, as an adaptation of the Russian techniques of psychoprophylaxis. In the Lamaze program the mother is conditioned, both mentally and physically, to suppress consciously the pain of uterine contractions. She learns conditioned responses, which she will use during labor. This method is based on the pavlovian conditioned-response theory.

The Lamaze method was introduced in France in 1951 and is used widely in that country. In 1960 it was introduced in the United States by Dr. Clement Yahia of Boston, where the method was first used. Since then it has gained increasing attention in this country.

Programs incorporating natural childbirth techniques are presently often called preparation-for-childbirth, education-for-childbirth, or training-for-childbirth programs. This change was brought about when it became apparent that the term "natural childbirth" suggested the idea of painless childbirth to many people. Some thought that labor would be without discomfort following preparation. They were strongly opposed to the use of analgesia during labor and delivery because they believed that the use of a pain-relieving medication was not a part of the program. If discomfort became severe enough to necessitate medication, it was often interpreted as failure to achieve a natural childbirth.

Another midcentury development in preparation for childbirth was the founding of local childbirth education organizations in various communities throughout the country, for the purpose of teaching relaxation techniques and exercises in preparation for childbirth. These organizations are composed largely of lay persons, primarily young couples. In 1960 local groups joined into a larger organization known as the International Childbirth Education Association (ICEA). The membership has expanded greatly and includes interested professional persons. The ICEA is thus a federation of parents' groups and professional individuals interested in family-centered maternity and infant care. The ICEA publishes a news bulletin containing pertinent information about new developments and new publications. Regional and international conferences are held. A board of consultants provides professional medical advice and professional persons, often nurses, teach preparation-for-childbirth classes.

Local childbirth education groups differ in organization and emphasis, but in general they stress education of both wife and husband in the physical and emotional aspects of pregnancy, labor, and delivery; physical preparation for pregnancy and labor; support during labor; the presence of the father at birth; rooming-in; and breast feeding.

In 1960 a group of physicians, nurses, physiotherapists, and parents founded the American Society for Psychoprophylaxis in Obstetrics (ASPO). ASPO is dedicated to extending the use of the Lamaze method of preparation for childbirth. The society is composed of three divisions—physicians, teachers, and parents, with a board of directors composed of members from each division. Chapters of the society have been formed in various parts of the United States.

The ASPO maintains an informational and referral service designed to help women obtain training, and it sponsors teacher training courses open to qualified nurses and physical therapists. Teaching materials are available from the society and it maintains a film rental and reference library.

Another organization devoted to family-centered maternity and infant care is the LaLeche League, organized in 1956 by a small group of mothers. Members of the league are mothers that are dedicated to helping other mothers successfully and happily breast-feed their babies. The league has expanded rapidly, with chapters across the nation. Their active members meet in small informal groups, in which mothers who have successfully nursed their babies encourage and assist expectant and new mothers. The league has published a book entitled *The Womanly Art of Breast Feeding* and also publishes a newsletter for exchange of news and views, practical hints on breast feeding, and reports on new research.

ROOMING-IN

Trends in infant care have gone through complete changes over the past 50 years. At the beginning of this century babies were born in the home, mother and baby roomed together, and the mother cared for the baby instinctively. The baby was breast-fed and allowed to eat when he wished, and he was held and rocked when it appeared he needed such care. The father had an important part in the care of mother and baby.

Early in the twentieth century infant care became increasingly strict, especially in the "scientific" 1920's, when everything was done according to schedule. Babies were fed on an inflexible schedule, given artificial feedings according to the latest nutritional knowledge, and allowed to cry for long periods of time, because picking them up would spoil them. All earlier methods of infant care were considered old-fashioned, and mothers were anxious to follow the latest scientific teachings. An era devoted to ultra-scientific care had arrived. More and more babies were being born in hospitals. The busy hospital made schedules seem even more important. There was little time to teach the mother about the care of her baby. She went home inexperienced, but with a set of rules to follow. The father was considered relatively unimportant, especially in the hospital situation.

Again, a change came about with a return to much of the earlier practice. This was a movement to "ancient processes in a scientific age." Schedules and routines became less important.

Thinking in terms of less rigidity in care of babies began in the late 1930's. The first organized effort to again change infant care began in 1942 when the Cornelian Corner was organized in Detroit, Michigan. This group was composed of a psychiatrist, a pediatrician, an obstetrician, a nurse, and workers in allied fields who planned to do research and education in child development and family life. They emphasized the importance of allowing each baby to follow his individual schedule since it is difficult for him to fit into a conventional one. They stressed the value of such permissiveness to the development of a wholesome personality. Rooming-in, breast-feeding, and self-demand feeding schedules were given special emphasis by the Cornelians. They believed that the first step in the development of a well-balanced, healthy adult was indulgent care as a baby.

Rooming-in[2] is a hospital arrangement by which the mother and baby are cared for in the same unit, and the father has the privilege of caring for the baby as much as he wishes, thus becoming closely acquainted with him. Rooming-in provides the mother with the advantages of hospital delivery and hospital care in as homelike an atmosphere as is possible to provide. This program focuses on the family, providing for the interrelation that comes from close association of mother, father, and baby.

Mothers began to request rooming-in, and professional support of this program increased. With growing concern over improving the care of the newborn infant, an attitude developed that at least the mothers who wanted their babies with them should have their requests granted. Separation of mother and baby and strict hospital nursery regulations had been instituted, at least in part, to improve infant health and reduce infant mortality. However, with overcrowding of nurseries and shortage of personnel, danger of cross-infection became a threat. It was felt that a return to rooming-in, with proper precautions, would restore the psychologic satisfaction of mother and baby and also give adequate protection against infection.

Rooming-in began with having the baby in the mother's room a part of each day. The George Washington University Hospital obstetric unit was designed to foster closer relationship between mother and baby. The mothers' rooms were planned around small nursery units. With the use of mobile bassinets, which could be taken to the mothers' bedside for certain periods of time, and with the nursery close enough for the mother to observe her baby through the glass window, the teaching of mothers was greatly improved. Four hospitals in Detroit, Michigan, cooperated with the Cornelian Corner by having babies rooming-in in single-room arrangements for at least a part of each day and in some instances for the entire 24-hour period. In 1946 a four-bed rooming-in unit was established on the University Service of the Grace–New Haven Community Hospital for study purposes. Since its early trial other hospitals have provided rooming-in, at least in part, or have made some arrangements for the

---

[2] The term "rooming-in" was first used by Dr. Arnold Gesell and Dr. Frances Ilg (Arnold Gesell and Frances L. Ilg, *Infant and Child in the Culture of Today*. Harper and Row, New York, 1943).

mother to have her baby in her room as she desires and for both parents to participate in the baby's care.

For rooming-in to be successful, interest and cooperation of the parents and hospital personnel are essential, and an attitude of family-centered care must prevail.

SUMMARY

At one time it was enough to know that mother and baby were alive shortly after delivery. Now it is recognized that the effects of childbearing are sometimes not apparent until months later. Maternity care is not now considered complete until all subsequent care needed by mother and baby has been given.

In less than 50 years the concept of maternity care has grown from attendance at delivery and a few days' rest afterward to supervision, care, and help from the moment the woman thinks she may be pregnant until a year after the baby is born. The early care was given by a midwife or doctor and untrained assistant. Now a whole group of trained and supervised workers is needed—physicians, dentists, nurses, licensed practical nurses, nurse-midwives, nurses' aides, social workers, mental hygienists, occupational therapists, nutritionists, and household helpers. Not all actually care for patients but are necessary as supervisors, advisers, or helpers to ensure adequate care of all maternity patients in a community.

Efforts to improve maternity care gradually become concerned with better teaching and practice in schools of medicine, midwifery, and nursing; increased supervision in hospitals; investigation of the circumstances of maternal deaths, and more recently fetal and neonatal deaths; continuing education courses to disseminate information of changes and developments; and regulation and control, by licensure and supervision, of doctors, nurses, midwives, and trained practical nurses. Adequate medical, hospital, laboratory, nursing, and social casework services are emphasized. Supervised household workers to provide relief from housekeeping responsibilities during pregnancy when necessary and during the postpartum period are advocated. Coordination of all services is urged so that each patient may have what she needs regardless of her economic status. The teaching of every man and woman of why women need maternity care and of what constitutes good care is stressed. This emphasis is given so that "women will seek it when they need it and citizens be willing to pay for it, both as individuals for personal service and as taxpayers for community services."

The emphasis today is on a family-centered approach to maternal and child care. Assisting the expectant family to understand and cope with the impact of pregnancy and parenthood becomes as important as providing for the physical needs of the mother and her baby.

Appendix 2

Minimum Standards for Public Protection of the Health of Mothers— 1919

The following minimum standards for protection of the maternity patient were formulated at the second White House Conference, held in 1919:

1. Maternity or prenatal centers sufficient to provide for all cases not receiving prenatal supervision from private physicians. The work of such a center should include:

   a. Complete examination by a physician as early in pregnancy as possible, including pelvic measurements, examination of heart, lungs, abdomen, and urine, and the taking of blood pressure; internal examination before seventh month in primiparae; examination of urine every four weeks during early months, at least every two weeks after sixth month, and more frequently if indicated; Wassermann test whenever possible, especially when indicated by symptoms.

   b. Instructions in hygiene of maternity and supervision throughout pregnancy, through at least monthly visits to a maternity center until the end of the sixth month, and every two weeks thereafter. Literature to be given to mother to acquaint her with the principles of infant hygiene.

   c. Employment of sufficient number of public health nurses to do home visiting and to give instructions to expectant mothers in hygiene of pregnancy and early infancy; to make visits and to care for patient in puerperium; and to see that every infant is referred to a children's health center.

   d. Confinement at home by a physician or a properly trained and qualified attendant, or in a hospital.

   e. Nursing service at home at the time of confinement and during the lying-period, or hospital care.

   f. Daily visits for five days, and at least two other visits during second week by physician or nurse from maternity center.

   g. At least ten days in bed after normal delivery, with sufficient household service for four to six weeks to allow mother to recuperate.

   h. Examination by physician six weeks after delivery before discharging patient.

Where these centers have not been established or where their immediate establishment is impracticable, as many as possible of these provisions here enumerated should be carried out by the community nurse, under the direction of the health officer or local physician.

2. Clinics, such as dental clinics and venereal-disease clinics, for needed treatment during pregnancy.
3. Maternity hospitals, or maternity wards in general hospitals, sufficient to provide care in all complicated cases and for all women wishing hospital care; free or part-payment

obstetrical care to be provided in every necessitous case at home or in a hospital.
4. All midwives to be required by law to show adequate training, and to be licensed and supervised.
5. Adequate income to allow the mother to remain in the home through the nursing period.
6. Education of general public as to problems presented by maternal and infant mortality and their solution.

Appendix 3

A Philosophy of Perinatal Care

One of the principal beliefs underlying perinatal care is recognition of the fact that a baby has a past history at birth—that of his genetic and family background and of his intrauterine environment. He also has a future that will be influenced by the care he receives in the perinatal period. Several persons have called attention to this philosophy. We quote from two of these, Charles P. Douglas, M.D., Professor and Chairman, Department of Obstetrics and Gynecology, University of London, Royal Free Hospital, London, England, and Effie O. Ellis, M.D., Co-Director, Quality of Life Center, City of Chicago, and Special Consultant on Community Health Affairs, National Foundation—March of Dimes.

Dr. Douglas writes[1]:

INSTRUCTIONS TO THE FETUS

Choose a young, healthy mother of good socioeconomic status who is over 64 inches tall, slender, Rh-positive, and has a regular menstrual cycle.

She must not smoke, take drugs, or seek medication. Her family background must be genetically impeccable, and she must seek good antenatal care and a safe place in which to deliver.

So order your own environment and request that you are not born either preterm or postterm. Let not your membranes rupture early, and, above all, enter the world head first with the minimum delay once the journey has started. Having arrived, breathe quickly before they cut your cord, and then ask to be directed to the intensive care unit!

By this you have the best chance to survive the risks of your prenatal life.

Dr. Effie Ellis's address to the inaugural meeting of the National Perinatal Association was abstracted and published in *Perinatal Press*.[2] Portions of the abstract read as follows:

In the first 100 years in the United States we worked for sheer survival. Our strength and understanding were dedicated to the tackling of the elements and the conquering of disease. In the second hundred years we were involved with the industrial revolution and the dramatization of technology and hardware. By the time of the 21st century, our minds should expand to consider the quality as well as the quantity of life.

Since recorded time, man has been concerned about himself. In the 1970's, the phrase "Quality of Life" came to represent consumer need for physician concern with the life of the individual. . . .

To this point, medicine has functioned as an intervention art rather than looking into how people develop. We must go back to the very beginning. Our

---

[1] Charles P. Douglas, Prenatal risks: An obstetrician's point of view, in *Risks in the Practice of Modern Obstetrics*, 2nd ed., edited by Silvio Aladjem. Mosby, St. Louis, Mo., 1975, Chapter 1, p. 1.

[2] V. H. Law, Quality of life—An abstract, *Perinatal Press*, 1(1):7 (Jan./Feb.) 1977. (894 Madison Ave., Memphis, Tennessee, 38163.)

concern must be multi-generational for the quality of life of the baby begins with the birth of the parents. Emphasizing prevention more than screening, the entire life span must be included. Medicine is but one aspect to be considered in health. The social, environmental and educational conditions must also become part of the evaluation.

Too many people are born without the opportunity to be born healthy. Not all of those people are in the traditional classifications of poor or poverty laden. Emotional considerations are vital.

Obstetricians and pediatricians have a crucial role in the determination of the productivity of the entire life span of an individual. In the early years—conception through 25 years—a lifetime must be planned. There is a great need for supportive services during this time. The middle years—25 to 65—involve growth and developmental tasks. The later years—65 and on—are the testing ground of perinatal endeavors. If a human being lives in this period without poverty of spirit, feeling important and loved until death, the perinatal work has been done well.

Appendix 4

THE PREGNANT PATIENT'S BILL OF RIGHTS

American parents are becoming increasingly aware that well-intentioned health professionals do not always have scientific data to support common American obstetrical practices and that many of these practices are carried out primarily because they are part of medical and hospital tradition. In the last forty years many artificial practices have been introduced which have changed childbirth from a physiological event to a very complicated medical procedure in which all kinds of drugs are used and procedures carried out, sometimes unnecessarily, and many of them potentially damaging for the baby and even for the mother. A growing body of research makes it alarmingly clear that every aspect of traditional American hospital care during labor and delivery must now be questioned as to its possible effect on the future well-being of both the obstetric patient and her unborn child.

One in every 35 children born in the United States today will eventually be diagnosed as retarded; in 75% of these cases there is no familial or genetic predisposing factor. One in every 10 to 17 children has been found to have some form of brain dysfunction or learning disability requiring special treatment. Such statistics are not confined to the lower socioeconomic group but cut across all segments of American society.

New concerns are being raised by childbearing women because no one knows what degree of oxygen depletion, head compression, or traction by forceps the unborn or newborn infant can tolerate before that child sustains permanent brain damage or dysfunction. The recent findings regarding the cancer-related drug diethylstilbestrol have alerted the public to the fact that neither the approval of a drug by the U.S. Food and Drug Administration nor the fact that a drug is prescribed by a physician serves as a guarantee that a drug or medication is safe for the mother or her unborn child. In fact, the American Academy of Pediatrics' Committee on Drugs has recently stated that there is no drug, whether prescription or over-the-counter remedy, which has been proven safe for the unborn child.

The Pregnant Patient has the right to participate in decisions involving her well-being and that of her unborn child, unless there is a clearcut medical emergency that prevents her participation. In addition to the rights set forth in the American Hospital Association's "Patient's Bill of Rights," (which has also been adopted by the New York City Department of Health) the Pregnant Patient, because she represents TWO patients rather than one, should be recognized as having the additional rights listed below.

1. *The Pregnant Patient has the right*, prior to the administration of any drug or procedure, to be informed by the health professional caring for her of any poten-

tial direct or indirect effects, risks or hazards to herself or her unborn or new-born infant which may result from the use of a drug or procedure prescribed for or administered to her during pregnancy, labor, birth or lactation.

2. *The Pregnant Patient has the right*, prior to the proposed therapy, to be in-formed, not only of the benefits, risks and hazards of the proposed therapy but also of known alternative therapy, such as available childbirth education classes which could help to prepare the Pregnant Patient physically and mentally to cope with the discomfort or stress of pregnancy and the experience of childbirth, thereby reducing or eliminating her need for drugs and obstetric intervention. She should be offered such information early in her pregnancy in order that she may make a reasoned decision.

3. *The Pregnant Patient has the right*, prior to the administration of any drug, to be informed by the health professional who is prescribing or administering the drug to her that any drug which she receives during pregnancy, labor and birth, no matter how or when the drug is taken or administered, may adversely affect her unborn baby, directly or indirectly, and that there is no drug or chemical which has been proven safe for the unborn child.

4. *The Pregnant Patient has the right* if Cesarean section is anticipated, to be in-formed prior to the administration of any drug, and preferably prior to her hospi-talization, that minimizing her and, in turn, her baby's intake of nonessential pre-operative medicine will benefit her baby.

5. *The Pregnant Patient has the right*, prior to the administration of a drug or procedure, to be informed of the areas of uncertainty if there is NO properly controlled follow-up research which has established the safety of the drug or procedure with regard to its direct and/or indirect effects on the physiological, mental and neurological development of the child exposed, via the mother, to the drug or procedure during pregnancy, labor, birth or lactation—(this would apply to virtually all drugs and the vast majority of obstetric procedures).

6. *The Pregnant Patient has the right*, prior to the administration of any drug, to be informed of the brand name and generic name of the drug in order that she may advise the health professional of any past adverse reaction to the drug.

7. *The Pregnant Patient has the right* to determine for herself, without pressure from her attendant, whether she will accept the risks inherent in the proposed therapy or refuse a drug or procedure.

8. *The Pregnant Patient has the right* to know the name and qualifications of the in-dividual administering a medication or procedure to her during labor or birth.

9. *The Pregnant Patient has the right* to be informed, prior to the administration of any procedure, whether that procedure is being administered to her for her or her baby's benefit (medically indicated) or as an elective procedure (for conve-nience, teaching purposes or research).

10. *The Pregnant Patient has the right* to be accompanied during the stress of labor and birth by someone she cares for, and to whom she looks for emotional comfort and encouragement.

11. *The Pregnant Patient has the right* after appropriate medical consultation to choose a position for labor and for birth which is least stressful to her baby and to herself.

12. *The Obstetric Patient has the right* to have her baby cared for at her bedside if her baby is normal, and to feed her baby according to her baby's needs rather than according to the hospital regimen.

13. *The Obstetric Patient has the right* to be informed in writing the name of the person who actually delivered her baby and the professional qualifications of that person. This information should also be on the birth certificate.

14. *The Obstetric Patient has the right* to be informed if there is any known or indicated aspect of her or her baby's care or condition which may cause her or her baby later difficulty or problems.

15. *The Obstetric Patient has the right* to have her and her baby's hospital medical records complete, accurate and legible and to have their records, including Nurses' Notes, retained by the hospital until the child reaches at least the age of majority, or, alternatively, to have the records offered to her before they are destroyed.

16. *The Obstetric Patient,* both during and after her hospital stay, has the right to have access to her complete hospital medical records, including Nurses' Notes, and to receive a copy upon payment of a reasonable fee and without incurring the expense of retaining an attorney.

It is the obstetric patient and her baby, not the health professional, who must sustain any trauma or injury resulting from the use of a drug or obstetric procedure. The observation of the rights listed above will not only permit the obstetric patient to participate in the decisions involving her and her baby's health care, but will help to protect the health professional and the hospital against litigation arising from resentment or misunderstanding on the part of the mother.

Endorsed by the International Childbirth Education Association

Clinical Laboratory
Values in Pregnancy

Table 1. Hematologic Changes During Pregnancy

	Nonpregnant	Pregnant
Complete blood count		
Hemoglobin, gm/100 ml	12–16	10–14
Hematocrit, %	37–47	32–42
Red cell volume, ml	1600	1900
Plasma volume, ml	2400	3700
Red blood cell indexes	Normal	Normal
White blood cells, total, /mm^3	4500–10,000	5000–15,000
Polymorphonuclear cells, %	54–62	60–85
Lymphocytes, %	38–46	15–40
Erythrocyte sedimentation rate, mm/hr	<20	30–90
Coagulation system		
Bleeding time	Normal	Normal
Clotting time	Normal	Normal
Platelets, /mm^3	175,000–250,000	200,000–350,000
Prothrombin time	Control± 3 sec	10% decrease
Fibrinogen, mg/100 ml	250	400
Factor VIII	Normal	3 × normal
Factors V, VII, IX, X	Normal	Moderate increase
Fibrinolytic activity	Normal	Moderate decrease
Erythropoietic system		
Serum iron, μg	75–150	65–120
Total iron-binding capacity, μg	250–450	300–500
Iron saturation, %	30–40	15–30
Vitamin B$_{12}$, folic acid, ascorbic acid	Normal	Moderate decrease

Table 2. Cardiovascular Changes During Pregnancy*

	Nonpregnant	Pregnant
Blood pressure, mmHg	120/80	114/65
Peripheral resistance, dyne/sec-cm^{-5}	120	100
Venous pressure, cmH$_2$O		
Femoral	9	24
Antecubital	8	8
Pulse, rate/min	70	80
Stroke volume, ml	65	75
Cardiac output, liters/min	4.5	6
Circulation time (arm-tongue), sec	15–16	12–14
Blood volume, ml		
Whole blood	4000	5600
Plasma	2400	3700
Red blood cell	1600	1900
Plasma renin, units/liter	3–10	10–80
Chest x-ray		
Transverse diameter of heart	Normal	1–2 cm increase
Left border of heart	Normal	Straightened
Cardiac volume	Normal	70 ml increase
Electrocardiogram	Normal	15° left axis deviation
V$_1$ and V$_2$	Normal	Inverted T wave
V$_4$	Normal	Low T
III	Normal	Q + inverted T
aVr	Normal	Small Q

*32 to 36 weeks' duration.

Table 3. Changes in Renal Function During Pregnancy*

	Nonpregnant	Pregnant
Renal blood flow, ml/min	900	1200
Renal plasma flow (PAH†), ml/min	500	700
Glomerular filtration rate (creatinine clearance), ml/min	80–120	110–180
Blood urea nitrogen, mg/100 ml	10–18	4–12
Creatinine, mg/100 ml	0.6–1.2	0.4–0.9
Uric acid, mg/100 ml	2.0–6.4	2.0–5.5
Phenolsulfonphthalein excretion	Normal	Delayed
Fishberg concentration test	1.023	Often less
Urine glucose	Negative	Present in 20% of patients
Intravenous pyelogram	Normal	Slight to moderate hydroureter and hydronephrosis; R>L

*32 to 36 weeks' duration.
† PAH, para-aminohippuric acid.

Tables 1, 2, and 3 reproduced with permission from David W. Brewer, Jr. and Richard H. Aubry, "The Physiology of Pregnancy," *Postgrad. Med.* 52(6):110–114 (Dec.) 1972 and 53(1):221–226 (Jan.) 1973.

Table 4. Additional Laboratory Values

	Nonpregnant	Pregnant
Blood sugar		
Fasting, mg/100 ml	70–80	65
2-hour postprandial, mg/100 ml	60–110	Under 140 after a 100 gm carbohydrate meal is considered normal
Serum proteins		
Total, gm/100 ml	6.7–8.3	5.5–7.5
Albumin, gm/100 ml	3.5–5.5	3.0–5.0
Globulin, total, gm/100 ml	2.3–3.5	3.0–4.0
Thyroid		
Protein-bound iodine μg/100 ml	4.0–8.0	6.5–12.0
Thyroxine, μg/100 ml	3.4–6.4	5.5–10.0
Triiodothyronine, percent	25–38	12–25
Free thyroxine, μg/100 ml	1.2–1.6	0.9–1.4

Appendix 6

Clinical Laboratory Values in the Newborn[*]

Constituent	Normal Range	Comments
pH	7.35–7.45 arterial, venous, or arterialized	Below 7.25 there is acidosis clinically
P_{CO_2}, mmHg	35–40 arterial, venous, or arterialized	45 is upper limit of normal
P_{O_2}, mmHg	50–80 arterial. capillary blood samples are not reliable	50 is lower limit of normal P_{O_2} should not exceed 100
Plasma bicarbonate, mEq/liter	20 to 25	
Base excess, mEq/liter	+4 to −4	
Hemoglobin, gm/100 ml	16–20 peripheral 14–17.0 venous	Less than 14.5 (capillary) Less than 13.0 (venous) } = anemia 22.0 or more (venous) = polycythemia
Hematocrit, %	48–60	45 or less = anemia 65 or greater (venous) = polycythemia
Red blood cells, mm^3	4,000,000 to 6,000,000	
Reticulocytes, %	3–4 at birth 1–3 at 4 days 0–1 by 7 days	
WBC, mm^3	9,000 to 30,000 15,000 = mean	

[*]These values are an overall average normal. Laboratory values will vary with the gestational age, the postnatal age, and the birth weight of the infant. Laboratory data may also vary with individual laboratories.

Constituent	Normal Range	Comments
Differential	Preponderance of polymorpho- nuclear neutrophils until day 3–4; then lymphocytes predominate	After 72 hours a neutro- phil count below 1,350 or over 8,800 should be regarded as sign of bacterial infection until proven otherwise †
Platelet count, mm³	100,000–300,000	
Serum bilirubin Total, mg/100 ml	5–12 after 48 hours and for no longer than one week	Above 12 = pathologic Daily increment in excess of 5 mg/100 ml − 24 hr = pathologic
Direct, mg/ 100 ml	0.0–1.0	Exceeding 1.0–2.0 = pathologic
Blood chemistry Blood sugar, mg/100 ml	40–100 in whole blood 5 mg/100 ml must be added if values are done on serum rather than whole blood	Hypoglycemia In full-term <30 in first 72 hours <40 after third day In low birth weight <20
Serum calcium, mg/100 ml mEq/liter	8–10 4–5	Below 7 mg/100 ml or 3.5 mEq/liter = hypocalcemia
Serum magnesium, mg/100 ml mEq/liter	1.5–2.8 1.5–2.5	<1.5 mg/100 ml = hypomagnesia
Serum sodium, mEq/liter	136–143	Below 130 = hyponatremia Above 150 = hypernatremia
Serum potassium, mEq/liter	3.8–6.5	Over 7.0 = hyperkalemia
Serum chloride, mEq/liter	95–105	
Total serum proteins, gm/100 ml	4.8–7.4 term 4.0–6.4 preterm	
Serum albumin, gm/100 ml	3.6–5.4 term 3.28–4.50 preterm	
Urine specific gravity	1.008–1.012	

† Frank A. Oski, Hematologic problems, in *Neonatology*, edited by Gordon B. Avery. Lippincott, Philadelphia, Pa., 1975, p. 415.

Appendix 7

Conversion Table for Newborn Weights

	OUNCES															
POUNDS	*0*	*1*	*2*	*3*	*4*	*5*	*6*	*7*	*8*	*9*	*10*	*11*	*12*	*13*	*14*	*15*
0	0	28	57	85	113	142	170	198	227	255	284	312	340	369	397	425
1	454	482	510	539	567	595	624	652	680	709	737	765	794	822	851	879
2	907	936	964	992	1021	1049	1077	1106	1134	1162	1191	1219	1247	1276	1304	1332
3	1361	1389	1418	1446	1474	1503	1531	1559	1588	1616	1644	1673	1701	1729	1758	1786
4	1814	1843	1871	1899	1928	1956	1985	2013	2041	2070	2098	2126	2155	2183	2211	2240
5	2268	2296	2325	2353	2381	2410	2438	2466	2495	2523	2552	2580	2608	2637	2665	2693
6	2722	2750	2778	2807	2835	2863	2892	2920	2948	2977	3005	3033	3062	3090	3119	3147
7	3175	3204	3232	3260	3289	3317	3345	3374	3402	3430	3459	3487	3515	3544	3572	3600
8	3629	3657	3686	3714	3742	3771	3799	3827	3856	3884	3912	3941	3969	3997	4026	4054
9	4082	4111	4139	4167	4196	4224	4253	4281	4309	4338	4366	4394	4423	4451	4479	4508
10	4536	4564	4593	4621	4649	4678	4706	4734	4763	4791	4820	4848	4876	4905	4933	4961
11	4990	5018	5046	5075	5103	5131	5160	5188	5216	5245	5273	5301	5330	5358	5387	5415
12	5443	5472	5500	5528	5557	5585	5613	5642	5670	5698	5727	5755	5783	5812	5840	5868
13	5897	5925	5954	5982	6010	6039	6067	6095	6124	6152	6180	6209	6237	6265	6294	6322
14	6350	6379	6407	6435	6464	6492	6521	6549	6577	6606	6634	6662	6691	6719	6747	6776
15	6804	6832	6861	6889	6917	6946	6974	7002	7031	7059	7088	7116	7144	7173	7201	7229

To convert pounds and ounces to grams, multiply the pounds by 453.6 and the ounces by 28.35 and add the two sums.
To convert grams into pounds and decimals of a pound, multiply the grams by 0.0022.
To convert grams into ounces, divide the grams by 28.35.

Appendix 8

Conversion Table for Newborn Lengths

Inches	Centimeters	Inches	Centimeters
10	25.4	17	43.2
10½	26.7	17½	44.5
11	27.9	18	45.7
11½	29.2	18½	47.0
12	30.5	19	48.3
12½	31.8	19½	49.5
13	33.0	20	50.8
13½	34.3	20½	52.1
14	35.6	21	53.3
14½	36.8	21½	54.6
15	38.1	22	55.9
15½	39.4	22½	57.2
16	40.6	23	58.4
16½	41.9	23½	59.7
		24	60.9

To convert inches to centimeters multiply inches by 2.54 or divide inches by 0.394.

To convert centimeters to inches multiply centimeters by 0.394 or divide centimeters by 2.54.

Appendix 9

Equivalent Temperature Readings of Celsius and Fahrenheit

°C	°F	°C	°F	°C	°F	°C	°F
0	32.0	35.8	96.4	37.4	99.3	39.0	102.2
		35.9	96.6	37.5	99.5	39.1	102.4
34.0	93.2	36.0	96.8	37.6	99.6	39.2	102.6
34.2	93.6	36.1	96.9	37.7	99.8	39.3	102.7
		36.2	97.2	37.8	100.0	39.4	102.9
34.4	93.9	36.3	97.3	37.9	100.2	39.5	103.1
34.6	94.3	36.4	97.5	38.0	100.4	39.6	103.3
		36.5	97.7	38.1	100.6	39.7	103.5
34.8	94.6	36.6	97.9	38.2	100.8	39.8	103.6
35.0	95.0	36.7	98.0	38.3	100.9	39.9	103.8
35.2	95.4	36.8	98.2	38.4	101.1	40.0	104.0
35.4	95.7	36.9	98.4	38.5	101.3		
		37.0	98.6	38.6	101.5	100	212
35.5	95.9	37.1	98.8	38.7	101.7		
35.6	96.1	37.2	99.0	38.8	101.8		
35.7	96.3	37.3	99.1	38.9	102.0		

1. To convert Celsius readings to Fahrenheit, multiply by 1.8 and add 32.
2. To convert Fahrenheit readings to Celsius, subtract 32 and divide by 1.8.

OR

3. To convert Celsius readings to Fahrenheit multiply by 9/5 and add 32.
4. To convert Fahrenheit readings to Celsius subtract 32 and multiply by 5/9.

Index

Heardman, Helen, 866
Health history, newborn, 481
  maternal, 167–70
Hearing of newborn, 463–64
Heartbeat of fetus, 164, 316–21
  auscultation, 325–31
  electrocardiography, 164, 321–25
Heartburn during pregnancy, 146, 205
Heart disease, congenital, 793–95
  pregnancy, 128, 676–78
Heart, embryo, 93, 101
  fetal, first heard, 164
    monitoring, 316–31
    rate, 164
  newborn, 427, 482
    abnormalities, 793–95
    physical assessment, 482, 491, 495
    rate, 427, 493
  pregnancy, 128–29
Heat loss and heat production in newborn, 432–34, 715–18
  prevention, 436–39, 715–18
Heat shield over baby, 717
Hegar's sign, 161
Hemangiomas, pregnancy, 134
Hematocrit, newborn, 428, 784
  pregnancy, 127, 171
Hematoma, newborn, head, 443
  vulvar and vaginal, after delivery, 696–97
Hematopoiesis, fetus, 93, 101, 102
  newborn, 429
Hemoconcentration, toxemia, 654, 656
Hemoglobin concentration, newborn, 428
  maternal, 127
Hemolytic disease of newborn, ABO blood group incompatibility, 646, 813
  RH factor incompatibility, 646–52, 809–14. *See also* Erythroblastosis fetalis
Hemorrhage, antepartum, 625–40
  intracranial, newborn, 835–37
  postpartum, 692–97
    causes, 693
    definition, 692–93
    hematomas of vulva and vagina as cause of, 696–97
    late (delayed), 693, 696
  subconjunctival, newborn, 501
Hemorrhoids, 207–208, 561
Heparin, 702
Hernia in newborn, diaphragmatic, 828
Heroin, 200, 822
Herpes virus infection, newborn, 671
  pregnancy, 671
Hexachlorophene, baby's bath, 453
  handwashing, 499
Hiccups, newborn, 439
High forceps operations, 404
High-risk infants, definition, 706
  identification, 706–709
  illnesses and abnormalities, 758
  LGA, 709, 752–54
  postterm, 748–52
  preterm, 707–44

SGA, 709, 744–48
High-risk pregnancy, assessment, 605–22
  medical complications, 668–86
  obstetric complications, 624–67
  other factors, 686–90
  screening for, 172–74
Hip, congenital dislocation, 484, 830–31
Hippocrates, 697, 855
History taking, antepartum, 167–72
  diet, 175–78
  family, 170, 687
  medical, 169
  menstrual, 167
  newborn, 481
  obstetric, 167
HMD (hyaline membrane disease). *See* Respiratory distress syndrome
Holmes, Oliver Wendell, 656, 698
Home delivery, 383
Hormonal feedback in reproductive cycles, 26–29, 34–36, 36–37, 38–39
Hormone(s), adrenal, fetal, 122
  in adolescence, 20–21
  maternal, 116, 125, 142, 143, 145, 151
  androgen, 20
  anterior pituitary, gonadotropic, 26–29, 34–36, 36–37, 38–39
  chorionic gonadotropin, 35–36, 67, 118
  chorionic growth hormone—prolactin, (CGP), 118
  estrogen, ovarian, 21, 22, 23, 24, 27–29, 30, 34, 122
    placental, 121–24, 142, 146, 151
  fetal production of, 84, 122
  follicle-stimulating (FSH), 26, 34–35, 39
  gonadotropin releasing factor (GnRF), 26, 38, 40
  human chorionic gonadotropin (HCG), 35–36, 67, 118, 162–64
  human chorionic sommatomammotropin (HCS), 118–20, 142, 151, 615
  human chorionic thyrotropin (HCT), 120
  human placental lactogen (HPL), 118, 615
  hypothalamus neurohormones (releasing factors), 26, 38, 40
  induced withdrawal bleeding as test for pregnancy, 164
  influence on breast development, 15, 115–16
  interstitial cell stimulating (ICSH), 39
  lactogen, human placental (HPL) 118, 615
  luteinizing (LH), 26–27, 34–35, 39
  melanocyte-stimulating (MSH), 147
  newborn's reactions to maternal influence, 456–57
  oral contraceptives, 595–97
  ovarian, 27–29. *See* Hormones, estrogen, progesterone
  parathyroid, in pregnancy, 124–25
  placental, 118–24
  placental transfer to and from fetus, 84
  posterior pituitary, 376–77
  progesterone, ovarian, 24, 27, 29, 31, 34–35, 120
    placental, 120–21, 142, 146, 151
  prolactin, pituitary, 125–26, 515, 553
  prostaglandins (PGs), 125, 258, 402
  relaxin, 116
  testosterone, 38–39